HISTOLOGY AND CELL BIOLOGY

An Introduction to Pathology

Second Edition

HISTOLOGY AND CELL BIOLOGY
An Introduction to Pathology

Second Edition

Abraham L. Kierszenbaum, M.D., Ph.D.
Professor and Chair
Department of Cell Biology and Anatomical Sciences
The Sophie Davis School of Biomedical Education/
The City University of New York Medical School
New York, New York

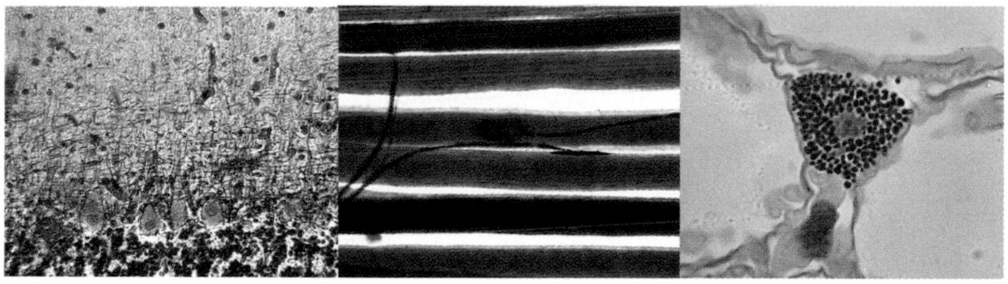

Back cover
1. Purkinje cells (cerebellum). Silver impregnation.
2. Neuromuscular junction. Motor end plates. Whole-mount preparation.
3. Mast cell. Metachromasia.

MOSBY
ELSEVIER

MOSBY
ELSEVIER

1600 John F. Kennedy Blvd.
Ste 1800
Philadelphia, PA 19103-2899

HISTOLOGY & CELL BIOLOGY: AN INTRODUCTION TO PATHOLOGY

ISBN-13: 978-0-323-04527-8
ISBN-10: 0-323-04527-8

Notice

Knowledge and best practice in this field are constantly changing. As new research and experience broaden our knowledge, changes in practice, treatment and drug therapy may become necessary or appropriate. Readers are advised to check the most current information provided (i) on procedures featured or (ii) by the manufacturer of each product to be administered, to verify the recommended dose or formula, the method and duration of administration, and contraindications. It is the responsibility of the practitioner, relying on their own experience and knowledge of the patient, to make diagnoses, to determine dosages and the best treatment for each individual patient, and to take all appropriate safety precautions. To the fullest extent of the law, neither the Publisher nor the Author assumes any liability for any injury and/or damage to persons or property arising out or related to any use of the material contained in this book.

The Publisher

Previous editions copyrighted 2002

Library of Congress Cataloging-in-Publication Data
Kierszenbaum, Abraham L.
Histology & cell biology : an introduction to pathology / Abraham L. Kierszenbaum.— 2nd ed.
p. ; cm.
Includes index.
ISBN 0-323-04527-8
1. Histology, Pathological. 2. Pathology, Cellular. I. Title. II. Title: Histology and cell biology.
[DNLM: 1. Pathology. 2. Cytology. 3. Histology. QZ 4 K47h 2007]
RB25.K54 2007
616.07—dc22
2006050557

Acquisitions Editor: Inta Ozols
Developmental Editor: Andrew Hall
Publishing Services Manager: Linda Van Pelt
Project Manager: Francisco Morales

Printed in Canada

Last digit is the print number: 9 8 7 6 5 4 3 2 1

DEDICATION

This book is dedicated with appreciation and love to Laura L. Tres, my academic colleague, research partner, best friend, spouse, and mother of our two daughters Adriana and Silvia.

To the beloved memory of my mother and my father, who now would understand why.

PREFACE

The second edition of this book contains new additions that strengthen the visual approach to learning histology within the context of cell biology introduced in the first edition. The combined histology–cell biology approach intends to prepare medical students for the contemporary molecular approach of learning pathology and clinical medicine. The practice of medicine changes gradually as new knowledge becomes known. Future physicians can find in this book the basis for continuing education to better help their patients by continuously integrating basic and clinical sciences.

The visual approach presented in this book emerged from over thirty-five years of experience teaching first pathology and then histology to medical students and from a need to communicate and reinforce relevant concepts to be mastered under increasing time constraints owing to changes in the basic science curriculum in most medical schools. The focal point of the visual approach is to provide medical students with an integrated method leading to the understanding of pathologic abnormalities. The cell biology component, although not complete, provides the necessary ingredients for integration with histology. Pathology students may find this book useful for refreshing basic concepts of histology and cell biology. Histology and pathology are visually oriented sciences, and the visual cues included in this book can facilitate interpretation opportunities in clinical practice.

Similar to the first edition, the second edition consists of six parts. Part I brings together histology and cell biology within the context of the basic tissues. Chapter 3, Cell Signaling, is an uncommon section in a histology book. It serves to unify the concept that the study of tissues and organs cannot be separated from physiology, biochemistry, and molecular biology. Parts II to VI present several organ systems grouped by their most relevant function for the purpose of integration. Instructors and students may find the grouping of organs useful for learning. In Part VI, Organ Systems: Reproductive System, the chapter headings depart from the traditional designation to emphasize prominent functions. All the information is presented in a clear, concise, and student-friendly manner using color graphics and photographs that are meant to be studied. In some cases the graphics reiterate the concise text; in others they add information complementing or extending the text. Several boxes dispersed in most of the chapters introduce students to clinical conditions based on new and evolving molecular knowledge. Each chapter concludes with *Essential Concepts*, a new section that highlights key issues to remember. Students may find the combined visual approach and *Essential Concepts* convenient for reviewing complex concepts and integrate them when the time of the board examinations arrives. Teachers may find the visual approach useful for delivering a lecture using the same or a different presentation sequence.

There are many people to be acknowledged and thanked. My thanks go to several classes of The Sophie Davis School of Biomedical Education/The City University of New York Medical School. They provided valuable feedback to make the message clearer and more consistent. The second edition is far better because of their insights and comments from a student's perspective. My colleagues Edward W. Gresik, Laura L. Tres, Wan-hua Amy Yu, and Young Kim, who worked with me throughout the years, provided suggestions and comments. Laura L. Tres reviewed every single line of text and illustrations. She made sure, in her natural and effective way, that changes were introduced to dispel doubts and possible misinterpretations. I am thankful for the numerous suggestions, comments, and encouragements offered by many colleagues from all over the world who used the first edition of this book. I also thank publishers who made available to students the Chinese, French, Japanese, and Portuguese editions. My special appreciation goes to the production team of Elsevier in the Philadelphia office and Andrew Vosburgh from Graphic World for their magnificent effort in making sure that the second edition met high publishing standards. Finally, I thank my family, in particular my wife Laura, for their patience and understanding during the many hours on the computer writing, revising, illustrating, and composing this second edition of *Histology and Cell Biology: An Introduction to Pathology.*

Abraham L. Kierszenbaum

CONTENTS

PART I | BASIC TISSUES AND INTEGRATED CELL BIOLOGY

Chapter 1 EPITHELIUM

Chapter 2 EPITHELIAL GLANDS

Chapter 3 CELL SIGNALING

Chapter 4 CONNECTIVE TISSUE

CONTENTS

CONTENTS

CONTENTS

CONTENTS

1. EPITHELIUM

Classification

The epithelium is a tightly cohesive sheet of cells that covers or lines body surfaces (for example, skin, intestine, secretory ducts) and forms the functional units of secretory glands (for example, salivary glands, liver). See **Box 1-A** for main characteristics of epithelia. The traditional classification and nomenclature of different types of epithelia are based on the **two-dimensional shape of cells as observed under the light microscope.**

Epithelia are classified into three major categories on the basis of the number of cell layers and the shape of the cells at the outermost layer:

1. **Simple epithelia** (Figure 1-1) are formed by only one layer of cells and are subdivided into **simple squamous**, **simple cuboidal**, and **simple columnar**, according to the height and width of the cells. The specific name **endothelium** is used for the simple epithelium lining the blood and lymphatic vessels. **Mesothelium** is the simple epithelium lining all body cavities (peritoneum, pericardium, and pleura).

2. **Stratified epithelia** (Figure 1-2) are composed of two or more cell layers. Stratified epithelia are subclassified according to the shape of the cells at the superficial or outer layer into **stratified squamous**, **stratified cuboidal**, and **stratified columnar**. Stratified squamous is the epithelium most frequently found and can be subdivided into **moderately keratinized** (also known as nonkeratinized) or **highly keratinized** types. The cells of the outer layer of a moderately keratinized squamous epithelium **can display nuclei** (for example, esophagus and vagina). **Nuclei are absent in the outer layer of the highly keratinized stratified squamous epithelium** (for example, the epidermis of the skin). The basal cells aligned along the basal lamina are mitotically active and replace the differentiating cells of the upper layers.

3. **Pseudostratified epithelia** (Figure 1-3) consist of basal and columnar cells resting on the basal lamina. Only the columnar cells reach the luminal surface, however. Because the nuclei of the basal and columnar cells are seen at different levels, one has the impression of a stratified epithelial organization. Within this category are the following:

1. The **pseudostratified columnar ciliated epithelium** of the trachea.

2. The **pseudostratified columnar epithelium with stereocilia** of the epididymis.

3. The **transitional epithelium** of the urinary passages, also referred to as **urothelium**. The urothelium also consists of basal and columnar or superficial cells. An important feature of this epithelium is that its height varies with distention and contraction of the organ (see Chapter 14, Urinary System).

Although this classification ignores specialized functional aspects of epithelia, the traditional classification is still useful from a descriptive point of view. We use the morphologic classification of epithelia as an introduction to a more contemporary view of this basic tissue: its **polarity**.

Epithelia line surfaces and cavities and have three domains (Figure 1-4):

1. The **apical domain** is exposed to the lumen or external environment.

2. The **lateral domain** faces neighboring epithelial cells linked to each other by cell adhesion molecules and junctional complexes.

3. The **basal domain** is associated with a **basal lamina** that separates the epithelium from underlying connective tissue. The basal lamina is reinforced by components of the connective tissue. The basal lamina–connective tissue complex is designated the **basement membrane**.

Epithelial cells are attached to each other by junctional complexes and adhe-

Box 1-A | **Main characteristics of epithelia**

- Epithelia derive from the ectoderm, mesoderm, and endoderm.
- Epithelia line and cover all body surfaces except the articular cartilage, the enamel of the tooth, and the anterior surface of the iris.
- The basic functions of epithelia are **protection** (skin), **absorption** (small and large intestine), **transport of material** at the surface (mediated by cilia), **secretion** (glands), **excretion** (tubules of the kidney), **gas exchange** (lung alveolus), and **gliding between surfaces** (mesothelium).
- Most epithelial cells renew continuously by mitosis.
- Epithelia lack a direct blood and lymphatic supply. Nutrients are delivered by diffusion.
- Epithelial cells have almost no free intercellular substances (in contrast to connective tissue).
- The cohesive nature of an epithelium is maintained by **cell adhesion molecules** and **junctional complexes**.
- Epithelia are anchored to a **basal lamina**. The basal lamina and connective tissue components cooperate to form the **basement membrane**.
- Epithelia have structural and functional **polarity**.

Figure 1-1. Simple epithelium

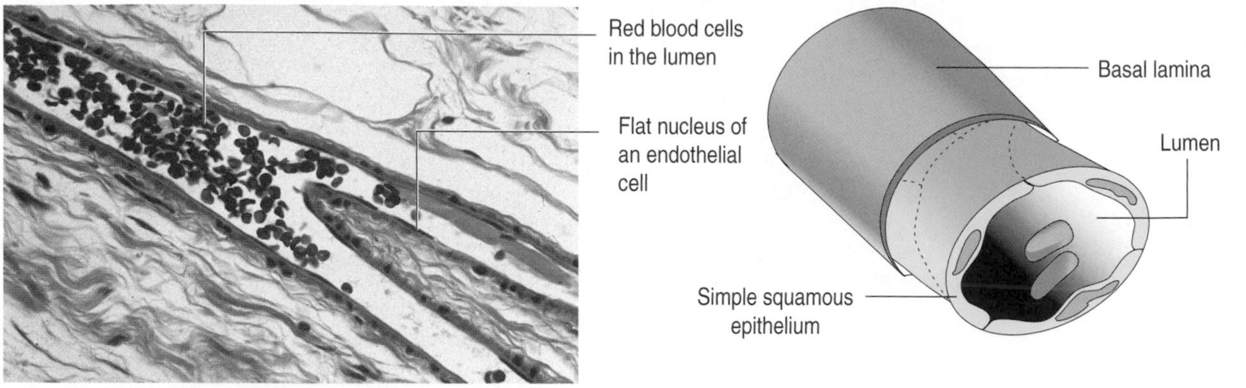

Simple squamous epithelium (endothelium)
The inner lining of all blood vessels consists of a single layer of squamous endothelial cells. The thinness of the simple squamous epithelial cells reflects their primary function in rapid exchange of substances between blood and tissue. A similar epithelium (called **mesothelium**) covers the peritoneum, pleura, and pericardium.

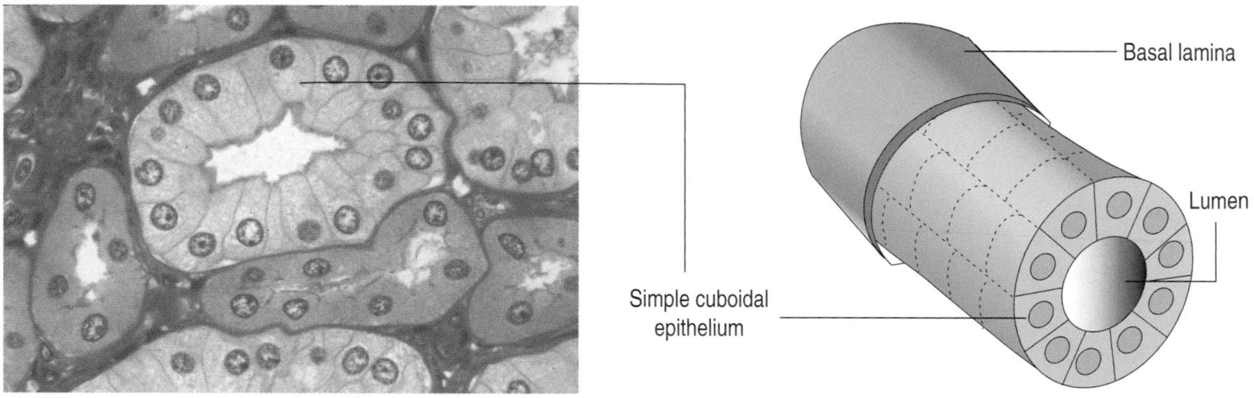

Simple cuboidal epithelium (collecting tubule, kidney)
The inner lining of kidney tubules and thyroid follicles consists of a single layer of cuboidal cells. Cuboidal cells are highly polarized and participate in absorption, secretion (thyroid gland), and active ion transport (kidney). Similar to the endothelium, a basal lamina attaches the cell to the subjacent connective tissue.

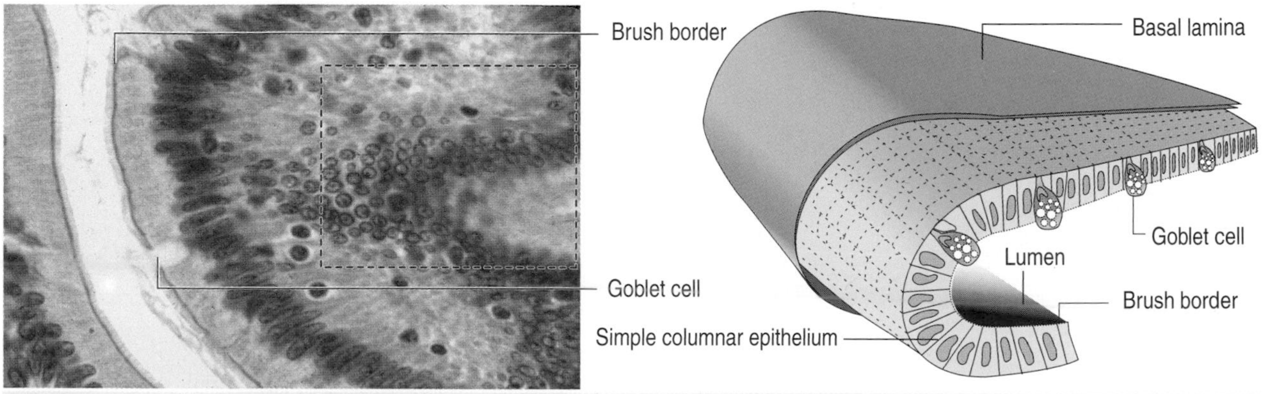

Simple columnar epithelium (small intestine)
The small intestine is lined by columnar epithelial cells with the nucleus in the basal portion of the cell. The apical domain contains finger-like projections called **microvilli** forming a **brush border**. Microvilli participate in the absorption of proteins, sugar, and lipids, which are released at the basolateral domain into the blood circulation for transport to the liver.
Columnar cells are oriented in different directions. The **box** indicates clusters of nuclei observed in a transverse section of the columnar epithelium through its most basal region. A transverse section passing through the apical region displays cytoplasmic profiles without visible nuclei.

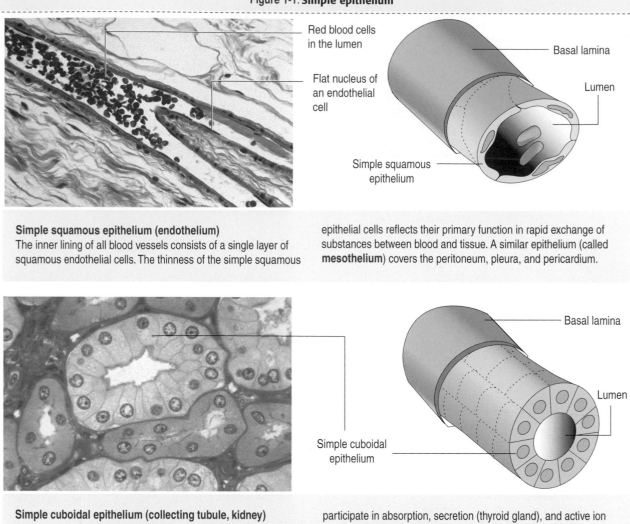

Figure 1-2. Stratified epithelium

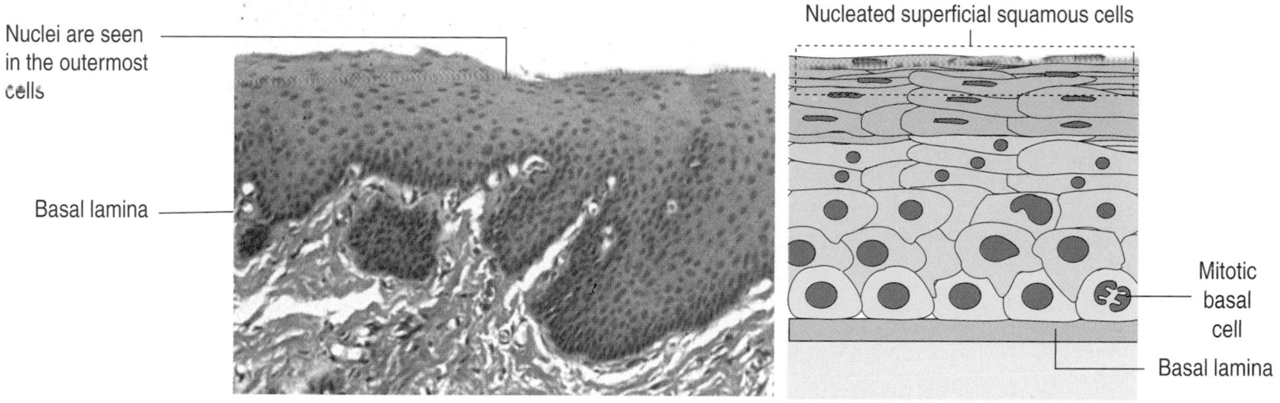

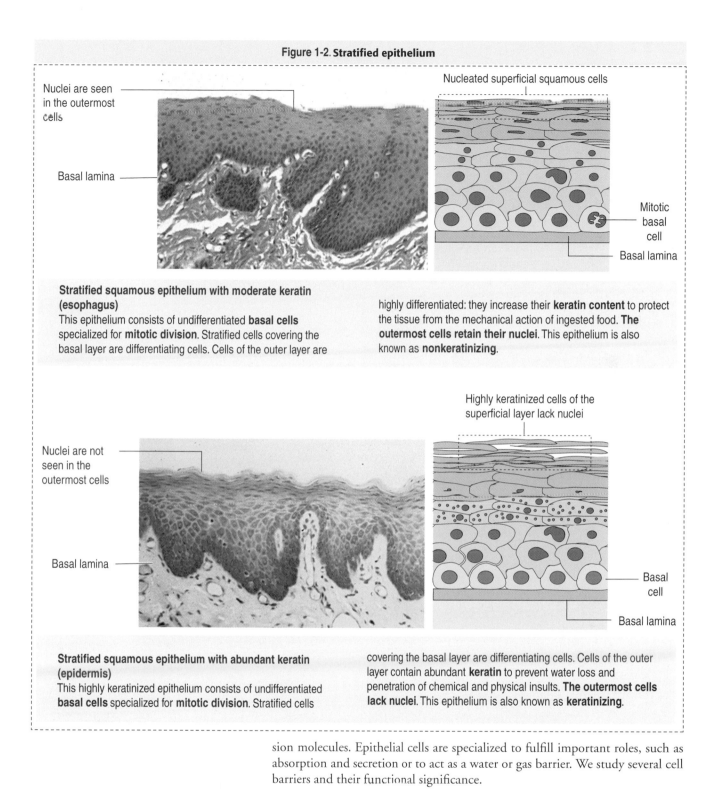

Nuclei are seen in the outermost cells
Basal lamina
Nucleated superficial squamous cells
Mitotic basal cell
Basal lamina

Stratified squamous epithelium with moderate keratin (esophagus)
This epithelium consists of undifferentiated **basal cells** specialized for **mitotic division**. Stratified cells covering the basal layer are differentiating cells. Cells of the outer layer are highly differentiated: they increase their **keratin content** to protect the tissue from the mechanical action of ingested food. **The outermost cells retain their nuclei.** This epithelium is also known as **nonkeratinizing**.

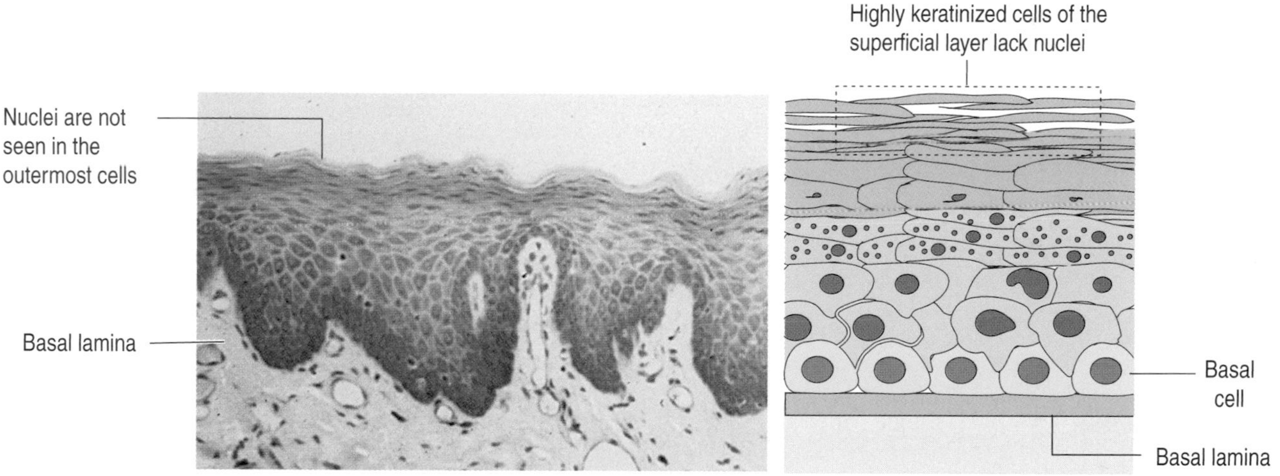

Highly keratinized cells of the superficial layer lack nuclei
Nuclei are not seen in the outermost cells
Basal lamina
Basal cell
Basal lamina

Stratified squamous epithelium with abundant keratin (epidermis)
This highly keratinized epithelium consists of undifferentiated **basal cells** specialized for **mitotic division.** Stratified cells covering the basal layer are differentiating cells. Cells of the outer layer contain abundant **keratin** to prevent water loss and penetration of chemical and physical insults. **The outermost cells lack nuclei.** This epithelium is also known as **keratinizing.**

sion molecules. Epithelial cells are specialized to fulfill important roles, such as absorption and secretion or to act as a water or gas barrier. We study several cell barriers and their functional significance.

Epithelial cell polarity

Epithelial cells have two major domains (Figure 1-4):

1. An **apical domain**
2. A **basolateral domain**

Each domain is defined by specific structural and functional characteristics. For example, the apical domain has structures important for the **protection** of the epithelial surface (such as **cilia** in the respiratory tract) or for the **absorption** of substances (such as **microvilli** in the intestinal epithelium).

Junctional complexes and **cell adhesion molecules** are present at the basolateral

Figure 1-3. Pseudostratified epithelium

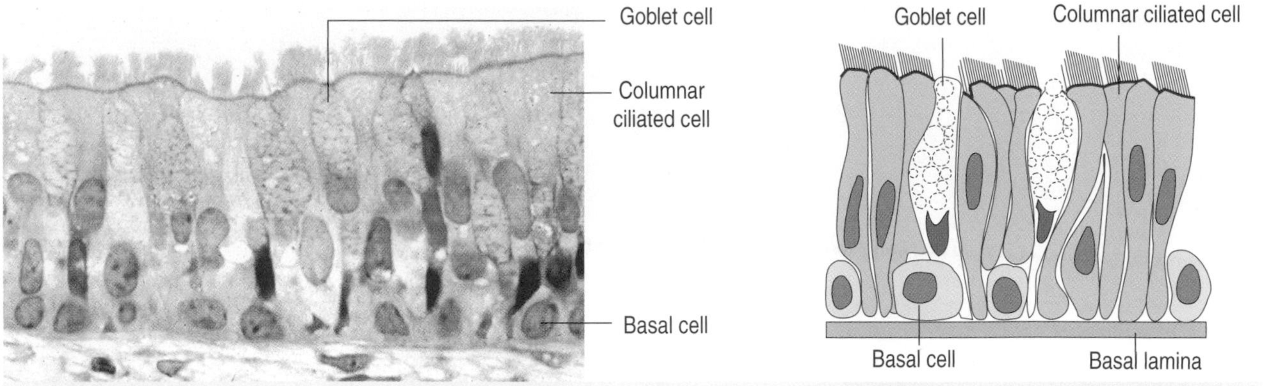
Goblet cell
Columnar ciliated cell
Basal cell
Goblet cell
Columnar ciliated cell
Basal cell
Basal lamina

Pseudostratified columnar ciliated epithelium (trachea)
This epithelium consists of three major cell types: (1) **Columnar cells** with **cilia** on their apical domain. (2) **Basal cells** anchored to the basal lamina. (3) **Goblet cells**, mucus-secreting epithelial cells. Columnar ciliated and goblet cells attach to the basal lamina and reach the lumen. Basal cells do not reach the lumen.

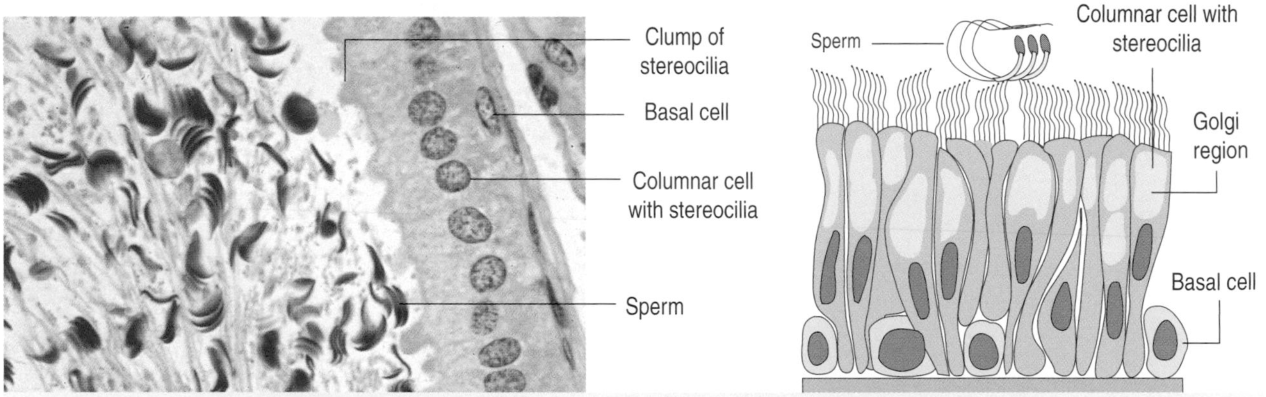
Clump of stereocilia
Basal cell
Columnar cell with stereocilia
Sperm
Sperm
Columnar cell with stereocilia
Golgi region
Basal cell

Pseudostratified columnar epithelium with stereocilia (epididymis)
The epididymal epithelium contains two major cell types. (1) **Columnar cells** with stereocilia and highly developed Golgi apparatus (called principal cells). (2) **Basal cells** attached to the basal lamina. Basal and principal cells are associated with the basal lamina. Only principal cells reach the lumen. Sperm can be visualized in the lumen.

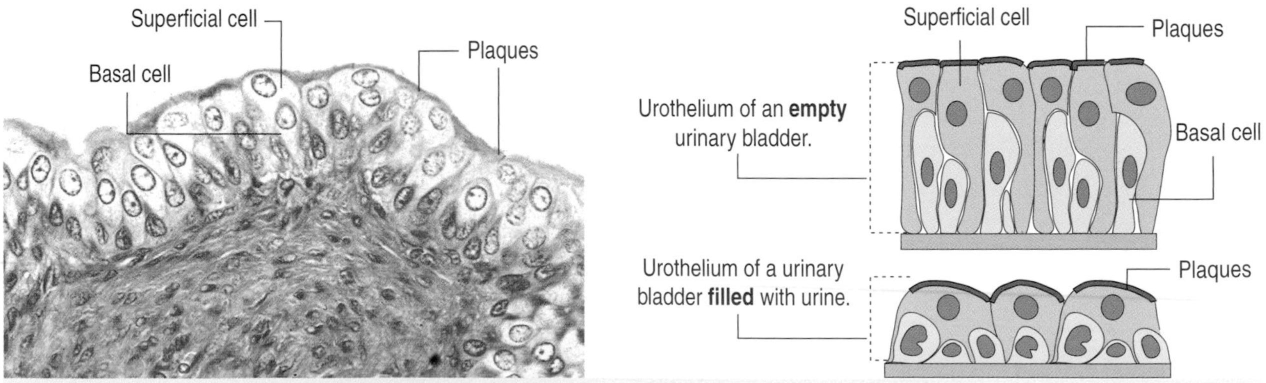
Superficial cell
Basal cell
Plaques
Superficial cell
Plaques
Urothelium of an empty urinary bladder.
Basal cell
Urothelium of a urinary bladder filled with urine.
Plaques

Transitional epithelium (urinary bladder)
The transitional epithelium, lining the urinary passages (also called **urothelium**), consists of two cell types. (1) **Columnar or superficial cells** extending from the basal lamina to the lumen. (2) **Basal cells** attached to the basal lamina. Essentially, the urothelium is a pseudostratified epithelium, although it has the appearance of a stratified squamous epithelium. A characteristic of the urothelium is that superficial cells respond to tensional forces —caused by urine—by changing their geometry and surface configuration. **Plaques** of aggregated proteins are found on the apical plasma membrane of the superficial cells.

domain to anchor epithelial cells to each other and to the basement membrane.

The **apical domain** of some epithelial cells can display three types of differentiation:

1. **Cilia**
2. **Microvilli**
3. **Stereocilia**

Cilia (singular, **cilium**; Figure 1-5) are motile cell projections originating from **basal bodies** anchored by **rootlets** to the apical portion of the cytoplasm. A basal body contains nine **triplet** microtubules in a **helicoid array** without a central microtubular component. By contrast, a cilium consists of an assembly called an **axoneme, formed by a central pair of microtubules surrounded by nine concentrically arranged microtubular pairs. This assembly is known as** the **9 + 2 microtubular doublet arrangement**. The axoneme is also a component of the sperm tail, or **flagellum**.

The trachea and the oviduct are lined by **ciliated** epithelial cells. In these epithelia, ciliary activity is important for the local defense of the respiratory system and for the transport of the fertilized egg to the uterine cavity.

Microvilli (singular, **microvillus**; see Figure 1-5) are finger-like cell projections of the apical epithelial cell surface containing a core of cross-linked microfilaments (a polymer of G-actin monomers). At the cytoplasmic end of the microvillus, bundles of **actin** and other proteins extend into the **terminal web**, a filamentous network of cytoskeletal proteins running parallel to the apical domain of the epithelial cell.

The intestinal epithelium and portions of the nephron in the kidney are lined by epithelial cells with microvilli forming a **brush border**. In general, a brush border indicates the **absorptive** function of the cell.

Stereocilia (singular, **stereocilium**; see Figure 1-5) are long and **branching** finger-like projections of the apical epithelial cell surface. Similar to microvilli, stereocilia contain a core of cross-linked actin with other proteins. **Stereocilia do not have axonemes.** Stereocilia are typical of the epithelial lining of the epididymis and contribute to the process of sperm maturation occurring in this organ.

Cell adhesion molecules and cell junctions

A sheet of epithelial cells forming the lining of the small intestine results from the tight attachment of similar cells to each other and to the **basal lamina**, a component of the extracellular matrix. **Cell adhesion molecules** enable interepithelial cell contact, and this contact is stabilized by specialized **cell junctions**. A

Figure 1–4. Domains of a polarized epithelial cell

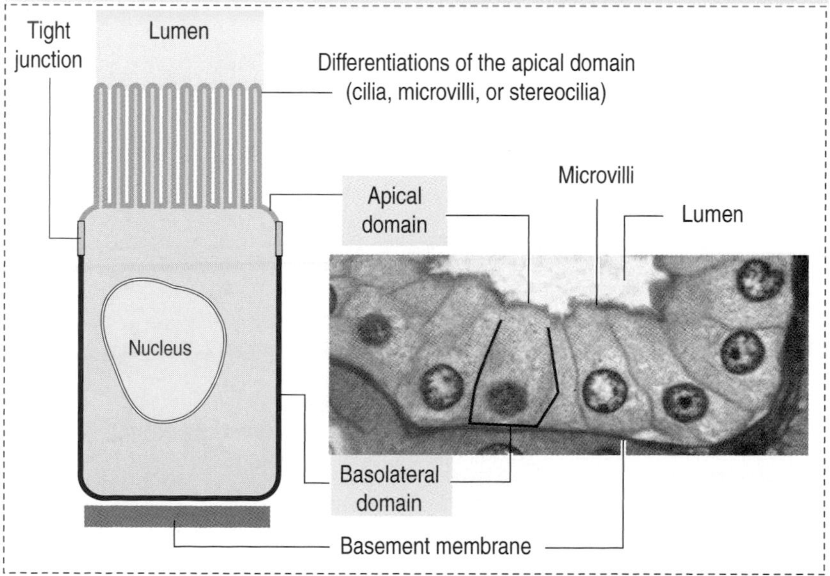
Tight junction
Lumen
Differentiations of the apical domain (cilia, microvilli, or stereocilia)
Microvilli
Apical domain
Lumen
Nucleus
Basolateral domain
Basement membrane

Figure 1–5. Apical differentiations of epithelial cells: cilia, microvilli and stereocilia

Cilium

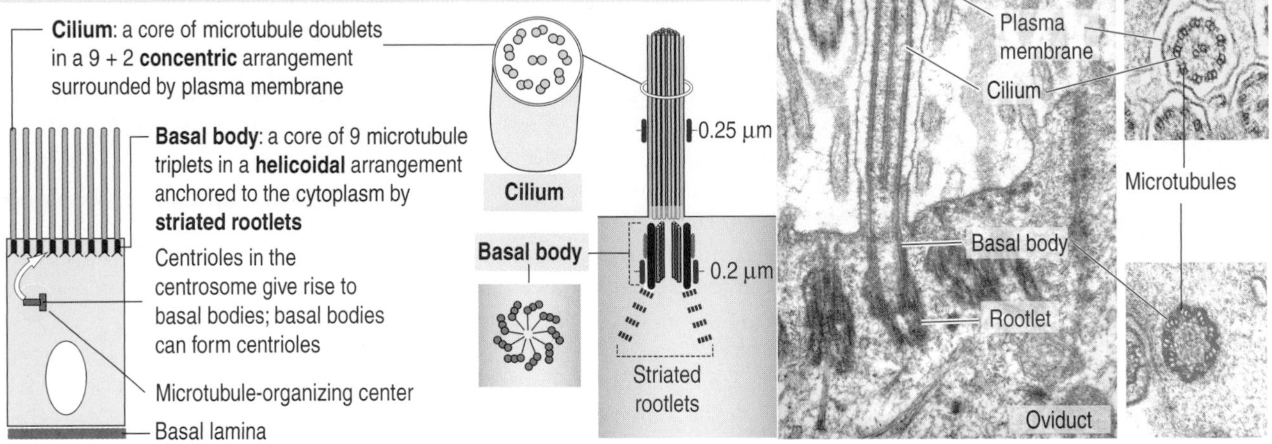

Cilium: a core of microtubule doublets in a 9 + 2 concentric arrangement surrounded by plasma membrane
Basal body: a core of 9 microtubule triplets in a helicoidal arrangement anchored to the cytoplasm by striated rootlets
Centrioles in the centrosome give rise to basal bodies; basal bodies can form centrioles
Microtubule-organizing center
Basal lamina
Cilium
Basal body
0.25 μm
0.2 μm
Striated rootlets
Plasma membrane
Cilium
Basal body
Rootlet
Oviduct
Microtubules

Cilia develop from **basal bodies** located in the apical domain of the cytoplasm. Basal bodies derive from **centrioles** with which they share a similar substructure: **nine peripheral microtubule triplets. Rootlets** anchor the basal body to the cytoplasm. Central microtubules are not present in basal bodies and centrioles. Centrioles, but not basal bodies, are surrounded by a dense material called the **microtubule-organizing center**. The cilium consists of a concentric array of nine microtubule doublets surrounding a central pair of microtubules (9 + 2 organization).

Microvillus

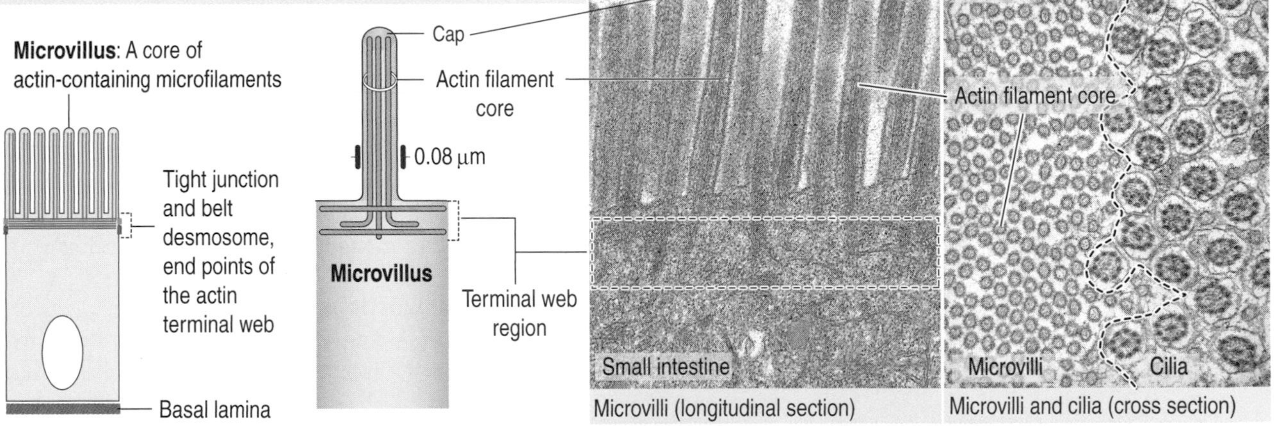

Microvillus: A core of actin-containing microfilaments
Tight junction and belt desmosome, end points of the actin terminal web
Basal lamina
Cap
Actin filament core
0.08 μm
Microvillus
Terminal web region
Small intestine
Microvilli (longitudinal section)
Oviduct
Actin filament core
Microvilli
Cilia
Microvilli and cilia (cross section)

Stereocilium

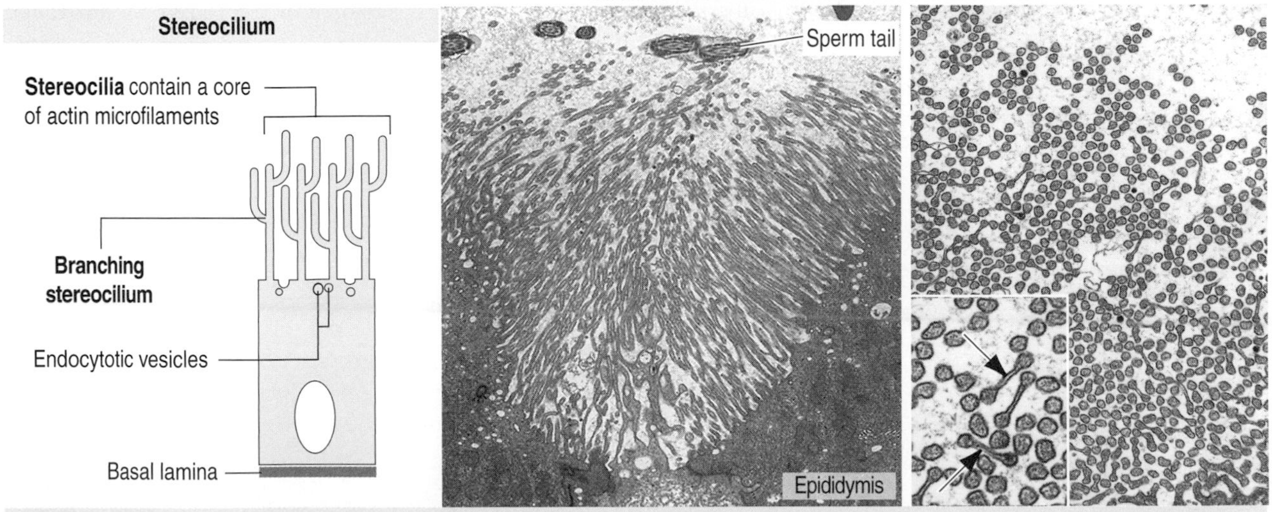

Stereocilia contain a core of actin microfilaments
Branching stereocilium
Endocytotic vesicles
Basal lamina
Sperm tail
Epididymis

Microvilli and **stereocilia** have the same substructure: A core of **actin microfilaments** and actin-associated proteins.
In the intestinal epithelium, actin extends into the **terminal web**, a network of cytoskeletal proteins in a collar-like arrangement at the apical domain of the cytoplasm. Although microvilli have comparable length, **stereocilia are longer and branch,** and the apical domain of the cell contains endocytotic vesicles. The bridges connecting adjacent stereocilia (red arrows) are indicators of their branching.

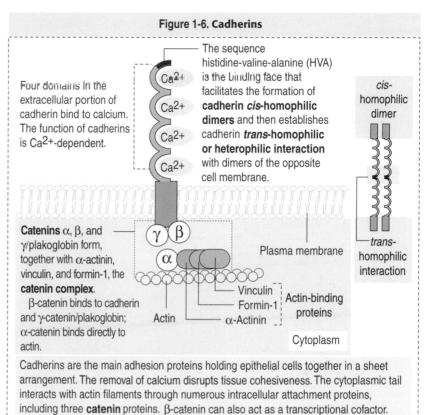

Figure 1-6. Cadherins

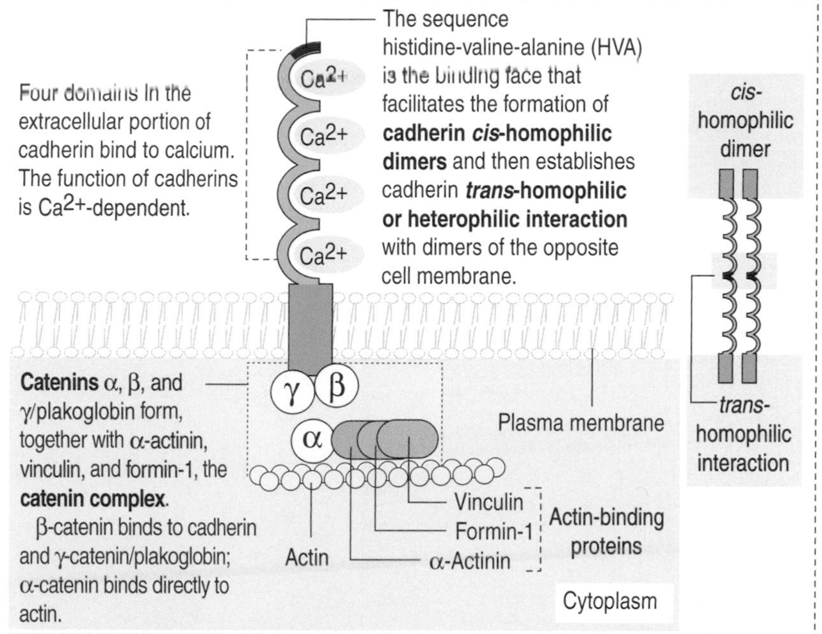

Four domains in the extracellular portion of cadherin bind to calcium. The function of cadherins is Ca2+-dependent.
Ca2+
Ca2+
Ca2+
Ca2+
The sequence histidine-valine-alanine (HVA) is the binding face that facilitates the formation of **cadherin *cis*-homophilic dimers** and then establishes cadherin ***trans*-homophilic or heterophilic interaction** with dimers of the opposite cell membrane.
cis-homophilic dimer
trans-homophilic interaction
Catenins α, β, and γ/plakoglobin form, together with α-actinin, vinculin, and formin-1, the **catenin complex**.
β-catenin binds to cadherin and γ-catenin/plakoglobin; α-catenin binds directly to actin.
γ
β
α
Plasma membrane
Vinculin
Formin-1
α-Actinin
Actin-binding proteins
Actin
Cytoplasm

Cadherins are the main adhesion proteins holding epithelial cells together in a sheet arrangement. The removal of calcium disrupts tissue cohesiveness. The cytoplasmic tail interacts with actin filaments through numerous intracellular attachment proteins, including three **catenin** proteins. β-catenin can also act as a transcriptional cofactor.

consequence of this arrangement is the apical and basolateral domain polarity of an epithelial sheet.

Although cell adhesion molecules and cell junctions are considered here within the framework of epithelia, nonepithelial cells also can use cell adhesion molecules and junctions to establish contact with each other, enabling cell-cell communication. A typical example of nonepithelial cells connected by specialized junctions is the cardiac muscle (see Chapter 7, Muscle Tissue).

There are two major classes of cell adhesion molecules (see Box 1-B):

1. **Ca^{2+}-dependent molecules**, including **cadherins** and **selectins**
2. **Ca^{2+}-independent molecules**, which compose the **immunoglobulin superfamily** and **integrins**

Many cells can use different cell adhesion molecules to mediate cell-cell attachment. Integrins are mainly involved in cell–extracellular matrix interactions. Cadherins and integrins establish a link between the internal cytoskeleton of a cell and the exterior of another cell (cadherins) or the extracellular matrix (integrins).

Cadherins (Figure 1-6) are a family of Ca^{2+}-dependent molecules with a major role in cell adhesion and morphogenesis. A loss of cadherins is associated with the acquisition of invasive behavior by tumor cells (**metastasis**) (see Chapter 4, Connective Tissue).

There are more than 40 different cadherins. **E-cadherin** is an epithelial cadherin found along the lateral cell surfaces and is responsible for the maintenance of most epithelial layers. The removal of calcium or the use of a blocking antibody to E-cadherin in epithelial cell cultures breaks down cell-cell attachment, and the formation of stabilizing junctions is disrupted. E-cadherin molecules form ***cis*-homophilic dimers** ("like-to-like"), which bind to dimers of the **same** or **different class of cadherins in the opposite cell membrane** (*trans*-homophilic or heterophilic ["like-to-unlike"] interaction). These forms of binding require the presence of calcium and result in a specialized zipper-like cell-cell adhesion pattern.

Box 1–B | **Cell adhesion molecules**

- Cell adhesion molecules can be classified as: Ca^{2+}-dependent and Ca^{2+}-independent.
- Ca^{2+}-dependent adhesion molecules include cadherins and selectins.
- Ca^{2+}-independent adhesion molecules include cell adhesion molecules of the immunoglobulin superfamily (CAMs) and integrins.
- Cadherins and CAMs display trans-homophilic interaction across the intercellular space.
- Integrins are the only cell adhesion molecules consisting of two subunits: α and β.
- Cadherins and integrins interact with F–actin through adapters (catenins for cadherins, and vinculin, talin, and α-actinin for integrins).

Figure 1-7. Selectins

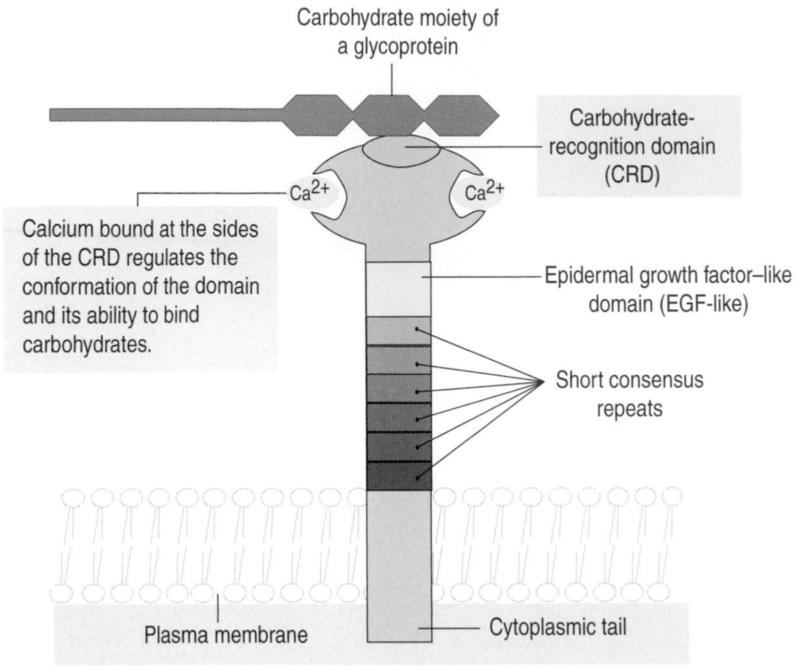

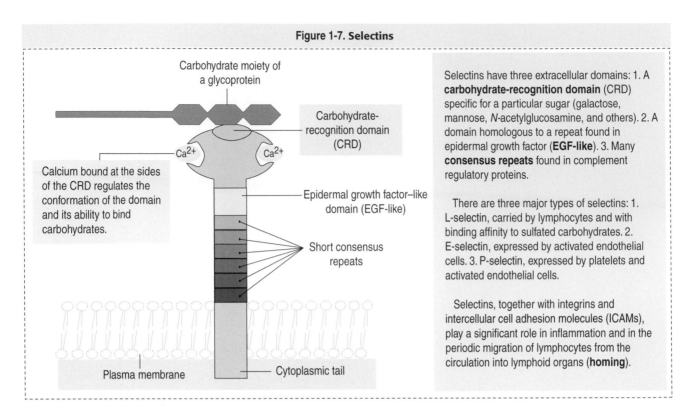

Carbohydrate moiety of a glycoprotein
Carbohydrate-recognition domain (CRD)
Ca2+
Ca2+
Calcium bound at the sides of the CRD regulates the conformation of the domain and its ability to bind carbohydrates.
Epidermal growth factor–like domain (EGF-like)
Short consensus repeats
Plasma membrane
Cytoplasmic tail

Selectins have three extracellular domains: 1. A **carbohydrate-recognition domain** (CRD) specific for a particular sugar (galactose, mannose, *N*-acetylglucosamine, and others). 2. A domain homologous to a repeat found in epidermal growth factor (**EGF-like**). 3. Many **consensus repeats** found in complement regulatory proteins.

There are three major types of selectins: 1. L-selectin, carried by lymphocytes and with binding affinity to sulfated carbohydrates. 2. E-selectin, expressed by activated endothelial cells. 3. P-selectin, expressed by platelets and activated endothelial cells.

Selectins, together with integrins and intercellular cell adhesion molecules (ICAMs), play a significant role in inflammation and in the periodic migration of lymphocytes from the circulation into lymphoid organs (**homing**).

N-cadherin is found in the central nervous system, the lens of the eye, and in skeletal and cardiac muscle. **P-cadherin** is observed in placenta (trophoblast).

The cytoplasmic domain of cadherins is linked to **actin** through intermediate proteins known collectively as the **catenin** (Latin *catena*, chain) **complex**. The complex includes **catenins** (α, β, and γ) and actin-binding proteins, such as α-actinin, vinculin, and formin-1, among others.

The catenin complex has at least three distinct roles in the function of cadherins: (1) catenins mediate a direct link to filamentous actin; (2) they interact with regulatory molecules of the actin cytoskeleton; and (3) they control the adhesive state of the extracellular domain of cadherins. The association of actin to the cadherin-catenin complex is essential for cell morphogenesis, changes in cell shape, and the establishment of cell polarity.

Members of the cadherin family also are present **between cytoplasmic plaques** of the zonula and the macula adherens. β-catenin plays a significant role in **colorectal carcinogenesis** (see Chapter 16, Lower Digestive Segment).

Selectins (Figure 1-7), similar to cadherins, are Ca^{2+}-dependent cell adhesion molecules. In contrast to cadherins, selectins bind to carbohydrates and belong to the group of **lectins** (Latin *lectum*, to select). Each selectin has a carbohydrate-recognition domain (CRD) with binding affinity to a **specific oligosaccharide** attached to a protein (glycoprotein) or a lipid (glycolipid). The molecular configuration of the CRD is controlled by calcium.

Selectins participate in the movement of **leukocytes** (Greek *leukos*, white, *kytos*, cell) circulating in blood (neutrophils, monocytes, B and T cells) toward tissues by **extravasation.** Extravasation is the essence of homing, a mechanism that enables leukocytes to escape from blood circulation and reach the sites of inflammation (see Figure 1-10). Homing also permits thymus-derived T cells to home in on peripheral lymph nodes (see Chapter 10, Immune-Lymphatic System).

The three major classes of cell surface selectins are as follows:

1. **P-selectin**, found in platelets and activated endothelial cells lining blood vessels
2. **E-selectin**, found on activated endothelial cells
3. **L-selectin**, found on leukocytes

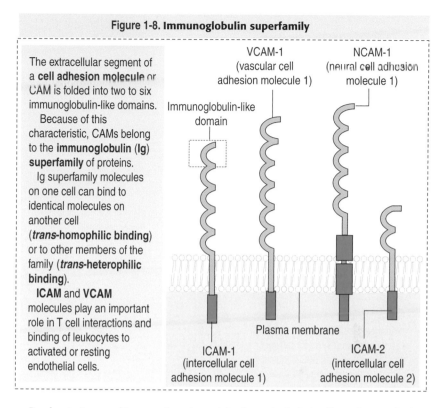

Figure 1-8. Immunoglobulin superfamily

The extracellular segment of a **cell adhesion molecule** or CAM is folded into two to six immunoglobulin-like domains.
Because of this characteristic, CAMs belong to the **immunoglobulin (Ig) superfamily** of proteins.
Ig superfamily molecules on one cell can bind to identical molecules on another cell (***trans*-homophilic binding**) or to other members of the family (***trans*-heterophilic binding**).
ICAM and **VCAM** molecules play an important role in T cell interactions and binding of leukocytes to activated or resting endothelial cells.

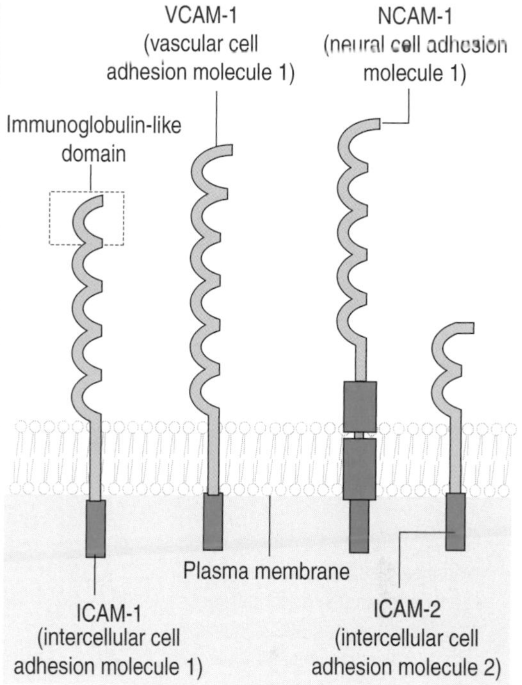
VCAM-1
(vascular cell
adhesion molecule 1)
NCAM-1
(neural cell adhesion
molecule 1)
Immunoglobulin-like
domain
Plasma membrane
ICAM-1
(intercellular cell
adhesion molecule 1)
ICAM-2
(intercellular cell
adhesion molecule 2)

P-selectin is stored in cytoplasmic vesicles in endothelial cells. When endothelial cells are activated by inflammatory signaling, P-selectin appears on the cell surface. On their surface, leukocytes contain **sialyl Lewis-x antigen**, a specific oligosaccharide ligand for P-selectin. P-selectin binding to the antigen slows down streaming leukocytes in blood, and they begin to roll along the endothelial cell surfaces. P-selectins get additional help from members of the immunoglobulin (Ig) superfamily and integrins to stabilize leukocyte attachment, leading to extravasation (see Figure 1-10).

N-CAM (for **neural cell adhesion molecule**) belongs to the Ig superfamily and mediates homophilic and heterophilic interactions. In contrast to cadherins and selectins, members of the Ig superfamily are Ca^{2+}-independent cell adhesion molecules and are encoded by a single gene. Members of the Ig superfamily are generated by the alternative messenger RNA (mRNA) splicing and have differences in glycosylation.

A conserved feature shared by all members of the Ig superfamily is an extracellular segment with one or more **folded domains characteristic of immunoglobulins** (Figure 1-8). Of particular interest is **CD4**, a member of the Ig superfamily and the receptor for the **human immunodeficiency virus type 1 (HIV-1)** in a subclass of lymphocytes known as T cells or helper cells. We discuss the significance of several members of the Ig superfamily in Chapter 10, Immune-Lymphatic System.

Other members of the Ig superfamily play important roles in the homing process during inflammation. Examples include **intercellular adhesion molecules 1** and **2 (ICAM-1** and **ICAM-2)** on endothelial cell surfaces. ICAM-1 is expressed when an inflammation is in progress to facilitate the transendothelial migration of leukocytes (see Chapter 6, Blood and Hematopoiesis).

Integrins (Figure 1-9) differ from cadherins, selectins, and members of the Ig superfamily in that integrins are **heterodimers** formed by two associated **α and β subunits** encoded by different genes. There are about 22 integrin heterodimers consisting of 17 forms of α subunits and 8 forms of β subunits.

Almost every cell expresses one or several integrins. Similar to cadherins, the cytoplasmic domain of β integrins is linked to **actin** filaments through **connecting proteins** (**talin**, **vinculin**, and **α-actinin**).

Figure 1-9. Integrins

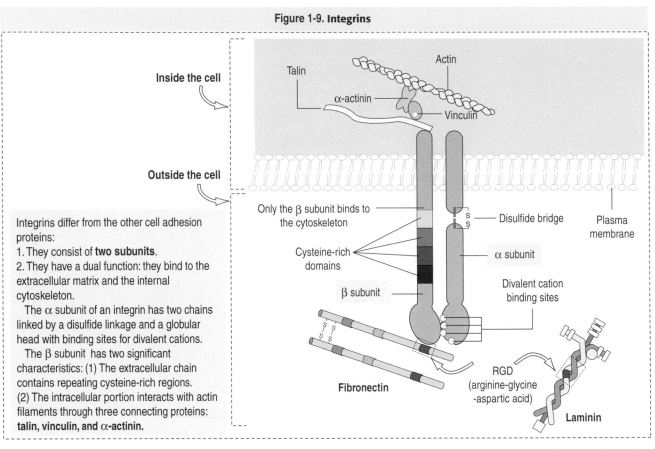

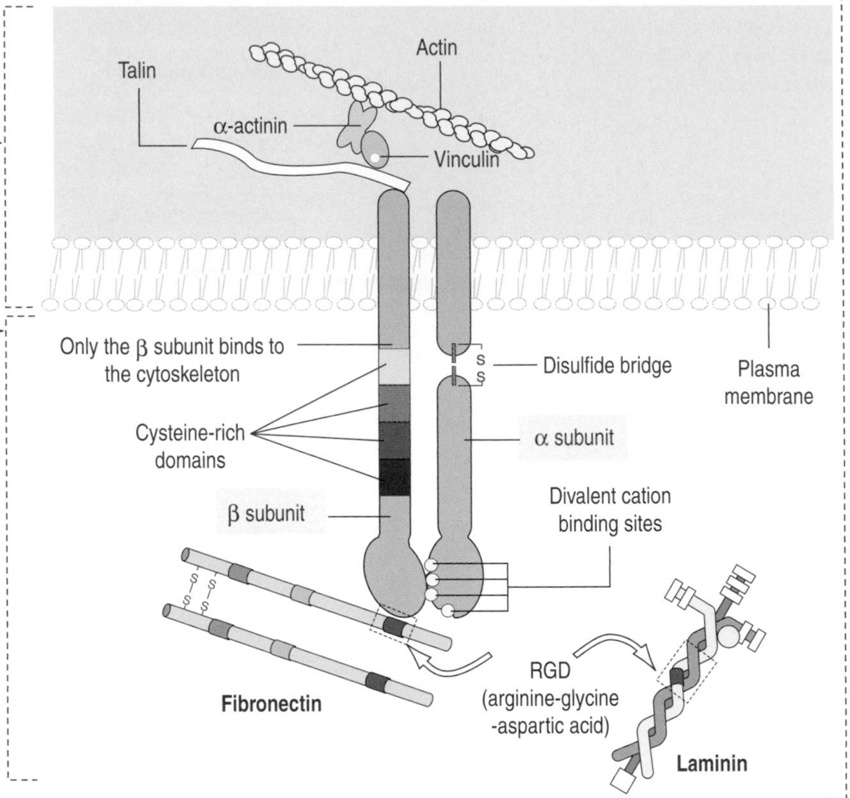
Inside the cell
Outside the cell
Talin
Actin
α-actinin
Vinculin
Only the β subunit binds to the cytoskeleton
S S
Disulfide bridge
Plasma membrane
Cysteine-rich domains
α subunit
β subunit
Divalent cation binding sites
Fibronectin
RGD (arginine-glycine -aspartic acid)
Laminin

Integrins differ from the other cell adhesion proteins:
1. They consist of **two subunits**.
2. They have a dual function: they bind to the extracellular matrix and the internal cytoskeleton.
The α subunit of an integrin has two chains linked by a disulfide linkage and a globular head with binding sites for divalent cations.
The β subunit has two significant characteristics: (1) The extracellular chain contains repeating cysteine-rich regions. (2) The intracellular portion interacts with actin filaments through three connecting proteins: **talin, vinculin, and α-actinin.**

The extracellular domain of integrins binds to the **tripeptide RGD (Arg-Gly-Asp)** sequence present in **laminin** and **fibronectin**, two major components of the **basement membrane**, a specific type of extracellular matrix. Laminin and fibronectin interact with various collagen types (including **type IV collagen**), **heparan sulfate proteoglycans**, and **entactin** (also called **nidogen**).

The integrin–extracellular matrix relationship is critical for cell migration to precise sites during embryogenesis and can be disrupted when cell motility is required. In addition to their role in cell-matrix interactions, integrins also mediate cell-cell interaction. Integrins containing β_2 subunits are expressed on the surface of leukocytes and mediate cell-cell binding. An example is the $\alpha_1\beta_2$ integrin heterodimer that binds to ligands on endothelial cell surfaces during the integrin phase (extravasation) of homing (Figure 1-10).

Integrins respond to intercellular events by changing their adhesive conformation with respect to molecules of the extracellular matrix. This response is known as **inside-out signaling**. In addition, integrins mediate a complex intracellular cascade in response to extracellular events.

ADAM proteins

The reversal of integrin mediated cell binding to the extracellular matrix can be disrupted by proteins called **ADAM** (for *a d*isintegrin *a*nd *m*etalloprotease). ADAMs have pivotal roles in fertilization, angiogenesis, neurogenesis, heart development, and cancer.

A typical ADAM protein (see Figure 1-11) contains an **extracellular domain** and an **intracellular domain.** The extracellular domain consists of several portions including a **disintegrin domain** and a **metalloprotease domain**.

1. A disintegrin domain binds to integrins and competitively prevents integrin-mediated binding of cells to laminin, fibronectin, and other extracellular matrix proteins.

2. A metalloprotease domain degrades matrix components and enables cell

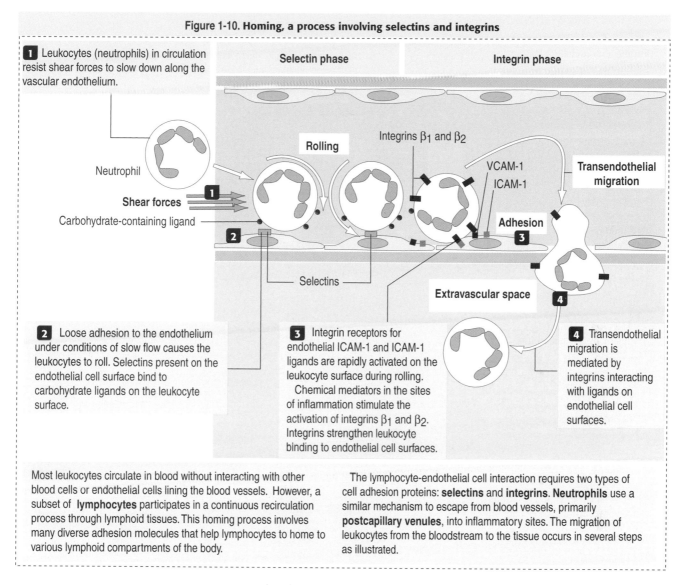

Figure 1-10. Homing, a process involving selectins and integrins

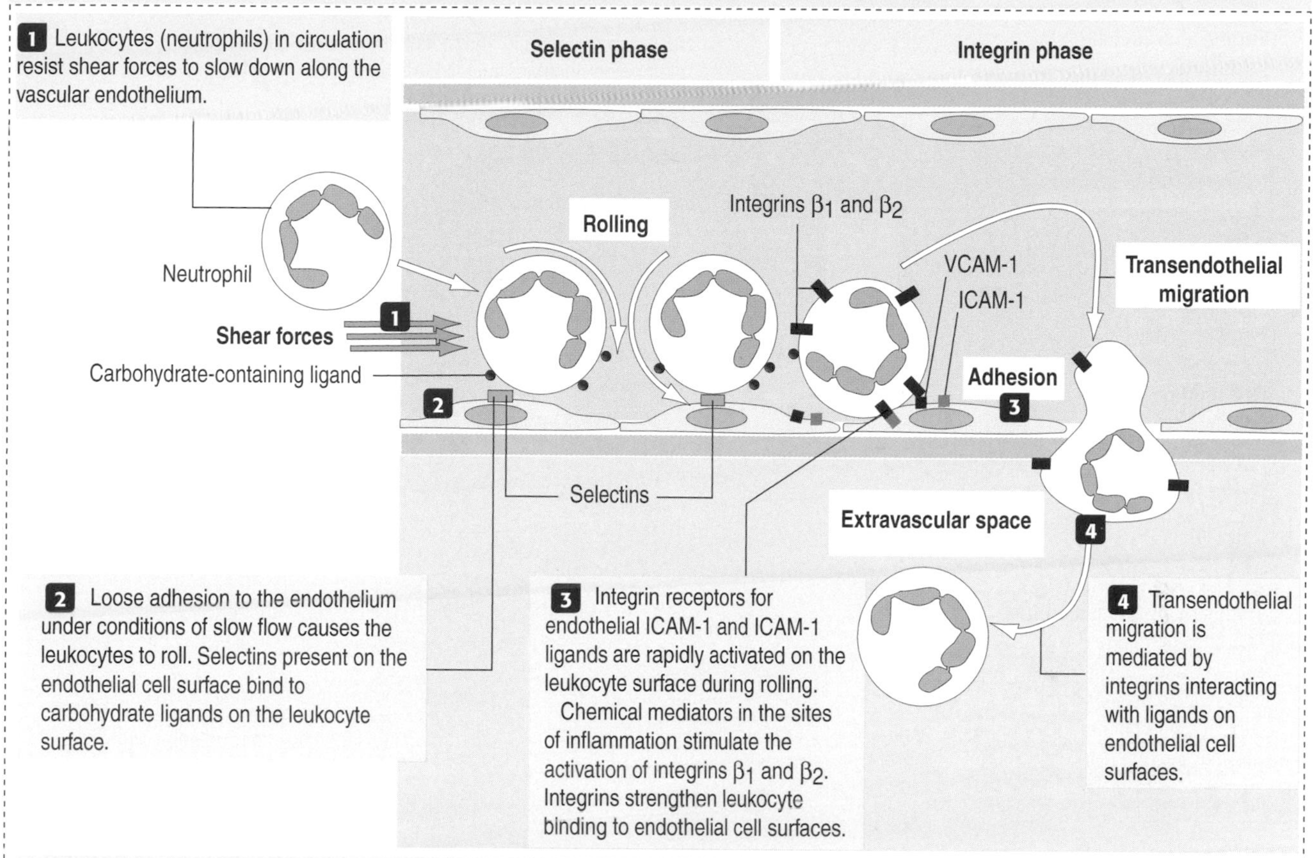
1 Leukocytes (neutrophils) in circulation resist shear forces to slow down along the vascular endothelium.
Selectin phase
Integrin phase
Neutrophil
Rolling
Integrins β1 and β2
VCAM-1
ICAM-1
Transendothelial migration
1
Shear forces
Carbohydrate-containing ligand
2
Adhesion
3
Selectins
Extravascular space
4
2 Loose adhesion to the endothelium under conditions of slow flow causes the leukocytes to roll. Selectins present on the endothelial cell surface bind to carbohydrate ligands on the leukocyte surface.
3 Integrin receptors for endothelial ICAM-1 and ICAM-1 ligands are rapidly activated on the leukocyte surface during rolling.
Chemical mediators in the sites of inflammation stimulate the activation of integrins β1 and β2. Integrins strengthen leukocyte binding to endothelial cell surfaces.
4 Transendothelial migration is mediated by integrins interacting with ligands on endothelial cell surfaces.

Most leukocytes circulate in blood without interacting with other blood cells or endothelial cells lining the blood vessels. However, a subset of **lymphocytes** participates in a continuous recirculation process through lymphoid tissues. This homing process involves many diverse adhesion molecules that help lymphocytes to home to various lymphoid compartments of the body.

The lymphocyte-endothelial cell interaction requires two types of cell adhesion proteins: **selectins** and **integrins**. **Neutrophils** use a similar mechanism to escape from blood vessels, primarily **postcapillary venules**, into inflammatory sites. The migration of leukocytes from the bloodstream to the tissue occurs in several steps as illustrated.

migration.

A significant function of ADAMs is **protein ectodomain shedding**, consisting of the proteolytic release of the ectodomain of a membrane protein cleaved adjacent to the plasma membrane. Ectodomain shedding targets for cleavage the **proinflammatory cytokine tumor necrosis factor-α** (TNF-α) and **all ligands of the epidermal growth factor receptor**. A released soluble ectodomain of a cytokine or growth factor can function at a distance from the site of cleavage (paracrine signaling). Ectodomain shedding of a receptor can inactivate the receptor by functioning as a decoy sequestering soluble ligands away from the plasma membrane-bound unoccupied receptor.

A defect in **TNF receptor 1** (TNFR1) shedding, determined by a mutation in the receptor cleavage site, causes a **periodic febrile syndrome** because of continuous availability of TNFR1 for TNF-α binding. Consequently, recurring fever occurs by increased inflammatory responses.

Cell junctions

Although cell adhesion molecules are responsible for cell-cell adhesion, cell junctions are necessary for providing stronger stability. In addition, the movement of solutes, ions, and water through an epithelial layer occurs **across** and **between** individual cell components. The **transcellular pathway** is controlled by numerous channels and transporters. The **paracellular pathway** is regulated by a continuous

Figure 1-11. **ADAM protein (a disintegrin and metalloprotease)**

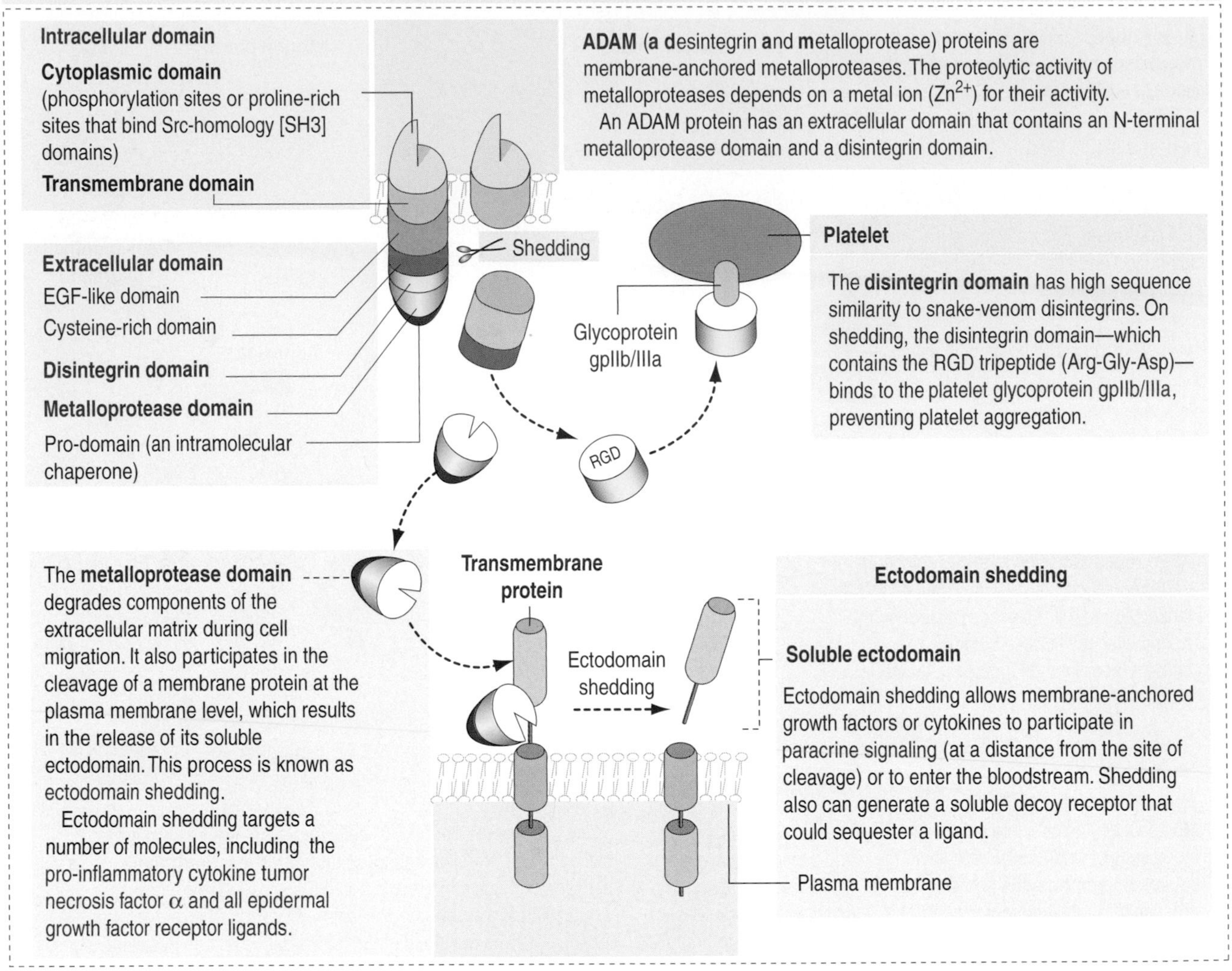

Intracellular domain
Cytoplasmic domain
(phosphorylation sites or proline-rich sites that bind Src-homology [SH3] domains)
Transmembrane domain
Extracellular domain
EGF-like domain
Cysteine-rich domain
Disintegrin domain
Metalloprotease domain
Pro-domain (an intramolecular chaperone)
Shedding
ADAM (a desintegrin and metalloprotease) proteins are membrane-anchored metalloproteases. The proteolytic activity of metalloproteases depends on a metal ion (Zn^{2+}) for their activity.
An ADAM protein has an extracellular domain that contains an N-terminal metalloprotease domain and a disintegrin domain.
Platelet
Glycoprotein gpIIb/IIIa
RGD
The disintegrin domain has high sequence similarity to snake-venom disintegrins. On shedding, the disintegrin domain—which contains the RGD tripeptide (Arg-Gly-Asp)—binds to the platelet glycoprotein gpIIb/IIIa, preventing platelet aggregation.
The metalloprotease domain degrades components of the extracellular matrix during cell migration. It also participates in the cleavage of a membrane protein at the plasma membrane level, which results in the release of its soluble ectodomain. This process is known as ectodomain shedding.
Ectodomain shedding targets a number of molecules, including the pro-inflammatory cytokine tumor necrosis factor α and all epidermal growth factor receptor ligands.
Transmembrane protein
Ectodomain shedding
Ectodomain shedding
Soluble ectodomain
Ectodomain shedding allows membrane-anchored growth factors or cytokines to participate in paracrine signaling (at a distance from the site of cleavage) or to enter the bloodstream. Shedding also can generate a soluble decoy receptor that could sequester a ligand.
Plasma membrane

intercellular contact or **cell junctions**. A deficiency in the cell junctions accounts for acquired and inherited diseases caused by inefficient epithelial barriers.

Cell junctions are **symmetrical** structures formed between two adjacent cells. There are three major classes of **symmetrical** cell junctions (Figure 1-12; see **Box 1-C**):

1. **Tight junctions**
2. **Anchoring junctions**
3. **Gap** or **communicating junctions**

Tight junctions (also called **occluding junctions**) (Figure 1-13) have two major functions:

1. They determine **epithelial cell polarity** by separating the apical domain from the basolateral domain and preventing the free diffusion of lipids and proteins between them.

2. They prevent the free passage of substances across an epithelial cell layer (**paracellular pathway barrier**).

Cell membranes of two adjacent cells come together at regular intervals to seal the apical intercellular space. These areas of close contact continue around the entire surface of the cell like a belt, forming anastomosing strips of the transmembrane proteins **occludin** and **claudin**. Occludin and claudin belong to the family of **tetraspanins** with four transmembrane domains, two outer loops and two short cytoplasmic tails.

Occludin interacts with four major **zonula occludin** (ZO) proteins: **ZO-1**,

Figure 1-12. Anchoring and communicating junctions

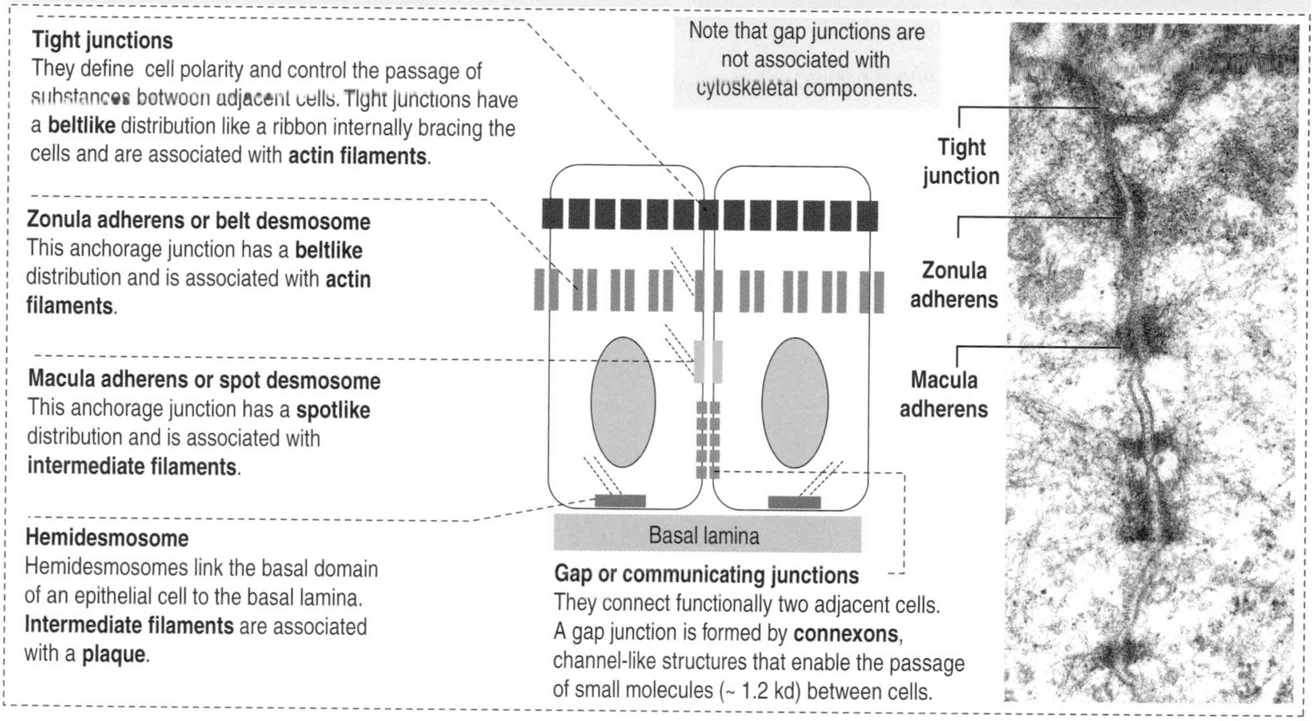
Tight junctions
They define cell polarity and control the passage of substances between adjacent cells. Tight junctions have a beltlike distribution like a ribbon internally bracing the cells and are associated with actin filaments.
Zonula adherens or belt desmosome
This anchorage junction has a beltlike distribution and is associated with actin filaments.
Macula adherens or spot desmosome
This anchorage junction has a spotlike distribution and is associated with intermediate filaments.
Hemidesmosome
Hemidesmosomes link the basal domain of an epithelial cell to the basal lamina. Intermediate filaments are associated with a plaque.
Note that gap junctions are not associated with cytoskeletal components.
Basal lamina
Gap or communicating junctions
They connect functionally two adjacent cells. A gap junction is formed by connexons, channel-like structures that enable the passage of small molecules (~ 1.2 kd) between cells.
Tight junction
Zonula adherens
Macula adherens

ZO-2, ZO-3, and **afadin**. **Claudin** (Latin *claudere*, to close), a family of 16 proteins forming linear fibrils in the tight junctions, confers barrier properties on the paracellular pathway. A mutation in the gene encoding **claudin 16** is the cause of a rare human **renal magnesium wasting syndrome** characterized by hypomagnesemia and seizures.

Two members of the Ig superfamily, **nectins** and **junctional adhesion molecules (JAMs)**, are present in tight junctions. Both form homodimers (*cis* homodimers) and then *trans* homodimers across the intercellular space. Nectins are connected to actin filaments through the protein **afadin**. The targeted deletion of the *afadin* gene in mice results in embryonic lethality. A mutation in the *nectin-1* gene is responsible for **cleft lip/palate and ectodermal dysplasia** (CLEPD1) of skin, hairs, nails, and teeth in humans. Nectin-2–deficient male mice are sterile.

Tight junctions can be visualized by **freeze-fracturing** a network of **branching and anastomosing sealing strands**. We discuss in Chapter 2, Epithelial Glands, the procedure of freeze-fracturing for the study of cell membranes.

Anchoring junctions are found below the tight junctions, usually near the apical surface of an epithelium. There are three classes of **anchoring junctions** (see Figures 1-12, 1-14, 1-16, and 1-17):

1. The **zonula adherens** or **belt desmosome**
2. The **macula adherens** or **spot desmosome**
3. The **hemidesmosome**

Similar to the tight junctions, the **zonula adherens** is a **beltlike junction**. The zonula adherens (Figure 1-14) is associated with **actin microfilaments**. This association is mediated by the interaction of **cadherins** (**desmocollins** and **desmogleins**) with **catenins** (α, β, and γ). The main desmogleins expressed in the epidermis of the skin are desmoglein 1 and desmoglein 3 (Figure 1-15).

The **macula adherens** (also called **desmosome**) is a **spotlike** junction associated with **keratin intermediate filaments** (also known as **tonofilaments**) extending from one spot to another on the lateral and basal cell surfaces of epithelial cells (Figure 1-16). Spot desmosomes provide strength and rigidity to an epithelial cell layer. Spot desmosomes are also present in the intercalated disks linking adjacent cardiocytes in heart (see Chapter 7, Muscle Tissue) and in the meninges lining

Figure 1-13. Molecular organization of tight junctions

Tight junctions are circumferential belts at the apical domain of epithelial cells and linking adjacent endothelial cells. Tight junctions seal the space between epithelial cells and regulate the passage of water and flux of ions between adjacent epithelial cells (**paracellular pathway**). Molecules across the cell follow a **transcellular pathway**.

Afadin-nectin complex is anchored to ZO-1. Nectins form *cis*-homodimers, which interact with each other (*trans*-homo interaction) through the extracellular region.

Junctional adhesion molecules (JAMs) are associated to afadin and ZO-1. JAMs *cis*-homodimers interact with each other (*trans*-homo interaction) and determine the formation of cell polarity.

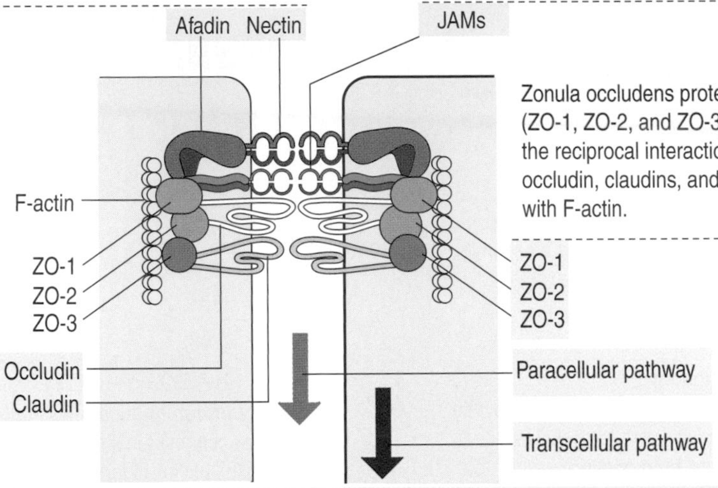

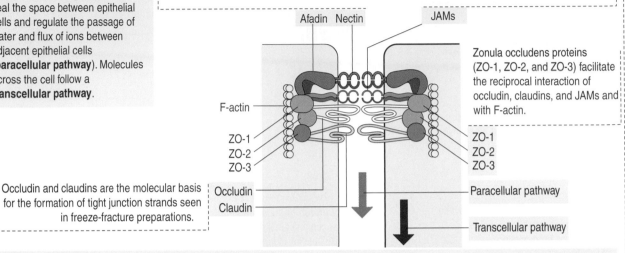

Zonula occludens proteins (ZO-1, ZO-2, and ZO-3) facilitate the reciprocal interaction of occludin, claudins, and JAMs and with F-actin.

Occludin and claudins are the molecular basis for the formation of tight junction strands seen in freeze-fracture preparations.

Nectins and JAMs are members of the immunoglobulin subfamily. Their structure is characterized by immunoglobulin loops, each stabilized by disulfide bonds. Nectins and JAMs *cis*-homodimers mediate *trans*-homo cell-cell adhesion.

Occludin and claudins are members of the tetraspanin family of proteins, containing four transmembrane domains, two loops and two cytoplasmic tails.

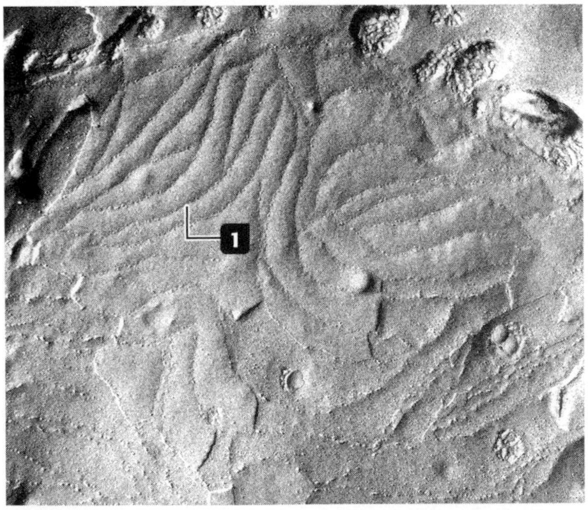

1 In **freeze-fracture preparations**, tight junctions appear as branching and **interconnected sealing ridges** forming a network near the apical domain of the cell. The ridges represent the transmembrane proteins **occludin** and **claudins** associated with the fractured protoplasmic face (PF).

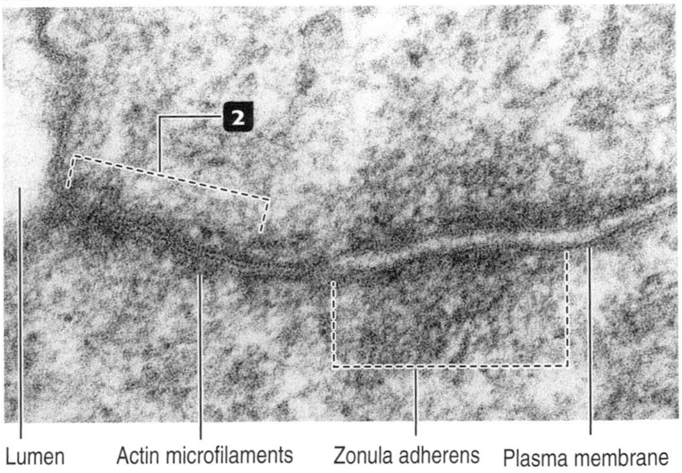

2 In thin sections, the intercellular space is occluded by **occludin**, **claudins**, **JAMs** and **nectins**. The **zonula adherens** or belt desmosome is usually found below tight junctions.

the outer surface of the brain and spinal cord.

In contrast to occluding junctions, adjacent cell membranes linked by zonula and macula adherens are separated by a relatively wide intercellular space. This space is occupied by the glycosylated portion of proteins of the **cadherin** family, **desmogleins** and **desmocollins**, anchored to **cytoplasmic plaques** containing **desmoplakin**, **plakoglobin** (γ-catenin), and **plakophilin**. The cytoplasmic plaques are attached to the cytosolic face of the plasma membrane. The interlocking of similar cadherins binds two cells together by Ca^{2+}-dependent homophilic or heterophilic interaction, as we have already seen. Inherited disorders of some of

Box 1–C | **Cell junctions**

• Cell junctions can be classified as **symmetrical** and **asymmetrical**. Symmetrical junctions include the tight junctions, the belt desmosome (zonula adherens), desmosomes (macula adherens), and gap junctions. The hemidesmosome is an asymmetrical junction
• **Tight junctions** contain occludin and claudin, belonging to the protein family of tetraspanins because four segments of each protein span the plasma membrane. An additional component is the afadin-nectin protein complex.
Junctional adhesion molecules (JAMs), zonula occludens (ZO) proteins ZO-1, ZO-2, and ZO-3 and F-actin are additional protein components. Tight junctions form a circumferential gasket that controls the paracellular pathway of molecules.
• **Zonula adherens** (belt desmosome) consists of a **plaque** that contains desmoplakin, plakoglobin (γ catenin), and plakophilin. Cadherins, mainly desmocollins and desmogleins dimers, and the afadin-nectin complex extend from the plaque to the extracellular space. A catenin complex links actin filaments to the plaque. Similar to tight junctions, the belt desmosome forms a circumferential gasket at the apical region of epithelial cells.
• **Macula adherens** (spot desmosome) are structurally comparable to the zonula adherens except that the afadin-nectin and catenin complexes are absent and intermediate filaments (tonofilaments), instead of actin filaments, are attached to the plaque.
• **Hemidesmosomes** consist of an outer **plate**—to which tonofilaments attach—and an outer **plaque**, linked by integrin $\alpha_6\beta_4$ and laminin 5 to the basal lamina.
• Tight junctions, the belt desmosome, spot desmosomes, and hemidesmosomes are anchoring junctions. **Gap junctions** are not anchoring junctions. Instead, gap junctions are communicating junctions linking adjacent cells. The basic unit of a gap junction is the connexon, formed by 6 connexin molecules surrounding a central channel.

Figure 1-14. Zonula adherens (belt desmosome)

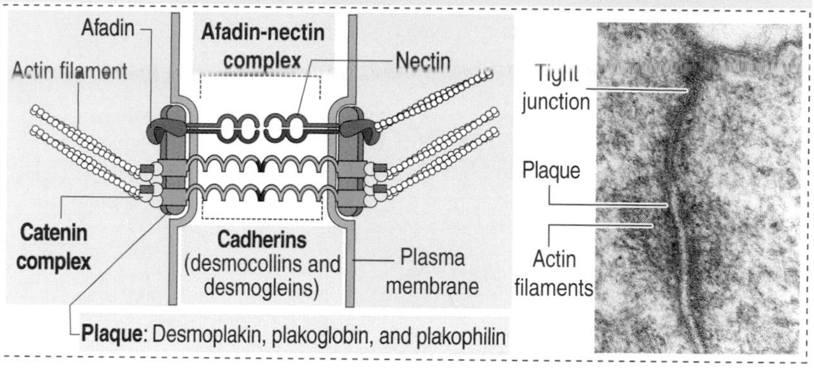

Afadin
Actin filament
Afadin-nectin complex
Nectin
Catenin complex
Cadherins (desmocollins and desmogleins)
Plasma membrane
Plaque: Desmoplakin, plakoglobin, and plakophilin
Tight junction
Plaque
Actin filaments

the desmosomal components are indicated in Figure 1-16.

The human desmosomal cadherins genes include four desmogleins and three desmocollins. Their cytoplasmic regions interact with plakoglobin and plakophilin. Desmoplakin interacts with the intermediate filaments keratin in epidermis, desmin in the intercalated disks, and vimentin in the meninges. **Desmoglein 1** and **desmoglein 3** maintain the cohesiveness of the epidermis, a stratified squamous epithelium. Autoantibodies to desmoglein 1 cause a blistering disease (disruption of cell adhesion) of the skin called **pemphigus foliaceus** (see Figure 1-15).

Hemidesmosomes are **asymmetrical** structures anchoring the basal domain of an epithelial cell to the underlying basal lamina (Figure 1-17).

Hemidesmosomes have a different organization compared with a macula adherens or desmosome. A hemidesmosome consists of the following:

1. An **inner cytoplasmic plate** associated with intermediate filaments (also called **keratins** or **tonofilaments**)

2. An **outer membrane plaque** linking the hemidesmosome to the basal lamina by **anchoring filaments** (composed of **laminin** 5) and **integrin** $\alpha_6\beta_4$

Although hemidesmosomes look like half-desmosomes, none of the biochemical components present in the desmosome is found in hemidesmosomes. Hemidesmosomes increase the overall stability of epithelial tissues by linking intermediate filaments of the cytoskeleton with components of the basal lamina. We consider additional details of the hemidesmosomes and their role in autoimmune diseases of the skin when we discuss the structure of intermediate filaments in the cytoskeleton section.

Gap junctions are symmetric communicating junctions formed by integral membrane proteins called **connexins. Six connexin monomers associate to form a connexon**, a hollow cylindrical structure that spans the plasma membrane. The

Figure 1-15. Desmogleins in skin disease: Pemphigus foliaceus

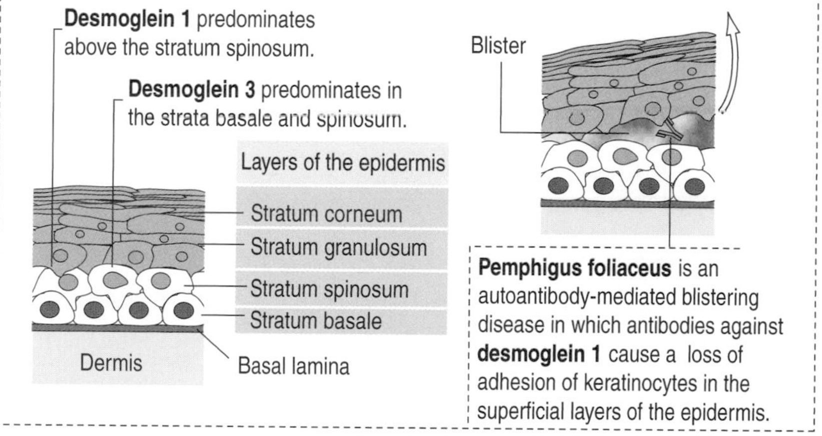

Desmoglein 1 predominates above the stratum spinosum.
Desmoglein 3 predominates in the strata basale and spinosum.
Layers of the epidermis
Stratum corneum
Stratum granulosum
Stratum spinosum
Stratum basale
Dermis
Basal lamina
Blister

Pemphigus foliaceus is an autoantibody-mediated blistering disease in which antibodies against **desmoglein 1** cause a loss of adhesion of keratinocytes in the superficial layers of the epidermis.

Figure 1-16. Macula adherens (spot desmosome)

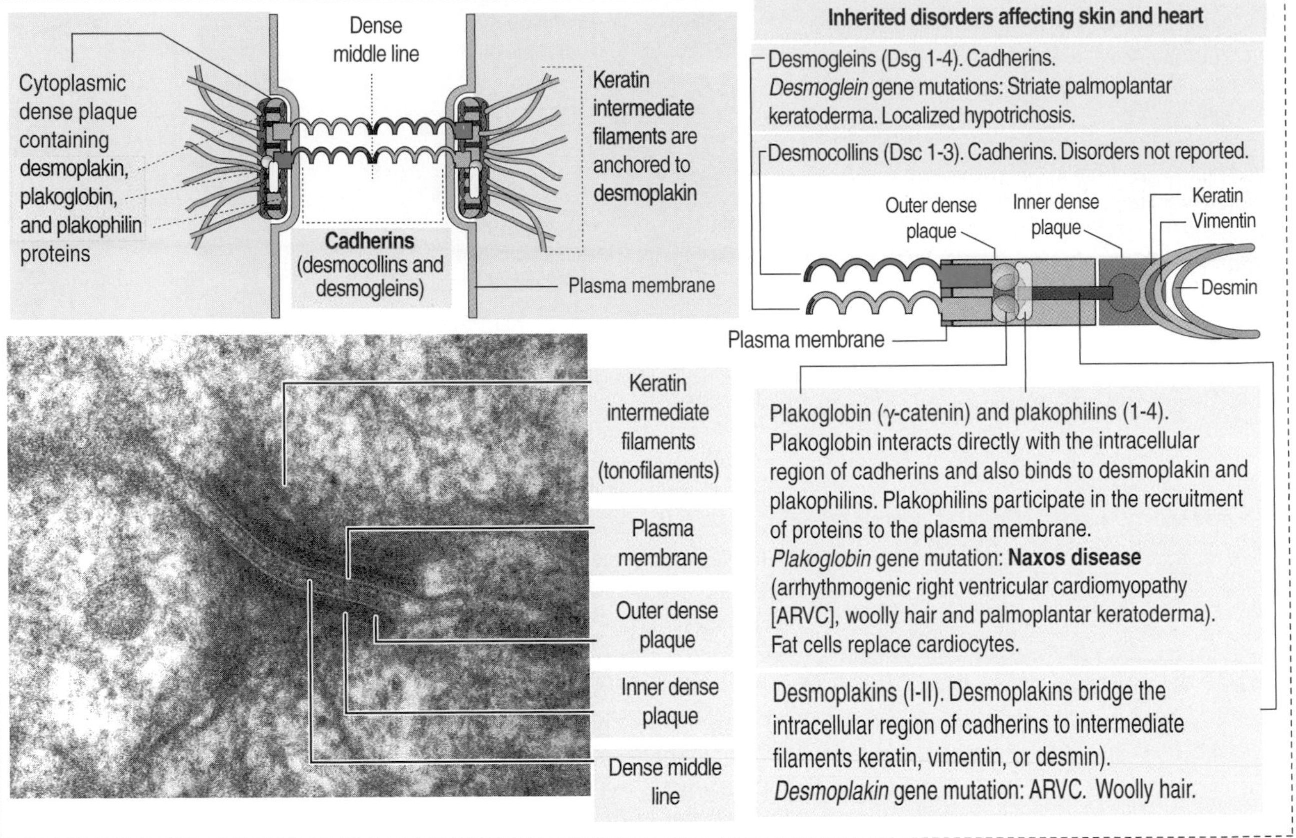
Dense middle line
Cytoplasmic dense plaque containing desmoplakin, plakoglobin, and plakophilin proteins
Keratin intermediate filaments are anchored to desmoplakin
Cadherins (desmocollins and desmogleins)
Plasma membrane
Inherited disorders affecting skin and heart
Desmogleins (Dsg 1-4). Cadherins.
Desmoglein gene mutations: Striate palmoplantar keratoderma. Localized hypotrichosis.
Desmocollins (Dsc 1-3). Cadherins. Disorders not reported.
Outer dense plaque
Inner dense plaque
Keratin
Vimentin
Desmin
Plasma membrane
Plakoglobin (γ-catenin) and plakophilins (1-4). Plakoglobin interacts directly with the intracellular region of cadherins and also binds to desmoplakin and plakophilins. Plakophilins participate in the recruitment of proteins to the plasma membrane.
Plakoglobin gene mutation: **Naxos disease** (arrhythmogenic right ventricular cardiomyopathy [ARVC], woolly hair and palmoplantar keratoderma). Fat cells replace cardiocytes.
Desmoplakins (I-II). Desmoplakins bridge the intracellular region of cadherins to intermediate filaments keratin, vimentin, or desmin).
Desmoplakin gene mutation: ARVC. Woolly hair.
Keratin intermediate filaments (tonofilaments)
Plasma membrane
Outer dense plaque
Inner dense plaque
Dense middle line

end-to-end alignment of connexons in adjacent cells provides a direct channel of communication (1.5 to 2 nm in diameter) between the cytoplasm of two adjacent cells (Figure 1-18). Connexons have a **clustering** tendency and can form patches about 0.3 mm in diameter.

These junctions facilitate the movement of molecules 1.2 nm in diameter (for example, Ca^{2+} and cyclic adenosine monophosphate [cAMP]) between cells. The connexon axial channels close when the concentration of Ca^{2+} is high. This junction is responsible for the chemical and electrical "**coupling**" between adjacent cells. A typical example is **cardiac muscle cells** connected by gap junctions to enable the transmission of electrical signals.

Figure 1-17. Hemidesmosome

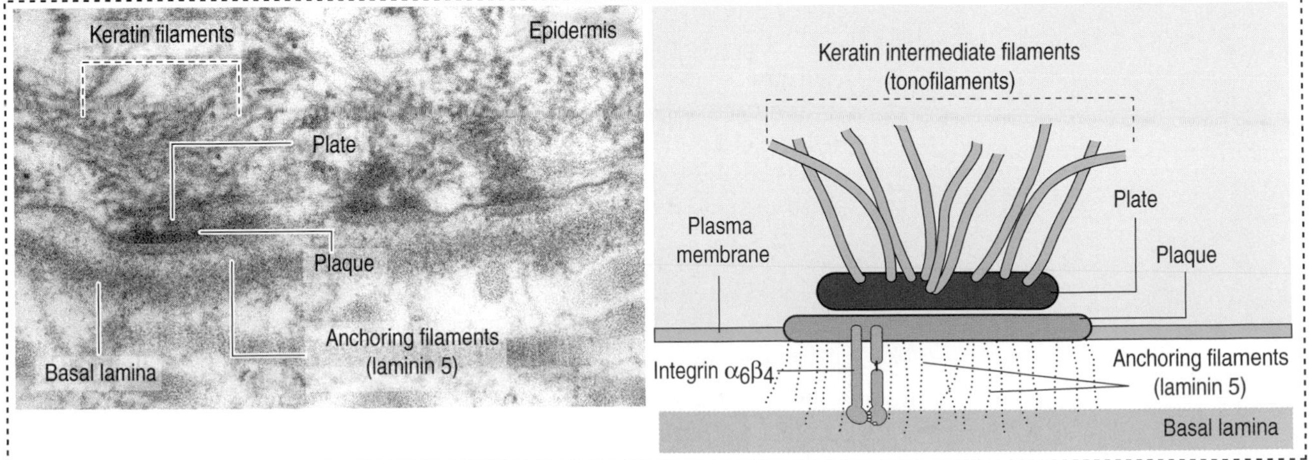
Keratin filaments
Epidermis
Plate
Plaque
Anchoring filaments (laminin 5)
Basal lamina
Keratin intermediate filaments (tonofilaments)
Plate
Plasma membrane
Plaque
Integrin α6β4
Anchoring filaments (laminin 5)
Basal lamina

Figure 1-18. Gap junctions

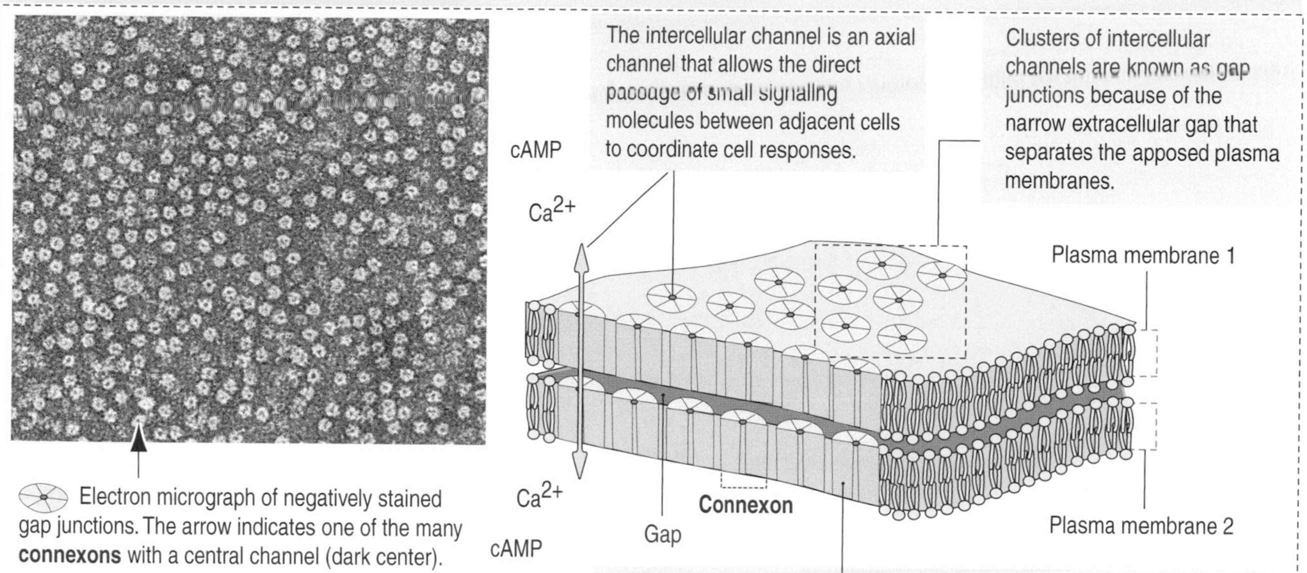
The intercellular channel is an axial channel that allows the direct passage of small signalling molecules between adjacent cells to coordinate cell responses.
Clusters of intercellular channels are known as gap junctions because of the narrow extracellular gap that separates the apposed plasma membranes.
cAMP
Ca2+
Plasma membrane 1
Ca2+
cAMP
Gap
Connexon
Plasma membrane 2

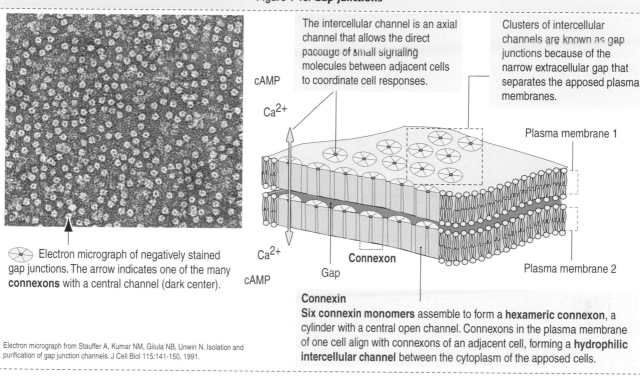

Electron micrograph of negatively stained gap junctions. The arrow indicates one of the many **connexons** with a central channel (dark center).

Connexin
Six connexin monomers assemble to form a **hexameric connexon**, a cylinder with a central open channel. Connexons in the plasma membrane of one cell align with connexons of an adjacent cell, forming a **hydrophilic intercellular channel** between the cytoplasm of the apposed cells.

Electron micrograph from Stauffer A, Kumar NM, Gilula NB, Unwin N. Isolation and purification of gap junction channels. J Cell Biol 115:141-150, 1991.

Clinical significance: Connexin mutations in human disease

Several diseases occur when genes encoding connexins are mutated. Mutations in the *connexin 26* (*Cx26*) **gene**, highly expressed in cells of the cochlea, are associated with **deafness**.

Mutations in the *connexin 32* (*Cx32*) gene are found in X-linked **Charcot-Marie-Tooth demyelinating neuropathy** resulting in progressive degeneration of peripheral nerves, characterized by distal muscle weakness and atrophy and impairment of deep tendon reflexes. Connexin 32 protein is expressed in Schwann cells, which are involved in the production of rolled myelin tubes around the axons in the peripheral nervous system (see Chapter 8, Nervous Tissue). Gap junctions couple different parts of the rolled myelin tubes of the *same Schwann cell*, rather than different cells. A loss of the functional axial channels in myelin leads to the demyelinating disorder. Mutations in the *connexin 50* (*Cx50*) gene are associated with **congenital cataracts**, leading to blindness.

Bone cells (osteoblasts/osteocytes) are connected by gap junctions and express connexin 43 (Cx43) and connexin 45 (Cx45) proteins. A deletion of the *Cx43* gene determines skeletal defects and delays in mineralization.

Laminin, fibronectin, and the basement membrane

Integrins mediate cell-matrix interactions by their binding affinity to the RGD domain in laminin and fibronectin (see Figure 1-9). **Laminin** and **fibronectin** are distinct proteins of the extracellular matrix and are associated with collagens, proteoglycans, and other proteins to organize a **basement membrane**, the supporting sheet of most epithelia.

The basement membrane consists of two components (Figure 1-19):

1. The **basal lamina**, a sheetlike extracellular matrix in direct contact with epithelial cell surfaces. The basal lamina results from the self-assembly of laminin molecules with type IV collagen, entactin, and proteoglycans.

2. A **reticular lamina**—formed by collagen fibers—supports the basal lamina and is continuous with the connective tissue.

The basal and reticular laminae can be distinguished by electron microscopy. Under the light microscope, the combined basal and reticular laminae receive the

Figure 1-19. **Basement membrane**

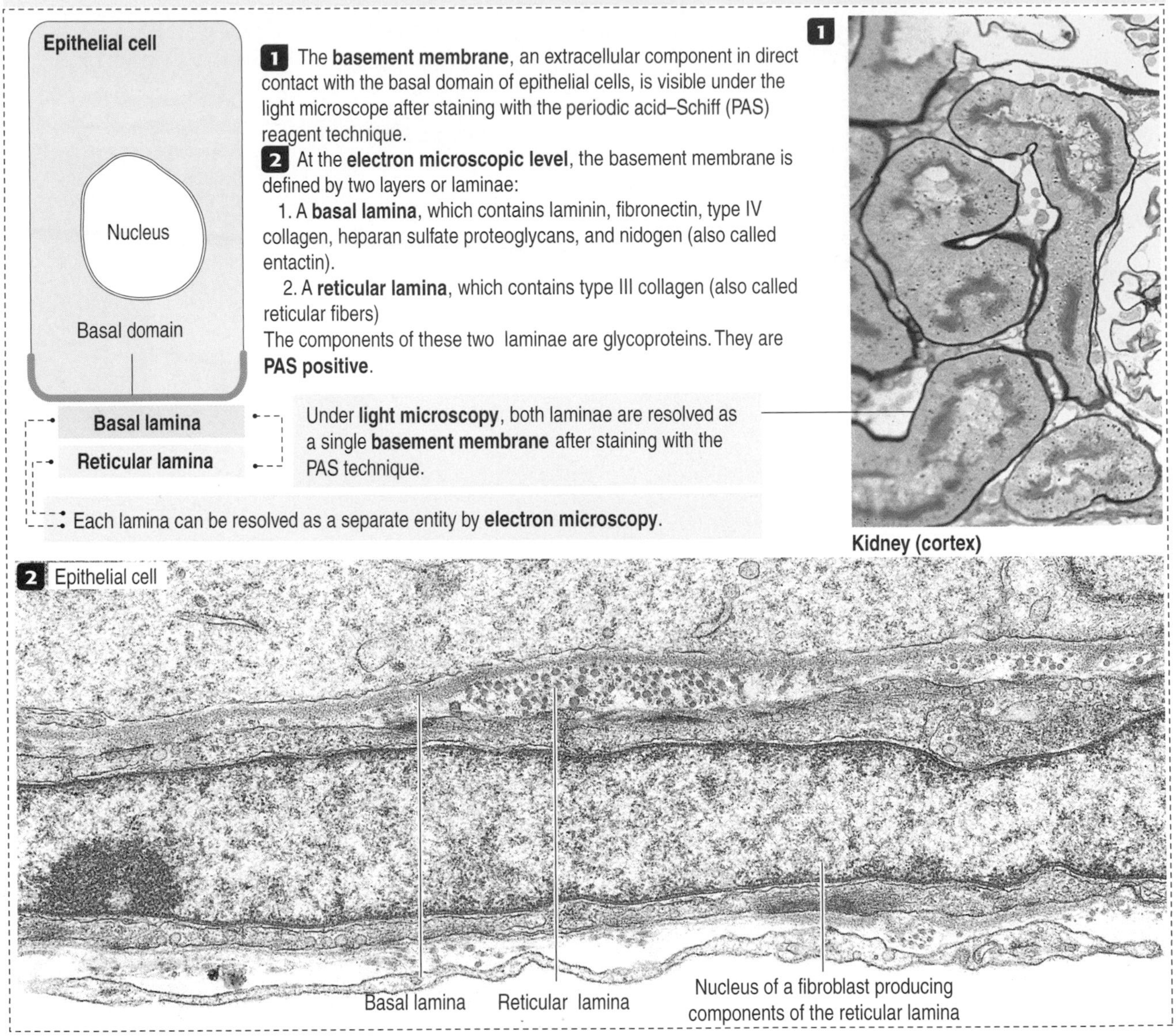

Epithelial cell
Nucleus
Basal domain
1 The basement membrane, an extracellular component in direct contact with the basal domain of epithelial cells, is visible under the light microscope after staining with the periodic acid–Schiff (PAS) reagent technique.
2 At the electron microscopic level, the basement membrane is defined by two layers or laminae:
1. A basal lamina, which contains laminin, fibronectin, type IV collagen, heparan sulfate proteoglycans, and nidogen (also called entactin).
2. A reticular lamina, which contains type III collagen (also called reticular fibers)
The components of these two laminae are glycoproteins. They are PAS positive.
Basal lamina
Reticular lamina
Under light microscopy, both laminae are resolved as a single basement membrane after staining with the PAS technique.
Each lamina can be resolved as a separate entity by electron microscopy.
1
Kidney (cortex)
2 Epithelial cell
Basal lamina
Reticular lamina
Nucleus of a fibroblast producing components of the reticular lamina

name of basement membrane, which can be recognized by the **periodic acid-Schiff (PAS)** stain (see Figure 1-19; see Box 1-D).

The basal lamina has specific functions in different tissues. The double basal lamina of the renal corpuscle constitutes the most important element of the **glomerular filtration barrier** during the initial step in the formation of urine (see Chapter 14, Urinary System).

In skeletal muscle, the basal lamina maintains the integrity of the tissue, and its disruption gives rise to **muscular dystrophies** (see Chapter 7, Muscle Tissue).

During the migration of primordial germinal cells, basal lamina components guide the migrating cells toward the gonadal ridge in preparation for the development of the gonads. The basal lamina not only provides support to epithelia, but also participates in other non-epithelial cell functions.

Laminin (Figure 1-20) is a cross-shaped protein consisting of three chains: the **α chain**, the **β chain**, and the **γ chain.** Laminin molecules can associate with each other to form a meshlike polymer. Laminin and **type IV collagen** are the major components of the basal lamina, and both are synthesized by epithelial cells resting on the lamina.

Laminin has binding sites for **nidogen** (also called entactin), **proteoglycans** (in

Box 1-D | Periodic acid–Schiff (PAS) reaction

- PAS is a widely used histochemical technique to show 1,2-glycol or 1,2-aminoalcohol groups, such as those present in glycogen, mucus, and glycoproteins.
- **Periodic acid**, an oxidant, converts these groups to **aldehydes**. The **Schiff reagent**, a colorless fuchsin, reacts with the aldehydes to form a characteristic **red-purple (magenta)** product.
- Some important PAS-positive structures are the **basement membrane, glycocalyx, mucus** produced by goblet cells, stored **glycoprotein hormones** in cells of the pituitary gland, and **collagens**.

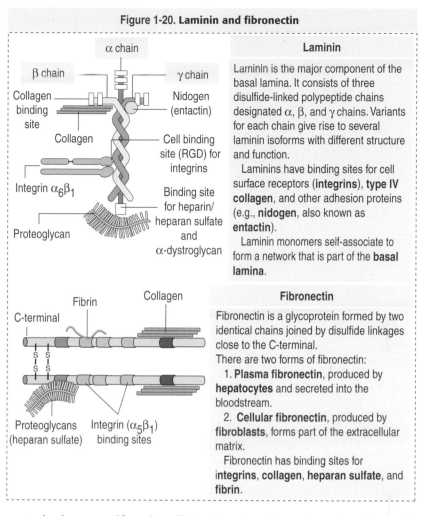

Figure 1-20. Laminin and fibronectin

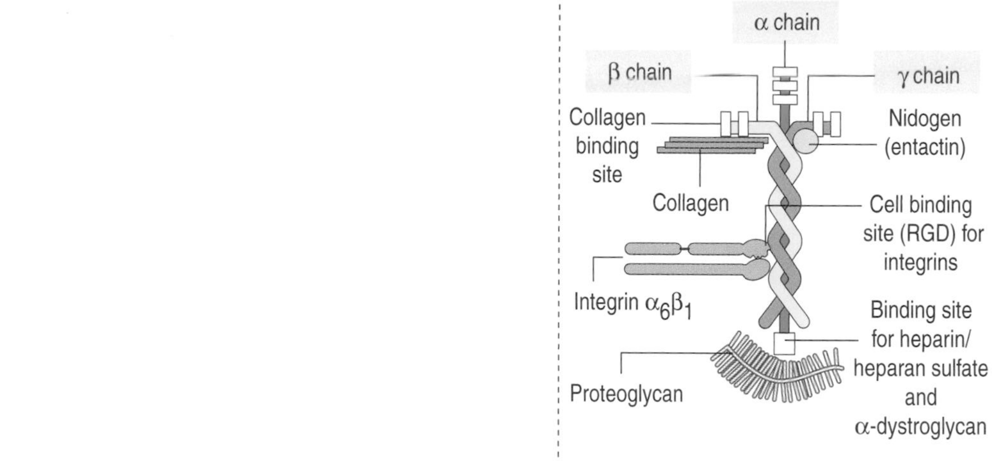

α chain
β chain
γ chain
Collagen binding site
Collagen
Nidogen (entactin)
Cell binding site (RGD) for integrins
Integrin $\alpha_6\beta_1$
Binding site for heparin/ heparan sulfate and α-dystroglycan
Proteoglycan

Laminin

Laminin is the major component of the basal lamina. It consists of three disulfide-linked polypeptide chains designated α, β, and γ chains. Variants for each chain give rise to several laminin isoforms with different structure and function.

Laminins have binding sites for cell surface receptors (**integrins**), **type IV collagen**, and other adhesion proteins (e.g., **nidogen**, also known as **entactin**).

Laminin monomers self-associate to form a network that is part of the **basal lamina**.

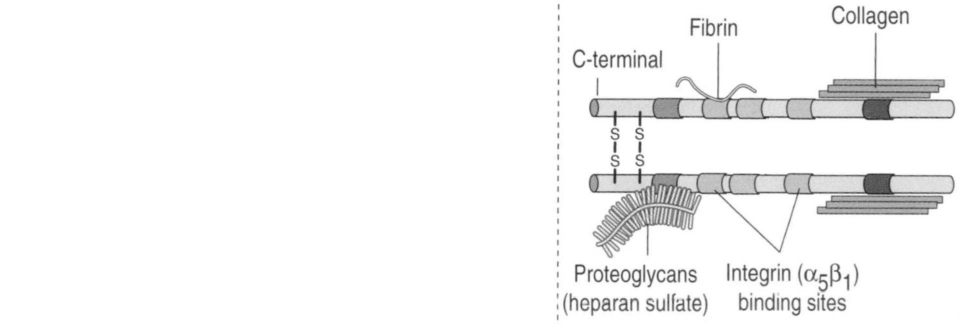

Fibrin
Collagen
C-terminal
S S
S S
Proteoglycans (heparan sulfate)
Integrin ($\alpha_5\beta_1$) binding sites

Fibronectin

Fibronectin is a glycoprotein formed by two identical chains joined by disulfide linkages close to the C-terminal.

There are two forms of fibronectin:

1. **Plasma fibronectin**, produced by **hepatocytes** and secreted into the bloodstream.
2. **Cellular fibronectin**, produced by **fibroblasts**, forms part of the extracellular matrix.

Fibronectin has binding sites for **integrins**, **collagen**, **heparan sulfate**, and **fibrin**.

particular, heparan sulfate, also called **perlecan**), **α-dystroglycan** (see Chapter 7, Muscle Tissue), and **integrins**.

Fibronectin (see Figure 1-20) consists of two protein chains cross-linked by disulfide bonds. Fibronectin is the main adhesion molecule of the extracellular matrix of the connective tissue and is produced by fibroblasts. Fibronectin has binding sites for **heparin** present in proteoglycans, several types of **collagens** (types I, II, III, and V), and **fibrin** (derived from fibrinogen during blood coagulation).

Fibronectin circulating in blood is synthesized in the liver by hepatocytes. It differs from fibronectin produced by fibroblasts in that it lacks one or two repeats (designated EDA and EDB for extra domain A and extra domain B) as a result of alternative mRNA splicing. Circulating fibronectin binds to fibrin, a component of the blood clot formed at the site of blood vessel damage. The RGD domain of immobilized fibronectin binds to integrin expressed on the surface of activated platelets, and the blood clot enlarges. We return to the topic of blood coagulation or hemostasis in Chapter 6, Blood and Hematopoiesis.

How cells interact with each other and with the basal lamina

Figure 1-21 summarizes the highlights of cell adhesion molecules and cell junctions. An epithelium is a continuous sheet of polarized cells supported by a basement membrane. The polarized nature of an epithelium depends on the tight junctions that separate the polarized cells into apical and basolateral regions. Tight junctions control the paracellular pathway of solutes, ions, and water. Tight junctions form a belt around the circumference of each cell.

Endothelial cells, the constituents of a simple squamous epithelium, are linked by tight and spot desmosomes tightly regulated to maintain the integrity of the

Figure 1-21. Summary of cell junctions and cell adhesion molecules

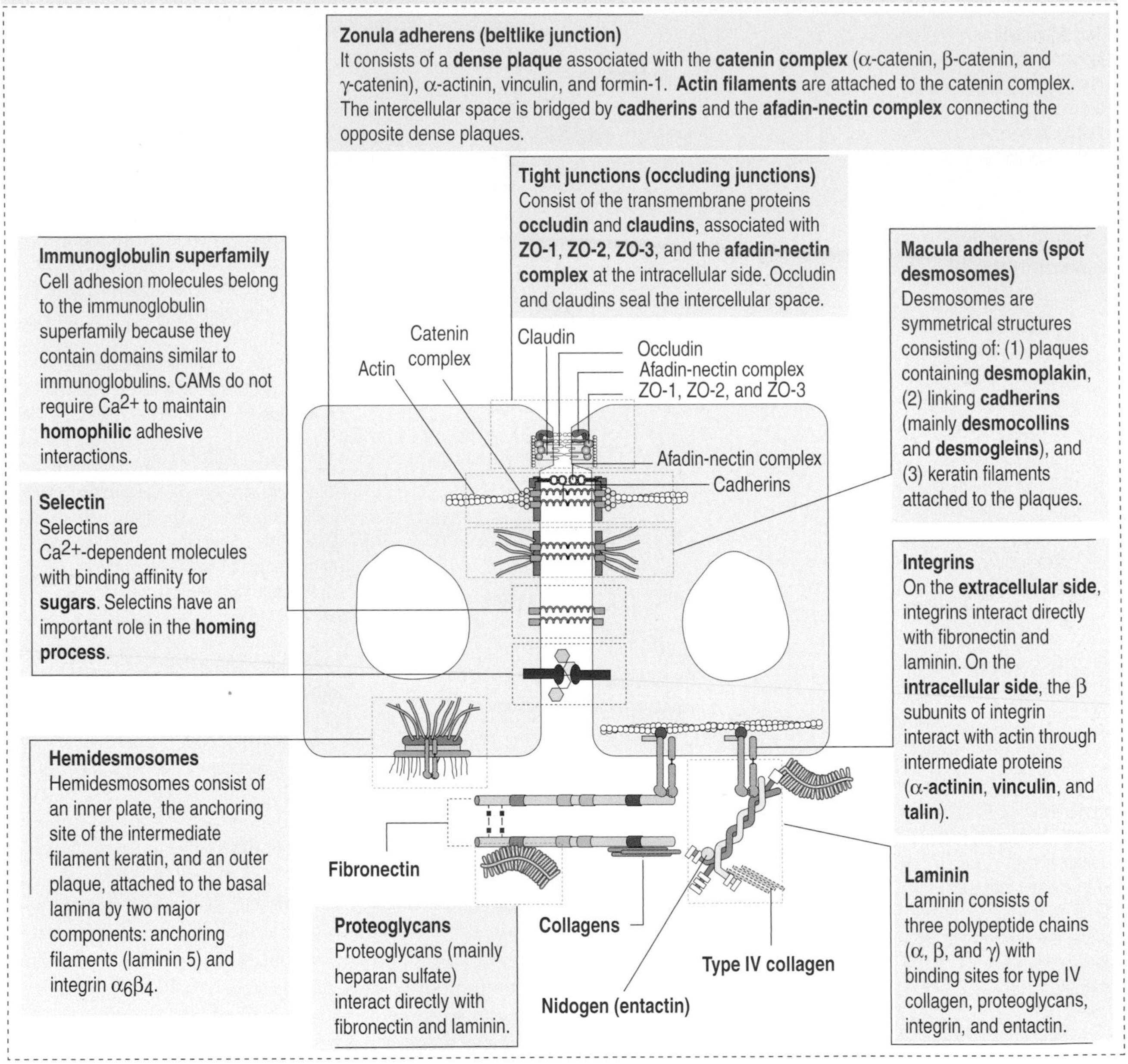
Zonula adherens (beltlike junction)
It consists of a dense plaque associated with the catenin complex (α-catenin, β-catenin, and γ-catenin), α-actinin, vinculin, and formin-1. Actin filaments are attached to the catenin complex. The intercellular space is bridged by cadherins and the afadin-nectin complex connecting the opposite dense plaques.
Tight junctions (occluding junctions)
Consist of the transmembrane proteins occludin and claudins, associated with ZO-1, ZO-2, ZO-3, and the afadin-nectin complex at the intracellular side. Occludin and claudins seal the intercellular space.
Immunoglobulin superfamily
Cell adhesion molecules belong to the immunoglobulin superfamily because they contain domains similar to immunoglobulins. CAMs do not require Ca2+ to maintain homophilic adhesive interactions.
Macula adherens (spot desmosomes)
Desmosomes are symmetrical structures consisting of: (1) plaques containing desmoplakin, (2) linking cadherins (mainly desmocollins and desmogleins), and (3) keratin filaments attached to the plaques.
Catenin complex
Actin
Claudin
Occludin
Afadin-nectin complex
ZO-1, ZO-2, and ZO-3
Afadin-nectin complex
Cadherins
Selectin
Selectins are Ca2+-dependent molecules with binding affinity for sugars. Selectins have an important role in the homing process.
Integrins
On the extracellular side, integrins interact directly with fibronectin and laminin. On the intracellular side, the β subunits of integrin interact with actin through intermediate proteins (α-actinin, vinculin, and talin).
Hemidesmosomes
Hemidesmosomes consist of an inner plate, the anchoring site of the intermediate filament keratin, and an outer plaque, attached to the basal lamina by two major components: anchoring filaments (laminin 5) and integrin α6β4.
Fibronectin
Laminin
Laminin consists of three polypeptide chains (α, β, and γ) with binding sites for type IV collagen, proteoglycans, integrin, and entactin.
Proteoglycans
Proteoglycans (mainly heparan sulfate) interact directly with fibronectin and laminin.
Collagens
Type IV collagen
Nidogen (entactin)

endothelium and protect the vessels from unregulated permeability, inflammation, and reactions leading to blood coagulation in the lumen (see Chapter 12, Cardiovascular System). Leukocytes reach the site of infection by attaching to endothelial cell surfaces and migrate across the endothelium into the underlying tissues by a mechanism called **diapedesis.** Leukocytes find their way through endothelial cell-cell junctions after docking to activated or resting endothelial cells by the endothelial cell adhesion molecules ICAM-1 and VCAM-1 (see Figure 1-8). ICAM-1 and VCAM-1 bind to β_2 and β_1 integrin subunits in leukocytes (see Figure 1-10).

The cohesive nature of the epithelium depends on three factors: cell junctions, cell adhesive molecules in general, and the interaction of integrins with the extracellular matrix, produced to a large extent by fibroblasts. The basal lamina is essential for the differentiation of epithelial cells during embryogenesis.

Note in Figure 1-21 that:

1. The basal domain of epithelial cells interacts with the basal lamina through hemidesmosomes and integrins. Hemidesmosomes, so called because of their

Figure 1-22. Immunocytochemistry

Two techniques are generally used: direct and indirect immunocytochemistry.
Immunocytochemistry requires that cells under study are made permeable, usually with a detergent, so that antibody molecules (immunoglobulins) can enter a cell and bind to an antigen.

Direct immunofluorescence

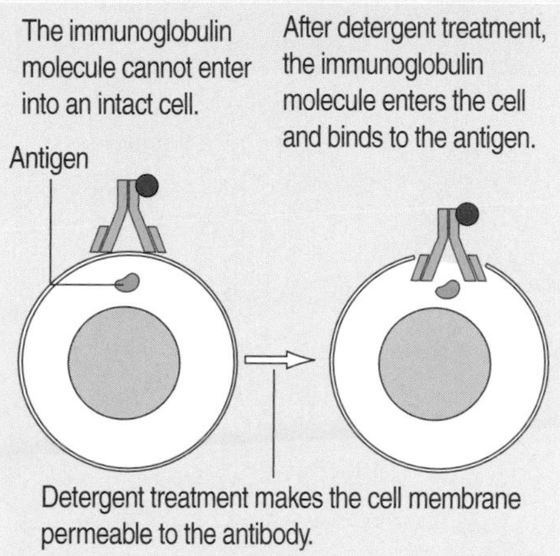

The immunoglobulin molecule cannot enter into an intact cell.
After detergent treatment, the immunoglobulin molecule enters the cell and binds to the antigen.
Antigen
Detergent treatment makes the cell membrane permeable to the antibody.

Direct immunocytochemistry involves a specific antibody or some agent with specific binding affinity to an antigen tagged with a visible marker. Visible markers attached to the immunoglobulin molecule can be a fluorescent dye such as **fluorescein** (green fluorescence) or **rhodamine** (red fluorescence). When examined with a fluorescence microscope, only labeled components are visible as bright, fluorescent structures. Direct immunofluorescence involves a single incubation step and provides a simple detection system.
Gold particles (electron-dense) attached to immunoglobulin molecules are convenient markers for immunocytochemistry at the electron microscopic level.

Indirect immunofluorescence

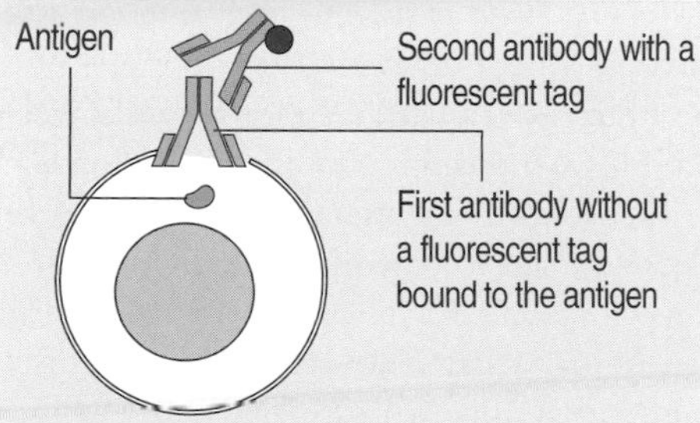

Antigen
Second antibody with a fluorescent tag
First antibody without a fluorescent tag bound to the antigen

Indirect immunocytochemistry involves a second antibody tagged with a visible marker. This second antibody binds to a nontagged first antibody specific for an antigen. The indirect method requires two separate incubations (one each for the first and second antibody) and is more specific for the identification of antigens.

appearance as half-desmosomes in electron micrographs, are anchored to the basal lamina ouside the cell and to a network of keratin intermediate filaments inside the cell through a plate-plaque complex. Mutations in hemidesmosome components cause severe skin blistering as a result of a rupture of the anchoring molecular integrity.

2. Integrins interact directly with laminin and fibronectin, in particular the RGD domain to which integrins bind. Inside the cell, integrins interact with actin microfilaments. Integrins connect the extracellular environment to the intracellular space. We have seen that some ADAM proteins can use their disintegrin domain to prevent integrin binding to extracellular matrix ligands.

3. Collagens and proteoglycans do not interact directly with the basal domain of epithelial cells. Instead, this interaction is mediated by laminin and fibronectin, which contain specific binding sites for collagens, proteoglycans, and entactin.

4. The lateral domains of adjacent epithelial cells and cardiocytes (myocardial muscle cells) communicate by gap junctions (not shown in Figure 1-21). In contrast to tight junctions and belt and spot desmosomes, gap junctions are not anchoring devices. They consist of intercellular channels connecting the cytoplasm of adjacent cells. They are communicating junctions.

5. Cadherins and the afadin-nectin complex are present in tight junctions and zonula adherens. Actin microfilaments are associated with these two junctions.

Cytoskeleton

Cytoskeleton is a three-dimensional network of proteins distributed throughout the cytoplasm of eukaryotic cells.

The cytoskeleton has roles in:

1. **Cell movement** (crawling of blood cells along blood-vessel walls, migration of fibroblasts during wound healing, and movement of cells during embryonic development).
2. **Support and strength for the cell.**
3. **Phagocytosis.**
4. **Cytokinesis.**
5. **Cell-cell and cell–extracellular matrix adherence.**
6. **Changes in cell shape.**

The components of the cytoskeleton were originally identified by **electron microscopy**. These early studies described a system of cytoplasmic "cables" that fell into three size groups, as follows:

1. **Microfilaments** (7 nm thick)
2. **Intermediate filaments** (10 nm thick)
3. **Microtubules** (25 nm in diameter)

Biochemical studies, involving the extraction of cytoskeletal proteins from cells with detergents and salts and in vitro translation of specific mRNA, showed that each class of filaments has a unique protein organization. When cytoskeletal proteins were purified, they were used as antigens for the production of antibodies. Antibodies are used as tools for the localization of the various cytoskeletal proteins in the cell. The **immunocytochemical localization** of cytoskeletal proteins (Figure 1-22) and **cell treatment with various chemical agents** disrupting the normal organization of the cytoskeleton have been instrumental in understanding the organization and function of the cytoskeleton.

Microfilaments

The main component of microfilaments is **actin**. Actin filaments are composed of globular monomers (**G-actin**, 42 kd), which polymerize to form helical and asymmetrical filaments (**F-actin**).

Actin is a versatile and abundant cytoskeletal component forming static and contractile bundles and filamentous networks specified by actin-binding proteins and their distinctive location and function in a cell. F-actin bundles are present in the microvilli of the intestinal (Figure 1-23) and kidney epithelial cells (brush

Figure 1-23. F-actin bundles form the core of intestinal villi

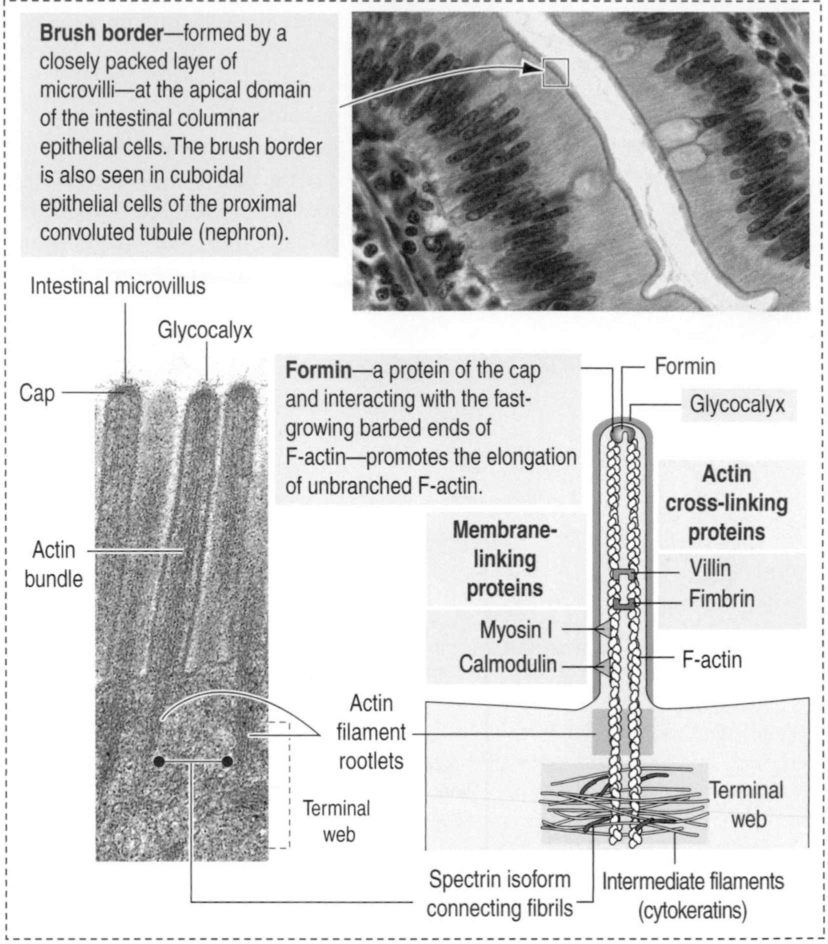

Brush border—formed by a closely packed layer of microvilli—at the apical domain of the intestinal columnar epithelial cells. The brush border is also seen in cuboidal epithelial cells of the proximal convoluted tubule (nephron).
Intestinal microvillus
Glycocalyx
Cap
Actin bundle
Formin—a protein of the cap and interacting with the fast-growing barbed ends of F-actin—promotes the elongation of unbranched F-actin.
Formin
Glycocalyx
Actin cross-linking proteins
Villin
Fimbrin
Membrane-linking proteins
Myosin I
Calmodulin
F-actin
Actin filament rootlets
Terminal web
Terminal web
Spectrin isoform connecting fibrils
Intermediate filaments (cytokeratins)

border) and the stereocilia from the hair cells of the inner ear.

We have already seen that the intracellular portion of the cell adhesion molecules cadherins and integrin β_1 interacts with F-actin through linker proteins (see Figures 1-6 and 1-9). As discussed in Chapter 6, Blood and Hematopoiesis, actin—together with spectrin—forms a filamentous network on the inner face of the red blood cell membrane that is crucial for maintaining the shape and integrity of red blood cells. **Spectrin** is a tetramer consisting of two distinct polypeptide chains (α and β).

Growth of actin filaments may occur at both ends; however, one end (the "**barbed end**" or **plus end**) grows faster than the other end (the "**pointed end**" or **minus end**). The names correspond to the arrowhead appearance of myosin head bound at an angle to actin. Actin filaments can branch in the **leading edge** (**lamellipodia**) of cells involved in either motility or interaction with other cell types. F-actin branching is initiated from the side of a preexisting actin filament by **Arp2/3** (for **actin-related protein**), an actin nucleating complex of seven proteins (Figure 1-24). As mentioned before, **formin** regulates the assembly of unbranched actin in cell protrusions such as the intestinal microvilli (see Figure 1-23).

Actin monomers have a binding site for adenosine triphosphate (**ATP**), which is hydrolyzed to adenosine diphosphate (**ADP**) as polymerization proceeds. **Actin polymerization is ATP-dependent** (see **Box 1-E**).

The kinetics of actin polymerization involves a mechanism known as **treadmilling: G-actin monomers added on the barbed end of the filament move, or treadmill, along the filament until they are lost by depolymerization at the pointed end** (see Figure 1-24). Four types of proteins control treadmilling (see Figure 1-24), as follows:

Figure 1-24. Role of actin binding proteins in the assembly and disassembly of F-actin

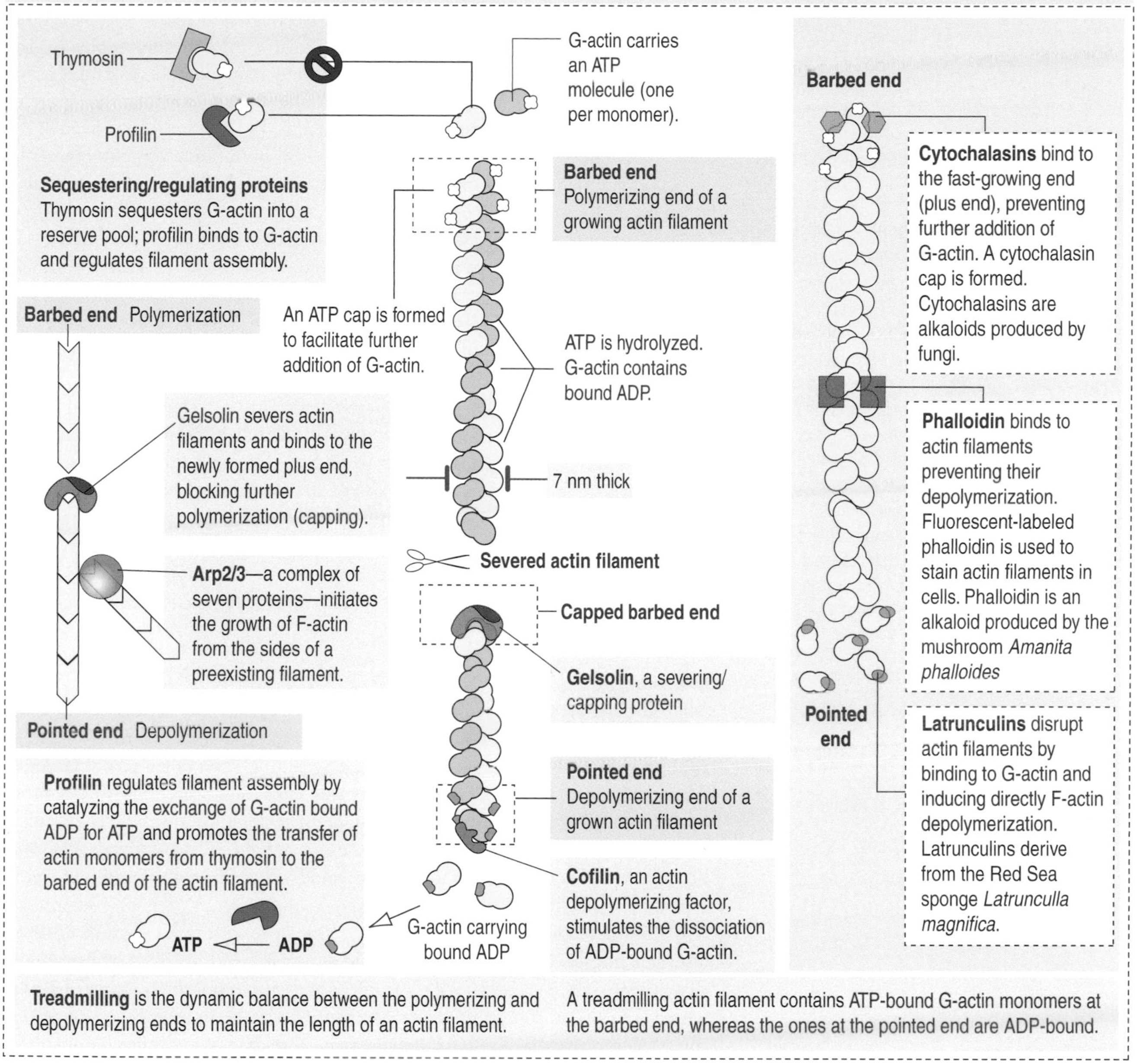

Thymosin
Profilin
G-actin carries an ATP molecule (one per monomer).
Barbed end
Sequestering/regulating proteins
Thymosin sequesters G-actin into a reserve pool; profilin binds to G-actin and regulates filament assembly.
Barbed end
Polymerizing end of a growing actin filament
Cytochalasins bind to the fast-growing end (plus end), preventing further addition of G-actin. A cytochalasin cap is formed. Cytochalasins are alkaloids produced by fungi.
Barbed end Polymerization
An ATP cap is formed to facilitate further addition of G-actin.
ATP is hydrolyzed. G-actin contains bound ADP.
Gelsolin severs actin filaments and binds to the newly formed plus end, blocking further polymerization (capping).
7 nm thick
Phalloidin binds to actin filaments preventing their depolymerization. Fluorescent-labeled phalloidin is used to stain actin filaments in cells. Phalloidin is an alkaloid produced by the mushroom Amanita phalloides
Arp2/3—a complex of seven proteins—initiates the growth of F-actin from the sides of a preexisting filament.
Severed actin filament
Capped barbed end
Gelsolin, a severing/capping protein
Pointed end Depolymerization
Pointed end
Latrunculins disrupt actin filaments by binding to G-actin and inducing directly F-actin depolymerization. Latrunculins derive from the Red Sea sponge Latrunculla magnifica.
Pointed end
Depolymerizing end of a grown actin filament
Profilin regulates filament assembly by catalyzing the exchange of G-actin bound ADP for ATP and promotes the transfer of actin monomers from thymosin to the barbed end of the actin filament.
Cofilin, an actin depolymerizing factor, stimulates the dissociation of ADP-bound G-actin.
ATP
ADP
G-actin carrying bound ADP
Treadmilling is the dynamic balance between the polymerizing and depolymerizing ends to maintain the length of an actin filament.
A treadmilling actin filament contains ATP-bound G-actin monomers at the barbed end, whereas the ones at the pointed end are ADP-bound.

Box 1-E | **Microfilaments**

- **Microfilaments** consist of G-actin, globular monomers, which polymerize in the presence of **ATP** into a long filamentous polymer, F-actin, that is 7 nm thick.
- F-actin has a distinct polarity: a barbed or polymerization end, and a pointed or depolymerizing end. Profilin has two roles: it severs F-actin and regulates F-actin assembly by catalyzing the exchange of G-actin bound ADP for ATP. Cofilin is a depolymerizing factor. The Arp2/3 complex initiates the branching of F-actin.
- Treadmilling, the dynamic balance between the polymerizing and depolymerizing ends of F-actin.

1. **Thymosin** (originally isolated from calf thymus and later found in most cell types and platelets) sequesters pools of G-actin monomers within cells.

2. **Profilin** suppresses nucleation of G-actin and promotes F-actin growth at the barbed end. Profilin can favor the assembly of monomeric G-actin into filaments by facilitating the exchange of bound ADP for ATP. **Only ATP-actin monomers** can be assembled into filaments.

3. **Cofilin** (also known as actin depolymerizing factor) triggers depolymerization of ADP-bound actin at the pointed end. Similar to profilin and thymosin, cofilin forms a dimeric complex with G-actin.

4. **Gelsolin** has a dual role: it is a **capping protein** and prevents the loss and addition of actin monomers, and it is a **severing protein**. In the presence of Ca^{2+}, gelsolin fragments actin filaments and remains bound to the barbed end, forming a cap that prevents further filament growth.

The assembly of G-actin monomers into filaments and the organization of these filaments into thick bundles are controlled by various types of **actin-binding or actin-related proteins.** A bundle of parallel nonbranching actin filaments, form-

Box 1-F | Wiskott-Aldrich syndrome

• The Arp2/3 complex is necessary for nucleating the assembly of branched networks of actin filaments. The function of phagocytic cells and platelets depends on a functional actin cytoskeleton.
• Numerous proteins activate the Arp2/3 complex. Without these proteins, the Arp2/3 complex is inactive.
• Two major proteins that bind and activate the Arp2/3 complex include the Wiskott-Aldrich syndrome protein (WASP) family, which consists of several members (WASP, neuronal WASP [N-WASP] and SCAR/WAVE1-3 (**s**uppressor of **cA**MP **r**eceptor/**WA**SP family **ve**rprolin-homologous protein 1-3). Additional members belong to the cortactin family, which includes cortactin and hematopoietic-specific protein.
• Mutations in the *WASP* gene, present in the X chromosome, are characterized by recurrent respiratory infections (defective function of T and B cells), a reduction in the number of platelets (thrombocytopenia) leading to increased susceptibility to bleeding, and eczema of the skin. Males but not females are affected by the Wiskott-Aldrich syndrome.

ing the core of the **microvillus**, is held together by actin-linking proteins, **villin** and **fimbrin**. Side arms of **myosin-I** and the Ca^{2+}-binding protein **calmodulin** anchor the bundle to the plasma membrane (see Figure 1-23).

Arp2/3 and additional regulatory proteins form a nucleation complex for the assembly of **branching actin filaments**. Branching actin filaments assemble at the leading edge of a cell during cell motility. In the microvillus, **formins** (proteins with highly conserved formin-homology domains, FH1 and FH2), instead of the Arp2/3 complex, seem to regulate the elongation of **nonbranching actin filaments**, while remaining attached to the barbed end (see **Box 1-E**). Formins are located at the tip of the microvillus, the **cap region** (see Figure 1-23).

Male patients with defects in proteins that activate the Arp2/3 complex—in particular a protein of the **Wiskott-Aldrich syndrome protein** (**WASP**) family—display recurrent respiratory infections because of hereditary immunodeficiency, thrombocytopenia (low platelet count) present from birth on and eczema of the skin after the first month of life (see **Box 1-F**). The mutation is inherited from the mother, a healthy carrier of the defective gene.

Microvilli and stereocilia are comparable structures, although they differ in length and the number of actin filaments: **intestinal microvilli** are 1 to 2 μm long, 0.1 μm wide, and consist of 20 to 30 bundled actin filaments; **stereocilia in hair cells of the inner ear** have a tapered shape at their base, the length range is 1.5 to 5.5 μm, and each actin bundle contains up to 900 actin filaments. Hair cells are extremely sensitive to mechanical displacement, and a slight movement of the stereocilium is amplified into changes in electric potential transmitted to the brain. We study hair cells of the inner ear in Chapter 9, Sensory Organs: Vision and Hearing.

Microtubules

Microtubules are composed of **tubulin dimers** (Figure 1-25; see **Box 1-G**). Each tubulin dimer consists of two tightly bound tubulin molecules: **α-tubulin** and **β-tubulin**. Tubulin subunits are arranged in longitudinal rows called **protofilaments**. Thirteen protofilaments associate side by side with each other to form a cylinder of **microtubules** with a hollow core. The diameter of a microtubule is **25 nm**.

Similar to actin filaments, microtubules are structurally **polarized**. Microtubules have a **plus end**, which grows more rapidly than the **minus end** (see Figure 1-25).

In contrast to actin filaments, most individual microtubules seem to undergo **alternate phases of slow growth and rapid depolymerization**. This process, called **dynamic instability**, consists of three major steps: (1) a **polymerization phase**, in which GTP-tubulin subunits add to the plus end of the microtubule and a **GTP cap** is assembled to facilitate further growth; (2) **release of hydrolyzed phosphate (Pi)** from tubulin-bound GTP; and (3) a **depolymerization phase**, in which GDP-tubulin subunits are released from the minus end at a fast rate. The polymerization-to-depolymerization transition frequency is known as *catastrophe*; the depolymerization-to-polymerization transition frequency is known as *rescue*.

Dynamic instability of microtubules can be modified by **microtubule-associated proteins**. Microtubule-associated proteins include **molecular motors** (**dynein** and **kinesin**) involved in organelle and molecular transport and **microtubule regulatory proteins**, such as **tau protein**, which prevent microtubule dynamic instability in axons; **CLIP-170**, usually found at the plus end of microtubules; and **stathmin/Op18**, a protein associated with microtubule disassembly in its unphosphorylated state and microtubule stability when phosphorylated. These basic concepts of microtubule-based transport are used later when we address specific cell types.

Centrosome, a microtubule-organizing center

The centrosome has three major functions: (1) it nucleates the polymerization of tubulin subunits into microtubules, (2) it organizes microtubules into functional

Box 1-G | **Microtubules**

- **Microtubules** consist of tubulin dimers, α and β, which polymerize in the presence of **GTP** into longitudinal rows of protofilaments. Thirteen protofilaments form a cylinder or microtubule 25 nm in diameter.
- Microtubules have a distinct polarity: a plus or polymerizing end and a minus or depolymerizing end.
- Microtubules undergo alternate phases of slow growth and rapid depolymerization, a process known as dynamic instability.
- Centrioles, basal bodies, and axonemes of cilia and flagella contain a precise array of microtubules.
- Kinesin and cytoplasmic dynein, two molecular motor proteins, use microtubules as tracks for the transport of vesicle and nonvesicle cargos.

Figure 1-25. Assembly of a microtubule

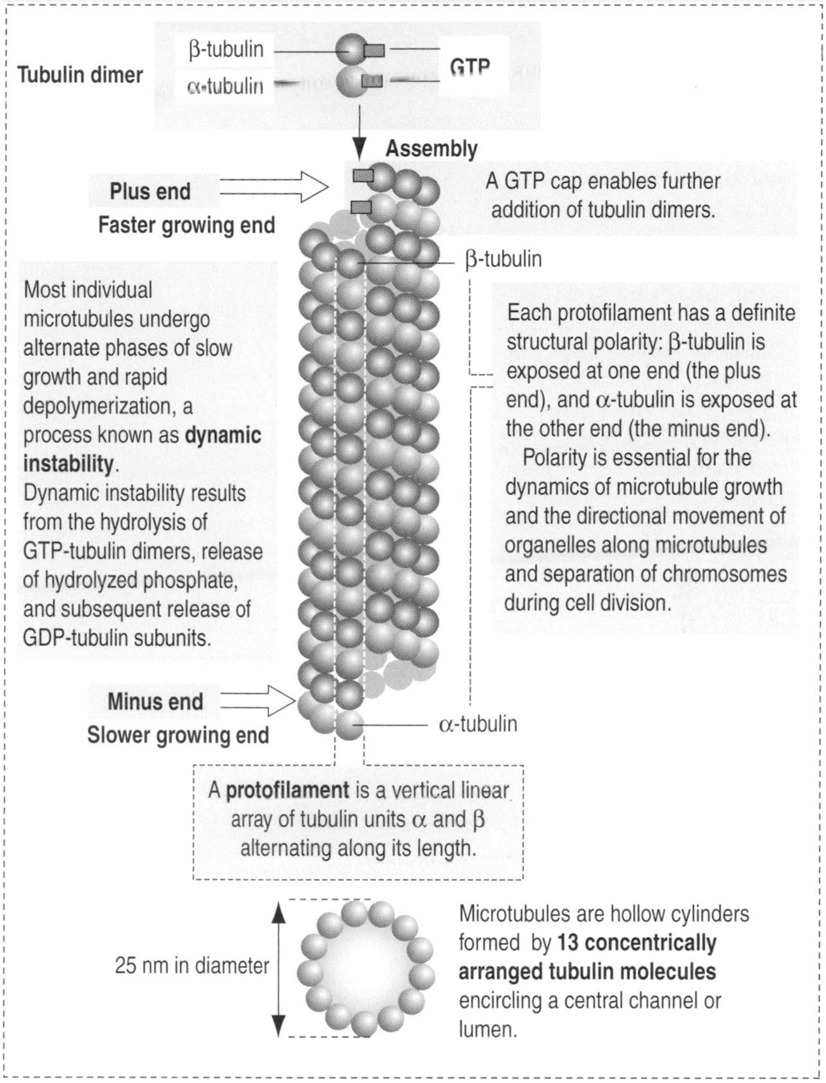

Tubulin dimer
β-tubulin
α-tubulin
GTP
Assembly
Plus end
Faster growing end
A GTP cap enables further addition of tubulin dimers.
β-tubulin
Most individual microtubules undergo alternate phases of slow growth and rapid depolymerization, a process known as dynamic instability.
Dynamic instability results from the hydrolysis of GTP-tubulin dimers, release of hydrolyzed phosphate, and subsequent release of GDP-tubulin subunits.
Each protofilament has a definite structural polarity: β-tubulin is exposed at one end (the plus end), and α-tubulin is exposed at the other end (the minus end).
Polarity is essential for the dynamics of microtubule growth and the directional movement of organelles along microtubules and separation of chromosomes during cell division.
Minus end
Slower growing end
α-tubulin
A protofilament is a vertical linear array of tubulin units α and β alternating along its length.
25 nm in diameter
Microtubules are hollow cylinders formed by 13 concentrically arranged tubulin molecules encircling a central channel or lumen.

units, and (3) it duplicates once every cell cycle.

Centrosomes consist of a **pair of centrioles** surrounded by **pericentriolar material**, an amorphous, electron-dense substance rich in proteins such as pericentrin and γ-tubulin. Centrioles give rise to structurally similar **basal bodies**, which are the outgrowth origin of cilia (see Figure 1-5) and flagella. A defect in the assembly of the basal body and cilia, caused by abnormal transport of ciliary proteins, results in the **Bardet-Biedl syndrome** (see **Box 1-H**).

Centrosomes are part of the **mitotic center**, which, together with the **mitotic spindle**, constitutes the **mitotic (or meiotic) apparatus** (Figure 1-26). A **centriole** is a small cylinder (0.2 μm wide and 0.4 μm long) composed of **nine microtubule triplets** in a helicoid array. In contrast to most cytoplasmic microtubules, which display dynamic instability, the centriolar microtubules are very stable.

During interphase, centrioles are oriented at right angles to each other. Before mitosis, centrioles replicate and form **two pairs**. During mitosis, each pair can be found at opposite poles of the cell, where they direct the formation of the **mitotic** or **meiotic spindle**.

There are three types of microtubules extending from the centrosomes: **radiating** or **astral microtubules**, anchoring each centrosome to the plasma membrane; **kinetochore microtubules**, attaching the chromosome-associated kinetochore to the centrosomes, and **polar microtubules**, extending from the two poles of the spindle where opposite centrosomes are located (Figure 1-26). If kinetochores fail

Box 1-H | **Bardet-Biedl syndrome**

- Bardet-Biedl syndrome (BBS) is a pleiotropic (multisystemic) disorder that includes age-related retinal dystrophy, obesity, polydactyly, renal dysplasia, reproductive tract abnormalities, and learning disabilities.
- BBS is a disorder of **basal bodies** and **cilia** resulting from a **defective microtubule-based transport function** (intraciliary transport) required for the assembly, maintenance, and function of basal bodies, cilia, and flagella (intraflagellar transport).
- Eight BBS genes (*BBS1-8*) have been identified. The degree of clinical variability in BBS is not fully explained.

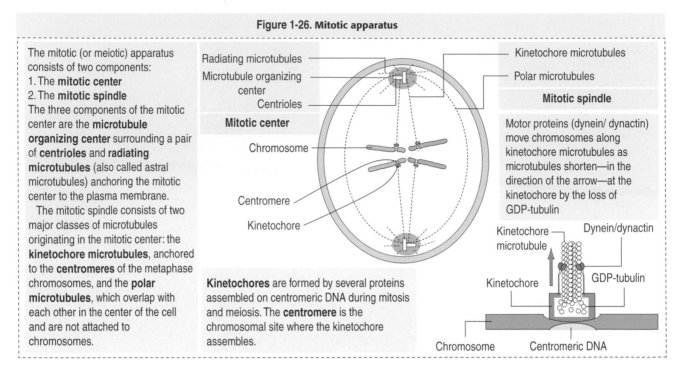

Figure 1-26. Mitotic apparatus

The mitotic (or meiotic) apparatus consists of two components:
1. The **mitotic center**
2. The **mitotic spindle**

The three components of the mitotic center are the **microtubule organizing center** surrounding a pair of **centrioles** and **radiating microtubules** (also called astral microtubules) anchoring the mitotic center to the plasma membrane.

The mitotic spindle consists of two major classes of microtubules originating in the mitotic center: the **kinetochore microtubules**, anchored to the **centromeres** of the metaphase chromosomes, and the **polar microtubules**, which overlap with each other in the center of the cell and are not attached to chromosomes.

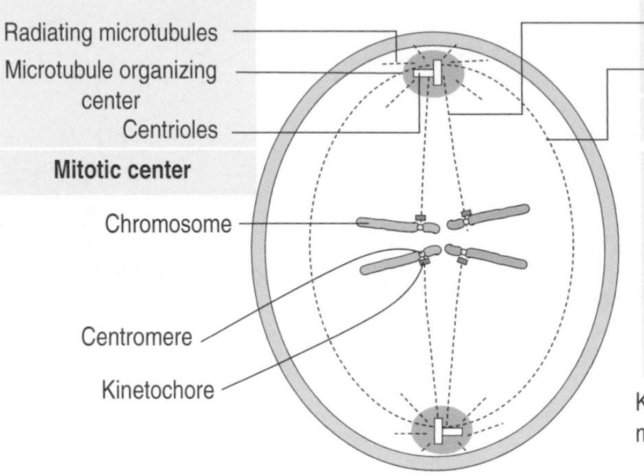

Kinetochores are formed by several proteins assembled on centromeric DNA during mitosis and meiosis. The **centromere** is the chromosomal site where the kinetochore assembles.

Motor proteins (dynein/ dynactin) move chromosomes along kinetochore microtubules as microtubules shorten—in the direction of the arrow—at the kinetochore by the loss of GDP-tubulin

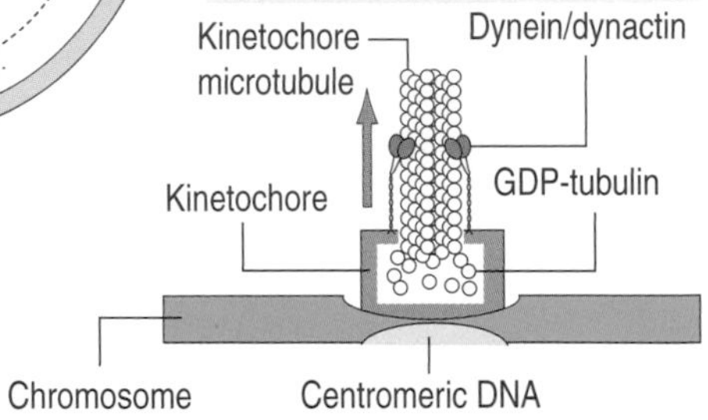

Box 1-I | **Difference between centromere and kinetochore**

- The terms centromere and kinetochore are often used synonymously, but do not mean the same.
- The **centromere** (not the centrosome) is the chromosomal site associated with microtubules of the spindle. Centromeres can be recognized cytologically as a narrow chromatin region on metaphase chromosomes known as **primary constriction** where centromeric DNA is present.
- The **kinetochore** consists of proteins assembled on the centromeric chromatin on sister chromatids. The assembly of the kinetochore depends exclusively on the presence of centromeric DNA sequences. The centromere and the kinetochore mediate attachment of the kinetochore microtubules of the spindle.

to assemble, chromosomes cannot segregate properly (see **Box 1-I**).

The **pericentriolar material** contains the **γ-tubulin ring complex** and numerous proteins, including **pericentrin**. Each γ-tubulin ring complex is the nucleation site or template for the assembly and growth of one microtubule. The centrioles do not have a direct role in the nucleation of microtubules in the centrosome. Tubulin dimers associate to the γ-tubulin ring by the α-tubulin subunit. Consequently, the minus end of each microtubule points to the centrosome; the plus end, the growing end, is oriented outward, free in the cytoplasm.

Microtubules in cilia and flagella

Cilia and flagella are motile cytoplasmic extensions containing a core of microtubules called the **axoneme** (Figure 1-27). The axoneme consists of nine peripheral microtubule doublets surrounding a central pair of microtubules. This arrangement is known as the **9 + 2** configuration (see **Box 1-J**).

Each peripheral doublet consists of a complete microtubule (called an **A tubule**, with **13 protofilaments**), sharing its wall with a second, partially completed microtubule (called a **B tubule**, with **10** to **11 protofilaments**). Extending inward from the A tubule are **radial spokes** that insert into an amorphous **inner sheath** surrounding the central microtubule pair. Adjacent peripheral doublets are linked by the protein **nexin**.

Projecting from the sides of the A tubule are sets of protein arms: the **inner** and **outer arms of dynein**, a microtubule-associated adenosine triphosphatase (ATPase). In the presence of ATP, the sliding of peripheral doublets relative to each other bends cilia and flagella. Sliding and bending of microtubules are the basic events of their motility.

Clinical significance: Microtubule-targeted drugs and sterility

Two groups of antimitotic drugs act on microtubules: **microtubule-destabilizing agents**, which inhibit microtubule polymerization, and **microtubule-stabilizing agents**, which affect microtubule function by suppressing dynamic instability.

The first group includes **colchicine**, **colcemid**, **vincristine**, and **vinblastine**, which bind to tubulin and inhibit microtubule polymerization, blocking mitosis. Colchicine is used clinically in the treatment of gout. Vincristine and vinblastine, from *Vinca* alkaloids isolated from the leaves of the periwinkle plant, have been

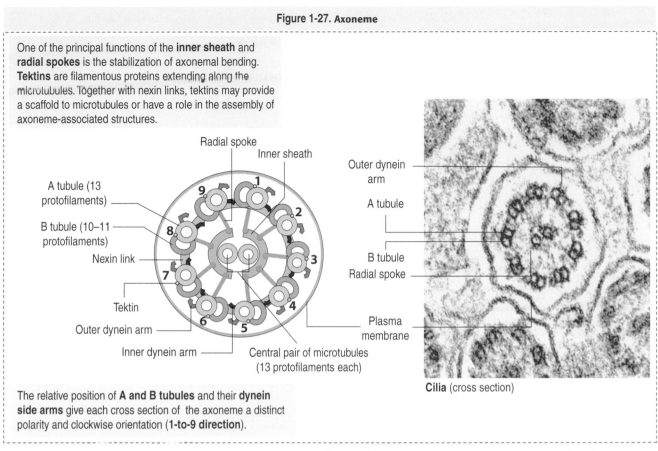

Figure 1-27. **Axoneme**

One of the principal functions of the **inner sheath** and **radial spokes** is the stabilization of axonemal bending. **Tektins** are filamentous proteins extending along the microtubules. Together with nexin links, tektins may provide a scaffold to microtubules or have a role in the assembly of axoneme-associated structures.

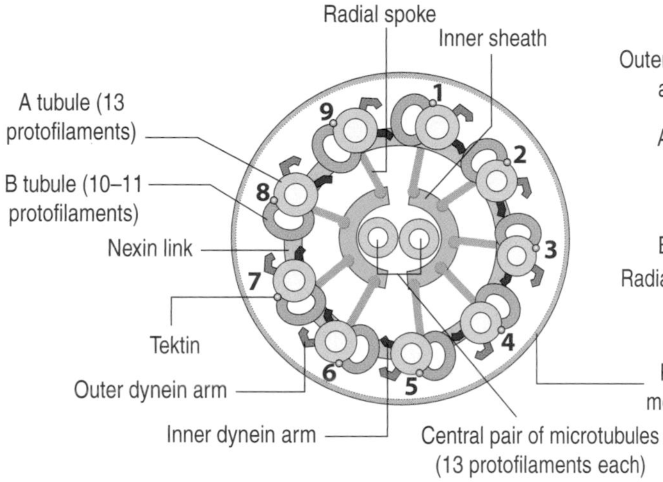

Radial spoke
Inner sheath
A tubule (13 protofilaments)
B tubule (10–11 protofilaments)
Nexin link
Tektin
Outer dynein arm
Inner dynein arm
Central pair of microtubules (13 protofilaments each)
1
2
3
4
5
6
7
8
9

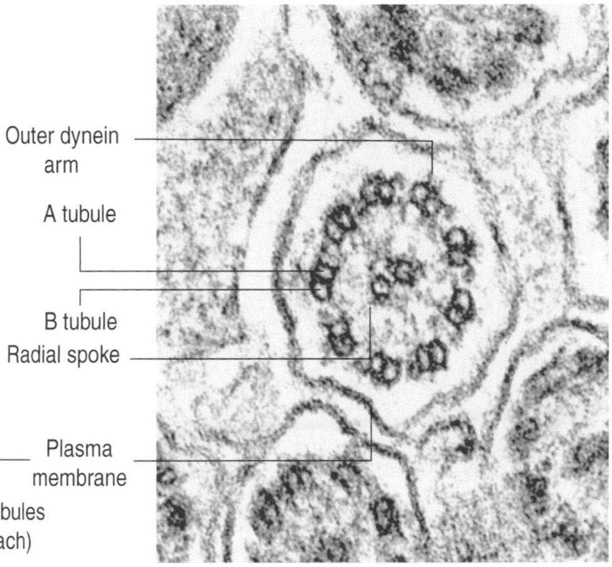

Outer dynein arm
A tubule
B tubule
Radial spoke
Plasma membrane

Cilia (cross section)

The relative position of **A and B tubules** and their **dynein side arms** give each cross section of the axoneme a distinct polarity and clockwise orientation (**1-to-9 direction**).

successfully used in childhood hematologic malignancies (leukemias). Neurotoxicity—resulting from the disruption of the microtubule-dependent axonal flow (loss of microtubules and binding of motor proteins to microtubules)—and myelosuppression are two side effects of microtubule-targeted drugs.

The second group includes **taxol** (isolated from the bark of the yew tree) with an opposite effect: It stabilizes microtubules instead of inhibiting their assembly (Figure 1-28). Paclitaxel (taxol) has been used widely to treat breast and ovarian cancer. Similar to *Vinca* alkaloids, its main side effects are neurotoxicity and suppression of hematopoiesis.

Kartagener's syndrome is an autosomal recessive disorder frequently associated with **bronchiectasis** (permanent dilation of bronchi and bronchioles) and **sterility** in men.

Kartagener's syndrome is the result of structural abnormalities in the axoneme (**defective or absent dynein**) that prevent mucociliary clearance in the airways (leading to persistent infections) and reduce sperm motility and egg transport in the oviduct (leading to sterility).

Box 1-J | **Major components of the ciliary and flagellar axonemes**

- Microtubules: Major component of the axoneme. Motor proteins use microtubules of the axoneme as tracks for intraciliary or intraflagellar cargo transport. Microtubule-based axonal transport also depends on motor proteins.
- Tektins: Intermediate filament-like proteins extending along the length of axonemal microtubules and, presumably, adding mechanical strength to the axoneme.
- Dynein arms: ATPase responsible for ciliary and flagellar movement. The heads are in contact with the adjacent outer microtubules at a periodic distance and move along them.
- Nexin links: A beltlike arrangement stabilizing the nine outer concentric pairs of microtubules.
- Radial spokes: Project from each of the nine outer microtubule doublets to the inner sheath surrounding the central pair.
- Inner sheath: A structure surrounding the central pair of microtubules, in contact with the globular end of the radial spokes.

Microtubules—cytoskeletal tracks for cargo transport powered by motor proteins

The transport of vesicles and nonvesicle cargos occurs along microtubules and F-actin. Specific molecular motors associate to microtubules and F-actin to mobilize cargos to specific intracellular sites. **Microtubule-based molecular motors include kinesin and cytoplasmic dynein** for the **long-range** transport of cargos. **F-actin–based molecular motors include unconventional myosin Va and VIIa** for the **short-range** transport of cargos. We discuss additional aspects of the F-actin–based cargo transport mechanism during the transport of **melanosomes** in Chapter 11, Integumentary System.

Three examples of microtubule-based cargo transport in mammalian systems are as follows (see **Box 1–K**):

Figure 1-28. Agents that prevent microtubular function

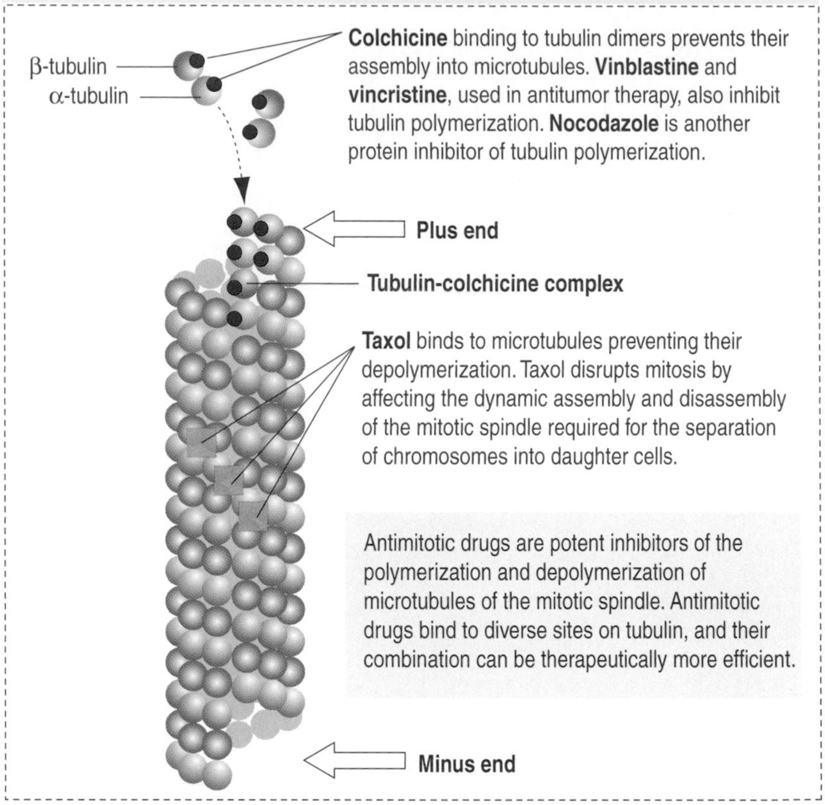

β-tubulin
α-tubulin
Colchicine binding to tubulin dimers prevents their assembly into microtubules. **Vinblastine** and **vincristine**, used in antitumor therapy, also inhibit tubulin polymerization. **Nocodazole** is another protein inhibitor of tubulin polymerization.
Plus end
Tubulin-colchicine complex
Taxol binds to microtubules preventing their depolymerization. Taxol disrupts mitosis by affecting the dynamic assembly and disassembly of the mitotic spindle required for the separation of chromosomes into daughter cells.
Antimitotic drugs are potent inhibitors of the polymerization and depolymerization of microtubules of the mitotic spindle. Antimitotic drugs bind to diverse sites on tubulin, and their combination can be therapeutically more efficient.
Minus end

1. **Axonemal transport**, including flagella (**intraflagellar transport**) and cilia (**intraciliary transport**) (Figure 1-29). During axonemal transport, particles are mobilized by kinesin and cytoplasmic dynein along the microtubule doublets of the axoneme. Defective axonemal transport results in the abnormal assembly of cilia and flagella, including **polycystic kidney disease**, **retinal degeneration**, **respiratory ciliary dysfunction**, and **lack of sperm tail development**. As indicated before (see **Box 1-H**), the **Bardet-Biedl syndrome** is a disorder caused by basal body/ciliary dysfunction secondary to a defective microtubule-based transport function.

2. **Axonal transport**, along the axon of neurons (see Figure 1-29).

3. **Intramanchette transport**, along microtubules of a transient microtubular structure, the manchette, assembled during the elongation of the spermatid head (see Chapter 20, Spermatogenesis).

Axonal transport

Axons are cytoplasmic extensions of neurons responsible for the conduction of neuronal impulses. Membrane-bound vesicles containing **neurotransmitters** produced in the cell body of the neuron travel to the terminal portion of the axon, where the content of the vesicle is released at the **synapse**.

Bundles of microtubules form tracks within the axon to carry these vesicles. Vesicles are transported by two motor proteins (see Figure 1-29):

1. **Kinesin**
2. **Cytoplasmic dynein**

Kinesins and **cytoplasmic dyneins** participate in two types of intracellular transport movements:

1. **Saltatory movement**, defined by the continuous and random movement of mitochondria and vesicles.

2. **Axonal transport**, a more direct intracellular movement of membrane-bound structures.

Box 1-K | Microtubule-based cargo transport by molecular motors

- Microtubules participate in the intracellular traffic of vesicles and nonvesicle materials or cargos.
- Molecular motor proteins, such as kinesin and cytoplasmic dynein, mediate the long-range transport of cargos, whereas short-range transport occurs on actin filaments.
- There are three major microtubule-based transport systems: 1. **axonemal transport**, including intraciliary transport and intraflagellar transport; 2. **axonal transport**; and 3. **intramanchette transport**.
- **Axonemal transport** is essential for the delivery of tubulin dimers and other molecules to the distal polymerization end of microtubules of cilia and flagella. Axonemes originate from basal bodies, centriole-derived, microtubule-containing structures.
- **Axonal transport** is crucial for the traffic of neurotransmitter-containing vesicles to neuronal synapses.
- **Intramanchette transport** is required for morphogenetic events during sperm development. The manchette is a transient microtubule-containing structure associated to a perinuclear ring that assembles during the elongation of the spermatid head and then disassembles.

Figure 1-29. Intraciliary transport and axonal transport

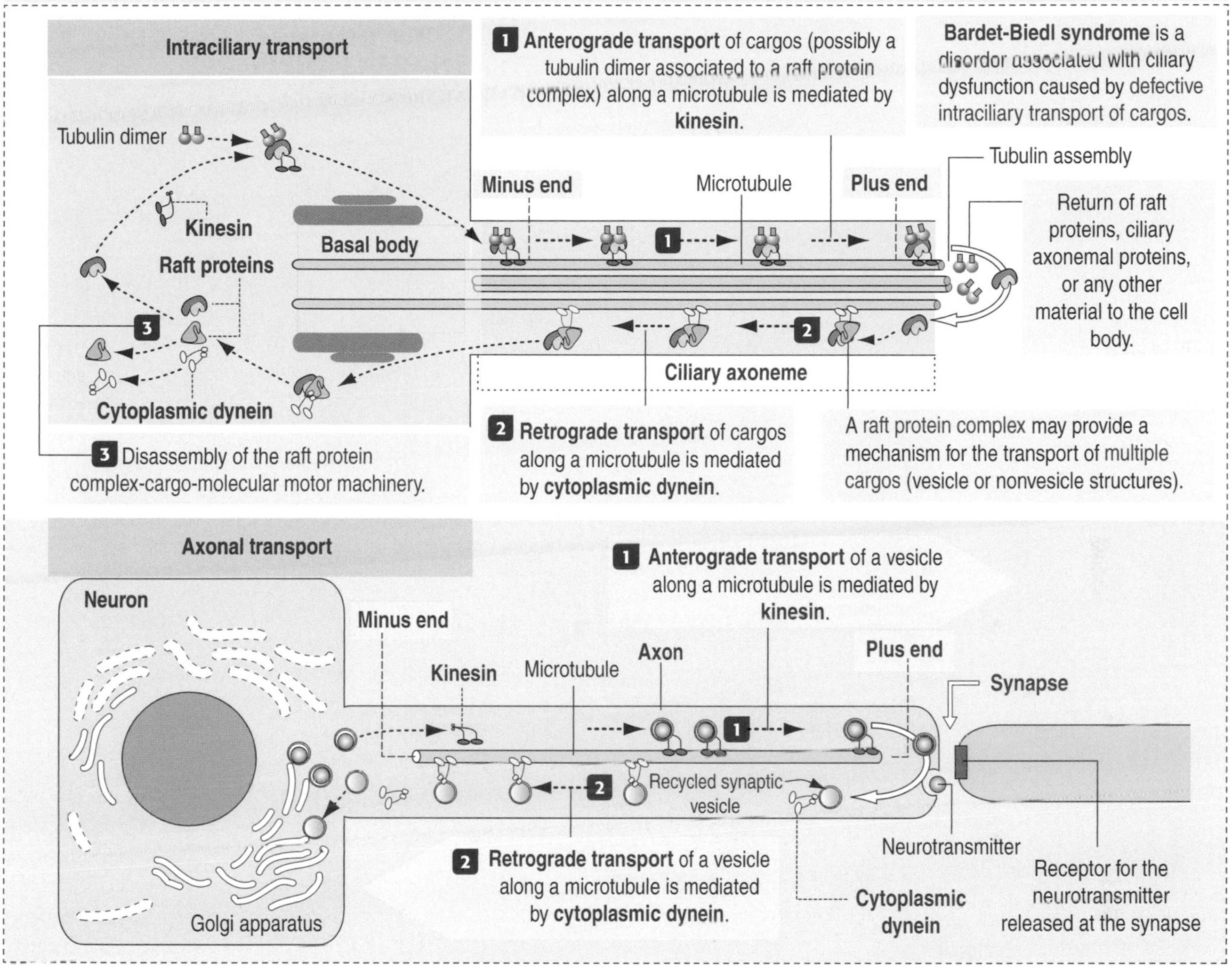
Intraciliary transport
1 Anterograde transport of cargos (possibly a tubulin dimer associated to a raft protein complex) along a microtubule is mediated by kinesin.
Bardet-Biedl syndrome is a disorder associated with ciliary dysfunction caused by defective intraciliary transport of cargos.
Tubulin dimer
Kinesin
Raft proteins
Basal body
Minus end
Microtubule
Plus end
Tubulin assembly
Return of raft proteins, ciliary axonemal proteins, or any other material to the cell body.
Ciliary axoneme
Cytoplasmic dynein
3 Disassembly of the raft protein complex-cargo-molecular motor machinery.
2 Retrograde transport of cargos along a microtubule is mediated by cytoplasmic dynein.
A raft protein complex may provide a mechanism for the transport of multiple cargos (vesicle or nonvesicle structures).
Axonal transport
Neuron
1 Anterograde transport of a vesicle along a microtubule is mediated by kinesin.
Minus end
Kinesin
Microtubule
Axon
Plus end
Synapse
Recycled synaptic vesicle
Neurotransmitter
Receptor for the neurotransmitter released at the synapse
Cytoplasmic dynein
2 Retrograde transport of a vesicle along a microtubule is mediated by cytoplasmic dynein.
Golgi apparatus

Kinesins and cytoplasmic dyneins have two ATP-binding heads and a tail. Energy derives from continuous ATP hydrolysis by ATPases present in the heads. The head domains interact with microtubules, and the tail binds to specific receptor binding sites on the surface of vesicles and organelles.

Kinesin uses energy from ATP hydrolysis to move vesicles from the cell body of the neuron toward the end portion of the axon (**anterograde transport**). Cytoplasmic dynein also uses ATP as an energy source to move vesicles in the opposite direction (**retrograde transport**).

Myosin family associates with F-actin to form contractile structures

Members of the myosin family of proteins bind and hydrolyze ATP to provide energy for their movement along actin filaments from the pointed (minus) end to the barbed (plus) end. **Myosin I** and **myosin II** are the predominant members of the myosin family (Figure 1-30; see **Box 1-L**).

Myosin I, regarded as an **unconventional** myosin, is found in all cell types and has only one head domain and a tail. The head is associated with a single light chain. The head interacts with actin filaments and contains ATPase, which enables myosin I to move along the filaments by binding, detaching, and rebinding. The tail binds to vesicles or organelles. When myosin I moves along an actin filament, the vesicle or organelle is transported. Myosin I molecules are smaller than myosin II molecules, lack a long tail, and do not form dimers.

Myosin II, a **conventional** myosin, is present in muscle and nonmuscle cells.

Figure 1-30. Classes of myosin molecules and how they work

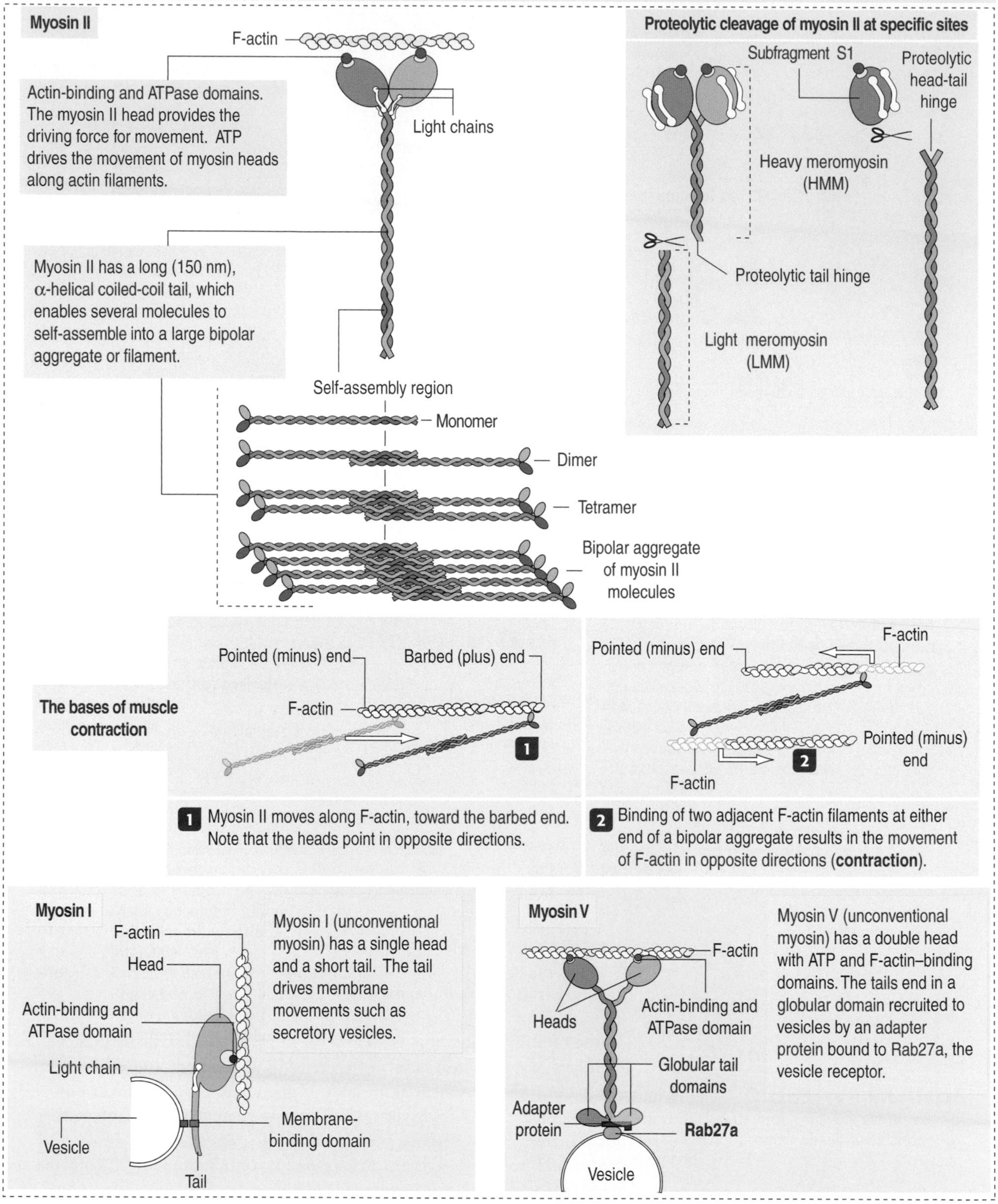

Myosin II
F-actin
Actin-binding and ATPase domains. The myosin II head provides the driving force for movement. ATP drives the movement of myosin heads along actin filaments.
Light chains
Myosin II has a long (150 nm), α-helical coiled-coil tail, which enables several molecules to self-assemble into a large bipolar aggregate or filament.
Self-assembly region
Monomer
Dimer
Tetramer
Bipolar aggregate of myosin II molecules
Proteolytic cleavage of myosin II at specific sites
Subfragment S1
Proteolytic head-tail hinge
Heavy meromyosin (HMM)
Proteolytic tail hinge
Light meromyosin (LMM)
The bases of muscle contraction
Pointed (minus) end
Barbed (plus) end
F-actin
1
Pointed (minus) end
F-actin
Pointed (minus) end
F-actin
2
1 Myosin II moves along F-actin, toward the barbed end. Note that the heads point in opposite directions.
2 Binding of two adjacent F-actin filaments at either end of a bipolar aggregate results in the movement of F-actin in opposite directions (contraction).
Myosin I
F-actin
Head
Actin-binding and ATPase domain
Light chain
Vesicle
Tail
Membrane-binding domain
Myosin I (unconventional myosin) has a single head and a short tail. The tail drives membrane movements such as secretory vesicles.
Myosin V
F-actin
Heads
Actin-binding and ATPase domain
Globular tail domains
Adapter protein
Rab27a
Vesicle
Myosin V (unconventional myosin) has a double head with ATP and F-actin–binding domains. The tails end in a globular domain recruited to vesicles by an adapter protein bound to Rab27a, the vesicle receptor.

Myosin II consists of a pair of identical molecules. Each molecule consists of an ATPase-containing head domain and a long rodlike tail. The tails of the dimer link to each other along their entire length to form a two-stranded coiled rod. The tail of myosin II self-assembles into dimers, tetramers, and a bipolar filament with the heads pointing away from the midline.

Box 1-L | Types of myosins

- Myosins are members of a large family of motor proteins that generate movement along actin filaments using energy from the hydrolysis of ATP.
- Two groups of myosins exist: **conventional myosin**, myosin II, which drives muscle contraction and contractile processes in nonmuscle cells, and **unconventional (nonmuscle) myosins**—myosin I and myosin V among others—involved in the movement of vesicle cargos inside cells.
- **Myosin II** consists of two polypeptides, each displaying a globular head attached to a tail coiled around the tail of its partner. The tails can self-assemble into bipolar filaments. Each head, which also contains a light chain, has an actin-binding site with ATPase activity stimulated by actin binding and regulated by the light chain.
- **Myosin I** is single-headed and has a tail shorter than myosin II. Myosin II is involved in vesicle transport along F-actin.
- **Myosin V** is double-headed with coiled double tails. The heads contain ATP and actin binding sites. The distal end of the tails is recruited by vesicles. The recruitment is mediated by the vesicle receptor Rab27a.
- Myosin V-Rab27a interaction plays a role in the transfer of melanosomes from melanocytes to keratinocytes. Defective transfer of melanosome from melanocytes to keratinocytes of the hair shaft by a mutation of *Rab27a* or *myosin Va* genes is the cause of **Griscelli syndrome** type I and II. Patients with Griscelli syndrome have silvery hair, partial albinism, occasional neurologic defects, and immunodeficiency.

The two heads—linked together but pointing in opposite directions—bind to adjacent actin filaments of opposite polarity. Each myosin head bound to F-actin moves toward the barbed (positive) end. Consequently, the two actin filaments are moved against each other, and contraction occurs (see Figure 1-30).

Heads and tails of myosin II can be cleaved by enzymes (trypsin or papain) into **light meromyosin (LMM)** and **heavy meromyosin (HMM)**. LMM forms filaments, but lacks ATPase activity and does not bind to actin. HMM binds to actin, is capable of ATP hydrolysis, and does not form filaments. HMM is responsible for generating force during muscle contraction. HMM can be cleaved further into two subfragments called **S1**. Each S1 fragment contains ATPase and light chains and binds actin.

Myosin V, an **unconventional** myosin, is double-headed with a coiled double tail. The head region binds to F-actin; the distal globular ends of the tails bind to **Rab27a**, a receptor on vesicle membranes. Myosin Va mediates vesicular transport along F-actin tracks. A specific example is the transport of melanosomes from melanocytes to keratinocytes, first along microtubules and later along F-actin.

Mutations in the *Rab27a* and *myosin Va* genes disrupt the F-actin transport of melanosomes. An example in humans is **Griscelli syndrome**, a rare autosomal recessive disorder characterized by pigment dilution of the hair caused by defects in melanosome transport and associated with disrupted T cell cytotoxic activity and neurologic complications.

Figure 1-31 summarizes the structural and functional characteristics of motor proteins.

Light-chain phosphorylation by myosin light-chain kinase

The self-assembly of myosin II and interaction with actin filaments in nonmuscle cells takes place in certain sites according to functional needs. These events are controlled by the enzyme **myosin light-chain kinase** (MLCK), which **phosphorylates one of the myosin light chains** (called the **regulatory light chain**) present on the myosin head. The activity of MLCK is regulated by the Ca^{2+}-binding protein **calmodulin** (Figure 1-32).

MLCK has a **catalytic domain** and a **regulatory domain**. When calmodulin and Ca^{2+} bind to the regulatory domain, the catalytic activity of the kinase is released. The MLCK–calmodulin–Ca^{2+} complex catalyzes the transfer of a phosphate group from ATP to the myosin light chain, and myosin cycles along F-actin to generate force and muscle contraction.

Phosphorylation of one of the myosin light chains results in two effects:

1. It exposes the actin-binding site on the myosin head. This step is essential for an interaction of the myosin head with the F-actin bundle.

2. It releases the myosin tail from its sticky attachment site near the myosin head. This step also is critical because only myosin II stretched tails can self-assemble and generate bipolar filaments, a requirement for muscle contraction (see Figure 1-31).

Figure 1-31. Comparison of motor proteins

	Myosin I	Myosin II	Kinesin	Cytoplasmic dynein
Number of heads	One	Two	Two	Two
Tail binds to	Cell membrane	Myosin II	Vesicle	Vesicle
Head binds to	**Actin**	**Actin**	**Microtubule**	**Microtubule**
Direction of head motion toward the	Barbed (plus) end	Barbed (plus) end	Plus end	Minus end

Figure 1-32. **Light-chain phosphorylation of myosin II in nonmuscle cells**

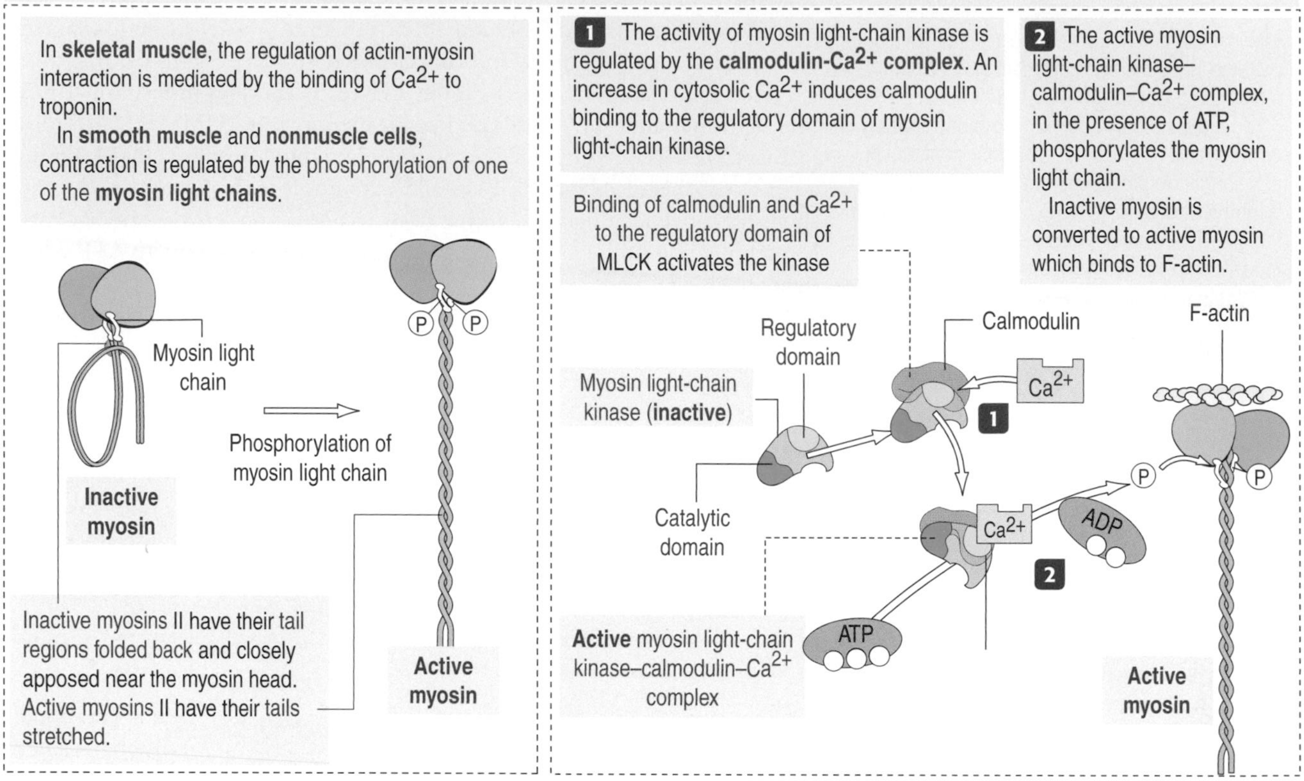

In **skeletal muscle**, the regulation of actin-myosin interaction is mediated by the binding of Ca^{2+} to troponin.
In **smooth muscle** and **nonmuscle cells**, contraction is regulated by the phosphorylation of one of the **myosin light chains**.
Myosin light chain
Phosphorylation of myosin light chain
Inactive myosin
Active myosin
Inactive myosins II have their tail regions folded back and closely apposed near the myosin head. Active myosins II have their tails stretched.
1 The activity of myosin light-chain kinase is regulated by the **calmodulin-Ca^{2+} complex**. An increase in cytosolic Ca^{2+} induces calmodulin binding to the regulatory domain of myosin light-chain kinase.
2 The active myosin light-chain kinase–calmodulin–Ca^{2+} complex, in the presence of ATP, phosphorylates the myosin light chain.
Inactive myosin is converted to active myosin which binds to F-actin.
Binding of calmodulin and Ca^{2+} to the regulatory domain of MLCK activates the kinase
Regulatory domain
Calmodulin
F-actin
Myosin light-chain kinase (**inactive**)
Catalytic domain
Active myosin light-chain kinase–calmodulin–Ca^{2+} complex
ATP
ADP
P

In smooth muscle cells, a **phosphatase** removes the phosphate group from myosin light chains. Skeletal muscle contraction does not require phosphorylation of the myosin light chains. We discuss additional details of muscle contraction when we study the muscle tissue (see Chapter 7, Muscle Tissue).

Intermediate filaments

Intermediate filaments (Figure 1-33) represent a heterogeneous group of structures so named because their diameter (10 nm) is intermediate between that of microtubules (25 nm) and microfilaments (7 nm). Intermediate filaments are the most stable cytoskeletal structures.

Detergent and salt treatments extract microfilament and microtubule components and leave intermediate filaments insoluble. All intermediate filaments have a common monomer consisting of a central α-helical rod flanked by head and tail domains (Figure 1-34).

The structure of the intermediate filament does not fluctuate between assembly and disassembly states similar to microtubules and microfilaments. In contrast to actin and tubulin, the assembly and disassembly of intermediate filament monomers are regulated by **phosphorylation**.

Intermediate filament protein monomers consist of three domains (see Figure 1-34): A central α-helical **rod domain** is flanked by a nonhelical N-terminal **head domain** and a C-terminal **tail domain**. During assembly, pairs of **dimers**—formed by the parallel alignment of monomers—associate into **tetramers** in a side-by-side but antiparallel orientation. About eight tetramers align end-to-end to form a **protofilament**. Pairs of protofilaments associate laterally to form a **protofibril**, and four protofibrils—a total of eight protofilaments—wind up to form a ropelike intermediate filament (see Figure 1-34). Intermediate filaments do not have the structural polarity seen in F-actin and microtubules. One end of an intermediate filament cannot be distinguished from another. Molecular motors associated to an intermediate filament would find it difficult to identify one direction from another.

Box 1-M | **Types of intermediate filament proteins**

- **Type I (acidic) and type II (basic)**
  Keratins (40-70 kd): Keratins assemble as type I and type II heteropolymers. Different keratin types are coexpressed in epithelial cells, hair, and nails. Keratin gene mutations occur in several skin diseases (blistering and epidermolysis diseases).
- **Type III** (can self-assemble as homopolymers)
  Vimentin (54 kd): Present in mesenchymal-derived cells.
  Desmin (53 kd): A component of Z disks of striated muscle and smooth muscle cells.
  Glial fibrillary acidic protein (GFAP 51 kd): Present in astrocytes.
  Peripherin (57 kd): A component of axons in the peripheral nervous system.
- **Type IV**
  Neurofilaments (NF): Three forms coexpressed and forming heteropolymers in neurons: NF-L (light, 60 to 70 kd), NF-M (medium, 105 to 110 kd) and NF-H (heavy, 135 to 150 kd).
  α-Internexin (66 kd): A component of developing neurons.
- **Type V**
  Lamin A and lamin B (60 to 70 kd, 63-68 kd): Present in the nuclear lamina associated to the inner layer of the nuclear envelope. Maintain the integrity of the nuclear envelope. A group of human diseases—laminopathies—is associated with *lamin A* gene (*LMNA*) mutations (see Box 1-K).

Figure 1-33. Fine structure of the major components of the cytoskeleton

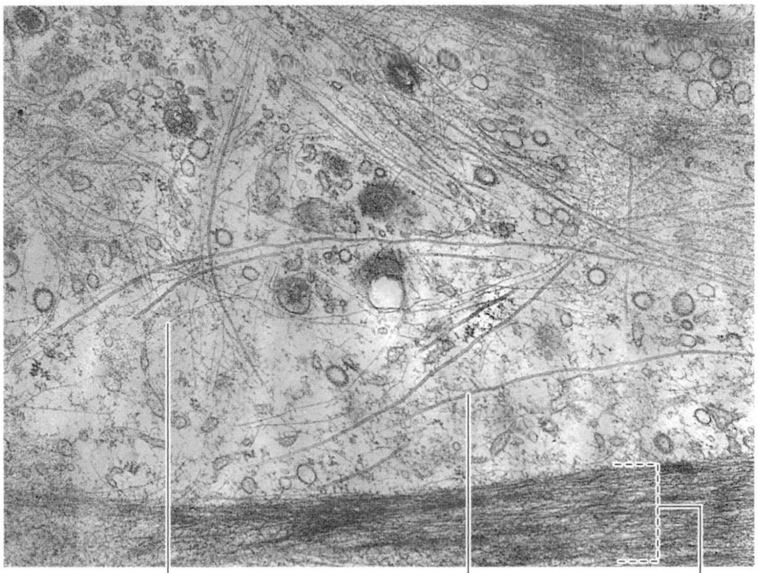

Intermediate filaments (10 nm thick)
Microtubules (25 nm thick)
Bundle formed by actin filaments (7 nm thick)

The major **function** of intermediate filaments is **to provide mechanical support for the cell**. Five major types of intermediate filament proteins have been identified on the basis of sequence similarities in the rod domain. They are referred to as **types** I through V (see **Box 1-M**). About 50 intermediate filament proteins have been reported so far.

Type I (acidic keratins) and type II (neutral to basic keratins). This class of proteins forms the intermediate filament cytoskeleton of **epithelial cells** (called **cytokeratins** to distinguish them from the keratins of hair and nails). Equal amounts of acidic (40 to 60 kd) and neutral-basic (50 to 70 kd) cytokeratins **combine** to form this type of intermediate filament protein. **Type I and type II intermediate filament keratins form tonofilaments associated with molecules present in the cytoplasmic plaques of desmosomes and hemidesmosomes** (see Figures 1-16 and 1-17). We come back to intermediate filament–binding proteins, such as **filaggrins**, when we discuss the differentiation of keratinocytes in the epidermis of the skin (Chapter 11, Integumentary System), and **plectin**, when we analyze the cytoskeletal protective network of skeletal muscle cells (Chapter 7, Muscle Tissue).

In the **epidermis** of the skin, the basal cells express keratins K5 and K14. The upper differentiating cells express keratins K1 and K10. In some regions of the epidermis, such as in the palmoplantar region, keratin K9 is found. Mutations in K5 and K14 cause hereditary blistering skin diseases belonging to the clinical type **epidermolysis bullosa simplex** (see below Clinical significance: Intermediate filaments and blistering diseases).

Type III. This group includes the following intermediate filament proteins:

Vimentin (54 kd) is generally found in cells of **mesenchymal origin**. In some cells, vimentin establishes a structural link between the plasma membrane and nuclear lamins.

Desmin (53 kd) is a component of **skeletal muscle cells** and is localized to the Z disk of the **sarcomere** (see Chapter 7, Muscle Tissue). This intermediate filament protein keeps individual contractile elements of the sarcomeres attached to the Z disk and plays a role in coordinating muscle cell contraction. Desmin is also found in **smooth muscle cells**.

Glial fibrillary acidic protein (GFAP) (51 kd) is observed in **astrocytes** and

Figure 1-34. **Assembly of an intermediate filament**

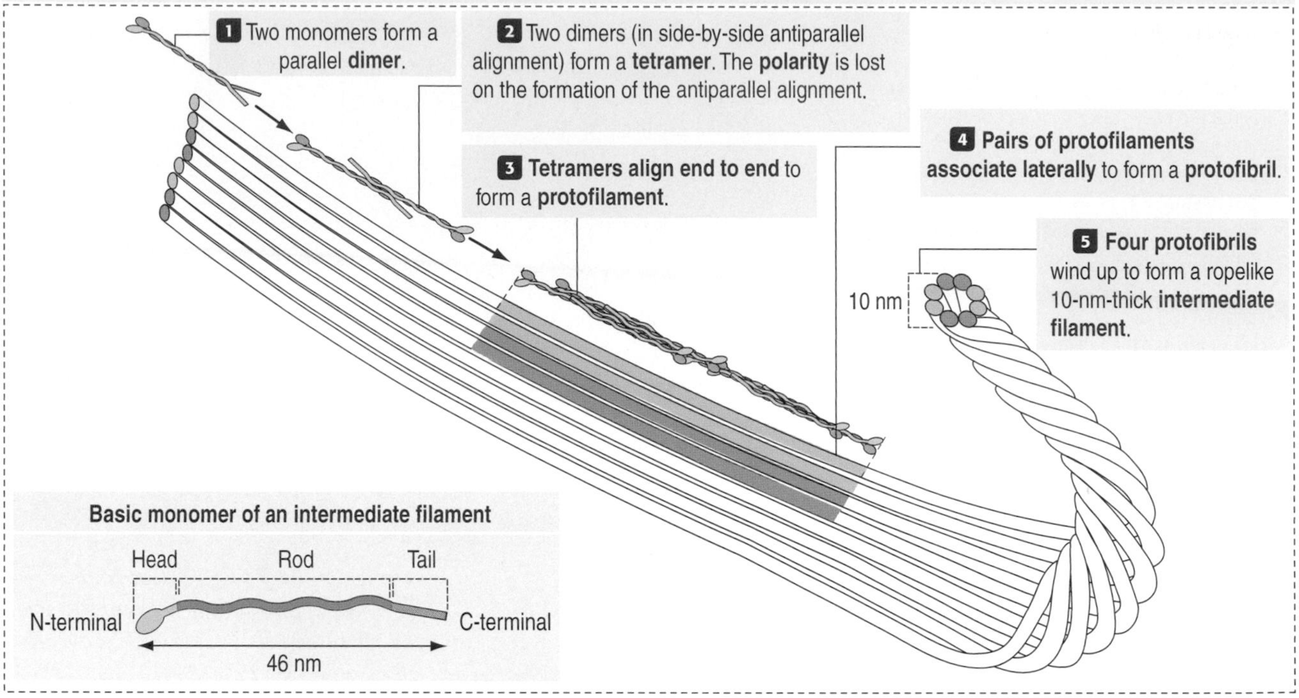

1 Two monomers form a parallel **dimer**.
2 Two dimers (in side-by-side antiparallel alignment) form a **tetramer**. The **polarity** is lost on the formation of the antiparallel alignment.
3 **Tetramers align end to end** to form a **protofilament**.
4 **Pairs of protofilaments associate laterally** to form a **protofibril**.
5 **Four protofibrils** wind up to form a ropelike 10-nm-thick **intermediate filament**.
10 nm
Basic monomer of an intermediate filament
Head
Rod
Tail
N-terminal
C-terminal
46 nm

some Schwann cells (see Chapter 8, Nervous Tissue).

Peripherin (57 kd) is a component of neurons of the peripheral nervous system and is coexpressed with neurofilament proteins (see Chapter 8, Nervous Tissue).

Type IV. Neurofilaments are the main components.

Neurofilaments (NFs) are found in axons and dendrites of **neurons**. Three types of proteins can be found in a neurofilament: **NF-L** (60 to 70 kd), **NF-M** (105 to 110 kd), and **NF-H** (135 to 150 kd), for low-molecular-weight, middle-molecular-weight, and high-molecular-weight neurofilaments.

α-Internexin (66 kd) is found predominantly in the central nervous system (particularly in the spinal cord and optic nerve).

Type V. Proteins of this group, the **nuclear lamins**, are encoded by three genes: *LMNA, LMNB1,* and *LMNB2.* **Lamin A** and **lamin C** arise from the alternative splicing of transcripts encoded by the ***LMNA*** gene. The ***LMNB1*** gene encodes **lamin B1** expressed in all somatic cells. The ***LMNB2*** gene encodes **lamin B2**, expressed in all somatic cells, and **lamin B3**, which is specific for spermatogenic cells.

Nuclear lamins (60 to 75 kd) **differ from the other intermediate filament proteins in that they organize an orthogonal meshwork—the nuclear lamina—** in association with the inner membrane of the nuclear envelope. Lamins provide mechanical support for the nuclear envelope and bind chromatin. Because of their clinical relevance, we come back to nuclear lamins and associated proteins when we discuss the organization of the nuclear envelope

A group of human diseases, known as **laminopathies**, are linked to defects in proteins of the nuclear envelope, including lamins (see **Box 1-N**). Numerous laminopathies affect cardiac and skeletal muscle, adipose tissue (**lipodystrophies**), and motor and sensory peripheral nerves.

Two hypotheses concerning the pathogenic mechanism of laminopathies have been considered:

1. The **gene expression hypothesis** regards lamin A and lamin C as essential for the correct tissue-specific expression of certain genes

2. The **mechanical stress hypothesis** proposes that a defect in lamin A and lamin C weakens the structural integrity of the nuclear envelope.

Box 1-N | **Clinical features of laminopathies**

- Classified into three distinct categories: muscular dystrophy, partial lipodystrophy, and neuropathy. Caused by lamin A or C mutations affecting skeletal and cardiac muscle and fat distribution.
- Emery-Dreifuss muscular dystrophy (phenotype inherited by autosomal dominant and recessive and X-linked mechanisms—the latter caused by mutations in *emerin* gene): Achilles tendon contractures, slow and progressive muscle weakness and wasting, cardiomyopathy with conduction defects.
- Limb girdle muscular dystrophy: Progressive muscle weakness of hip girdle and proximal arm and muscle of the leg. Dilated cardiomyopathy.
- Charcot-Marie-Tooth disorder type 2B1: Motor and sensory deficit neuropathy distal in the upper limbs and proximal and distal in the lower limbs. *Note*: X-linked Charcot-Marie-Tooth type 1 disease also displays motor and sensory neuropathies of the peripheral nervous system, but is caused by a mutation in the *connexin23* (*Cx23*) gene expressed in Schwann cells. It affects myelin.
- Dunnigan-type familial partial lipodystrophy: Becomes evident at puberty with a loss of subcutaneous fat from trunk and limbs and accumulation of fat in the face and neck.

During mitosis, the **phosphorylation** of lamin **serine residues** causes a transient disassembly of the meshwork, followed by a breakdown of the nuclear envelope into small fragments. At the end of mitosis, lamins are **dephosphorylated**, and the lamin meshwork and the nuclear envelope reorganize. See the cell nucleus section concerning the mechanism of phosphorylation and dephosphorylation of lamins during the cell cycle.

Hemidesmosomes and intermediate filaments

Hemidesmosomes are specialized junctions observed in basal cells of the stratified squamous epithelium attaching to the basement membrane (Figure 1-35). **Inside the cell**, the proteins **BPAG1** (for **bullous pemphigoid antigen 1**) and **plectin** (members of the **plakin family** of cross-linker proteins) are associated to **intermediate filaments** (also called **tonofilaments**). Plectin connects intermediate filaments to the integrin subunit β_4.

On the extracellular side, integrin $\alpha_6\beta_4$, **BPAG2** (for **bullous pemphigoid antigen 2**) and **laminin 5**, a protein present in specialized structures called **anchoring filaments**, link hemidesmosomes to the basal lamina. The plakin-related protein BPAG1 associates to BPAG2, a transmembrane protein with an extracellular collagenous domain. Putting all things together, BPAG1 constitutes a bridge between the transmembrane protein BPAG2 and intermediate filaments. If this bridge is disrupted, as in bullous pemphigoid, the epidermis becomes detached from the basal lamina anchoring sites. BPAG1 and BPAG2 were discovered in patients with bullous pemphigoid, an autoimmune disease.

Clinical significance: Intermediate filaments and blistering diseases

Bullous pemphigoid is an autoimmune blistering disease similar to **pemphigus vulgaris** (called "pemphigoid"). Blisters or bullae develop at the epidermis-dermis junction when circulating immunoglobulin G (IgG) cross-reacts with bullous pemphigoid antigen 1 or 2. IgG-antigen complexes lead to the formation of complement complexes (C3, C5b, and C9), which damage the attachment of hemidesmosomes and perturb the synthesis of anchoring proteins by basal cells (Figure 1-36).

The production of local toxins causes the degranulation of mast cells and release of chemotactic factors attracting eosinophils. Enzymes released by eosinophils cause blisters or bullae.

Intermediate filaments strengthen the cellular cytoskeleton. The expression of mutant keratin genes results in the **abnormal assembly of keratin filaments**, which **weakens the mechanical strength of cells** and causes inherited skin diseases, as shown in Figure 1-37:

1. **Epidermolysis bullosa simplex** (EBS), characterized by skin blisters after minor trauma. EBS is determined by **keratin 5** and **14** mutant genes.
2. **Epidermolytic hyperkeratosis** (EH), in which patients have excessive keratinization of the epidermis owing to mutations of **keratin 1** and **10** genes.
3. **Epidermolytic plantopalmar keratoderma** (EPPK), a skin disease producing fragmentation of the epidermis of palms and soles, caused by a mutation of the **keratin 9** gene.

Cell nucleus, nuclear envelope, and nuclear pore complex

The mammalian cell nucleus consists of three major components: (1) the **nuclear envelope**, (2) **chromatin**, and (3) the **nucleolus**. The **nuclear envelope** consists of two concentric membranes separated by a perinuclear space. The **inner nuclear membrane** is associated with the **nuclear lamina (see Box 1-O)**, **chromatin**, and **ribonucleoproteins**. The **outer nuclear membrane** is continuous with the membranes of the endoplasmic reticulum and can be associated with ribosomes.

The **nuclear pore complex** has a **tripartite structure**, composed of a **central cylindrical body** placed between **inner** and **outer octagonal rings**, each consisting

Figure 1-35. **Structure and composition of a hemidesmosome**

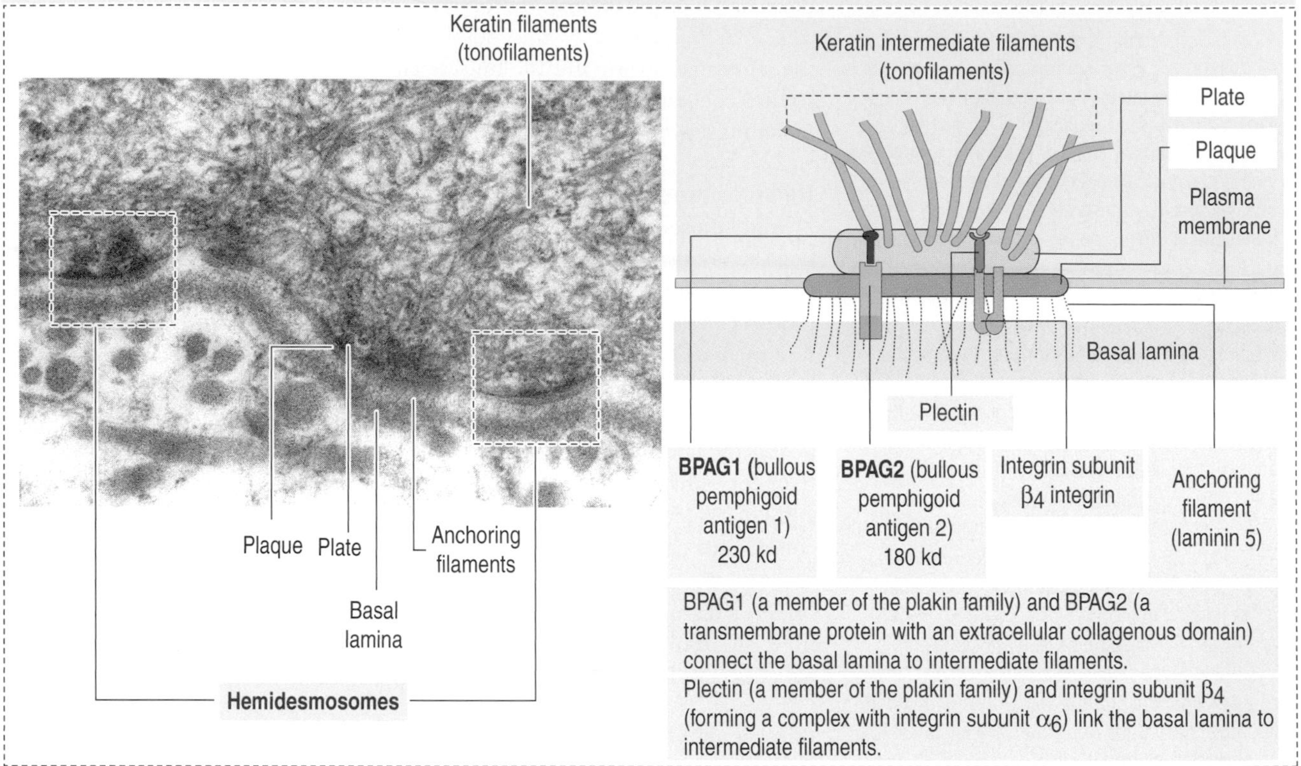

Keratin filaments (tonofilaments)
Plaque
Plate
Anchoring filaments
Basal lamina
Hemidesmosomes
Keratin intermediate filaments (tonofilaments)
Plate
Plaque
Plasma membrane
Basal lamina
Plectin
BPAG1 (bullous pemphigoid antigen 1) 230 kd
BPAG2 (bullous pemphigoid antigen 2) 180 kd
Integrin subunit β4 integrin
Anchoring filament (laminin 5)
BPAG1 (a member of the plakin family) and BPAG2 (a transmembrane protein with an extracellular collagenous domain) connect the basal lamina to intermediate filaments.
Plectin (a member of the plakin family) and integrin subunit β4 (forming a complex with integrin subunit α6) link the basal lamina to intermediate filaments.

of eight protein particles. The central cylinder consists of a central plug and eight radiating **spokes** (Figure 1-38). The exact role of individual nuclear pore complex proteins in nucleocytoplasmic trafficking is unclear.

Nuclear pore complexes embedded in the nuclear envelope establish bidirectional communication gates for the trafficking of macromolecules between the cytoplasm and the nucleus. Small molecules (less than 40 to 60 kd) can diffuse through the nuclear pore complex. Proteins of any size, containing a **nuclear localization amino acid sequence** *(*NLS, Pro-Lys-Lys-Lys-Arg-Lys-Val*)*, can be

Figure 1-36. **Pathogenesis of bullous pemphigoid, an autoimmune disease**

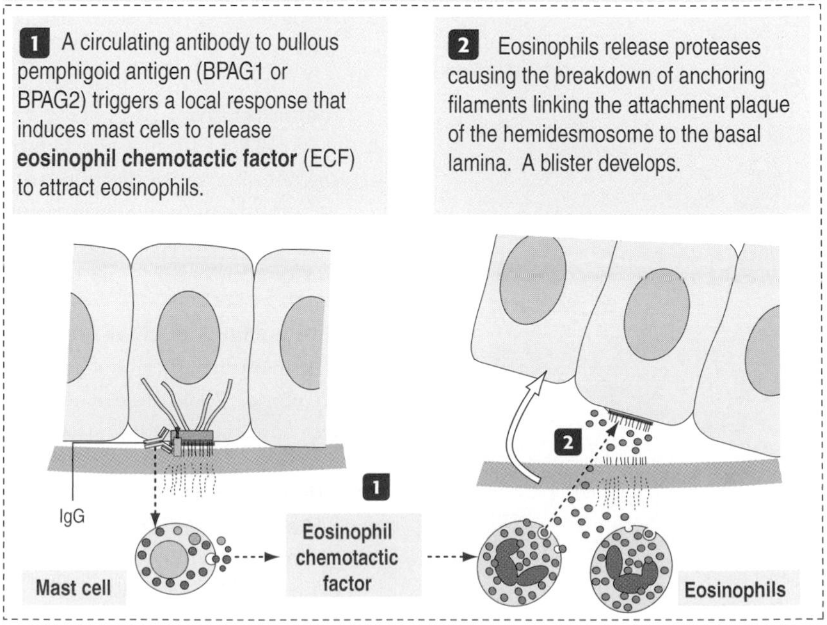

1 A circulating antibody to bullous pemphigoid antigen (BPAG1 or BPAG2) triggers a local response that induces mast cells to release **eosinophil chemotactic factor** (ECF) to attract eosinophils.
2 Eosinophils release proteases causing the breakdown of anchoring filaments linking the attachment plaque of the hemidesmosome to the basal lamina. A blister develops.
IgG
Mast cell
Eosinophil chemotactic factor
Eosinophils

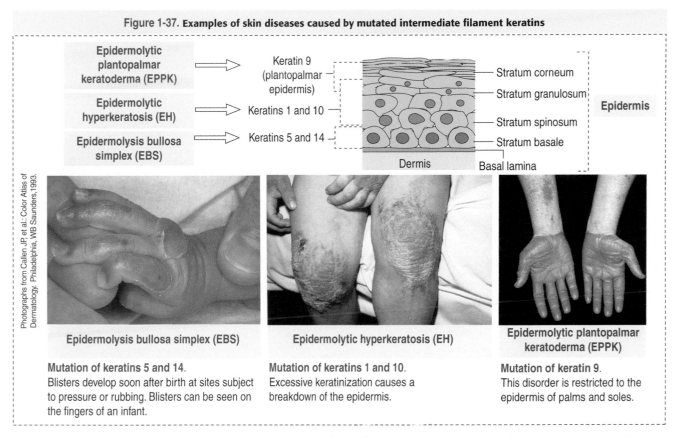

Figure 1-37. **Examples of skin diseases caused by mutated intermediate filament keratins**

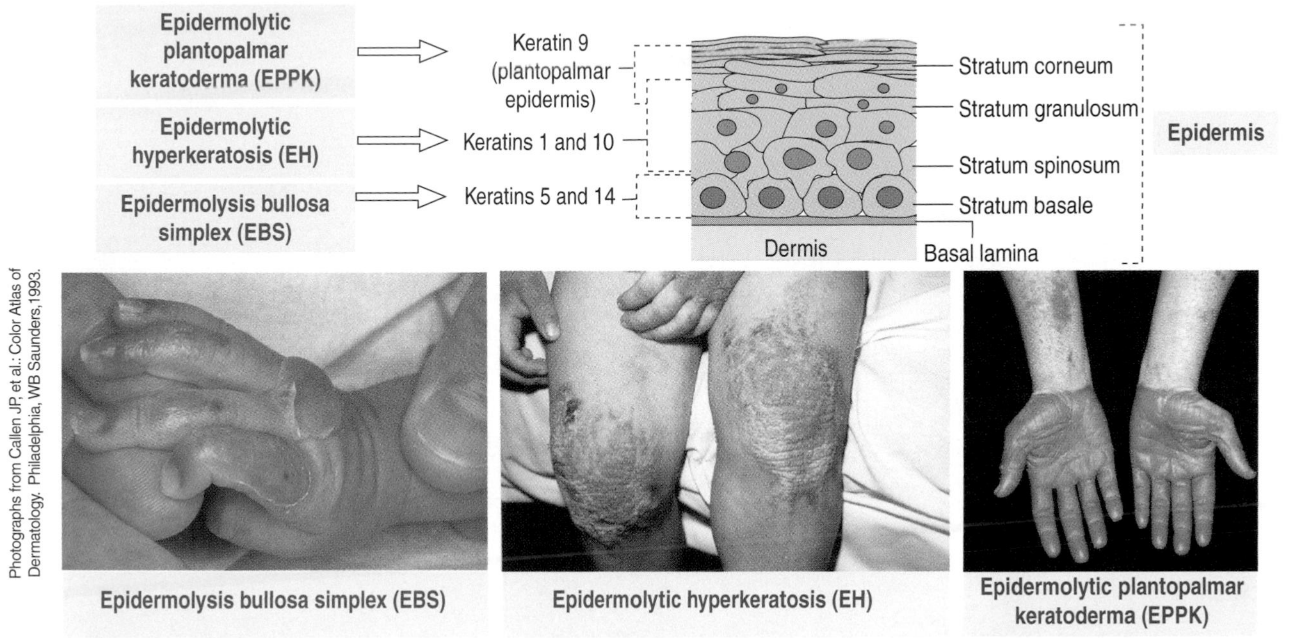
Epidermolytic plantopalmar keratoderma (EPPK)
Epidermolytic hyperkeratosis (EH)
Epidermolysis bullosa simplex (EBS)
Keratin 9 (plantopalmar epidermis)
Keratins 1 and 10
Keratins 5 and 14
Stratum corneum
Stratum granulosum
Stratum spinosum
Stratum basale
Epidermis
Dermis
Basal lamina
Epidermolysis bullosa simplex (EBS)
Epidermolytic hyperkeratosis (EH)
Epidermolytic plantopalmar keratoderma (EPPK)

Photographs from Callen JP, et al.: Color Atlas of Dermatology. Philadelphia, WB Saunders, 1993.

Mutation of keratins 5 and 14.
Blisters develop soon after birth at sites subject to pressure or rubbing. Blisters can be seen on the fingers of an infant.

Mutation of keratins 1 and 10.
Excessive keratinization causes a breakdown of the epidermis.

Mutation of keratin 9.
This disorder is restricted to the epidermis of palms and soles.

imported into the nucleus, however, by an energy-dependent mechanism (requiring ATP and GTP).

Ran-GTPase regulates nucleocytoplasmic transport

Protein nuclear import/export is controlled by **Ran** (for Ras-like nuclear GTPase), **a small GTPase of the Ras superfamily** that dictates the directionality of nucleocytoplasmic transport.

Ran shuttles across the nuclear pores and accumulates inside the nucleus by an active transport mechanism (Figure 1-39).

1. **In the nucleus**, a high concentration of Ran-GTP is achieved by **RCC1**, a GDP-GTP exchanger protein bound to chromatin. Ran-GTP determines the dissociation of imported proteins containing **NLS** by binding to **importin** β, the transporter receptor protein.

2. **In the opposite direction, from the nucleus to the cytoplasm**, binding of Ran-GTP to the carrier protein **exportin/Crm1** facilitates the assembly of complexes containing proteins with **nuclear export sequence** (**NES**).

3. **In the cytoplasm**, Ran-GTP is converted to Ran-GDP by Ran-GTPase, which is activated by two cooperating proteins: **Ran-GAP** (Ran-GTPase-activating protein) and **RanBP** (Ran-GTP binding protein). Consequently, the exported protein is dissociated from its transporter receptor protein exportin/Crm1 and Ran-GTP. Importin and exportins are recycled by transport back across the nuclear pore complex.

Ran-GTPase also has a role in the assembly of the mitotic spindle.

Chromatin

Chromatin is defined as particles or "beads" (called **nucleosomes**) on a double-stranded DNA string (Figure 1-40). Each nucleosome consists of a **histone octamer core** and about two turns of DNA wound around the histone core. The histone octamer contains two molecules each of H2A, H2B, H3, and H4 histones. H1 histone cross-links the DNA molecule wrapped around the octamer.

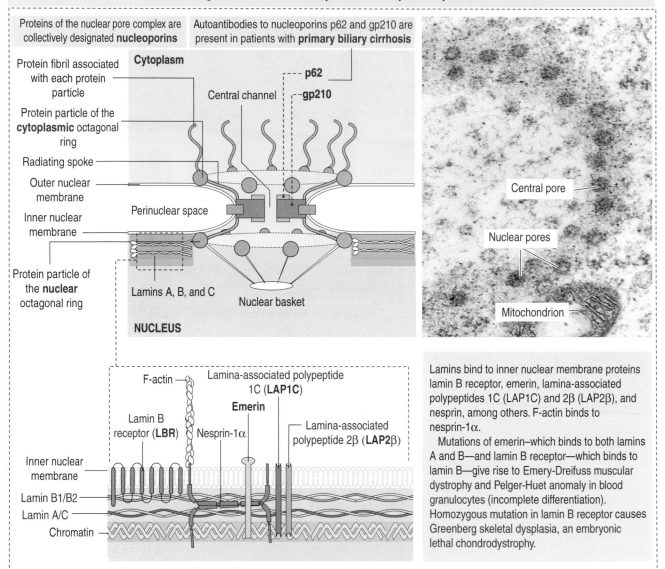

Figure 1-38. Nuclear envelope and nuclear pore complex

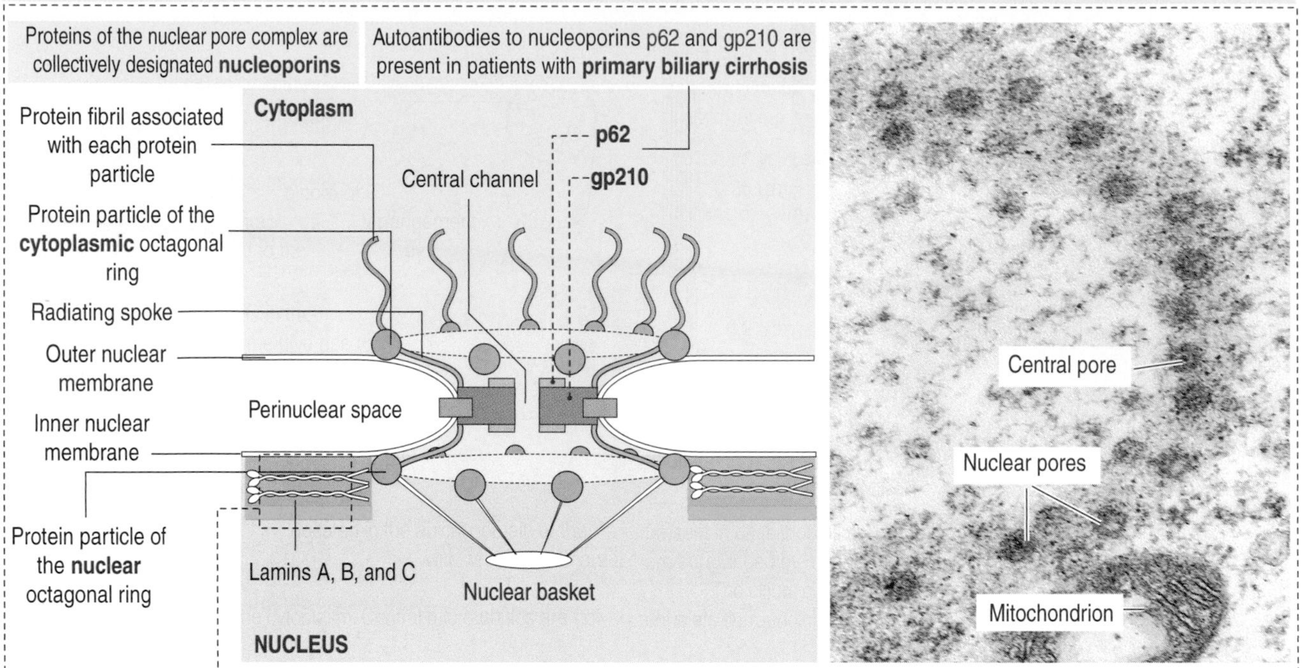

Proteins of the nuclear pore complex are collectively designated **nucleoporins**
Autoantibodies to nucleoporins p62 and gp210 are present in patients with **primary biliary cirrhosis**
Cytoplasm
Protein fibril associated with each protein particle
p62
Central channel
gp210
Protein particle of the **cytoplasmic** octagonal ring
Radiating spoke
Outer nuclear membrane
Perinuclear space
Inner nuclear membrane
Protein particle of the **nuclear** octagonal ring
Lamins A, B, and C
Nuclear basket
NUCLEUS
Central pore
Nuclear pores
Mitochondrion

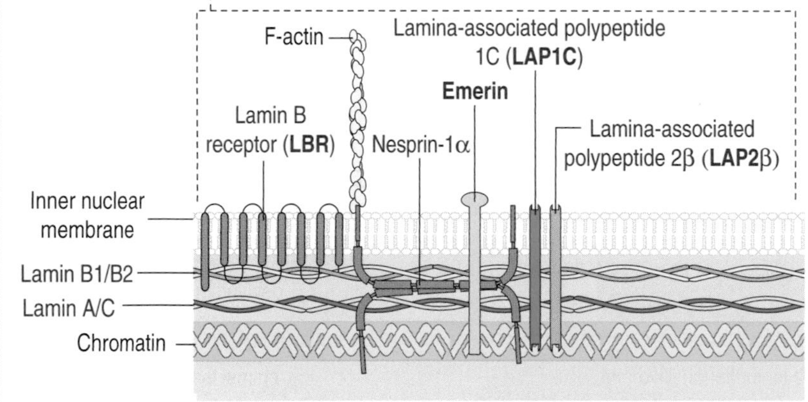

F-actin
Lamina-associated polypeptide 1C (**LAP1C**)
Emerin
Lamin B receptor (**LBR**)
Nesprin-1α
Lamina-associated polypeptide 2β (**LAP2β**)
Inner nuclear membrane
Lamin B1/B2
Lamin A/C
Chromatin

Lamins bind to inner nuclear membrane proteins lamin B receptor, emerin, lamina-associated polypeptides 1C (LAP1C) and 2β (LAP2β), and nesprin, among others. F-actin binds to nesprin-1α.

Mutations of emerin–which binds to both lamins A and B—and lamin B receptor—which binds to lamin B—give rise to Emery-Dreifuss muscular dystrophy and Pelger-Huet anomaly in blood granulocytes (incomplete differentiation). Homozygous mutation in lamin B receptor causes Greenberg skeletal dysplasia, an embryonic lethal chondrodystrophy.

Chromatin is packed in separate chromosomes that can be visualized during mitosis (or meiosis). During interphase (phases G_1, S, and G_2 of the cell cycle), individual chromosomes cannot be identified as such, but are present in a diffuse or noncondensed state.

Diffuse chromatin, called **euchromatin** ("good chromatin"), is transcriptionally (RNA synthesis) active and represents about 10% of total chromatin. Euchromatin is the site of synthesis on **nonribosomal RNAs**, including **mRNA** and **transfer RNA (tRNA)** precursors. **All mature RNA species derive from precursors of larger molecular mass.** Condensed chromatin, called **heterochromatin** ("different chromatin"), is transcriptionally inactive and represents about 90% of total chromatin (Figure 1-41).

Dosage compensation: Inactivation of one of the X chromosomes

The random inactivation of one of the two X chromosomes in every **female somatic** cell is known as **dosage compensation. Both X chromosomes in the germinal cell line (oocytes) remain active.** The inactivation is random because either the paternal or the maternal X chromosome is inactivated. The choice remains nonrandom for all subsequent cell descendants. The transcriptional inactivation of one of the two X chromosomes is observed in the trophoblast on

Figure 1-39. **Ran GTPase directs nucleocytoplasmic transport**

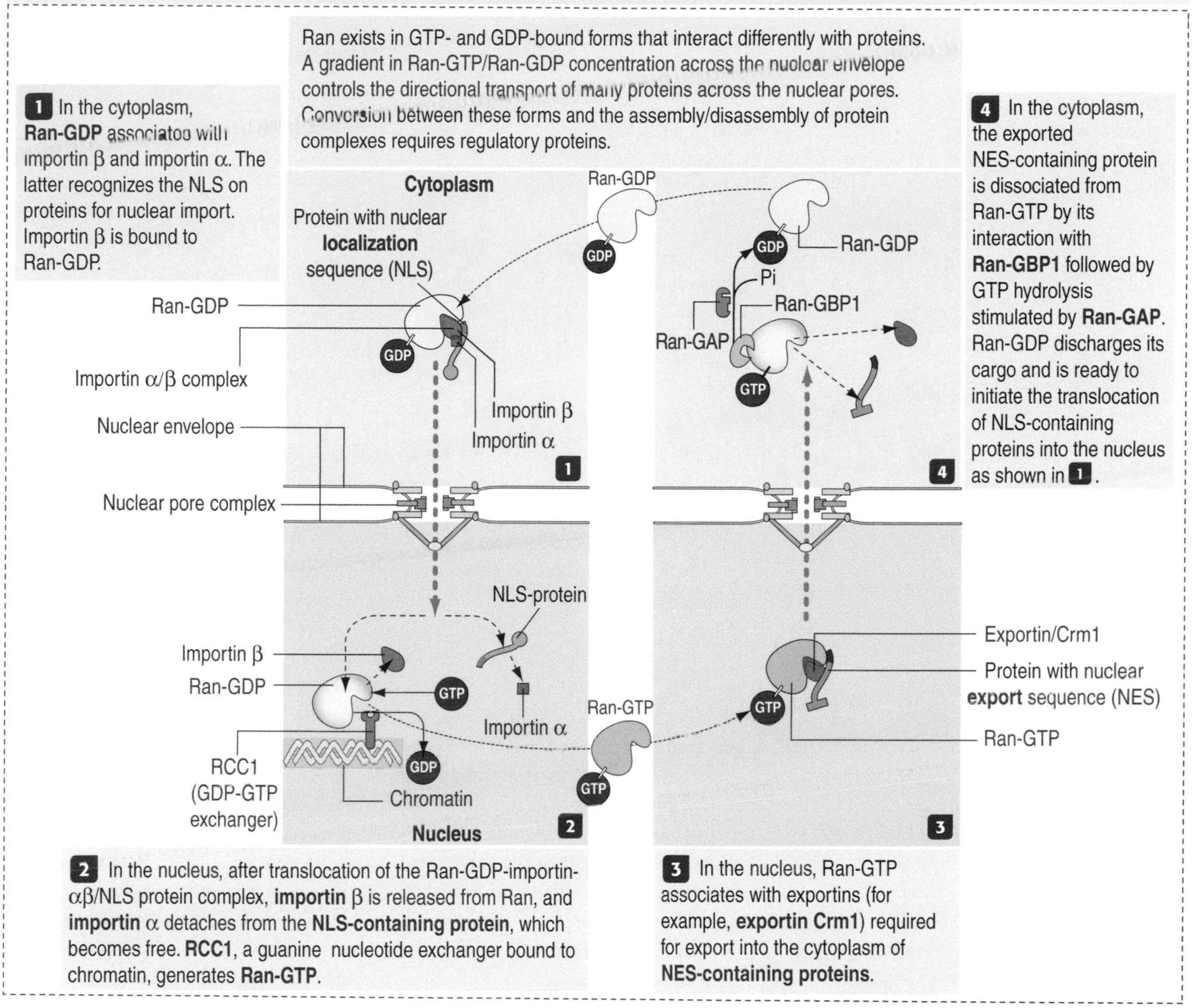
Ran exists in GTP- and GDP-bound forms that interact differently with proteins. A gradient in Ran-GTP/Ran-GDP concentration across the nuclear envelope controls the directional transport of many proteins across the nuclear pores. Conversion between these forms and the assembly/disassembly of protein complexes requires regulatory proteins.
1 In the cytoplasm, Ran-GDP associates with importin β and importin α. The latter recognizes the NLS on proteins for nuclear import. Importin β is bound to Ran-GDP.
Cytoplasm
Protein with nuclear localization sequence (NLS)
Ran-GDP
GDP
Importin α/β complex
Importin β
Importin α
Nuclear envelope
Nuclear pore complex
NLS-protein
Importin β
Ran-GDP
GTP
Importin α
Ran-GTP
RCC1 (GDP-GTP exchanger)
Chromatin
Nucleus
2 In the nucleus, after translocation of the Ran-GDP-importin-αβ/NLS protein complex, importin β is released from Ran, and importin α detaches from the NLS-containing protein, which becomes free. RCC1, a guanine nucleotide exchanger bound to chromatin, generates Ran-GTP.
3 In the nucleus, Ran-GTP associates with exportins (for example, exportin Crm1) required for export into the cytoplasm of NES-containing proteins.
Exportin/Crm1
Protein with nuclear export sequence (NES)
Ran-GTP
Pi
Ran-GBP1
Ran-GAP
4 In the cytoplasm, the exported NES-containing protein is dissociated from Ran-GTP by its interaction with Ran-GBP1 followed by GTP hydrolysis stimulated by Ran-GAP. Ran-GDP discharges its cargo and is ready to initiate the translocation of NLS-containing proteins into the nucleus as shown in 1.

day 12 after fertilization and on day 16 in the embryo.

In humans, the inactivated X chromosome is recognized by the presence of the **Barr body**, a heterochromatin mass observed adjacent to the nuclear envelope or in the form of a **drumstick** in polymorphonuclear leukocytes (see Figure 1-41). If a cell has more than two X chromosomes, the extra X chromosomes are inactivated, and more than one Barr body is visualized.

Box 1-O | Nuclear lamina

- Lamins, type V intermediate filament proteins, are the main components of the nuclear lamina.
- Lamins bind to proteins of the inner nuclear membrane, including emerin (with eight transmembrane spans), lamin B receptor, lamina-associated polypeptides 1 and 2β, and nesprin-1α, a protein with several spectrin-like repeats that binds lamin A and emerin (see Figure 1-38).
- Lamins and their associated proteins have roles in chromatin organization, spacing of nuclear pore complexes, and reassembly of the nucleus after cell division.
- Mutations of lamins and lamin-binding proteins cause various diseases (called laminopathies) (see **Box 1-L**). Hutchinson-Gilford progeria syndrome (premature aging) is caused by a mutation in lamin A.

Nucleolus

The **nucleolus** is the site of synthesis of **ribosomal RNA (rRNA)** and **assembly or ribosomal subunits.** The nucleolus houses several proteins, including **fibrillarin** and **nucleolin**, required for pre-rRNA processing. In addition, the nucleolus contains **nucleostemin**, a protein unrelated to ribosomal biogenesis. Nucleolin and nucleostemin are shuttling proteins; they relocalize from the nucleolus to the nucleoplasm where they interact with **protein p53**, a protector of DNA damage by preventing DNA replication in response to genomic stress. We come back to p53 later (see Figure 1-52).

Essentially, the nucleolus is a multifunctional nuclear structure consisting of stable proteins involved in ribosomal synthesis and molecules shuttling between the nucleolus and nucleoplasm to fulfill non-nucleolar functions.

The nucleolus is a large spherical nuclear structure consisting of three major

Figure 1-40. **Structure of the chromatin fiber: the nucleosome**

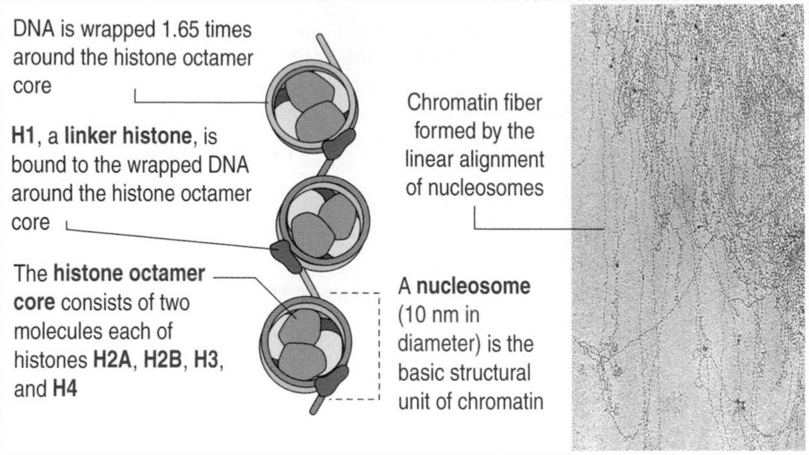

DNA is wrapped 1.65 times around the histone octamer core
H1, a **linker histone**, is bound to the wrapped DNA around the histone octamer core
The **histone octamer core** consists of two molecules each of histones **H2A**, **H2B**, **H3**, and **H4**
Chromatin fiber formed by the linear alignment of nucleosomes
A **nucleosome** (10 nm in diameter) is the basic structural unit of chromatin

structural components (Figure 1-42; see **Box 1-P**):

1. A **fibrillar center** (corresponding to chromatin containing repeated rRNA genes and the presence of **RNA polymerase I** and **signal recognition particle [SRP] RNA**).

2. A dense **fibrillar component** (where nascent rRNA is present and undergoing some of its processing). **Fibrillarin** and **nucleolin** are found in the fibrillar dense component.

3. **A granular component** (where the assembly of ribosomal subunits—containing **18S rRNA** [small subunit] and **28S rRNA** [large subunit]—is completed). **Nucleostemin**, a protein unrelated to ribosomal biogenesis, coexists with the granular components.

The nucleolus dissociates during mitosis, then reappears at the beginning of the G_1 phase. More than one nucleolar mass, each representing the product of a chromosome with a **nucleolar organizing region** (**NOR**), can be observed in the nucleus. In some cells with an extended interphase, such as neurons, a single large nucleolus is organized by the fusion of several nucleolar masses.

The active process of rRNA synthesis can be visualized at the electron microscopic level (Figure 1-43) by spreading the contents of nuclei of cells with hundreds of nucleoli (e.g., amphibian oocytes). **rRNA genes** can be seen as repeating **gene units** along the chromatin axis, like "Christmas trees," pointing in the same direction and separated by nontranscribed **spacers**. The entire rRNA gene region is covered by more than 100 **RNA polymerase I** molecules synthesizing an equivalent number of **fibrils**, each with a terminal **granule**.

Each fibril represents an rRNA precursor (45S) **ribonucleoprotein molecule** oriented perpendicularly to the chromatin axis similar to the branches of a tree. The **45S rRNA** precursor is detached from the chromatin axis and cleaved into **28S**, **18S**, and **5.8S rRNAs**.

The 18S rRNA and associated proteins form the **small ribosomal subunit**. The 28S and 5.8S, together with 5S rRNA made outside the nucleolus, and associated proteins form the **large ribosomal subunit**.

The mRNA precursor is transcribed by RNA polymerase II, and the tRNA precursor is transcribed by RNA polymerase III.

Figure 1-41. **X chromosome inactivation**

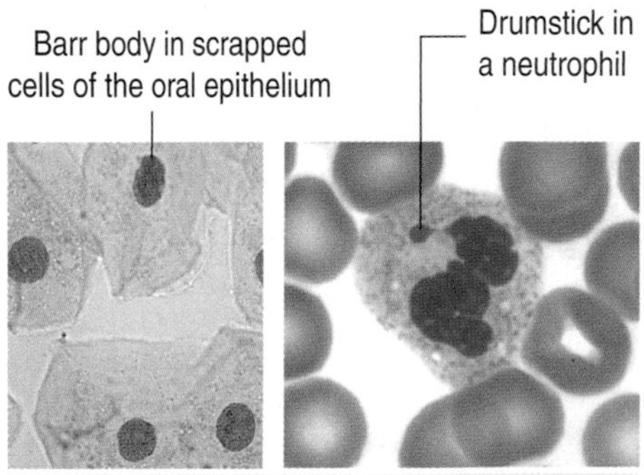

Barr body in scrapped cells of the oral epithelium
Drumstick in a neutrophil

Dosage compensation

The inactive X chromosome remains condensed during most of the interphase of the cell cycle.

It is visualized as a densely stained chromatin mass (**Barr body** or X chromatin) in a variable number of nuclei (about 30%-80%) of a normal female. A small **drumstick** is observed in 1%-10% of neutrophils in the female.

The inactivation of one of the X chromosomes is **random** (paternal or maternal X chromosome).

If a cell has more than two X chromosomes, the extra ones are inactivated and the maximum number of Barr bodies per nucleus will be one less than the total number of X chromosomes in the karyotype.

Localization of nucleic acids

Cytochemistry and **autoradiography** (Figure 1-44) provide information about the cellular distribution and synthesis of nucleic acids. The **Feulgen reaction is specific for the localization of DNA (see Box 1-Q)**. Basic dyes, such as toluidine blue, stain DNA and RNA (**see Box 1-R**) . Pretreatment with deoxyribonuclease (DNAse) and ribonuclease (RNAse) defines the distribution sites of DNA and RNA by selective removal of one of the nucleic acids.

Figure 1-42. Components of the nucleus and nucleolus

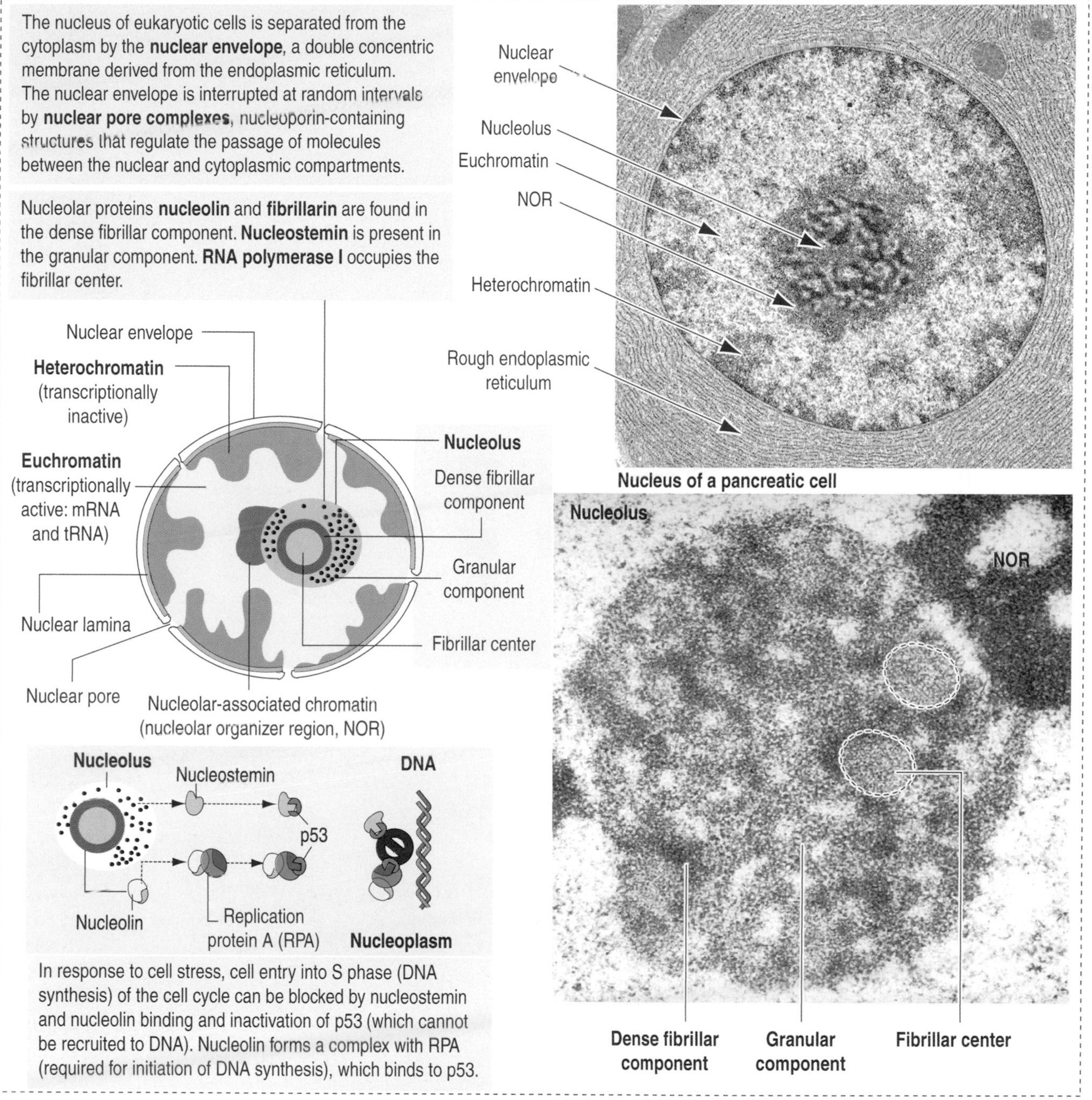
Nuclear envelope
Nucleolus
Euchromatin
NOR
Heterochromatin
Rough endoplasmic reticulum
Nucleus of a pancreatic cell
Nuclear envelope
Heterochromatin
(transcriptionally inactive)
Euchromatin
(transcriptionally active: mRNA and tRNA)
Nuclear lamina
Nuclear pore
Nucleolar-associated chromatin
(nucleolar organizer region, NOR)
Nucleolus
Dense fibrillar component
Granular component
Fibrillar center
Nucleolus
Nucleostemin
DNA
p53
Nucleolin
Replication protein A (RPA)
Nucleoplasm
Nucleolus
NOR
Dense fibrillar component
Granular component
Fibrillar center

The nucleus of eukaryotic cells is separated from the cytoplasm by the **nuclear envelope**, a double concentric membrane derived from the endoplasmic reticulum. The nuclear envelope is interrupted at random intervals by **nuclear pore complexes**, nucleoporin-containing structures that regulate the passage of molecules between the nuclear and cytoplasmic compartments.

Nucleolar proteins **nucleolin** and **fibrillarin** are found in the dense fibrillar component. **Nucleostemin** is present in the granular component. **RNA polymerase I** occupies the fibrillar center.

In response to cell stress, cell entry into S phase (DNA synthesis) of the cell cycle can be blocked by nucleostemin and nucleolin binding and inactivation of p53 (which cannot be recruited to DNA). Nucleolin forms a complex with RPA (required for initiation of DNA synthesis), which binds to p53.

Autoradiography and **radiolabeled precursors** for one of the nucleic acids can determine the timing of their synthesis. In this technique, a radioactive precursor of DNA ([^{3}H]thymidine) or RNA ([^{3}H]uridine) is exposed to living cells. As a result of exposure to the radiolabel, any synthesized DNA or RNA contains the precursor. The radioactivity is detected by coating the cells with a thin layer of a photographic emulsion. Silver-containing crystals of the emulsion are exposed to structures of the cell containing radioactive DNA or RNA. After development of the emulsion, silver grains indicate the location of the labeled structures. This approach has been used extensively for determining the duration of several phases of the cell cycle.

Cell cycle

The cell cycle is defined as **the interval between two successive mitotic divisions**

Figure 1-43. **Processing of ribosomal RNA**

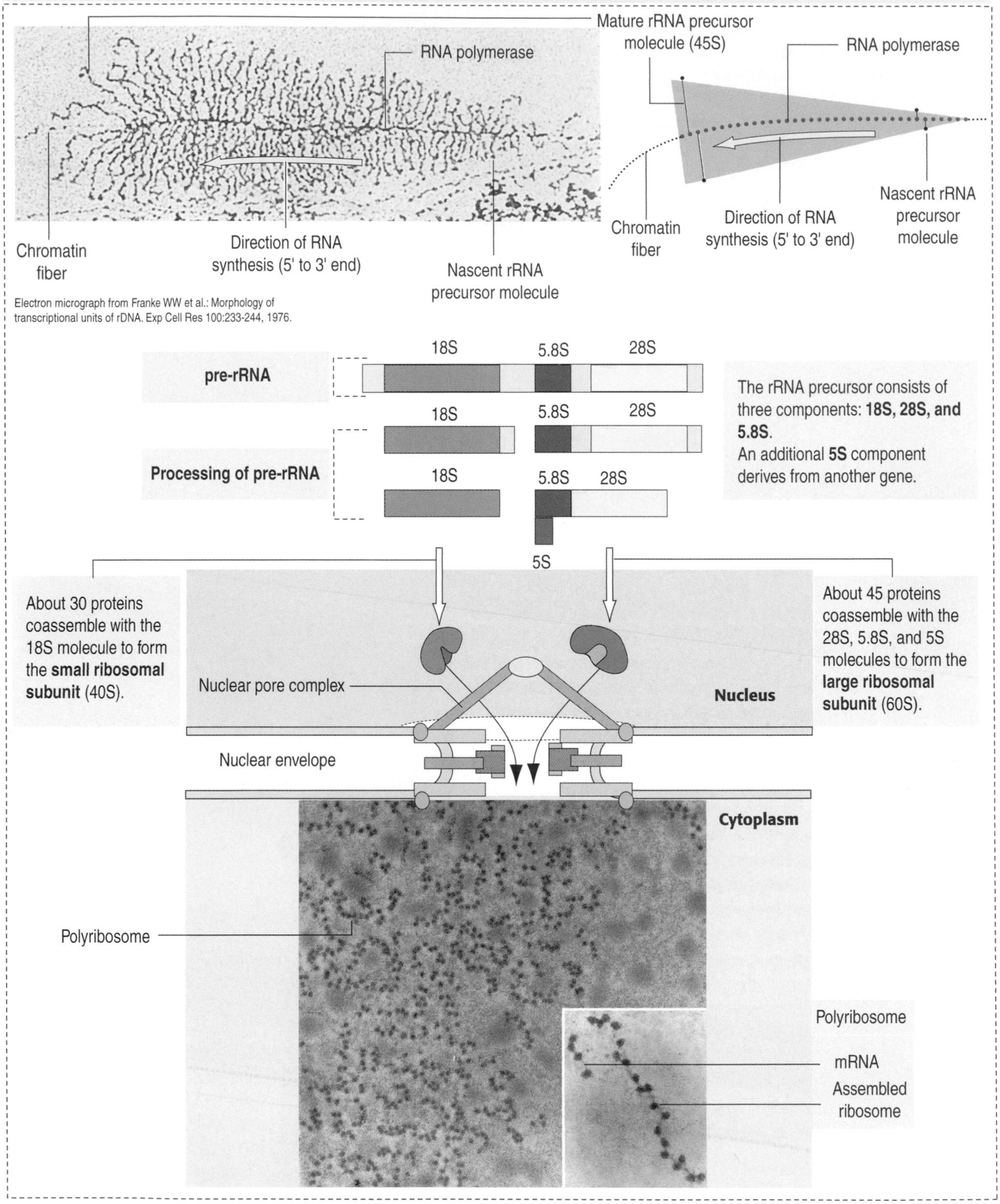

Mature rRNA precursor molecule (45S)
RNA polymerase
RNA polymerase
Chromatin fiber
Direction of RNA synthesis (5' to 3' end)
Nascent rRNA precursor molecule
Chromatin fiber
Direction of RNA synthesis (5' to 3' end)
Nascent rRNA precursor molecule
Electron micrograph from Franke WW et al.: Morphology of transcriptional units of rDNA. Exp Cell Res 100:233-244, 1976.
pre-rRNA
18S
5.8S
28S
Processing of pre-rRNA
5S
The rRNA precursor consists of three components: 18S, 28S, and 5.8S.
An additional 5S component derives from another gene.
About 30 proteins coassemble with the 18S molecule to form the small ribosomal subunit (40S).
About 45 proteins coassemble with the 28S, 5.8S, and 5S molecules to form the large ribosomal subunit (60S).
Nuclear pore complex
Nucleus
Nuclear envelope
Cytoplasm
Polyribosome
Polyribosome
mRNA
Assembled ribosome

resulting in the production of two daughter cells (Figure 1-45). The cell cycle is traditionally divided into two major phases: (1) **interphase** and (2) **mitosis** (also known as the **M phase**).

The most relevant event of interphase is the **S phase**, when the DNA in the nucleus is replicated. S phase is preceded by an interval or **gap** called the G_1

Figure 1-44. Localization of nucleic acids

Feulgen reaction

1 **Hydrolysis with hydrochloric acid** forms aldehyde groups on deoxyribose (DNA sugar) but not ribose (RNA sugar).

2 DNA-containing chromatin stains purple because aldehyde groups reacting with the colorless **Schiff's reagent** yield a **purple product**.

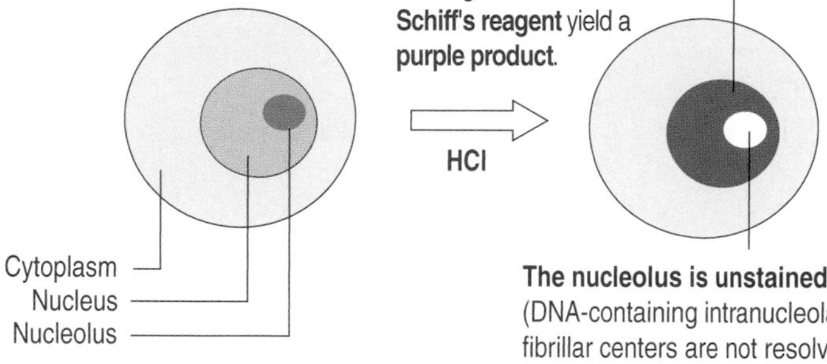

HCl
Cytoplasm
Nucleus
Nucleolus

The nucleolus is unstained (DNA-containing intranucleolar fibrillar centers are not resolved with the light microscope).

Autoradiography

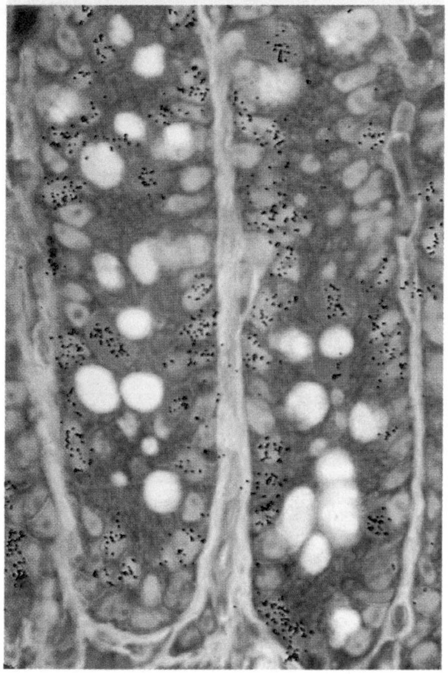

This autoradiogram illustrates the uptake of **[³H]thymidine** by nuclei of intestinal epithelial cells (duodenum).

The radiolabeled precursor was injected into an experimental animal, which was sacrificed 24 hours later.

Histologic sections were coated with a photographic emulsion and exposed in the dark for 48 hours.

Development of the photographic emulsion followed by staining of the section reveals the localization of silver grain (black dots) on some nuclei that were passing through the S phase (DNA synthesis) of their cell cycle.

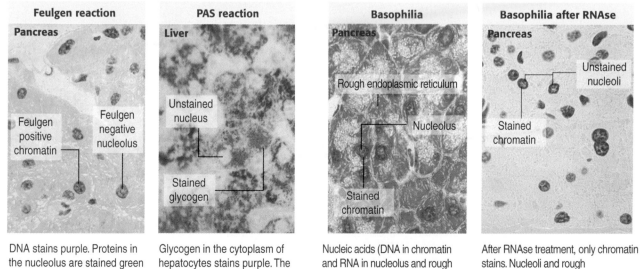

Basophilia

1 **Toluidine blue**, a basic dye, binds to the negatively charged phosphate groups on DNA and RNA. Chromatin (DNA), the nucleolus (RNA), and ribosomes attached to the endoplasmic reticulum (RNA) stain blue. These structures are **basophilic**.

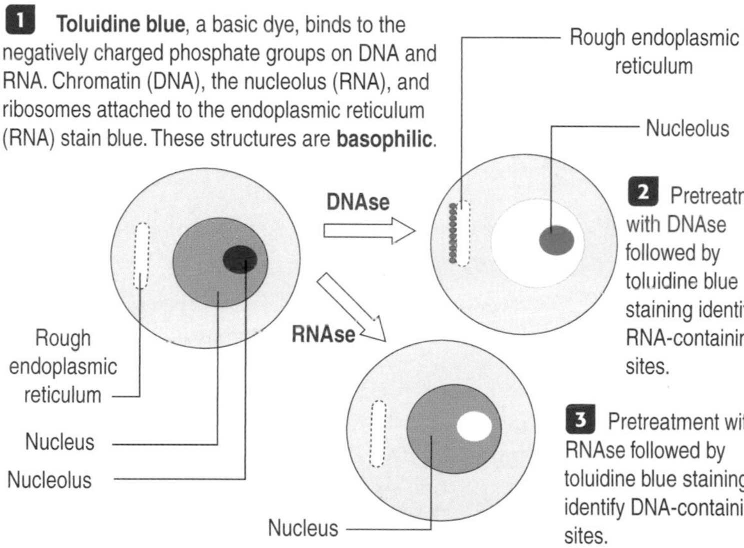

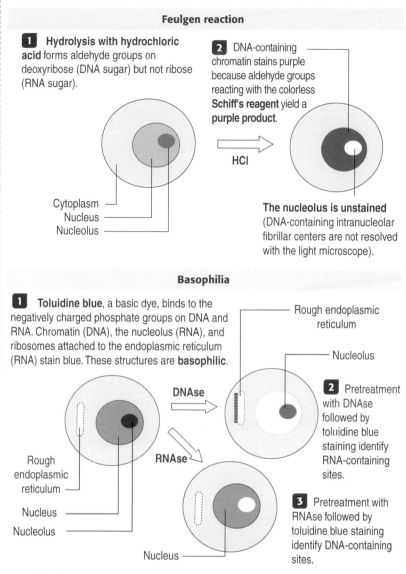

Rough endoplasmic reticulum
Nucleolus
DNAse
RNAse
Rough endoplasmic reticulum
Nucleus
Nucleolus
Nucleus

2 Pretreatment with DNAse followed by toluidine blue staining identify RNA-containing sites.

3 Pretreatment with RNAse followed by toluidine blue staining identify DNA-containing sites.

Feulgen reaction

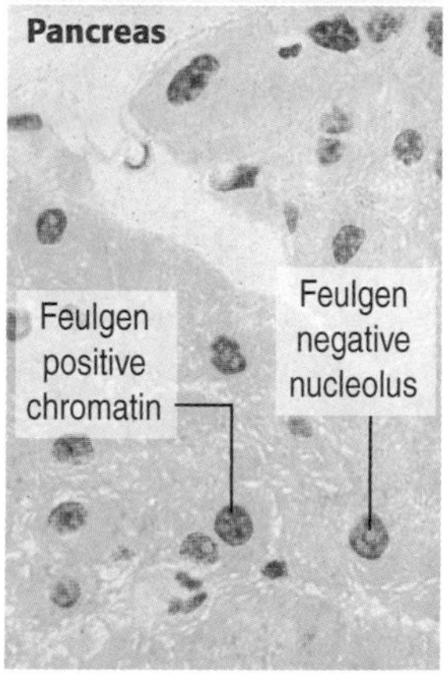

Pancreas
Feulgen positive chromatin
Feulgen negative nucleolus

DNA stains purple. Proteins in the nucleolus are stained green with a contrast dye.

PAS reaction

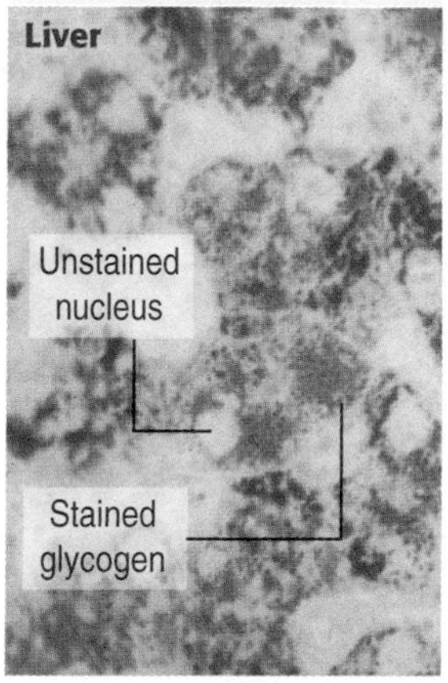

Liver
Unstained nucleus
Stained glycogen

Glycogen in the cytoplasm of hepatocytes stains purple. The nucleus is unstained.

Basophilia

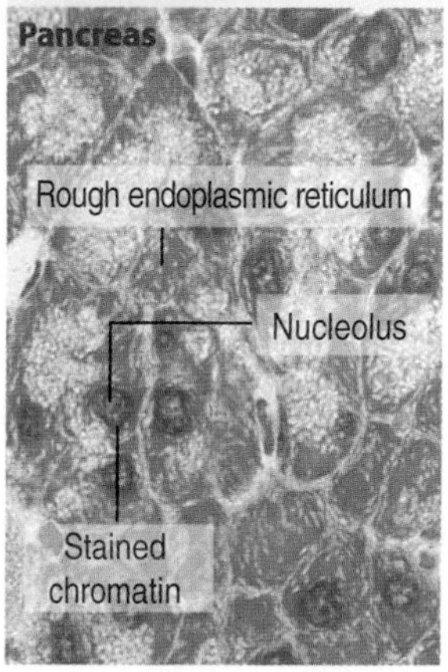

Pancreas
Rough endoplasmic reticulum
Nucleolus
Stained chromatin

Nucleic acids (DNA in chromatin and RNA in nucleolus and rough endoplasmic reticulum) are stained.

Basophilia after RNAse

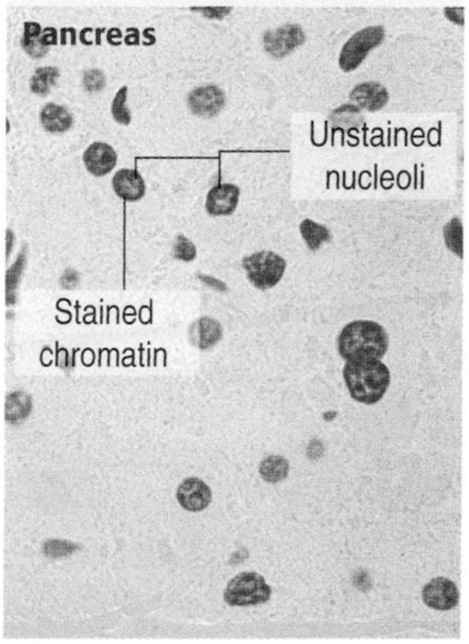

Pancreas
Unstained nucleoli
Stained chromatin

After RNAse treatment, only chromatin stains. Nucleoli and rough endoplasmic reticulum are not stained.

Box 1-P | **Nucleolus**

- The nucleolus is the site of synthesis, processing, and modification of pre-rRNA and initial preribosomal assembly. It also houses proteins unrelated to ribosome synthesis and shuttling between the nucleolus and the nucleoplasm to serve specific functions.
- The nucleolus consists of three components: (1) fibrillar centers; (2) a dense fibrillar component surrounding the fibrillar centers; and (3) a granular component. Pre-rRNA synthesis occurs at the interface between the fibrillar centers and the surrounding dense fibrillar component. Nascent pre-rRNA transcripts extend into the dense fibrillar component and migrate to the granular component where processing, modification, and preribosomal assembly occur.
- The fibrillar centers contain chromatin and transcription factors, including RNA polymerase I. The dense fibrillar component, the site of initial pre-rRNA processing, contains small ribonucleoproteins involved in RNA modification. The granular component accounts for about 75% of the nucleolar mass; the granules correspond to preribosomes.
- The nucleolus disappears during mitotic prophase and reassembles at the end of telophase at specific chromosomal regions named nucleolar-organizer regions (NORs).

Box 1-Q | **PAS and Feulgen reactions**

- Both reactions use the **Schiff reagent**.
- In the **PAS reaction, periodic acid** forms aldehyde groups in sugars of glycoproteins by an **oxidation process.**
- In the **Feulgen reaction, hydrochloric acid** forms aldehyde groups in deoxyribose by **hydrolysis**.

Box 1-R | **Basophilia and acidophilia**

Many cytologic stains use **acidic** and **basic** dyes.

- **Basic** or **cationic dyes** have positively charged color radicals forming electrostatic linkages with acidic groups (e.g., phosphate groups in nucleic acids). **Toluidine blue** is a cationic dye that binds to phosphate groups in DNA and RNA to give a blue color. DNA and RNA are considered to be **basophilic** (having binding affinity for a basic dye).
- **Acidic** or **anionic dyes** have negatively charged color radicals establishing electrostatic linkages with basic groups. **Eosin** is an anionic dye that stains many basic proteins. Basic proteins are considered to be **acidophilic** (having affinity for an acidic dye).

phase. The beginning of mitosis is preceded by the **G_2 phase**, a phase in which the cell ensures that DNA replication is completed before starting the M phase. Essentially, G_1 and G_2 phases provide time for cell growth before and after DNA synthesis. Cell growth is required for doubling the cell mass in preparation for cell division.

Cells in G_1 can make a commitment to DNA replication and enter the S phase or stop their progression into the following S phase. If a cell does not enter the S phase, it remains in a **resting state** known as **G_0**, where it can remain for days, months, or years before reentering the cell cycle.

In a more contemporary view, the cycle is regarded as the coordinated progression and completion of three separate cycles:

1. A **cytoplasmic cycle**, consisting of the sequential activation of **cyclin-dependent protein kinases** in the presence of **cyclins.**
2. A **nuclear cycle,** in which DNA is replicated and chromosomes condense in preparation for cell division.
3. A **centrosome cycle**, consisting of the duplication of the two centrioles, called mother and daughter centrioles, and assembly of pericentriolar proteins in preparation for the organization of the mitotic spindle curing mitosis or meiosis (see Figure 1-45). Recall from our previous discussion on the centrosome as a microtubule organizing center that **γ-tubulin ring** complexes are microtubule-nucleating complexes interacting with the protein **pericentrin** in the pericentriolar material. If this interaction is disrupted, the cell cycle is arrested during the G_2-M phase transition, and the cell undergoes programmed cell death or apoptosis. **Basal bodies**, the origin site of cilia and flagella, derive from centrioles.

The activities of cyclin-dependent protein kinases–cyclin complexes coordinate the timed progression of the nuclear and centrosome cycles (see **Box 1-S**).

Control of the cell cycle by cyclins and cyclin-dependent protein kinases

Two types of proteins regulate the cell cycle: **cyclins** and **cyclin-dependent protein kinases (Cdk)**. Cyclins bind to **Cdk**, which phosphorylate selected proteins. The cyclic assembly, activation, and disassembly of the cyclin-Cdk2 complex drive the cell cycle to completion.

Phosphorylation of Cdk2 is crucial for its protein kinase activity. In its unphosphorylated state, Cdk2—bound or unbound to cyclin—does not have kinase activity. When phosphorylation occurs, a conformational change of Cdk2 enables interaction or activation of the already bound cyclin partner. This interaction exposes the **substrate binding surface** of the Cdk2-cyclin complex, resulting in a significant increase in the binding affinity of the complex for protein substrates.

Figure 1-46 provides additional details on how the phosphorylation and dephosphorylation of specific amino acids regulate the activity of the cyclin B-Cdk2 complex during the cell cycle.

Two cyclin-Cdk2 complexes are important to remember:

1. A **G_1 cyclin–Cdk2 complex** (known as **start kinase**), which triggers cell entry into the S phase after passing **checkpoint 1**, just before the S phase.
2. A **mitotic cyclin B–Cdk2 complex** (known as **M-phase promoting factor, MPF**), formed gradually during the G_2 phase to activate distinct substrates to initiate mitosis, after forcing the cell to pass through **checkpoint 2**, just before mitosis.

Analysis of the dynamics of the cell cycle: Autoradiography and FACS

The various phases of the cell cycle can be studied by autoradiography. Cells in the S phase can be recognized by detecting the synthesis of DNA using [^{3}H]thymidine as a radiolabeled precursor. Cells can be stained through the developed emulsion layer to determine the precise localization sites of the overlapping silver grains.

The time progression of cells through the different phases of the cell cycle can be estimated using both brief and prolonged [^{3}H]thymidine pulses. The number of

Figure 1-45. Phases of the cell cycle

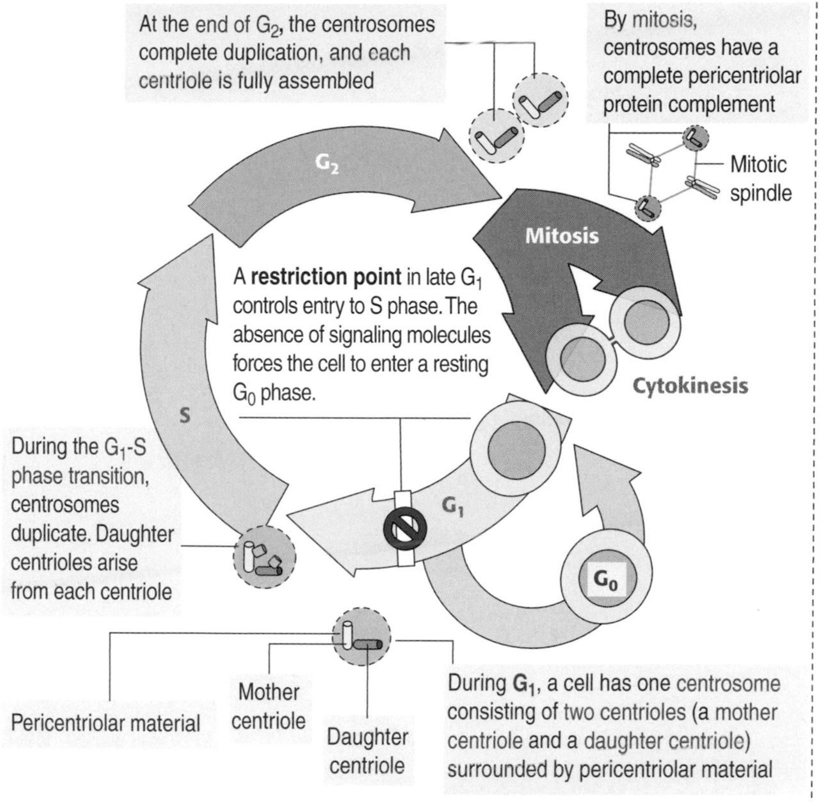
At the end of G_2, the centrosomes complete duplication, and each centriole is fully assembled
By mitosis, centrosomes have a complete pericentriolar protein complement
G_2
Mitotic spindle
Mitosis
A **restriction point** in late G_1 controls entry to S phase. The absence of signaling molecules forces the cell to enter a resting G_0 phase.
Cytokinesis
S
During the G_1-S phase transition, centrosomes duplicate. Daughter centrioles arise from each centriole
G_1
G_0
Pericentriolar material
Mother centriole
Daughter centriole
During G_1, a cell has one centrosome consisting of two centrioles (a mother centriole and a daughter centriole) surrounded by pericentriolar material

Cell division in eukaryotic cells: the nuclear cycle and centrosome cycle

The cell cycle is divided into **four phases**: G_1 (gap 1), S, G2 (gap 2), and mitosis. Mitosis is followed in most cases by cytokinesis. DNA replication occurs during the S phase and can be detected by **autoradiography** using [^{3}H]thymidine as a precursor.

The **duration of the phases of the cell cycle** varies. The mitotic phase is the shortest (about 1 hour for a total cycle time of 24 hours). The G_1 phase is the longest (about 11 hours). The S phase is completed within 8 hours; G_2 in about 4 hours.

Some cells stop cell division or divide occasionally to replace cells lost by injury or cell death. These cells leave the G_1 phase of the cell cycle and become quiescent by entering the so-called **G_0 phase**. Although G_0 cells are metabolically active, they have lost their proliferation potential unless appropriate extracellular signals enable their reentry to the cell cycle.

Box 1-S | **Cell cycle**

- Cell division requires the coordination of three cycles: cytoplasmic cycle, nuclear cycle, and centrosome cycle. The centrosome cycle plays a role in regulating the cytoplasmic and nuclear cycles.
- The **cytoplasmic cycle** depends on the availability of cyclins activated and deactivated by cyclin-dependent kinases (Cdks). Cdk inhibitors inactivate Cdk-cyclin complexes. Cdk inhibitors are upregulated at the transcriptional level to arrest, if necessary, the cytoplasmic and nuclear cycle.
- The **nuclear cycle** involves DNA duplication and chromosomal condensation. **Cdk2** phosphorylation of a protein complex bound to the origin of DNA replication recruits DNA polymerase to initiate and complete DNA synthesis in S-phase. **Cdk1** phosphorylation triggers chromosomal condensation (mediated by **histone H3** phosphorylation) and breakdown of the nuclear envelope (determined by nuclear lamin phosphorylation).
- During the **centrosome cycle**, the two centrioles of a centrosome duplicate during S-phase after phosphorylation of centrosome substrates by **Cdk2**. Daughter centrioles derive from each centriole.
- Cdks are involved in the coordination of the cytoplasmic, nuclear, and centrosome cycle.
- Cdk2 activity is required to initiate DNA replication and centriolar duplication.

cells radiolabeled during interphase (generally about 30%) represent the **labeling index** of the S phase. The fraction of radiolabeled cells seen in mitosis (**mitotic index**) indicates that the radiolabeled precursor, which entered the cell during the S phase, progressed through the G_2 phase into M phase.

An alternative to autoradiography is the measurement of **DNA content** (**C value**1.5 pg per haploid cell) using a **fluorescence-activated cell sorter** (**FACS**). Cells are stained with a fluorescent dye, which binds to DNA. The amount of fluorescence detected by the FACS is equivalent to the amount of DNA in each cell (for example, 2C in G_1; 4C at the end of S phase; 4C during G_2).

Breakdown and reassembly of the nuclear envelope

The disassembly of the nuclear envelope occurs at the end of the mitotic and meiotic prophase. It involves the fragmentation of the nuclear envelope, the dissociation of the nuclear pore complexes, and the depolymerization of the nuclear lamina (Figure 1-47).

The nuclear lamina is composed of type V intermediate filament proteins, **lamins A, B, and C**, which associate with each other to form the nuclear lamina.

Figure 1-46. Regulation of the cell cycle

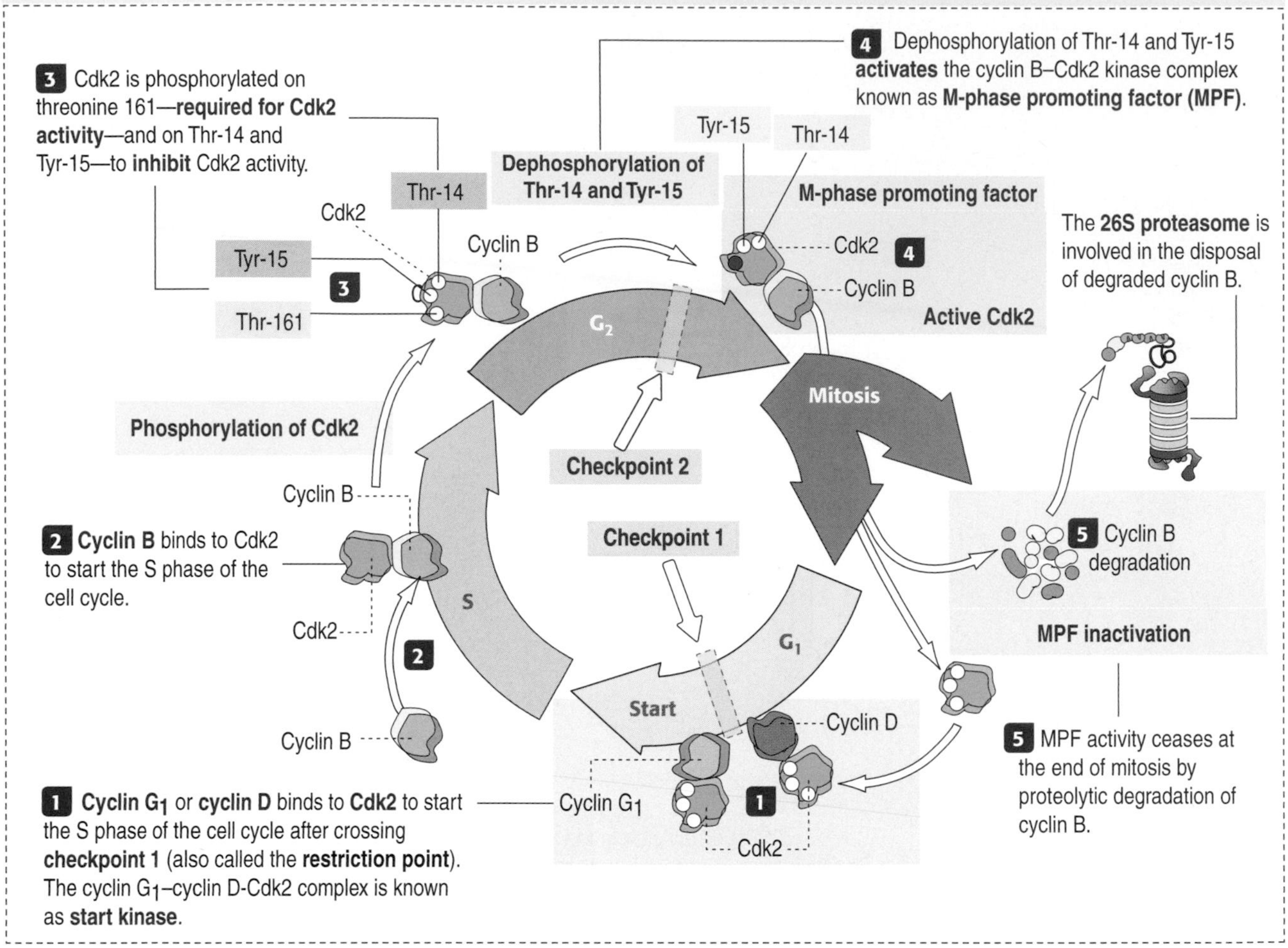
3 Cdk2 is phosphorylated on threonine 161—required for Cdk2 activity—and on Thr-14 and Tyr-15—to inhibit Cdk2 activity.
4 Dephosphorylation of Thr-14 and Tyr-15 activates the cyclin B–Cdk2 kinase complex known as M-phase promoting factor (MPF).
Tyr-15
Thr-14
Dephosphorylation of Thr-14 and Tyr-15
M-phase promoting factor
Thr-14
Cdk2
Cyclin B
Tyr-15
3
Thr-161
Cdk2
4
Cyclin B
Active Cdk2
The 26S proteasome is involved in the disposal of degraded cyclin B.
G2
Mitosis
Phosphorylation of Cdk2
Checkpoint 2
Cyclin B
Checkpoint 1
5 Cyclin B degradation
2 Cyclin B binds to Cdk2 to start the S phase of the cell cycle.
S
Cdk2
2
G1
MPF inactivation
Start
Cyclin D
Cyclin B
5 MPF activity ceases at the end of mitosis by proteolytic degradation of cyclin B.
Cyclin G1
1
Cdk2
1 Cyclin G1 or cyclin D binds to Cdk2 to start the S phase of the cell cycle after crossing checkpoint 1 (also called the restriction point). The cyclin G1–cyclin D-Cdk2 complex is known as start kinase.

Phosphorylation of lamins—catalyzed first by **protein kinase C** and later by **cyclin B–activated Cdk2 protein kinase**—results in the disassembly of the nuclear lamina. In addition, the components of the nuclear pore complex, the nucleoporins, and the membranous cisternae of the endoplasmic reticulum also disperse. The endoplasmic reticulum is the nuclear membrane reservoir for nuclear envelope reassembly.

During anaphase, nucleoporins and three transmembrane protein components of the inner nuclear membrane—**lamina-associated polypeptide** 2β, **lamin B receptor**, and **emerin**—attach to the surface of the chromosomes (chromatin). Then, cisternae of the endoplasmic reticulum are recruited by nucleoporins and inner nuclear membrane proteins, and the nuclear envelope is rebuilt by the end of telophase.

A final step in the reconstruction of the nuclear envelope is the dephosphorylation of lamin B by **protein phosphatase 1**. Dephosphorylated lamin B associates with lamins A and C to form the nuclear lamina before cytokinesis. This sequence of events stresses the impact of gene mutations affecting the expression of lamin A or lamin-binding proteins (see **Box 1-M**) as causes of laminopathies.

Tumor-suppressor genes

Not only Cdk-cyclin complexes control the progresssion and completion of the cell cycle. Tissues use two strategies to restrict cell proliferation:

1. By limiting mitogenic factors, such as platelet-derived growth factor (PDGF) and fibroblast-growth factor (FGF), which **stimulate cell growth**.
2. By regulatory genes that actively **suppress proliferation.** These genes, called **suppressor genes**, control normal cell proliferation.

Figure 1-47. Assembly and disassembly of the nuclear envelope

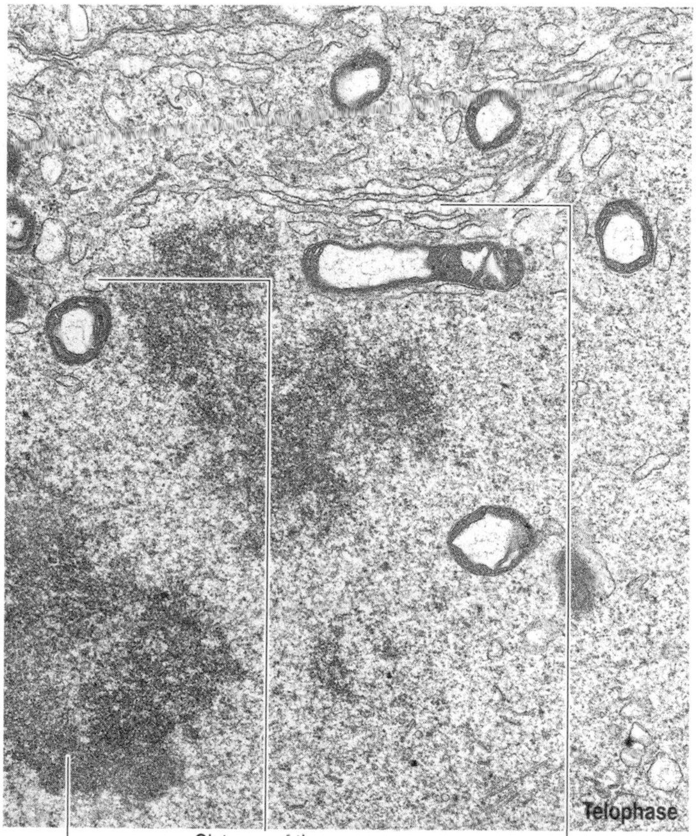

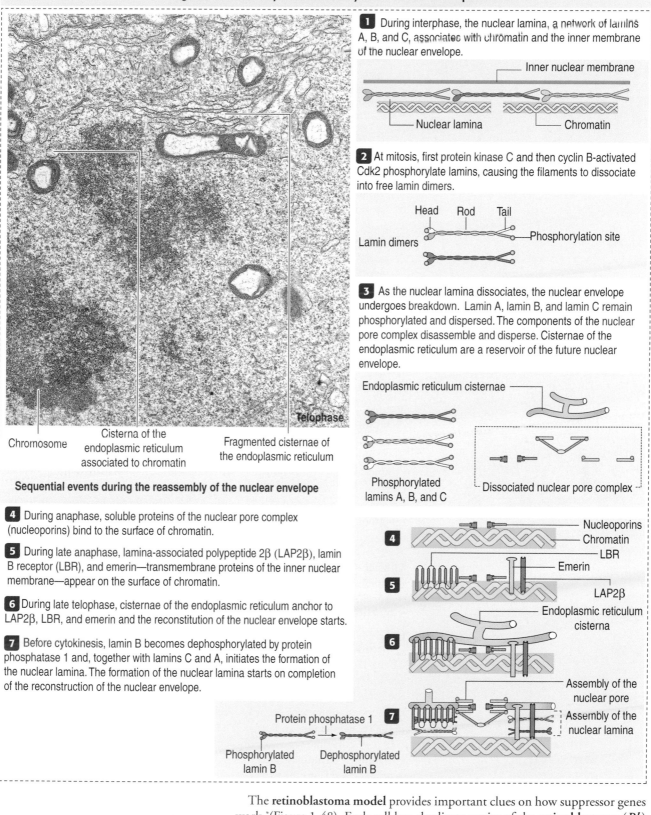

1 During interphase, the nuclear lamina, a network of lamins A, B, and C, associates with chromatin and the inner membrane of the nuclear envelope.

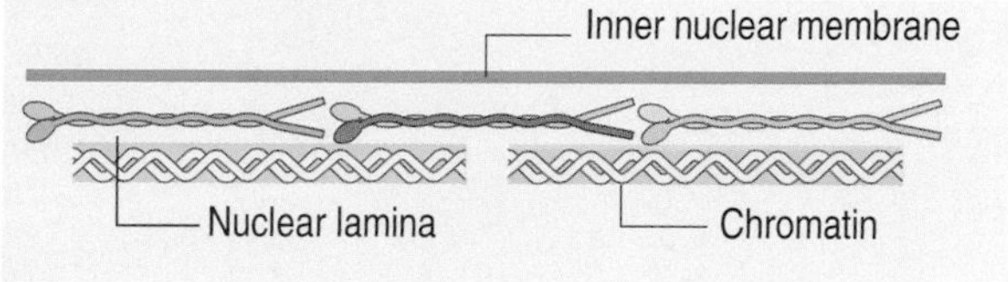

2 At mitosis, first protein kinase C and then cyclin B-activated Cdk2 phosphorylate lamins, causing the filaments to dissociate into free lamin dimers.

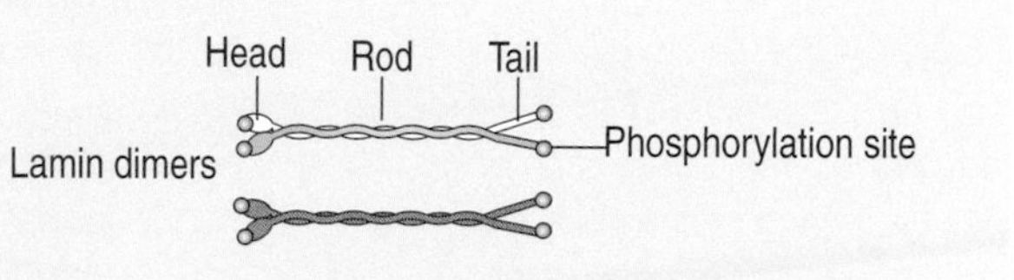

3 As the nuclear lamina dissociates, the nuclear envelope undergoes breakdown. Lamin A, lamin B, and lamin C remain phosphorylated and dispersed. The components of the nuclear pore complex disassemble and disperse. Cisternae of the endoplasmic reticulum are a reservoir of the future nuclear envelope.

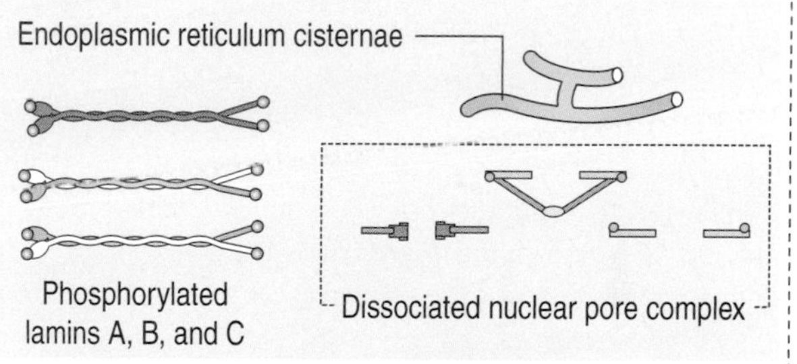

Sequential events during the reassembly of the nuclear envelope

4 During anaphase, soluble proteins of the nuclear pore complex (nucleoporins) bind to the surface of chromatin.

5 During late anaphase, lamina-associated polypeptide 2β (LAP2β), lamin B receptor (LBR), and emerin—transmembrane proteins of the inner nuclear membrane—appear on the surface of chromatin.

6 During late telophase, cisternae of the endoplasmic reticulum anchor to LAP2β, LBR, and emerin and the reconstitution of the nuclear envelope starts.

7 Before cytokinesis, lamin B becomes dephosphorylated by protein phosphatase 1 and, together with lamins C and A, initiates the formation of the nuclear lamina. The formation of the nuclear lamina starts on completion of the reconstruction of the nuclear envelope.

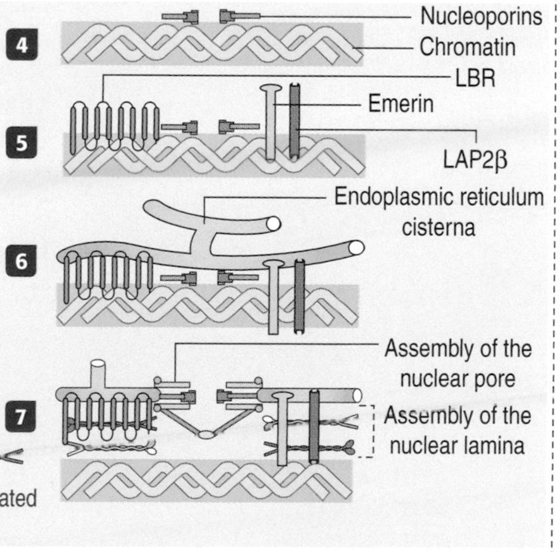

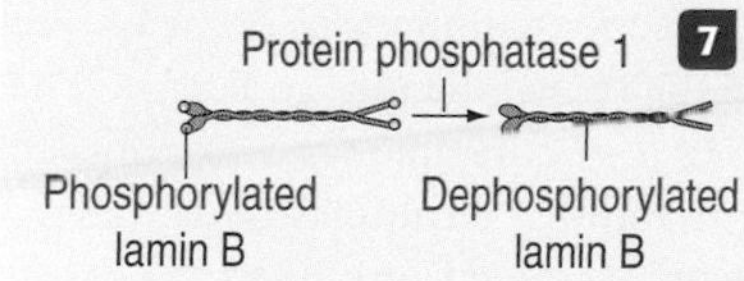

The **retinoblastoma model** provides important clues on how suppressor genes work (Figure 1-48). Each cell has duplicate copies of the **retinoblastoma (*Rb*) gene** as a safety backup. When the **two copies** of the ***Rb*** gene are mutated, an abnormal **Rb protein** induces cancerous growth of retinal cells.

When a single copy of the *Rb* gene pair is mutated, the remaining *Rb* gene copy functions normally and suppresses unregulated cell proliferation unless a second

Figure 1-48. **Rb protein, an inhibitor of cell cycle progression**

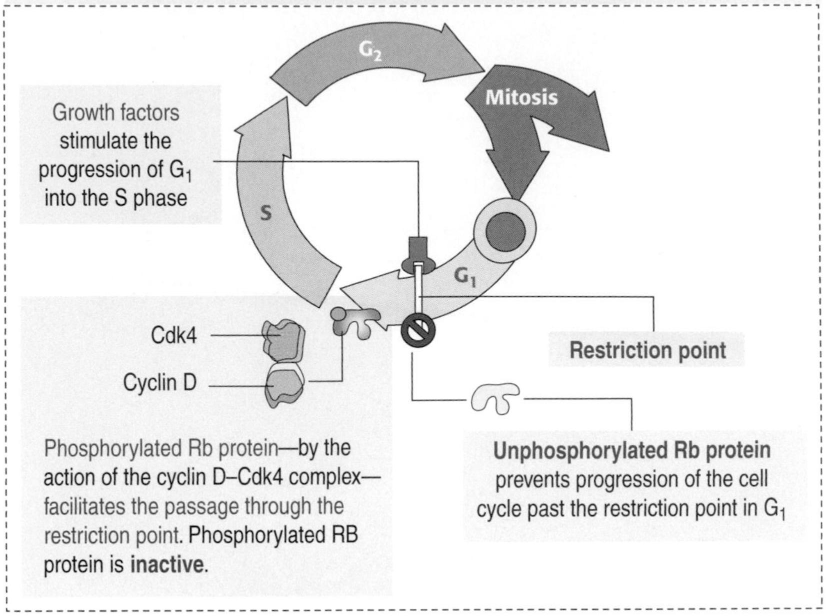

G2
Mitosis
Growth factors stimulate the progression of G1 into the S phase
S
G1
Cdk4
Cyclin D
Restriction point
Phosphorylated Rb protein—by the action of the cyclin D–Cdk4 complex—facilitates the passage through the restriction point. Phosphorylated RB protein is inactive.
Unphosphorylated Rb protein prevents progression of the cell cycle past the restriction point in G1

mutation occurs. In children with only a single intact *Rb* gene copy, all cells of the developing embryo grow normally. Late in gestation, during the development of the eye and its retina, retinal cells may lose the normal copy of the *Rb* gene, and a retinoblastoma develops.

The *Rb* gene specifies a **nuclear protein** involved in regulating the activity of a group of proteins—**transcription factors**—involved in DNA synthesis and cell cycle progression. When Rb protein is **dephosphorylated**, it binds to transcription factors. Although the Rb protein–transcription factor complex can bind to target genes, the activity of the transcription factors is repressed.

When Rb protein is **phosphorylated** by the **Cdk4–cyclin D** complex, it dissociates from the transcription factor complex, which activates specific gene expression (Figure 1-49). Phosphorylated Rb protein switches transcription factors from suppression to activation required for DNA synthesis and progression of the cell cycle.

Clinical significance: Retinoblastoma gene and other suppressor genes

Retinoblastoma tumors occur early in life and are seldom seen after age 5 or 6 years. The disease often runs in families. In such families, this tumor may affect half of the offspring. Children with the **familial form** of retinoblastoma usually have multiple tumor sites growing in both eyes.

A second type of retinoblastoma, the **sporadic form**, is seen in children whose parents have no history of the disease. Once cured, these patients, as adults, do not transmit the disease to the next generation. Children with the sporadic retinoblastoma are genetically normal at fertilization, but during embryonic development two somatic mutations occur in a cell lineage, giving rise to the photoreceptors of the retina: the rods and cones. The resulting **double-mutated *Rb*** genes induce cells to proliferate into a retinoblastoma.

In **familial retinoblastoma**, the fertilized egg already carries a single mutant *Rb* gene, acquired from the sperm or egg. All cells derived from the zygote carry this mutation, including the cells of the retina. The remaining normal *Rb* gene must undergo a mutation to reach the double-mutated condition required for tumor formation. Each of the retinal cells is primed for tumorigenesis, and a single event triggers the malignant tumor.

Retinoblastoma is only one of several tumors that arise through loss or inactivation of critical genes. **Wilms tumor** of the kidney is caused by the loss of a

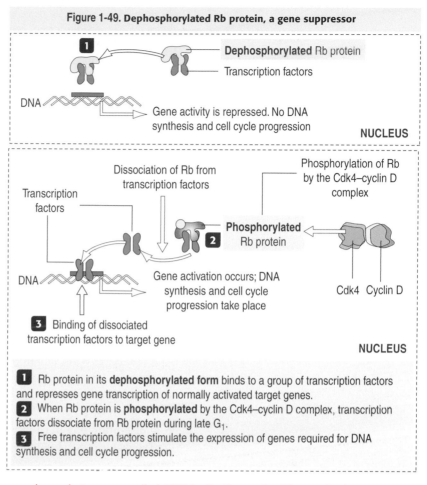

Figure 1-49. Dephosphorylated Rb protein, a gene suppressor

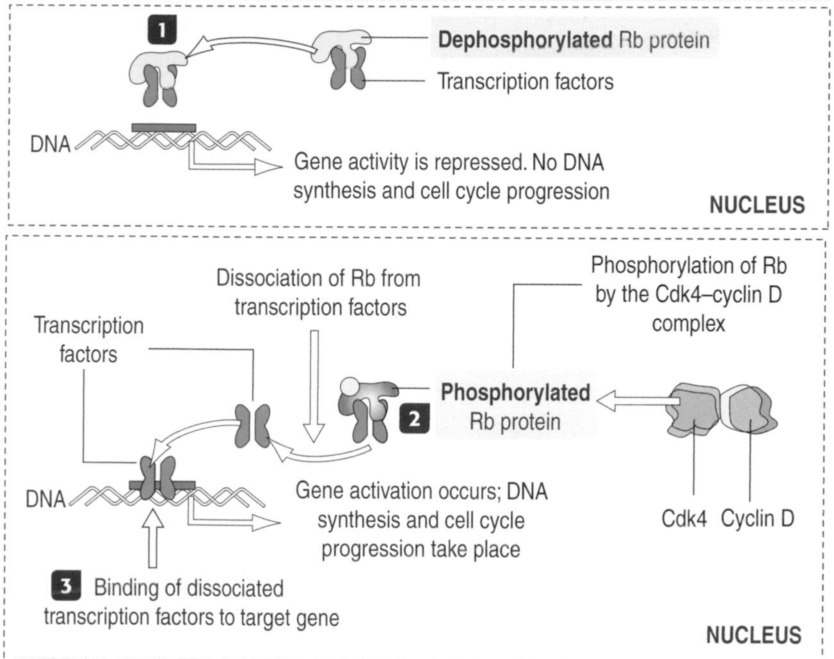
1
Dephosphorylated Rb protein
Transcription factors
DNA
Gene activity is repressed. No DNA synthesis and cell cycle progression
NUCLEUS
Dissociation of Rb from transcription factors
Phosphorylation of Rb by the Cdk4–cyclin D complex
Transcription factors
Phosphorylated Rb protein
2
DNA
Gene activation occurs; DNA synthesis and cell cycle progression take place
Cdk4
Cyclin D
3 Binding of dissociated transcription factors to target gene
NUCLEUS

1 Rb protein in its **dephosphorylated form** binds to a group of transcription factors and represses gene transcription of normally activated target genes.
2 When Rb protein is **phosphorylated** by the Cdk4–cyclin D complex, transcription factors dissociate from Rb protein during late G_1.
3 Free transcription factors stimulate the expression of genes required for DNA synthesis and cell cycle progression.

growth-regulating gene, called *WT-1*. Similar to the *Rb* gene, both copies must be mutated before a cell begins to grow out of control.

One suppressor gene that does not fit easily into this model is *p53*, the most frequently mutated gene in human tumors (leukemias, lymphomas, brain tumors, and breast cancer among others). The *p53* gene encodes the **p53 protein**, a tetramer that binds to a specific sequence of DNA involved in the transcriptional control of certain genes.

A mutation that affects one of the four subunits of **p53** may compromise the function of the remaining three subunits. In contrast to the mutations that affect most other suppressor genes by knocking out gene function completely, the *p53* mutations can result in either mild or aggressive growth.

In Chapter 16, Lower Digestive Segment, we study the tumor-suppressor ***adenomatous polyposis coli (APC)*** gene responsible for a hereditary form of colon cancer (**familial adenomatous polyposis**) derived from the malignant transformation of some of the many **polyps** (benign tumors) observed in individuals affected by this condition.

Mitosis

Mitosis is preceded by the duplication of a pair of centrioles, each of which moves toward opposite sites of the nucleus to organize a **centrosome**. The primary function of the centrosome is the formation and maintenance of the **mitotic spindle** consisting of microtubules. Because of this function, the centrosome is also called the **microtubule-organizing center** (**MOC**). About 1000 new microtubules can be generated per minute on each centrosome using a pool of tubulin dimers derived from disassembled cytoplasmic microtubules.

As we have seen, the initiation of mitosis is triggered by the **mitotic cyclin–Cdk2 protein complex** (mitotic phase promoting factor, [MPF]) at the end of G_2 (at

checkpoint 2). The mitotic cyclin–Cdk2 complex is inactivated by destruction of the mitotic cyclin. This event results in the arrest of protein phosphorylation and rapid removal of inorganic phosphate from proteins by specific phosphatases.

Mitosis is divided into four substages: **prophase**, **metaphase**, **anaphase**, and **telophase**. The highlights of mitosis are summarized in Figure 1-50.

Telomerase, senescence, and tumor growth

Somatic cells can undergo a limited number of cell divisions, after which they enter a state of **senescence**. In contrast, tumor cells have an unlimited life span required for the formation of a tumor. In vitro studies using cultured cells have provided a model for the study of the biological clock of normal somatic cells.

The **telomeres** are the ends of chromosomes formed by a stretch of repeated nucleotide sequences (Figure 1-51). Telomeres are responsible for maintaining chromosomal integrity and represent the cellular biological clock. When DNA polymerases fail to copy the chromosomal ends, telomeres decrease in size with every cell division. Cellular senescence occurs when the telomeres shorten to a point at which the integrity of a chromosome cannot be maintained.

The length of the telomeres in male and female germinal cells and hematopoietic stem cells is protected by the enzyme **telomerase**, a ribonucleoprotein with reverse transcriptase activity that uses an RNA template to maintain the length of the telomeres. Telomerase is not present in somatic cells.

Most tumor cells express high levels of telomerase. Telomerase contains a catalytic subunit, called hTERT, which induces malignant transformation. The development of specific hTERT inhibitors is in progress to prevent tumoral cell growth.

Role of protein p53 in chemotherapy and drug resistance

Chemotherapy and radiotherapy are effective in the treatment of metastatic tumors. Chemotherapeutic agents can:

1. Chemically cross-link DNA (alkylating agents).
2. Inhibit enzymes required for DNA synthesis (nucleotide analogues).
3. Affect microtubules of the mitotic spindle (taxol, vinblastine) (see page 28).

These agents are usually administered in combination, during short periods or continuously, depending on the sensitivity of the type of tumor and avoiding toxic effects on highly sensitive organs, such as the bone marrow, intestinal epithelium, kidneys, and nervous system.

There are two kinds of resistance of tumors to chemotherapeutic agents:

1. **Intrinsic resistance** (tumors typically refractory to many agents—melanoma, liver cancer, renal cell carcinoma).

2. **Acquired resistance** (tumors becoming resistant to chemotherapy, after initial sensitivity).

One form of acquired resistance is caused by genes of the **multidrug-resistance (*mdr*) gene family** (Figure 1-52). These genes encode ATP-dependent pumps involved in the transport of large organic compounds. We see the ***mdr*** gene family of proteins again in Chapter 17, Digestive Glands, when we discuss the mechanism of bile secretion by hepatocytes.

The most studied gene involved in resistance to cancer chemotherapy is ***mdr-1***. Repeated exposure to certain chemotherapeutic agents correlates with overexpression of ***mdr-1*** and increased export of antitumoral agents when they enter the tumor cell.

DNA damage induced by chemotherapy and radiotherapy—**genotoxic stress**—triggers the activation of **p53**, a transcription factor tetramer that destroys terminally damaged cells through the activation of a cell death program, or **apoptosis** (see **Box 1-T**). In **normal cells**, genotoxic stress leads to the *inhibition* of **Mdm2** (for **m**ouse **d**ouble **m**inute 2) allowing activation of p53 and continuation of normal growth and development (Figure 1-52).

Figure 1-50. Phases of mitosis

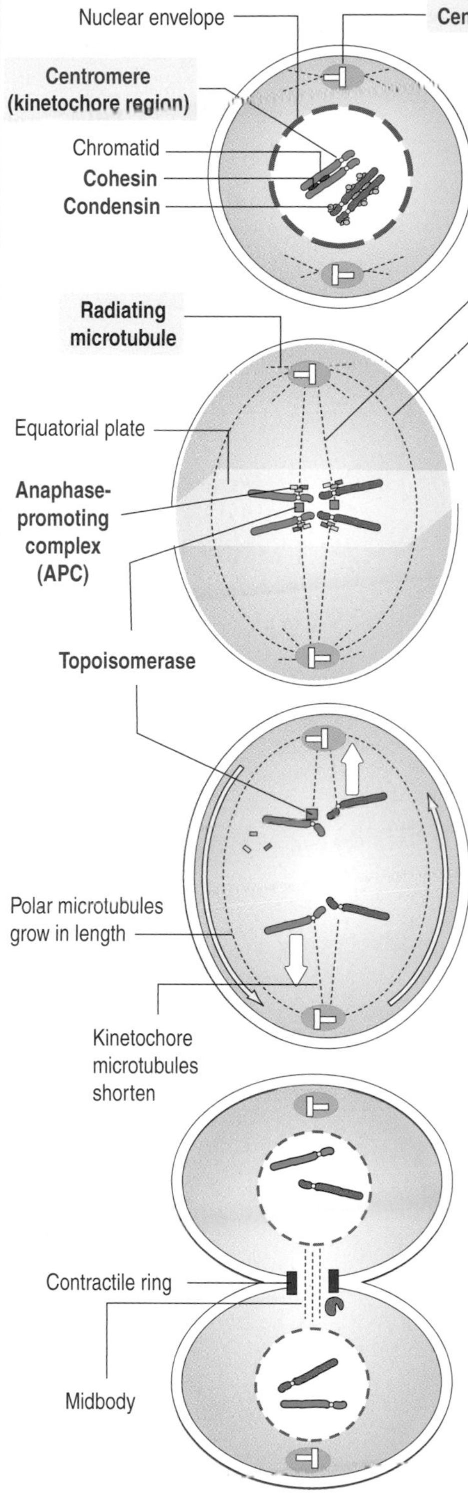

Prophase

1. A **centrosome** starts the organization of the **mitotic spindle**.
2. The nuclear envelope breaks down when **lamins phosphorylate**.
3. Replicated chromosomes condense. Each chromosome consists of two identical **chromatids** (called **sister chromatids**) held together at the **centromere** or primary constriction of the chromosome. A chromatin-binding protein, called **cohesin**, links sister chromatids to each other. **Condensin** at the periphery of the chromatids compacts chromatin.

Metaphase

1. The **kinetochore** develops at the centromeric region. The kinetochore is a structural specialization of the surface of the chromosome into which microtubules insert. Microtubules extending from the centrosome to the kinetochore are **kinetochore microtubules**.
2. Chromosomes align at the **equatorial plate** (also called the **metaphase plate**).
3. Microtubules extending from one cell pole to the other are **polar microtubules**. **Radiating microtubules** project from the centrosome. They are not attached to the kinetochore.
4. During metaphase, two opposing but balanced forces maintain the chromosomes at the equatorial plate. **Kinetochore microtubules** pull chromosomes toward one of the poles; **radiating microtubules** stabilize the centrosome by anchoring to the plasma membrane.
5. The **anaphase-promoting complex**, **APC**, disassembles when the attachment of kinetochore microtubules to the kinetochore is correct. If the kinetochore is not attached to the microtubules, the APC arrests the mitotic cycle at metaphase by delaying cyclin activity.

Anaphase

1. Sister chromatids separate by the synchronous detachment of the centromeres.
2. **Topoisomerase**, an enzyme present in the kinetochore region, frees entangled chromatin fibers to facilitate the separation of the sister chromatids.
3. Chromatids are pulled to opposite poles by two independent but coincidental processes: (1) The kinetochore microtubules shorten and chromatids move away from the equatorial plane toward their respective poles. This step is usually referred to as **anaphase A**. (2) The cell poles separate by the elongation of the polar microtubules. This step is known as **anaphase B**.
4. **Aneuploidy** (abnormal chromosomal number) can result from improper allocation of the two chromatids of a chromosome to the two daughter cells. Failure of the kinetochore microtubules to attach to the kinetochore can block the onset of anaphase. A checkpoint mechanism operates at the kinetochore to prevent aneuploidy.

Telophase

1. The nuclear envelope gradually reforms; **lamins dephosphorylate** and assemble the nuclear lamina.
2. Chromosomes decondense.
3. A transient **contractile ring**, composed of actin and myosin, develops during **cytokinesis** around the equatorial region and contracts to separate the two daughter cells by a process called **abscission** (from Latin *abscindo*, to cut away from).
4. Residual microtubules can be found in the core of the contractile ring. They form a structure known as the **midbody**.
5. Radiating, kinetochore, and polar microtubules disappear.

Mdm2 is a **ubiquitin ligase** that binds to p53 and facilitates its ubiquitin-dependent degradation in the cytoplasm by the **26S proteasome** (see Figure 3-14 in Chapter 3, Cell Signaling). Mdm2 inhibition (for example, by **ARF**—for **a**lternate **r**eading **f**rame—a 14-kd protein) allows p53 to activate its tumor-suppressor functions. Mdm2 exerts a similar inhibitory effect on retinoblastoma tumor-suppressor protein (Rb protein). The protein levels of ARF, Mdm2, and p53 are not abundant in genotoxic stress-free cells. The half-life of p53 is only

Figure 1-51. **Telomeres, telomerase, and senescence**

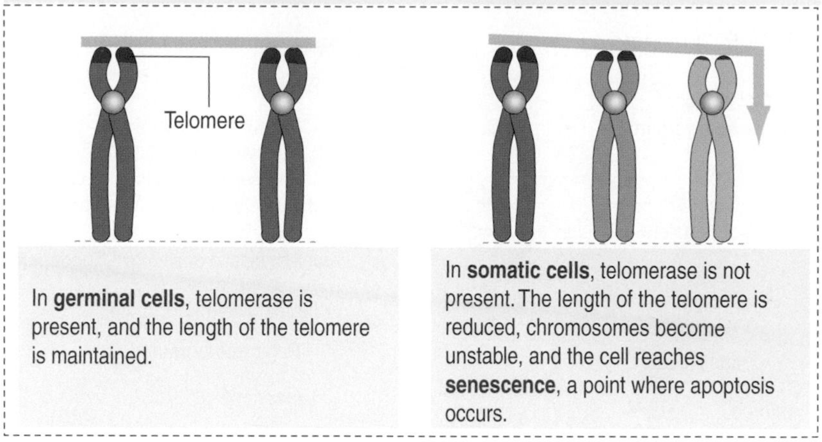

Telomere
In **germinal cells**, telomerase is present, and the length of the telomere is maintained.
In **somatic cells**, telomerase is not present. The length of the telomere is reduced, chromosomes become unstable, and the cell reaches **senescence**, a point where apoptosis occurs.

10 to 15 minutes.

In **cancer cells**, three possible mechanisms may prevent apoptotic cell destruction after genotoxic stress:

1. Mdm2 is unable to inhibit p53 tumor-suppressive function.
2. A mutational inactivation affects p53 function.
3. The apoptotic cascade has been disrupted (e.g., a loss in the activation of caspase 9).

Mutations of the *TP53* gene—which encodes the p53 protein—are observed in 50% of human cancers. The loss of *TP53* gene expression by an autosomal dominant mutation is responsible for a multicancer phenotype known as **Li-Fraumeni syndrome** (see **Box 1-U**). ***p53* is a tumor-suppressor gene**. The

Figure 1-52. **Cancer chemotherapy and p53 activity**

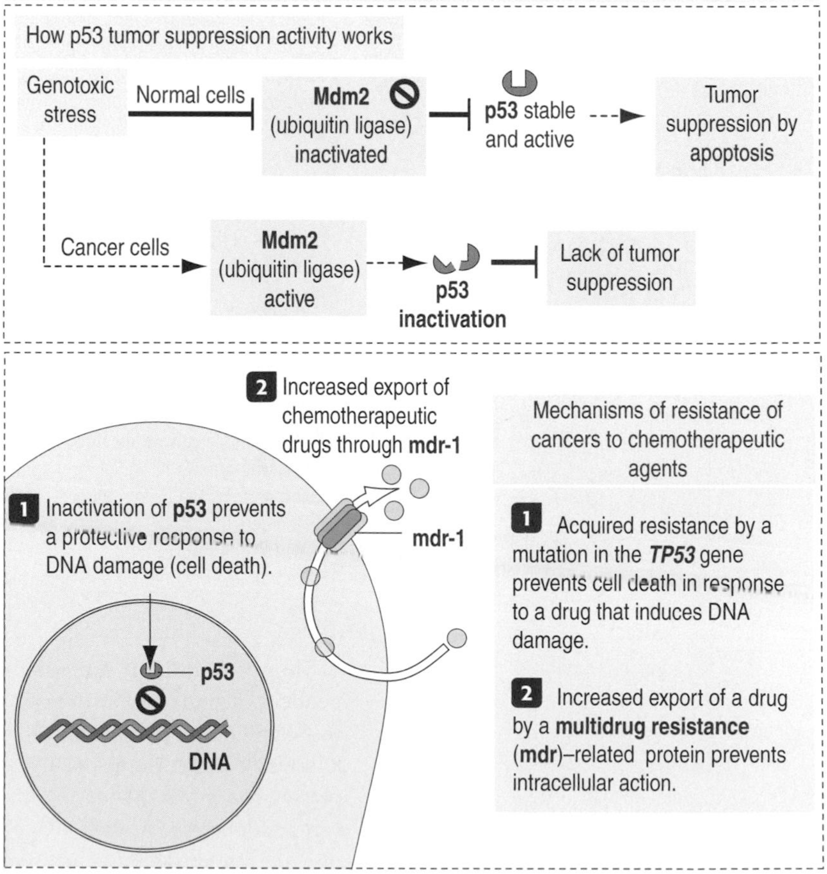

How p53 tumor suppression activity works
Genotoxic stress
Normal cells
Mdm2 (ubiquitin ligase) inactivated
p53 stable and active
Tumor suppression by apoptosis
Cancer cells
Mdm2 (ubiquitin ligase) active
p53 inactivation
Lack of tumor suppression
2 Increased export of chemotherapeutic drugs through **mdr-1**
1 Inactivation of **p53** prevents a protective response to DNA damage (cell death).
mdr-1
p53
DNA
Mechanisms of resistance of cancers to chemotherapeutic agents
1 Acquired resistance by a mutation in the ***TP53*** gene prevents cell death in response to a drug that induces DNA damage.
2 Increased export of a drug by a **multidrug resistance (mdr)**–related protein prevents intracellular action.

Box 1-T | **p53, a tumor-suppressor protein**

- The tumor-suppressor protein p53 protects the integrity of DNA in response to harmful stress, called genotoxic stress.
- The protective function depends on the ability of p53 to induce programmed cell death or apoptosis or arrest cell cycle activities when a cell undergoes genotoxic stress.
- How does p53 work? As a transcription factor, p53 controls the transcriptional activation of proapoptotic genes and the inactivation of antiapoptotic genes. By this mechanism, a cell affected by genotoxic stress is eliminated.
- What can go wrong? A loss of p53 function may occur by a mutation of the *TP53* gene—which encodes p53—or by an abnormal signaling pathway controlling p53 function (see Figure 1-52).
- Why is p53 important? Cancer cells are highly sensitive to apoptotic signals, but can survive if there is a loss of p53 function.

Figure 1-53. **Nomenclature of human chromosomes: normal and abnormal karyotype**

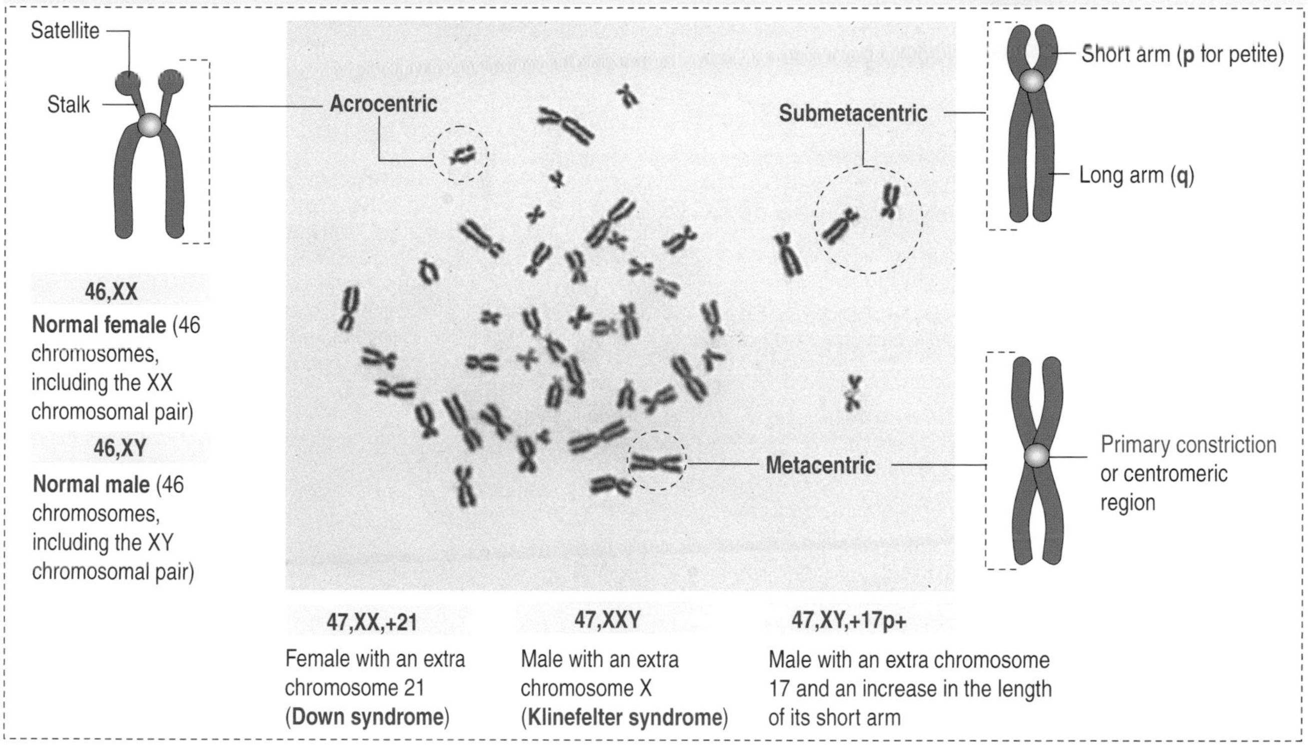

Satellite
Stalk
Acrocentric
Submetacentric
Short arm (**p** for petite)
Long arm (**q**)
Metacentric
Primary constriction or centromeric region
46,XX
Normal female (46 chromosomes, including the XX chromosomal pair)
46,XY
Normal male (46 chromosomes, including the XY chromosomal pair)
47,XX,+21
Female with an extra chromosome 21 (**Down syndrome**)
47,XXY
Male with an extra chromosome X (**Klinefelter syndrome**)
47,XY,+17p+
Male with an extra chromosome 17 and an increase in the length of its short arm

inactivation of p53 activity is disrupted in drug-resistant cancer cells (see Figure 1-52). Loss of p53 expression is observed in human cancer cells, and clinical studies suggest that inactivation of p53 expression correlates with resistance to chemotherapeutic agents.

Pharmacologic agents binding to Mdm2 could stabilize and increase the levels of p53 in cancer cells to exert a tumor-suppressor activity through its death-inducing functions. We discuss in detail the mechanism of programmed cell death or apoptosis in Chapter 3, Cell Signaling.

Karyotyping

There are **22 pairs of autosomes** and **one pair of sex chromosomes (XX or XY) in the human**. Chromosomes can be classified according to the length and position of the centromere into seven groups, identified by the letters A to G.

In the notation of human cytogenetics, the total number of chromosomes (46) is followed by the total number of sex chromosomes (Figure 1-53). A **normal male** is identified as **46,XY** (46 chromosomes, including the XY chromosomal pair) and a female as **46,XX** (46 chromosomes, including the XX chromosomal pair).

Extra autosomes are indicated by placing the number of the extra chromosomes after the sex chromosomes with a plus (+) sign. 47,XX+21 is the karyotype of a female with trisomy 21 (**Down syndrome**). A male with an extra X chromosome is symbolized as 47,XXY.

A plus or minus sign is placed following a chromosome symbol to indicate the increase or decrease in arm length.

The letter **p** symbolizes the **short arm** and **q** the **long arm**. 47,XY,+17p+ **identifies a male with 47 chromosomes, including an additional chromosome 17, with an increase in the length of its short arm.**

Box 1-U | **Li-Fraumeni syndrome**

- Li-Fraumeni syndrome (**LFS**) is an autosomal dominant condition characterized by a predisposition to cancer.
- Several types of cancer develop in a young individual (less than 45 years old): brain tumors, breast tumors (40% of the tumors in females), acute leukemia, and soft tissue and bone sarcomas.
- LFS syndrome is caused by a mutation of the tumor-suppressor gene encoding p53, a transcription factor with a cell cycle regulatory function.
- The incidence of LFS is low. Although the initial cancer can be successfully treated in affected children, there is a significant risk in the subsequent development of a second primary malignant tumor.

• Epithelium is one of the four basic tissues. The three additional basic tissues are connective tissue, muscle tissue, and nervous tissue.

Epithelia can be classified into three major groups based on (1) the number of cell layers (one layer: simple epithelium; more than one layer: stratified epithelium), (2) the shape of the cells (squamous epithelium, cuboidal epithelium, and columnar epithelium), and (3) the shape of the cells at the outermost layer (stratified squamous epithelium, stratified cuboidal epithelium, and stratified columnar epithelium). The stratified squamous epithelium can be subdivided into moderately keratinized (usually called nonkeratinized) and highly keratinized types. The name endothelium identifies the simple squamous epithelium lining blood and lymphatic vessels. The name mesothelium is used to describe the simple squamous or cuboidal lining of serosa (peritoneum, pleura, and pericardium). Tumors originated in the mesothelium are called **mesotheliomas**.

• An important cytoskeletal component of epithelial cells are keratin proteins (cytokeratins). The pathologist looks for the presence of keratins to determine the epithelial origin of a tumor (called **carcinoma**, in contrast to connective tissue–derived tumors called **sarcomas**).

• An intermediate type is the pseudostratified epithelium, in which all the cells are in contact with the basal lamina, but not all of them reach the lumen. The transitional epithelium, or urothelium, lining the urinary passages, can be regarded as a pseudostratified epithelium, although it has the appearance of a stratified squamous epithelium. The outermost cells of the urothelium of the urinary bladder have the property of changing their geometry and surface configuration in response to tensional forces exerted by urine.

• A refinement in the classification of selected epithelia relies on apical differentiations, such as cilia, microvilli, and stereocilia. A pseudostratified epithelium with cilia is seen along the respiratory tract and the oviduct. Simple cuboidal epithelium of specific segments of the nephron and the simple columnar epithelium of the small intestine contain microvilli forming a brush border along the apical domain. Stereocilia are seen in the epithelial lining of the epididymis and hair cells of the inner ear.

Epithelial cells organize layers of cells that are closely linked by specialized plasma membrane–associated structures, such as tight junctions, anchoring junctions (belt and spot desmosomes and hemidesmosomes), and gap junctions.

• Epithelial cells are highly polarized. They have an apical domain and a basolateral domain. The boundaries of the domains are defined by the distribution of junctions and their components, the polarized distribution of the actin cytoskeleton, and the presence of a basement membrane at the basal surface.

• The apical domain of some epithelial cells displays differentiations projecting into the lumen. The apical differentiations can be motile (cilia) and nonmotile (microvilli and stereocilia). Motile cilia contain an axoneme, formed by a concentric array of nine microtubule doublets surrounding a central pair. Cilia originate from a basal body—a centriolar derivative—inserted in the apical plasma membrane. In contrast to the axoneme, the basal body and the centriole are formed by nine microtubule triplets in a helicoid arrangement. There are no central microtubules in basal bodies and centrioles. The nonmotile microvilli and stereocilia contain an actin microfilament core. Microvilli have a uniform length. Stereocilia are longer, their length is variable, and, in the epididymal epithelium, they have a tendency to branch.

• The position and stability of the epithelial cell layer are maintained by cell adhesion molecules and cell junctions.

• Cell adhesion molecules can be classified as Ca^{2+}-dependent and Ca^{2+}-independent. Cadherins and selectins are Ca^{2+}-dependent. Cell adhesion molecules (CAMs) of the immunoglobulin-like family and integrins are Ca^{2+}-independent. In contrast to cadherins, selectins, and CAMs, integrins consist of two subunits, α and β, forming a heterodimer.

Cadherins constitute homophilic *cis*-homodimers (like-to-like), which interact through the extracellular domain with similar or different dimers present in the adjacent epithelial cell (forming *trans*-homodimers or *trans*-heterodimers [like to unlike]). The intracellular domain of cadherins interacts with the catenin complex consisting of catenins α, β, and γ. The catenin complex interacts with filamentous actin through adapter proteins (α-actinin, vinculin, and formin-1).

Selectins bind carbohydrate ligands through their carbohydrate recognition domain. Selectins play an important role in homing, the transendothelial migration of neutrophils, lymphocytes, and macrophages during **inflammation** and deposit of fatty streaks in the subendothelial space of blood vessels during **early atherosclerotic lesions**.

The extracellular immunoglobulin-like domain of CAMs binds to identical (homotypic binding) or different molecules (heterotypic binding) on another adjacent cell. The CAM CD4 is the receptor of HIV-1 in T cells (helper cells).

Integrins are heterodimers formed by two associated subunits, α and β. The extracellular domain of the integrin subunit β binds to laminin and fibronectin, two components of the basal lamina. Proteoglycans and collagens bind to laminin and fibronectin to form the reticular lamina. The intracellular domain of integrins binds to filamentous actin through the adapter proteins α-actinin, vinculin, and talin. Integrins establish a link between the extracellular matrix and the internal cytoskeleton.

• The basement membrane is a PAS-positive structure present at the basal domain of epithelial cells. It consists of a basal lamina and a reticular lamina, which can be defined by electron microscopy. The pathologist looks for the integrity of the basal lamina to determine if growing malignant epithelial cells are restricted to the epithelial layer (carcinoma in situ) or have invaded the underlying connective tissue where blood and lymphatic vessels are present.

• Related to the function of integrins are the ADAM proteins. The disintegrin domain of selected ADAMs can block integrin-binding affinities. The metalloprotease domain of ADAMs can participate in the shedding of the extracellular domain of plasma membrane–anchored growth factors, cytokines, and receptors. ADAMs have roles in angiogenesis, fertilization, neurogenesis, and cancer.

• Cell junctions not only maintain the mechanical integrity of the epithelium but also can function as signaling structures reporting cell position and are able to modulate cell growth or programmed cell death (apoptosis). Intercellular junctions can be symmetrical, such as tight junctions, belt desmosomes (zonula adherens), spot desmosomes (macula adherens) and gap junctions, or asymmetrical, such as hemidesmosomes.

• Tight junctions consist of two transmembrane proteins—the tetraspanins occludin and claudin—and two immunoglobulin-like proteins—junctional adhesion molecules (JAMs) and nectins. Nectins are associated to the protein afadin forming the afadin-nectin complex. JAMs and nectins form dimers (called *cis*-dimers) and dimers inserted in the opposing plasma membrane interact with each other (*trans*-dimers).

The adapter proteins zonula occludens ZO-1, ZO-2, and ZO-3 link occludin, claudins, JAMs, and the afadin-nectin complex to actin microfilaments. Claudins constitute the backbone of tight junction strands visualized on freeze-fracture electron micrographs.

Tight junctions constitute a circumferential fence separating the apical domain from the basolateral domain. Materials can cross epithelial and endothelial cellular sheets by two distinct pathways: the transcellular pathway and the paracellular pathway. Tight junctions regulate the paracellular transport of ions and molecules in a charge-dependent and size-dependent fashion.

Similar to tight junctions, zonula adherens (belt desmosome) also have a circumferential distribution and interact with filamentous actin. A distinctive feature is the presence of a plaque containing desmoplakin, plakoglobin (γ-catenin), and plakophilin. Cadherins (desmocollins and desmogleins) and the afadin-nectin complex link the plasma membranes of adjacent epithelial cells. The intracellular region of cadherins interacts with actin through the catenin complex.

Macula adherens (spot desmosome) provides strength and rigidity to the epithelial cell layer, particularly in the stratified squamous epithelium, and links adjacent cardiocytes as a component of the intercalated disk. In contrast to the belt desmosome, spot desmosomes are spotlike. The plaque—which contains desmoplakin, plakoglobin, and plakophilin—is the insertion site of intermediate filament keratins (called tonofilaments) or desmin (intercalated disk). The intermediate filament-binding protein in the plaque is desmoplakin. The catenin complex is not present. Desmocollins and desmogleins are the predominant cadherins.

Hemidesmosomes are asymmetrical anchoring junctions found at the basal region of epithelial cells. Hemidesmosomes consist of two components: an inner plate, associated to intermediate filaments, and an outer plaque anchoring the hemidesmosome to the basal lamina by anchoring filaments (laminin 5).

Gap junctions are symmetrical communicating junctions (instead of anchoring junctions). Gap junctions consist of clusters of intercellular channels connecting the cytoplasm of adjacent cells. There are more than 20 connexin monomers, each identified by the assigned molecular mass. Six connexin monomers form a connexon inserted into the plasma membrane. Connexons pair with their counterparts in the plasma membrane of an adjacent cell and form an axial intercellular channel allowing the cell-to-cell diffusion of ions and small molecules. A mutation in *connexin32* (*Cx32*) gene in the myelin-producing Schwann cell is the cause of the X-chromosome–linked **Charcot-Marie-Tooth disease**, a demyelinating disorder of the peripheral nervous system.

• The basement membrane consists of two components: a basal lamina, in direct contact with the epithelial basal cell surface, and a reticular lamina, formed by fibronectin and collagen fibers and continuous with the connective tissue. The basal lamina consists of laminin, type IV collagen, entactin, and proteoglycans. The basal lamina is an important component of the glomerular filtration barrier in the kidney. A basal lamina covers the surface of muscle cells and contributes to maintaining the integrity of the skeletal muscle fiber during contraction. A disruption of the basal lamina–cell muscle relationship gives rise to **muscular dystrophies**. The basement membrane can be recognized by light microscopy by the PAS stain.

• The cytoskeleton consists of microfilaments (7 nm thick), microtubules (25 nm in diameter), and intermediate filaments (10 nm in diameter). The basic unit of a microfilaments is the G-actin monomer. The ATP-dependent polymerization of monomers forms a 7-nm-thick F-actin filament. Monomers added on the barbed end of the filament move, or treadmill, along the filament until they detach by depolymerization at the pointed end.

Motor proteins, such as myosin Va, transport vesicle cargos along F-actin. Defective myosin Va is the cause of **Griscelli syndrome**, a disorder in the transport of melanosomes from melanocytes to keratinocytes in the epidermis. Patients with Griscelli syndrome have silvery hair, partial albinism, occasional neurological defects, and immunodeficiency.

F-actin associated with myosin II forms the contractile structures of skeletal and cardiac muscle cells. They represent the myofilament components of myofibrils. Myofibrils, consisting of a linear chain of sarcomeres, are the basic contractile unit found in the cytoplasm of striated muscle cells.

Microtubules are composed of tubulin dimers, α and β tubulin. Tubulin dimers arranged longitudinally form protofilaments. Thirteen protofilaments associate side-by-side with each other to form a microtubule. Microtubules undergo alternate phases of slow growth and rapid depolymerization, a process called dynamic instability. The polymerization of tubulin subunits is GTP-dependent.

Microtubules organize the centrosome, a structure consisting of a pair of centrioles surrounded by a pericentriolar matrix. Each centriole consists of nine triplets of microtubules arranged in a helicoid manner. Centrioles duplicate during the cell cycle in preparation for the assembly of the mitotic spindle during cell division. Centrioles give rise to basal bodies, the origin site of cilia.

The mitotic apparatus consists of a mitotic center, represented by the centrosome, and the mitotic spindle, consisting of three types of microtubules: (1) radial microtubules, (2) kinetochore microtubules, and (3) polar microtubules. Kinetochore microtubules attach to the kinetochore, a cluster of proteins associated with the centromere, the primary constriction of a chromosome. Centrosome and centromere sound alike but they represent two different structures.

Microtubules are a target of **cancer chemotherapy** with the purpose of blocking cell division of tumor cells by destabilizing or stabilizing dynamic instability. Derivatives of *Vinca* alkaloids and taxol have been widely used.

The axoneme consists of nine microtubule doublets in a concentric array, surrounding a central pair of microtubules. Each doublet consists of a tubule A, consisting of 13 protofilaments and closely attached to tubule B, formed by 10 to 11 microtubules. Axonemes are present in cilia and flagella of the sperm tail. Dynein arms, an ATPase, are linked to tubule A. ATPase hydrolyzes ATP to use energy for the sliding of microtubules, the basis for ciliary and flagellar movement.

Microtubules provide tracks for motor proteins transporting vesicle and nonvesicle cargos within the cell. Molecular motors, such as kinesin and cytoplasmic dynein, mediate the transport of cargos. There are three major microtubule-based transport systems: axonemal transport, which includes intraciliary and intraflagellar transport; axonal transport; and intramanchette transport, a transient structure involved in sperm development.

Bardet-Biedl syndrome, a disorder of basal bodies and cilia resulting from defective intraciliary transport, is characterized by retinal dystrophy, obesity, polydactyly, renal dysplasia, reproductive tract abnormalities, and learning disabilities.

Kartagener's syndrome, a disorder of axonemes of defective or absent dynein arms, is associated with bronchiectasis and infertility (reduced sperm motility and egg transport in the oviduct).

Intermediate filaments are formed by monomers displaying a central coiled-coil flanked by globular regions. In contrast to F-actin and microtubules, the assembly of intermediate filaments is regulated by phosphorylation-dephosphorylation.

There are several types of intermediate filaments, including type I and type II keratins (markers of epithelial cells), vimentin (present in mesenchymal-derived cells), desmin (abundant in muscle cells), glial fribrillary acidic protein (a marker of glial cells), neurofilaments (found in neurons), and lamins (forming the nuclear lamina associated to the inner layer of the nuclear envelope).

Disorders of keratins cause **blistering diseases** of the skin. Defective gene expression of lamins causes a group of diseases called **laminopathies** affecting muscle tissue (e.g., **Emery-Dreifuss muscular dystrophy**), nervous tissue (**Charcot-Marie-Tooth disease type 2B1**) and adipose tissue (**Dunnigan-type familial lipodystrophy**).

• The cell nucleus consists of the nuclear envelope, chromatin, and the nucleolus. The nuclear envelope has nuclear pores, a tripartite structure consisting of inner and outer octagonal rings and a central cylindrical body. Nuclear pores contain several proteins called nucleoporins. Ran-GTPase regulates nucleocytoplasmic transport across nuclear pores by enabling the passage of proteins with a nuclear import sequence bound to a protein complex of importins α and β and Ran-GDP. In the nucleus, Ran-GDP is converted to Ran-GTP by RCCl, a GDP-GTP exchanger and the importin-imported protein complex is dissociated. Ran-GTP associates with exportins, and proteins with a nuclear export sequence are transported to the cytoplasm. Ran-GTP interacts with Ran-GBP1, and is converted to Ran-GDP by hydrolysis stimulated by Ran-GAP. The cargo is discharged, and Ran-GDP is ready to initiate another transport cycle.

Two forms of chromatin exist: heterochromatin (transcriptionally inactive) and euchromatin (transcriptionally active). One of the two X chromosomes in every female somatic cell remains condensed, a process known as dosage compensation. The condensed X chromosome can be visualized as a mass of heterochromatin adjacent to the nuclear envelope (called Barr body) and in the form of a drumstick in polymorphonuclear leukocytes.

The nucleolus consists of a fibrillar center (chromatin containing repeat rRNA genes, RNA polymerase I, and SRP); a dense fibrillar component (containing the proteins fibrillarin and nucleolin); and a granular component (the assembly sites of ribosomal subunits).

Staining techniques and autoradiography can determine the localization of nucleic acids in cells. The Feulgen reaction detects DNA. Basic dyes can localize DNA and RNA. RNAse and DNAse cell pretreatment can define the identity of the basophilic staining. Autoradiography is based on the administration of a radiolabeled precursor to living cells. Radioactive sites can be traced using a photographic emulsion, which after developing and fixation, produces silver grain in sites where the radiolabeled precursor is localized. This procedure enables the study of the cell cycle and the detection of sites involved in protein synthesis, glycosylation, and transport. Fluorescence-activated cell sorting enables the identification and separation of cell types using cell surface markers, and the study of the cell cycle based on the content of DNA.

• Cell cycle is defined as the interval between two successive cell divisions (mitotic and meiotic) resulting in the production of two daughter cells. Traditionally, the cell cycle consists of two major phases: (1) interphase and (2) mitosis (or meiosis). Interphase consists of the S phase (DNA synthesis), preceded by the G1 phase and followed by the G2 phase.

The phases of mitosis are:

1. Prophase (the centrosomes organize the mitotic spindle; lamins phosphorylate; each chromosome consists of sister chromatids held together at the centromere; the protein cohesin holds together the noncentromeric regions; condensin compacts the chromatin).
2. Metaphase (kinetochore microtubules attach to the kinetochore present in each chromosome; chromosomes align at the equatorial plate; the anaphase-promoting complex disassembles if the attachment of the kinetochore microtubules is correct).
3. Anaphase (topoisomerase frees entangled chromatin fibers; chromatids separate from each other and move closer to their respective poles—anaphase A—and cell poles separated by the action of polar microtubules—anaphase B).
4. Telophase (lamins dephosphorylate and the nuclear envelope is reassembled; chromosomes decondense; a contractile ring [actin-myosin] develops during cytokinesis; microtubules of the spindle disappear).

In a more contemporary view, the cell cycle consists of three distinct cycles: (1) cytoplasmic cycle (sequential activation of cyclin-dependent protein kinases; (2) nuclear cycle (DNA replication and chromosome condensation); and (3) centrosome cycle (duplication of the two centrioles—mother and daughter centrioles—in preparation for assembly of the mitotic apparatus).

Karyotyping is the structural and numerical analysis of metaphase chromosomes. A normal male has a chromosomal complement 46,XY (46 chromosomes, including the XY chromosomal pair; a normal female has 46,XX (46 chromosomes, including the XX chromosomal pair). Depending on the position of the centromere or primary constriction, chromosomes are classified as metacentric, submetacentric, and acrocentric.

Cyclin-dependent protein kinases control the progression and completion of the cell cycle. Tumor-suppressor proteins control cell cycle progression. Dephosphorylated Rb protein, a tumor-suppressor, binds to transcription factors and represses gene activity. Transcription factors dissociate from phosphorylated Rb protein and stimulate cell cycle progression. **Retinoblastoma**, a malignant tumor of the eye, is observed when the *Rb* gene is mutated.

Another tumor-suppressor protein is p53, a transcription factor with a cell cycle regulatory function. Mutations of the *p53* gene are seen in patients with leukemias, lymphomas, and brain tumors. p53 has a protective cell function: it can induce apoptosis or arrest the cell cycle when the cell undergoes harmful stress (called **genotoxic stress**). Mutations of the *p53* gene prevent this protective function.

Li-Fraumeni syndrome is caused by a mutation of the *p53* gene. Young patients have a predisposition to cancer (brain tumors, breast tumors, acute leukemia, and soft tissue and bone sarcomas).

Breakdown of the nuclear envelope occurs at the end of prophase. It involves the fragmentation of the nuclear envelope, dissociation of nuclear pore complexes, and phosphorylation of lamins (depolymerization). Reassembly of the nuclear envelope involves the dephosphorylation of lamins by a protein phosphatase.

Telomeres are the end regions of chromosomes formed by a stretch of repeated nucleotide sequences. When DNA polymerase fails to copy the chromosomal ends, telomeres decrease in length with every cell division until the integrity of the chromosome cannot be maintained. Male and female germinal cells can protect the telomeres by the enzyme telomerase, which is not present in somatic cells. Most tumor cells express telomerase.

2. EPITHELIAL GLANDS

Development of epithelial glands

Most glands develop as epithelial outgrowths into the underlying connective tissue (Figure 2-1). **Exocrine glands** remain connected to the surface of the epithelium by an excretory duct that transports the secretory product to the outside. **Endocrine glands lack an excretory duct**, and their product is released into the blood circulation.

Typically, endocrine glands are surrounded by fenestrated capillaries and commonly store the secretions they synthesize and release after stimulation by chemical or electrical signals. Exocrine and endocrine glands can be found together (for example, in pancreas), as separate structures in endocrine organs (thyroid, parathyroid), or as single cells (enteroendocrine cells). Endocrine glands will be studied later in Chapter 18, Neuroendocrine System, and Chapter 19, Endocrine System.

Figure 2-1. **Development of exocrine and endocrine glands**

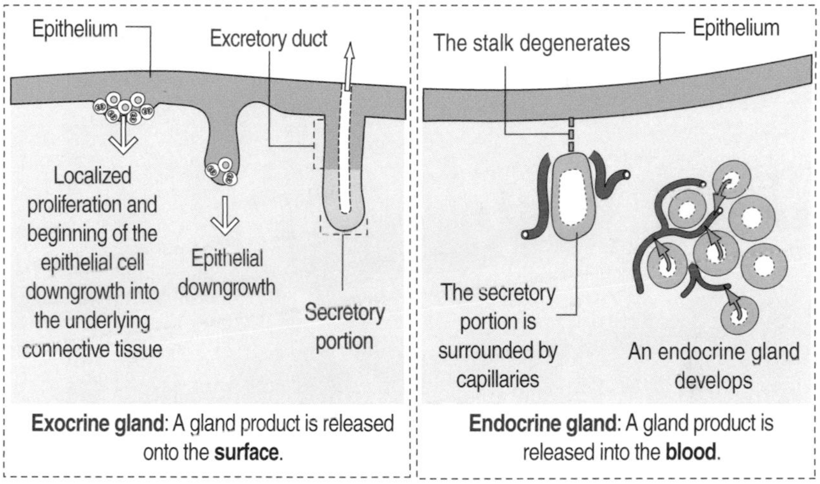

Epithelium
Excretory duct
Localized proliferation and beginning of the epithelial cell downgrowth into the underlying connective tissue
Epithelial downgrowth
Secretory portion
Exocrine gland: A gland product is released onto the **surface**.
The stalk degenerates
Epithelium
The secretory portion is surrounded by capillaries
An endocrine gland develops
Endocrine gland: A gland product is released into the **blood**.

Classification of epithelial glands

Glands are classified according to the type of **excretory duct** into **simple** and **branched** (also called **compound**) glands. The gland can be **simple** (Figure 2-2) when the excretory duct is **unbranched** or **branched** when the excretory duct subdivides (Figure 2-3).

Figure 2-2. **Simple glands**

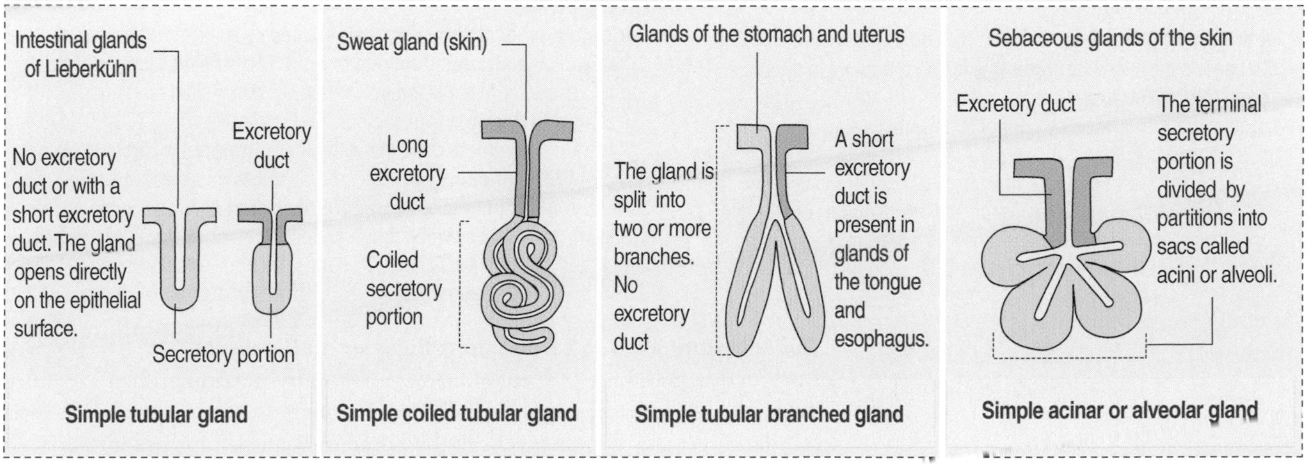

Intestinal glands of Lieberkühn
Excretory duct
No excretory duct or with a short excretory duct. The gland opens directly on the epithelial surface.
Secretory portion
Simple tubular gland
Sweat gland (skin)
Long excretory duct
Coiled secretory portion
Simple coiled tubular gland
Glands of the stomach and uterus
The gland is split into two or more branches. No excretory duct
A short excretory duct is present in glands of the tongue and esophagus.
Simple tubular branched gland
Sebaceous glands of the skin
Excretory duct
The terminal secretory portion is divided by partitions into sacs called acini or alveoli.
Simple acinar or alveolar gland

Figure 2-3. **Glands with branched ducts**

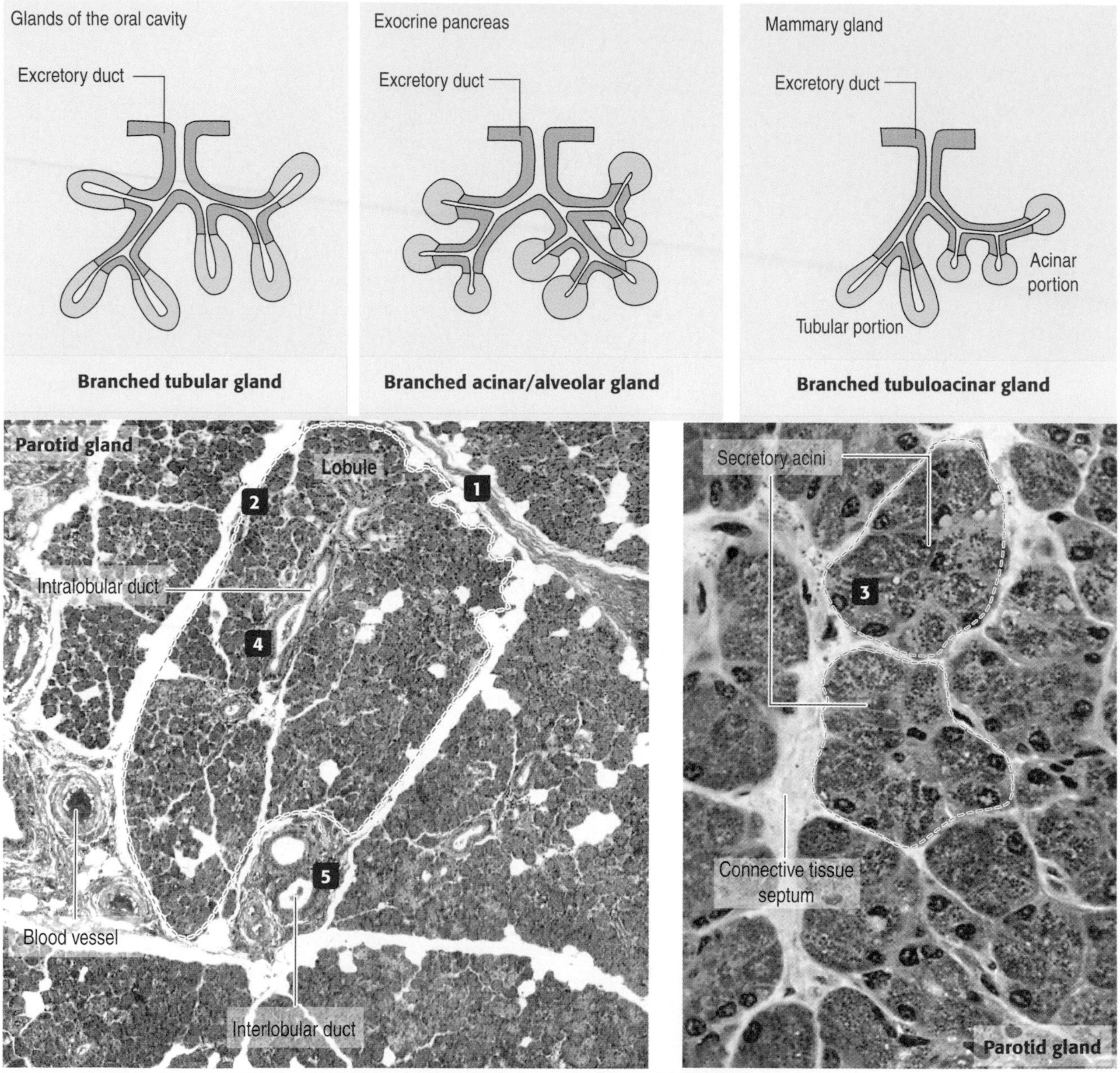

Glands of the oral cavity
Excretory duct
Branched tubular gland
Exocrine pancreas
Excretory duct
Branched acinar/alveolar gland
Mammary gland
Excretory duct
Acinar portion
Tubular portion
Branched tubuloacinar gland
Parotid gland
Lobule
1
2
Intralobular duct
4
5
Blood vessel
Interlobular duct
Secretory acini
3
Connective tissue septum
Parotid gland

General organization of a branched (compound) gland

A **branched gland** is surrounded by a connective tissue capsule that sends partitions or **septa** 1 inside the gland to organize large units called **lobes** (not shown).

Lobes are subdivided by connective tissue into small subunits called **lobules** 2.

A branched gland consists of a varying number of secretory units classified according to their morphology as **tubular**, **acinar** 3, or **tubuloacinar**. The secretion drains into an excretory duct located within the lobule (**intralobular duct** 4). Generally, the **intralobular excretory ducts** are formed by an **intercalated duct** followed by a **striated duct** (not shown). The striated duct—present only in salivary glands—drains into an excretory duct continuous with an **intralobular duct** (not shown).

Intralobular ducts combine with other **intralobular ducts** to form an **interlobular duct** 5. **Interlobular ducts** combine with other **interlobular ducts** to form an **intralobar duct** of larger diameter (not shown). **Intralobar ducts** converge to form a **lobar duct**. See Figure 2-4, and Chapter 17, Digestive Glands, for additional information.

The secretory portion can be unicellular or multicellular

An **exocrine gland** has two components: a **secretory portion** and an **excretory duct**. The **secretory portion** of a gland may be composed of one cell type (**unicellular**, for example, **goblet cells** in the respiratory epithelium and intestine) or

Figure 2-4. Histologic overview of a compound salivary gland

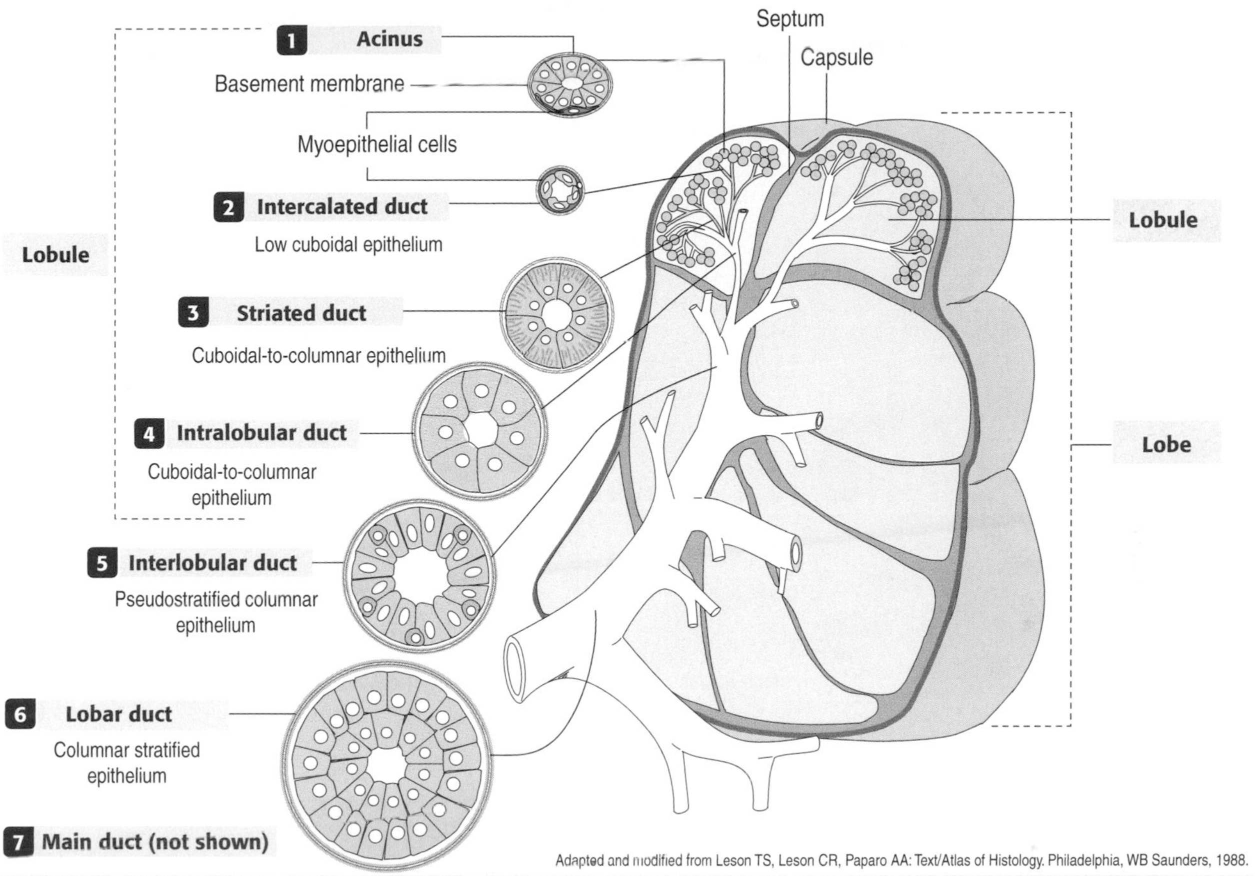

1 Acinus
Basement membrane
Myoepithelial cells
2 Intercalated duct
Low cuboidal epithelium
3 Striated duct
Cuboidal-to-columnar epithelium
4 Intralobular duct
Cuboidal-to-columnar epithelium
5 Interlobular duct
Pseudostratified columnar epithelium
6 Lobar duct
Columnar stratified epithelium
7 Main duct (not shown)
Lobule
Septum
Capsule
Lobule
Lobe

Adapted and modified from Leson TS, Leson CR, Paparo AA: Text/Atlas of Histology. Philadelphia, WB Saunders, 1988.

All **branched exocrine glands** contain epithelial components (secretory acini and ducts) called **parenchyma**, and supporting connective tissue, including blood vessels and nerves, the **stroma.**

The gland is enclosed by a connective tissue **capsule** that branches inside the gland forming **septa** (singular *septum*) that subdivide the parenchyma.

In large branched glands, the parenchyma is anatomically subdivided into **lobes**. Adjacent lobes are separated by an **interlobar septum**. A lobe is formed by **lobules**, separated from each other by a thin **interlobular septum**.

Septa support the major branches of the **excretory duct**. **Interlobular ducts** extend along **interlobular septa**; **interlobar ducts** extend along **interlobar septa**. However, **intralobular ducts** lie within lobules and are surrounded by little connective tissue.

Intralobular ducts are lined by a **simple cuboidal-to-columnar epithelium**, whereas the epithelial lining of **interlobular ducts** is pseudostratified columnar. **Lobar ducts** are lined by a **stratified columnar epithelium**.

many cells (**multicellular**).

According to the **shape** of the secretory portion (see Figures 2-2 and 2-3), glands can be **tubular**, **coiled**, or **alveolar** (Latin *alveolus,* small hollow sac; plural *alveoli*), also called **acinar** (Latin *acinus,* grape; plural *acini*).

Tubular glands are found in the large intestine. The sweat glands of the skin are typical coiled glands. The sebaceous gland of the skin is an example of an alveolar gland.

Shape of the secretory portion

Glands can be classified as **simple tubular** or **simple alveolar** (or acinar) according to the **shape of the secretory portion.** In addition, tubular and alveolar secretory portions can coexist with branching excretory ducts; the gland is called **a branched (or compound) tubulo-alveolar** (or acinar) gland (for example, the salivary glands). The mammary gland is an example of a branched alveolar gland.

A branched gland (Figure 2-4) is surrounded by a **capsule. Septa** or **trabeculae** extend from the capsule into the glandular tissue. Large septa divide the gland

Figure 2-5. Histologic differences between submandibular, sublingual, and parotid glands

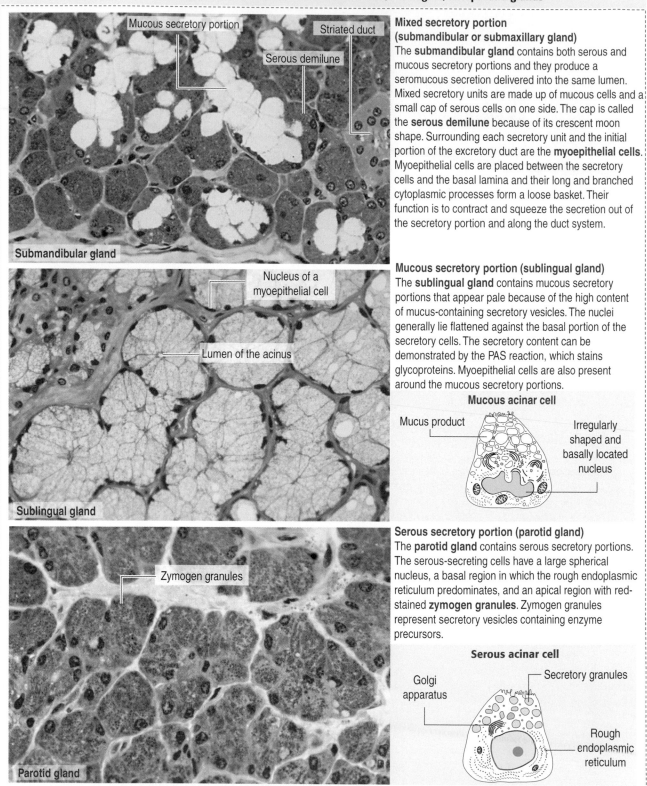

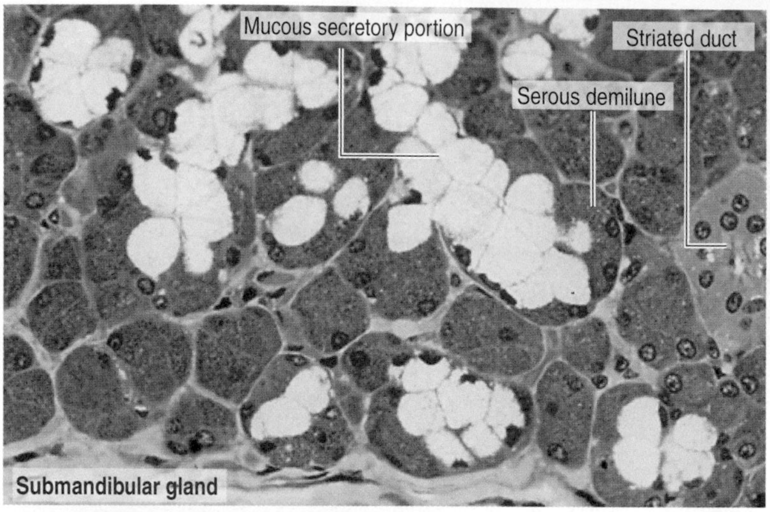
Mucous secretory portion
Striated duct
Serous demilune
Submandibular gland

Mixed secretory portion (submandibular or submaxillary gland)
The **submandibular gland** contains both serous and mucous secretory portions and they produce a seromucous secretion delivered into the same lumen. Mixed secretory units are made up of mucous cells and a small cap of serous cells on one side. The cap is called the **serous demilune** because of its crescent moon shape. Surrounding each secretory unit and the initial portion of the excretory duct are the **myoepithelial cells**. Myoepithelial cells are placed between the secretory cells and the basal lamina and their long and branched cytoplasmic processes form a loose basket. Their function is to contract and squeeze the secretion out of the secretory portion and along the duct system.

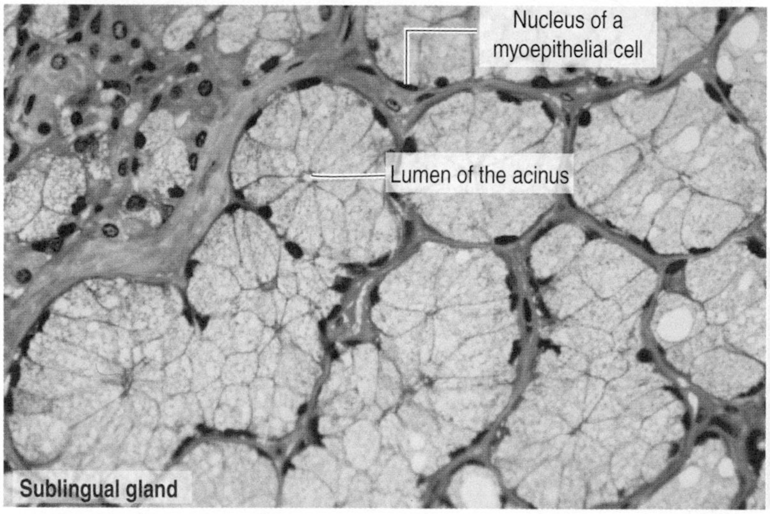
Nucleus of a myoepithelial cell
Lumen of the acinus
Sublingual gland

Mucous secretory portion (sublingual gland)
The **sublingual gland** contains mucous secretory portions that appear pale because of the high content of mucus-containing secretory vesicles. The nuclei generally lie flattened against the basal portion of the secretory cells. The secretory content can be demonstrated by the PAS reaction, which stains glycoproteins. Myoepithelial cells are also present around the mucous secretory portions.

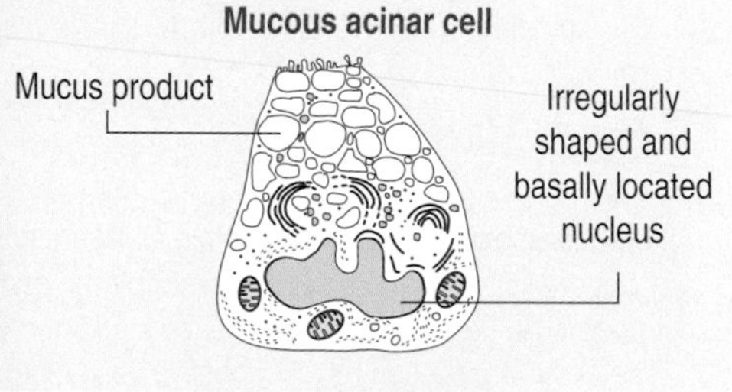
Mucous acinar cell
Mucus product
Irregularly shaped and basally located nucleus

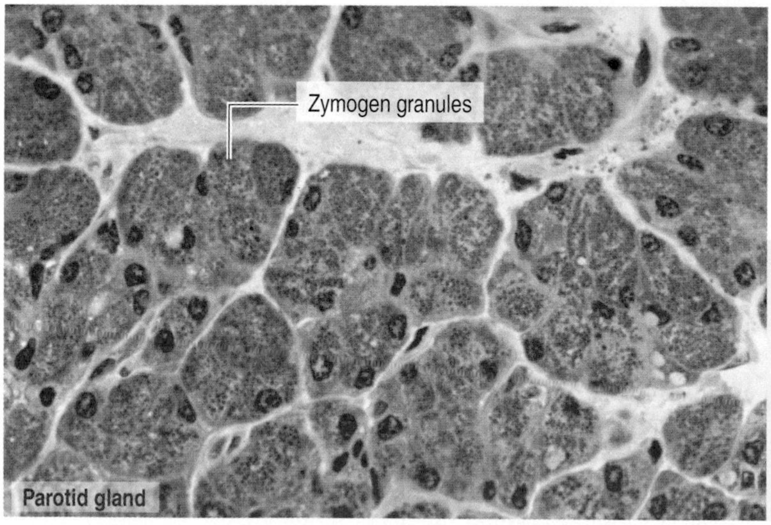
Zymogen granules
Parotid gland

Serous secretory portion (parotid gland)
The **parotid gland** contains serous secretory portions. The serous-secreting cells have a large spherical nucleus, a basal region in which the rough endoplasmic reticulum predominates, and an apical region with red-stained **zymogen granules**. Zymogen granules represent secretory vesicles containing enzyme precursors.

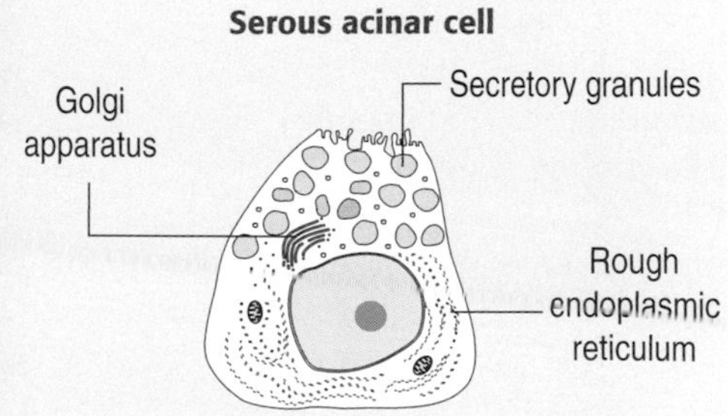
Serous acinar cell
Golgi apparatus
Secretory granules
Rough endoplasmic reticulum

into a number of **lobes.** Branches from the septa separating adjacent lobes divide the lobes into smaller compartments called **lobules.**

During development, a main excretory duct gives rise to branches that lie either between (**interlobar**) or within lobes (**intralobar**). Small branches derived from each of these ducts generate small subdivisions that constitute the **lobule**

Figure 2-6. Mechanisms of glandular secretion

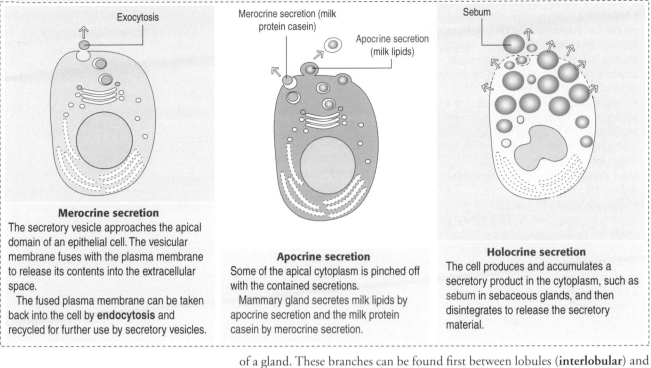

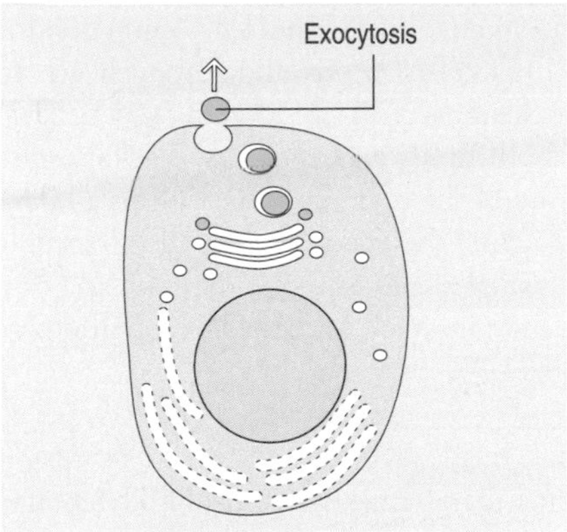

Merocrine secretion

The secretory vesicle approaches the apical domain of an epithelial cell. The vesicular membrane fuses with the plasma membrane to release its contents into the extracellular space.

The fused plasma membrane can be taken back into the cell by **endocytosis** and recycled for further use by secretory vesicles.

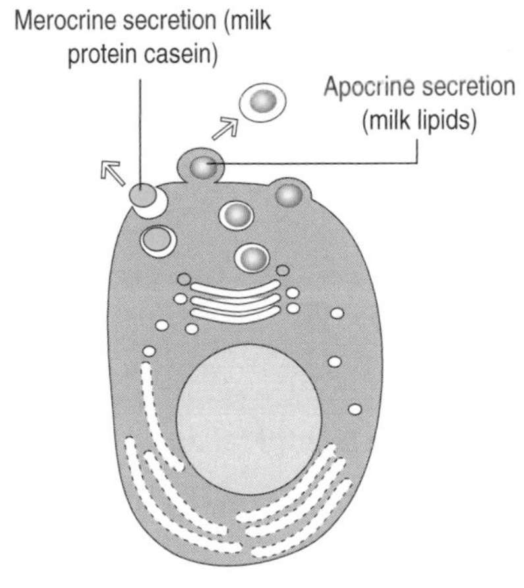

Apocrine secretion

Some of the apical cytoplasm is pinched off with the contained secretions.

Mammary gland secretes milk lipids by apocrine secretion and the milk protein casein by merocrine secretion.

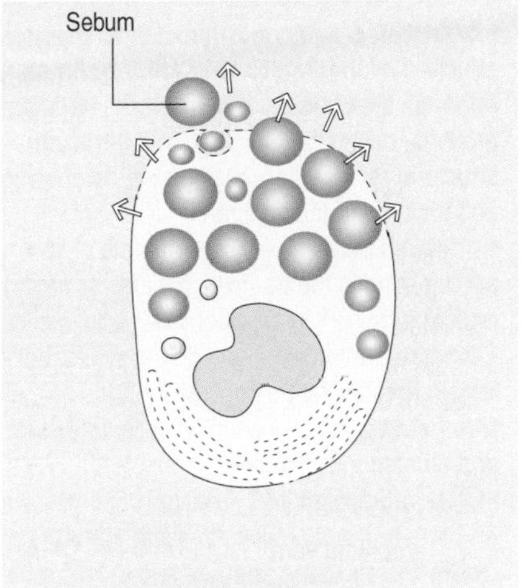

Holocrine secretion

The cell produces and accumulates a secretory product in the cytoplasm, such as sebum in sebaceous glands, and then disintegrates to release the secretory material.

of a gland. These branches can be found first between lobules (**interlobular**) and within lobules (**intralobular**). Additional details are presented in Chapter 17, Digestive Glands.

Type of secretion

Based on the type of secretion, exocrine glands can be classified as **mucous glands**, when their products are rich in **glycoproteins** and water; **serous glands**, with secretions enriched with **proteins** and water; and **mixed glands**, which contain both mucous and serous cells (Figure 2-5).

Mechanism of secretion

Exocrine glands can also be classified on the basis of **how the secretory product is released** (Figure 2-6).

In **merocrine secretion** (Greek *meros*, part; *krinein*, to separate), the product is released by **exocytosis**. Secretory granules are enclosed by a membrane that fuses with the apical plasma membrane during discharge or exocytosis. An example is the secretion of zymogen granules by the pancreas.

In **apocrine secretion** (Greek *apoknino*, to separate), the release of the secretory product involves **partial loss of the apical portion of the cell.** An example is the secretion of **lipids** by epithelial cells of the mammary gland. **Proteins** secreted by epithelial cells of the mammary gland follow the merocrine pathway (exocytosis).

In **holocrine secretion** (Greek *holos*, all), the secretory product constitutes **the entire cell and its product**. An example is the sebaceous glands of the skin, which produce a secretion called **sebum**.

Cytomembranes: Plasma membrane

A review of major concepts of cytomembranes and organelles (lysosomes and mitochondria) and their clinical relevance is presented in this chapter. Epithelial glands are a convenient topic for this integration. We initiate the review by addressing the structural and biochemical characteristics of the plasma membrane. Additional information related to plasma membrane–mediated cell signaling is presented in Chapter 3, Cell Signaling.

Box 2-A | **Lipid rafts**

- A lipid raft is a region of the plasma membrane enriched in **cholesterol** and **sphingolipids.** Although the classical lipid raft lacks structural proteins, others are enriched in a particular structural protein that modifies the composition and function of the lipid raft.
- **Caveolin** proteins are components of lipid rafts participating in the traffic of vesicles or **caveolae** (see Figure 7-21 in Chapter 7, Muscle Tissue). Caveolae are found in several cell types, particularly in fibroblasts, adipocytes, endothelial cells, type I alveolar cells, epithelial cells, and smooth and striated muscle cells.
- Other protein families, in addition to the **caveolin protein family** (caveolin-1, -2, and -3), can modify the structure and function of lipid rafts. These proteins include **flotillins**, **glycosphingolipid-linked proteins**, and **Src tyrosine kinases**.
- Lipid rafts can participate in cell signaling by concentrating or separating specific membrane-associated proteins in unique lipid domains.

The **plasma membrane** determines the structural and functional boundaries of a cell. Intracellular membranes, called **cytomembranes**, separate diverse cellular processes into compartments known as **organelles.** The nucleus, mitochondria, and lysosomes are membrane-bound organelles; lipids and glycogen are not membrane-bound and are known as **inclusions.**

The plasma membrane consists of both **lipids** and **proteins**. The phospholipid bilayer is the fundamental structure of the membrane and forms a bilayer barrier between two aqueous compartments: the extracellular and intracellular compartments. Proteins are embedded within the phospholipid bilayer and carry out specific functions of the plasma membrane such as cell-cell recognition and selective transport of molecules (see Box 2-A).

Phospholipid bilayer

The four major phospholipids of plasma membranes are **phosphatidylcholine, phosphatidylethanolamine, phosphatidylserine,** and **sphingomyelin** (Figure 2-7). They represent more than half the lipid of most membranes. A fifth phospholipid, **phosphatidylinositol**, is localized to the inner leaflet of the plasma membrane.

In addition to phospholipids, the plasma membrane of animal cells contains **glycolipids** and **cholesterol.** Glycolipids, a minor membrane component, are found in the outer leaflet, with the carbohydrate moieties exposed on the cell surface.

Cholesterol, a major membrane constituent, is present in about the same amounts as are phospholipids. Cholesterol, a rigid ring structure, does not form a membrane but is inserted into the phospholipid bilayer to modulate membrane fluidity by restricting the movement of phospholipid fatty acid chains at high temperatures.

Cholesterol is not present in bacteria.

Two general aspects of the phospholipid bilayer are important to remember:

1. **The structure of phospholipids accounts for the function of membranes as**

Figure 2-7. **Structure of the plasma membrane**

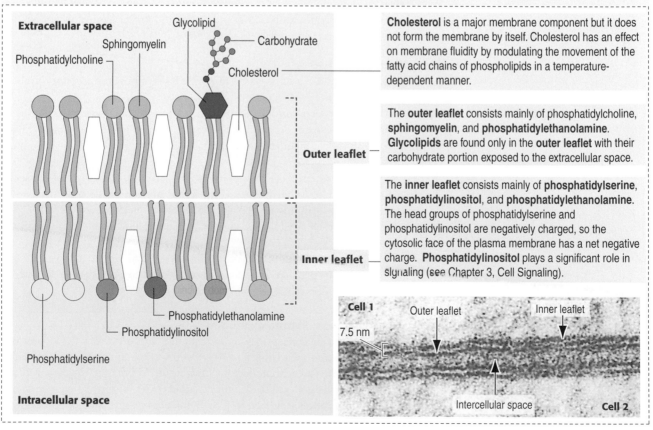

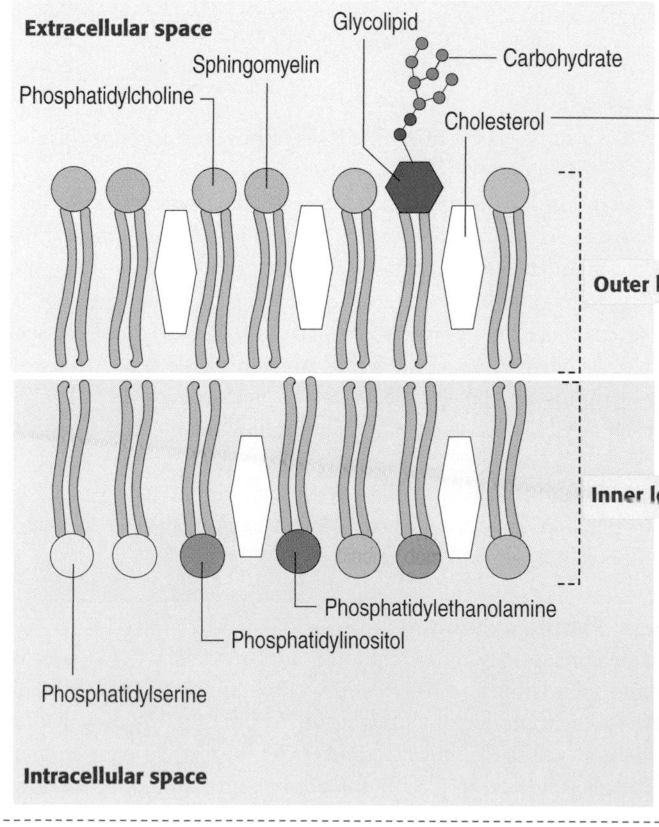

Cholesterol is a major membrane component but it does not form the membrane by itself. Cholesterol has an effect on membrane fluidity by modulating the movement of the fatty acid chains of phospholipids in a temperature-dependent manner.

The **outer leaflet** consists mainly of phosphatidylcholine, **sphingomyelin**, and **phosphatidylethanolamine. Glycolipids** are found only in the **outer leaflet** with their carbohydrate portion exposed to the extracellular space.

The **inner leaflet** consists mainly of **phosphatidylserine, phosphatidylinositol**, and **phosphatidylethanolamine.** The head groups of phosphatidylserine and phosphatidylinositol are negatively charged, so the cytosolic face of the plasma membrane has a net negative charge. **Phosphatidylinositol** plays a significant role in signaling (see Chapter 3, Cell Signaling).

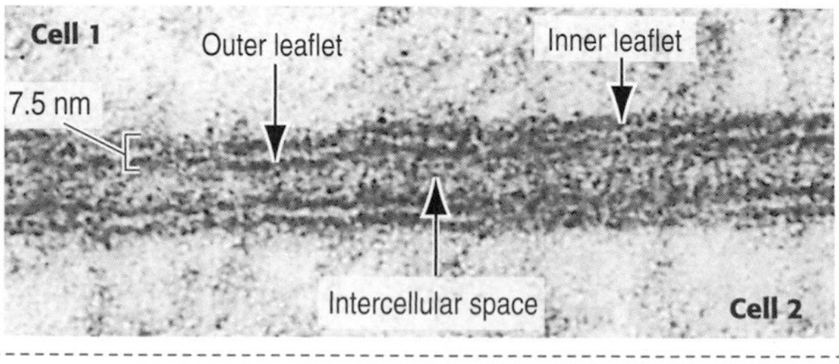

Box 2-B | Glycocalyx

- The extracellular domain of a plasma membrane is generally glycosylated by the carbohydrate portions of glycolipids and transmembrane glycoproteins. The surface of the cell is, therefore, covered by a carbohydrate coat, known as the **glycocalyx**.
- The glycocalyx protects the cell surface and facilitates cell-cell interactions. An appropriate example is the mechanism of **homing**, a process allowing leukocytes to leave blood vessels and mediate inflammatory responses. As you recall, the initial step in adhesion between endothelial cells and leukocytes is mediated by **selectins**, a family of transmembrane proteins which recognize specific sugars on the cell surface.

barriers between two aqueous compartments. The hydrophobic fatty acid chains in the interior of the phospholipid bilayer are responsible for the membranes being impermeable to water-soluble molecules.

2. **The phospholipid bilayer is a viscous fluid.** The long hydrocarbon chains of the fatty acids of most phospholipids are loosely packed and can move in the interior of the membrane. Therefore, phospholipids and proteins can diffuse laterally within the membrane to perform critical membrane functions.

Membrane proteins

Most plasma membranes consist of about 50% lipid and 50% protein (Figure 2-8). The carbohydrate component of glycolipids and glycoproteins represents 5% to 10% of the membrane mass. The surface of a plasma membrane is coated by a **glycocalyx** (see Box 2-B).

According to the **fluid mosaic model** of the membrane structure, membranes are two-dimensional fluids in which proteins are inserted into lipid bilayers. It is difficult for membrane proteins and phospholipids to switch back and forth between the inner and outer leaflets of the membrane. However, because they exist in a fluid environment, both proteins and lipids are able to diffuse laterally through the plane of the membrane. However, not all proteins can diffuse freely; the mobility of membrane proteins is limited by their association with the cytoskeleton.

Restrictions in the mobility of membrane proteins are responsible for the polarized nature of epithelial cells, divided into distinct **apical** and **basolateral domains** that differ in protein composition and function. Tight junctions between adjacent epithelial cells (discussed in Chapter 1, Epithelium) not only seal the space between cells but also serve as barriers to the diffusion of proteins and lipids between the apical and basolateral domains.

Two major classes of membrane-associated proteins are recognized: **peripheral proteins** and **integral membrane proteins.**

Peripheral membrane proteins are not inserted into the hydrophobic interior of the membrane but are, instead, indirectly associated with membranes through protein-protein ionic bond interactions, which are disrupted by solutions of **high**

Figure 2-8. Peripheral and integral proteins of the plasma membrane

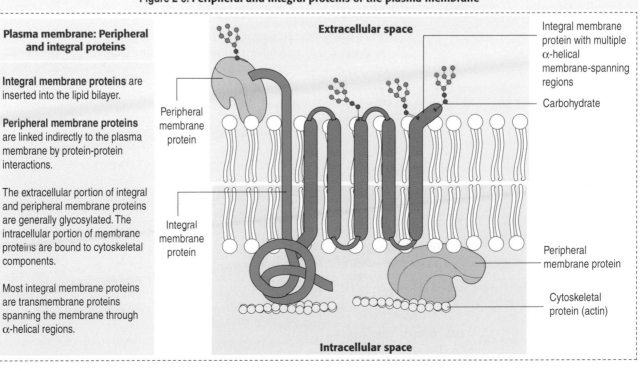

Plasma membrane: Peripheral and integral proteins

Integral membrane proteins are inserted into the lipid bilayer.

Peripheral membrane proteins are linked indirectly to the plasma membrane by protein-protein interactions.

The extracellular portion of integral and peripheral membrane proteins are generally glycosylated. The intracellular portion of membrane proteins are bound to cytoskeletal components.

Most integral membrane proteins are transmembrane proteins spanning the membrane through α-helical regions.

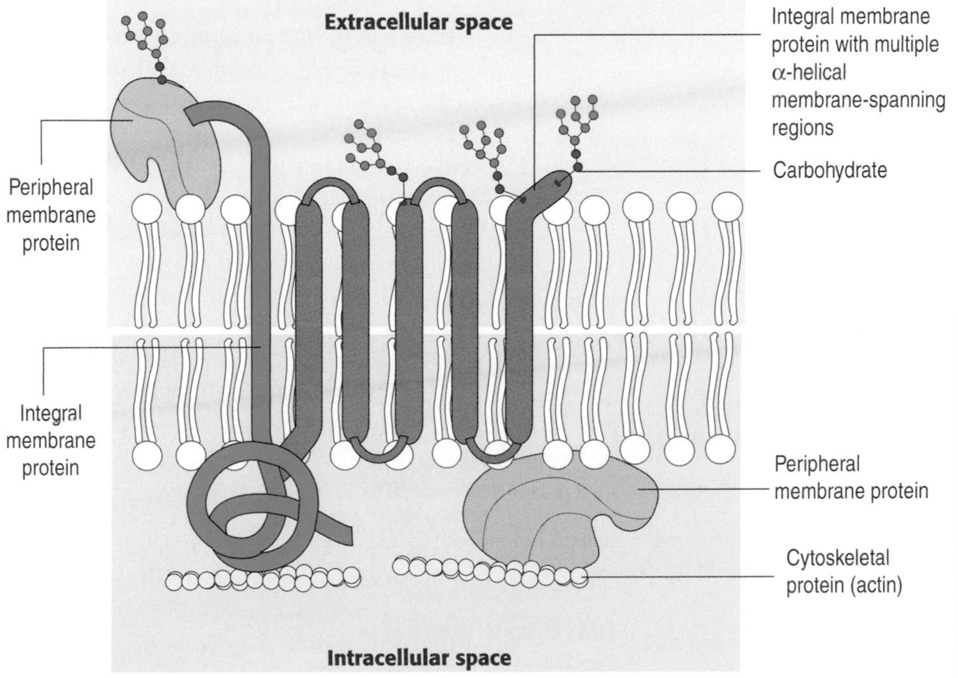

Figure 2-9. **Freeze-fracturing: Difference between surface and face**

Freeze-fracture of a cell membrane splits the bilayer into two leaflets. Each leaflet has a surface and a face. The surface of each leaflet faces either the extracellular surface (ES) or intracellular or protoplasmic surface (PS). The extracellular and protoplasmic faces (EF and PF) are artificially produced by splitting the membrane bilayer along its hydrophobic core. After membrane fracture, membrane proteins remain associated to the protoplasmic membrane leaflet and appear as particles in the PF replica. The region once occupied by the protein shows a complementary pit in the EF replica.

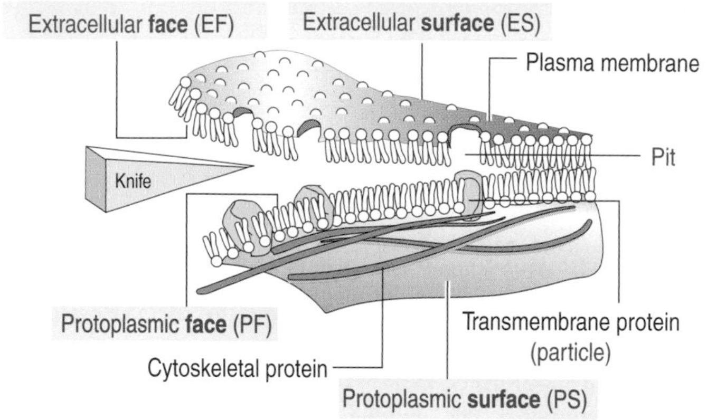

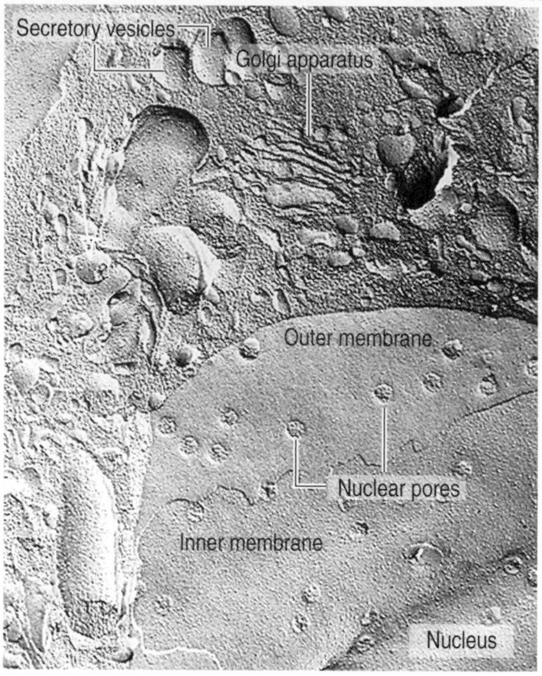

salt concentration or **extreme pH**.

Portions of integral membrane proteins are inserted into the lipid bilayer. They can only be released by solubilization using **detergents**. Detergents are chemical agents that contain both hydrophobic and hydrophilic groups. The **hydrophobic domains** of the detergent penetrate the membrane lipids and bind to the membrane-inserted hydrophobic portion of the protein. The **hydrophilic domains** combine with the protein, forming aqueous-soluble detergent-protein complexes.

Numerous integral proteins are **transmembrane proteins**, spanning the lipid bilayer, with segments exposed on both sides of the membrane. Transmembrane proteins can be visualized by the **freeze-fracture technique**.

Freeze-fracturing: Difference between a surface and a face

The **freeze-fracture technique** is valuable for the visualization of intramembranous proteins with the electron microscope. This technique provided the first evidence for the presence of transmembrane proteins in the plasma membrane and cytomembranes.

Specimens are frozen at liquid nitrogen temperature (–196°C) and "split" with a knife (under high vacuum) along the hydrophobic core of the membrane. As a result, two complementary halves, corresponding to each membrane bilayer, are produced. Each membrane half has a **surface** and a **face.** The face is artificially produced during membrane splitting.

A replica of the specimen is generated by evaporating a very thin layer of a heavy metal (generally platinum with a thickness of 1.0 to 1.5 nm) at a 45° angle to produce a contrasting shadowing effect. The platinum replica is then detached from the real specimen by floating it on a water surface, mounted on a metal grid, and examined under the electron microscope.

Figure 2-9 indicates the nomenclature for the identification of surfaces and faces in electron micrographs of freeze-fracture preparations.

The **surface** of the plasma membrane exposed to the **extracellular space** is labeled ES, for **extracellular surface**. The **surface** of the plasma membrane exposed to the **cytoplasm** (also called protoplasm) is labeled **PS**, for **protoplasmic surface**.

The **face** of the membrane leaflet looking to the **extracellular space** (the exocy-

Figure 2-10. Transporters

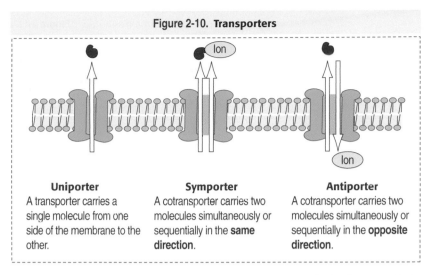

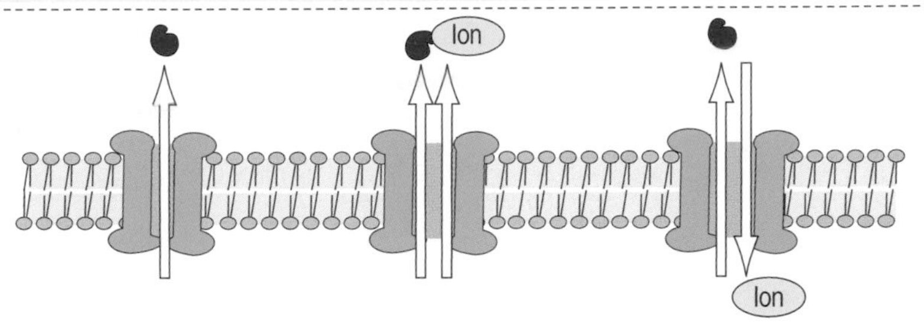

Uniporter
A transporter carries a single molecule from one side of the membrane to the other.

Symporter
A cotransporter carries two molecules simultaneously or sequentially in the **same direction**.

Antiporter
A cotransporter carries two molecules simultaneously or sequentially in the **opposite direction**.

toplasmic leaflet in the illustration) is labeled **EF**, for **extracellular face**. Similarly, the face of the leaflet facing the **protoplasmic space** (identified as a protoplasmic leaflet) is **PF**, for **protoplasmic face**.

Now that we have an understanding of what surface and face represent, remember that **faces** are chemically **hydrophobic** and **surfaces** are chemically **hydrophilic**. One last point: Note that a transmembrane protein stays with the protoplasmic leaflet, leaving a complementary **pit** in the opposite exocytoplasmic leaflet. Why? Cytoskeletal components may be directly or indirectly attached to the tip of the protein exposed to the cytoplasmic side and will not let go.

Transporter and channel proteins

Most biological molecules cannot diffuse through the phospholipid bilayer. Specific transport proteins, such as **carrier proteins** and **channel proteins**, mediate the selective passage of molecules across the membrane, thus allowing the cell to control its internal composition.

Molecules (such as **oxygen** and **carbon dioxide**) can cross the plasma membrane down their concentration gradient by dissolving first in the phospholipid bilayer and then in the aqueous environment at the cytosolic or extracellular side of the membrane. This mechanism, known as **passive diffusion**, does not involve membrane proteins. Lipid substances can also cross the bilayer.

Other biological molecules (such as **glucose**, **charged molecules**, and **small ions**—H^+, Na^+, K^+, and Cl^-) are unable to dissolve in the hydrophobic interior of the phospholipid bilayer. They require the help of specific **transport proteins** (Figure 2-10) and **channel proteins**, which facilitate the diffusion of most biological molecules.

Similar to passive diffusion, **facilitated diffusion** of biological molecules **is determined by concentration and electrical gradients across the membrane**. However, facilitated diffusion requires one of the following:

1. **Carrier proteins**, which can bind specific molecules to be transported.
2. **Channel proteins**, forming open gates through the membrane.

Carrier proteins transport sugars, amino acids, and nucleosides. Channel proteins are ion channels involved in the rapid transport of ions (faster transport than carrier proteins), are **highly selective of molecular size and electrical charge**, and **are not continuously open.**

Some channels open in response to the binding of a signaling molecule and are called **ligand-gated channels**. Other channels open in response to changes in electric potential across the membrane and are called **voltage-gated channels**.

Internal environment of the cell

The **endoplasmic reticulum** is an interconnected network of membrane-bound

Figure 2-11. **Intracellular compartments**

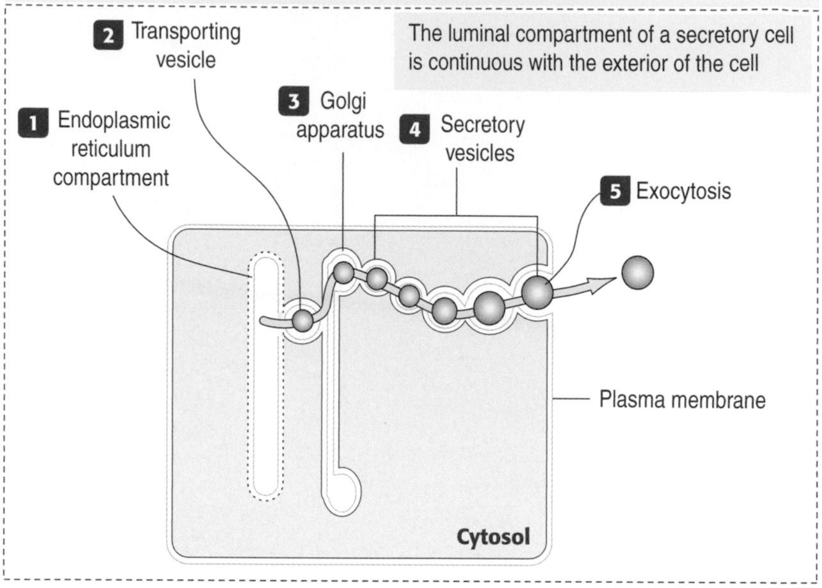

channels within the cytoplasm, part of the **cytomembrane** system and distinct from the **plasma membrane**.

The endoplasmic reticulum system, consisting of **cisternae** (flat sacs), **tubules**, and **vesicles**, divides the cytoplasm into two compartments:

1. The **luminal** or **endoplasmic compartment**.
2. The **cytoplasmic** or **cytosolic compartment**.

Products released into the luminal compartment of the rough endoplasmic reticulum are transported to the Golgi apparatus by a transporting vesicle and eventually to the exterior of the cell by exocytosis. One can visualize the sequence in which the lumen of the cytomembrane system is interconnected and remains as such in an imaginary stage; you can visualize that the **luminal compartment of a secretory cell is continuous with the exterior of the cell** (Figure 2-11). The surrounding space is the cytosolic compartment in which soluble proteins, cytoskeletal components, and organelles are present.

Now, let us imagine that we can visualize the membrane of each component of the cytomembrane system as consisting of two leaflets (Figure 2-12):

1. The **exocytoplasmic leaflet** (facing the extracellular space).
2. The **protoplasmic leaflet** (facing the cytosolic compartment).

Let us also imagine that exocytoplasmic and protoplasmic leaflets form a continuum. During the **freeze-fracturing process,** the knife fractures the membrane as it jumps from one fracture plane to the other across the hydrophobic core and splits membranes into two leaflets. The knife cannot stay with a single membrane because cytomembrane-bound organelles occupy different levels and have random orientations within the cell. This randomness will be apparent during the examination of the replica.

The sample may contain a combination of exocytoplasmic and protoplasmic leaflets which, in turn, can expose surfaces and faces. Membrane proteins tend to remain associated with the cytoplasmic (protoplasmic) leaflet and appear as **particles on the PF** (protoplasmic face). A shallow **complementary pit is visualized in the EF** (exocytoplasmic face).

Endoplasmic reticulum

The **rough endoplasmic reticulum** is recognized under the light microscope as a diffuse basophilic cytoplasmic structure called **ergastoplasm**.

The rough endoplasmic reticulum is involved in the synthesis of proteins, carried out by their attached **ribosomes** (Figure 2-13), and in the addition of

Figure 2-12. Leaflets of cytomembranes and plasma membrane

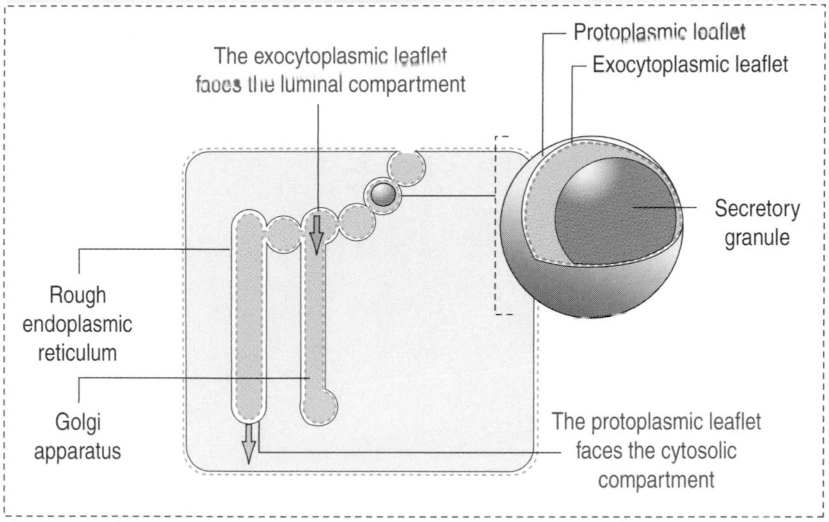

oligosaccharides to many proteins. Most proteins exit the rough endoplasmic reticulum in vesicles transported to the *cis* portion of the Golgi apparatus (see Figures 2-16 and 2-17). Other proteins are retained by the rough endoplasmic reticulum to participate in the initial steps of protein synthesis (see Figure 2-15). The retained proteins contain the targeting sequence Lys-Asp-Glu-Leu (KDEL) at the C-terminal. A lack of the KDEL sequence marks proteins for transport to the Golgi apparatus.

The **smooth endoplasmic reticulum** lacks ribosomes and is generally in proximity to deposits of glycogen and lipids in the cytoplasm. The smooth endoplasmic reticulum has an important role in **detoxification reactions** required for the conversion of harmful lipid-soluble or water-insoluble substances into water-soluble compounds more convenient for discharge by the kidney. It also participates in **steroidogenesis** (see Chapter 19, Endocrine System).

Rough endoplasmic reticulum and protein synthesis and sorting

The role of the rough endoplasmic reticulum in protein synthesis and sorting was demonstrated by incubating pancreatic acinar cells in a medium containing radiolabeled amino acids and localizing radiolabeled proteins by autoradiography. The secretory pathway taken by secretory proteins includes the following sequence: rough endoplasmic reticulum, to Golgi apparatus, to secretory vesicles, to the extracellular space or lumen (Figure 2-14). Plasma membrane and lysosomal proteins also follow the sequence of rough endoplasmic reticulum to Golgi apparatus but are retained within the cell.

Proteins targeted to the nucleus, mitochondria, or peroxisomes are synthesized on free ribosomes and then released into the cytosol. In contrast, proteins for secretion or targeted to the endoplasmic reticulum, Golgi apparatus, lysosomes, or plasma membrane are synthesized by membrane-bound ribosomes and then transferred to the rough endoplasmic reticulum as protein synthesis progresses.

Ribosomes attach to the endoplasmic reticulum under the guidance of the amino acid sequence of the polypeptide chain being synthesized. Ribosomes synthesizing proteins for secretion are directed to the endoplasmic reticulum by a signal sequence at the growing end of the polypeptide chain.

The mechanism by which secretory proteins are directed to the endoplasmic reticulum is explained by the **signal hypothesis** (Figure 2-15).

Golgi apparatus and the protein sorting pathways

The Golgi apparatus is a cellular organelle highly developed in secretory cells. Its main function is the **addition of oligosaccharides to proteins and lipids.**

Figure 2-13. Rough endoplasmic reticulum

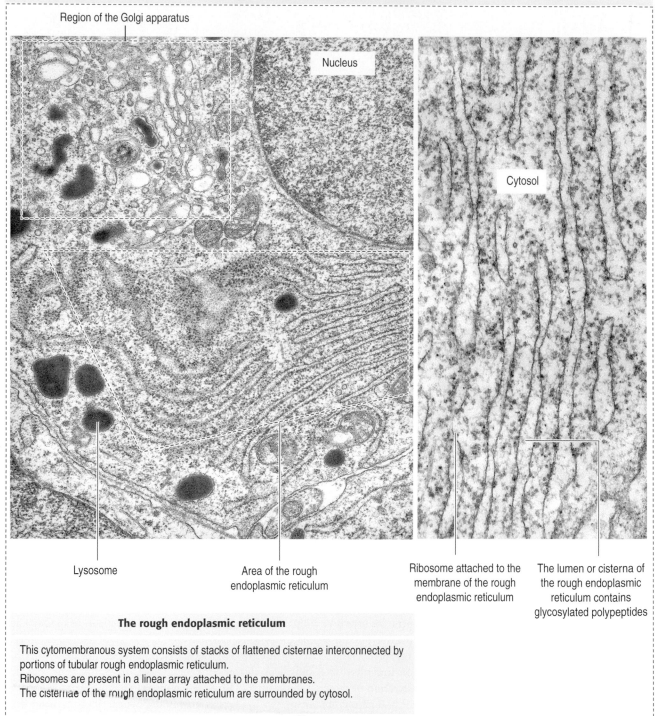

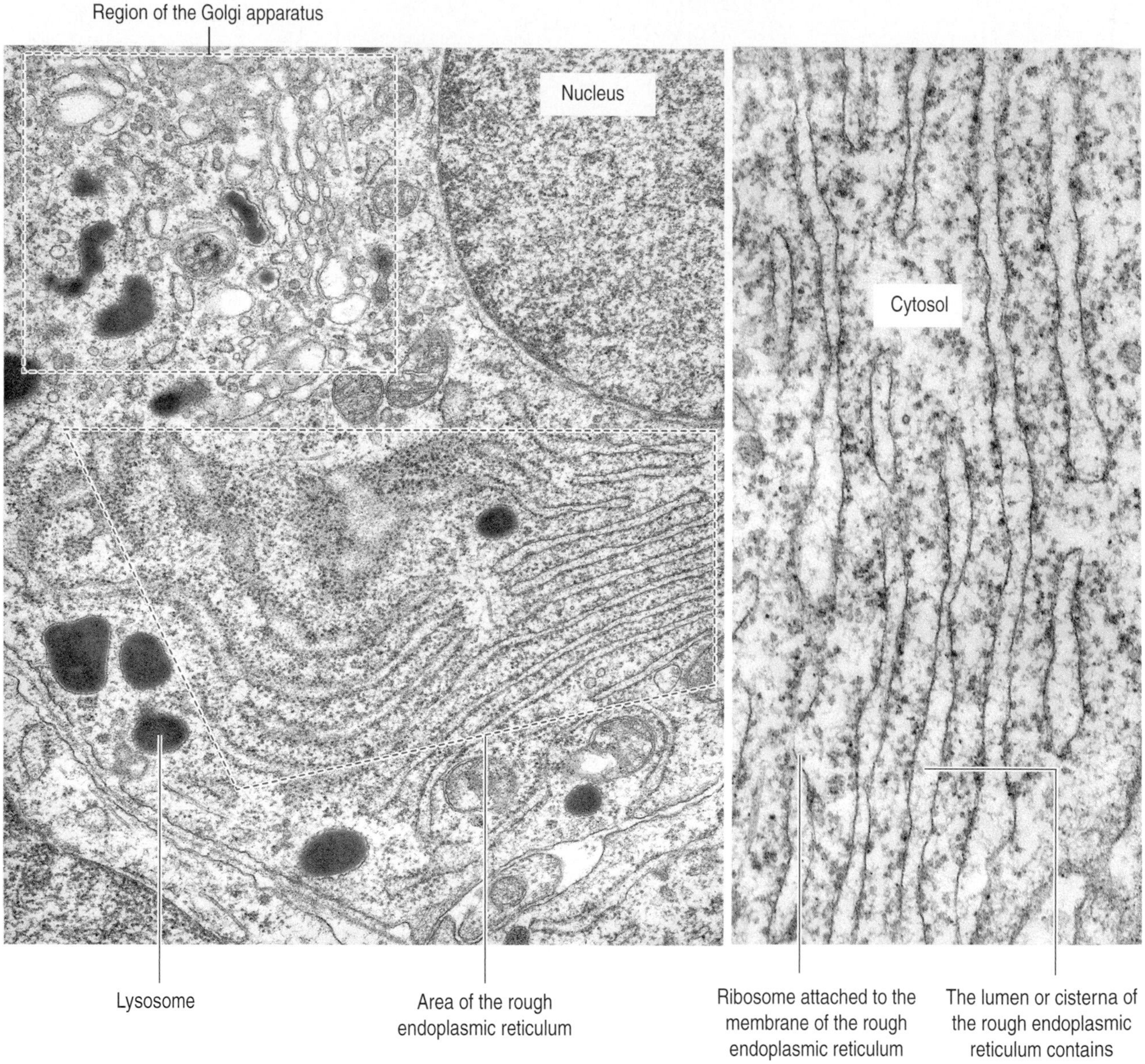
Region of the Golgi apparatus
Nucleus
Cytosol
Lysosome
Area of the rough endoplasmic reticulum
Ribosome attached to the membrane of the rough endoplasmic reticulum
The lumen or cisterna of the rough endoplasmic reticulum contains glycosylated polypeptides

The rough endoplasmic reticulum

This cytomembranous system consists of stacks of flattened cisternae interconnected by portions of tubular rough endoplasmic reticulum.
Ribosomes are present in a linear array attached to the membranes.
The cisternae of the rough endoplasmic reticulum are surrounded by cytosol.

The opposite site of the Golgi stack, the *trans* or **exit face**, known as the ***trans*-Golgi network**, gives rise to vesicles that exit the stack for various destinations. A **medial compartment** of stacks links the *cis* and *trans* compartments (Figures 2-16 and 2-17).

Functional differences between the *cis*, medial, and *trans* compartments of the Golgi apparatus are indicated by the presence of specific **glycosyltransferases** in each compartment. Glycosyltransferases are enzymes that transfer sugars to terminal portions of the oligosaccharide chains of glycoproteins and glycolipids.

Glycosyltransferases can be demonstrated by **cytochemical reactions**, by providing an enzyme substrate that gives rise to a visible product after enzymatic

Figure 2-14. **Protein synthesis, transport, and secretion by exocrine pancreatic cells**

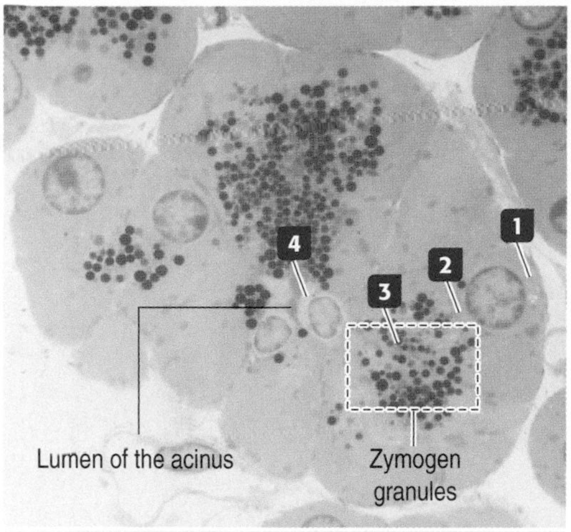

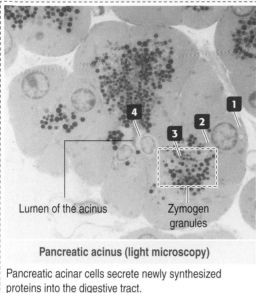

Pancreatic acinus (light microscopy)

Pancreatic acinar cells secrete newly synthesized proteins into the digestive tract.

When cells were labeled with a radioactive amino acid to trace the intracellular pathway of the secreted proteins, it was found by autoradiography that, after a 3-minute labeling, newly synthesized proteins were localized in the rough endoplasmic reticulum 1.

Later on, the radiolabeled proteins were found to translocate to the Golgi apparatus 2 and then, within secretory vesicles as zymogen granules 3, to the plasma membrane and the extracellular space 4.

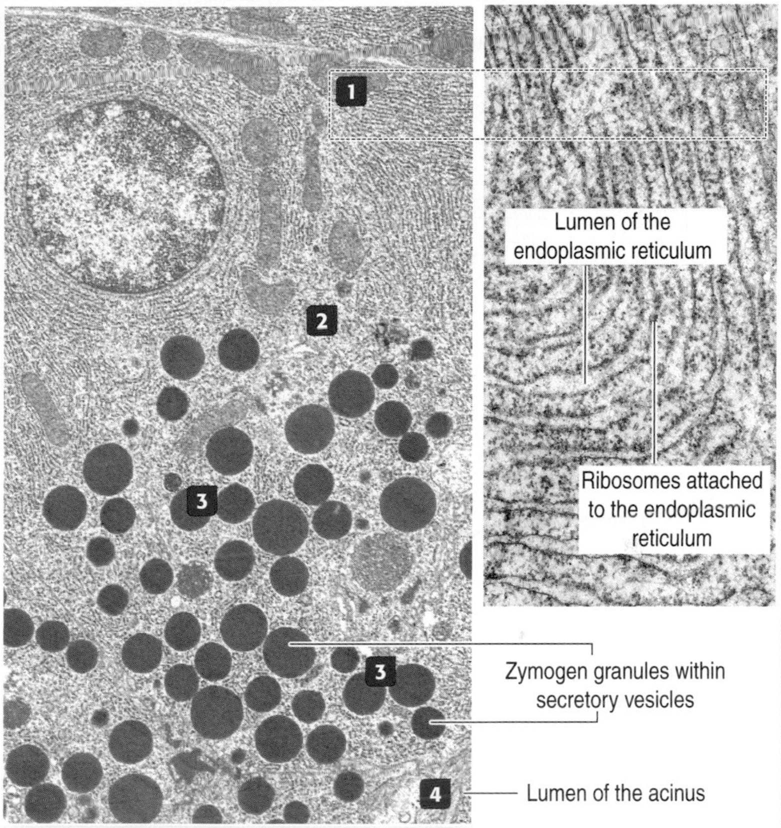

Pancreatic acinar cells (electron microscopy)

activity, or by **immunocytochemistry**, using specific antibodies.

The glycosylation pathway can be traced by **electron microscopic autoradiography** using [^{3}H]**fucose**, a carbohydrate present only at the terminal portion of the oligosaccharide chain.

Secretory products can be released from the cell (**exocytosis**) by two mechanisms:

1. **By continuous exocytosis.**
2. **By selective exocytosis of stored secretory granules.**

Continuous exocytosis does not require a triggering signal (for example, the secretion of immunoglobulins by plasma cells). This mechanism is known as the **constitutive secretory pathway**. In the second mechanism, selective exocytosis, cell products are released under control of a chemical or electrical signal (for example, the secretion of hormones by cells of the anterior hypophysis). This mechanism is called the **regulated secretory pathway**.

Not all cell products are released by exocytosis. Some products remain within the cell after being "sorted" by the Golgi apparatus.

Lysosomal hydrolases are synthesized in the rough endoplasmic reticulum, transported to the *cis*-Golgi, and finally sorted to **lysosomes**. This sorting mechanism involves two important steps (Figure 2-18):

1. The insertion of **mannose-6-phosphate (M6P)** into oligosaccharides attached to glycoproteins destined to lysosomes.

2. The presence of the **transmembrane M6P receptor protein** in the transporting vesicle.

By this mechanism, M6P-containing lysosomal enzymes are separated from other glycoproteins in vesicles with the M6P receptor. After being transported to a clathrin-coated transporting vesicle, lysosomal enzymes dissociate from

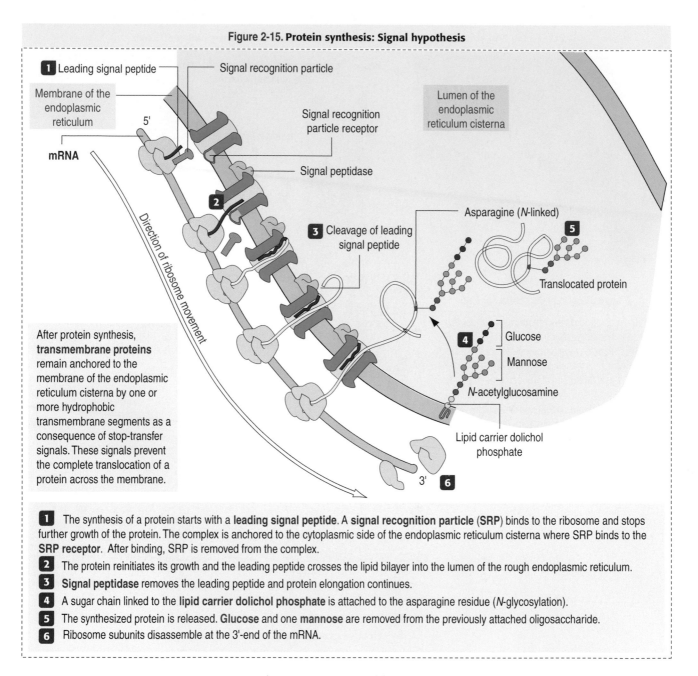

Figure 2-15. Protein synthesis: Signal hypothesis

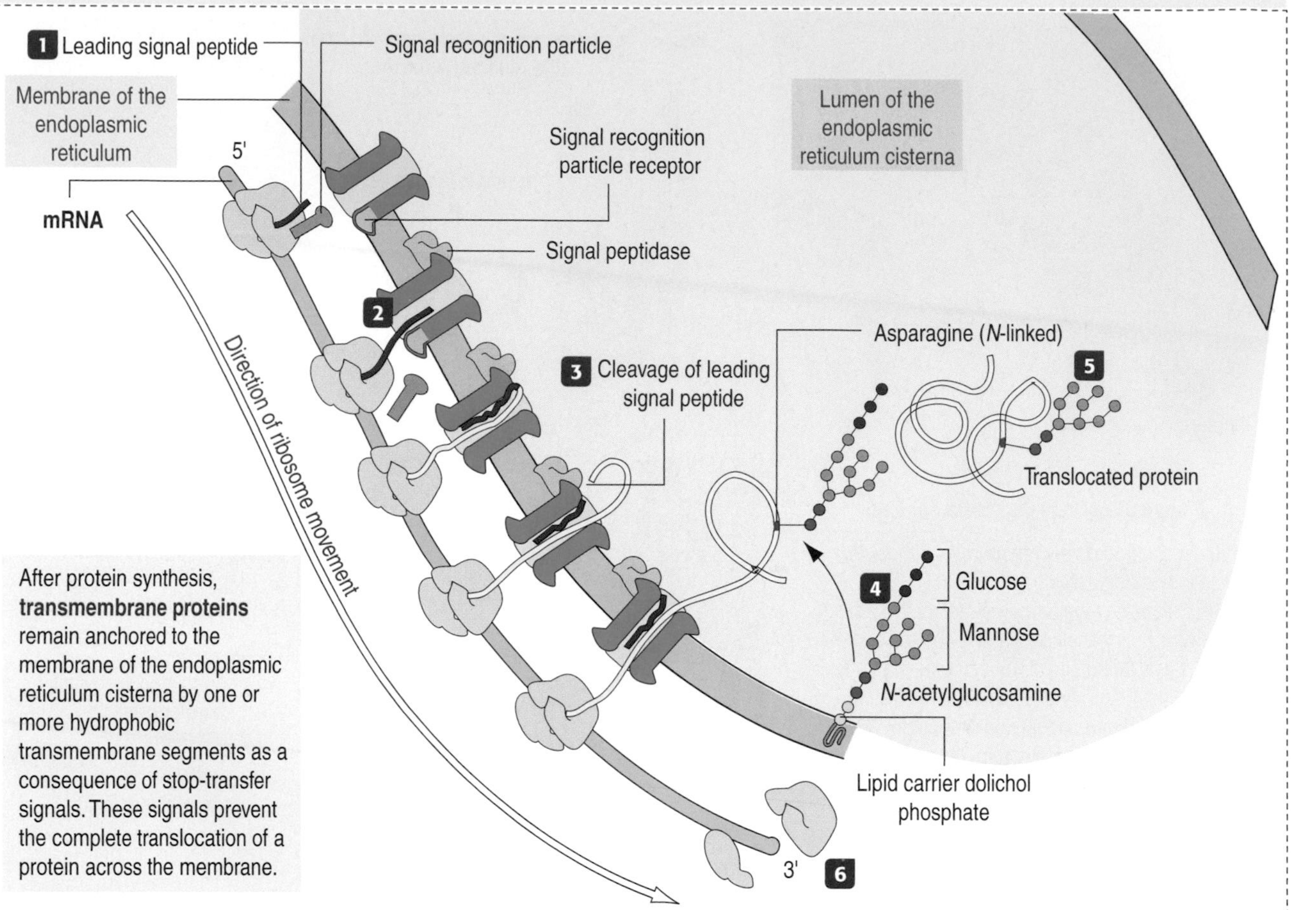

1 Leading signal peptide
Signal recognition particle
Membrane of the endoplasmic reticulum
5'
mRNA
Signal recognition particle receptor
Lumen of the endoplasmic reticulum cisterna
Signal peptidase
2
Direction of ribosome movement
3 Cleavage of leading signal peptide
Asparagine (*N*-linked)
5
Translocated protein
4
Glucose
Mannose
N-acetylglucosamine
Lipid carrier dolichol phosphate
3'
6

After protein synthesis, **transmembrane proteins** remain anchored to the membrane of the endoplasmic reticulum cisterna by one or more hydrophobic transmembrane segments as a consequence of stop-transfer signals. These signals prevent the complete translocation of a protein across the membrane.

1 The synthesis of a protein starts with a **leading signal peptide**. A **signal recognition particle** (**SRP**) binds to the ribosome and stops further growth of the protein. The complex is anchored to the cytoplasmic side of the endoplasmic reticulum cisterna where SRP binds to the **SRP receptor**. After binding, SRP is removed from the complex.

2 The protein reinitiates its growth and the leading peptide crosses the lipid bilayer into the lumen of the rough endoplasmic reticulum.

3 **Signal peptidase** removes the leading peptide and protein elongation continues.

4 A sugar chain linked to the **lipid carrier dolichol phosphate** is attached to the asparagine residue (*N*-glycosylation).

5 The synthesized protein is released. **Glucose** and one **mannose** are removed from the previously attached oligosaccharide.

6 Ribosome subunits disassemble at the 3'-end of the mRNA.

the M6P receptor and become surrounded by a membrane to form a **primary lysosome.** Membranes containing free M6P receptor are returned to the Golgi apparatus for **recycling.**

Lysosomes

Two types of lysosomes are recognized: **primary lysosomes** (Figure 2-19), defined as the primary storage site of lysosomal hydrolases, and **secondary lysosomes**, regarded as lysosomes engaged in a catalytic process.

The plasma membrane can internalize extracellular particles and fluids using vesicles resulting from the invagination of the membrane by a process called **endocytosis.** The reverse process, called **exocytosis**, represents transport to the outside of products processed or synthesized by the cell.

Endocytosis involves two major types of vesicles:

1. **Phagocytic clathrin-independent vesicles**, used to internalize particles (for example, virus or bacteria).
2. **Clathrin-coated vesicles**, to take in small macromolecules.

Figure 2-16. The Golgi apparatus: Exocytosis and lysosomal pathways

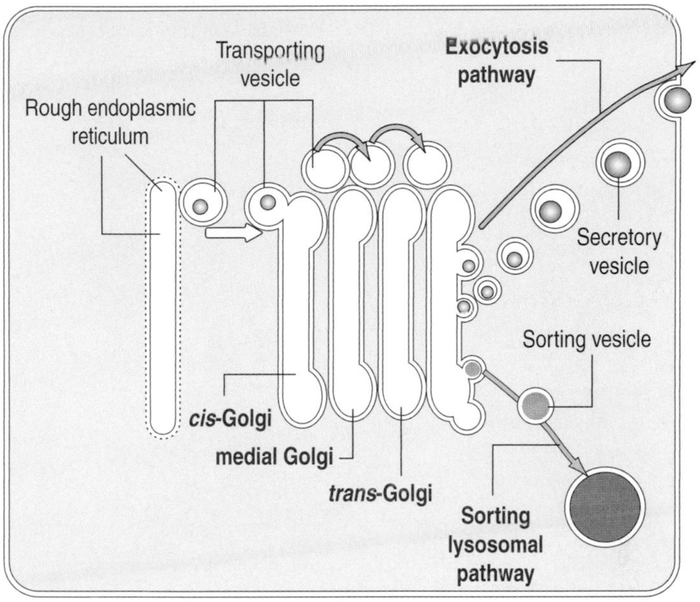

The Golgi apparatus

First described in 1898 by Camillo Golgi (1843-1926) in neurons impregnated with silver salts, this structure consists of orderly stacks of flattened disklike cisternae and associated vesicles.

The cisterna closest to the endoplasmic reticulum is the ***cis* face**, whereas the cisterna closest to the apical domain of the cell is the ***trans* face**. The **medial region** is the site where most protein glycosylation occurs. The membranes of the Golgi apparatus are devoid of ribosomes.

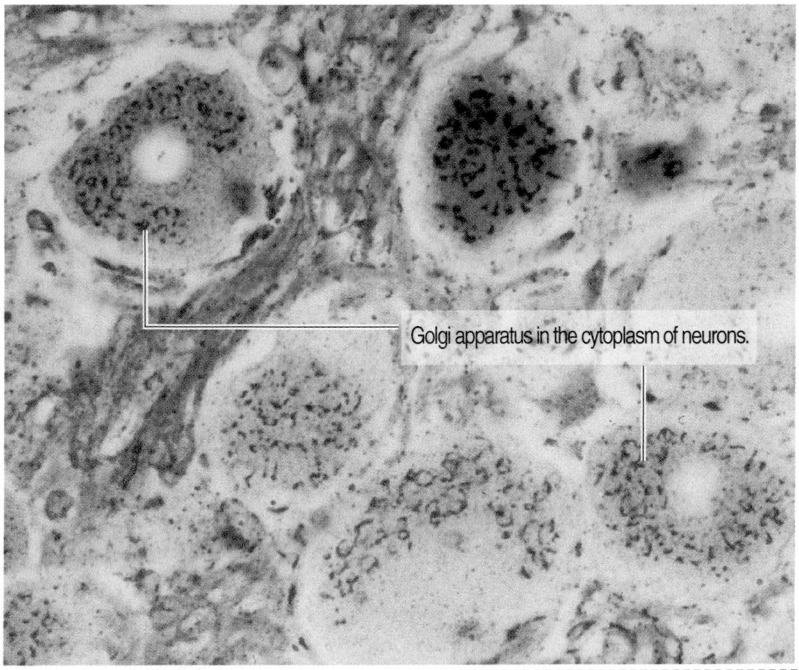

The internalization of fluids, known as **pinocytosis**, involves vesicles known as **caveolae** coated by a protein called **caveolin.**

Endocytosis has two important roles:

1. **To bring material into the cell.**
2. **To recycle the plasma membrane.**

Figure 2-17. **Compartments of the Golgi apparatus**

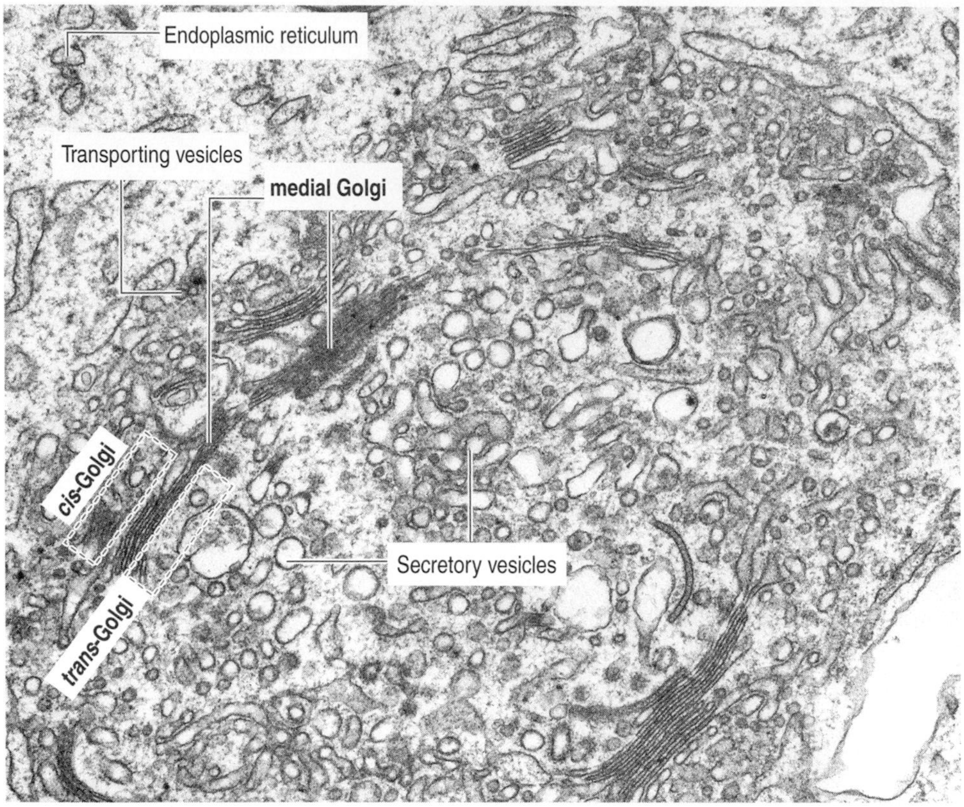
Endoplasmic reticulum
Transporting vesicles
medial Golgi
cis-Golgi
trans-Golgi
Secretory vesicles

The **Golgi apparatus** is visualized under the electron microscope as a series of curved flattened saccules stacked upon one another. The ends of the saccules are dilated and can form spherical vesicles. The saccules and vesicles contain proteins being glycosylated for further secretion or sorting.

The Golgi apparatus consists of three major functionally distinct compartments:
1. The ***cis*-Golgi** is the entry site to the Golgi apparatus of products derived from the endoplasmic reticulum.
2. The **medial Golgi** (formed by stacked saccules) is the site where most glycosylation takes place.
3. The ***trans*-Golgi** is the distribution or sorting site of products for transport to lysosomes or secretion (exocytosis).

Receptor-mediated endocytosis: The uptake of cholesterol

The internalization of a **ligand** (such as low-density lipoprotein [LDL] cholesterol, transferrin, polypeptide hormones, or growth factors) by a cell requires a specific **membrane receptor** (Figure 2-20).

LDL carries about 75% of the cholesterol and circulates in blood for about 2 to 3 days. Approximately 70% of LDL is cleared from blood by cells containing

Figure 2-18. **Golgi apparatus: Lysosomal sorting pathways**

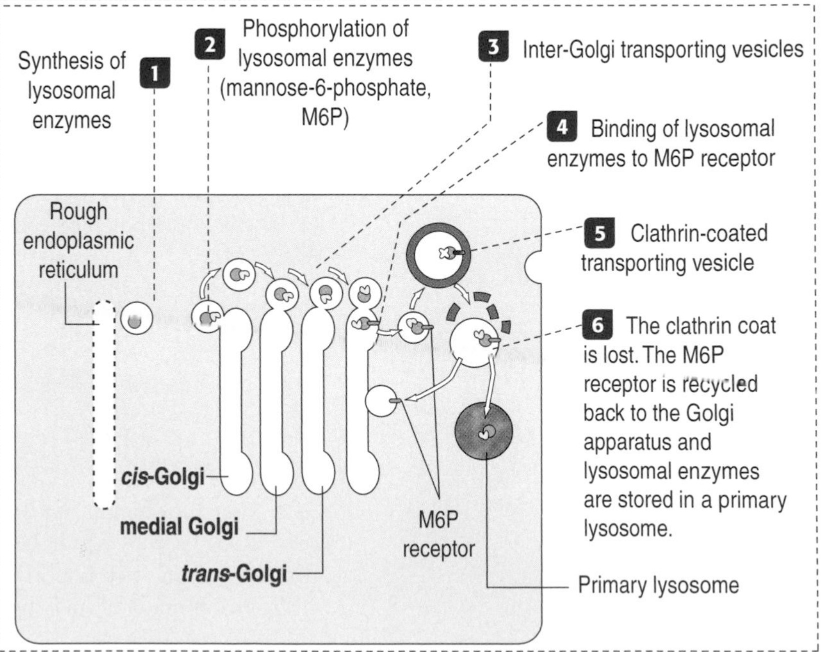
1 Synthesis of lysosomal enzymes
2 Phosphorylation of lysosomal enzymes (mannose-6-phosphate, M6P)
3 Inter-Golgi transporting vesicles
4 Binding of lysosomal enzymes to M6P receptor
5 Clathrin-coated transporting vesicle
6 The clathrin coat is lost. The M6P receptor is recycled back to the Golgi apparatus and lysosomal enzymes are stored in a primary lysosome.
Rough endoplasmic reticulum
cis-Golgi
medial Golgi
trans-Golgi
M6P receptor
Primary lysosome

Figure 2-19. **Types of lysosomes**

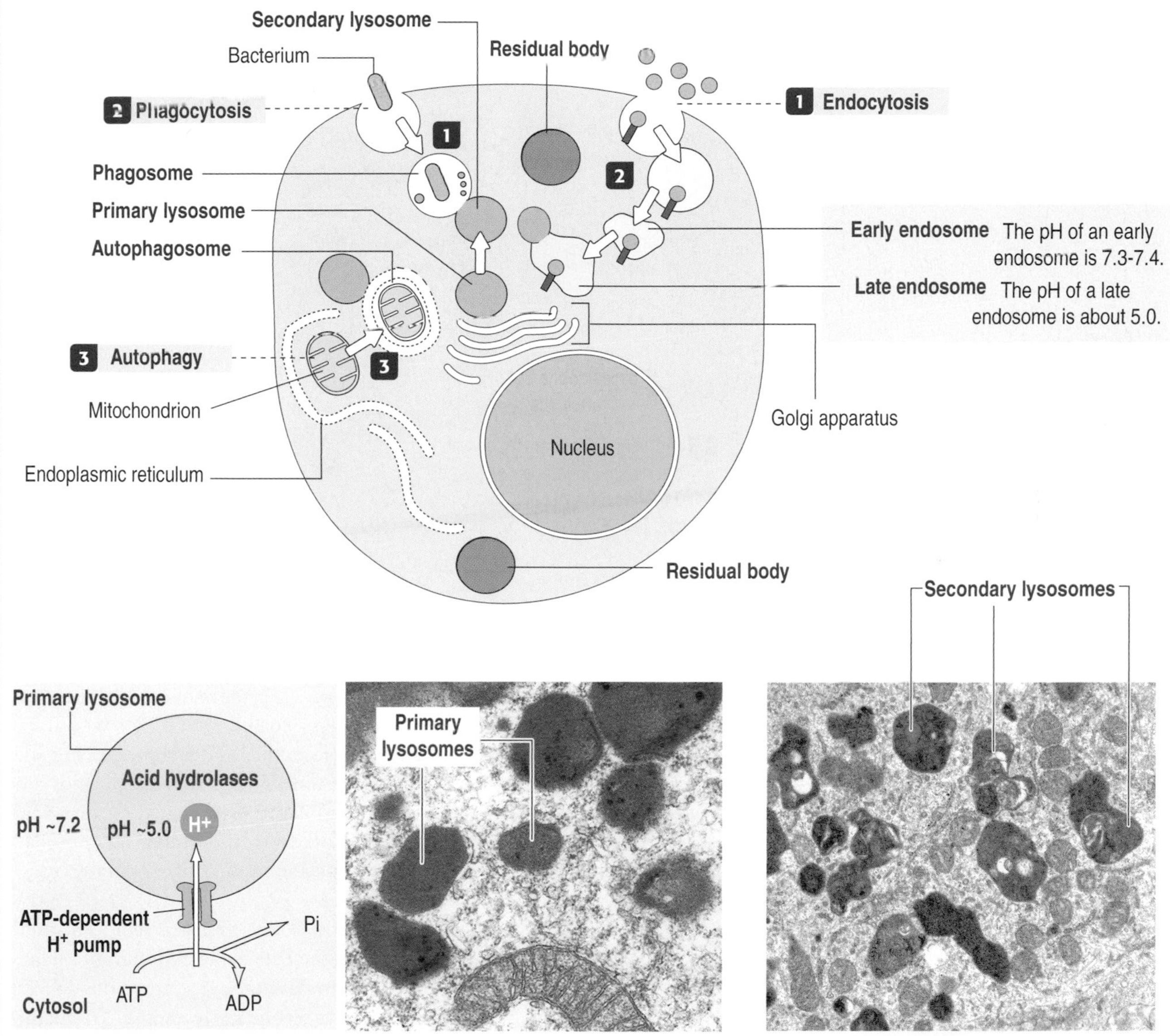

Lysosomes

Lysosomes are organelles which contain about 40 types of hydrolytic enzymes active in an acidic environment (~ pH 5.0). Their function is to degrade proteins, nucleic acids, oligosaccharides, and phospholipids.

The surrounding membrane has three characteristics:

1. It separates hydrolytic enzymes from the cytosol.
2. It harbors transport proteins (**lysosomal glycoprotein A and B**) that translocate breakdown products from the lysosome into the cytosol (amino acids, sugars, and nucleotides).
3. It contains an **ATP-dependent H^+ pump** to maintain an acidic intralysosomal environment.

There are three major pathways for the intracellular degradation of materials. Extracellular particles can be taken up by phagocytosis and endocytosis. Aged intracellular components are degraded by autophagy.

1 Endocytosis: The material that is endocytosed is delivered to an early endosome and then to a late endosome. The membrane of a late endosome contains the H^+ pump, the early endosome does not. A primary lysosome fuses with the late endosome to begin its catalytic function. Endocytosis is characteristic of receptor-mediated endocytosis of polypeptide hormones and growth factors.

2 Phagocytosis: The material that is phagocytosed is enclosed within a phagosome which then fuses with a lysosome. Abundant phagosomes are observed in macrophages.

3 Autophagy: Autophagy starts with the endoplasmic reticulum enclosing an aged cell component to form an autophagosome which then fuses with a lysosome and its content is digested. Autophagy plays a significant role in tissue remodeling during differentiation. A **residual body** is a structure containing partially digested material.

Figure 2-20. **Cholesterol uptake**

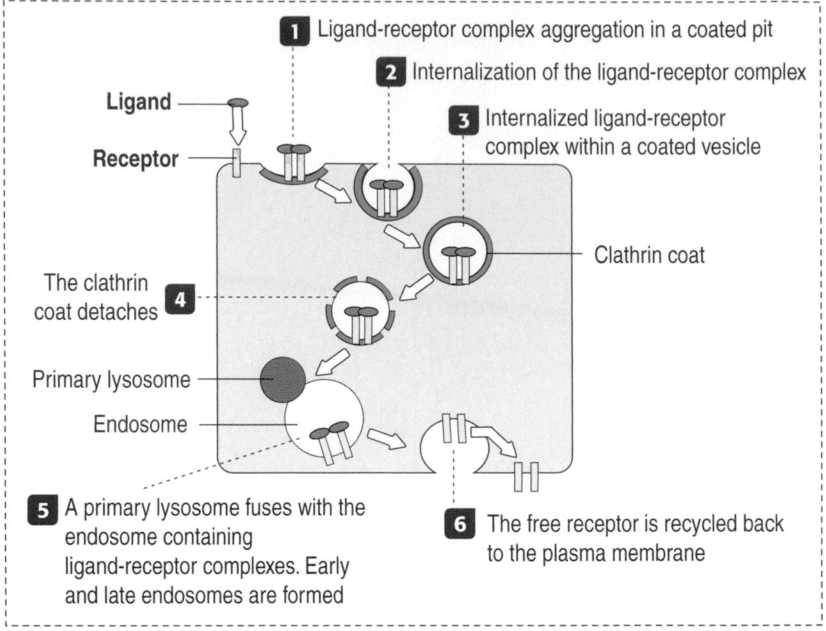

1 Ligand-receptor complex aggregation in a coated pit
2 Internalization of the ligand-receptor complex
3 Internalized ligand-receptor complex within a coated vesicle
Ligand
Receptor
Clathrin coat
The clathrin coat detaches 4
Primary lysosome
Endosome
5 A primary lysosome fuses with the endosome containing ligand-receptor complexes. Early and late endosomes are formed
6 The free receptor is recycled back to the plasma membrane

LDL receptors; the remainder is removed by a scavenger pathway using a receptor-independent mechanism.

The **receptor-ligand complex** (for example, LDL bound to its receptor) is internalized by a process called **receptor-mediated endocytosis**. This process involves the assembly of the protein **clathrin** on the cytoplasmic side of the plasma membrane which forms a coated crater called a **coated pit**.

The function of clathrin is to concentrate receptor-ligand complexes in a small surface area of the plasma membrane. Receptors with their bound ligands move by lateral diffusion in the plane of the lipid bilayer. The coated pit invaginates to form a **coated vesicle**, which pinches off from the plasma membrane to transport receptor-ligand complexes to a specific intracellular pathway, usually an **endosome**.

After internalization, the clathrin coat of the coated vesicle is removed and the uncoated vesicle fuses with a larger vesicle, the endosome, with an internal low pH. In this acidic environment, LDL detaches from the receptor and is delivered to a **primary lysosome**, which changes into a **secondary lysosome**.

The LDL receptor is recycled back to the plasma membrane, the LDL particle is degraded by lysosomal enzymes, and free cholesterol is released into the cytosol.

Cholesterol is required for the synthesis of steroid hormones, the production of bile acids in liver hepatocytes, and the synthesis of cell membranes.

Clinical significance: Familial hypercholesterolemia. Lysosomal storage disorders

Familial hypercholesterolemia is characterized by an elevation of LDL cholesterol, the predominant cholesterol transport protein in the plasma. The primary defect is a **mutation in the gene encoding the LDL receptor**, required for the internalization of dietary cholesterol by most cells. High levels of LDL cholesterol in blood plasma lead to the formation of **atherosclerotic plaques** in the coronary vessels, a common cause of **myocardial infarction**.

Patients with familial hypercholesterolemia have three types of defective receptors:

1. LDL receptors incapable of binding LDL cholesterol.
2. LDL receptors that bind LDL cholesterol but at a reduced capacity.
3. LDL receptors that can bind LDL cholesterol normally but are incapable of

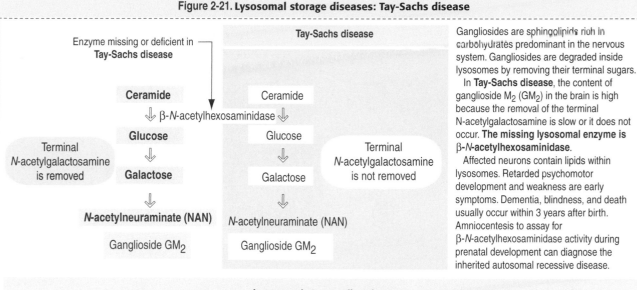

Figure 2-21. Lysosomal storage diseases: Tay-Sachs disease

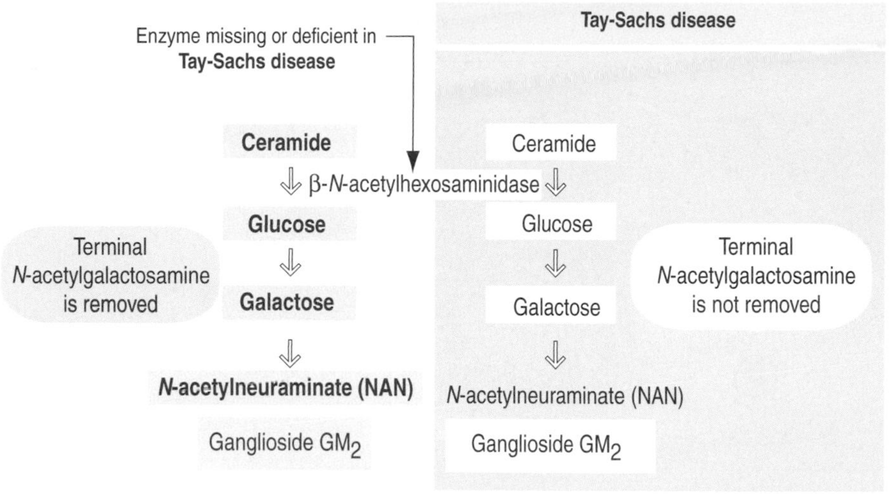
Tay-Sachs disease
Enzyme missing or deficient in
Tay-Sachs disease
Ceramide
Ceramide
β-N-acetylhexosaminidase
Glucose
Glucose
Terminal
N-acetylgalactosamine
is removed
Galactose
Galactose
Terminal
N-acetylgalactosamine
is not removed
N-acetylneuraminate (NAN)
N-acetylneuraminate (NAN)
Ganglioside GM2
Ganglioside GM2

Gangliosides are sphingolipids rich in carbohydrates predominant in the nervous system. Gangliosides are degraded inside lysosomes by removing their terminal sugars.

In **Tay-Sachs disease**, the content of ganglioside M_2 (GM_2) in the brain is high because the removal of the terminal N-acetylgalactosamine is slow or it does not occur. **The missing lysosomal enzyme is β-*N*-acetylhexosaminidase**.

Affected neurons contain lipids within lysosomes. Retarded psychomotor development and weakness are early symptoms. Dementia, blindness, and death usually occur within 3 years after birth. Amniocentesis to assay for β-*N*-acetylhexosaminidase activity during prenatal development can diagnose the inherited autosomal recessive disease.

Lysosomal storage disorders

The hydrolytic enzymes within lysosomes are involved in the breakdown of sphingolipids, glycoproteins, and glycoproteins into soluble products. These molecular complexes can derive from the turnover of intracellular organelles or enter the cell by phagocytosis.

A number of genetic diseases lacking lysosomal enzymes result in the progressive accumulation within the cell of partially degraded insoluble products. This condition leads to clinical conditions known as **lysosomal storage disorders**.

These disorders include broad categories depending on the major accumulating insoluble product and the substrate for the defective lysosomal enzyme.

The **deficient breakdown of sphingolipids** is the cause of:

1. **Gaucher's disease**, characterized by defective activity of a **glucocerebrosidase**, resulting in the accumulation of glucocerebrosides in the spleen and central nervous system.
2. **Niemann-Pick disease**, defined by a defective **sphingomyelinase**, leading to the accumulation of sphingomyelin and cholesterol in the spleen and central nervous system.
3. **Tay-Sachs disease**, characterized by a deficiency of **β-*N*-acetylhexosaminidase**, resulting in the accumulation of gangliosides in the central nervous system.

The **diagnosis** of these three lysosomal storage disorders is based on the detection of enzymatic activity in leukocytes and cultured fibroblasts of the patients.

internalization.

Lysosomal storage disorders or **diseases** are caused by the progressive accumulation of cell membrane components within cells because of a hereditary deficiency of enzymes required for their breakdown. An example is **Tay-Sachs disease** (Figure 2-21).

Vesicular transport

A continual process of **budding** and **fusion** of **transport vesicles** mobilizes products from the rough endoplasmic reticulum to the Golgi apparatus, between membranous stacks of the Golgi apparatus, and from the Golgi apparatus to other components of the cytomembrane system. The vesicular transport pathway can internalize cholesterol by a receptor-mediated endocytosis mechanism involving inward budding of clathrin-coated pits and vesicles.

The vesicular transport mechanism involves two types of coated vesicles (Figure 2-22):

1. **Clathrin-coated vesicles**, transporting products from the Golgi apparatus to lysosomes, and endocytic vesicles, carrying products from the exterior of the cell to lysosomes (for example, cholesterol).

2. **COP-coated vesicles** (COP stands for coat protein), transporting products between stacks of the Golgi apparatus (**COPI-coated vesicles**), and from the rough endoplasmic reticulum to the Golgi apparatus (**COPII-coated vesicles**).

Adaptins mediate the binding of clathrin to the vesicular membrane as well as select specific molecules to be trapped in a vesicle. For example, an adaptin

Figure 2-22. Vesicular transport

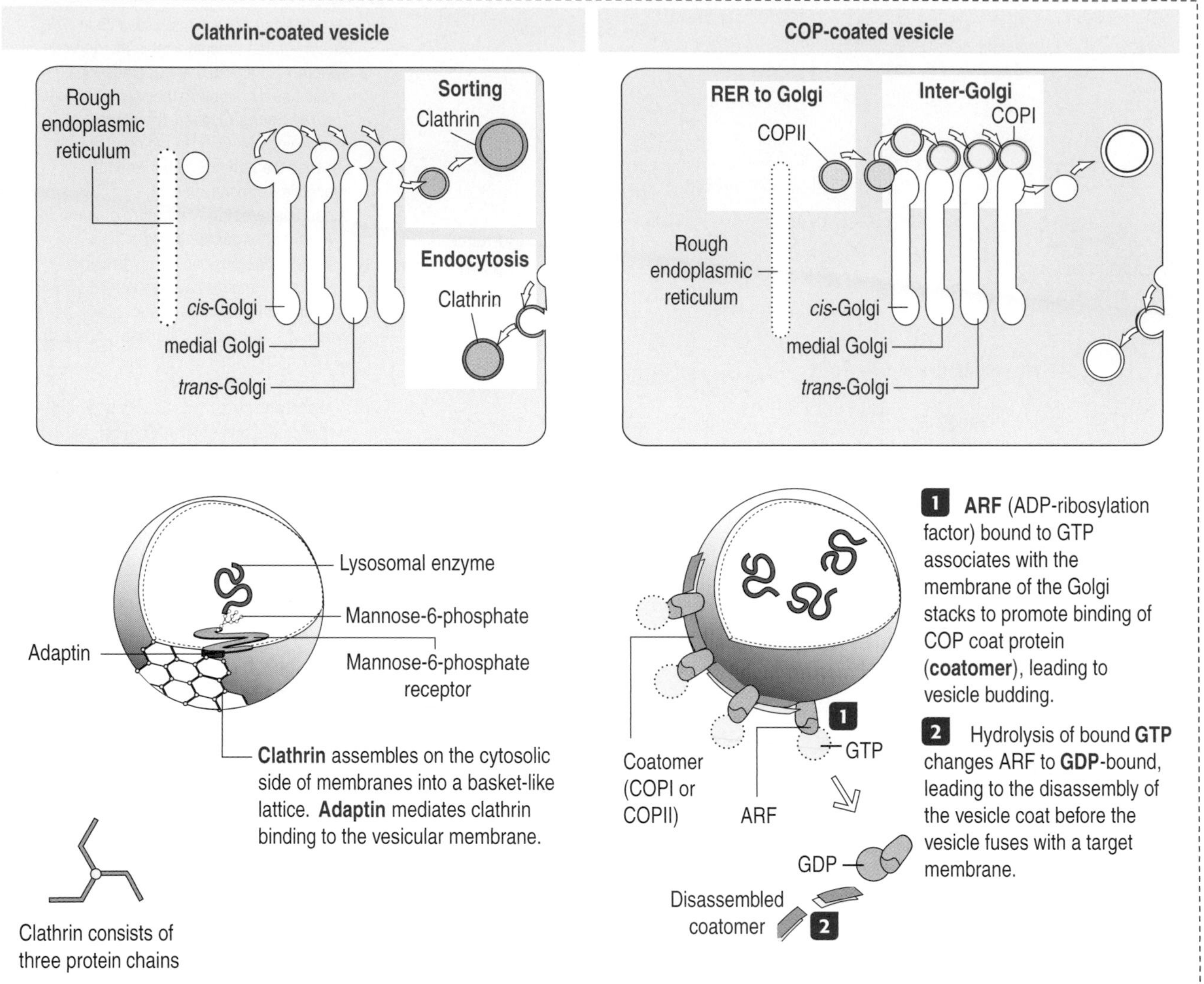

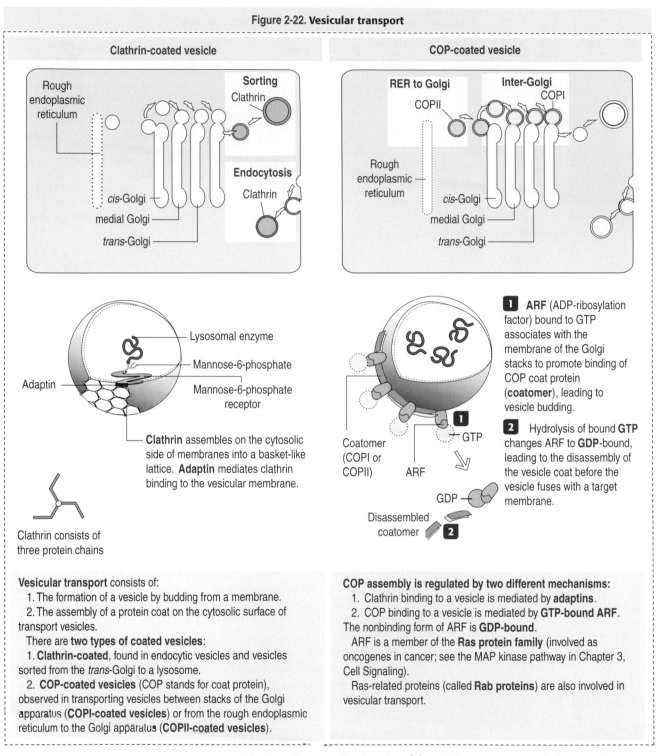

Clathrin-coated vesicle
Rough endoplasmic reticulum
Sorting
Clathrin
Endocytosis
Clathrin
cis-Golgi
medial Golgi
trans-Golgi
COP-coated vesicle
RER to Golgi
COPII
Inter-Golgi
COPI
Rough endoplasmic reticulum
cis-Golgi
medial Golgi
trans-Golgi
Lysosomal enzyme
Mannose-6-phosphate
Adaptin
Mannose-6-phosphate receptor
Clathrin assembles on the cytosolic side of membranes into a basket-like lattice. Adaptin mediates clathrin binding to the vesicular membrane.
Clathrin consists of three protein chains
1 ARF (ADP-ribosylation factor) bound to GTP associates with the membrane of the Golgi stacks to promote binding of COP coat protein (coatomer), leading to vesicle budding.
2 Hydrolysis of bound GTP changes ARF to GDP-bound, leading to the disassembly of the vesicle coat before the vesicle fuses with a target membrane.
1
GTP
Coatomer (COPI or COPII)
ARF
GDP
Disassembled coatomer
2

Vesicular transport consists of:

1. The formation of a vesicle by budding from a membrane.
2. The assembly of a protein coat on the cytosolic surface of transport vesicles.

There are **two types of coated vesicles**:

1. **Clathrin-coated**, found in endocytic vesicles and vesicles sorted from the *trans*-Golgi to a lysosome.
2. **COP-coated vesicles** (COP stands for coat protein), observed in transporting vesicles between stacks of the Golgi apparatus (**COPI-coated vesicles**) or from the rough endoplasmic reticulum to the Golgi apparatus (**COPII-coated vesicles**).

COP assembly is regulated by two different mechanisms:

1. Clathrin binding to a vesicle is mediated by **adaptins**.
2. COP binding to a vesicle is mediated by **GTP-bound ARF**. The nonbinding form of ARF is **GDP-bound**.

ARF is a member of the **Ras protein family** (involved as oncogenes in cancer; see the MAP kinase pathway in Chapter 3, Cell Signaling).

Ras-related proteins (called **Rab proteins**) are also involved in vesicular transport.

binds to the cytosolic domain of the M6P receptor to guide lysosomal enzymes into clathrin-coated vesicles for lysosomal sorting.

A guanosine triphosphate (GTP)-binding protein called **ARF** (for adenosine diphosphate [ADP]-ribosylation factor), is required for the assembly of COPI and COPII molecules to form a protein coat called a **coatomer** on the cytosolic side of a transporting vesicle. When GTP is converted to guanosine diphosphate (GDP) by hydrolysis, the coatomer dissociates from the vesicle just before the vesicle fuses with a target membrane. ARF is related to **Ras proteins**, a group of oncogene proteins also regulated by the alternate binding of GTP and GDP (see the MAP kinase pathway in Chapter 3, Cell Signaling).

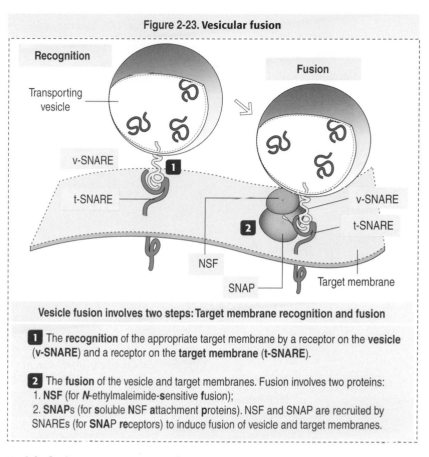

Figure 2-23. Vesicular fusion

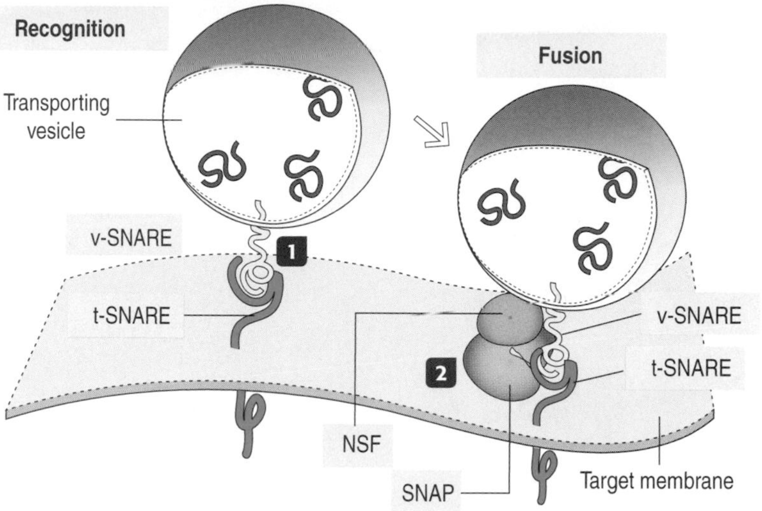

Vesicle fusion involves two steps: Target membrane recognition and fusion

1 The **recognition** of the appropriate target membrane by a receptor on the **vesicle (v-SNARE)** and a receptor on the **target membrane (t-SNARE)**.

2 The **fusion** of the vesicle and target membranes. Fusion involves two proteins:
1. **NSF** (for ***N***-ethylmaleimide-**s**ensitive **f**usion);
2. **SNAPs** (for **s**oluble NSF **a**ttachment **p**roteins). NSF and SNAP are recruited by SNAREs (for **SNA**P **re**ceptors) to induce fusion of vesicle and target membranes.

Vesicle fusion to a target membrane

The fusion of a transporting vesicle to a target membrane (Figure 2-23) requires:

1. The **recognition of the specific target membrane** (for example, a transporting vesicle containing lysosomal enzymes fuses with the membrane of a lysosome).

2. The **vesicle and target membranes fuse** to deliver the transported product.

Vesicle fusion is mediated by two interacting cytosolic proteins: **NSF** (for *N*-ethylmaleimide-sensitive fusion) and **SNAPs** (for soluble NSF attachment proteins). NSF and SNAP bind to specific membrane receptors called SNARE (for SNAP receptors). SNAREs are present on the transporting vesicle (v-SNARE) and target membranes (t-SNARE) and represent **docking proteins.** Following docking, the SNARE complex recruits NSF and SNAPs to produce the fusion of the vesicle and target membranes.

Mitochondria

The mitochondrion (Greek *mito*, thread; *chondrion*, granule) is a highly compartmentalized organelle. The primary function of mitochondria is to house the enzymatic machinery for oxidative phosphorylation resulting in the production of ATP and the release of energy from the metabolism of molecules.

Mitochondria consist of outer and inner membranes separated by an intermembrane space (Figure 2-24). The inner membrane folds into partitions or cristae. Cristae project into the mitochondrial matrix. Cristae contain the **electron transport chain** and **adenosine triphosphate (ATP) synthase.**

Most of the enzymes of the **tricarboxylic acid cycle** (TCA, also called Krebs cycle) and other oxidation pathways are located in the mitochondrial matrix. As you have studied in your Biochemistry course, the TCA cycle is responsible for more than two thirds of the ATP produced from fuel (fatty acids and pyruvate) oxidation.

Figure 2-24. **Mitochondria**

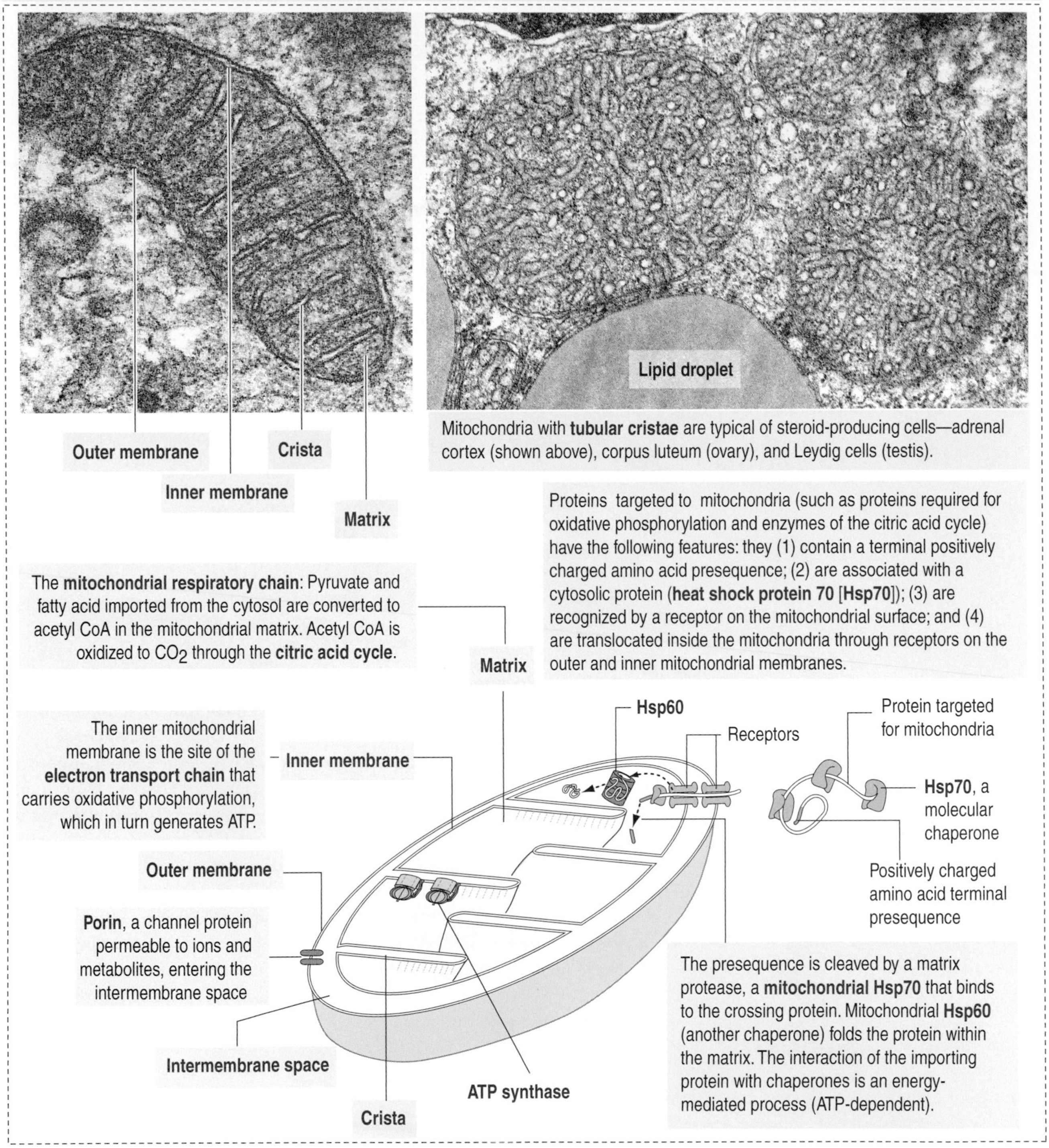

Outer membrane
Crista
Inner membrane
Matrix
Lipid droplet
Mitochondria with **tubular cristae** are typical of steroid-producing cells—adrenal cortex (shown above), corpus luteum (ovary), and Leydig cells (testis).
Proteins targeted to mitochondria (such as proteins required for oxidative phosphorylation and enzymes of the citric acid cycle) have the following features: they (1) contain a terminal positively charged amino acid presequence; (2) are associated with a cytosolic protein (**heat shock protein 70 [Hsp70]**); (3) are recognized by a receptor on the mitochondrial surface; and (4) are translocated inside the mitochondria through receptors on the outer and inner mitochondrial membranes.
The **mitochondrial respiratory chain**: Pyruvate and fatty acid imported from the cytosol are converted to acetyl CoA in the mitochondrial matrix. Acetyl CoA is oxidized to CO_2 through the **citric acid cycle**.
Matrix
Hsp60
Receptors
Protein targeted for mitochondria
The inner mitochondrial membrane is the site of the **electron transport chain** that carries oxidative phosphorylation, which in turn generates ATP.
Inner membrane
Hsp70, a molecular chaperone
Outer membrane
Positively charged amino acid terminal presequence
Porin, a channel protein permeable to ions and metabolites, entering the intermembrane space
The presequence is cleaved by a matrix protease, a **mitochondrial Hsp70** that binds to the crossing protein. Mitochondrial **Hsp60** (another chaperone) folds the protein within the matrix. The interaction of the importing protein with chaperones is an energy-mediated process (ATP-dependent).
Intermembrane space
ATP synthase
Crista

The pathway for oxidation of fatty acids generates **acetyl coenzyme A (acetyl CoA)**, a substrate for the TCA cycle. The oxidation of acetyl CoA and the conservation of energy as **nicotinamide adenine dinucleotide** (**NADH**) and **flavin adenine dinucleotide** FAD(2H) is critical for the production of ATP in most of the tissues. The electron and oxygen carriers NADH and FAD(2H) donate electron to oxygen through the electron transport chain and ATP is generated by oxidative phosphorylation.

The supply of fuels and ATP utilization may change, but cells can maintain a constant level of ATP (ATP homeostasis). The rate of the TCA cycle corresponds to the rate of the electron transport chain, and the latter is regulated by the rate

Figure 2-25. ATP synthase

ATP synthase is an enzyme complex that synthesizes ATP from ADP and inorganic phosphate. It consists of an **F0 portion** associated to the inner mitochondrial membrane and a stalk and headpiece (**F1 portion**) extending into the mitochondrial matrix.

The **F0 portion**, attached to a shaft, consists of **12 C subunits** forming a channel through which protons cross the inner mitochondrial membrane.

The **F1 portion** is composed of three αβ subunit pairs. Each β subunit contains a catalytic site for ATP synthesis.

The F1 portion is kept stationary by a long protein—β subunit—connecting a δ subunit—associated to the headpiece—to subunit A in the inner mitochondrial membrane.

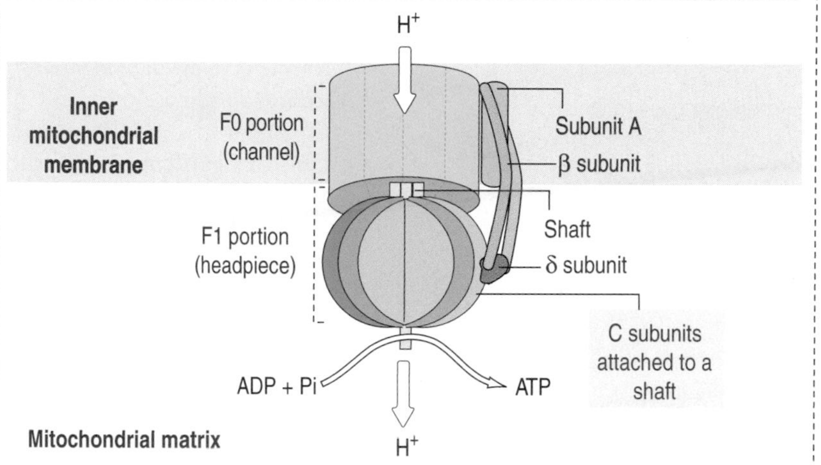

H+
Inner mitochondrial membrane
F0 portion (channel)
Subunit A
β subunit
F1 portion (headpiece)
Shaft
δ subunit
C subunits attached to a shaft
ADP + Pi
ATP
Mitochondrial matrix
H+

of consumption of ATP and the ATP/ADP ratio.

The TCA cycle is essential for the production of energy from cellular respiration. If the TCA cycle is impaired, ATP cannot be generated from fuel oxidation and TCA cycle precursors will build up. A disruption of pyruvate oxidation in the TCA cycle will result in a decrease in lactate that may lead to **lactic acidosis**.

The **outer mitochondrial membrane** contains **porin**, a membrane channel protein that enables the free diffusion of ions and metabolites into the intermembrane space. The **inner mitochondrial membrane** contains **cardiolipin**, a phospholipid (see Box 2-C).

Multiple copies of mitochondrial circular DNA, tRNAs, and ribosomes are present in the matrix. Although most mitochondrial proteins are encoded by genes in the cell nucleus, some are encoded by mitochondrial DNA, and DNA mutations can cause severe abnormalities. Mitochondrial DNA encodes 13 polypeptides that are subunits of proteins required for oxidative phosphorylation.

Enzyme proteins transported to the matrix must cross the outer and inner mitochondrial membranes. **Targeting polypeptide signals** and **chaperones** (**Hsp60** and **Hsp70**) enable proteins to reach the matrix (see Figure 2-24).

ATP synthase (Figure 2-25), a multisubunit complex enzyme that generates ATP, consists of an inner membrane component, **F0 portion**, and a stalk and headpiece (**F1 portion**) projecting into the mitochondrial matrix. The F0 portion, consisting of 12 **C subunits** and an **A subunit**, forms a **rotor** that is attached to a **shaft**. The F1 headpiece is composed of three αβ subunit pairs; the β subunit contains a catalytic site for ATP synthesis. The influx of protons turns the rotor as the newly synthesized ATP is released.

Mitochondria also participate in **programmed cell death** or **apoptosis** and in **steroidogenesis,** the production of steroid hormones.

Concerning apoptosis, mitochondria contain **procaspases-2, -3 and -9** (precursors of proteolytic enzymes), **apoptosis initiation factor** (AIF), and **cytochrome c**. The release of these proteins in the cytosol initiates apoptosis. We come back

Box 2-C | Mitochondria

- Mitochondria are surrounded by a double membrane: the outer mitochondrial membrane and the inner mitochondrial membrane separated by the intermembrane space.
  The outer membrane is permeable and contains channels formed by proteins (porins); the inner membrane is less permeable and contains the phospholipid cardiolipin.
- The inner mitochondrial membrane is folded into cristae extending into the mitochondrial matrix.
- Enzymes of the tricarboxylic acid cycle and mitochondrial DNA are located in the mitochondrial matrix. Enzymes of the electron transport pathway and oxidative phosphorylation are localized in the inner mitochondrial membrane.
- Mitochondria with numerous cristae are present in cardiac muscle and steroid-producing cells.

to mitochondria and apoptosis in Chapter 3, Cell Signaling.

Concerning steroidogenesis, mitochondrial membranes contain enzymes involved in the synthesis of the steroids aldosterone, cortisol, and androgens. We discuss the participation of mitochondria in steroid production in Chapter 19, Endocrine System, and Chapter 20, Spermatogenesis.

The **uncoupling proteins** (**UCPs**) are members of the superfamily of mitochondrial anion-carrier proteins and are present in the mitochondrial inner membrane. UCPs mediate the regulated discharge of protons (called **proton leak**) resulting in the release of heat. Proton leak (movement of the proton H^+) across the mitochondrial inner membrane occurs spontaneously or is mediated by proteins, such as UCP-1. UCP-1 uncouples the processes of electron transport/proton-gradient generation from the process of ATP synthesis. The energy derived from oxidized substrates is released as heat by dissipating the proton gradient.

UCP-1 is present in the mitochondrial inner membrane of brown adipocytes. Its role is to mediate regulated **thermogenesis** in response to cold exposure (see section on adipose tissue in Chapter 4, Connective Tissue).

Clinical significance: Mitochondrial inheritance

Mitochondria are transmitted by the mother (**maternal inheritance**). Both males and females can be affected by mitochondrial diseases, but males never transmit the disorder. **Males do not transmit mitochondria at fertilization.**

Myoclonic epilepsy with ragged red fibers (MERRF) is characterized by generalized muscle weakness, loss of coordination (**ataxia**), and multiple seizures. The major complications are respiratory and cardiac failure because the respiratory and cardiac muscles are affected.

Histologic preparations of muscle biopsies of individuals with MERRF display a peripheral red-stained material corresponding to **aggregates of abnormal mitochondria**, giving a ragged appearance to red muscle fibers. **MERRF is caused by a point mutation in a mitochondrial DNA gene encoding tRNA for lysine.** An abnormal tRNA causes a deficiency in the synthesis of two complexes of the oxidative phosphorylation chain (complexes I and IV). Consequently, neurons and muscle cells, highly dependent on mitochondrial oxidative phosphorylation, are the most affected.

Three maternally inherited mitochondrial diseases affect males more severely than females:

1. About 85% of individuals affected by **Leber's hereditary optic neuropathy** (LHON) are male. The disease is confined to the eye. Individuals suffer a sudden loss of vision in the second and third decades of life.
2. **Pearson marrow-pancreas syndrome** (anemia and mitochondrial myopathy observed in childhood).
3. **Male infertility**. Almost all the energy for sperm motility derives from mitochondria.

Peroxisomes

Peroxisomes are membrane-bound structures (Figure 2-26). They are assembled from proteins synthesized on free ribosomes and then imported into peroxisomes. Peroxisomes contain about 50 different enzymes. **Catalase**, a major peroxisomal enzyme, decomposes hydrogen peroxide into water or is utilized to oxidize other organic compounds (uric acid, amino acids, and fatty acids). The oxidation of fatty acids by mitochondria and peroxisomes provides metabolic energy.

Peroxisomes participate in the biosynthesis of lipids. Cholesterol and dolichol are synthesized in both peroxisomes and endoplasmic reticulum. In liver, peroxisomes are involved in the synthesis of **bile acids** (derived from cholesterol).

Peroxisomes contain enzymes involved in the synthesis of **plasmalogens**, phospholipids in which one of the hydrocarbon chains is linked to glycerol by an ether bond (instead of an ester bond). Plasmalogens are membrane components

Figure 2-26. Peroxisome

1 Proteins for peroxisomes are synthesized by free cytosolic ribosomes and then transported into peroxisomes. Phospholipids and membrane proteins are also imported to peroxisomes from the endoplasmic reticulum.

2 Proteins are targeted to the interior of the peroxisome by targeting amino acid signals (mainly Ser-Lys-Leu at the C-terminal). Other amino acid signals target proteins to the peroxisome membrane. Targeting amino acid signals are not cleaved.

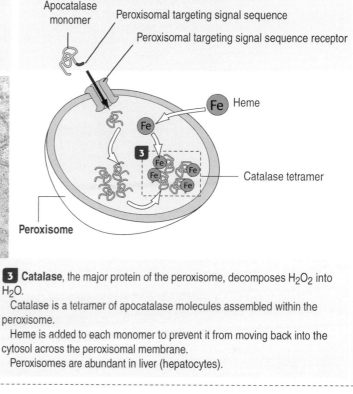

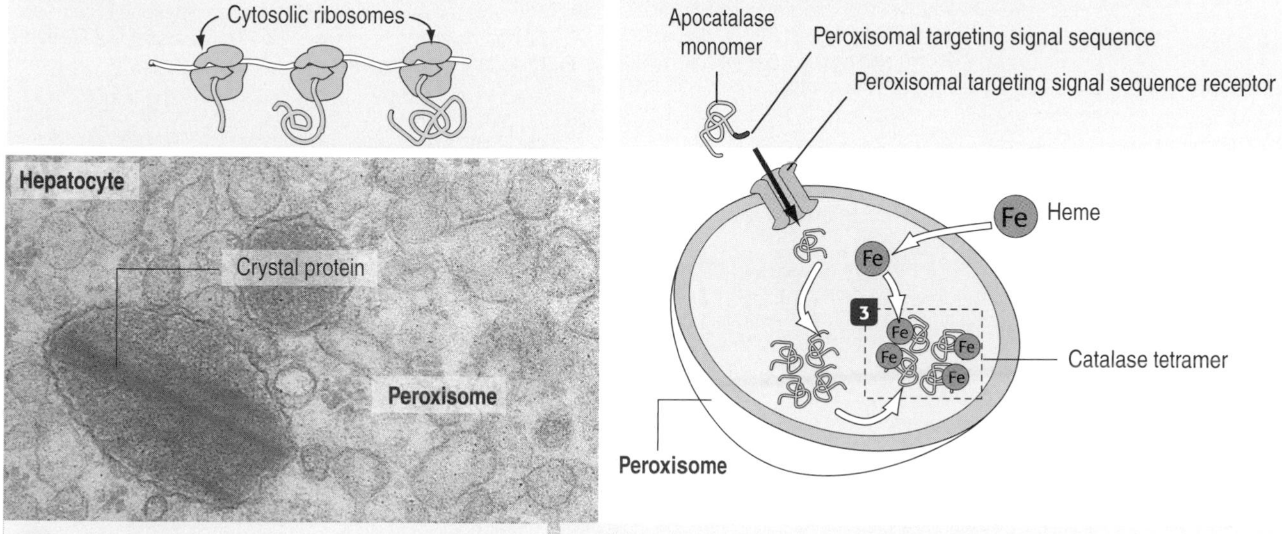

Cytosolic ribosomes
Hepatocyte
Crystal protein
Peroxisome
Apocatalase monomer
Peroxisomal targeting signal sequence
Peroxisomal targeting signal sequence receptor
Fe
Heme
3
Catalase tetramer
Peroxisome

4 **Zellweger syndrome** is a lethal condition caused by the defective assembly of peroxisomes due to the lack of transport of enzyme proteins (but not membrane proteins) into the peroxisome.

Newly synthesized peroxisomal enzymes remain in the cytosol and eventually are degraded. Cells in patients with Zellweger syndrome contain **empty peroxisomes**.

3 **Catalase**, the major protein of the peroxisome, decomposes H_2O_2 into H_2O.

Catalase is a tetramer of apocatalase molecules assembled within the peroxisome.

Heme is added to each monomer to prevent it from moving back into the cytosol across the peroxisomal membrane.

Peroxisomes are abundant in liver (hepatocytes).

of heart and brain.

Clinical significance: Zellweger syndrome

Zellweger syndrome (see Figure 2-26) is a rare, congenital disease, lethal within the first year of life. It belongs to the group of **leukodystrophies**, affecting myelin formation in axons of the brain. Zellweger syndrome is characterized by a **reduction or absence of peroxisomes** in hepatocytes, and cells of the kidney and brain. Multiple peroxisomal proteins, called **peroxins**, fail to be imported into peroxisomes.

The primary defect is the mutation of the *PXR1* (peroxisome receptor 1) gene encoding the receptor on the surface of peroxisomes for peroxisome-targeted enzymes that are required for cellular lipid metabolism and metabolic oxidations. The clinical characteristics include **hepatomegalia** (enlargement of the liver), **high levels of iron and copper in blood**, and **defective vision.** Affected children may show at birth muscle hypotonicity, an inability to move, and a failure to suck or swallow. A diagnostic test is the measurement of plasma **very-long-chain fatty acid (VLCFA)** concentrations, regarded as an indicator of defects in the peroxisomal fatty acid metabolism.

Epithelial glands
There are two types of glands: exocrine glands secrete their products through ducts onto an internal or external space. Endocrine glands secrete their products into the blood and lack ducts.

• There are different types of exocrine glands: Unicellular (a single cell, for example, the goblet cell of the intestinal or respiratory epithelium) and multicellular glands. Multicellular glands form the parenchyma of organs such as the pancreas and the prostate.

• Exocrine glands have two components: the secretory units, whose cells synthesize and secrete a product called secretion, and the excretory ducts, that transport the secretion to an epithelial surface.

• Glands with a single unbranched duct are called simple glands. Larger glands have a branched duct system and are called branched or compound glands. Branched glands are surrounded by a connective tissue capsule that sends partitions or septa into the mass of the gland which becomes partitioned into lobes. Thinner septa partition lobes into smaller units called lobules.

• A simple gland can be straight, coiled, or branched. The gland is called simple tubular, simple coiled, or simple branched tubular. A gland with a secretory unit with a rounded form is called simple acinar or alveolar gland. The secretory unit can be tubular and the gland is called simple tubular.

• In a branched acinar gland, the acini are lined by secretory cells surrounding a narrow lumen. The acinar cellular organization can be part of the wall of short tubular ducts and also form their endings. The gland is then called branched tubuloacinar gland (for example, mammary gland).

• Glands can secrete mucus (mucous glands), proteins (serous glands), or a combination of mucus and proteins (mixed glands). Mixed glands contain both mucous and serous cells, the latter forming a crescentic region (serous demilunes) capping the acini.

• When a gland releases its product by exocytosis, it is called merocrine gland (such as the pancreas). A gland in which the apical region of a cell is pinched off and released into the lumen, is called apocrine gland (an example is the mammary gland). When the whole cell is released and is part of the secretion, the gland is called holocrine gland (such as the sebaceous glands of the skin).

Cytomembranes and the plasma membrane. Intracellular membranes, called cytomembranes, separate diverse cellular processes into compartments. Cytomembranes are components of the endoplasmic reticulum and Golgi apparatus. The nucleus, mitochondria, lysosomes, and peroxisomes are bound by cytomembranes and are called organelles. The nucleus and mitochondria are surrounded by a double membrane; lysosomes and peroxisomes are surrounded by a single membrane. Lipids and glycogen are not membrane-bound and are called inclusions.

• The plasma membrane is the structural and functional boundary of a cell. It separates the intracellular environment from the extracellular space.

The plasma membrane consists of lipids and proteins. Phospholipids form a bilayer consisting of outer and inner leaflets. Cholesterol is inserted into the phospholipid bilayer and modulates membrane fluidity.

Integral membrane proteins are transmembrane proteins spanning the lipid bilayer through α-helical regions. Peripheral membrane proteins are indirectly linked to the plasma membrane by protein-protein interactions. Peripheral membrane proteins exposed to the cytosol interact with cytoskeletal components. The extracellular portion of integral and peripheral membrane proteins is generally glycosylated. A glycocalyx coats the surface of most epithelial cells.

• Freeze-fracture combined with electron microscopy enables the visualization of intramembranous proteins. A frozen and fractured specimen is used to produce a thin metal replica of the two surfaces of a membrane and its two artificial faces.

The lipid bilayer membranes are frozen at liquid nitrogen temperature (−196°C) and "split" along the middle of the hydrophobic core. As a result, two complementary halves of a membrane are produced and the hydrophobic face exposed.

Each half or monolayer of the membrane has a surface and a face. The original monolayer facing the extracellular environment exhibits a surface designated extracellular surface (ES); the corresponding area facing the hydrophobic core of the membrane becomes the extracellular face (EF) and was created artificially after "splitting" the membrane. The original monolayer facing the intracellular or protoplasmic environment has a surface called the protoplasmic surface (PS); the corresponding area facing the hydrophobic core is the protoplasmic face (PF).

Membrane proteins tend to remain associated to the cytoplasmic or protoplasmic leaflet and appear as particles in on the P fracture face (PF). Pits complementary to the particles and representing the space once occupied by the protein, are present on the E fracture face (EF).

• **Transporters** include carrier proteins and channel proteins. They mediate the selective passage of molecules across the cell membrane. Gases (such as oxygen and carbon dioxide) can cross membranes by passive diffusion. Glucose, electrically charged molecules, and small ions require transport proteins and channel proteins for facilitated diffusion across a membrane.

Channel proteins can be ligand-gated channels (which open upon ligand binding) or voltage-gated channels (which open in response to changes in electric potential across the membrane).

• Cytomembranes, represented in part by the endoplasmic reticulum and Golgi apparatus, establish a continuum between intracellular compartments and the extracellular space. The lumen of cisternae, tubules, and vesicles is continuous with the extracellular space. The membranous wall separates the luminal compartment from the cytosolic compartment. Products released into the lumen of the endoplasmic reticulum are transported to the Golgi apparatus by transporting vesicles and eventually to the cell exterior by exocytosis. Imagine that there is a continuum in this secretory sequence and that all the luminal spaces are virtually interconnected and continuous with the cell exterior. The freeze-fracture technique takes advantage of this virtual arrangement if you consider that the splitting knife can jump from the exocytoplasmic leaflet of a membrane-bound vesicle to the exocytoplasmic leaflet of the plasma membrane exposed to the environment.

• The cytomembranes of the endoplasmic reticulum can be associated with ribosomes (rough endoplasmic reticulum) or lack ribosomes (smooth endoplasmic reticulum). The rough endoplasmic reticulum participates in protein synthesis and transport to the Golgi apparatus. The smooth endoplasmic reticulum is generally adjacent to glycogen deposits and lipid droplets (nonmembrane-bound inclusions). Proteins targeted to the nucleus, mitochondria, or peroxisomes are synthesized on free ribosomes and released in the cytosol.

• The **Golgi apparatus** is involved in the attachment of oligosaccharides to proteins and lipids involving glycosyltransferases. It consists of three compartments: (1) a *cis* compartment, the receiving site; (2) a medial compartment, the site where most glycosylation occurs; and (3) a *trans* compartment, the exit and sorting site.

Golgi-derived products can be released from the cell by exocytosis or sorted to lysosomes. Exocytosis can be continuous and does not require a triggering signal. This form of secretion is called constitutive secretion. Exocytosis under control of a chemical or electrical signal is called facultative secretion. The sorting mechanism of lysosomes involves two steps: (1) the insertion of mannose-6-phosphate (M6P) into glycoproteins destined to lysosomes; and (2) the presence of the transmembrane M6P receptor protein in the membrane of the transporting vesicle. This mechanism separates M6P-containing lysosomal enzymes from other glycoproteins.

• Lysosomes are organelles surrounded by a single membrane. Two types of **lysosomes** are recognized: primary lysosomes, the primary storage of lysosomal enzymes, and secondary lysosomes, engaged in a catalytic process. Lysosomes target internalized extracellular material for degradation through the activity of lysosomal hydrolytic enzymes operating at an acidic pH (5.0).

Lysosomal storage disorders occur when hereditary deficiency in lysosomal enzymes prevents the normal breakdown of cell components. Examples are **Tay-Sachs disease** (accumulation of ganglioside GM_2 in the brain), **Gaucher's disease** (accumulation of glucocerebrosides in the spleen and central nervous system), and **Niemann-Pick disease** (accumulation of sphingomyelin in the spleen and central nervous system).

Internalization occurs by the process of endocytosis. The reverse process is called exocytosis. Endocytosis involves the internalization of virus or bacteria by phagocytosis using clathrin-independent vesicles and the uptake of small macromolecules utilizing clathin-coated vesicles.

Receptor-mediated endocytosis of a ligand requires a plasma membrane receptor. The ligand-receptor complex is internalized by the process of receptor-mediated endocytosis. This process involves: (1) the formation of a clathrin-coated pit (to concentrate ligand-receptor complexes in a small surface area); (2) the invagination of the coated pit to form a coated vesicle; (3) the pinching off of the coated vesicle from the plasma membrane; (4) transport of the vesicle to an endosome; (5) removal of the clathrin coat before fusion of the vesicle with the endosome; and (6) recycling back of the receptor-containing vesicle to the plasma membrane.

This transport mechanism is defective in **familial hypercholesterolemia** because of a mutation in the gene encoding the receptor for the ligand low-density lipoprotein (LDL). High levels of cholesterol in blood plasma result in the formation of atheromas in the intima of blood vessels.

• The fusion of a vesicle to a target membrane requires: (1) recognition of a specific target membrane site; and (2) the vesicle-membrane fusion. Vesicle fusion is mediated by two interacting cytosolic proteins: NSF (for *N*-ethylmaleimide-sensitive fusion) and SNAP (for soluble NSF attachment protein). NSF and SNAP bind to specific membrane receptors called SNARE (for SNAP receptors). SNARE ligands on the membrane of the transporting vesicle (vesicle-SNARE, v-SNARE) and the target membrane receptor (target-SNARE, t-SNARE) are responsible for docking the vesicle to the target membrane. Following docking, NSF and SNAP are recruited to produce fusion.

• Mitochondria are organelles surrounded by a double membrane. The outer mitochondrial membrane is separated by an intermembrane space from the inner mitochondrial membrane. The inner membrane folds into cristae extending into the mitochondrial matrix. Cristae contain the electron transport chain and adenosine triphosphate (ATP) synthase. The mitochondrial matrix contains most of the enzymes of the tricarboxylic acid cycle, (also called the Krebs cycle).

Mitochondria participate in apoptosis (programmed cell death), steroidogenesis, and thermogenesis in brown fat.

Mitochondria are transmitted by the mother (maternal inheritance). Males do not transmit mitochondria at fertilization. Both males and females can be affected by mitochondrial disease, but males never transmit the disorder.

Myoclonic epilepsy with ragged red fibers (MERRF) presents with muscle weakness, loss of coordination (ataxia), and multiple sizures. MERRF is caused by a mutation in a mitochondrial DNA gene encoding lysine tRNA.

Maternally inherited mitochondrial diseases affecting males more severely than females are **Leber's hereditary optic neuropathy** (LHON), **Pearson marrow-pancreas syndrome**, and **male infertility**.

• Peroxisomes are organelles surrounded by a single membrane. Peroxisomes contain catalase, an enzyme that decomposes hydrogen peroxide into water and oxidizes organic compounds. Peroxisomes are involved in the synthesis of bile acids and biosynthesis of lipids.

Zellweger syndrome is determined by the failure of peroxisomal enzymes to be imported from the cytosol into the peroxisome. This condition is lethal.

3. CELL SIGNALING

Cells respond to extracellular signals produced by other cells or by themselves. This mechanism, called **cell signaling**, allows cell-cell communication and is necessary for the functional regulation and integration of multicellular organisms. Our discussion in this chapter not only provides the basis for understanding normal cell function but serves also as an introduction to the role of abnormal cell signaling in human disease.

Signaling molecules are either **secreted** or **expressed at the cell surface** of one cell. Signaling molecules can bind to receptors on the surface of another cell or the same cell.

Different types of signaling molecules transmit information in multicellular organisms, and their mechanisms of action on their target cells can be diverse. Some signaling molecules can act on the cell surface after binding to cell surface receptors; others can cross the plasma membrane and bind to intracellular receptors in the cytoplasm and nucleus.

When a signaling molecule binds to its receptor, it initiates a cascade of intracellular reactions to regulate critical functions such as **cell proliferation, differentiation, movement, metabolism**, and **behavior**. Because of their critical role in the control of normal cell growth and differentiation, signaling molecules have acquired significant relevance in cancer research.

Box 3-A | **Paracrine cell signaling**

- **Paracrine signaling molecules** include four major families of proteins: 1. The **fibroblast growth factor (FGF) family**. 2. The **Hedgehog family**. 3. The **wingless (Wnt) family**. 4. The **transforming growth factor β (TGF-β) superfamily**.
- Each of these signaling proteins can bind to one or more receptors. Mutations of genes encoding these proteins may lead to abnormal cell-cell interaction.
- The first member of the **Hedgehog family** was isolated in a *Drosophila* mutant with bristles in a naked area in the normal fly. The most widely found hedgehog homolog in vertebrates is **sonic hedgehog (Shh)**. Shh participates in the development of the neural plate and neural tube (see Chapter 8, Nervous Tissue). Shh binds to a transmembrane protein encoded by the ***patched*** gene and suppresses transcription of genes encoding members of the Wnt and TGF-β families and inhibits cell growth. Mutation of the patched homolog in humans (***PTC***) causes the **Gorlin syndrome** (rib abnormalities, cyst of the jaw, and basal cell carcinoma, a form of skin cancer).
- The **Wnt family** of genes is named after the *Drosophila* gene ***wingless***. In vertebrates, *Wnt* genes encode secretory glycoproteins that specify the dorsal-ventral axis and formation of brain, muscle, gonads, and kidneys.
- The **TGF-β superfamily** encodes protein forming **homodimers** and **heterodimers**. Members of this superfamily include the TGF-β family itself, the **bone morphogenetic protein (BMP) family**, the **activin family**, and the **vitellogenin 1 (Vg1) family**. Mutations in a member of the BMP family, **cartilage-derived morphogenetic protein-1 (CDMP1)** causes skeletal abnormalities. Vg1 is a signaling molecule determining the left-right axis in embryos.

Cell signaling mechanisms

Five major types of cell-cell signaling are considered (Figure 3-1):

1. **Endocrine cell signaling** involves a signaling molecule, called a **hormone**, secreted by an **endocrine cell and transported through the circulation to act on distant target cells**. An example is the steroid hormone testosterone produced in the testes, that stimulates the development and maintenance of the male reproductive tract.
2. **Paracrine cell signaling** is mediated by a signaling molecule acting **locally** to regulate the behavior of a **nearby cell**. An example is the action of **neurotransmitters** produced by nerve cells and released at a **synapse**. See Box 3-A for a summary of the four major families of paracrine signaling molecules.
3. **Autocrine cell signaling** is defined by **cells responding to signaling molecules that they themselves produce.** A classic example is the response of cells of the immune system to foreign antigens or growth factors that trigger their own proliferation and differentiation. Abnormal autocrine signaling leads to the unregulated growth of cancer cells.
4. **Neurotransmitter cell signaling**, a specific form of paracrine signaling.
5. **Neuroendocrine cell signaling**, a specific form of endocrine signaling.

Mechanisms of action of cell signaling molecules

Cell signaling molecules exert their action after binding to receptors expressed by their target cells. Target cells, in turn, can determine either a **negative** or **positive feedback** action to regulate the release of the targeting hormone (Figure 3-2).

Cell receptors can be expressed on the **cell surface** of the target cells. Some receptors are **intracellular proteins** in the **cytosol** or the **nucleus** of target cells. Intracellular receptors require that the signaling molecules **diffuse across the plasma membrane** (Figure 3-3).

Steroid hormones (Box 3-B) belong to this class of signaling molecules. Steroid hormones are synthesized from **cholesterol** and include **testosterone, estrogen, progesterone**, and **corticosteroids**.

Testosterone, estrogen, and progesterone are **sex steroids** and are produced

Figure 3-1. Mechanisms of hormone action

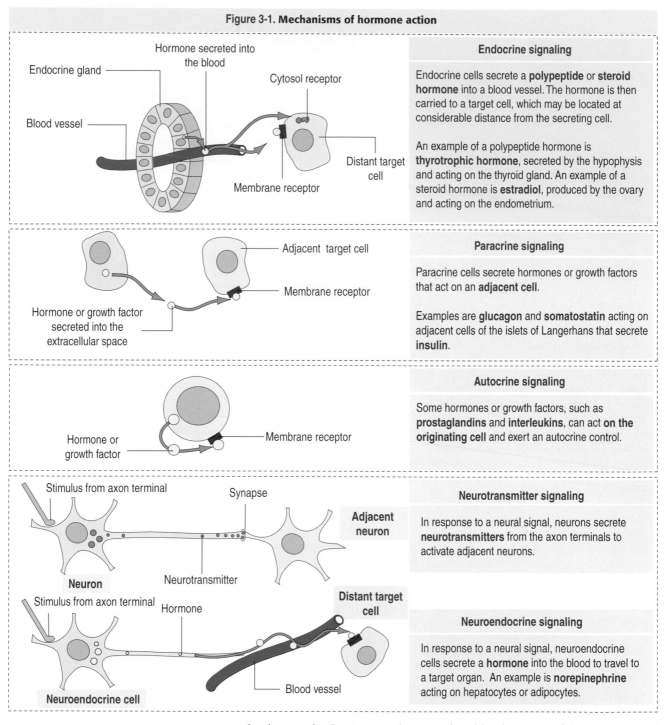

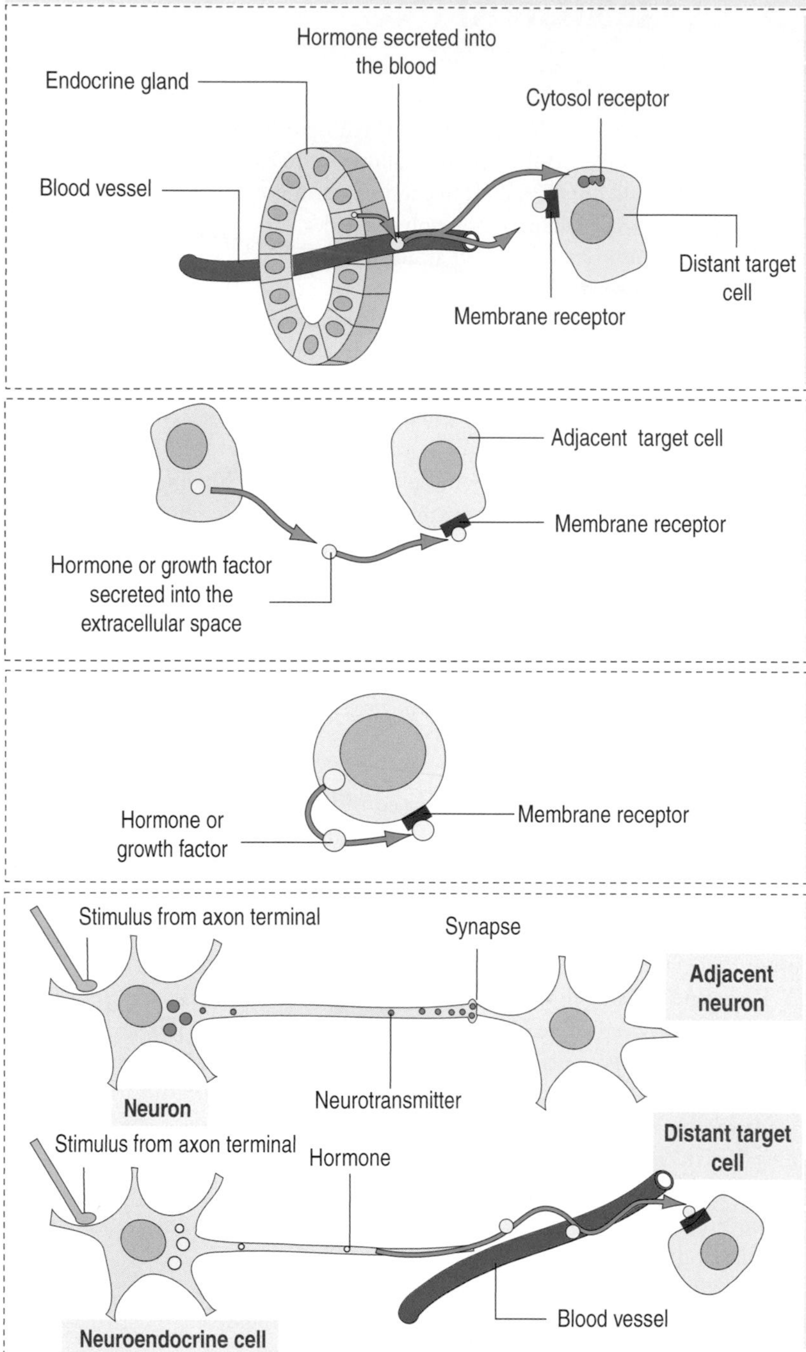

Endocrine signaling

Endocrine cells secrete a **polypeptide** or **steroid hormone** into a blood vessel. The hormone is then carried to a target cell, which may be located at considerable distance from the secreting cell.

An example of a polypeptide hormone is **thyrotrophic hormone**, secreted by the hypophysis and acting on the thyroid gland. An example of a steroid hormone is **estradiol**, produced by the ovary and acting on the endometrium.

Paracrine signaling

Paracrine cells secrete hormones or growth factors that act on an **adjacent cell**.

Examples are **glucagon** and **somatostatin** acting on adjacent cells of the islets of Langerhans that secrete **insulin**.

Autocrine signaling

Some hormones or growth factors, such as **prostaglandins** and **interleukins**, can act **on the originating cell** and exert an autocrine control.

Neurotransmitter signaling

In response to a neural signal, neurons secrete **neurotransmitters** from the axon terminals to activate adjacent neurons.

Neuroendocrine signaling

In response to a neural signal, neuroendocrine cells secrete a **hormone** into the blood to travel to a target organ. An example is **norepinephrine** acting on hepatocytes or adipocytes.

Box 3-B | **Steroid hormones**

- They derive from **cholesterol**.
- They bind mainly to **intracellular receptors** in the cytosol and nucleus.
- They circulate in blood **bound to a protein**.
- They are **nonpolar** molecules.
- Steroid hormones **are not stored in the producing endocrine cell**.
- Steroid hormones **can be administered orally** and are readily absorbed in the gastrointestinal tract.

by the gonads. Corticosteroids are produced by the cortex of the adrenal gland and include two major classes: **glucocorticoids**, which stimulate the production of glucose, and **mineralocorticoids**, which act on the kidney to regulate water and salt balance.

There are three cell signaling molecules that are structurally and functionally distinct from steroids but act on target cells by binding to intracellular receptors after entering the cell by diffusion across the plasma membrane. They include **thyroid hormone** (produced in the thyroid gland to regulate development and metabolism), **vitamin D_3** (regulates calcium metabolism and bone growth), and **retinoids** (synthesized from vitamin A to regulate development).

Steroid receptors are members of the **steroid receptor superfamily**. They act as transcription factors through their DNA binding domains, which have transcrip-

Figure 3-2. **Feedback**

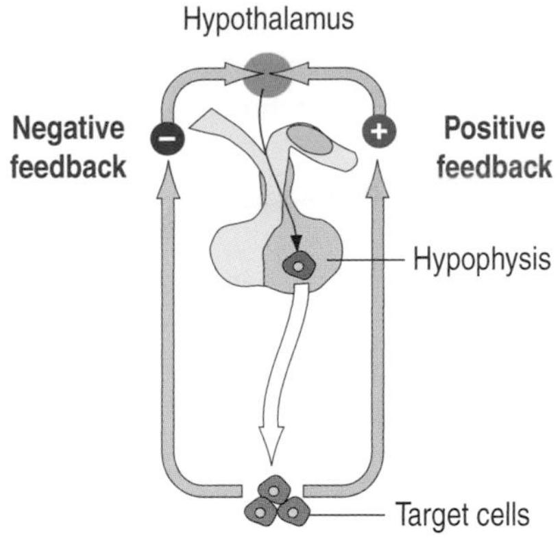

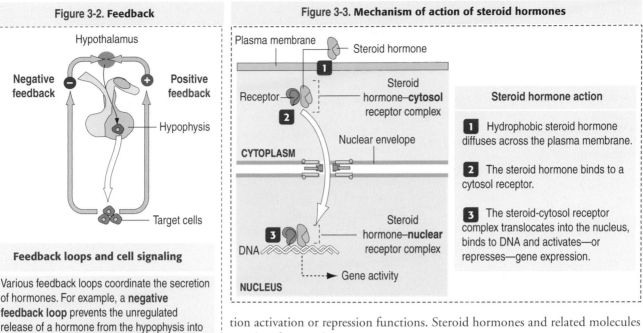

Hypothalamus
Negative feedback
Positive feedback
Hypophysis
Target cells

Feedback loops and cell signaling

Various feedback loops coordinate the secretion of hormones. For example, a **negative feedback loop** prevents the unregulated release of a hormone from the hypophysis into the blood circulation when the target cell or tissue may be nonresponsive.

A **positive feedback loop** (more rarely) occurs when the hypophysis senses a decrease in the blood levels of a hormone produced by the target cell or tissue. See Chapter 19, Endocrine System, for additional details.

Figure 3-3. **Mechanism of action of steroid hormones**

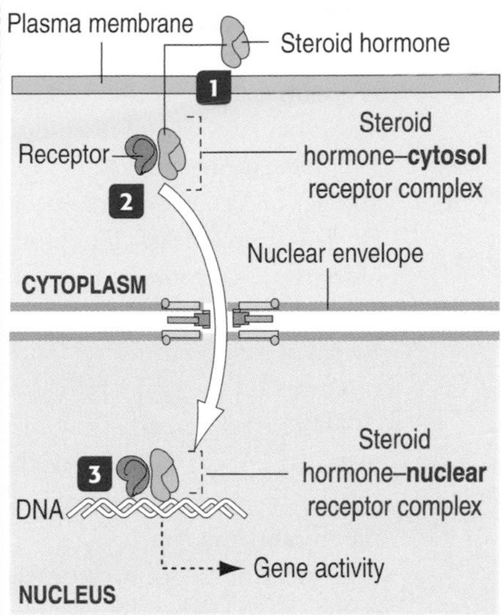

Plasma membrane
Steroid hormone
1
Receptor
2
Steroid hormone–**cytosol** receptor complex
Nuclear envelope
CYTOPLASM
3
DNA
Steroid hormone–**nuclear** receptor complex
Gene activity
NUCLEUS

Steroid hormone action

1 Hydrophobic steroid hormone diffuses across the plasma membrane.

2 The steroid hormone binds to a cytosol receptor.

3 The steroid-cytosol receptor complex translocates into the nucleus, binds to DNA and activates—or represses—gene expression.

tion activation or repression functions. Steroid hormones and related molecules can therefore regulate gene expression.

In the **androgen insensitivity syndrome** (also known as the **testicular feminization syndrome** [**Tfm**]), there is a mutation in the gene expressing the **testosterone receptor** such that the receptor cannot bind the hormone, and hence the cells do not respond to the hormone. Although genetically male, the individual develops the secondary sexual characteristics of a female. We discuss the androgen insensitivity syndrome in Chapter 21, Sperm Transport and Maturation.

Nitric oxide

Nitric oxide is a signaling molecule. It is a simple gas synthesized from the amino acid **arginine** by the enzyme **nitric oxide synthase**. It acts as a paracrine signaling molecule in the nervous, immune, and circulatory systems. Like steroid hormones, nitric oxide can diffuse across the plasma membrane of its target cells. Unlike steroids, nitric oxide does not bind to an intracellular receptor to regulate transcription. Instead, **it regulates the activity of intracellular target enzymes**.

The following are relevant characteristics of nitric oxide:

1. It is an unstable molecule with a limited half-life (seconds).
2. It has local effects.
3. A well-defined function of nitric oxide signaling is the **dilation of blood vessels**. For example, the release of the neurotransmitter acetylcholine from nerve cell endings in the blood vessel muscle cell wall stimulates the release of nitric oxide from endothelial cells.

Nitric oxide increases the activity of the second messenger cyclic guanosine monophosphate (cGMP; see later in this section) in smooth muscle cells, which then causes cell muscle relaxation and blood vessel dilation. **Nitroglycerin, a pharmacologic agent used in the treatment of heart disease, is converted to nitric oxide, which increases heart blood flow by dilation of the coronary blood vessels.**

Box 3-C | **Peptide hormones**

- They are synthesized as **precursor molecules** (prohormones).
- They are stored in **membrane-bound secretory vesicles**.
- They are generally **water soluble** (polar).
- They circulate in blood as **unbound molecules**.
- Peptide hormones **cannot be administered orally**.
- They usually bind to **cell surface receptors**.

Cell signaling molecules bind to cell surface receptors

A large variety of signaling molecules bind to cell surface receptors. Several groups are recognized:

1. **Peptides** (Box 3-C): This group includes **peptide hormones** (insulin, glucagon, and hormones secreted by the hypophysis), **neuropeptides**, secreted by neurons (**enkephalins** and **endorphins**, which decrease pain responses in the central nervous system), and **growth factors**, which control cell growth and

Box 3-D | Eicosanoids

1. They **derive from polyunsaturated fatty acids** with 18, 20, and 22 carbons.
2. **Arachidonic acid** is the main precursor.
3. This group includes **prostaglandins**, **leukotrienes**, **thromboxanes**, and **prostacyclin**.
4. They have primary **autocrine** and **paracrine** actions.
5. The **synthesis of eicosanoids is regulated by hormones**.
6. They usually bind to **cell surface receptors**.

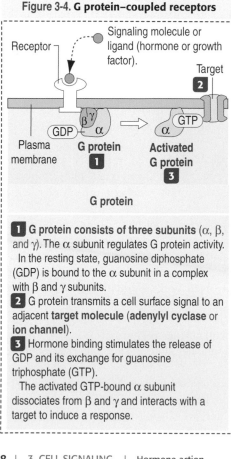

Figure 3-4. G protein–coupled receptors

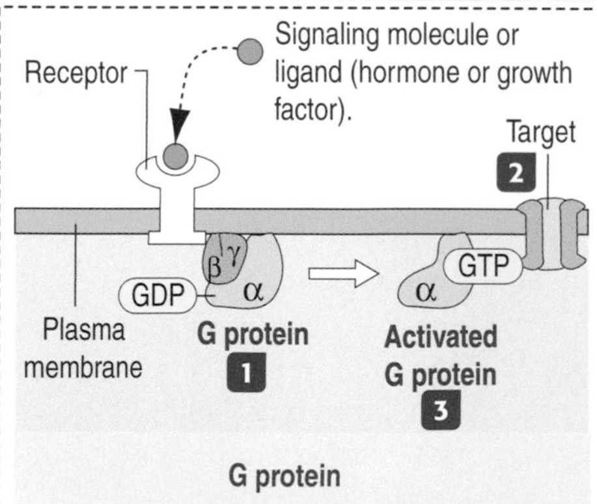

Signaling molecule or ligand (hormone or growth factor).
Receptor
Target
2
GDP
β γ
α
GTP
α
Plasma membrane
G protein
1
Activated G protein
3
G protein

1 **G protein consists of three subunits** (α, β, and γ). The α subunit regulates G protein activity. In the resting state, guanosine diphosphate (GDP) is bound to the α subunit in a complex with β and γ subunits.
2 G protein transmits a cell surface signal to an adjacent **target molecule** (**adenylyl cyclase** or **ion channel**).
3 Hormone binding stimulates the release of GDP and its exchange for guanosine triphosphate (GTP).
The activated GTP-bound α subunit dissociates from β and γ and interacts with a target to induce a response.

differentiation (**nerve growth factor** [NGF]; **epidermal growth factor** [EGF]; **platelet-derived growth factor** [PDGF]; and **cytokines**).

NGF is a member of a family of peptides called **neurotrophins**, which regulate the development and viability of neurons. EGF stimulates cell proliferation and is essential during embryonic development and in the adult. PDGF is stored in blood platelets and released during clotting.

2. **Neurotransmitters**: These cell signaling molecules are released by neurons and act on cell surface receptors present in neurons or other type of target cells (such as muscle cells). This group includes **acetylcholine**, **dopamine**, **epinephrine** (adrenaline), **serotonin**, **histamine**, **glutamate**, and **γ-aminobutyric acid** (GABA). The release of neurotransmitters from neurons is triggered by an **action potential**. Released neurotransmitters diffuse across the **synaptic cleft** and bind to surface receptors on the target cells.

There are differences that distinguish the **mechanism of action of neurotransmitters**. For example, **acetylcholine is a ligand-gated ion channel**. It induces a change in conformation of ion channels to control ion flow across the plasma membrane in target cells.

As we will see soon, neurotransmitter receptors can be associated to G proteins, a class of signaling molecules linking cell surface receptors to intracellular responses.

Some neurotransmitters have a **dual function**. For example, epinephrine (produced in the medulla of the adrenal gland) can act as a neurotransmitter and as a hormone to induce the breakdown of glycogen in muscle cells.

3. **Eicosanoids and leukotrienes**: These are lipid-containing cell-signaling molecules that, **in contrast to steroids, bind to cell surface receptors** (Box 3-D).

Prostaglandins, **prostacyclin**, **thromboxanes**, and **leukotrienes** are members of this group of molecules. They stimulate blood platelet aggregation, inflammatory responses, and smooth muscle contraction.

Eicosanoids are synthesized from **arachidonic acid**. During the synthesis of prostaglandins, arachidonic acid is converted to **prostaglandin H_2** by the enzyme **prostaglandin synthase**. This enzyme is inhibited by **aspirin** and **anti-inflammatory drugs**. **Inhibition of prostaglandin synthase by aspirin reduces pain, inflammation, platelet aggregation, and blood clotting** (prevention of strokes).

Pathways of intracellular signaling by cell surface receptors

When a cell-signaling molecule binds to a specific receptor, it activates a series of **intracellular targets located downstream of the receptor**. Several molecules associated with receptors have been identified:

1. **G protein–coupled receptors** (guanine nucleotide–binding proteins): Members of a large family of **G proteins** (more than 1000 proteins) are present at the inner leaflet of the plasma membrane (Figure 3-4).

When a signaling molecule or **receptor ligand** binds to the extracellular portion of a cell surface receptor, its cytosolic domain undergoes a conformational change that enables binding of the receptor to a G protein. This contact activates the G protein, which then dissociates from the receptor and triggers an intracellular signal to an enzyme or ion channel. We return to the G protein when we discuss the cyclic adenosine monophosphate (cAMP) pathway.

2. **Tyrosine kinases as receptor proteins** (Figure 3-5): These surface receptors are themselves enzymes that phosphorylate substrate proteins on **tyrosine** residues. **EGF, NGF, PDGF, insulin, and several growth factors are receptor protein tyrosine kinases.** Most of the receptor protein tyrosine kinases consist of single polypeptides, although the insulin receptor and other growth factors consist of a pair of polypeptide chains.

Binding of a ligand (a growth factor) to the extracellular domain of these receptors induces **receptor dimerization** that results in **receptor autophosphorylation** (the two polypeptide chains phosphorylate one another). The autophosphoryla-

Figure 3-5. Tyrosine kinases

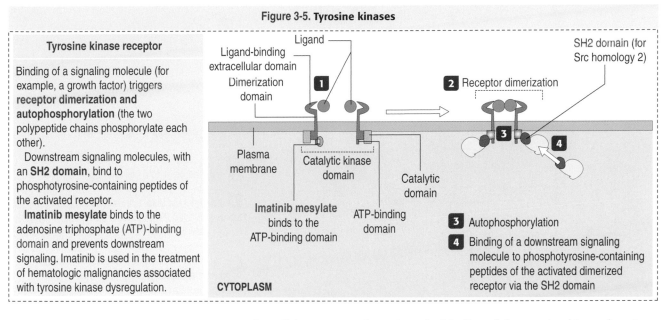

Tyrosine kinase receptor

Binding of a signaling molecule (for example, a growth factor) triggers **receptor dimerization and autophosphorylation** (the two polypeptide chains phosphorylate each other).

Downstream signaling molecules, with an **SH2 domain**, bind to phosphotyrosine-containing peptides of the activated receptor.

Imatinib mesylate binds to the adenosine triphosphate (ATP)-binding domain and prevents downstream signaling. Imatinib is used in the treatment of hematologic malignancies associated with tyrosine kinase dysregulation.

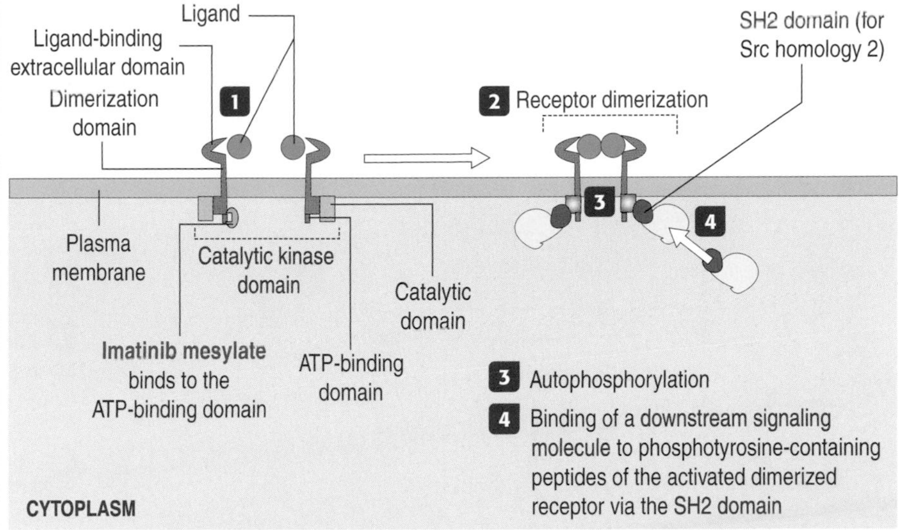

tion of the receptors determines the binding of the tyrosine kinase domain to downstream signaling molecules. Downstream signaling molecules bind to phosphotyrosine residues through domains called **SH2 domains** (for Src homology 2). *Src* (for **sarcoma**) is a gene present in the tumor-producing Rous sarcoma virus and encodes a protein that functions as a protein tyrosine kinase.

3. **Cytokine receptors:** This family of receptors stimulates **intracellular protein tyrosine kinases**, which **are not intrinsic components of the receptor**. A growth factor ligand induces the dimerization and cross-phosphorylation of the associated tyrosine kinases. Activated kinases phosphorylate the receptors, providing binding sites for downstream signaling molecules that contain the SH2 domain.

The cytokine receptor–associated tyrosine kinases belong to two families: the ***Src* family** and the **Janus kinase family** (JAK).

4. **Receptors linked to other enzymes** (**protein tyrosine phosphatases** and **protein serine and threonine kinases**): Some receptors associate with protein tyrosine phosphatases to remove phosphate groups from phosphotyrosine residues. Therefore, **they regulate the effect of protein tyrosine kinases by arresting signals initiated by protein tyrosine phosphorylation.**

Members of the **transforming growth factor-β** (**TGF-β**) family are protein kinases that phosphorylate serine and threonine residues (rather than tyrosine). TGF-β inhibits the proliferation of their target cells. Like tyrosine kinase and cytokine receptors, binding of ligand to the TGF-β receptor induces receptor dimerization and the cytosolic protein serine or threonine kinase domain cross-phosphorylates the polypeptide chains of the receptor.

Clinical significance: Tyrosine kinases, targets for therapeutic agents

There are two main classes of tyrosine kinases: (1) **receptor tyrosine kinases** are transmembrane proteins with a ligand-binding extracellular domain and a catalyic intracellular kinase domain (see Figure 3-5), and (2) **nonreceptor tyrosine kinases** found in the cytosol, nucleus, and inner side of the plasma membrane.

The transmembrane receptor kinase subfamily belongs to the PDGF family, which includes c-kit. The subfamily of nonreceptor tyrosine kinases includes the **Src family**, the **Fujinami poultry sarcoma/feline sarcoma** (Fps/Fes), and **Fes-related** (Fer) subfamily.

In the absence of a ligand, receptor tyrosine kinases are unphosphorylated and monomeric. The nonreceptor tyrosine kinase is maintained in an inactive state by cellular inhibitor proteins. Activation occurs when the inhibitors are dissociated or by recruitment to transmembrane receptors that trigger autophosphorylation.

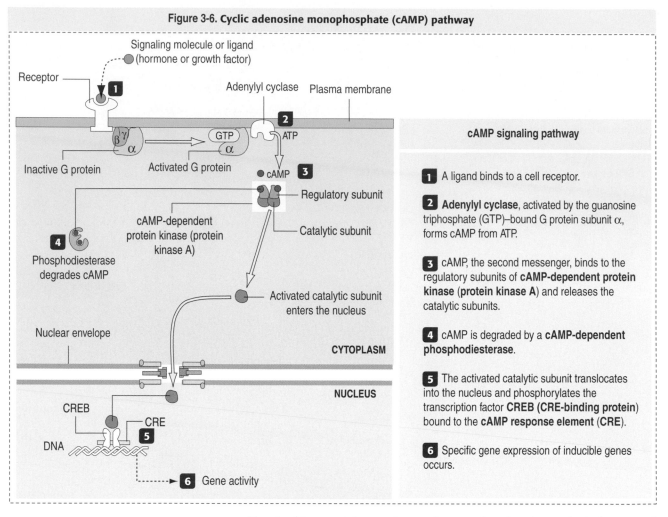

Figure 3-6. Cyclic adenosine monophosphate (cAMP) pathway

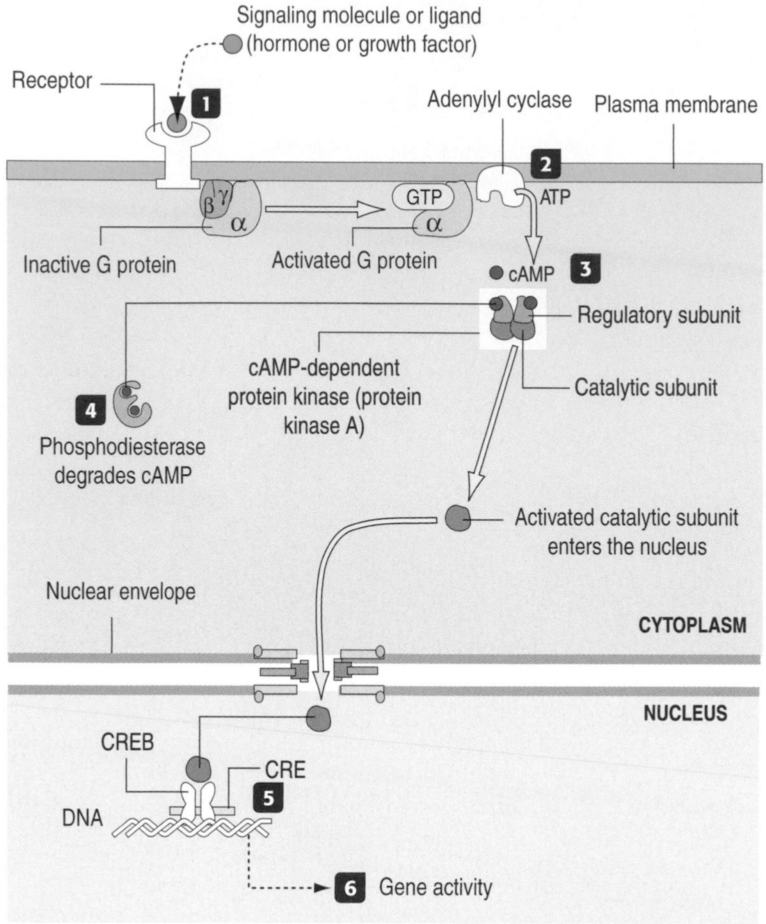

Signaling molecule or ligand
(hormone or growth factor)
Receptor
1
Adenylyl cyclase
Plasma membrane
2
GTP
ATP
β γ
α
α
Inactive G protein
Activated G protein
cAMP
3
Regulatory subunit
cAMP-dependent protein kinase (protein kinase A)
Catalytic subunit
4
Phosphodiesterase degrades cAMP
Activated catalytic subunit enters the nucleus
Nuclear envelope
CYTOPLASM
NUCLEUS
CREB
CRE
5
DNA
6
Gene activity

cAMP signaling pathway

1 A ligand binds to a cell receptor.

2 **Adenylyl cyclase**, activated by the guanosine triphosphate (GTP)–bound G protein subunit α, forms cAMP from ATP.

3 cAMP, the second messenger, binds to the regulatory subunits of **cAMP-dependent protein kinase** (**protein kinase A**) and releases the catalytic subunits.

4 cAMP is degraded by a **cAMP-dependent phosphodiesterase**.

5 The activated catalytic subunit translocates into the nucleus and phosphorylates the transcription factor **CREB (CRE-binding protein)** bound to the **cAMP response element** (**CRE**).

6 Specific gene expression of inducible genes occurs.

Tyrosine kinase activity terminates when tyrosine phosphatases hydrolyze tyrosyl phosphates and by induction of inhibitory molecules.

The activity of tyrosine kinases in cancer cells can be disrupted by a protein that determines unregulated autophosphorylation in the absence of a ligand, by disrupting autoregulation of the tyrosine kinase, or by overexpression of receptor tyrosine kinase and/or its ligand. Abnormal activation of tyrosine kinases can stimulate the proliferation and anticancer drug resistance of malignant cells.

Tyrosine kinase activity can be inhibited by **imatinib mesylate**, a molecule that binds to the adenosine triphosphate (ATP)–binding domain of the tyrosine kinase catalytic domain. Imatinib can induce hematologic remission in patients with chronic myeloid leukemia and in tumors caused by activated receptor tyrosine kinase PDGF receptor (chronic myelomonocytic leukemia) and c-kit (systemic mastocytosis and mast cell leukemias). Imatinib has been successfully used in the treatment of gastrointestinal solid tumors.

Major pathways of intracellular cell signaling

Upon ligand binding, most cell surface receptors stimulate intracellular target enzymes to **transmit and amplify a signal**. An amplified signal can be propagated to the nucleus to regulate gene expression in response to an external cell stimulus.

The major intracellular signaling pathways include the cAMP and cGMP pathways, the phospholipase C–Ca^{2+} pathway, the **NF-κB** (for nuclear factor involved in the transcription of the κ light chain gene in B lymphocytes) transcription factor pathway, the Ca^{2+}-calmodulin pathway, the **MAP** (for mitogen-activated protein) kinase pathway, and the **JAK-STAT** (for signal transducers and activators of transcription) pathway.

The cAMP pathway

The intracellular signaling pathway mediated by **cAMP** was discovered in 1958 by Earl Sutherland while studying the action of **epinephrine**, a hormone that breaks down glycogen into glucose before muscle contraction.

When epinephrine binds to its receptor, there is an increase in the intracellular concentration of cAMP. cAMP is formed from adenosine triphosphate (ATP) by the action of the enzyme **adenylyl cyclase** and degraded to adenosine monophosphate (AMP) by the enzyme **cAMP phosphodiesterase**. This mechanism led to the concept of a **first messenger** (epinephrine) mediating a cell-signaling effect by a **second messenger**, cAMP. The epinephrine receptor is linked to adenylyl cyclase by G protein, which stimulates cyclase activity upon epinephrine binding.

The intracellular signaling effects of cAMP (Figure 3-6) are mediated by the enzyme **cAMP-dependent protein kinase** (or **protein kinase A**). **In its inactive form, protein kinase A is a tetramer composed of two regulatory subunits** (to which cAMP binds) **and two catalytic subunits**. Binding of cAMP results in the **dissociation of the catalytic subunits**. Free catalytic subunits can phosphorylate **serine residues** on target proteins.

In the epinephrine-dependent regulation of glycogen metabolism, protein kinase A phosphorylates two enzymes:

1. **Phosphorylase kinase**, which in turn phosphorylates glycogen phosphorylase to break down glycogen into glucose-1-phosphate.
2. **Glycogen synthase**, which is involved in the synthesis of glycogen. Phosphorylation of glycogen synthase prevents the synthesis of glycogen.

Note that an elevation of cAMP results in two distinct events: the breakdown of glycogen and, at the same time, a blockage of further glycogen synthesis. Also note that the binding of epinephrine to a single receptor leads to a signal amplification mechanism during intracellular signaling mediated by many molecules of cAMP. cAMP signal amplification is further enhanced by the phosphorylation of many molecules of phosphorylase kinase and glycogen synthase by the catalytic subunits dissociated from protein kinase A. It is important to realize that protein phosphorylation can be rapidly reversed by **protein phosphatases** present in the cytosol and as transmembrane proteins. These protein phosphatases can terminate responses initiated by the activation of kinases by removing phosphorylated residues.

cAMP also has an effect on the transcription of specific target genes that contain a regulatory sequence called the **cAMP response element** (**CRE**). Catalytic subunits of protein kinase A enter the nucleus after dissociation from the regulatory subunits. Within the nucleus, catalytic subunits phosphorylate a transcription factor called **CRE-binding protein** (**CREB**), which activates cAMP-inducible genes.

Finally, cAMP effects can be direct, independent of protein phosphorylation. An example is the direct regulation of **ion channels in the olfactory epithelium**. **Odorant receptors** in sensory neurons of the nose are linked to G protein, which stimulates adenylyl cyclase to increase intracellular cAMP.

cAMP does not stimulate protein kinase A in sensory neurons but acts directly to open Na^+ channels in the plasma membrane to initiate membrane depolarization and nerve impulses.

The cGMP pathway

cGMP is also a second messenger. It is produced from guanosine triphosphate (GTP) by guanylate cyclase and degraded to GMP by a phosphodiesterase. Guanylate cyclases are activated by nitric oxide and peptide signaling molecules.

The best characterized role of cGMP is in photoreceptor rod cells of the retina, where it converts light signals to nerve impulses. Chapter 9, Sensory Organs: Vision and Hearing, in the eye section, provides a detailed description of this cell signaling process.

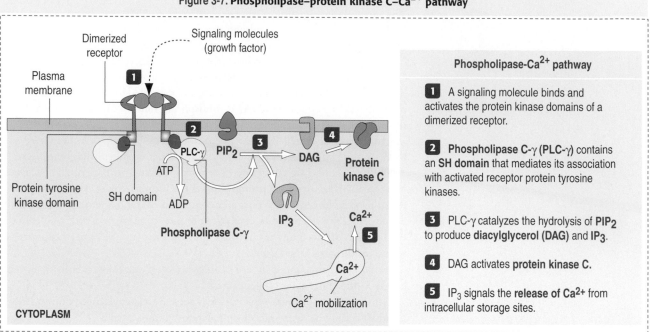

Figure 3-7. **Phospholipase–protein kinase C–Ca^{2+} pathway**

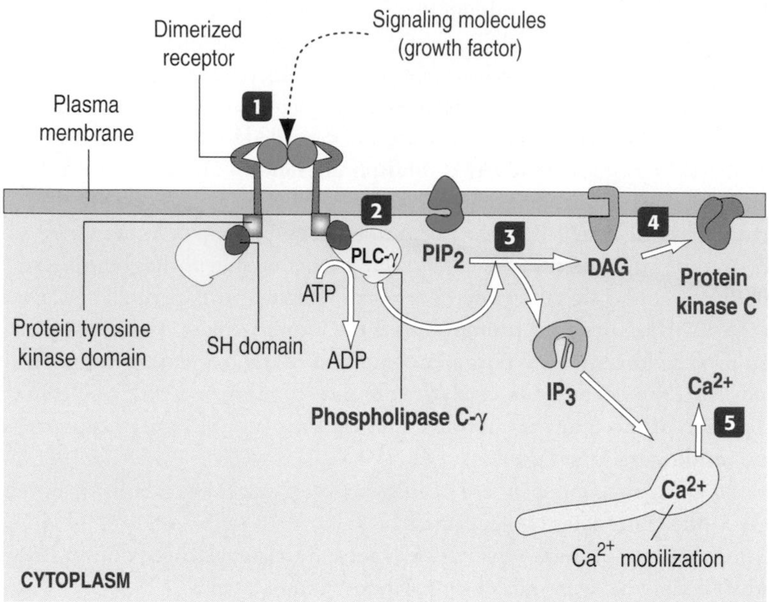

Phospholipase-Ca^{2+} pathway

1 A signaling molecule binds and activates the protein kinase domains of a dimerized receptor.

2 **Phospholipase C-γ (PLC-γ)** contains an **SH domain** that mediates its association with activated receptor protein tyrosine kinases.

3 PLC-γ catalyzes the hydrolysis of **PIP_2** to produce **diacylglycerol (DAG)** and **IP_3**.

4 DAG activates **protein kinase C.**

5 IP_3 signals the **release of Ca^{2+}** from intracellular storage sites.

Phospholipase C–Ca^{2+} pathway

Another second messenger involved in intracellular signaling derives from the phospholipid **phosphatidylinositol 4,5-bisphosphate** (PIP_2) present in the inner leaflet of the plasma membrane (Figure 3-7).

The hydrolysis of PIP_2 by the enzyme **phospholipase C (PLC)**—stimulated by a number of hormones and growth factors—produces two second messengers: **diacylglycerol** and **inositol 1,4,5-trisphosphate** (IP_3).

These two messengers stimulate two downstream signaling pathway cascades: **protein kinase C** and **Ca^{2+} mobilization.**

Two forms of PLC exist: **PLC-β** and **PLC-γ**. PLC-β is activated by G protein. PLC-γ contains SH2 domains that enable association with receptor protein tyrosine kinases. Tyrosine phosphorylation increases PLC-γ activity, which in turn stimulates the breakdown of PIP_2.

Diacylglycerol, derived from PIP_2 hydrolysis, activates members of the **protein kinase C** family (**protein serine and threonine kinases**).

Phorbol esters are tumor growth–promoting agents acting, like diacylglycerol, by stimulation of protein kinase C activities. Protein kinase C activates other intracellular targets such as protein kinases of the **MAP kinase pathway** to produce the phosphorylation of transcription factors leading to changes in gene expression and cell proliferation.

NF-κB transcription factor pathway

NF-κB is a transcription factor involved in immune responses in several cells and is stimulated by protein kinase C (Figure 3-8).

In its **inactive state**, the NF-κB protein heterodimer is bound to the **inhibitory subunit** I-κB and the complex is retained in the cytoplasm. The phosphorylation of I-κB—triggered by I-κB kinase—leads to the destruction of I-κB by the 26S proteasome and the release of NF-κB. The free NF-κB heterodimer translocates into the nucleus to activate gene transcription in response to immunologic and inflammatory signaling.

Ca^{2+}–calmodulin pathway

Although the second messenger diacylglycerol remains associated with the plasma membrane, the other second messenger IP_3, derived from PIP_2, is released into

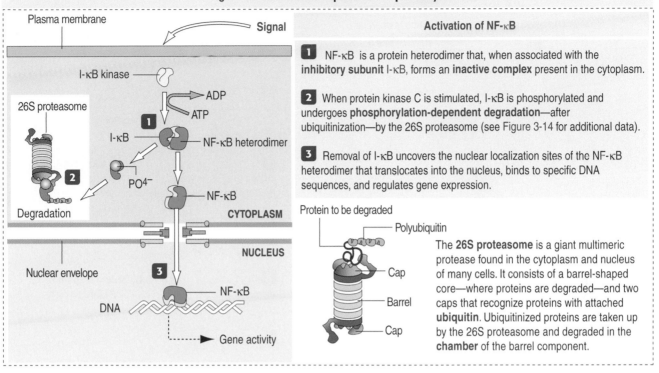

Figure 3-8. NF-κB transcription factor pathway

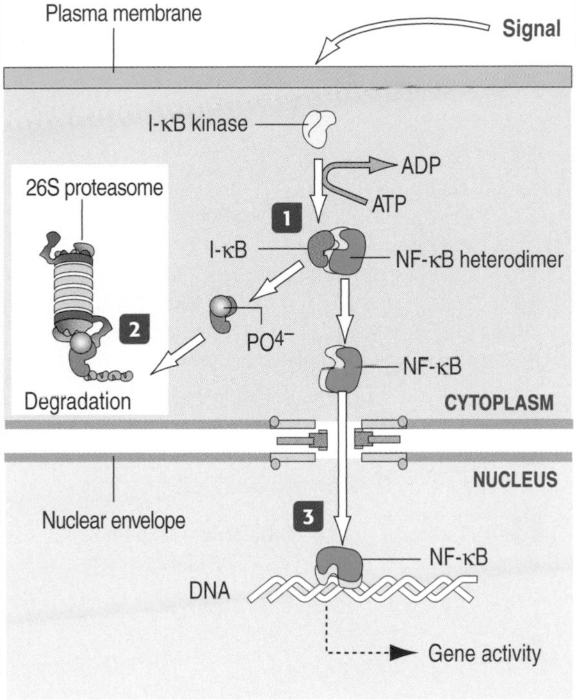

Activation of NF-κB

1 NF-κB is a protein heterodimer that, when associated with the **inhibitory subunit** I-κB, forms an **inactive complex** present in the cytoplasm.

2 When protein kinase C is stimulated, I-κB is phosphorylated and undergoes **phosphorylation-dependent degradation**—after ubiquitinization—by the 26S proteasome (see Figure 3-14 for additional data).

3 Removal of I-κB uncovers the nuclear localization sites of the NF-κB heterodimer that translocates into the nucleus, binds to specific DNA sequences, and regulates gene expression.

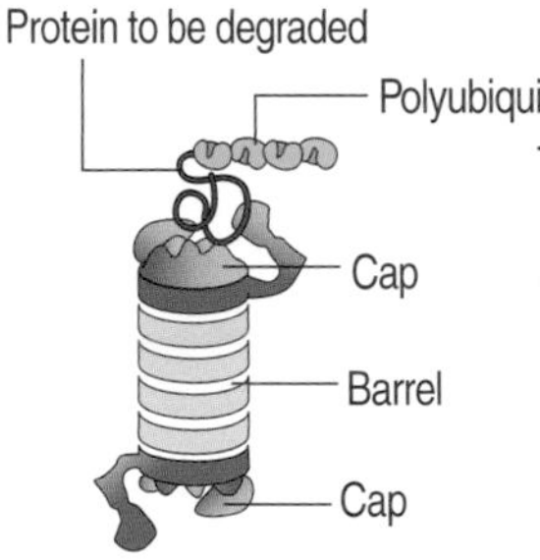

The **26S proteasome** is a giant multimeric protease found in the cytoplasm and nucleus of many cells. It consists of a barrel-shaped core—where proteins are degraded—and two caps that recognize proteins with attached **ubiquitin**. Ubiquitinized proteins are taken up by the 26S proteasome and degraded in the **chamber** of the barrel component.

the cytosol to activate ion pumps and free Ca^{2+} from intracellular storage sites. High cytosolic Ca^{2+} concentrations (from a basal level of 0.1 μM to an increased 1.0 μM concentration after cytosolic release) activate several Ca^{2+}-dependent protein kinases and phosphatases.

Calmodulin is a Ca^{2+}-dependent protein that is activated when the Ca^{2+} concentration increases to 0.5 μM. Ca^{2+}-calmodulin complexes bind to a number of cytosolic target proteins to regulate cell responses. Note that **Ca^{2+} is an important second messenger** and that its intracellular concentration can be increased not only by its release from intracellular storage sites but also by increasing the entry of Ca^{2+} into the cell from the extracellular space.

MAP kinase pathway

This pathway involves evolutionarily conserved protein kinases (yeast to humans) with roles in cell growth and differentiation. **MAP kinases** are protein serine and threonine kinases activated by growth factors and other signaling molecules (Figure 3-9).

A well-characterized form of MAP kinase is the ERK family. Members of the **ERK** (for extracellular signal–regulated kinase) family act **through either protein tyrosine kinase or G protein–associated receptors.** Both cAMP and Ca^{2+}-dependent pathways can stimulate or inhibit the ERK pathway in different cell types.

The activation of ERK is mediated by two protein kinases: **Raf**, a protein serine or threonine kinase, which, in turn, activates a second kinase called **MEK** (for MAP kinase or ERK kinase). Stimulation of a growth factor receptor leads to the activation of the GTP-binding protein **Ras** (for rat sarcoma virus), which interacts with Raf. Raf phosphorylates and activates MEK, which then activates ERK by phosphorylation of serine and threonine residues. ERK then phosphorylates nuclear and cytosolic target proteins.

In the nucleus, activated ERK phosphorylates the transcription factors **Elk-1** (for E-26-like protein 1) and **serum response factor** (**SRF**), which recognize the regulatory sequence called **serum response element** (**SRE**).

In addition to ERK, mammalian cells contain two other MAP kinases called **JNK** and **p38 MAP kinases.** Cytokines and ultraviolet irradiation stimulate JNK

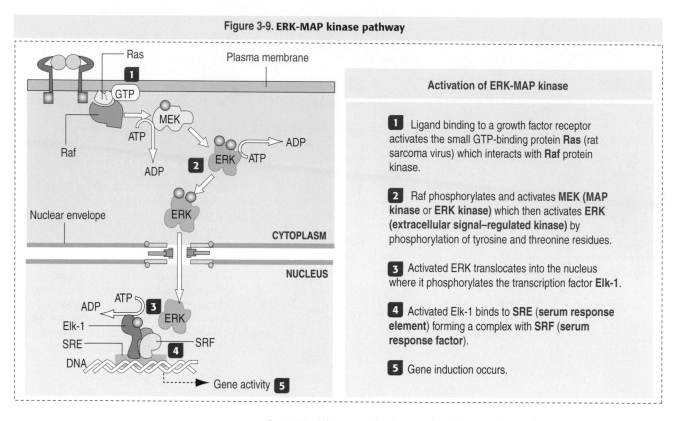

Figure 3-9. ERK-MAP kinase pathway

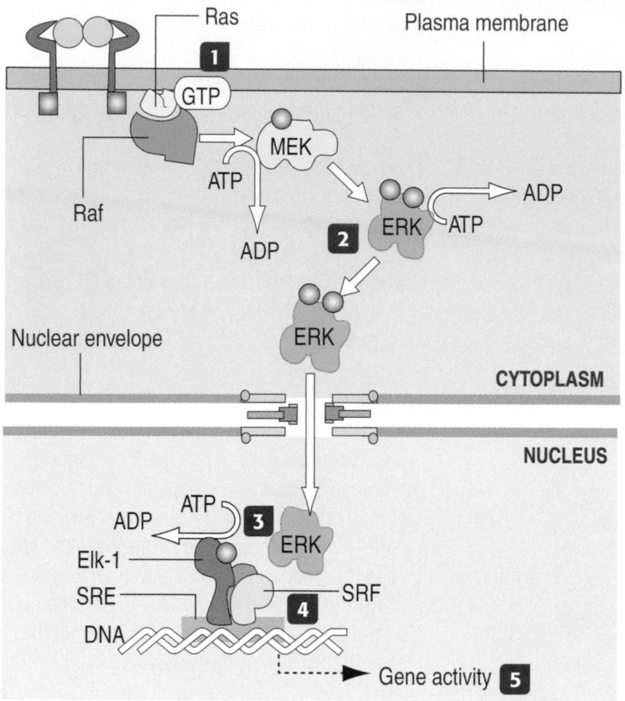

Activation of ERK-MAP kinase

1 Ligand binding to a growth factor receptor activates the small GTP-binding protein **Ras** (rat sarcoma virus) which interacts with **Raf** protein kinase.

2 Raf phosphorylates and activates **MEK (MAP kinase** or **ERK kinase)** which then activates **ERK (extracellular signal–regulated kinase)** by phosphorylation of tyrosine and threonine residues.

3 Activated ERK translocates into the nucleus where it phosphorylates the transcription factor **Elk-1**.

4 Activated Elk-1 binds to **SRE (serum response element)** forming a complex with **SRF (serum response factor)**.

5 Gene induction occurs.

and p38 MAP kinase activation mediated by small GTP-binding proteins different from Ras. These kinases are not activated by MEK but by a distinct dual kinase called **MKK** (for MAP kinase kinase).

A key element in the ERK pathway are the **Ras proteins**, a group of oncogenic proteins of tumor viruses that cause sarcomas in rats. Mutations in the Ras gene have been linked to human cancer. **Ras proteins are guanine nucleotide–binding protein with functional properties similar to the G protein α subunits** (activated by **GTP** and inactivated by guanosine diphosphate [**GDP**]).

A difference with G protein is that Ras proteins do not associate with $\beta\gamma$ subunits. Ras is activated by **guanine nucleotide exchange factors** to facilitate the release of GDP in exchange for GTP. The activity of the Ras-GTP complex is terminated by GTP hydrolysis, which is stimulated by **GTPase-activating proteins.**

In human cancers, mutation of *Ras* genes results in a breakdown failure of GTP and, therefore, the mutated Ras protein remains continuously in the active GTP-bound form.

JAK-STAT pathway

The preceding MAP kinase pathway links the cell surface to the nucleus signaling mediated by a protein kinase cascade leading to the phosphorylation of transcription factors.

The **JAK-STAT pathway** provides a close connection between protein tyrosine kinases and transcription factors by directly affecting transcription factors (Figure 3-10).

STAT (for **signal transducers and activators of transcription**) **proteins** are transcription factors with an SH2 domain and are present in the **cytoplasm** in an inactive state. Stimulation of a receptor by ligand binding recruits STAT proteins, which bind to the cytoplasmic portion of receptor-associated **JAK protein tyrosine kinase** through their SH2 domain and become phosphorylated. Phosphorylated STAT proteins then dimerize and translocate into the nucleus, where they activate the transcription of target genes.

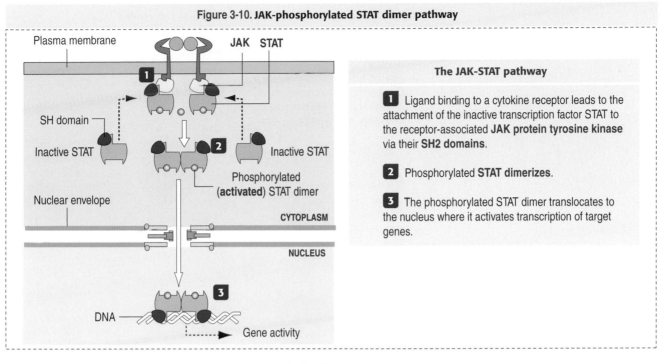

Figure 3-10. **JAK-phosphorylated STAT dimer pathway**

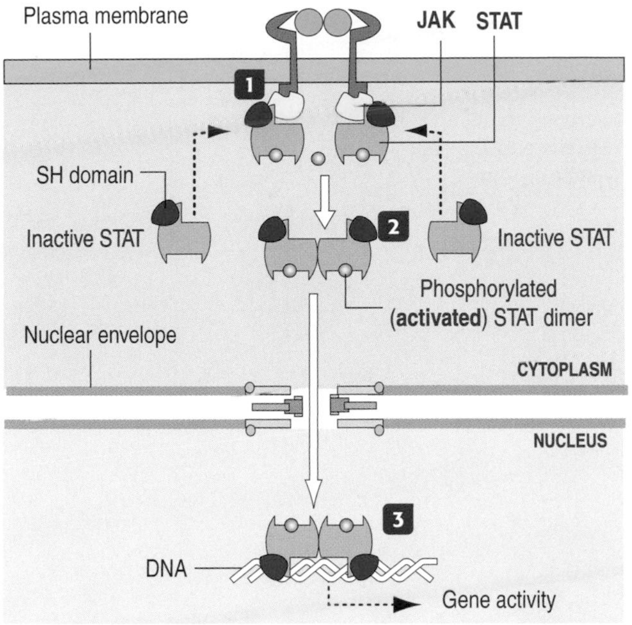
Plasma membrane
JAK
STAT
1
SH domain
Inactive STAT
2
Inactive STAT
Phosphorylated
(activated) STAT dimer
Nuclear envelope
CYTOPLASM
NUCLEUS
3
DNA
Gene activity

The JAK-STAT pathway

1 Ligand binding to a cytokine receptor leads to the attachment of the inactive transcription factor STAT to the receptor-associated **JAK protein tyrosine kinase** via their **SH2 domains**.

2 Phosphorylated **STAT dimerizes**.

3 The phosphorylated STAT dimer translocates to the nucleus where it activates transcription of target genes.

Transcription factor genes: *SOX9*

Genes encoding proteins that turn on (activate) or turn off (repress) other genes are called transcription factors. Many transcription factors have common DNA-binding domains and can also activate or repress a single target gene as well as other genes (a cascade effect). Therefore, mutations affecting genes encoding transcription factor have **pleiotropic effects** (Greek *pleion,* more; *trope*, a turning toward).

Examples of transcription factor genes include homeobox-containing genes, high mobility group (HMG)-box–containing genes, and the T-box family.

The HMG domain of Sox proteins can bend DNA, and facilitate the interaction of enhancers with a distantly located promoter region of a target gene. Several *SOX* genes act in different developmental pathways. For example, Sox9 protein is expressed in the gonadal ridges of both sexes but is upregulated in males and downregulated in females before gonadal differentiation. Sox9 also regulates chondrogenesis and the expression of type II collagen (see Chapter 4, Connective Tissue). Mutations of the *SOX9* gene cause skeletal defects (campomelic dysplasia), and sex reversal (XY females).

Stem cells, a multipotent cell population

Cells in the body show a remarkable range in ability to divide and grow. Some cells (for example, nerve cells and erythrocytes) reach a mature, differentiated state and usually do not divide. Such cells are referred to as **postmitotic cells**. Other cells, called **stem cells**, show continuous division throughout life (for example, epithelial cells lining the intestine and stem cells that give rise to the various blood cell types).

Many other cells are intermediate between these two extremes and remain quiescent most of the time but can be triggered to divide by appropriate signals. Liver cells are an example. If the liver is damaged, cell division can be triggered to compensate for the lost cells.

Stem cells have three properties: **self-renewal**, **proliferation**, and **differentiation**.

Stem cells have the potential to generate a large number of mature cells continuously throughout life. When stem cells divide by mitosis, some of the progeny differentiates into a specific cell type. Other progeny remains as stem cells (Figure

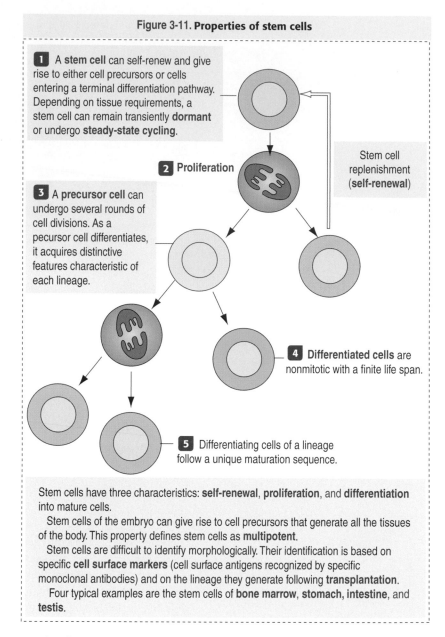

Figure 3-11. Properties of stem cells

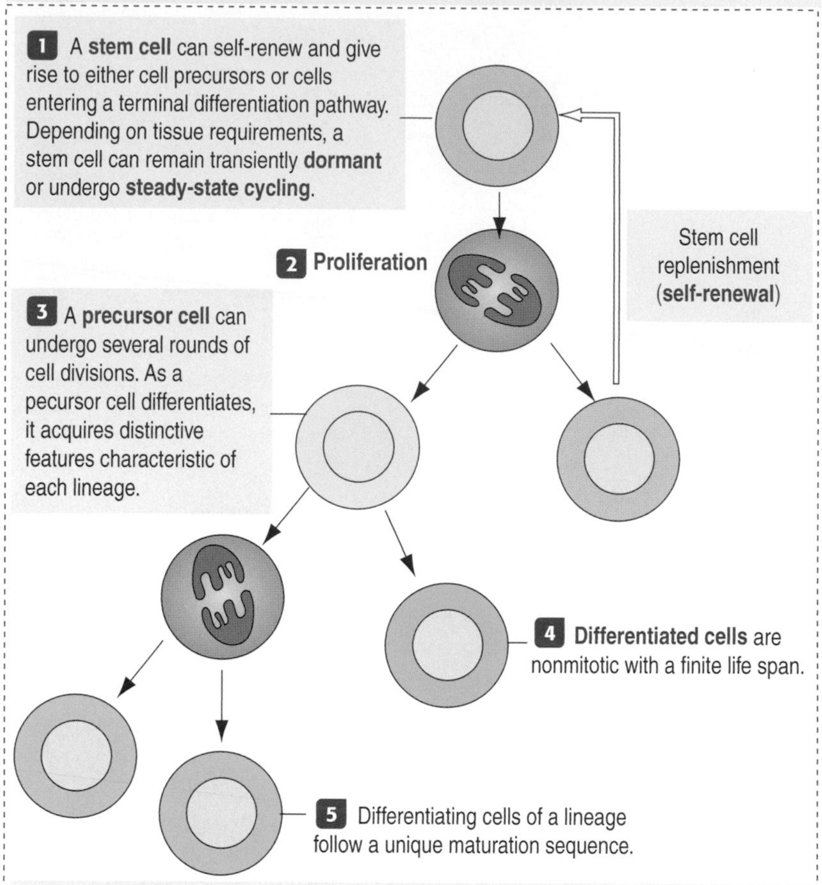
1 A **stem cell** can self-renew and give rise to either cell precursors or cells entering a terminal differentiation pathway. Depending on tissue requirements, a stem cell can remain transiently **dormant** or undergo **steady-state cycling**.
2 Proliferation
Stem cell replenishment (self-renewal)
3 A **precursor cell** can undergo several rounds of cell divisions. As a pecursor cell differentiates, it acquires distinctive features characteristic of each lineage.
4 **Differentiated cells** are nonmitotic with a finite life span.
5 Differentiating cells of a lineage follow a unique maturation sequence.

Stem cells have three characteristics: **self-renewal**, **proliferation**, and **differentiation** into mature cells.

Stem cells of the embryo can give rise to cell precursors that generate all the tissues of the body. This property defines stem cells as **multipotent**.

Stem cells are difficult to identify morphologically. Their identification is based on specific **cell surface markers** (cell surface antigens recognized by specific monoclonal antibodies) and on the lineage they generate following **transplantation**.

Four typical examples are the stem cells of **bone marrow**, **stomach, intestine**, and **testis**.

3-11). The intestinal epithelium, the epidermis of the skin, the hematopoietic system, and spermatogenic cells of the seminiferous epithelium share this property. We discuss in detail the significance of stem cells in each of these tissues in the appropriate chapters. Following stress and injury, other tissues, such as liver, muscle, and the nervous system, can regenerate mature cells.

For example, it has been shown that bone marrow stem cells can produce muscle tissue as well as hematopoietic tissue in an appropriate host system (see Chapter 7, Muscle Tissue). Cultured stem cells of the central nervous system are capable of hematopoiesis in transplanted irradiated mouse recipients.

Recall that embryonic stem cells, forming the **inner cell mass (embryoblast)** of the early embryo (the blastocyst), give rise to all the tissues and organs except the placenta. Embryonic stem cells provide an experimental source of medically useful differentiating tissues such as pancreatic islets for the treatment of diabetes, skin for the treatment of burns and wounds, regenerating cartilage for the treatment of arthritis, and endothelial cells for the repair of blood vessels affected by arteriosclerosis. A potential complication is that embryonic stem cells injected into mature mice develop an embryonic tumor called a **teratoma**.

In vitro cell proliferation, senescence, and telomerase

Cell culture techniques have been a powerful tool for examining the factors that regulate cell growth and for comparing the properties of normal and cancer cells.

Many cells grow in tissue culture, but some are much easier to grow than others. Culture medium contains **salts**, **amino acids**, **vitamins**, and a source of energy such as **glucose**. In addition, most cells require a number of **hormones** or **growth factors** for sustained culture and cell division. These factors are usually provided by addition of **serum** to the culture medium.

For some cell types the components supplied by serum have been identified, and these cells can be grown in **serum-free, hormone and growth factor–supplemented medium**. Some of these factors are hormones, such as insulin. A number of growth factors have been identified, for example, EGF, fibroblast growth factor (FGF), and PDGF.

When normal cells are placed in culture in the presence of adequate nutrients and growth factors, they will grow until they cover the bottom of the culture dish, forming a monolayer. Further cell division then ceases. This is called **density-dependent inhibition of growth**. The cells become quiescent but can be triggered to enter the cell cycle and divide again by an additional dose of growth factor or by replating at a lower cell density.

Cells cultured from a tissue can be kept growing and dividing by regularly replating the cells at lower density once they become confluent. After about 50 cell divisions, however, the cells begin to stop dividing and the cultures become **senescent**. The number of divisions at which this occurs depends on the age of the individual from which the initial cells were taken. Cells from an embryo will thus keep growing longer than cells taken from an adult.

In our discussion of mitosis (see Figure 1-51 in Chapter 1, Epithelium), we call attention to the role of **telomerase**, an enzyme that maintains the ends of chromosomes, or **telomeres**.

In normal cells, insufficient telomerase activity limits the number of mitotic divisions and forces the cell into **senescence**, defined as the finite capacity for cell division. **Telomere shortening and the limited life span of a cell are regarded as potent tumor suppressor mechanisms**. Most human tumors express **human telomerase reverse transcriptase** (**hTERT**). The ectopic expression of hTERT in primary human cells confers endless growth in culture. The use of telomerase inhibitors in cancer patients is currently being pursued.

Occasionally cells that would normally stop growing become altered and appear to become **immortal**. Such cells are called a **cell line**. Cell lines are very useful experimentally and still show most of the phenotype and growth characteristics of the original cells.

An additional change known as **transformation** is associated with the potential for **malignant growth**. Transformed cells no longer show normal growth control and have many alterations, such as **anchorage-independent growth**. Normal cells can grow when anchored to a solid substrate.

Cells in culture can be transformed by **chemical carcinogens** or by **infection with certain viruses** (tumor viruses). Tumor viruses will also cause tumors in certain host animals, but in different species they may cause ordinary infections. Cancer cells cultured from tumors also show the characteristics of transformation. We will discuss at the end of this chapter the role of retroviruses in carcinogenesis.

Apoptosis or programmed cell death

Cell death occurs by necrosis or apoptosis. Under normal physiologic conditions, cells deprived of survival factors, damaged, or senescent commit suicide through an orderly regulated cell death program called **apoptosis** (Greek *apo*, off; *ptosis*, fall).

Apoptosis (Figure 3-12) is different from **necrosis**. Necrosis is a nonphysiologic

Figure 3-12. **Programmed cell death or apoptosis**

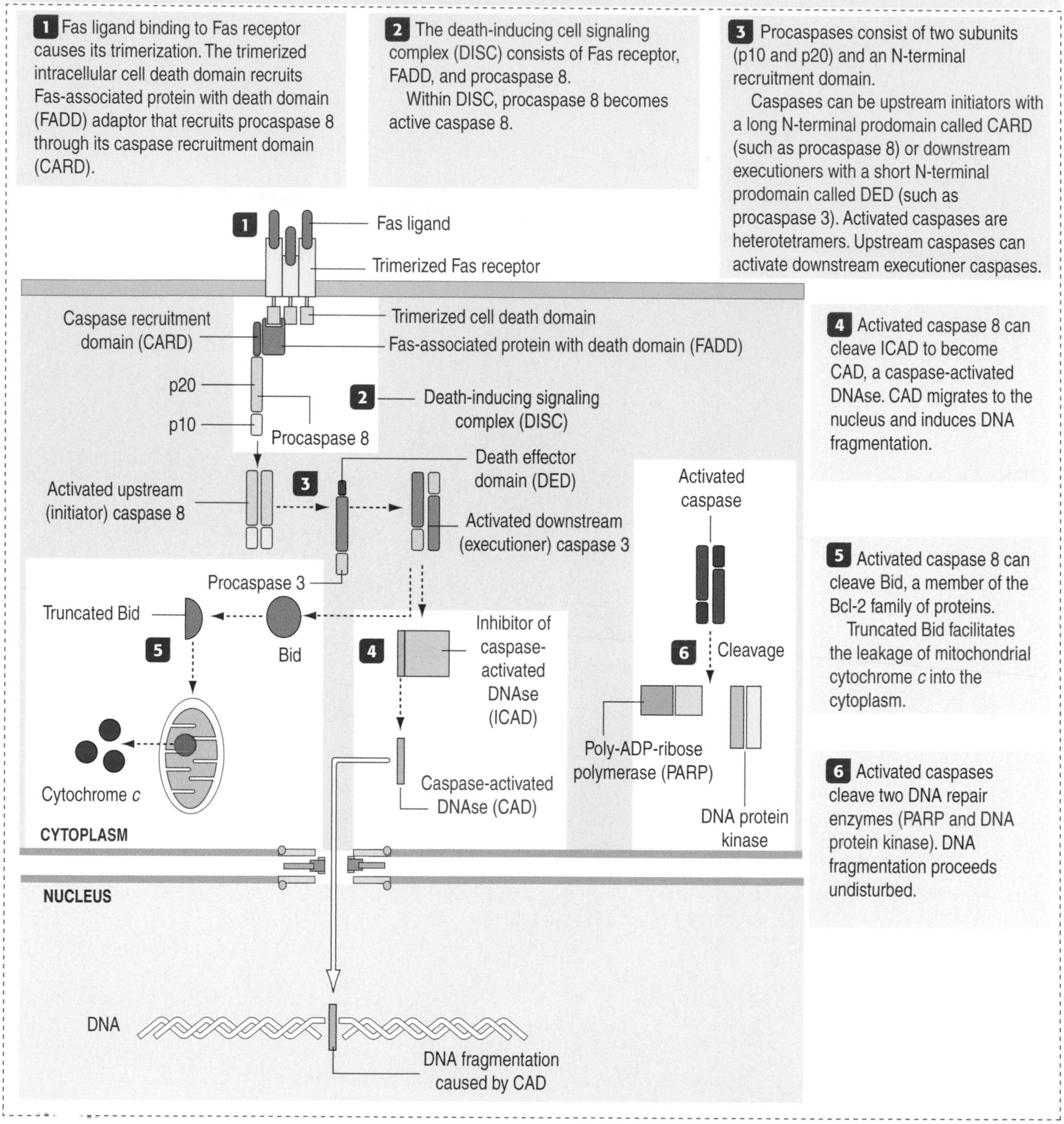

1 Fas ligand binding to Fas receptor causes its trimerization. The trimerized intracellular cell death domain recruits Fas-associated protein with death domain (FADD) adaptor that recruits procaspase 8 through its caspase recruitment domain (CARD).
2 The death-inducing cell signaling complex (DISC) consists of Fas receptor, FADD, and procaspase 8.
Within DISC, procaspase 8 becomes active caspase 8.
3 Procaspases consist of two subunits (p10 and p20) and an N-terminal recruitment domain.
Caspases can be upstream initiators with a long N-terminal prodomain called CARD (such as procaspase 8) or downstream executioners with a short N-terminal prodomain called DED (such as procaspase 3). Activated caspases are heterotetramers. Upstream caspases can activate downstream executioner caspases.
Fas ligand
Trimerized Fas receptor
Caspase recruitment domain (CARD)
Trimerized cell death domain
Fas-associated protein with death domain (FADD)
p20
p10
Procaspase 8
Death-inducing signaling complex (DISC)
Death effector domain (DED)
Activated upstream (initiator) caspase 8
Activated downstream (executioner) caspase 3
Procaspase 3
Truncated Bid
Bid
Cytochrome c
CYTOPLASM
NUCLEUS
Inhibitor of caspase-activated DNAse (ICAD)
Caspase-activated DNAse (CAD)
Activated caspase
Cleavage
Poly-ADP-ribose polymerase (PARP)
DNA protein kinase
DNA
DNA fragmentation caused by CAD
4 Activated caspase 8 can cleave ICAD to become CAD, a caspase-activated DNAse. CAD migrates to the nucleus and induces DNA fragmentation.
5 Activated caspase 8 can cleave Bid, a member of the Bcl-2 family of proteins.
Truncated Bid facilitates the leakage of mitochondrial cytochrome c into the cytoplasm.
6 Activated caspases cleave two DNA repair enzymes (PARP and DNA protein kinase). DNA fragmentation proceeds undisturbed.

process that occurs after acute injury (for example, in an ischemic stroke). Necrotic cells lyse and release cytoplasmic and nuclear contents into the environment, thus triggering an inflammatory reaction.

Cells undergoing apoptosis lose intercellular adhesion, fragment the chromatin, and break down into small blebs called **apoptotic bodies**. Apoptotic bodies are phagocytosed by macrophages and inflammation does not occur.

Apoptotic cell death is observed during fetal development. For example, the formation of fingers and toes of the fetus requires the elimination by apoptosis of the tissue between them. During fetal development of the central nervous system, an excess of neurons, eliminated later by apoptosis, is required to establish appropriate connections or synapses between them (see Chapter 8, Nervous Tissue). Mature granulocytes in peripheral blood have a life span of 1 to 2 days before undergoing apoptosis. The clonal selection of T cells in the thymus (to eliminate self-reactive lymphocytes to prevent autoimmune diseases; see Chapter 10, Immune-Lymphatic System) and cellular immune responses involve apoptosis.

What a nematode worm told us about apoptosis

The genetic and molecular mechanisms of apoptosis emerged from studies of the nematode worm *Caenorhabditis elegans*, in which 131 cells are precisely killed and 959 remain. In this worm, four genes are required for the orderly cell death program: *ced-3* (for cell death defective-3), *ced-4*, *egl-1* (for egg laying-1), and *ced-9*. The products of the first three genes mediate cell death. The gene *ced-9* is an inhibitor of apoptosis.

The proteins encoded by these four genes in the worm are found in vertebrates. Protein ced-3 is homologous to **caspases**, ced-4 corresponds to **Apaf-1** (for **apoptotic protease activating factor-1**), ced-9 to **Bcl-2** (for B-cell leukemia-2), and egl-1 is homologous to Bcl-2 homology region 3 (BH3)-only proteins.

External signals trigger apoptosis: Fas receptor/Fas ligand

External and internal signals determine cell apoptosis. External signals bind to cell surface receptors (for example, tumor necrosis factor-α and Fas ligand). Internal signals (for example, the release of cytochrome *c* from mitochondria) can trigger cell death.

Fas receptor (also known as APO-1 or CD95) is a cell membrane protein that belongs to the **tumor necrosis factor** (TNF) **receptor family**. Fas receptor has an intracellular cell death domain. **Fas ligand** binds to Fas receptor and causes its **trimerization**. Fas ligand initiates programmed cell death by binding to the **Fas receptor** and triggers a cell signaling cascade consisting of the sequential activation of **procaspases** into active **caspases**. The trimerized cell death domain recruits procaspase 8 through the **FADD** (for **Fas-associated protein with death domain**) adaptor and forms a **DISC** (for **death-inducing signaling complex**). DISC consists of Fas receptor, FADD, and procaspase 8.

Procaspase 8 autoactivated at DISC becomes active caspase 8. Active caspase 8 can do two things:

1. It can process procaspase 3 to active caspase 3, which can cleave several cellular proteins, including **ICAD** (for **inhibitor of CAD**) giving rise to CAD. **CAD** (for **caspase-activated DNAse**) is released from ICAD, translocates to the cell nucleus, and breaks down chromosomal DNA.

2. Caspase 8 can cleave **Bid**, a proapoptotic member of the Bcl-2 family. The truncated Bid translocates to mitochondria to release cytochrome *c* into the cytoplasm.

As we will discuss in Chapter 10, Immune-Lymphatic System, a cytotoxic T cell destroys a target cell (for example, a virus-infected cell) by first binding to the target cell and then releasing Fas ligand. Fas ligand binds to Fas receptor on the surface of the target cell and triggers the cell death cascade.

Caspases, initiators and executioners of cell death

Caspases (for **cysteine aspartic acid–specific proteases**) exist as inactive precursors (procaspases), which are activated to produce directly or indirectly cellular morphologic changes during apoptosis.

Procaspases consist of two subunits (**p10** and **p20**) and an N-terminal recruitment domain (see Figure 3-12). Activated caspases are heterotetramers consisting of two p10 subunits and two p20 subunits derived from two procaspases.

Caspases can be **upstream initiators** and **downstream executioners.** Upstream initiators are activated by the cell-death signal (for example, Fas ligand or TNF-α). Upstream initiator caspases activate downstream caspases, which directly mediate cell destruction.

Completion of the cell death process occurs when executioner caspases activate

Figure 3-13. Role of mitochondria in apoptosis

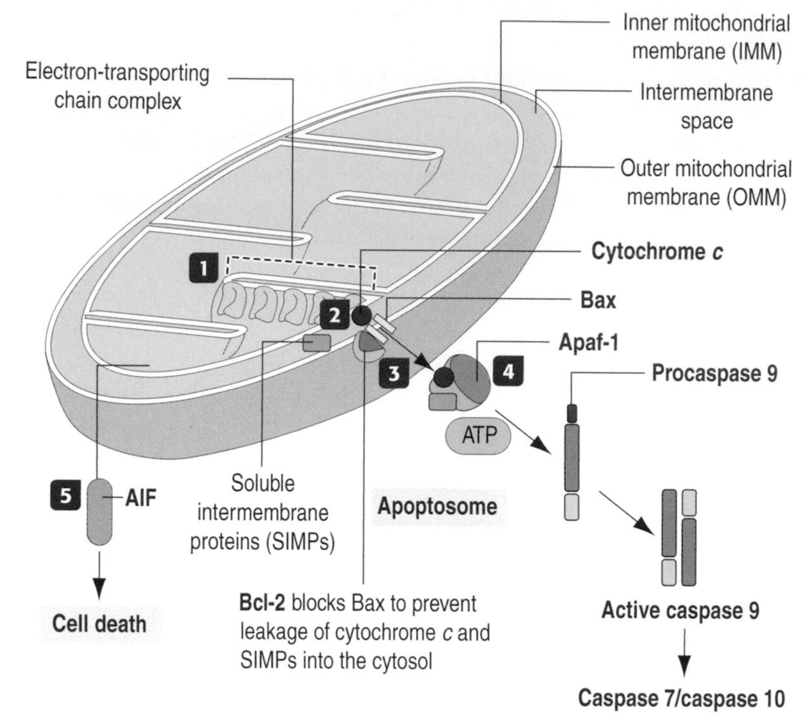

Cytochrome *c* in apoptosis

1 Cytochrome c shuttles electrons between respiratory chain complexes III and IV. If cytochrome *c* is not present, electron flow stops and ATP synthesis does not occur.
2 Cytochrome *c* is located between the IMM and OMM.
3 **Antiapoptotic Bcl-2** blocks **Bax** which facilitates the release of **cytochrome *c*** and **SIMPs**.
4 During apoptosis, **cytochrome *c* and SIMPs are released across the OMM and interact with apoptosis protease activating factor-1** (**Apaf-1**) to form the **apoptosome** (together with **ATP** and **procascapse 9**).
Apaf-1 activates procaspase 9. Caspase 9 activates caspase 7 and caspase 10 leading to the proteolytic destruction of the cell.
5 **Apoptosis-inducing factor (AIF)** is a mitochondrial protein that can be released into the cytoplasm, migrate to the cell nucleus, bind to DNA and trigger DNA fragmentation in the absence of caspases.

the DNA degradation machinery. Caspases cleave two DNA repair enzymes (**poly-ADP–ribose polymerase** [PARP], and **DNA protein kinase**), and unrestricted fragmentation of chromatin occurs.

As you realize, the key event in caspase-mediated cell death is the regulation of the activation of **initiator caspases.**

Upstream (initiator) procaspases include procaspases 8, 9, and 10 with a **long** N-terminal prodomain called **CARD** (for **caspase-recruiting domain**). Downstream (executioner) procaspases comprise procaspases 3, 6, and 7 with a **short** N-terminal prodomain called **DED** (for **death-effector domain**).

Caspase activation takes place when a caspase-specific regulatory molecule (for example, FADD) binds to the CARD/DED domain. Caspase activation may become out of control and destroy the cell. To prevent this uncontrolled event, inhibitors of apoptosis are available to interact with modulators of cell death, thus preventing unregulated caspase activation.

Bcl-2 regulates the release of mitochondrial cytochrome c through Bax

Cytochrome *c* is a component of the mitochondria electron-transporting chain involved in the production of ATP, and also a trigger of the caspase cascade.

The cell death pathway can be activated when cytochrome *c* is released from the mitochondria into the cytoplasm. How does cytochrome *c* leave mitochondria? To answer this question, we need to consider aspects of members of the **Bcl-2 family.**

Bcl-2 family members can have **proapoptotic** or **antiapoptotic** activities. **Bcl-2 and Bcl-xL have antiapoptotic activity. Bax, Bak, Bid, and Bad are proapoptotic proteins.** Bcl-2 is associated with the outer mitochondrial membrane of viable cells and prevents Bax from punching holes in the outer mitochondrial membrane, causing cytochrome *c* to leak out. As you see, a balance between proapoptotic Bax and antiapoptotic Bcl-2 proteins controls the release of cytochrome *c*.

In the cytoplasm, leaking cytochrome *c*, in the presence of ATP, **soluble internal membrane proteins** (**SIMPs**), and procaspase 9, binds to Apaf-1 to form a complex called an **apoptosome**.

The apoptosome determines the activation of **caspase 9**, an upstream initiator of apoptosis (Figure 3-13). Caspase 9 activates caspase 3 and caspase 7, leading to cell death.

You can gather from this discussion that external activators such as Fas ligand and TNF-α, and the internal release of cytochrome *c* are two key triggers of apoptosis. However, **AIF** (for **apoptosis-inducing factor**) is a protein of the intermitochondrial membrane space that can be released into the cytoplasm, migrate to the nucleus, bind to DNA, and trigger cell destruction without participation of caspases.

Clinical significance of apoptosis: Apoptosis in the immune system

Mutations in the *Fas receptor*, *Fas ligand*, or *caspase 10* genes can cause **autoimmune lymphoproliferative syndrome** (**ALPS**). ALPS is characterized by the accumulation of mature lymphocytes in lymph nodes and spleen causing **lymphoadenopathy** (enlargement of lymph nodes) and **splenomegaly** (enlargement of the spleen), and the existence of autoreactive lymphocyte clones producing autoimmune conditions such as **hemolytic anemia** (caused by destruction of red blood cells) and **thrombocytopenia** (reduced number of platelets).

Clinical significance of apoptosis: Neurodegenerative diseases

Neurologic diseases are examples of the mechanism of cell death. For example, an **ischemic stroke** can cause an **acute neurologic disease** in which necrosis and activation of caspase 1 are observed. Necrotic cell death occurs in the center of the infarction, where the damage is severe. Apoptosis may be observed at the periphery of the infarction, because the damage is not severe due to collateral blood circulation. Pharmacologic treatment with caspase inhibitors can reduce tissue damage leading to neurologic improvement.

Caspase activation is associated with the fatal progression of **chronic neurodegenerative diseases. Amyotrophic lateral sclerosis** (ALS) and **Huntington's disease** are two examples.

ALS consists in the progressive loss of motor neurons in brain, brainstem, and spinal cord. A mutation in the gene encoding **superoxide dismutase 1** (***SID1***) has been identified in patients with familial ALS. Activated caspase 1 and caspase 3 have been found in spinal cord samples of patients with ALS. Motor neurons and axons die and reactive microglia and astrocytes are present. We come back to ALS in Chapter 9, Nervous Tissue.

Huntington's disease is an autosomal dominant neurodegenerative disease characterized by a movement disorder (**Huntington's chorea**). The disease is caused by a mutation in the protein **huntingtin**. Huntingtin protein fragments accumulate and aggregate in the neuronal nucleus and transcription of the *caspase 1* gene is upregulated. Caspase 1 activates caspase 3 and both caspases cleave the allelic wild-type form of huntingtin, which becomes depleted. As the disease progresses, Bid is activated and releases mitochondrial cytochrome *c*. Apoptosomes are assembled and further caspase activation leads to neuronal death.

Three major cellular mechanisms are involved in proteolysis

In addition to the **procaspase-caspase pathway** activated by Fas ligand (see Figure 3-12), the intracellular degradation of residual or misfolded proteins (**proteolysis**) can occur by the classic **endosomal-lysosomal pathway** (see Figure 2-19), the apoptosis pathway (see Figure 3-12), and the **ubiquitin-proteasome pathway** (Figure 3-14). We have already seen that the endosomal-lysosomal mechanism operates within a membrane-bound acidic compartment. In contrast, the procaspase-caspase pathway and the ubiquitin-proteasome pathway carry out proteolysis in the cytosol.

The ubiquitin–26S proteasome pathway involves four successive regulated steps:

Figure 3-14. **Three proteolytic mechanisms**

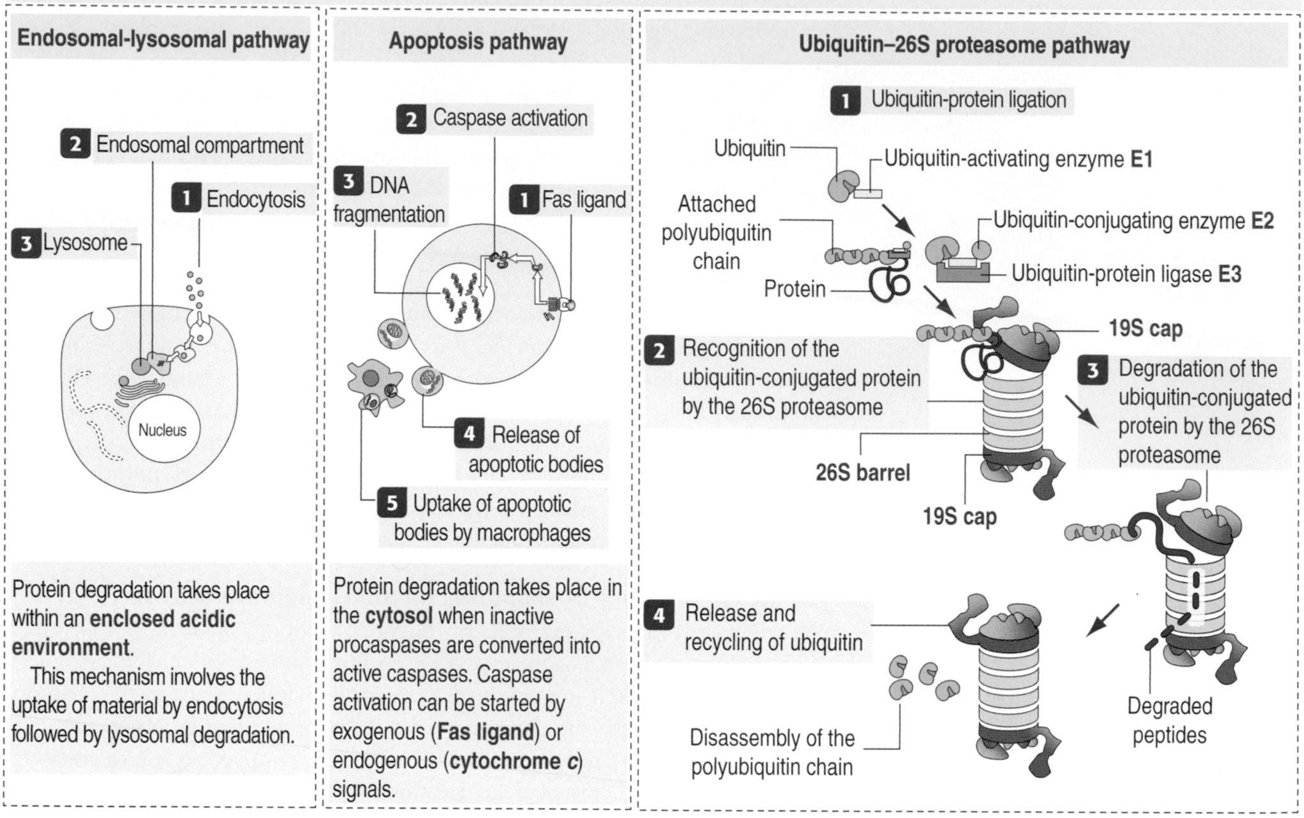

Endosomal-lysosomal pathway
2 Endosomal compartment
1 Endocytosis
3 Lysosome
Nucleus
Protein degradation takes place within an enclosed acidic environment.
This mechanism involves the uptake of material by endocytosis followed by lysosomal degradation.
Apoptosis pathway
2 Caspase activation
3 DNA fragmentation
1 Fas ligand
4 Release of apoptotic bodies
5 Uptake of apoptotic bodies by macrophages
Protein degradation takes place in the cytosol when inactive procaspases are converted into active caspases. Caspase activation can be started by exogenous (Fas ligand) or endogenous (cytochrome c) signals.
Ubiquitin–26S proteasome pathway
1 Ubiquitin-protein ligation
Ubiquitin
Ubiquitin-activating enzyme E1
Attached polyubiquitin chain
Ubiquitin-conjugating enzyme E2
Protein
Ubiquitin-protein ligase E3
19S cap
2 Recognition of the ubiquitin-conjugated protein by the 26S proteasome
3 Degradation of the ubiquitin-conjugated protein by the 26S proteasome
26S barrel
19S cap
4 Release and recycling of ubiquitin
Disassembly of the polyubiquitin chain
Degraded peptides

1. The attachment of a chain of ubiquitin molecules to a protein substrate by an enzymatic cascade. First, **E1**, the ubiquitin-activating enzyme, activates ubiquitin in the presence of ATP to form a thioester bond. **E2**, the ubiquitin-conjugating enzyme, uses the thioester bond to conjugate activated ubiquitin to the target protein. E2 transfers the activated ubiquitin to a lysine residue of the substrate with the help of **E3**, a specific ubiquitin-protein ligase. This process is repeated several times to generate a long polyubiquitin chain attached to the substrate protein destined for degradation in the **26S proteasome**.

2. Recognition of the ubiquitin-conjugated protein by the 26S proteasome. A protein subunit (designated S5a) in the 19S cap of the proteasome acts as a receptor for the polyubiquitin chain.

3. Degradation of the ubiquitin-conjugated protein into oligopeptides in the 26S barrel, the inner proteolytic chamber of the proteasome, in the presence of ATP.

4. The release and recycling of ubiquitin.

The 26S proteasome is a giant (~2000 kd) multimeric protease present in the nucleus and cytoplasm. Structurally, the 26S proteasome consists of a barrel-shaped core capped by two structures that recognize ubiquitinated proteins. Protein degradation occurs within a chamber of the barrel-shaped core. Proteins degraded by the 26S proteasome include molecules involved in the regulation of the cell cycle (cyclins), transcription factors, and the processing of antigens involved in the activation of inflammatory and immune responses.

Box 3-E | **Proto-oncogenes and oncogenes**

A **proto-oncogene** is a normal gene encoding a regulatory protein of the cell cycle, cell differentiation, or a cell-signaling pathway. Proto-oncogenic proteins mimic growth factors, hormone receptors, G proteins, intracellular enzymes, and transcription factors.

An **oncogene** is a **mutated proto-oncogene** that encodes an **oncoprotein** able to disrupt the normal cell cycle and to cause cancer.

Proto-oncogenes and oncogenes are designated by an **italicized three-letter** name. An oncogene present in a virus has the prefix **v**. A proto-oncogene present in a cell has the prefix **c**.

A protein encoded by a proto-oncogene or oncogene has the same three-letter designation as the proto-oncogene or oncogene. However, the letters are not italicized and the first letter is capitalized.

Antioncogenes are also called **tumor suppressor genes.** A loss of activity of a tumor suppressor gene product results in constitutive activation of cell growth.

Proto-oncogenes and oncogenes

Genes that cause cancer are called **oncogenes** (Greek *onkos*, bulk, mass; *genos*, birth). Most oncogenes originate from **proto-oncogenes** (Greek *prōtos*, first). Proto-oncogenes (Box 3-E) are involved in the **four basic regulatory mechanisms of cell growth** by expressing **growth factors**, **growth factor receptors**, **signal transduction molecules**, and **nuclear transcription factors**.

An oncogene results from the mutation of a proto-oncogene. Oncogenes express constantly active products leading to unregulated cell growth and differentiation. A cell becomes **transformed** when it changes from regulated to unregulated growth.

Although most animal viruses destroy the cells they infect, several types of viruses are able to establish a long-term infection, in which the cell is not killed. This stable virus–host cell interaction perpetuates the viral information in the cell, usually by direct insertion into cellular DNA.

The first oncogenes to be identified came from the study of **retroviruses**. All vertebrate animals, including humans, inherit genes related to retroviral genes and transmit them to their progeny. These are called **endogenous proviruses**, whereas those that infect a cell are called **exogenous proviruses**.

Cancer viruses isolated from every type of vertebrate animal induce a wide variety of tumors and belong to several virus types: **RNA-containing tumor viruses**, called **retroviruses**, and **DNA-containing tumor viruses**, including the **polyomaviruses**, the **papillomaviruses**, the **adenoviruses**, and the **herpesviruses**.

RNA-containing retroviruses have a distinct cell cycle. In the initial stages of infection, the **viral RNA** is **copied into DNA** by the viral enzyme **reverse transcriptase**. Once synthesized, the viral DNA molecule is transported into the nucleus and inserted randomly as a **provirus** at any one of the available sites of host chromosomal DNA. Proviruses contain signals for the regulation of their own viral genes, but such signals can be transmitted to the proto-oncogene, forcing it to produce larger than normal amounts of RNA and a protein.

Retroviruses and polyomaviruses have received the most attention because they carry one or two genes that have specific cancer-inducing properties: so-called **viral oncogenes**. Retroviruses and polyomaviruses like cellular genes, are subject to mutations. A group of such mutants of **Rous sarcoma virus** (**RSV**; species of origin: chicken) has proved useful for determining the role of the **viral** gene v-*src*. The *src*-like sequences in normal cells constitute a **cellular** gene called **c-*src***, a **proto-oncogene**.

The **viral *src*** derives directly from the **cellular *src***. A precursor of RSV seems to have acquired a copy of c-*src* during infection of a chicken cell. **c-src is harmless but its close relative v-src causes tumors and transform cells after RSV infection.** A chicken fibroblast produces about 50 times more src RNA and protein than an uninfected fibroblast containing only the c-*src* gene. The c-*src* gene assumed great significance when it was recognized that many other retroviruses carry oncogenes, often different from v-*src*. Each of these genes is also derived from a distinct, normal cellular precursor.

The classification of genes as proto-oncogenes is based on the understanding that mutant forms of these genes participate in the development of cancer (see Box 3-F). However, proto-oncogenes serve different biochemical functions in the control of normal growth and development. They can also undergo a variety of mutations that convert them to dominant genes capable of inducing cancers in the absence of viruses.

RSV-infected cells produce a 60-kd protein. This protein was identified as the product that the **v-*src* gene** uses to transform cells. It was designated **$p60^{v\text{-}src}$**. This protein can function as a **protein kinase** and, within a living cell, many proteins can be phosphorylated by **Src kinase** activity. The target for phosphorylation is **tyrosine** residues.

Cell transformation by the v-*src* oncogene causes a tenfold increase in total cellular phosphotyrosine in cellular target proteins restricted to the inner side of the **cell membrane**. Many other proteins encoded by proto-oncogenes or involved in control of cell growth function like the Src protein, such as protein kinases, are often specific for tyrosine.

Box 3-F | **Proto-oncogenes and tumor suppressor proteins in human cancers**

Chronic myelogenous leukemia: The **c-*abl*** proto-oncogene translocated from chromosome 9 to chromosome 22 (called the Philadelphia chromosome) encodes a fusion protein with constitutive active tyrosine kinase activity.

Burkitt's lymphoma: The **c-*myc*** proto-oncogene is translocated from chromosome 8 to chromosome 14. This translocation places *c-myc* under the control of an active immunoglobulin locus (immunoglobulin heavy-chain gene, Cm) and detached from its normal regulatory elements. Burkitt's lymphoma is endemic in some parts of Africa and affects mainly children or young adults. It generally involves the maxilla or mandible. It responds to chemotherapy.

p53: Inactivation of this **tumor suppressor protein**, a transcription factor expressed in response to DNA damage (see Figure 1-52), is associated with 50% to 60% of human cancers. Inactive p53 enables the progression of cells containing damaged DNA through the cell cycle.

• Cell signaling is the mechanism by which cells respond to chemical signals. Signaling molecules are either secreted or expressed on the cell surface of cells. When a signaling molecule binds to its receptor, it initiates intracellular reactions to regulate cell proliferation, differentiation, cell movements, metabolism, and behavior.

• There are several cell signaling mechanisms. (1) Endocrine signaling involves a hormone secreted by an endocrine cell and transported through blood circulation to act on a distant target. (2) Paracrine signaling is mediated by molecules acting locally to regulate the function of a neighboring cell. (3) Autocrine signaling consists in cells responding to signaling molecules that are produced by themselves. (4) Neurotransmitter signaling is a specific form of paracrine signaling involving neurons and neurotransmitter molecules released at a synapse. (5) Neuroendocrine signaling consists in a neuroendocrine cell releasing a hormone into the bloodstream in response to a stimulus released from an axon terminal.

• Hormones can be protein hormones (for example, insulin, neuropeptides secreted by neurons, and growth factors) or steroid hormones (for example, cholesterol-derived testosterone, estrogen, progesterone, and corticosteroids). Protein hormones bind to a cell surface receptor. Steroid hormones bind to cytosol and nuclear receptors. Nonsteroid signaling molecules, such as thyroid hormone, vitamin D_3, and retinoids (vitamin A), bind to intracellular receptors.

Several specific signaling molecules exist. (1) Epinephrine can be a neurotransmitter and also a hormone released into the bloodstream. (2) Eicosanoids and leukotrienes (derived from arachidonic acid) are lipid-containing signaling molecules which bind to cell surface receptors.

• Nitric oxide is a signaling molecule of very short half-life (seconds). Nitric oxide is synthesized from arginine by the enzyme nitric oxide synthase. Nitric oxide can diffuse across the plasma membrane but it does not bind to a receptor. Its major function is the regulation of the activity of intracellular enzymes. One of the relevant functions of nitric oxide is the dilation of blood vessels. Nitroglycerin, an agent used in the treatment of heart disease, is converted to nitric oxide, which increases heart blood flow by dilation of the coronary artery.

• After binding to a receptor, hormones activate intracellular targets downstream of the receptor.

1. G protein–coupled receptor consists of three subunits (α, β, and γ) forming a complex. The α subunit binds GDP (guanosine diphosphate) and regulates G protein activity. When a signaling molecule binds to its receptor, the α subunit of the associated G protein dissociates, releases GDP, and binds GTP (guanosine triphosphate) to activate an adjacent target molecule.

2. Tyrosine kinases can be a transmembrane protein or present in the cytosol. The first form is called tyrosine kinase receptor; the second form is known as nonreceptor tyrosine kinase. Binding of a ligand to tyrosine kinase receptor produces its dimerization resulting in autophosphorylation of the intracellular domain. Downstream molecules with SH2 (Src homology 2) domains bind to the catalytic kinase domain of tyrosine kinase receptor. The activity of tyrosine kinase receptor can be disrupted by inducing unregulated autophosphorylation in the absence of a ligand. Tyrosine kinase activity can be inhibited by imatinib mesylate, a molecule with binding affinity to the adenosine triphosphate (ATP)-binding domain of the catalytic domain. Imatinib is used in the treatment of **chronic myeloid leukemia, chronic myelomonocytic leukemia, systemic mastocytosis, and mast cell leukemias.**

3. Cytokine receptors are a family of receptors that stimulate intracellular protein tyrosine kinases, which are not intrinsic components of the receptor. Ligand binding to cytokine receptors triggers receptor dimerization and cross-phosphorylation of the associated tyrosine kinases. Members of the cytokine receptor–associated tyrosine kinase family are the Src family and the Janus kinase family (JAK).

4. Receptors can be linked to enzymes such as protein tyrosine phosphatases and protein serine and threonine kinases. Tyrosine phosphatases remove tyrosine phosphate groups from phosphotyrosine and arrest signaling started by tyrosine phosphorylation. Members of the transforming growth factor-β (TGF-β) family are protein kinases that phosphorylate serine and threonine residues. Ligand binding to TGF-β induces receptor dimerization and the serine- or threonine-containing intracellular domain of the receptor cross-phosphorylates the polypeptide chains of the receptor.

• Following ligand binding, most receptors activate intracellular enzymes to transmit and amplify a signal.

1. The cAMP (cyclic adenosine monophosphate) pathway results from the formation of cAMP (known as a second messenger) from ATP by the enzyme adenylyl cyclase. The intracellular effects of cAMP are mediated by cAMP-dependent protein kinase (also known as protein kinase A). Inactive cAMP-dependent protein kinase is a tetramer composed of two regulatory subunits (the binding site of cAMP) and two catalytic subunits. The enzyme phosphodiesterase degrades cAMP. Upon cAMP binding, the catalytic subunits dissociate and each catalytic subunit phosphorylates serine residues on target proteins or migrates to the cell nucleus.

In the cell nucleus, the catalytic subunit phosphorylates the transcription factor CREB (CRE-binding protein) bound to CRE (the cAMP response element), and specific gene activity is induced.

2. The cGMP (cyclic guanosine monophosphate) pathway utilizes guanylate cyclase to produce cGMP which is degraded by a cGMP-dependent phosphodiesterase. Photoreceptors of the retina utilize cGMP to convert light signals to nerve impulses.

3. The phospholipase C–Ca^{2+} pathway consists in the production of second messengers from the phospholipid phosphatidylinositol 4.5-bisphosphate (PIP_2). Hydrolysis of PIP_2 by phospholipase C (PLC) produces two second messengers: diacylglycerol and inositol 1,4,5-triphosphate (IP_3). Diacylglycerol and IP_3 stimulate protein kinase C (protein serine and threonine kinases) and the mobilization of Ca^{2+}. Protein kinase C activates protein kinases of the MAP (mitogen activated protein) kinase pathway to phosphorylate transcription factors.

4. The NF-κB (for nuclear factor involved in the transcription of the κ light chain gene in B lymphocytes) transcription factor pathway is stimulated by protein kinase C and is involved in immune responses. When inactive, the NF-κB heterodimer is bound to the inhibitory subunit I-κB and remains in the cytoplasm. Phosphorylation of I-κB, triggered by I-κB kinase, results in the destruction of I-κB by the 26S proteasome and the nuclear translocation of the NF-κB heterodimer to activate gene transcription.

5. The Ca^{2+}-calmodulin pathway consists in the activation of calmodulin, a Ca^{2+}-dependent protein, when Ca^{2+} concentration increases and binds to calmodulin. You should note that the phospholipase C–Ca^{2+} and Ca^{2+}-calmodulin pathway regulates Ca^{2+} concentration by Ca^{2+} release from intracellular storage as well as entry into the cell from the extracellular space.

6. The MAP kinase pathway involves serine and threonine MAP kinases. The extracellular signal–regulated kinase (ERK)

family is a MAP kinase acting through either tyrosine kinase or G protein–associated receptors. The activation of ERK is mediated by two protein kinases: Raf and MEK (MAP kinase or ERK kinase). Raf interacts with rat sarcoma virus (Ras) protein, a key element of the group of oncogenic proteins.

Raf phosphorylates MEK which activates ERK, and then phosphorylated ERK activates nuclear (Elk-1) and cytosolic target proteins. Two other MAP kinases are JNK and p38 MAP kinases.

7. The JAK-STAT pathway regulates transcription factors. Signal transducer and activators of transcription (STAT) proteins are transcription factors with an SH2 domain and present in the cytoplasm in an inactive state. Ligand binding to a cytokine receptor determines the attachment of STAT to the receptor associated Janus kinase (JAK), a tyrosine kinase, through their SH2 domain. Phosphorylated STAT dimerizes and translocates to the cell nucleus to activate gene transcription.

• Transcription factors activate and inactivate genes. Sox9 is a transcription factor that regulates chondrogenesis (cartilage growth). Mutations of the *Sox9* gene cause campomelic dysplasia (skeletal defects) and sex reversal (XY females).

• Stem cells have three properties: self-renewal, proliferation, and differentiation. Stem cells can give rise to cell precursors that generate tissues of the body. Stem cells are present in the intestinal epithelium, the epidermis of the skin, the hematopoietic tissue, and spermatogenic cells. Stem cells are recognized by the expression of cell surface markers and by the cells they produce following culture or transplantation.

• Cell culture procedures demonstrate that: (1) cells stop growing when they cover entirely the surface of a culture dish. This is called density-dependent inhibition of growth. (2) Cultured cells can continue growing until they stop dividing. The cells have become senescent. Telomerases maintain the end of the chromosomes, the telomeres. Insufficient telomerase activity forces cells into senescence.

Telomere shortening is a potent tumor suppressor mechanism. Most tumors express human telomerase reverse transcriptase (hTERT) and growth in culture is endless. Cells become immortal. Such cells can establish a cell line. (3) Transformed cells have a malignant growth potential and exhibit anchorage-independent growth. In contrast, normal cells grow attached to a substrate.

• Apoptosis or programmed cell death can be determined by external and internal signals. An external signal is the Fas ligand which binds to the Fas receptor. An internal signal is the leakage of cytochrome *c* from mitochondria. The end point is the activation of procaspases to caspases, the initiators and executors of cell death.

A defect in the activity of Fas receptor, Fas ligand, and caspases can cause the **autoimmune lymphoproliferative syndrome (ALPS)**, characterized by the abnormal and excessive accumulation of lymphocytes in lymph nodes and spleen.

Aberrant activation of caspases is associated with neurodegenerative disease, such as **amyotrophic lateral sclerosis (ALS)** and **Huntington's disease.**

• The proteolysis of residual and misfolded proteins can occur by the classic endosomal-lysosomal pathway, the apoptosis pathway, and the ubiquitin–26S proteasome pathway. The first pathway takes place within a membrane-bound acidic compartment. The last two occur predominantly in the cytosol. The apoptosis pathway involves caspases; the ubiquitin–26S proteasome pathway requires the attachment of a polyubiquitin chain to proteins marked for degradation by the 26S proteasome.

• Proto-oncogenes express growth factors, growth factor receptors, signal transduction molecules, and nuclear transcription factors. An oncogene results from the mutation of a proto-oncogene. Oncogenes determine unregulated cell growth and a cell then becomes transformed. The first oncogenes to be identified were the retroviruses (RNA-containing viruses) with cancer-inducing properties (viral oncogenes). DNA-containing viruses (polyomaviruses, the papillomaviruses, the adenoviruses, and the herpesviruses) can induce tumors. The chicken cell Rous sarcoma virus (RSV) includes the viral gene *v-src*. The proto-oncogene equivalent in normal cells is *c-src*. The *v-src* gene encodes the protein $p60^{v\text{-}src}$, which functions as a tyrosine protein kinase. Cell transformation by the *v-src* oncogene results in a significant increase in total cell phosphotyrosine.

4. CONNECTIVE TISSUE

Classification

The connective tissue provides the **supportive** and **connecting** framework (or **stroma**) for all the other tissues of the body. The connective tissue is formed by **cells** and the **extracellular matrix (ECM)**. The ECM represents a combination of **collagens**, **noncollagenous glycoproteins**, and **proteoglycans (ground substance)** surrounding the cells of connective tissue. The cells of the connective tissue have important roles in the **storage of metabolites**, **immune and inflammatory responses**, and **tissue repair after injury**.

Unlike epithelial cells, which are almost free of intercellular material, **connective tissue cells are widely separated by components of the ECM**. In addition, epithelial cells lack direct blood and lymphatic supply, whereas connective tissue is directly supplied by blood and lymphatic vessels and nerves.

Connective tissue can be classified into three major groups (Figure 4-1): **embryonic connective tissue**, **adult connective tissue**, and **special connective tissue**.

Embryonic connective tissue is a loose tissue formed during early embryonic development. This type of connective tissue, found primarily in the **umbilical cord**, consists predominantly of a **hydrophilic ECM** and therefore has a jelly-like consistency. Because of this consistency, it is also called **mucoid connective tissue** or **Wharton's jelly**.

Adult connective tissue has considerable structural diversity because **the proportion of cells to fibers and of ground substance varies from tissue to tissue**. This variable cell-to-ECM ratio is the basis for the subclassification of adult connective tissue into two types of connective tissue proper:

1. **Loose** (or **areolar**) connective tissue.
2. **Dense connective tissue.**

Loose connective tissue contains **more cells than collagen fibers** and is generally found in the **mucosa** and **submucosa** of various organs and surrounding blood vessels, nerves, and muscles. This type of connective tissue facilitates dissection as performed by anatomists, pathologists, and surgeons.

Dense connective tissue contains **more collagen fibers than cells**. When the collagen fibers are preferentially oriented—as in tendons, ligaments, and the cornea—the tissue is called **dense regular connective tissue**. When the collagen fibers are **randomly oriented**—as in the dermis of the skin—the tissue is called dense irregular connective tissue.

In addition, **reticular** and **elastic fibers** predominate in irregular connective tissue.

Reticular connective tissue contains reticular fibers, which form the **stroma** of organs of the lymphoid-immune system (for example, lymph nodes and spleen), the hematopoietic bone marrow, and the liver. This type of connective tissue provides a delicate meshwork to allow passage of cells and fluid.

Elastic connective tissue contains irregularly arranged **elastic fibers** in ligaments of the vertebral column or concentrically arranged **sheets** or **laminae** in the wall of the aorta. This type of connective tissue provides **elasticity**.

The **special connective tissue** comprises types of connective tissue with special properties not observed in the embryonic or adult connective tissue proper. There are four types of special connective tissue (Figure 4-2):

1. **Adipose tissue.**
2. **Cartilage.**
3. **Bone.**
4. **Hematopoietic tissue (bone marrow).**

Figure 4-1. Classification of connective tissue

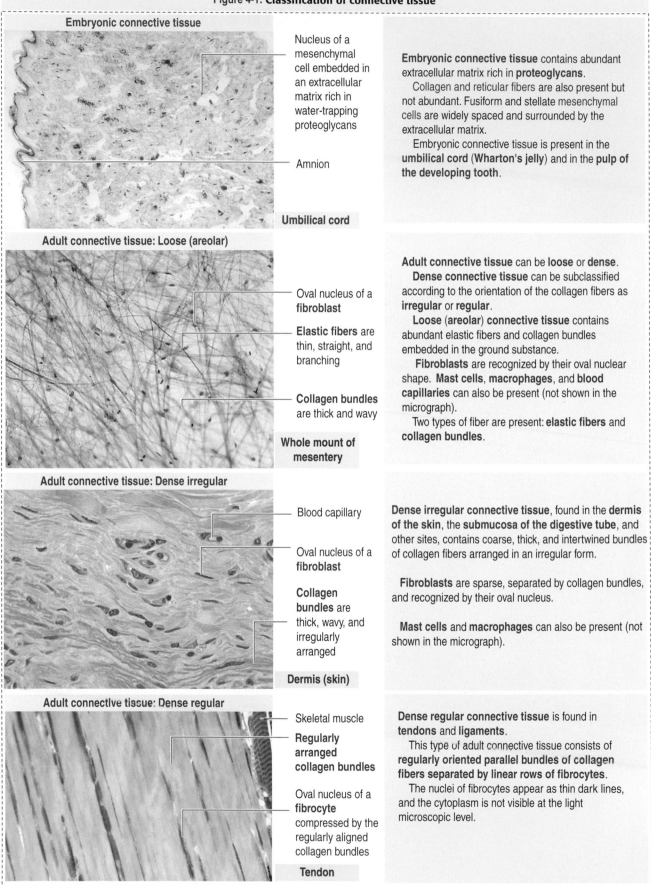

Embryonic connective tissue

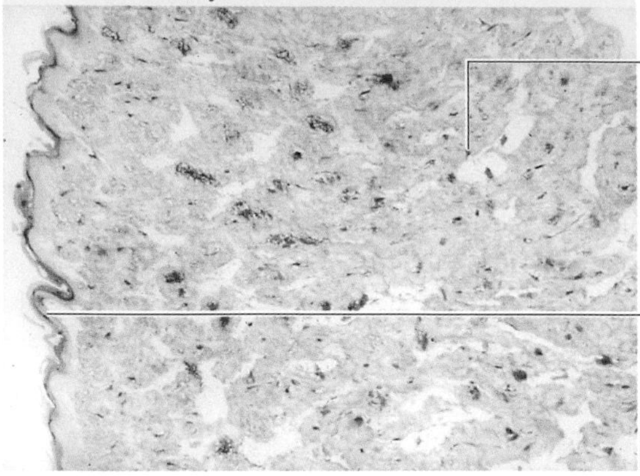
Nucleus of a mesenchymal cell embedded in an extracellular matrix rich in water-trapping proteoglycans
Amnion

Umbilical cord

Embryonic connective tissue contains abundant extracellular matrix rich in **proteoglycans**.

Collagen and reticular fibers are also present but not abundant. Fusiform and stellate mesenchymal cells are widely spaced and surrounded by the extracellular matrix.

Embryonic connective tissue is present in the **umbilical cord (Wharton's jelly)** and in the **pulp of the developing tooth**.

Adult connective tissue: Loose (areolar)

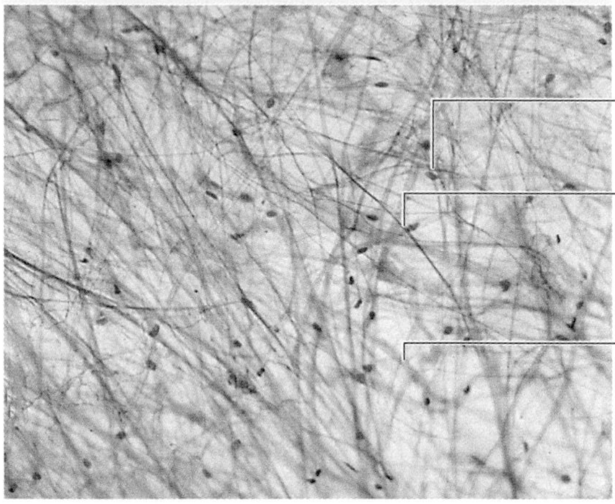
Oval nucleus of a **fibroblast**
Elastic fibers are thin, straight, and branching
Collagen bundles are thick and wavy

Whole mount of mesentery

Adult connective tissue can be **loose** or **dense**.

Dense connective tissue can be subclassified according to the orientation of the collagen fibers as **irregular** or **regular**.

Loose (areolar) connective tissue contains abundant elastic fibers and collagen bundles embedded in the ground substance.

Fibroblasts are recognized by their oval nuclear shape. **Mast cells**, **macrophages**, and **blood capillaries** can also be present (not shown in the micrograph).

Two types of fiber are present: **elastic fibers** and **collagen bundles**.

Adult connective tissue: Dense irregular

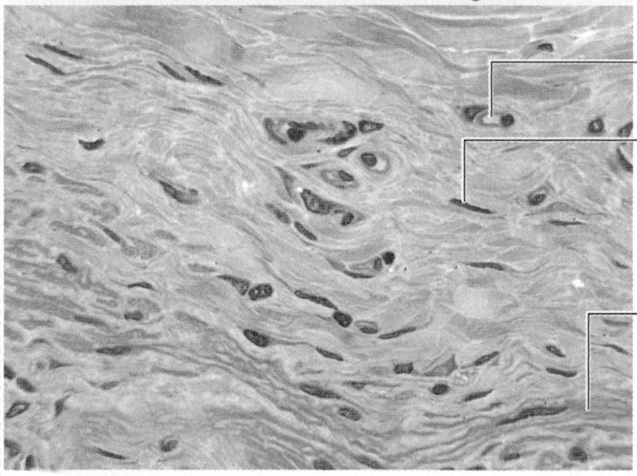
Blood capillary
Oval nucleus of a **fibroblast**
Collagen bundles are thick, wavy, and irregularly arranged

Dermis (skin)

Dense irregular connective tissue, found in the **dermis of the skin**, the **submucosa of the digestive tube**, and other sites, contains coarse, thick, and intertwined bundles of collagen fibers arranged in an irregular form.

Fibroblasts are sparse, separated by collagen bundles, and recognized by their oval nucleus.

Mast cells and **macrophages** can also be present (not shown in the micrograph).

Adult connective tissue: Dense regular

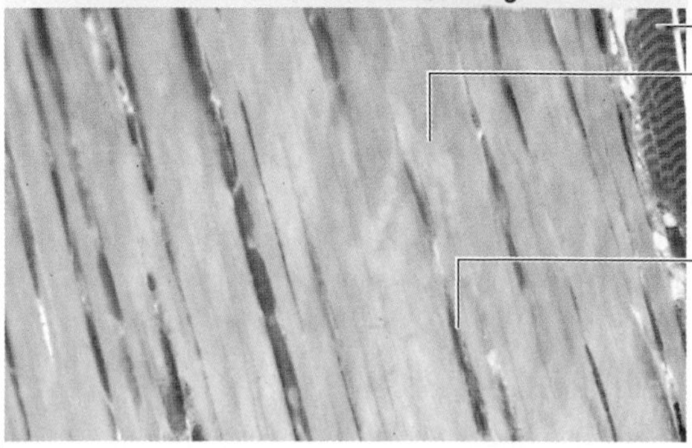
Skeletal muscle
Regularly arranged collagen bundles
Oval nucleus of a **fibrocyte** compressed by the regularly aligned collagen bundles

Tendon

Dense regular connective tissue is found in **tendons** and **ligaments**.

This type of adult connective tissue consists of **regularly oriented parallel bundles of collagen fibers separated by linear rows of fibrocytes**.

The nuclei of fibrocytes appear as thin dark lines, and the cytoplasm is not visible at the light microscopic level.

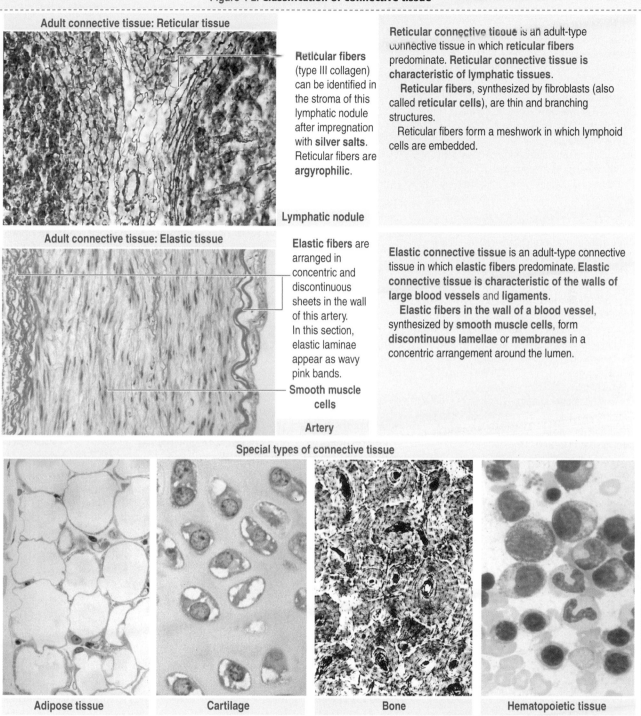

Figure 4-2. Classification of connective tissue

Adult connective tissue: Reticular tissue

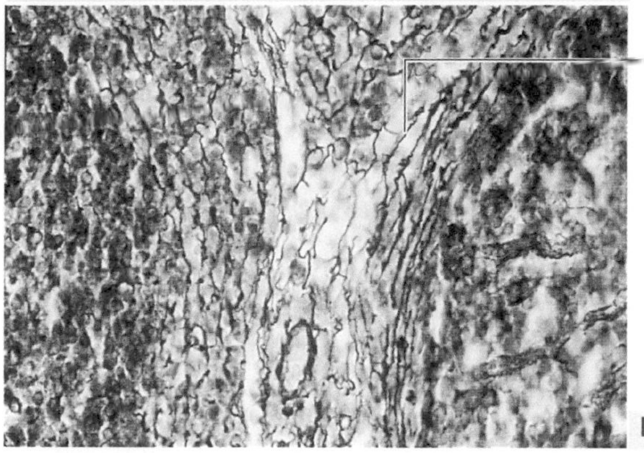
Reticular fibers (type III collagen) can be identified in the stroma of this lymphatic nodule after impregnation with **silver salts**. Reticular fibers are **argyrophilic**.
Lymphatic nodule

Reticular connective tissue is an adult-type connective tissue in which **reticular fibers** predominate. **Reticular connective tissue is characteristic of lymphatic tissues.**

Reticular fibers, synthesized by fibroblasts (also called **reticular cells**), are thin and branching structures.

Reticular fibers form a meshwork in which lymphoid cells are embedded.

Adult connective tissue: Elastic tissue

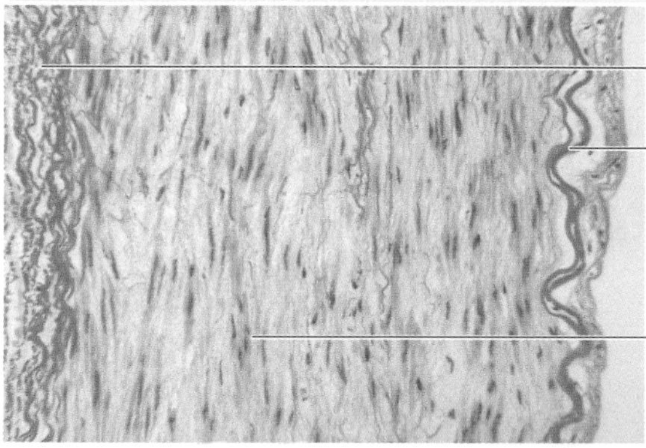
Elastic fibers are arranged in concentric and discontinuous sheets in the wall of this artery.
In this section, elastic laminae appear as wavy pink bands.
Smooth muscle cells
Artery

Elastic connective tissue is an adult-type connective tissue in which **elastic fibers** predominate. **Elastic connective tissue is characteristic of the walls of large blood vessels** and **ligaments**.

Elastic fibers in the wall of a blood vessel, synthesized by **smooth muscle cells**, form **discontinuous lamellae** or **membranes** in a concentric arrangement around the lumen.

Special types of connective tissue

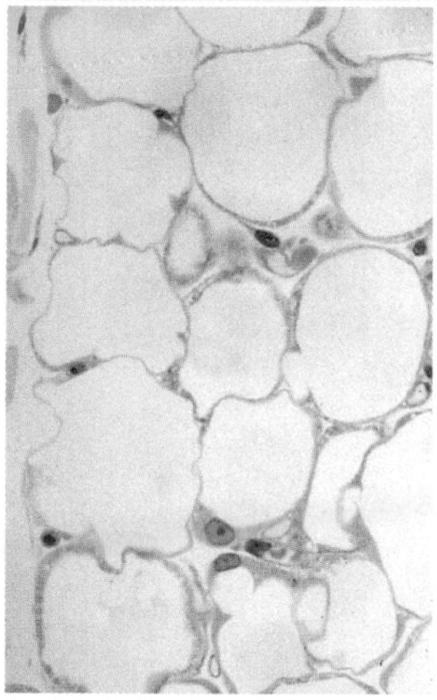
Adipose tissue

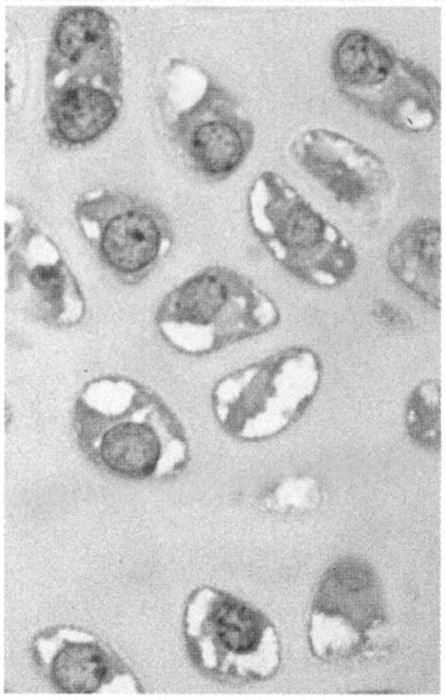
Cartilage

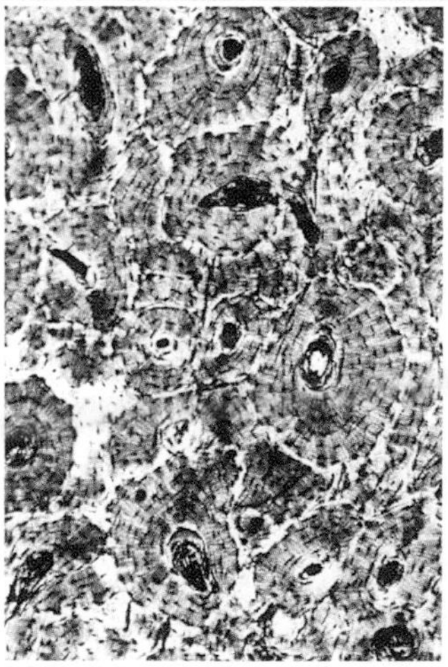
Bone

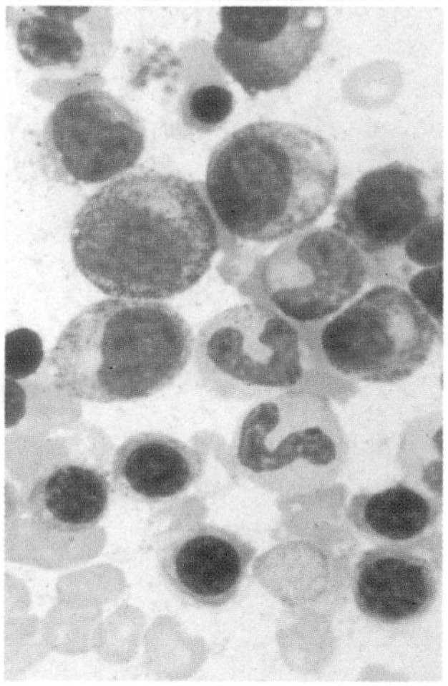
Hematopoietic tissue

Adipose tissue has more cells (called **adipose cells** or **adipocytes**) than collagen fibers and ground substance. This type of connective tissue is the most significant energy storage site of the body.

The **hematopoietic tissue** is found in the marrow of selected bones. This type of connective tissue is discussed in Chapter 6, Blood and Hematopoiesis.

Cartilage and bone are also regarded as **special connective tissue** but are traditionally placed in separate categories. Essentially, cartilage and bone are dense connective tissues with specialized cells and ground substance. An important difference is that cartilage has a **noncalcified ECM**, whereas the ECM of bone is

Box 4-A | **Distribution of collagen**

- **Type I collagen**
Present in **bone**, **tendon**, **dentin**, and **skin** as banded fibers with a transverse periodicity of 64 nm. This type of collagen provides tensile strength.
- **Type II collagen**
Observed in **hyaline** and **elastic cartilage** as fibrils thinner than type I collagen.
- **Type III collagen**
Present in the **reticular lamina of basement membranes**, as a component of reticular fibers. This is the first collagen type synthesized during wound healing and then is replaced by type I collagen.
Reticular fibers can be better recognized after impregnation with silver salts because reticular fibers are **argyrophilic** (silver-loving; Greek *argyros*, silver). Reticular fibers—and collagens in general—are glycoproteins and can be recognized with the **periodic acid–Schiff (PAS) reaction** because of their carbohydrate content.
Silver impregnation is a valuable tool in pathology for the recognition of distortions in the distribution of reticular fibers in alterations of lymphoid organs.
- **Type IV collagen**
Present in the **basal lamina**. This type of collagen does not form bundles. Single molecules of type IV collagen bind to one of the type IV collagen-binding sites of laminin.
- **Type V collagen**
Observed in **amnion** and **chorion** in the fetus and in muscle and tendon sheaths. **This type of collagen does not form banded fibrils.**

Box 4-B | **Cell types making collagen**

- The so-called **reticular cell** is a fibroblast that synthesizes reticular fibers containing type III collagen. Reticular fibers form the stroma of bone marrow and lymphoid organs.
- **The osteoblast (bone), chondroblast (cartilage), and odontoblast (teeth) also synthesize collagen.** These cell types are fibroblast equivalents in their respective tissues. Therefore, the synthesis of collagen is not limited to the fibroblast in connective tissue. In fact, **epithelial cells synthesize type IV collagen.**
- **A fibroblast may simultaneously synthesize more than one type of collagen.**
- **Smooth muscle cells**, found in the wall of arteries, intestine, the respiratory bronchial tree, and uterus, **can synthesize types I and III collagen.**

calcified. These two types of specialized connective tissue fulfill weight-bearing and mechanical functions that are discussed later (see Cartilage and Bone).

Cell components of connective tissue

The four major cell components of connective tissue are the **fibroblast**, the **macrophage**, the **mast cell**, and the **plasma cell**.

Under light microscopy, the **fibroblast** appears as a spindle-shaped cell with an elliptical nucleus. The cytoplasm is very thin and generally not resolved by the light microscope. Under **electron microscopy**, the fibroblast shows the typical features of a protein-secreting cell: a well-developed rough endoplasmic reticulum and a Golgi apparatus.

The fibroblast synthesizes and continuously secretes mature proteoglycans and glycoproteins and the precursor molecules of various types of collagens and elastin. Different types of collagen proteins and proteoglycans can be recognized as components of the **basement membrane**. As you remember, **type IV collagen is found in the basal lamina** and **type III collagen** appears in the **reticular lamina** as a component of **reticular fibers** (see Boxes 4-A and 4-B). Heparan sulfate proteoglycans and the glycoprotein fibronectin are two additional products of the fibroblast that appear in the basement membrane. The protein collagen is a component of collagen and reticular fibers. However, elastic fibers do not contain collagen.

Collagen: Synthesis, secretion, and assembly

Collagens are generally divided into two categories: **fibrillar collagens** (forming fibrils with a characteristic banded pattern), and **nonfibrillar collagens** (see Box 4-C).

The synthesis of collagen starts in the rough endoplasmic reticulum (RER) following the typical pathway of synthesis for export from the cell (Figure 4-3).

Preprocollagen is synthesized with a **signal peptide** and released as **procollagen** within the cisterna of the RER. **Procollagen** consists of three polypeptide a chains, lacking the signal peptide, assembled in a **triple helix.**

Hydroxyproline and **hydroxylysine** are typically observed in collagen. Hydroxylation of proline and lysine residues occurs in the RER and requires ascorbic acid (vitamin C) as a cofactor. Inadequate wound healing is characteristic of **scurvy**, caused by vitamin C deficiency.

Packaging and secretion of **procollagen** take place in the Golgi apparatus. Upon secretion of procollagen, the following three events occur in the extracellular space:

1. Enzymatic (**procollagen peptidase**) removal of most of the nonhelical endings of procollagen to give rise to soluble **tropocollagen** molecules.
2. Self-aggregation of tropocollagen molecules by a stepwise overlapping process to form **collagen fibrils.**
3. Cross-linking of tropocollagen molecules, leading to the formation of **collagen fibers. Lysyl oxidase** catalyzes cross-links between tropocollagens.

Groups of collagen fibers orient along the same axis to form **collagen bundles.** The formation of collagen bundles is guided by proteoglycans and other glycoproteins, including **FACIT** (for fibril-associated collagens with interrupted triple helices) collagens.

Clinical significance: Ehlers-Danlos syndrome

Ehlers-Danlos syndrome is clinically characterized by **hyperelasticity of the skin** (Figure 4-4) and **hypermobility of the joints**. The major defect resides in the connective tissue. Several clinical subtypes are observed. They are classified by the degree of severity and the mutations in the collagen genes. For example, the type IV form of Ehlers-Danlos syndrome—caused by a mutation in the *COL3A1* gene—is associated with severe vascular alterations leading to the development

Figure 4-3. Synthesis of collagen

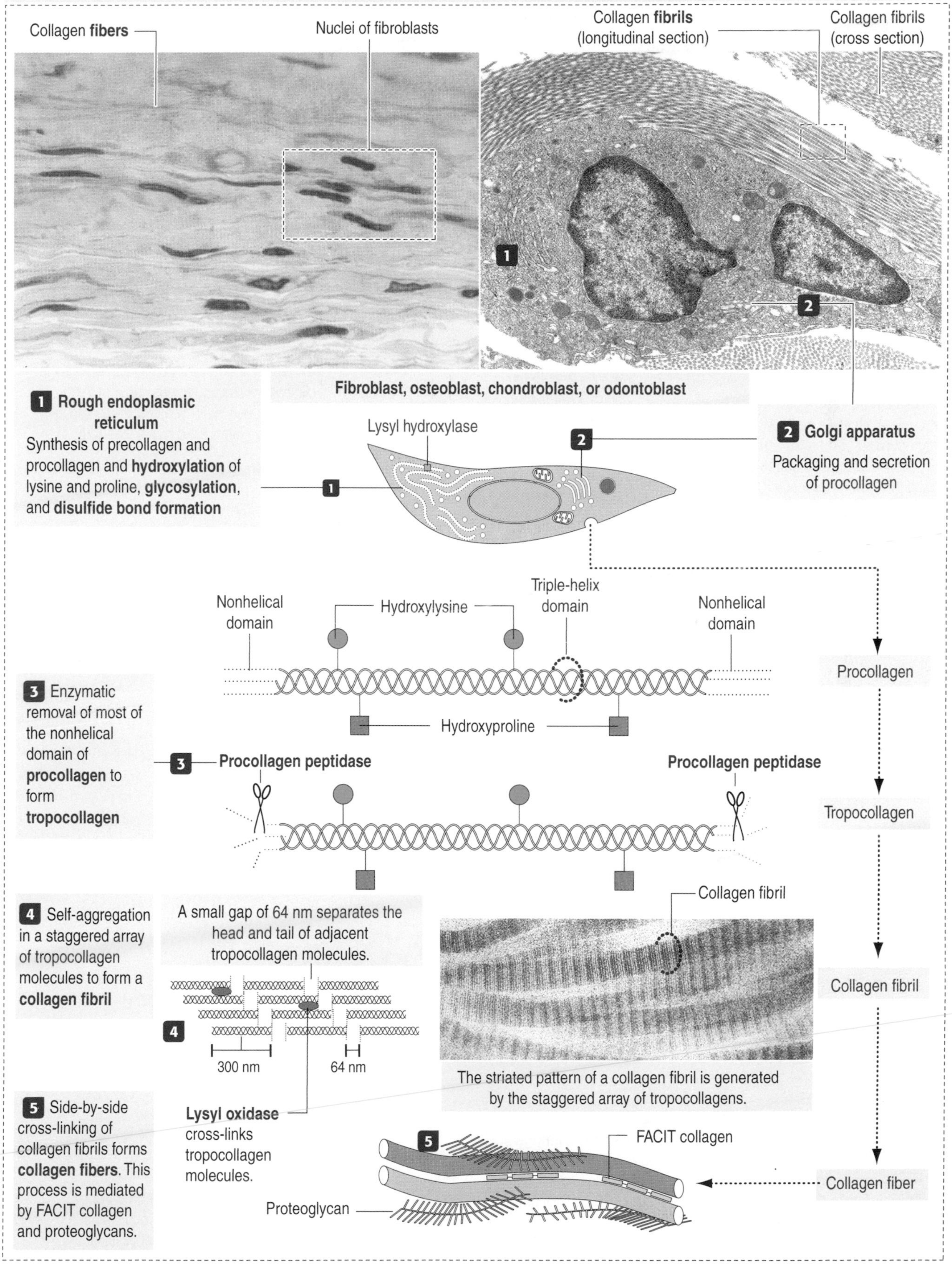

Collagen fibers
Nuclei of fibroblasts
Collagen fibrils (longitudinal section)
Collagen fibrils (cross section)
1
2
Fibroblast, osteoblast, chondroblast, or odontoblast
1 Rough endoplasmic reticulum
Synthesis of precollagen and procollagen and hydroxylation of lysine and proline, glycosylation, and disulfide bond formation
Lysyl hydroxylase
2 Golgi apparatus
Packaging and secretion of procollagen
Nonhelical domain
Hydroxylysine
Triple-helix domain
Nonhelical domain
Procollagen
Hydroxyproline
3 Enzymatic removal of most of the nonhelical domain of procollagen to form tropocollagen
3 Procollagen peptidase
Procollagen peptidase
Tropocollagen
4 Self-aggregation in a staggered array of tropocollagen molecules to form a collagen fibril
A small gap of 64 nm separates the head and tail of adjacent tropocollagen molecules.
Collagen fibril
Collagen fibril
4
300 nm
64 nm
The striated pattern of a collagen fibril is generated by the staggered array of tropocollagens.
5 Side-by-side cross-linking of collagen fibrils forms collagen fibers. This process is mediated by FACIT collagen and proteoglycans.
Lysyl oxidase cross-links tropocollagen molecules.
5
FACIT collagen
Collagen fiber
Proteoglycan

Box 4-C | **Characteristics of collagens**

- Collagen is a three-chain fibrous protein in which the chains coil around each other (called a coiled-coil structure) like the strands of a rope. This triple-helix molecular organization generates a protein with considerable tensile strength.
- In **fibrillar collagen** (types I, II, III, and V), the completely processed molecule contains one triple helix, which accounts for almost the entire length of each molecule. Multiple triple helices of collagen fibers are aligned end-to-end and side-by-side in a regular arrangement. As a result, collagen fibers form dark and light periodic bands observed with the electron microscope.
- In **nonfibrillar collagens**, such as **type IV collagen,** several shorter triple-helical segments are separated by nontriple-helical domains and the N-terminal and C-terminal globular domains are not cleaved during protein processing.
- **Collagens form aggregates** (fibrils, fibers, or bundles) either alone or with extracellular matrix components. **Collagen fibrils and fibers** can be visualized with the electron microscope but not with the light microscope. **Collagen bundles** can be identified with the light microscope.

Figure 4-4. **Ehlers-Danlos syndrome**

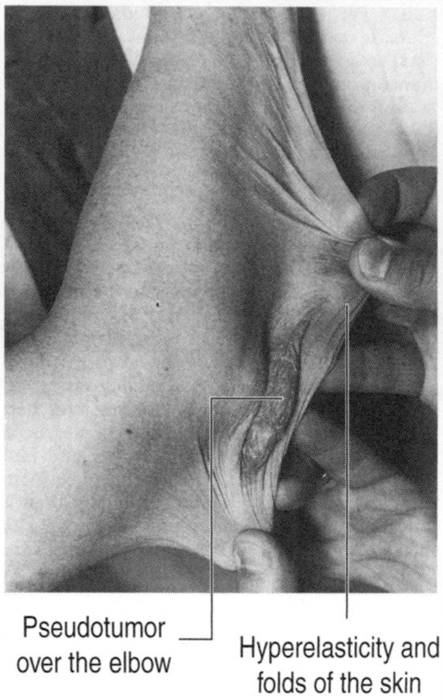
Pseudotumor over the elbow
Hyperelasticity and folds of the skin

Steinmann B, et al.: The Ehlers-Danlos syndrome. In ConnectiveTissue and its Heritable Disorders. New York, Wiley-Liss, 1993.

Ehlers-Danlos syndrome

An inherited defect in the **procollagen peptidase**–triggered removal of the nonhelical endings of procollagen results in the formation of defective collagen fibrils.

Another form of the syndrome involves a mutation of the gene encoding the enzyme **lysyl hydroxylase,** required for the post-translational modification of lysine into hydroxylysine. **Lysyl oxidase** stabilizes the staggered array of tropocollagen molecules by catalyzing the formation of aldol cross-links between hydroxylysine side chains. Defective hydroxylation of lysine decreases the strength of the collagen molecule in Ehlers-Danlos syndrome.

This syndrome can be divided into several clinically distinct subtypes, most of them characterized by **joint dislocation** (hip and other large joints) and **hyperelasticity of the skin.**

of varicose veins and spontaneous rupture of major arteries. A deficiency in the synthesis of type III collagen, prevalent in the walls of blood vessels, is the major defect. Type VII Ehlers-Danlos syndrome displays congenital dislocation of the hips and marked joint hypermobility. Mutations in the *COL1A1* and *COL1A2* genes (Figure 4-5), encoding type I collagen, disrupt the cleavage site at the N-terminal of the molecule and affect the conversion of procollagen to collagen in some individuals.

Elastic fibers: Synthesis, secretion, and assembly

Like collagen, the synthesis of elastic fibers involves both the RER and the Golgi

Figure 4-5. **Pathology of collagen: Molecular defects**

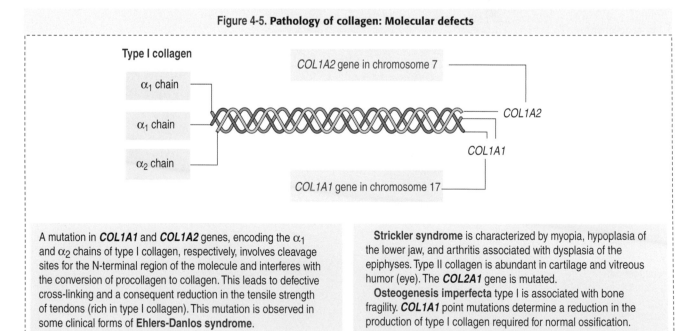

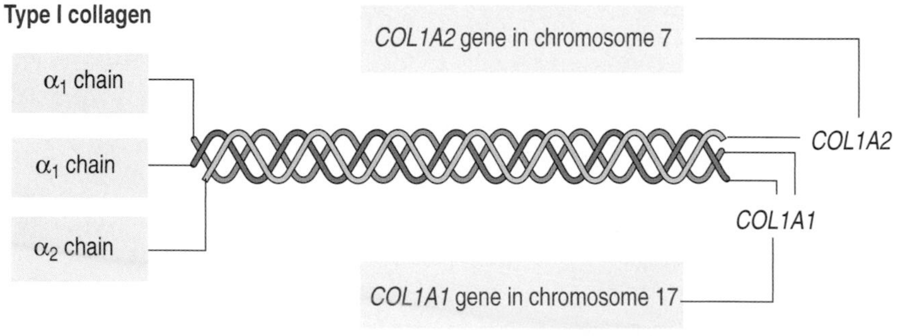
Type I collagen
COL1A2 gene in chromosome 7
α_1 chain
α_1 chain
α_2 chain
COL1A2
COL1A1
COL1A1 gene in chromosome 17

A mutation in ***COL1A1*** and ***COL1A2*** genes, encoding the α_1 and α_2 chains of type I collagen, respectively, involves cleavage sites for the N-terminal region of the molecule and interferes with the conversion of procollagen to collagen. This leads to defective cross-linking and a consequent reduction in the tensile strength of tendons (rich in type I collagen). This mutation is observed in some clinical forms of **Ehlers-Danlos syndrome**.

Strickler syndrome is characterized by myopia, hypoplasia of the lower jaw, and arthritis associated with dysplasia of the epiphyses. Type II collagen is abundant in cartilage and vitreous humor (eye). The ***COL2A1*** gene is mutated.

Osteogenesis imperfecta type I is associated with bone fragility. ***COL1A1*** point mutations determine a reduction in the production of type I collagen required for normal ossification.

Figure 4-6. **Synthesis of elastic fibers**

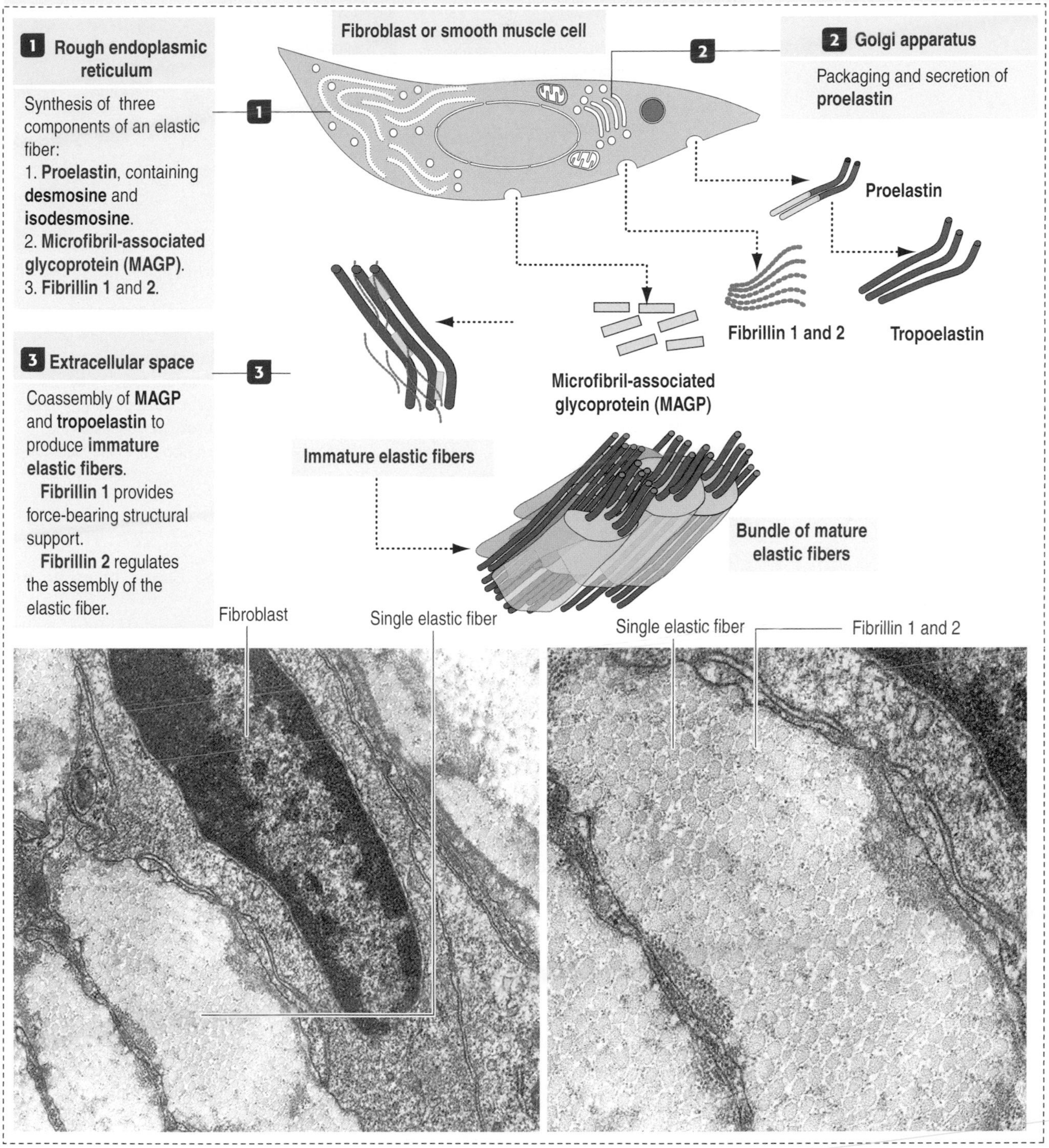

1 Rough endoplasmic reticulum
Synthesis of three components of an elastic fiber:
1. Proelastin, containing desmosine and isodesmosine.
2. Microfibril-associated glycoprotein (MAGP).
3. Fibrillin 1 and 2.
Fibroblast or smooth muscle cell
2 Golgi apparatus
Packaging and secretion of proelastin
Proelastin
Fibrillin 1 and 2
Tropoelastin
Microfibril-associated glycoprotein (MAGP)
3 Extracellular space
Coassembly of MAGP and tropoelastin to produce immature elastic fibers.
Fibrillin 1 provides force-bearing structural support.
Fibrillin 2 regulates the assembly of the elastic fiber.
Immature elastic fibers
Bundle of mature elastic fibers
Fibroblast
Single elastic fiber
Single elastic fiber
Fibrillin 1 and 2

apparatus (Figure 4-6).

Elastic fibers are synthesized by the **fibroblast** (in skin and tendons), the **chondroblast**, the **chondrocyte** (in elastic cartilage of the auricle of the ear, epiglottis, larynx, and auditory tubes), and **smooth muscle cells** (in large blood vessels like the aorta and in the respiratory tree).

Proelastin, the precursor of elastin, is secreted as **tropoelastin.** In the extracellular space, tropoelastin interacts with **fibrillin** to organize **immature elastic fibers**, which aggregate to form **mature elastic fibers.** Elastin contains two characteristic but uncommon amino acids: **desmosine** and **isodesmosine.** These amino acids are responsible for cross-linking mature elastic fibers and

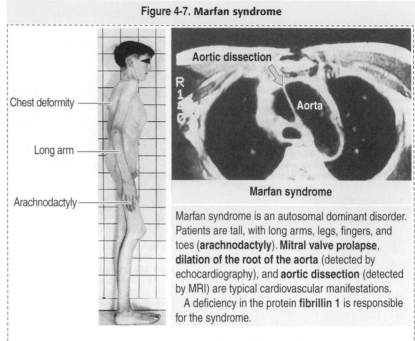

Figure 4-7. Marfan syndrome

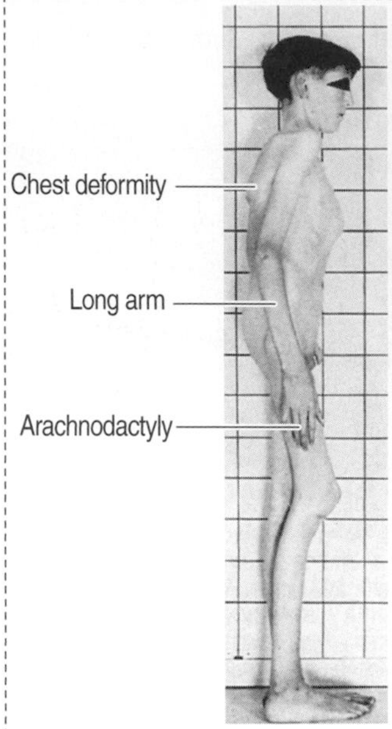

Chest deformity
Long arm
Arachnodactyly

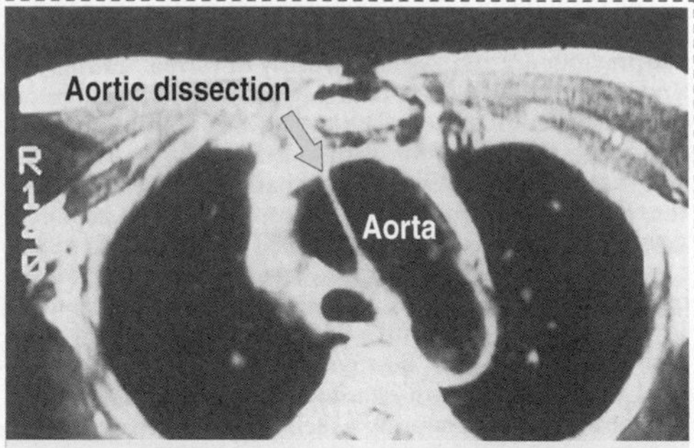

Aortic dissection
Aorta

Marfan syndrome

Marfan syndrome is an autosomal dominant disorder. Patients are tall, with long arms, legs, fingers, and toes (**arachnodactyly**). **Mitral valve prolapse**, **dilation of the root of the aorta** (detected by echocardiography), and **aortic dissection** (detected by MRI) are typical cardiovascular manifestations.

A deficiency in the protein **fibrillin 1** is responsible for the syndrome.

Patient with Marfan syndrome from McKusick VA: Heritable Disorders of Connective Tissue, 4th ed. St. Louis, Mosby, 1972.
MRI from Pyeritz RE: The Marfan syndrome, Royce PM, Steinmann B (eds): In Connective Tissue and its Heritable Disorders. New York, Wiley-Liss, 1993.

enable their stretching and recoil, like rubber bands. **Elastic fibers do not contain collagen.**

Under the light microscope, elastic fibers stain black or dark blue with **orcein**, a natural dye obtained from lichens.

Under the electron microscope, a cross section of an elastic fiber shows a dense core of elastin surrounded by microfibrils containing a number of **microfibril-associated glycoproteins** (MAGPs) and **fibrillin**. Fibrillin is a 35-kd glycoprotein.

Clinical significance: Marfan syndrome

Marfan syndrome is an autosomal dominant disorder in which the elastic tissue is weakened. Defects are predominantly observed in three systems: the **ocular**, **skeletal**, and **cardiovascular systems**. The **ocular defects** include **myopia** and **detached lens** (ectopia lentis). The skeletal defects (Figure 4-7) include long and thin arms and legs (**dolichostenomelia**), hollow chest (**pectus excavatum**), scoliosis, and elongated fingers (**arachnodactyly**). Cardiovascular abnormalities are life-threatening. Patients with Marfan syndrome display **prolapse of the mitral valve** and **dilation of the ascending aorta**. Dilation of the aorta leads to dissecting aneurysm (Greek *aneurysma*, widening) or rupture. Medical treatment, such as administration of β-adrenergic blockers to reduce the force of systolic contraction in order to diminish stress on the aorta, and limited heavy exercise increase the survival rate of patients with Marfan syndrome.

Defects observed in Marfan syndrome are caused by abnormalities in the connective tissue, which becomes too elastic, with poor recoiling. In the skeletal system, the periosteum, a relatively rigid layer covering the bone, is abnormally elastic and does not provide an oppositional force during bone development, resulting in skeletal defects.

A mutation of the fibrillin 1 gene on chromosome 15 is responsible for Marfan syndrome. Fibrillin is present in the aorta, suspensory ligaments of the lens (see Chapter 9, Sensory Organs: Vision and Hearing), and the periosteum (see Bone).

A homologous fibrillin 2 gene is present on chromosome 5. Mutations in the fibrillin 2 gene cause a disease called congenital contractural arachnodactyly.

Figure 4-8. Macrophage

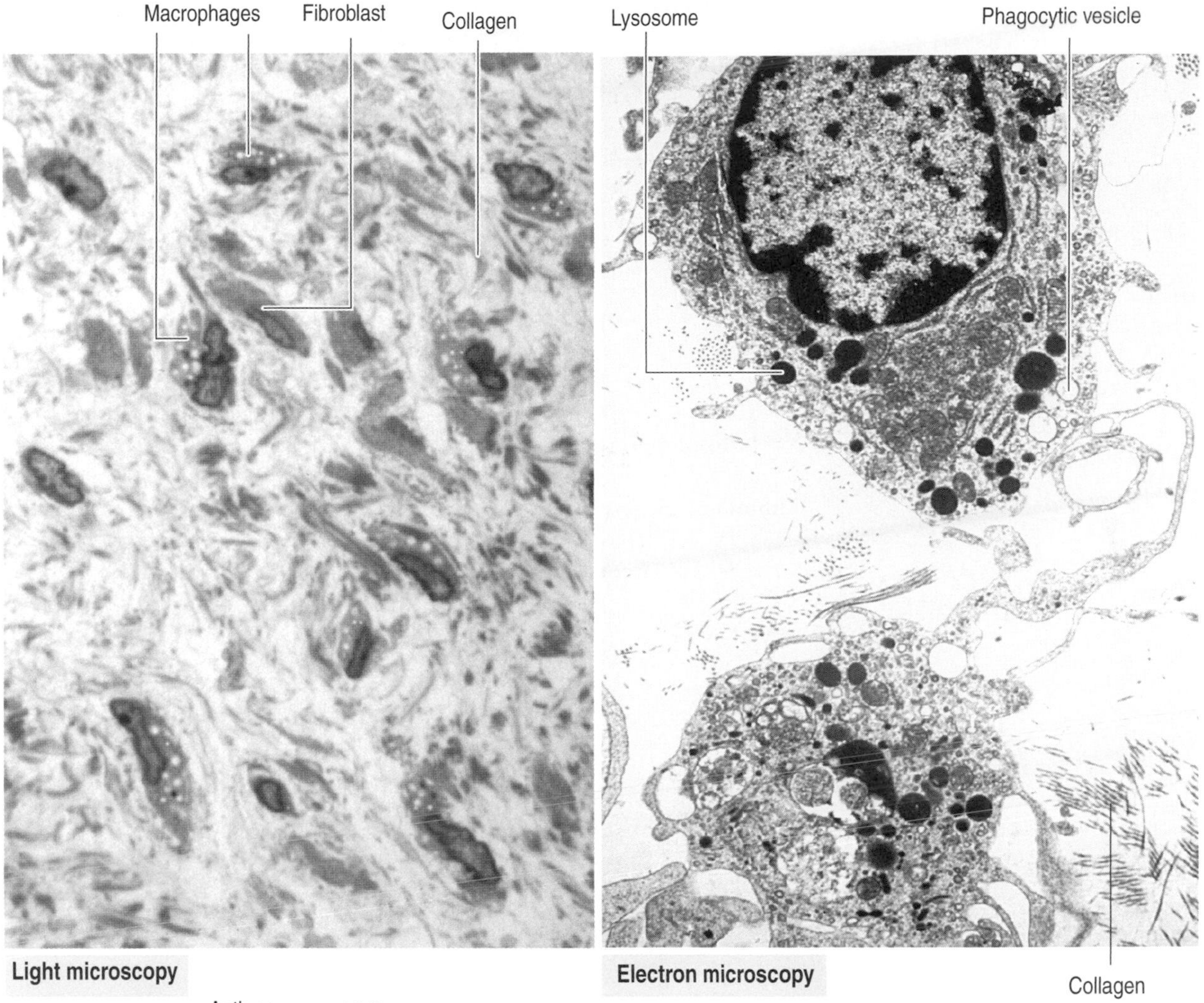

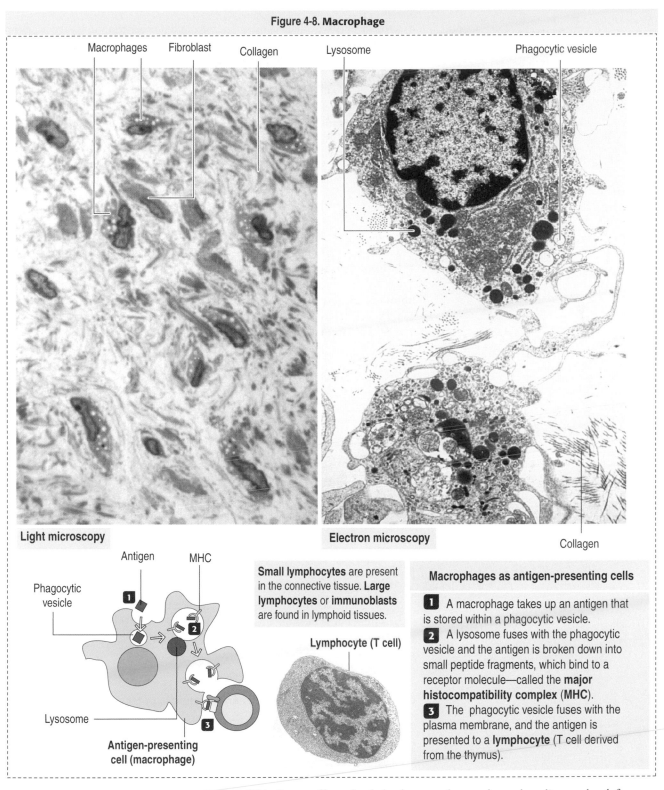

Macrophages
Fibroblast
Collagen
Lysosome
Phagocytic vesicle
Light microscopy
Electron microscopy
Collagen

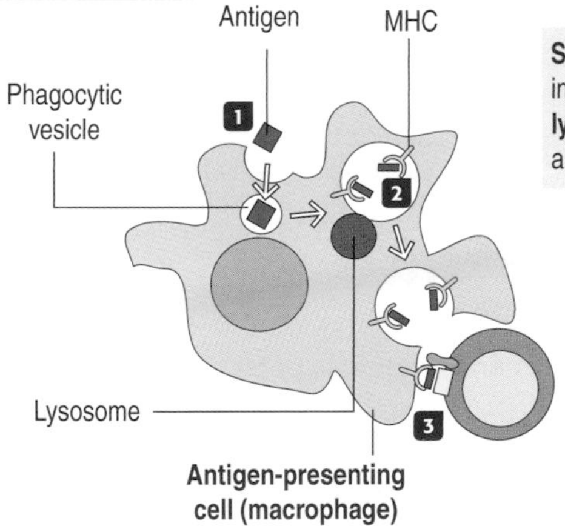

Antigen
MHC
Phagocytic vesicle
1
2
3
Lysosome
Antigen-presenting cell (macrophage)

Small lymphocytes are present in the connective tissue. **Large lymphocytes** or **immunoblasts** are found in lymphoid tissues.

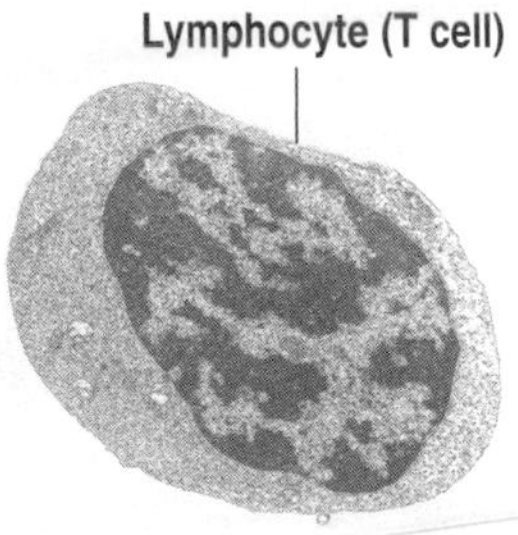

Lymphocyte (T cell)

Macrophages as antigen-presenting cells

1 A macrophage takes up an antigen that is stored within a phagocytic vesicle.
2 A lysosome fuses with the phagocytic vesicle and the antigen is broken down into small peptide fragments, which bind to a receptor molecule—called the **major histocompatibility complex** (**MHC**).
3 The phagocytic vesicle fuses with the plasma membrane, and the antigen is presented to a **lymphocyte** (T cell derived from the thymus).

This disease affects the skeletal system, but ocular and cardiovascular defects are not observed.

More than 100 different fibrillin mutations have been observed. One mutation of the fibrillin 1 gene can decrease fibrillin synthesis and diminish the deposition of this glycoprotein in the ECM. Another mutation prevents the assembly of microfibrils or coassembly of defective fibrillin with normal fibrillin protein produced by a normal allele in the heterozygote.

Box 4-D | **Metachromasia**

• The granules of the mast cell have a staining property known as **metachromasia** (Greek *meta*, beyond; *chroma*, color).
• After staining with a metachromatic dye, such as **toluidine blue**, the mast cell granules stain with a color that is different from the color of the dye (purple-red instead of blue).
• This phenomenon is determined by a change in the electronic structure of the dye molecule after binding to the granular material. In addition, mast cell granules are PAS positive because of their glycoprotein nature.

Macrophage

Macrophages have **phagocytic** properties and derive from monocytes, cells formed in the bone marrow (Figure 4–8).

Monocytes circulate in blood and migrate into the connective tissue, where they differentiate into macrophages. Macrophages have specific names in certain organs; for example, they are called **Kupffer cells** in the liver, **osteoclasts** in bone, and **microglial cells** in the central nervous system. Macrophages migrate to the site of inflammation, attracted by certain mediators, particularly C5a (a member of the complement cascade; see Chapter 10, Immune-Lymphatic System).

Macrophages in the connective tissue have the following structural features:

1. They contain abundant **lysosomes** required for the breakdown of phagocytic materials.

2. Active macrophages have numerous **phagocytic vesicles** (or **phagosomes**) for the transient storage of ingested materials.

3. The nucleus has an irregular outline.

Macrophages of the connective tissue have three major functions:

1. **To turn over senescent fibers and ECM material.**

2. The **presentation of antigens to lymphocytes as part of inflammatory and immunologic responses** (see Chapter 10, Immune-Lymphatic System).

3. **Production of cytokines** (for example, **interleukin-1**, an activator of helper T cells, and **tumor necrosis factor-α**, an inflammatory mediator).

Mast cell

Like macrophages, **mast cells originate in the bone marrow** from precursor cells lacking cytoplasmic granules. When mast cell precursors migrate into the connective tissue or the lamina propria of mucosae, they proliferate and accumulate cytoplasmic granules. **Mast cells and basophils circulating in blood derive from the same progenitor in the bone marrow.**

The **mast cell** is the source of **vasoactive mediators** contained in **cytoplasmic granules** (Figure 4-9). These granules contain **histamine**, **heparin**, and **chemotactic mediators** to attract monocytes, neutrophils, and eosinophils circulating in blood to the site of mast cell activation. Leukotrienes are vasoactive products of mast cells. **Leukotrienes are not present in granules; instead, they are released from the cell membrane of the mast cells as metabolites of arachidonic acid.**

There are two populations of mast cells: **mucosal mast cells** (found predominantly in intestine and lung), and **connective tissue mast cells.**

Connective tissue mast cells differ from mucosal mast cells in the number and size of **metachromatic** (see Box 4-D) cytoplasmic granules, which tend to be more abundant in connective tissue mast cells. Although these two cell populations have the same cell precursor, the definitive structural and functional characteristics of mast cells depend on the site of differentiation (mucosa or connective tissue).

Clinical significance: Mast cells and allergic hypersensitivity reactions

The secretion of specific vasoactive mediators plays an important role in the regulation of vascular permeability and bronchial smooth muscle tone during **allergic hypersensitivity reactions** (for example, in **asthma**, **hay fever**, and **eczema**).

The surface of **mast cells** and **basophils** contains immunoglobulin E (IgE) receptors. Antigens bind to two adjacent IgE receptors and the mast cell becomes IgE-sensitized. An IgE-sensitized mast cell releases Ca^{2+} from intracellular storage sites and the content of the cytoplasmic granules is rapidly discharged by a process known as **degranulation.**

The release of histamine during asthma (Greek *asthma*, panting) causes dyspnea (Greek *dyspnoia*, difficulty with breathing) triggered by the histamine-induced spasmodic contraction of the smooth muscle surrounding the bronchioles and the hypersecretion of goblet cells and mucosal glands of bronchi.

Figure 4-9. **Mast cell**

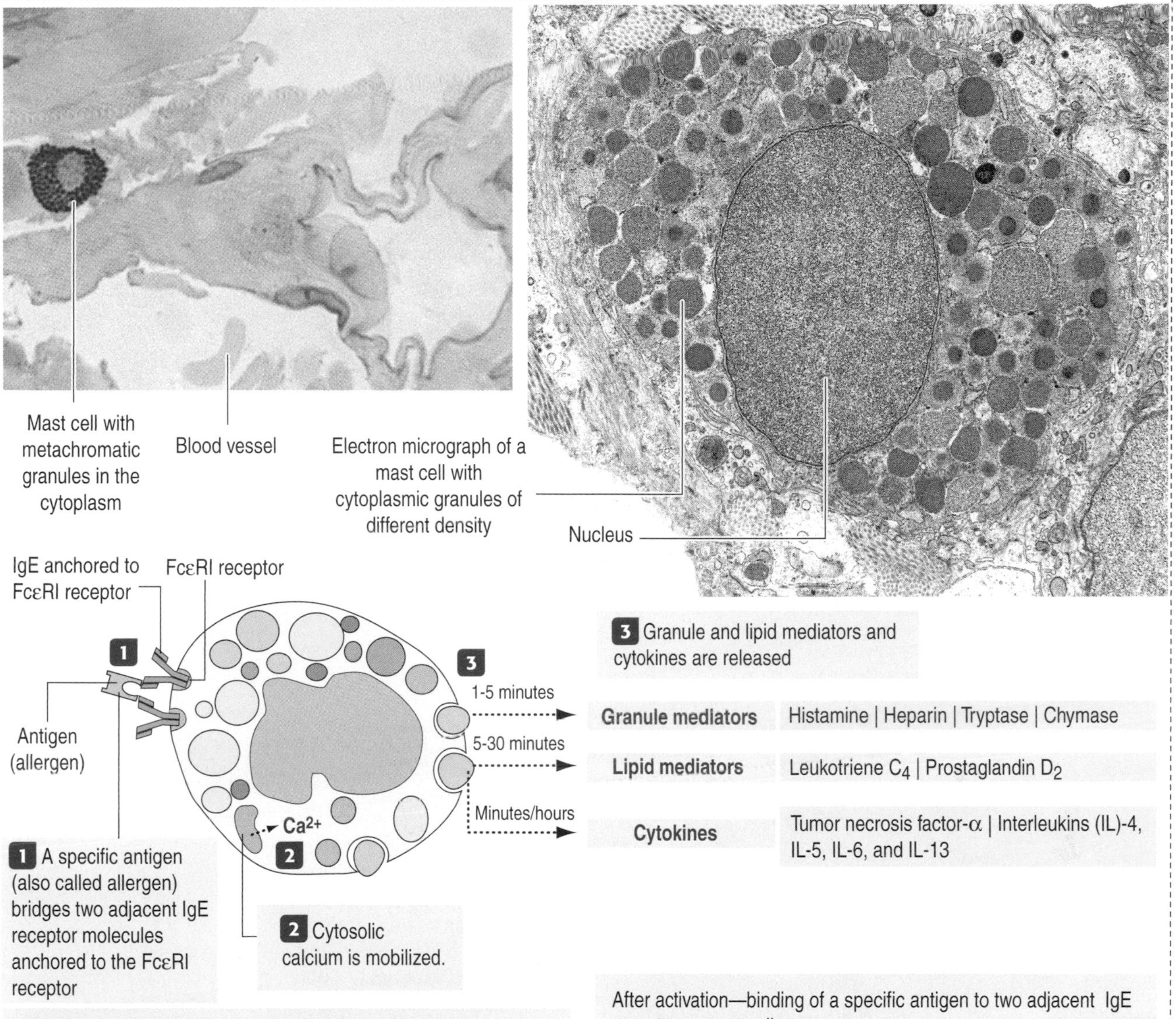

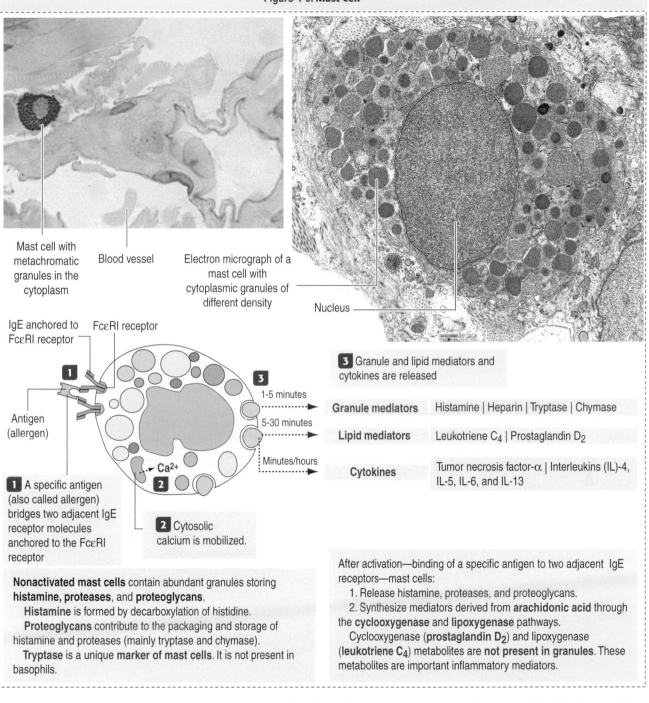

Mast cell with metachromatic granules in the cytoplasm
Blood vessel
Electron micrograph of a mast cell with cytoplasmic granules of different density
Nucleus
IgE anchored to FcεRI receptor
FcεRI receptor
1
Antigen (allergen)
Ca2+
2
3
1-5 minutes
5-30 minutes
Minutes/hours
3 Granule and lipid mediators and cytokines are released
Granule mediators
Histamine | Heparin | Tryptase | Chymase
Lipid mediators
Leukotriene C4 | Prostaglandin D2
Cytokines
Tumor necrosis factor-α | Interleukins (IL)-4, IL-5, IL-6, and IL-13
1 A specific antigen (also called allergen) bridges two adjacent IgE receptor molecules anchored to the FcεRI receptor
2 Cytosolic calcium is mobilized.

Nonactivated mast cells contain abundant granules storing **histamine, proteases**, and **proteoglycans**.

Histamine is formed by decarboxylation of histidine.

Proteoglycans contribute to the packaging and storage of histamine and proteases (mainly tryptase and chymase).

Tryptase is a unique **marker of mast cells**. It is not present in basophils.

After activation—binding of a specific antigen to two adjacent IgE receptors—mast cells:

1. Release histamine, proteases, and proteoglycans.
2. Synthesize mediators derived from **arachidonic acid** through the **cyclooxygenase** and **lipoxygenase** pathways.

Cyclooxygenase (**prostaglandin D_2**) and lipoxygenase (**leukotriene C_4**) metabolites are **not present in granules**. These metabolites are important inflammatory mediators.

During **hay fever**, histamine increases vascular permeability leading to edema (excessive accumulation of fluid in intercellular spaces).

Mast cells in the connective tissue of skin release leukotrienes that induce increased vascular permeability associated with **urticaria** (Latin *urtica*, stinging nettle), a transient swelling in the dermis of the skin.

Plasma cell

The plasma cell, which derives from the differentiation of **B lymphocytes** (also called **B cells**), synthesizes and secretes a single class of immunoglobulin (Figure 4-10). We discuss in Chapter 10, Immune-Lymphatic System, details of the origin of plasma cells.

Immunoglobulins are glycoproteins, and therefore plasma cells have the three

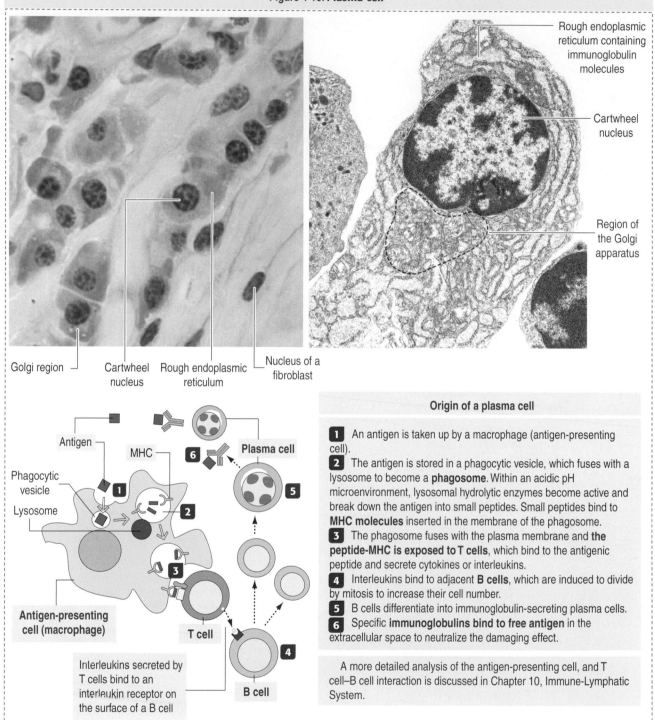

Figure 4-10. Plasma cell

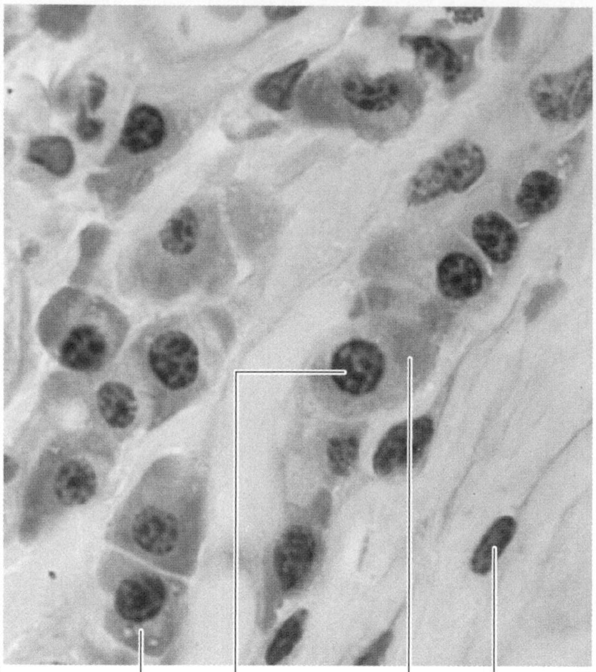

Golgi region
Cartwheel nucleus
Rough endoplasmic reticulum
Nucleus of a fibroblast

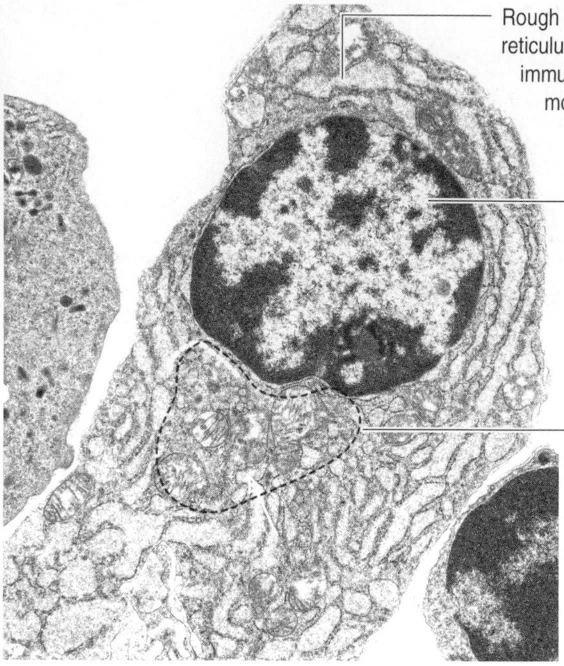

Rough endoplasmic reticulum containing immunoglobulin molecules
Cartwheel nucleus
Region of the Golgi apparatus

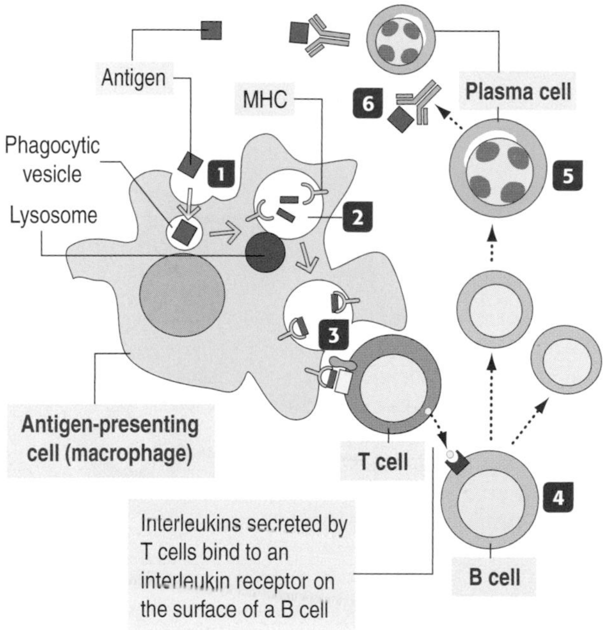

Antigen
MHC
Plasma cell
Phagocytic vesicle
Lysosome
1
2
3
4
5
6
Antigen-presenting cell (macrophage)
T cell
B cell
Interleukins secreted by T cells bind to an interleukin receptor on the surface of a B cell

Origin of a plasma cell

1 An antigen is taken up by a macrophage (antigen-presenting cell).

2 The antigen is stored in a phagocytic vesicle, which fuses with a lysosome to become a **phagosome**. Within an acidic pH microenvironment, lysosomal hydrolytic enzymes become active and break down the antigen into small peptides. Small peptides bind to **MHC molecules** inserted in the membrane of the phagosome.

3 The phagosome fuses with the plasma membrane and **the peptide-MHC is exposed to T cells**, which bind to the antigenic peptide and secrete cytokines or interleukins.

4 Interleukins bind to adjacent **B cells**, which are induced to divide by mitosis to increase their cell number.

5 B cells differentiate into immunoglobulin-secreting plasma cells.

6 Specific **immunoglobulins bind to free antigen** in the extracellular space to neutralize the damaging effect.

A more detailed analysis of the antigen-presenting cell, and T cell–B cell interaction is discussed in Chapter 10, Immune-Lymphatic System.

structural characteristics of cells active in protein synthesis and secretion:

1. A well-developed **rough endoplasmic reticulum.**
2. An extensive **Golgi apparatus.**
3. A prominent **nucleolus.**

At the light microscopic level, most of the cytoplasm of a plasma cell is basophilic because of the large amount of ribosomes associated with the endoplasmic reticulum. A clear area near the nucleus is slightly **acidophilic** and represents the Golgi apparatus. The nucleus has a characteristic cartwheel configuration created by the particular distribution of heterochromatin.

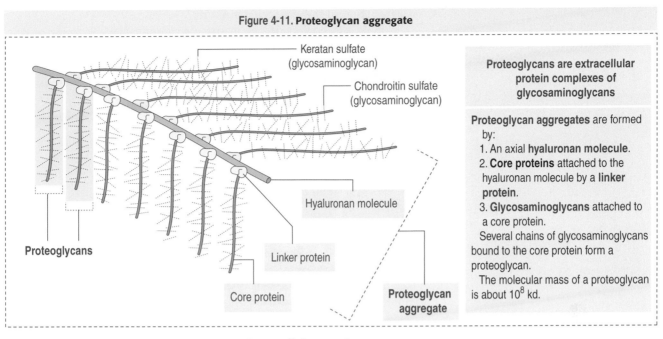

Figure 4-11. **Proteoglycan aggregate**

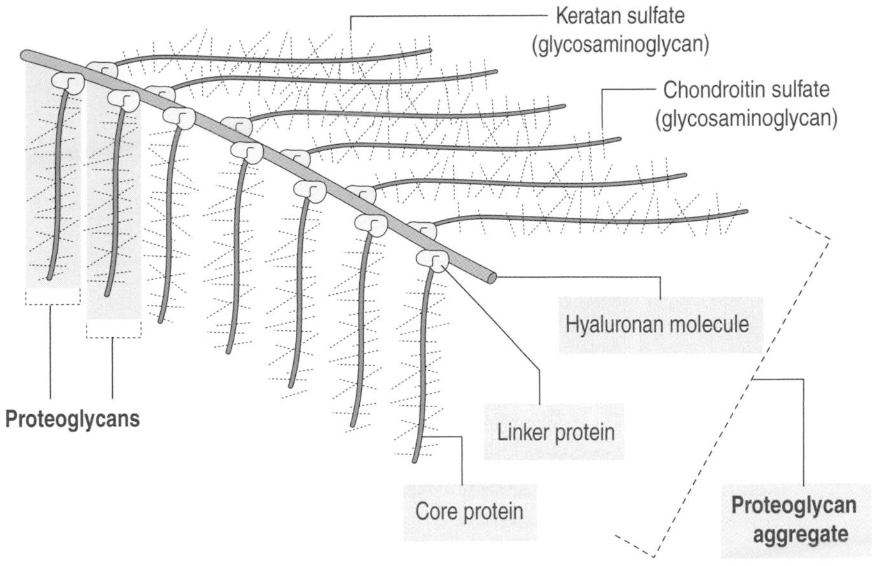

Proteoglycans are extracellular protein complexes of glycosaminoglycans

Proteoglycan aggregates are formed by:
1. An axial **hyaluronan molecule.**
2. **Core proteins** attached to the hyaluronan molecule by a **linker protein.**
3. **Glycosaminoglycans** attached to a core protein.

Several chains of glycosaminoglycans bound to the core protein form a proteoglycan.

The molecular mass of a proteoglycan is about 10^8 kd.

Extracellular matrix

The ECM is a combination of **collagens**, **noncollagenous glycoproteins**, and **proteoglycans** surrounding cells and fibers of the connective tissue.

Recall that the **basement membrane** contains several ECM components such as **laminin**, **fibronectin**, various types of **collagen**, and **heparan sulfate proteoglycan**. In addition, epithelial and nonepithelial cells have receptors for ECM constituents. An example is the family of **integrins** with binding affinity for laminin and fibronectin. Integrins interact with the cytoskeleton, strengthening cell interactions with the ECM by establishing focal contacts or modifying cell shape or adhesion.

Several noncollagenous glycoproteins of the ECM mediate interactions with cells and regulate the assembly of ECM components. Noncollagenous glycoproteins have a widespread distribution in several connective tissues, although cartilage and bone contain specific types of noncollagenous glycoproteins. We study them later when we discuss the processes of **chondrogenesis** (formation of cartilage) and **osteogenesis** (bone formation).

Proteoglycan aggregates (Figure 4-11) are the major components of the ECM. Each proteoglycan consists of **glycosaminoglycans (GAGs)**, proteins complexed with polysaccharides. GAGs are linear polymers of disaccharides with sulfate residues. GAGs control the biological functions of proteoglycans by establishing links with cell surface components, growth factors, and other ECM constituents.

Different types of GAGs are attached to a **core protein** to form a proteoglycan. The core protein, in turn, is linked to a **hyaluronan molecule** by a **linker protein.** The hyaluronan molecule is the axis of a **proteoglycan aggregate.** Proteoglycans are named according to the prevalent GAG (for example, **proteoglycan chondroitin sulfate, proteoglycan dermatan sulfate, proteoglycan heparan sulfate**).

The **embryonic connective tissue** of the umbilical cord (**Wharton's jelly**) is predominantly ECM material surrounding the two umbilical arteries and the single umbilical vein. Proteoglycans have extremely high charge density and, therefore, significant osmotic pressure. These attributes enable a connective tissue bed to resist compression because of the very high swelling capacity of these molecules. The umbilical blood vessels, crucial elements for fetal-maternal fluid, gas, and nutritional exchange, are surrounded by a proteoglycan-enriched type of connective tissue to provide resistance to compression.

Degradation of the extracellular matrix

The ECM can be degraded by **matrix metalloproteinases**, a family of zinc-dependent proteases **secreted as latent precursors (zymogens)** proteolytically activated in the ECM. The activity of matrix metalloproteinases in the extracellular space can be specifically inhibited by **tissue inhibitors of metalloproteinases (TIMPs)**.

The expression of matrix metalloproteinase genes is regulated by cytokines, growth factors, and cell contact with the ECM.

The degradation of the ECM occurs normally during the development, growth, and repair of tissues. However, excessive degradation of the ECM is observed in several pathologic conditions such as rheumatoid arthritis, osteoarthritis, and diseases of the skin. Tumor invasion, metastasis, and tumor angiogenesis require the participation of matrix metalloproteinases whose expression increases in association with tumorigenesis.

Members of the family of matrix metalloproteinases include:

1. **Collagenases**. Collagenases 1, 2 and 3 can degrade types I, II, III, and V collagens. Collagenase 1 is synthesized by fibroblasts, chondrocytes (cartilage), keratinocytes (epidermis), monocytes and macrophages, hepatocytes (liver), and tumor cells. Collagenase 2 is stored in cytoplasmic granules of polymorphonuclear leukocytes and released in response to a stimulus. Collagenase 3 can degrade several collagens (types I, II, III, IV, IX, X, and XI), laminin and fibronectin, and other ECM components.

2. **Stromelysins** (1, 2, and metalloelastase), which degrade basement membrane components (type IV collagen and fibronectin) and elastin.

3. **Gelatinases A** and **B** can degrade type I collagen. Gelatinases are produced by alveolar macrophages.

4. **Membrane-type matrix metalloproteinases** are produced by tumor cells.

Matrix metalloproteinases are a target of therapeutic intervention to inhibit tumor invasion and metastasis. We come back to this topic in Chapter 23, Fertilization, Placentation, and Lactation, when we discuss the early stages of embryo implantation in the endometrial stroma or decidua.

Clinical significance: Molecular biology of tumor invasion

Invasion and metastasis are two important events of carcinoma (Greek *karkinoma*, from *karkinos*, crab, cancer + *oma*, tumor), a tumor derived from epithelial tissues. **Adenoma** is a structurally benign tumor of epithelial cell origin lacking invasive and metastatic properties. Malignant carcinomas may arise from benign adenomas. For example, a small benign adenoma or **polyp** of the colon can become an invasive carcinoma.

Sarcoma (Greek *sarx,* flesh + *oma*) is a tumor derived from the connective tissues (muscle, bone, cartilage) and mesodermal cells. For example, fibrosarcoma derives from fibroblasts and osteosarcoma originates from bone.

Invasion is defined by the **breakdown of the basement membrane** by tumor cells and implies the transition from precancer to cancer. **Metastasis** is the spread of tumor cells throughout the body through blood and lymphatic vessels, generally leading to death. Figure 4-12 illustrates and describes the initial events of tumor cell invasion.

Many carcinomas produce members of the matrix metalloproteinase family to digest various types of collagen as we have seen in the preceding section. Normal tissues produce tissue inhibitors of metalloproteinases that are neutralized by carcinoma cells. Tumors that behave aggressively are capable of overpowering the protease inhibitors.

One critical event during metastasis is angiogenesis, the development of blood vessels. Blood vessels supply oxygen and nutrients required for tumor growth. Angiogenesis is stimulated by tumor cells, in particular the proliferation of capillary endothelial cells forming new capillaries in the tumoral growth.

Figure 4-12. Tumor invasion and metastasis

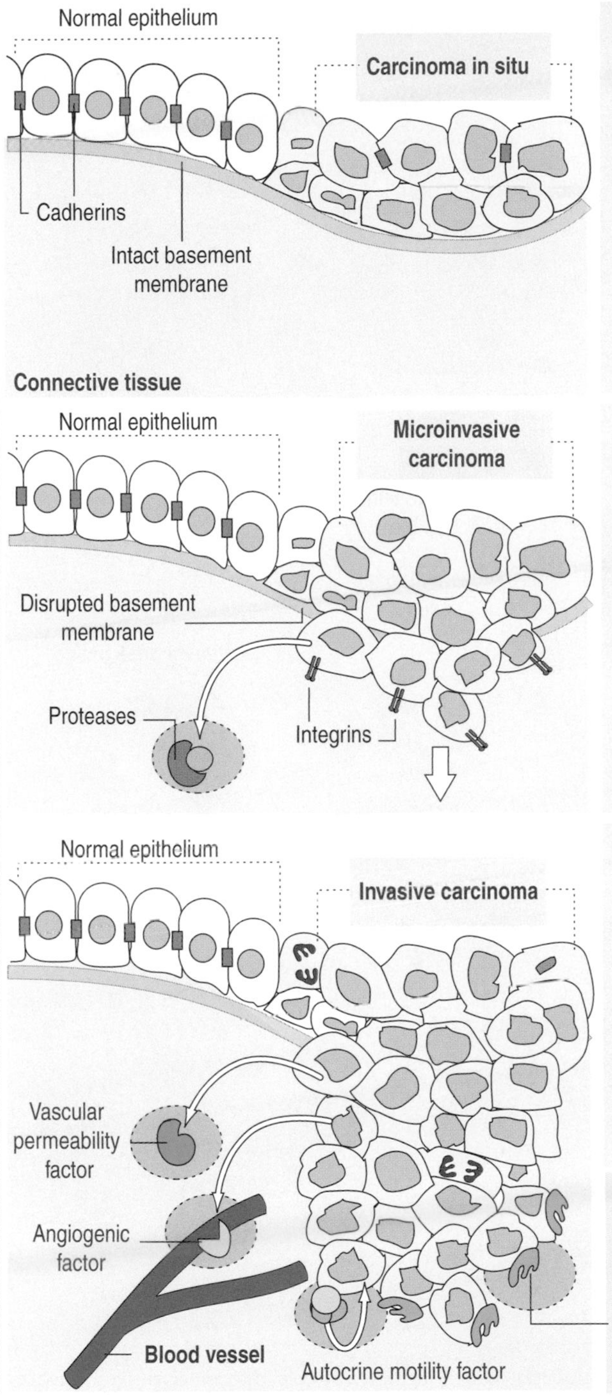

Tumor cells have not invaded the basement membrane and remain confined within the epithelial layer. This stage is known as **carcinoma in situ.**

The expression of cell adhesion molecules, such as **cadherins**, decreases. This decrease weakens the cohesive nature of the intraepithelial tumor cells, and **microinvasion** starts when the basement membrane breaks down.

Collagenase IV, released by invading tumor cells, dissolves the basement membrane and allows tumor cells to invade the subjacent connective tissue. Other proteases, such as **plasminogen activator**, **collagenases I**, **II**, and **III**, **cathepsins**, and **hyaluronidase**, destroy noncollagenous glycoproteins and proteoglycans, enabling further advancement of tumor cells into the destroyed connective tissue.

Invading tumor cells overexpress **integrins** (laminin and fibronectin receptors) to facilitate cell attachment and progression in the connective tissue. Tumor cells generally invade along pathways that provide low resistance, such as connective tissue.

As tumor cells start their **invasive phase**, they secrete:

1. **Autocrine motility factors** (to direct the motion of the advancing tumor cells).
2. **Vascular permeability factors** (to enable plasma proteins and nutritional factors to accumulate).
3. **Angiogenic factor** (to increase the vascularity and nutritional support of the growing tumor). See Chapter 12, Cardiovascular System, for a discussion of tumor angiogenesis.

Because newly formed blood vessels are connected with the general circulation, tumor cells can rapidly enter the blood vessels and disseminate to distant tissues. This event is known as **metastasis**.

Mammary tumor cells express **CXC chemokine receptor 4** (**CXCR4**) on their surface. When tumor cells migrate across the wall of blood and lymphatic vessels, they are stalled in vascular beds producing high levels of the CXCR4 ligand **CXCL12**, which is expressed on the surface of **endothelial cells**. CXCL12 binding to CXCR4 induces migration of tumor cells into the surrounding normal tissue where they form a metastatic tumor.

In Chapter 12, Cardiovascular System, we discuss the mechanism of action and targets of endostatin and angiostatin, two new proteins that inhibit angiogenesis.

Adipose tissue or fat

There are two classes of adipose tissue:

1. **White fat**, the major **reserve of long-term energy**.
2. **Brown fat**, which serves primarily to **dissipate energy** instead of storing it.

Similar to fibroblasts, the primitive **preadipocyte** derives from a mesenchymal

Figure 4-13. Adipogenesis

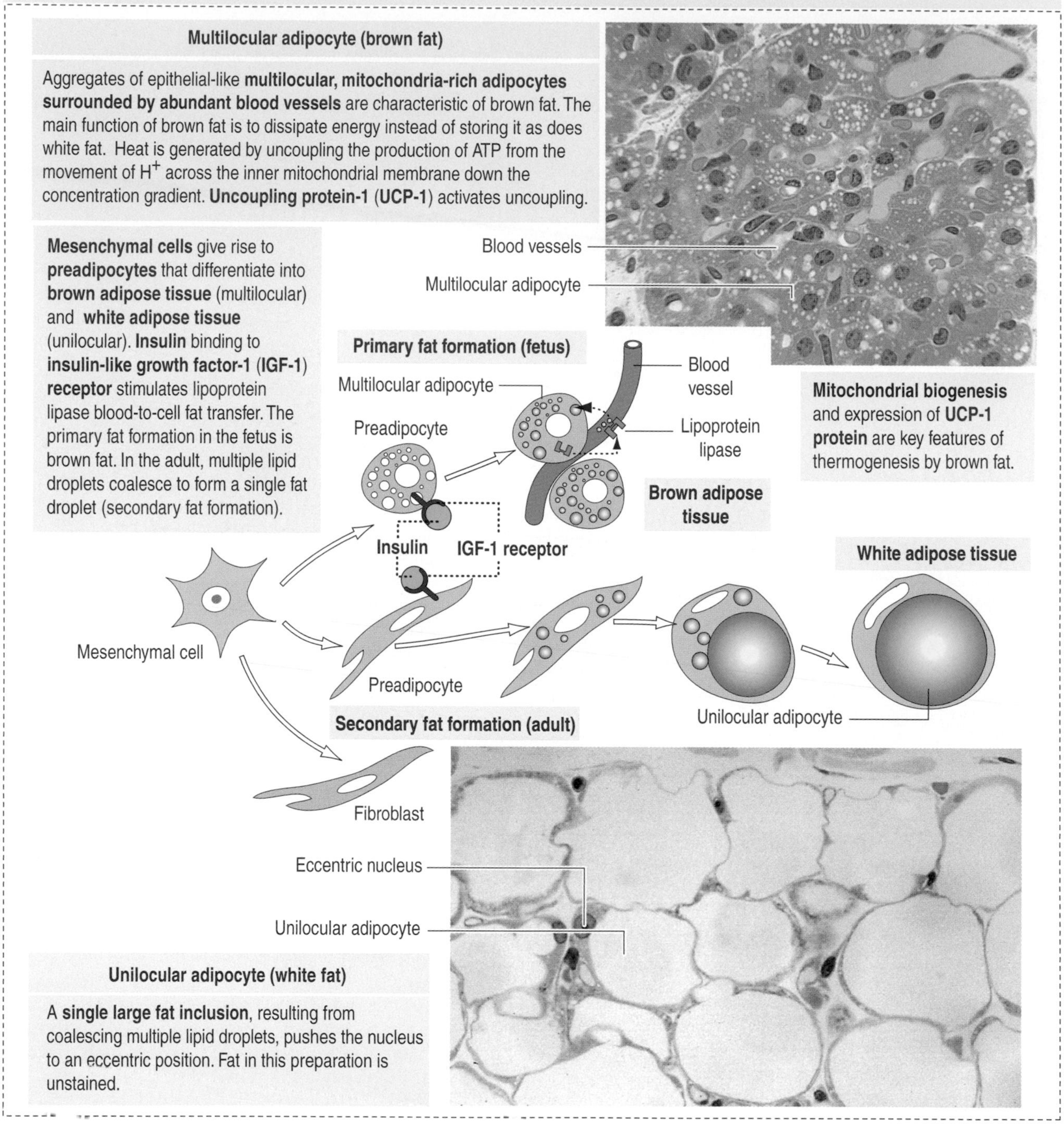
Multilocular adipocyte (brown fat)
Aggregates of epithelial-like **multilocular, mitochondria-rich adipocytes surrounded by abundant blood vessels** are characteristic of brown fat. The main function of brown fat is to dissipate energy instead of storing it as does white fat. Heat is generated by uncoupling the production of ATP from the movement of H^+ across the inner mitochondrial membrane down the concentration gradient. **Uncoupling protein-1** (**UCP-1**) activates uncoupling.
Blood vessels
Multilocular adipocyte
Mesenchymal cells give rise to **preadipocytes** that differentiate into **brown adipose tissue** (multilocular) and **white adipose tissue** (unilocular). **Insulin** binding to **insulin-like growth factor-1** (**IGF-1**) **receptor** stimulates lipoprotein lipase blood-to-cell fat transfer. The primary fat formation in the fetus is brown fat. In the adult, multiple lipid droplets coalesce to form a single fat droplet (secondary fat formation).
Primary fat formation (fetus)
Multilocular adipocyte
Preadipocyte
Blood vessel
Lipoprotein lipase
Brown adipose tissue
Mitochondrial biogenesis and expression of **UCP-1 protein** are key features of thermogenesis by brown fat.
Insulin
IGF-1 receptor
White adipose tissue
Mesenchymal cell
Preadipocyte
Secondary fat formation (adult)
Unilocular adipocyte
Fibroblast
Eccentric nucleus
Unilocular adipocyte
Unilocular adipocyte (white fat)
A **single large fat inclusion**, resulting from coalescing multiple lipid droplets, pushes the nucleus to an eccentric position. Fat in this preparation is unstained.

cell precursor. Preadipocytes can follow two cell differentiation pathways: one pathway results in the formation of white fat; the other generates brown fat. Adipogenesis occurs during both the prenatal and postnatal states of the individual and is reduced as age increases.

Under the influence of **insulin**—bound to **insulin-like growth factor-1 (IGF-1) receptor**—preadipocytes synthesize **lipoprotein lipase** and begin to accumulate fat in small droplets. Small droplets fuse to form a single large lipid-storage droplet, a characteristic of mature unilocular (Latin *unus*, single; *loculus*, small place) **adipocytes** (also called **adipose cell**) (Figure 4-13). The single lipid-storage droplet pushes the nucleus to an eccentric position and the adipocyte assumes a "signet-ring" appearance. **In histologic sections, capillaries appear as single structures that may contain blood cell elements, whereas adipocytes**

Figure 4-14. **Regulation of adipocyte function**

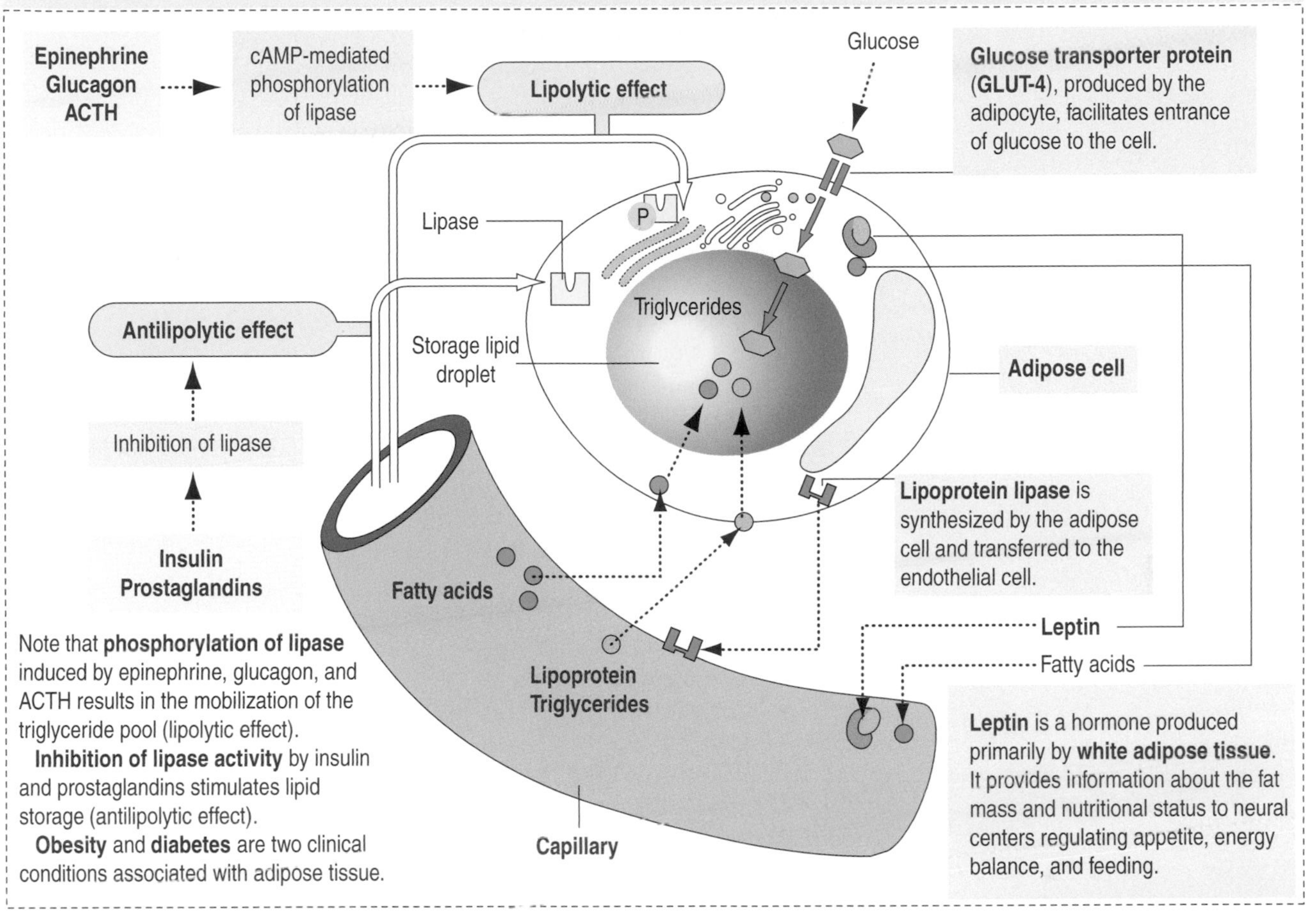
Epinephrine
Glucagon
ACTH
cAMP-mediated phosphorylation of lipase
Lipolytic effect
Glucose
Glucose transporter protein (GLUT-4), produced by the adipocyte, facilitates entrance of glucose to the cell.
Lipase
P
Triglycerides
Antilipolytic effect
Storage lipid droplet
Adipose cell
Inhibition of lipase
Insulin
Prostaglandins
Fatty acids
Lipoprotein lipase is synthesized by the adipose cell and transferred to the endothelial cell.
Leptin
Fatty acids
Note that **phosphorylation of lipase** induced by epinephrine, glucagon, and ACTH results in the mobilization of the triglyceride pool (lipolytic effect).
Inhibition of lipase activity by insulin and prostaglandins stimulates lipid storage (antilipolytic effect).
Obesity and **diabetes** are two clinical conditions associated with adipose tissue.
Lipoprotein
Triglycerides
Leptin is a hormone produced primarily by **white adipose tissue.** It provides information about the fat mass and nutritional status to neural centers regulating appetite, energy balance, and feeding.
Capillary

Box 4-E | **Fat in histologic sections**

- Fat is usually dissolved by solvents (xylene) used during paraffin embedding. Only the nucleus and a narrow cytoplasmic rim, surrounding a central empty space, can be visualized.
- Fat that is fixed and stained with osmium tetroxide appears brown. This reagent is also used for the visualization of lipid-rich myelin in nerves (see Chapter 8, Nervous Tissue).
- Alcoholic solutions of fat-soluble dyes (such as Sudan III or Sudan black) can also be used for the detection of fat in frozen sections.

form aggregates.

Lipid droplets contain about 95% triglycerides rich in carotene, a lipid-soluble pigment that gives the so-called white fat a yellowish color. **Each lipid droplet is in direct contact with the cytosol and is not surrounded by a cytomembrane.** Therefore, lipid droplets can be classified as cell **inclusions** (see Box 4-E).

The **main function of white fat is storage of energy.** Unlike brown fat, white fat responds slightly to cold and acts as an **insulator.** The blood supply to white fat, mainly capillaries, is not as extensive as in brown fat. Adipose tissue also insulates the body against heat loss, fills spaces, and cushions certain anatomic parts, behaving as a shock-absorber in the soles of the feet, around the kidneys, and in the orbit around the eye. Most adipose tissues form at sites where loose connective tissue is present, such as the subcutaneous layer—or hypodermis—of the skin.

The **storage of lipids** by mature adipocytes are regulated by **insulin** and **prostaglandins.** The **breakdown and release of lipids** is regulated by **epinephrine**, **glucagon**, and **adrenocorticotropic hormone** (ACTH) (Figure 4-14). Adipose tissue is innervated by the sympathetic nervous system.

Preadipocytes can differentiate into mature **multilocular** (Latin *multus*, many; *loculus*, small place) **adipocytes of brown fat** in the fetus and newborn. Brown fat is found in the neck, shoulders, back, perirenal, and para-aortic regions of the body. Brown fat is mostly lost during childhood. Brown fat is supplied by abundant blood vessels and sympathetic adrenergic nerve fibers. Lipochrome pigment and abundant mitochondria, rich in cytochromes, give this type of fat a brownish color.

As stated initially, the main function of brown fat is to dissipate energy in the form of heat (thermogenesis) in cold environments as a protective mechanism in the newborn. Thermogenesis by brown fat cells has two requirements (see Figure 4-13):

1. Mitochondrial biogenesis.
2. The expression of the transporter **uncoupling protein-1 (UCP-1)**.

As we briefly mentioned in Chapter 2, Epithelial Glands, in our discussion on UCP transporters in mitochondria, UCP-1 dissipates the proton gradient established across the inner mitochondrial membrane when electrons pass along the respiratory chain. Thermogenesis takes place because UCP-1 allows the reentry of protons down their concentration gradient into the mitochondrial matrix and uncouples respiration from ATP production.

Clinical significance: Obesity

Obesity is a disorder of energy balance. It occurs when energy intake exceeds energy expenditure. Protection against obesity without consideration of energy intake results in an increase in circulating levels of triglycerides, and excessive accumulation of fat in liver (**steatosis**). The metabolic activities of adipocytes have very significant clinical consequences. An increase in visceral adiposity is associated with a higher risk of insulin resistance (see Chapter 19, Endocrine System), **dyslipidemia** (alteration in blood fat levels), and cardiovascular disease.

One of the secreted products of adipocytes is **leptin**, a 16-kd protein encoded by the *ob* **gene**. Leptin is released into the circulation and acts peripherally to regulate body weight. Leptin acts on hypothalamic targets involved in appetite and energy balance. Leptin-deficient mice (*ob/ob*) are obese and infertile. Both conditions are reversible with leptin administration.

The leptin receptor in hypothalamic target cells shares sequence homology with cytokine receptors. During inflammation, the release of the cytokines **interleukin-1** and **tumor necrosis factor-α** increases leptin in serum, an indication that leptin interacts with cytokines to influence responses to infection and inflammatory reactions. Infections, injury, and inflammation upregulate leptin gene expression and serum protein levels. As we discuss later, leptin has a role in bone formation.

Cartilage

Like the fibroblast and the adipocytes, the **chondroblast** derives from a mesenchymal cell. Chondroblasts contain lipids and glycogen, a well-developed RER (basophilic cytoplasm), and Golgi apparatus. The proliferation of chondroblasts results in growth of the cartilage.

Similar to typical connective tissue, the **cartilage consists of cells and ECM surrounded by the perichondrium.** The perichondrium is formed by a layer of undifferentiated cells that can differentiate into chondroblasts.

In contrast to typical connective tissue, the cartilage is **avascular** and cells receive nutrients by diffusion through the ECM. At all ages, chondrocytes have significant nutritional requirements. Although they rarely divide in the adult cartilage, they continuously synthesize molecules to replace a constantly turned-over ECM, in particular, proteoglycans (Figure 4-15; see Box 4-F).

Box 4-F | Cartilage repair after injury

- Cartilage has a modest repair capacity. Cartilage injuries frequently result in the formation of **repair cartilage** from the perichondrium.
- This repair cartilage contains undifferentiated cells with a potential to differentiate into chondrocytes that synthesize components of the cartilage matrix.
- The repair cartilage has a matrix composition intermediate between hyaline and fibrous cartilage (for example, it contains both type I and II collagen).

Growth of cartilage (chondrogenesis)

Cartilage grows by two mechanisms (Figures 4-16 and 4-17):

1. By **interstitial growth** (from chondrocytes **within the cartilage**; see Figure 4-16).
2. By **appositional growth** (from undifferentiated cells **at the surface of the cartilage or perichondrium**; see Figure 4-17).

During chondrogenesis, chondroblasts produce and deposit **type II collagen** fibers and ECM (**hyaluronic acid** and **GAGs**, mainly chondroitin sulfate and keratan sulfate) until chondroblasts are separated and trapped within spaces in

Figure 4-15. **Chondrocytes and the surrounding matrix**

Chondrocytes

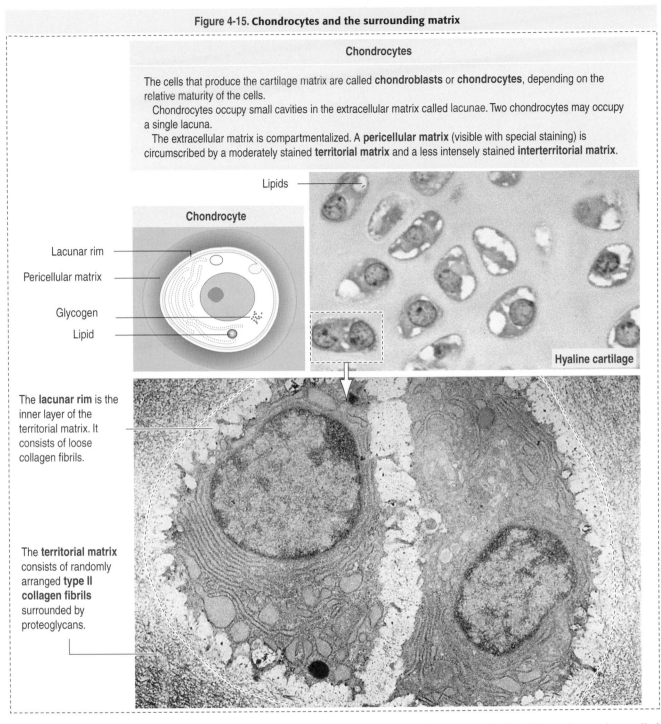

The cells that produce the cartilage matrix are called **chondroblasts** or **chondrocytes**, depending on the relative maturity of the cells.

Chondrocytes occupy small cavities in the extracellular matrix called lacunae. Two chondrocytes may occupy a single lacuna.

The extracellular matrix is compartmentalized. A **pericellular matrix** (visible with special staining) is circumscribed by a moderately stained **territorial matrix** and a less intensely stained **interterritorial matrix.**

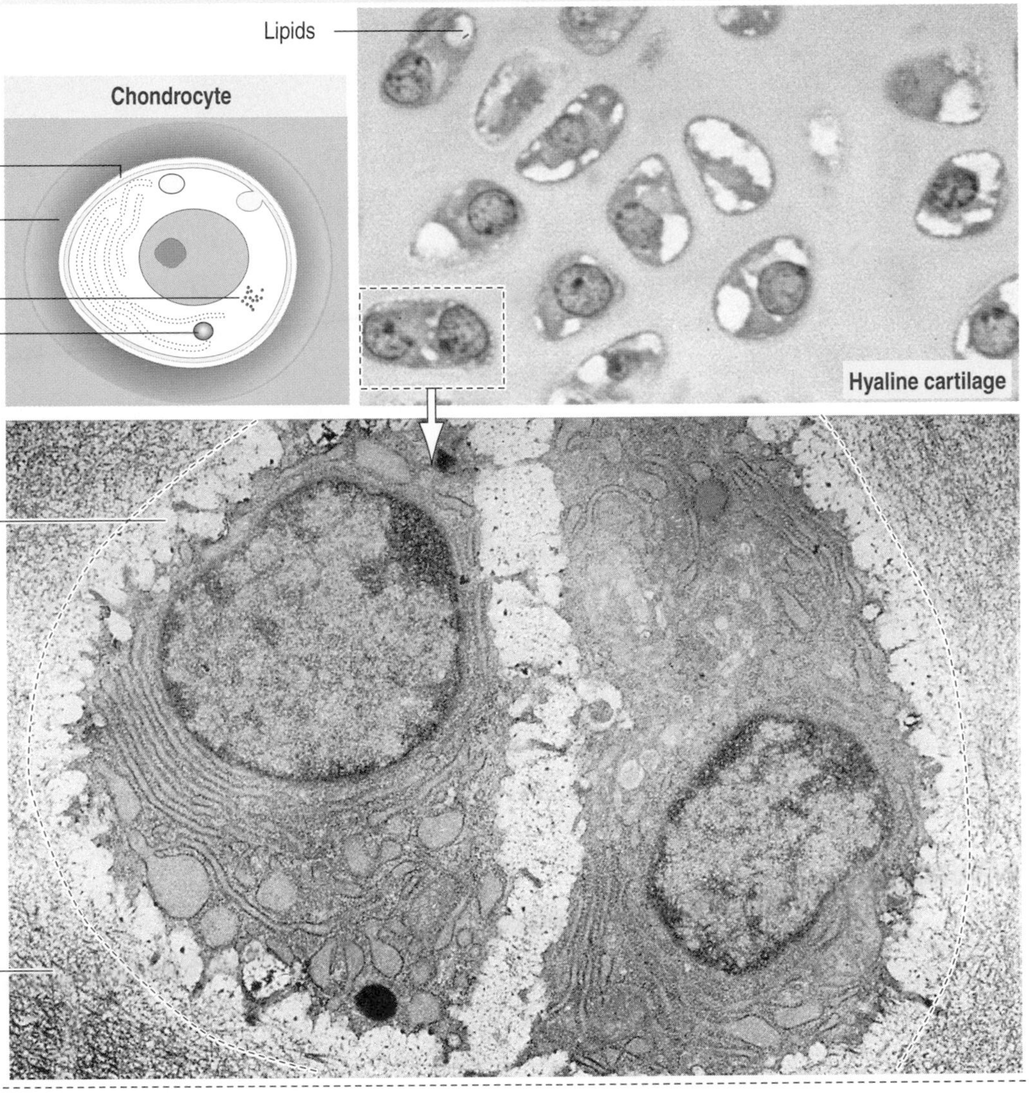
Lipids
Chondrocyte
Lacunar rim
Pericellular matrix
Glycogen
Lipid
Hyaline cartilage
The **lacunar rim** is the inner layer of the territorial matrix. It consists of loose collagen fibrils.
The **territorial matrix** consists of randomly arranged **type II collagen fibrils** surrounded by proteoglycans.

the matrix called **lacunae** (Latin *lacuna*, small lake). The cells are then called **chondrocytes**. The space between the chondrocyte and the wall of the lacuna seen in histologic preparations is an artifact of fixation.

The matrix in close contact with each chondrocyte forms a bluish (with hematoxylin and eosin), metachromatic (see Box 4-D), or PAS-positive basket-like structure called the **territorial matrix**.

Each cluster of chondrocytes (known as an **isogenous group**) enveloped by the territorial matrix is separated by a wide but pale **interterritorial matrix.**

Types of cartilage

There are three major types of cartilage (Figure 4-18):

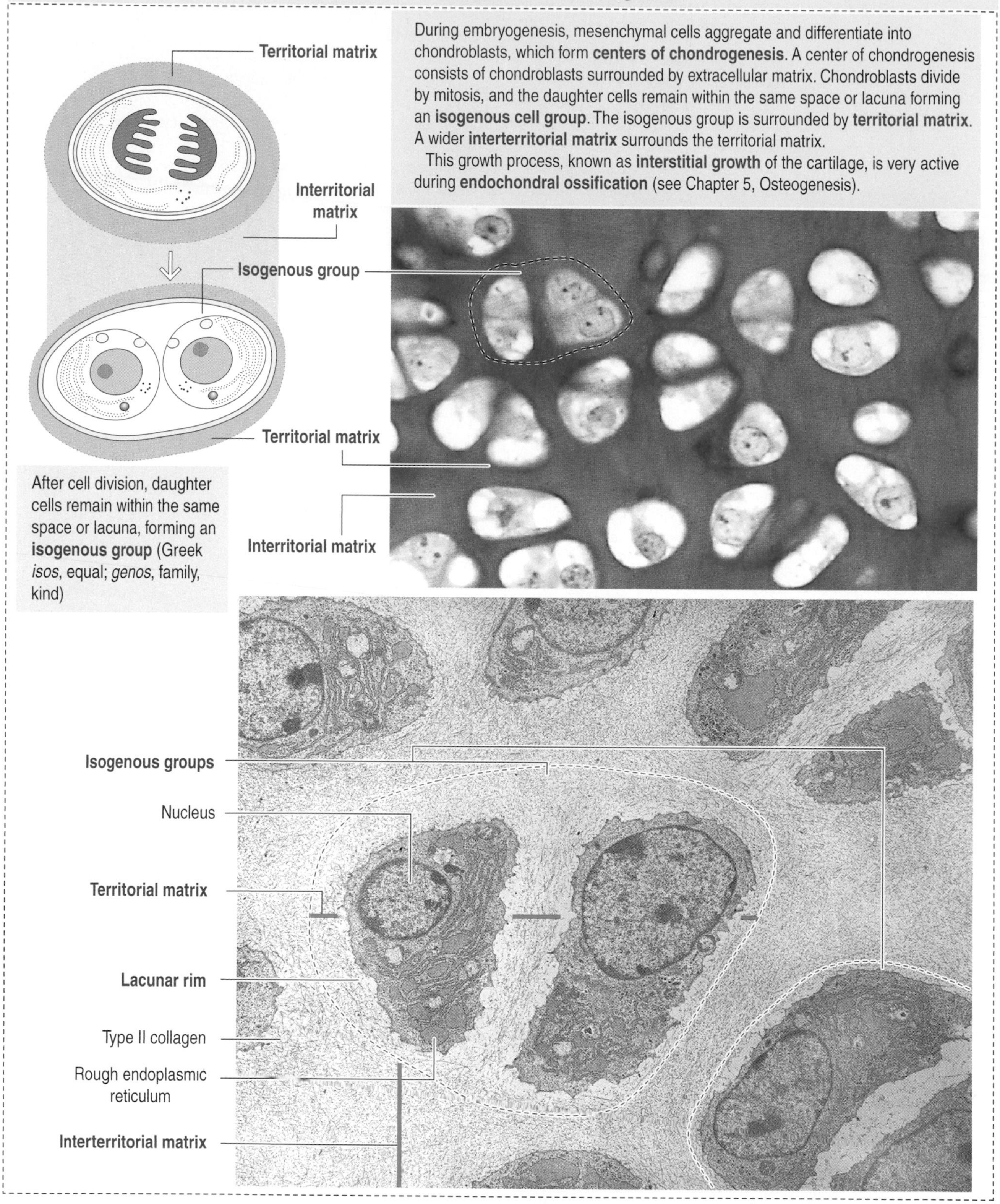
During embryogenesis, mesenchymal cells aggregate and differentiate into chondroblasts, which form **centers of chondrogenesis**. A center of chondrogenesis consists of chondroblasts surrounded by extracellular matrix. Chondroblasts divide by mitosis, and the daughter cells remain within the same space or lacuna forming an **isogenous cell group**. The isogenous group is surrounded by **territorial matrix**. A wider **interterritorial matrix** surrounds the territorial matrix.
This growth process, known as **interstitial growth** of the cartilage, is very active during **endochondral ossification** (see Chapter 5, Osteogenesis).
Territorial matrix
Interritorial matrix
Isogenous group
Territorial matrix
Interritorial matrix
After cell division, daughter cells remain within the same space or lacuna, forming an **isogenous group** (Greek *isos*, equal; *genos*, family, kind)
Isogenous groups
Nucleus
Territorial matrix
Lacunar rim
Type II collagen
Rough endoplasmic reticulum
Interterritorial matrix

Figure 4-16. Chondrogenesis: Interstitial growth

1. **Hyaline cartilage.**
2. **Elastic cartilage.**
3. **Fibrocartilage.**

Hyaline cartilage is the most widespread cartilage in humans. Its name derives from the clear appearance of the matrix (Greek *hyalos,* glass).

In the fetus, hyaline cartilage forms most of the skeleton before it is reabsorbed

Figure 4-17. Chondrogenesis: Appositional growth

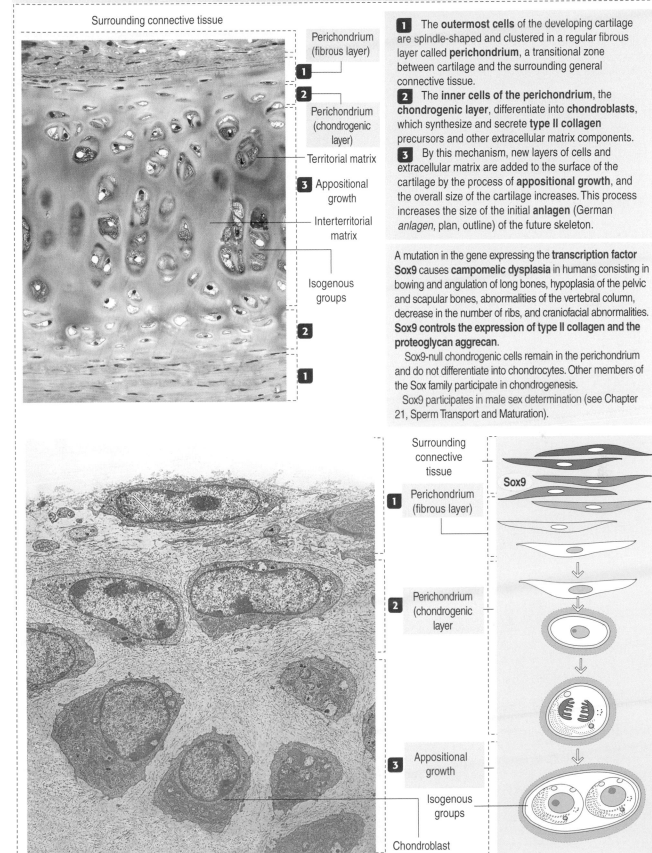

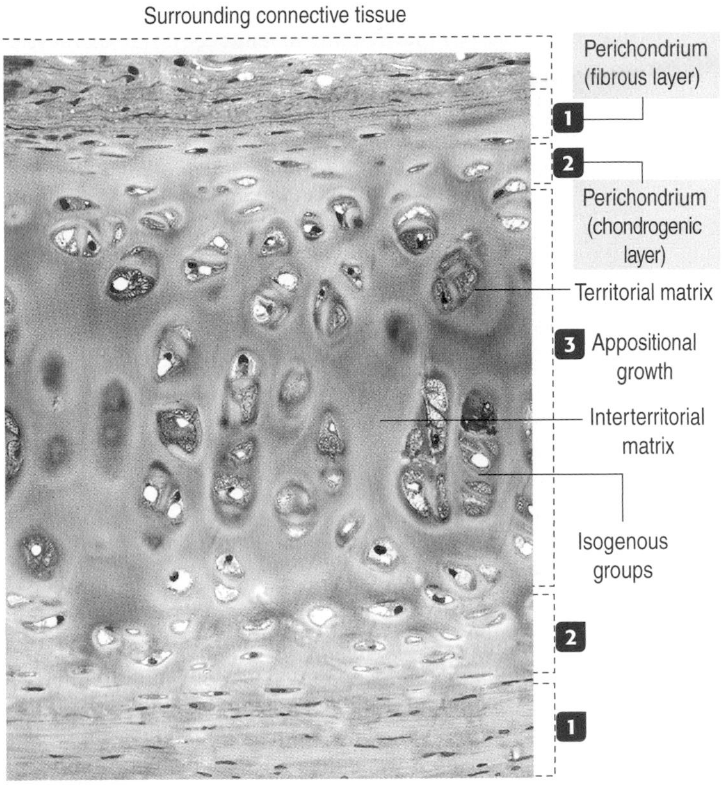

Surrounding connective tissue
Perichondrium (fibrous layer)
1
2
Perichondrium (chondrogenic layer)
Territorial matrix
3 Appositional growth
Interterritorial matrix
Isogenous groups
2
1

1 The **outermost cells** of the developing cartilage are spindle-shaped and clustered in a regular fibrous layer called **perichondrium**, a transitional zone between cartilage and the surrounding general connective tissue.

2 The **inner cells of the perichondrium**, the **chondrogenic layer**, differentiate into **chondroblasts**, which synthesize and secrete **type II collagen** precursors and other extracellular matrix components.

3 By this mechanism, new layers of cells and extracellular matrix are added to the surface of the cartilage by the process of **appositional growth**, and the overall size of the cartilage increases. This process increases the size of the initial **anlagen** (German *anlagen*, plan, outline) of the future skeleton.

A mutation in the gene expressing the **transcription factor Sox9** causes **campomelic dysplasia** in humans consisting in bowing and angulation of long bones, hypoplasia of the pelvic and scapular bones, abnormalities of the vertebral column, decrease in the number of ribs, and craniofacial abnormalities. **Sox9 controls the expression of type II collagen and the proteoglycan aggrecan.**

Sox9-null chondrogenic cells remain in the perichondrium and do not differentiate into chondrocytes. Other members of the Sox family participate in chondrogenesis.

Sox9 participates in male sex determination (see Chapter 21, Sperm Transport and Maturation).

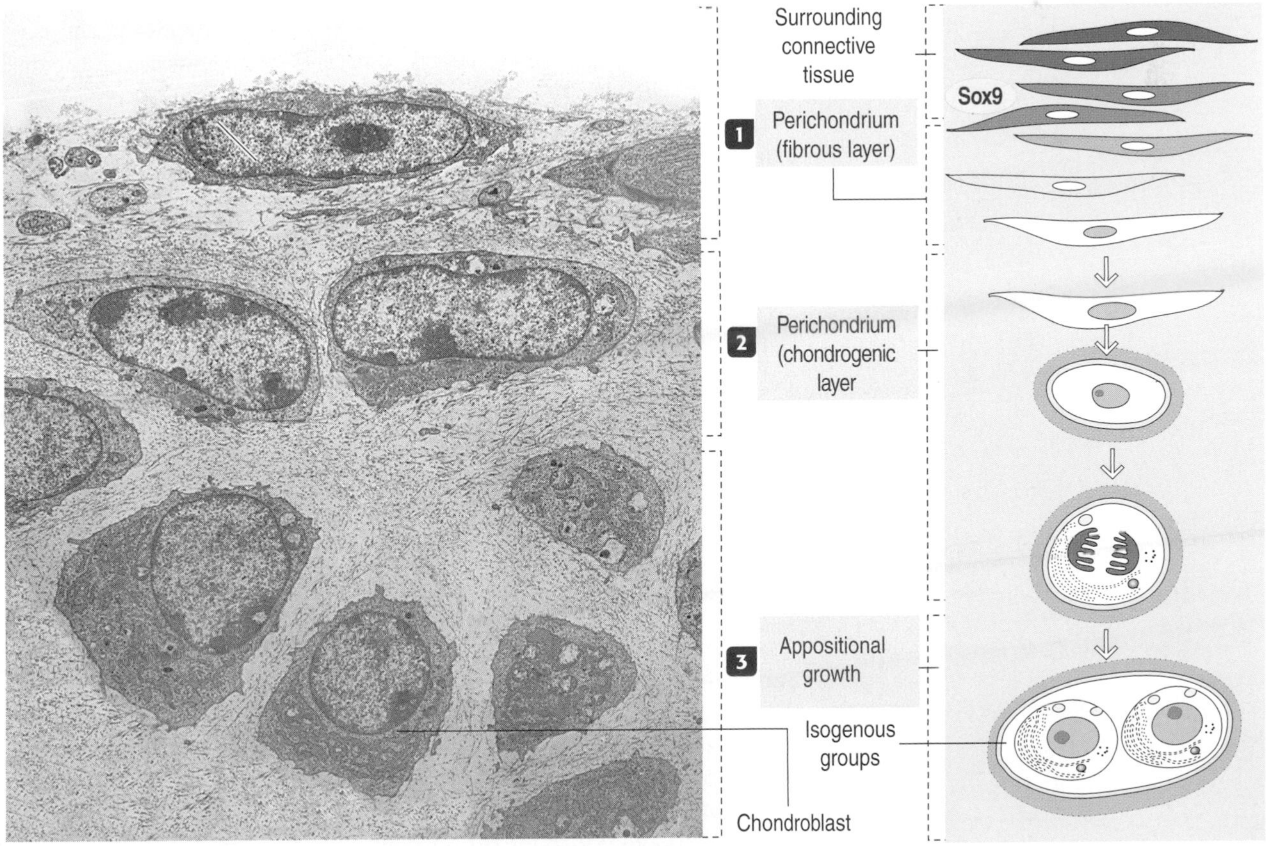

Surrounding connective tissue
Sox9
1 Perichondrium (fibrous layer)
2 Perichondrium (chondrogenic layer
3 Appositional growth
Isogenous groups
Chondroblast

Box 4-G | Cartilage repair after injury

- The specialized extracellular matrix of hyaline cartilage has a dual role:
  1. It acts like a **shock absorber**, because of its stiffness and elasticity.
  2. It provides a **lubricated surface for movable joints**.

  The lubrication fluid (hyaluronic acid, immunoglobulins, lysosomal enzymes, collagenase in particular, and glycoproteins) is produced by the **synovial lining of the capsule of the joint**.
- The analysis of the **synovial fluid** is valuable in the diagnosis of joint disease.

Box 4-H | How chondrocytes survive

- In **cartilage**, chondroblasts and chondrocytes are sustained by diffusion of nutrients and metabolites through **the aqueous phase of the extracellular matrix**.
- In **bone**, deposits of calcium salts in the matrix prevent the diffusion of soluble solutes, which thus must be transported from blood vessels to osteocytes through **canaliculi** (see Bone).

and replaced by bone by a process known as **endochondral ossification.**

In adults, hyaline cartilage persists as the nasal, laryngeal, tracheobronchial, and costal cartilage. **The articular surface of synovial joints** (knee, shoulder) **is hyaline cartilage and does not participate in endochondral ossification.** Articular surfaces are not lined by an epithelium.

The hyaline cartilage contains:

1. **Cells** (chondrocytes).
2. **Fibers** (**type II collagen** synthesized by chondrocytes).
3. **ECM** (also synthesized by chondrocytes).

Chondrocytes have the structural characteristics of a protein-secreting cell (well-developed RER and Golgi apparatus, and large nucleolus) and store lipids and glycogen in the cytoplasm. Chondrocytes are coated by a pericellular matrix, surrounded by the territorial and interterritorial matrices, respectively. A lacunar rim separates the cell from the territorial matrix.

The surface of hyaline cartilage is covered by the **perichondrium**, a fibrocellular layer that is continuous with the periosteal cover of the bone and that blends into the surrounding connective tissue. **Articular cartilage lacks a perichondrium.**

The perichondrium consists of two layers:

1. An **outer fibrous layer**, which contains bundles of type I collagen and elastin.
2. An **inner layer**, called the **chondrogenic layer**, formed by flat chondrocytes aligned tangentially to the margin of the cartilage.

The ECM contains hyaluronic acid, proteoglycans (rich in the GAGs chondroitin sulfate and keratan sulfate), and a high water content (70% to 80% of its weight). **Aggrecan** is a large proteoglycan characteristic of cartilage (see Boxes 4-G and 4-H).

The **transcription factor Sox9** is required for expression of cartilage-specific ECM components such as type II collagen and the proteoglycan aggrecan. Sox9 activates the expression of collagen by the *COL2A1* gene. A lack of Sox9 expression prevents the chondrogenic layer to differentiate into chondrocytes. Mutations in the *Sox9* gene cause the rare and severe dwarfism **campomelic dysplasia** (Figure 4-17).

The structure of the **elastic cartilage** is similar to that of hyaline cartilage except that the ECM contains abundant **elastic fibers** synthesized by chondrocytes. Elastic cartilage is found in the auricle of the external ear, a major portion of the epiglottis, and some of the laryngeal cartilages. The specialized matrix of the cartilage has remarkable flexibility and the ability to regain its original shape after deformation.

Unlike hyaline cartilage, **fibrocartilage** is opaque, the matrix contains **type I collagen fibers**, the **ECM has a low concentration of proteoglycans and water**, and **it lacks a perichondrium.**

Fibrocartilage has great tensile strength and forms part of the intervertebral disk, pubic symphysis, and sites of insertion of tendon and ligament into bone.

The fibrocartilage is sometimes difficult to distinguish from dense regular connective tissue of some regions of tendons and ligaments. Fibrocartilage is distinguished by **characteristic chondrocytes within lacunae, forming short columns** (in contrast to flattened fibroblasts or fibrocytes lacking lacunae, surrounded by the dense connective tissue and ECM).

Bone

Bone is a rigid inflexible connective tissue in which the ECM has become impregnated with salts of calcium and phosphate by a process called mineralization. Bone is highly vascularized and metabolically very active.

The functions of bone are:

1. **Support and protection for the body and its organs.**
2. **A reservoir for calcium and phosphate ions.**

Figure 4-18. Types of cartilage

Hyaline cartilage

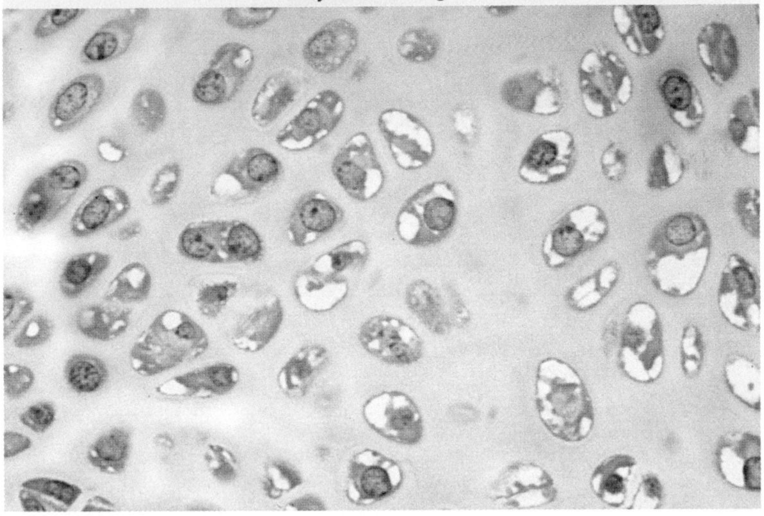

Hyaline cartilage has the following features:

It is **avascular**.

It is surrounded by **perichondrium** (except in articular cartilage). The perichondrium has an **outer fibrous layer**, an **inner chondrogenic layer**, and **blood vessels**.

It consists of chondrocytes surrounded by territorial and interterritorial matrices containing **type II collagen** interacting with proteoglycans.

It occurs in the **temporary skeleton of the embryo**, **articular cartilage**, and the **cartilage of the respiratory tract** (nose, larynx, trachea, and bronchi) and costal cartilages.

Elastic cartilage

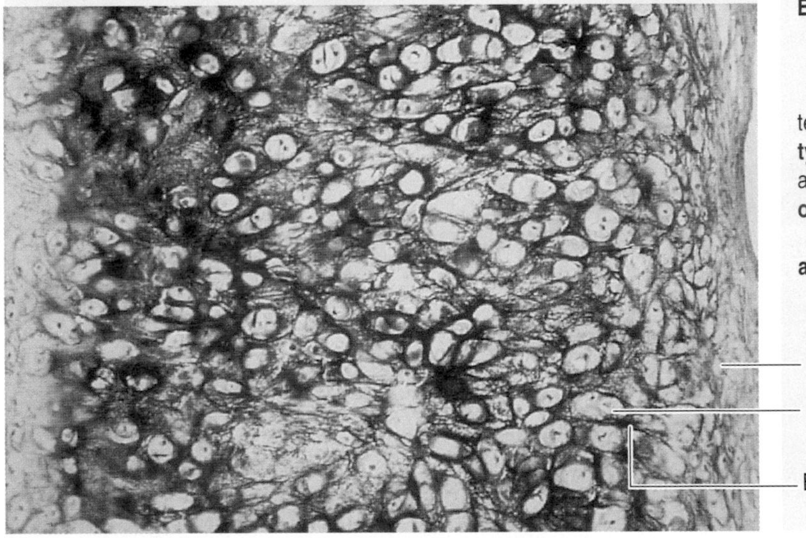
Perichondrium
Chondrocytes
Elastic fibers

Elastic cartilage has the following features:

It is **avascular**.

It is surrounded by **perichondrium**.

It consists of chondrocytes surrounded by territorial and interterritorial matrices containing **type II collagen** interacting with proteoglycans and **elastic fibers**, which can be stained by **orcein** for light microscopy.

It occurs in the **external ear**, **epiglottis**, and **auditory tube**.

Fibrocartilage

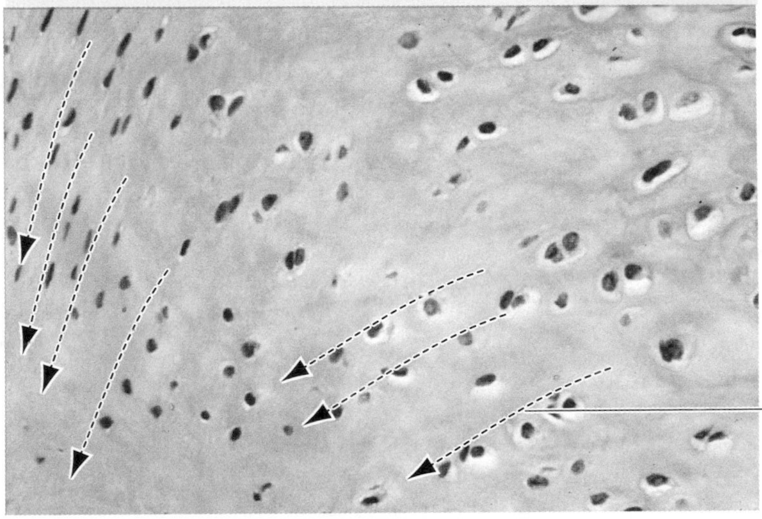
Chondrocytes aligned along the lines of stress

Fibrocartilage has the following features:

It is generally **avascular**.

It **lacks a perichondrium**.

It consists of **chondrocytes** and **fibroblasts** surrounded by **type I collagen** and a less rigid extracellular matrix. Fibrocartilage is considered an intermediate tissue between hyaline cartilage and dense connective tissue.

It predominates in the **intervertebral disks**, **articular disks of the knee, mandible**, **sternoclavicular joints**, and **pubic symphysis**.

Figure 4-19. **General architecture of a long bone**

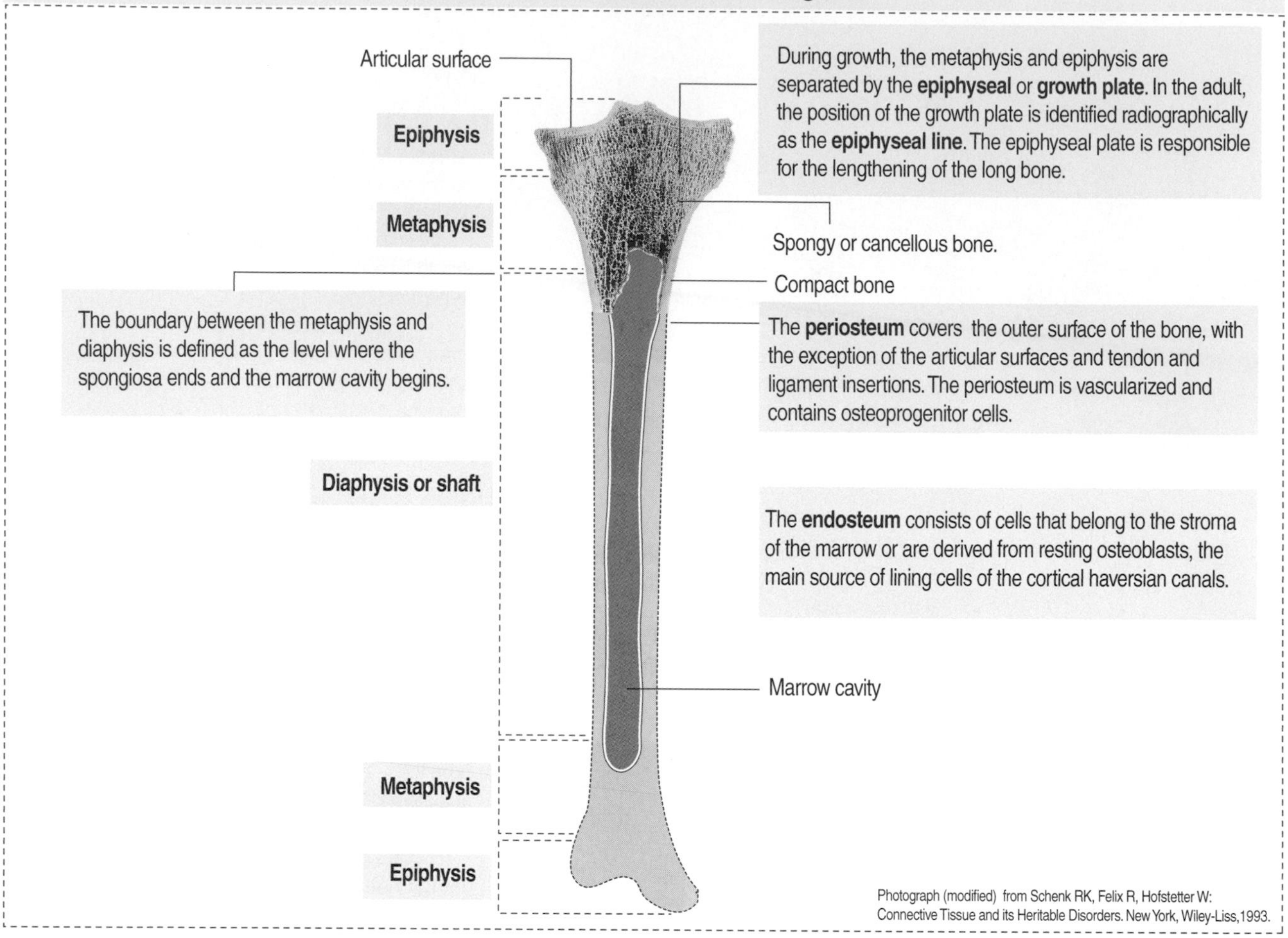

Articular surface
Epiphysis
Metaphysis
The boundary between the metaphysis and diaphysis is defined as the level where the spongiosa ends and the marrow cavity begins.
Diaphysis or shaft
Metaphysis
Epiphysis
During growth, the metaphysis and epiphysis are separated by the **epiphyseal** or **growth plate.** In the adult, the position of the growth plate is identified radiographically as the **epiphyseal line.** The epiphyseal plate is responsible for the lengthening of the long bone.
Spongy or cancellous bone.
Compact bone
The **periosteum** covers the outer surface of the bone, with the exception of the articular surfaces and tendon and ligament insertions. The periosteum is vascularized and contains osteoprogenitor cells.
The **endosteum** consists of cells that belong to the stroma of the marrow or are derived from resting osteoblasts, the main source of lining cells of the cortical haversian canals.
Marrow cavity

Photograph (modified) from Schenk RK, Felix R, Hofstetter W: Connective Tissue and its Heritable Disorders. New York, Wiley-Liss, 1993.

Classification of bone

Based on its gross appearance (Figure 4-19), two forms of bone are distinguished:

1. Compact bone.
2. Spongy or cancellous bone.

Compact bone appears as a solid mass. Spongy bone consists of a network of bony spicules or trabeculae delimiting spaces occupied by the bone marrow.

In long bones, such as the femur, the shaft or diaphysis consists of compact bone forming a hollow cylinder with a central marrow space, called the medullary or marrow cavity.

The ends of the long bones, called epiphyses, consist of spongy bone covered by a thin layer of compact bone. In the growing individual, epiphyses are separated from the shaft or diaphysis by a cartilaginous epiphyseal plate, connected to the diaphysis by spongy bone. A tapering transitional region, called the metaphysis, connects the epiphysis and the diaphysis. Both the epiphyseal plate and adjacent spongy bone represent the growth zone, responsible for the increase in length of the growing bone.

The articular surfaces, at the ends of the long bones, are covered by hyaline cartilage, the articular cartilage. Except on the articular surfaces and at the insertion site of tendons and ligaments, most bones are surrounded by the periosteum, a layer of specialized connective tissue with osteogenic potential.

The marrow cavity of the diaphysis and the spaces within spongy bone are lined by endosteum, also with osteogenic potential.

Two types of bone are identified on the basis of the microscopic organization of the ECM:

Figure 4-20. Haversian system or osteon

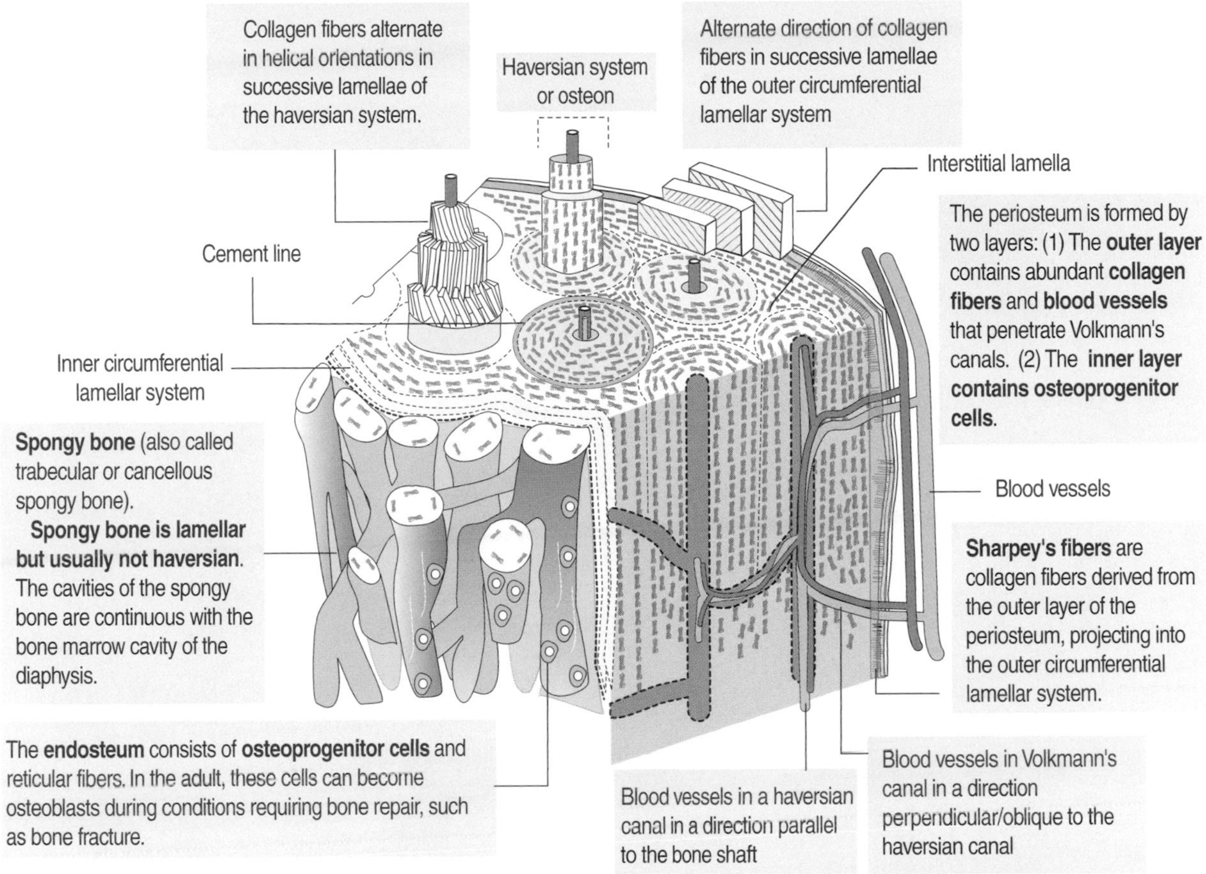

Collagen fibers alternate in helical orientations in successive lamellae of the haversian system.
Haversian system or osteon
Alternate direction of collagen fibers in successive lamellae of the outer circumferential lamellar system
Interstitial lamella
Cement line
The periosteum is formed by two layers: (1) The **outer layer** contains abundant **collagen fibers** and **blood vessels** that penetrate Volkmann's canals. (2) The **inner layer contains osteoprogenitor cells**.
Inner circumferential lamellar system
Spongy bone (also called trabecular or cancellous spongy bone).
Spongy bone is lamellar but usually not haversian. The cavities of the spongy bone are continuous with the bone marrow cavity of the diaphysis.
Blood vessels
Sharpey's fibers are collagen fibers derived from the outer layer of the periosteum, projecting into the outer circumferential lamellar system.
The **endosteum** consists of **osteoprogenitor cells** and reticular fibers. In the adult, these cells can become osteoblasts during conditions requiring bone repair, such as bone fracture.
Blood vessels in a haversian canal in a direction parallel to the bone shaft
Blood vessels in Volkmann's canal in a direction perpendicular/oblique to the haversian canal

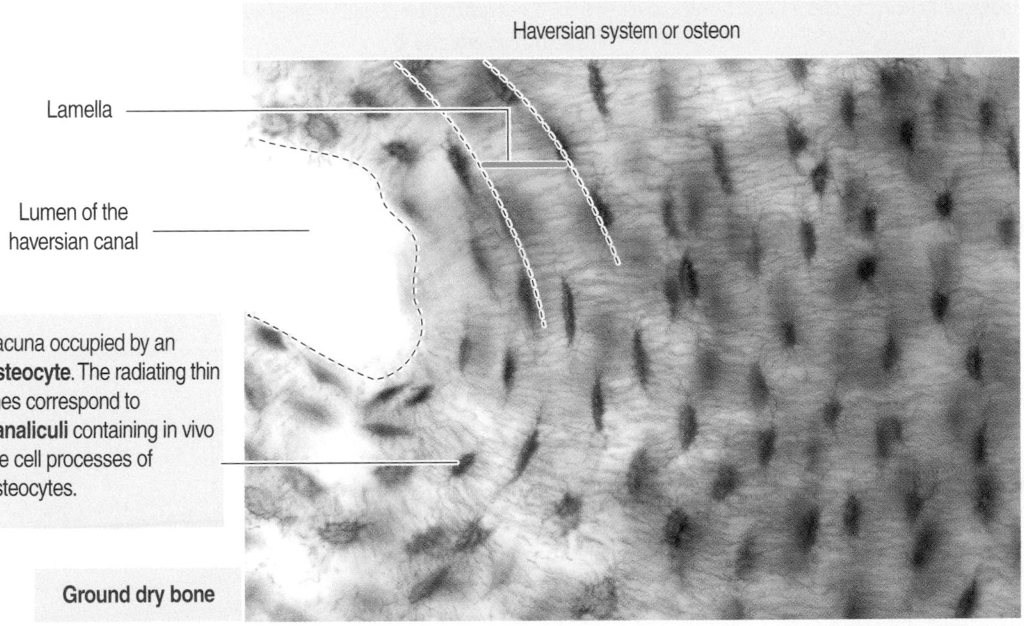

Haversian system or osteon
Lamella
Lumen of the haversian canal
Lacuna occupied by an **osteocyte**. The radiating thin lines correspond to **canaliculi** containing in vivo the cell processes of osteocytes.
Ground dry bone

1. **Lamellar bone**, typical of the mature or compact bone.
2. **Woven bone**, observed in the developing bone.

The **lamellar bone** consists of **lamellae**, largely composed of **bone matrix**, a mineralized substance deposited in layers or lamellae, and osteocytes, each one occupying a cavity or **lacuna** with radiating and branching **canaliculi** that

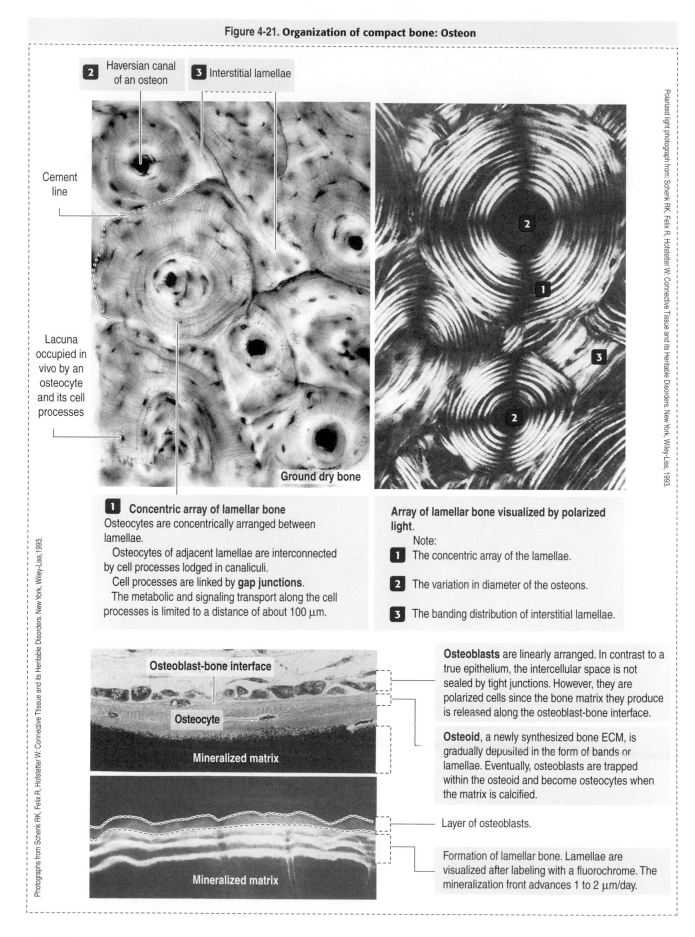

Figure 4-21. Organization of compact bone: Osteon

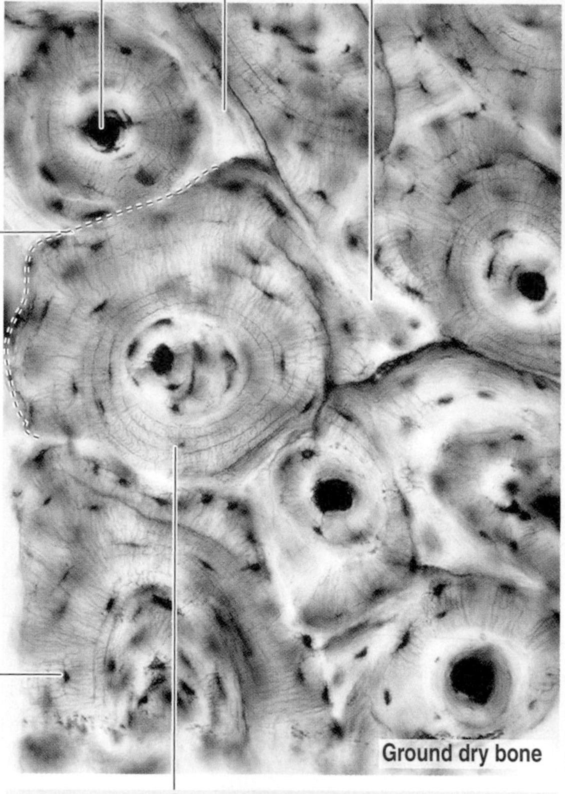

2 Haversian canal of an osteon
3 Interstitial lamellae
Cement line
Lacuna occupied in vivo by an osteocyte and its cell processes
Ground dry bone

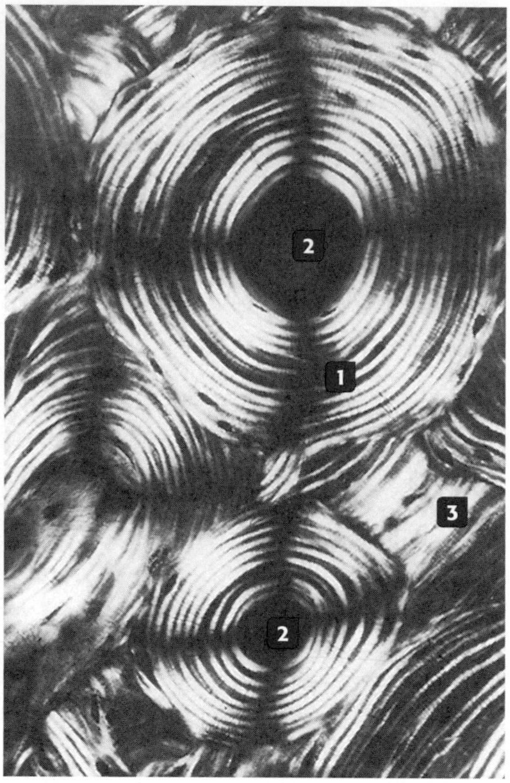

2
1
3
2

Polarized light photograph from: Schenk RK, Felix R, Hofstetter W: Connective Tissue and its Heritable Disorders. New York, Wiley-Liss, 1993.

1 Concentric array of lamellar bone
Osteocytes are concentrically arranged between lamellae.

Osteocytes of adjacent lamellae are interconnected by cell processes lodged in canaliculi.

Cell processes are linked by **gap junctions**.

The metabolic and signaling transport along the cell processes is limited to a distance of about 100 μm.

Array of lamellar bone visualized by polarized light.

Note:

1 The concentric array of the lamellae.

2 The variation in diameter of the osteons.

3 The banding distribution of interstitial lamellae.

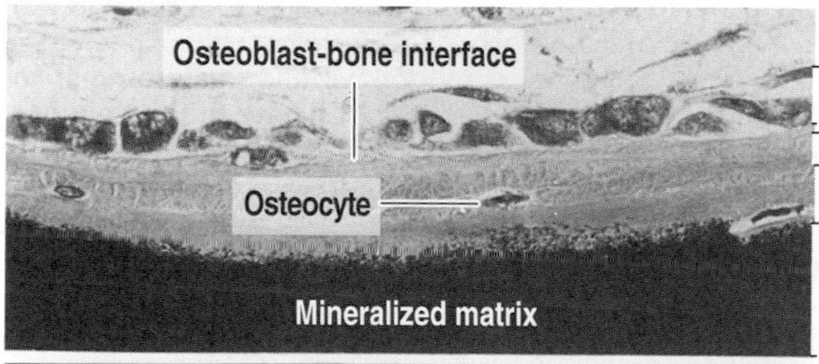

Osteoblast-bone interface
Osteocyte
Mineralized matrix

Osteoblasts are linearly arranged. In contrast to a true epithelium, the intercellular space is not sealed by tight junctions. However, they are polarized cells since the bone matrix they produce is released along the osteoblast-bone interface.

Osteoid, a newly synthesized bone ECM, is gradually deposited in the form of bands or lamellae. Eventually, osteoblasts are trapped within the osteoid and become osteocytes when the matrix is calcified.

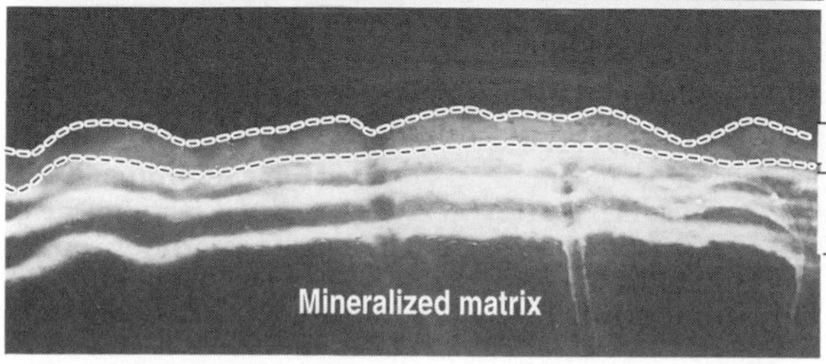

Mineralized matrix

Layer of osteoblasts.

Formation of lamellar bone. Lamellae are visualized after labeling with a fluorochrome. The mineralization front advances 1 to 2 μm/day.

Photographs from Schenk RK, Felix R, Hofstetter W: Connective Tissue and its Heritable Disorders. New York, Wiley-Liss, 1993.

Figure 4-22. Osteocytes are connected to each other by cell processes

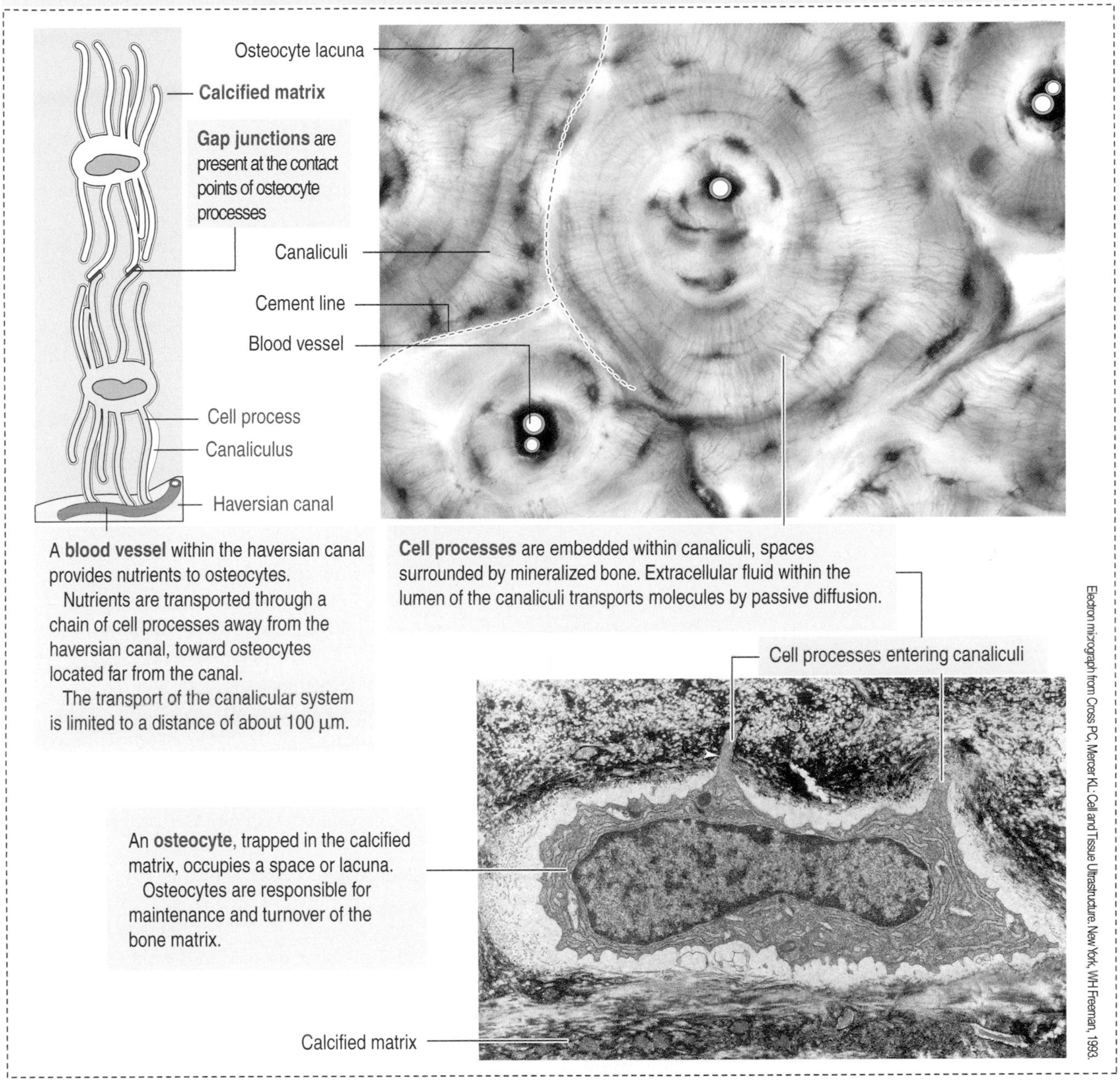
Osteocyte lacuna
Calcified matrix
Gap junctions are present at the contact points of osteocyte processes
Canaliculi
Cement line
Blood vessel
Cell process
Canaliculus
Haversian canal
A blood vessel within the haversian canal provides nutrients to osteocytes.
Nutrients are transported through a chain of cell processes away from the haversian canal, toward osteocytes located far from the canal.
The transport of the canalicular system is limited to a distance of about 100 μm.
Cell processes are embedded within canaliculi, spaces surrounded by mineralized bone. Extracellular fluid within the lumen of the canaliculi transports molecules by passive diffusion.
Cell processes entering canaliculi
An osteocyte, trapped in the calcified matrix, occupies a space or lacuna.
Osteocytes are responsible for maintenance and turnover of the bone matrix.
Calcified matrix

Electron micrograph from Cross PC, Mercer KL: Cell and Tissue Ultrastructure. New York, WH Freeman, 1993.

penetrate the lamellae of adjacent lacunae.

The lamellar bone displays four distinct patterns (Figure 4-20):

1. The **osteons** or **haversian systems**, formed by concentrically arranged lamellae around a longitudinal vascular channel.

2. The **interstitial lamellae**, observed between osteons and separated from them by a thin layer known as the **cement line**.

3. The **outer circumferential lamellae**, visualized at the external surface of the compact bone under the periosteum.

4. The **inner circumferential lamellae**, seen on the internal surface subjacent to the endosteum.

The **vascular channels** in compact bone have two orientations with respect to the lamellar structures:

1. The longitudinal capillaries and postcapillary venules, running in the center of the osteon within a space known as the **haversian canal** (Figures 4-20 to 4-22).

2. The haversian canals are connected with one another by transverse or oblique canals known as **Volkmann's canals**, containing blood vessels from the marrow and some from the periosteum.

Periosteum and endosteum

During embryonic and postnatal growth, the periosteum consists of an **inner layer of bone-forming cells** (**osteoblasts**) in direct contact with the bone. The inner layer is the **osteogenic layer**. In the adult, the periosteum contains inactive connective tissue cells that retain their osteogenic potential in case of bone injury and repair.

The **outer layer** is rich in blood vessels, some of them entering Volkmann's canals, and thick anchoring collagen fibers, called **Sharpey's fibers**, that penetrate the outer circumferential lamellae deep in the bone (see Figure 4-20).

The **endosteum** consists of squamous cells and connective tissue fibers covering the spongy walls housing the bone marrow and extending into all the cavities of the bone, including the haversian canals.

Bone matrix

The **bone matrix** consists of organic (35%) and inorganic (65%) components. The organic bone matrix contains **type I collagen fibers** (90%); **proteoglycans**, enriched in **chondroitin sulfate**, **keratan sulfate**, and **hyaluronic acid**; and **noncollagenous proteins**. The **inorganic component of the bone** is represented predominantly by deposits of **calcium phosphate** with the crystalline characteristics of **hydroxyapatite**. The crystals are distributed along the length of collagen fibers through an assembly process assisted by noncollagenous proteins.

Type I collagen is the predominant protein of the bone matrix. In mature lamellar bone, collagen fibers have a highly ordered arrangement with changing orientations with respect to the axis of the haversian canal in successive concentric lamellae (see Figure 4-20).

Noncollagenous matrix proteins include **osteocalcin**, **osteopontin**, and **osteonectin**, synthesized by osteoblasts and with unique properties in the mineralization of bone.

Osteocalcin and osteopontin synthesis increases following stimulation with the active vitamin D metabolite, 1α,25-dihydroxycholecalciferol. Osteocalcin inhibits osteoblast function.

Osteonectin is not exclusively an osteoblast product and is present in tissues undergoing remodeling and morphogenesis.

Bone sialoprotein is also a bone matrix component.

As we later discuss in greater detail, **osteoprotegerin**, **RANKL**, and **macrophage colony-stimulating factor** are products of osteoblasts required for regulating the differentiation of osteoclasts.

Cellular components of bone

Actively growing bone contains cells of two different lineages:

1. The **osteoblast lineage**, which includes the osteoprogenitor cells and derived osteoblasts and osteocytes.

2. The **osteoclast lineage**.

Osteoprogenitor cells are of mesenchymal origin and have the properties of **stem cells**: the **potential for proliferation** and a **capacity to differentiate**. Osteoprogenitor cells give rise to osteoblasts by a regulatory mechanism involving growth and transcription factors and are present in the inner layer of the periosteum and the endosteum. Osteoprogenitor cells persist throughout postnatal life as bone-lining cells; they are reactivated in the adult during the repair of bone fractures and other injuries.

Osteoblasts differentiate into osteocytes after they are trapped inside lacunae

Figure 4-23. Function of the osteoblast

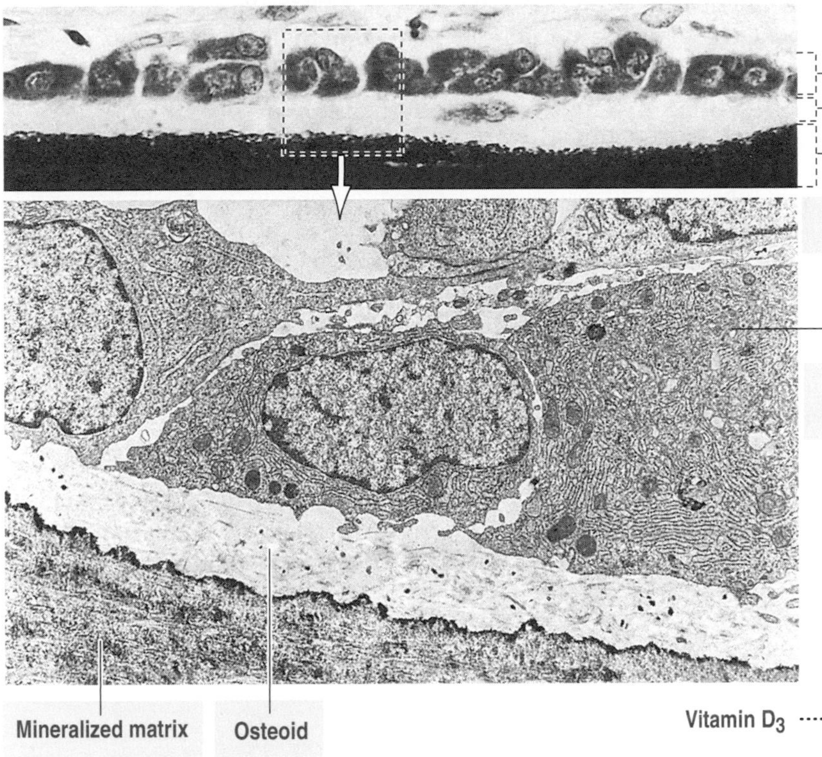

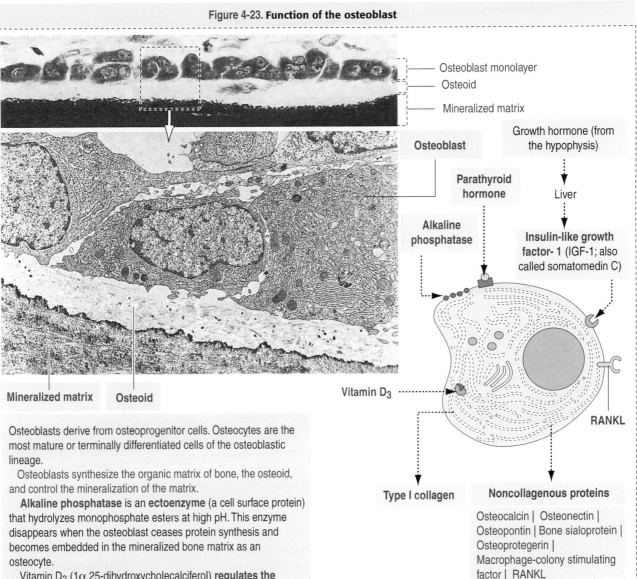

Osteoblast monolayer
Osteoid
Mineralized matrix
Mineralized matrix
Osteoid

Photographs from Schenk RK, Felix R, Hofstetter W: Connective Tissue and its Heritable Disorders. New York, Wiley-Liss, 1993.

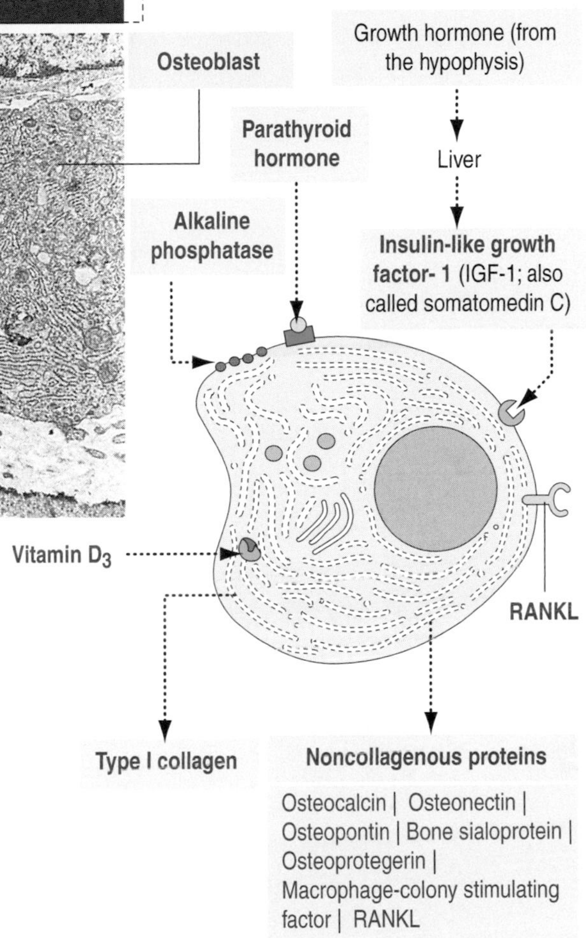

Osteoblast
Growth hormone (from the hypophysis)
Parathyroid hormone
Liver
Alkaline phosphatase
Insulin-like growth factor- 1 (IGF-1; also called somatomedin C)
Vitamin D3
RANKL
Type I collagen
Noncollagenous proteins
Osteocalcin | Osteonectin | Osteopontin | Bone sialoprotein | Osteoprotegerin | Macrophage-colony stimulating factor | RANKL

Osteoblasts derive from osteoprogenitor cells. Osteocytes are the most mature or terminally differentiated cells of the osteoblastic lineage.

Osteoblasts synthesize the organic matrix of bone, the osteoid, and control the mineralization of the matrix.

Alkaline phosphatase is an **ectoenzyme** (a cell surface protein) that hydrolyzes monophosphate esters at high pH. This enzyme disappears when the osteoblast ceases protein synthesis and becomes embedded in the mineralized bone matrix as an osteocyte.

Vitamin D_3 (1α,25-dihydroxycholecalciferol) **regulates the expression of osteocalcin**, a protein with high binding affinity for hydroxyapatite.

Growth hormone stimulates the production of **IGF-1** in hepatocytes. IGF-1 stimulates the growth of long bones at the level of the epiphyseal plates.

The major protein products of an osteoblast are:

1. **Type 1 collagen. Osteoid** consists of type I collagen and proteoglycans. As a typical protein-producing cell, the osteoblast has a well-developed rough endoplasmic reticulum.

2. Several **noncollagenous proteins.** They include: **RANKL,** the ligand for receptor for activation of nuclear factor kappa B (RANK)—present in osteoclast precursor cells; **osteocalcin**—required for bone mineralization; **osteopontin**—to mediate the formation of the sealing zone; **bone sialoprotein**—to mediate binding of osteoblasts to the extracellular matrix through integrins.

within the mineralized matrix they produce. Their differentiation involves the participation of two transcription factors: Cbfa1/Runx2 and osterix (see Box 4-I).

The osteoclast lineage derives from the monocyte-macrophage population in the bone marrow.

Osteoblasts and osteocytes

Osteoblasts are epithelial-like cells with cuboidal or columnar shapes, forming a monolayer covering all sites of active bone formation. Osteoblasts are highly polarized cells: they deposit **osteoid**, the **nonmineralized organic matrix of the bone**, along the osteoblast-bone interface. Osteoblasts initiate and control the subsequent mineralization of the osteoid.

In electron micrographs, osteoblasts display the typical features of cells actively engaged in protein synthesis, glycosylation, and secretion. Their specific products are **type I collagen**, **osteocalcin**, **osteopontin**, and **bone sialoprotein** (Figure 4-23). Osteoblasts give a strong cytochemical reaction for **alkaline phosphatase** that disappears when the cells become embedded in the matrix as osteocytes. In addition, osteoblasts produce growth factors, in particular members of the **bone morphogenetic protein family**, with bone-inductive activities.

When bone formation is completed, osteoblasts flatten out and transform into osteocytes. Osteocytes are highly branched cells with their body occupying small spaces between lamellae, called lacunae. Small channels, the canaliculi, course through the lamellae and interconnect neighboring lacunae. Adjacent cell processes, found within canaliculi, are connected by **gap junctions** (see Figure 4-22). Nutrient materials diffuse from a neighboring blood vessel, within the haversian canal, through the canaliculi into the lacunae. As you can see, the dense network of osteocytes depends not only on intracellular communication across gap junctions but also on the mobilization of nutrients and signaling molecules along the extracellular environment facilitated by canaliculi running from lacuna to lacuna.

The life of an osteocyte depends on this nutrient diffusion process and the life of the bone matrix depends on the osteocyte. Osteocytes can remain alive for years provided vascularization is continuous.

In compact bone, 4 to 20 lamellae are concentrically arranged around the haversian canal; they contain a blood vessel, either a capillary or a postcapillary venule.

Clinical significance: Osteoblast to osteocyte differentiation

Osteoblasts derive from a pluripotent mesenchymal cell that is also the precursor of muscle cells, adipocytes, fibroblasts, and chondroblasts.

The differentiation of the osteoblast is controlled by growth and transcription factors. Several members of the **bone morphogenetic protein (BMP) family** and **transforming growth factor-β** can regulate the embryonic development and differentiation of the osteoblast.

Osteoblast-specific genes modulate the differentiation of the osteoblast progeny (Figure 4-24): ***Cbfa1/Runx2*** (a member of the core-binding factor family) encodes a **transcription factor** that induces the differentiation of osteoblasts and controls the expression of osteocalcin. Cbfa1/Runx2 is the earliest and most specific indicator of osteogenesis and its expression is induced by **BMP7**, followed by the expression of osteocalcin and osteopontin. **Osteocalcin** is a specific secretory protein expressed only in terminally differentiated osteoblasts under the control of Cbfa1/Runx2 (see Box 4-I).

Cbfa1/Runx2-deficient mice develop to term and have a skeleton consisting of cartilage. There is no indication of osteoblast differentiation or bone formation in these mice. In addition, Cbfa1/Runx2-deficient mice lack osteoclasts. As we will discuss soon, osteoblasts produce proteins that regulate the formation of osteoclasts.

Consistent with the skeletal observations in the Cbfa1/Runx2-deficient mice is a condition in humans known as **cleidocranial dysplasia** (**CCD**). CCD is characterized by hypoplastic clavicles, delayed ossification of sutures of certain skull bones, and mutations in the *Cbfa1/Runx2* gene.

Leptin, a peptide synthesized by **adipocytes** with binding affinity to its receptor in the hypothalamus, regulates bone formation by a central mechanism. Although details of the leptin-hypothalamic control mechanism are unknown, mice deficient in leptin or its receptor have a considerably higher bone mass than wild-type mice. In fact, patients with generalized **lipodystrophy** (absence of adipocytes and white fat) exhibit **osteosclerosis** (increased bone hardening) and accelerated bone growth.

Box 4-I | How osteocytes differentiate

- The osteoblast to osteocyte differentiation process requires the activation of two transcription factors: **Cbfa1/Runx2** (for core binding factor a1/runt homeodomain protein 2) and **osterix**.
- We have already seen that chondrogenesis involves the transcription factor **Sox9** (see Figure 4-17). We discuss in Chapter 5, Ossification, that Cbfa1/Runx2 controls the conversion of proliferating chondrocytes to hypertrophic chondrocytes, an event that is prevented by Sox9.
- The transcription factors Sox9, Cbfa1/Runx2, and osterix (the latter specific for osteoblast to osteocyte differentiation) play critical roles in the development of the skeleton.
- Mutations in genes encoding these transcription factors are the genetic basis of skeletal diseases. For example, a total lack of expression of the *Cbfa1/Runx2* gene determines that the entire skeleton consists only of cartilage.

Figure 4-24. **Osteoblast differentiation**

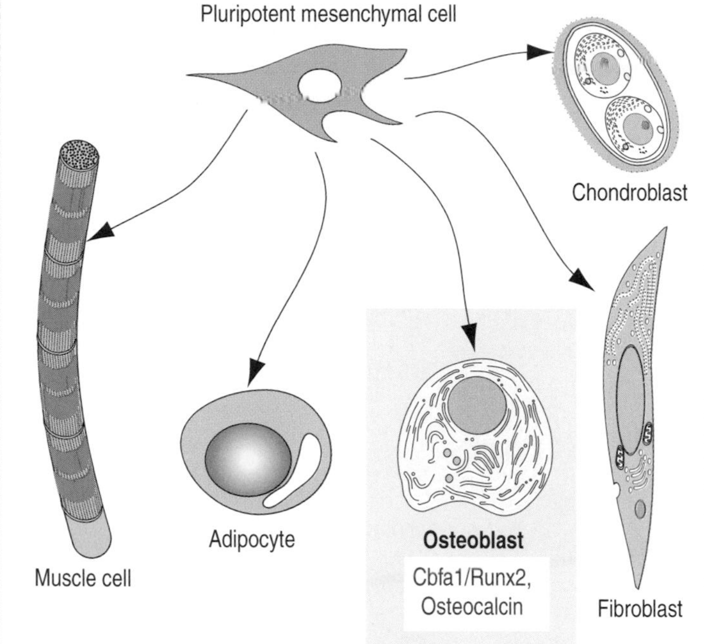

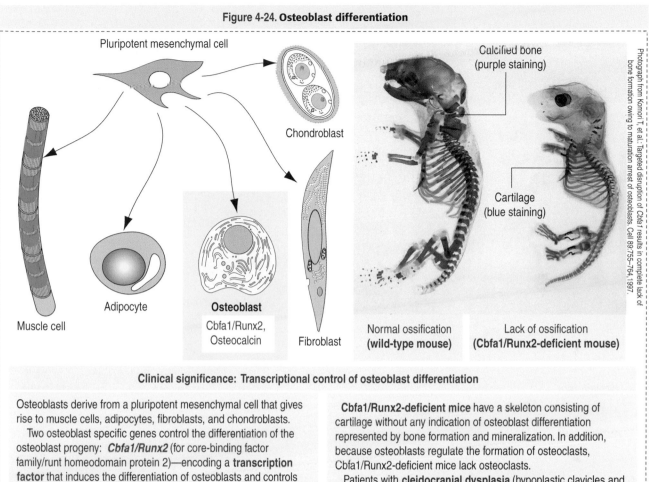

Pluripotent mesenchymal cell
Chondroblast
Muscle cell
Adipocyte
Osteoblast
Cbfa1/Runx2,
Osteocalcin
Fibroblast

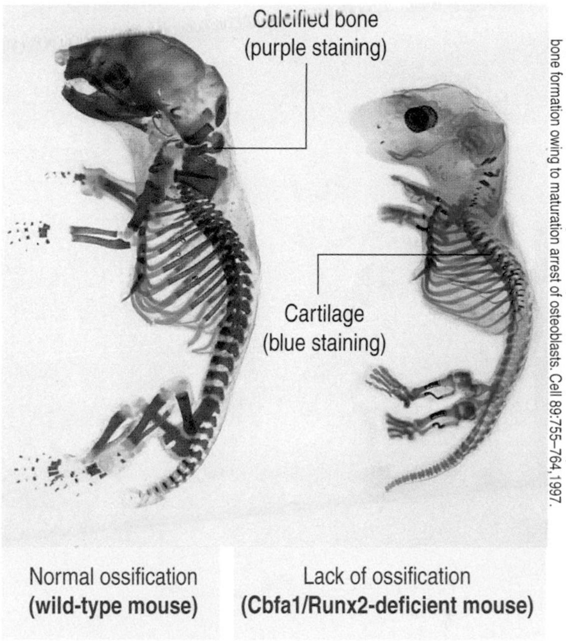

Calcified bone
(purple staining)
Cartilage
(blue staining)
Normal ossification
(wild-type mouse)
Lack of ossification
(Cbfa1/Runx2-deficient mouse)

Photograph from Komori T, et al.: Targeted disruption of *Cbfa1* results in complete lack of bone formation owing to maturation arrest of osteoblasts. Cell 89:755–764,1997.

Clinical significance: Transcriptional control of osteoblast differentiation

Osteoblasts derive from a pluripotent mesenchymal cell that gives rise to muscle cells, adipocytes, fibroblasts, and chondroblasts.

Two osteoblast specific genes control the differentiation of the osteoblast progeny: ***Cbfa1/Runx2*** (for core-binding factor family/runt homeodomain protein 2)—encoding a **transcription factor** that induces the differentiation of osteoblasts and controls the expression of osteocalcin, a specific secretory protein expressed only in terminally differentiated osteocytes.

Cbfa1/Runx2-deficient mice have a skeleton consisting of cartilage without any indication of osteoblast differentiation represented by bone formation and mineralization. In addition, because osteoblasts regulate the formation of osteoclasts, Cbfa1/Runx2-deficient mice lack osteoclasts.

Patients with **cleidocranial dysplasia** (hypoplastic clavicles and delayed ossification of sutures of certain skull bones) have a *Cbfa1/Runx2* type of gene mutation.

Osteoclasts

Osteoclasts do not belong to the osteoprogenitor cell lineage. Instead, osteoclasts derive from the **monocyte-macrophage progenitor cell lineage** in the bone marrow, which diverges into the **osteoclast progenitor pathway**.

The osteoclast precursor cells are **monocytes**, which reach the bone through the blood circulation and fuse into multinucleated cells with as many as 30 nuclei to form osteoclasts by a process regulated by osteoblasts and stromal cells of the bone marrow.

After attachment to the target bone matrix, osteoclasts generate a secluded acidic environment required for bone resorption. Bone resorption involves first the dissolution of the inorganic components of the bone (**bone demineralization**) mediated by H^+-ATPase (adenosine triphosphatase) within an acidic environment, followed by enzymatic degradation of the organic matrix (type I collagen and noncollagenous proteins) by the protease cathepsin K.

Osteoclasts play an essential role in **bone remodeling and renewal.** This process involves removal of bone matrix at several sites, followed by its replacement with new bone by osteoblasts.

The osteoclast is a large (up to 100 μm in diameter) and highly polarized cell that occupies a shallow concavity called **Howship's lacuna** or the **subosteoclastic compartment** (Figures 4-25 and 4-26).

The cytoplasm of the osteoclast is very **rich in mitochondria** and **acidified vesicles**. The membrane of the acidified vesicles contains H^+-ATPase; mitochondria are the source of adenosine triphosphate (ATP) to drive the

Figure 4-25. Function of the osteoclast

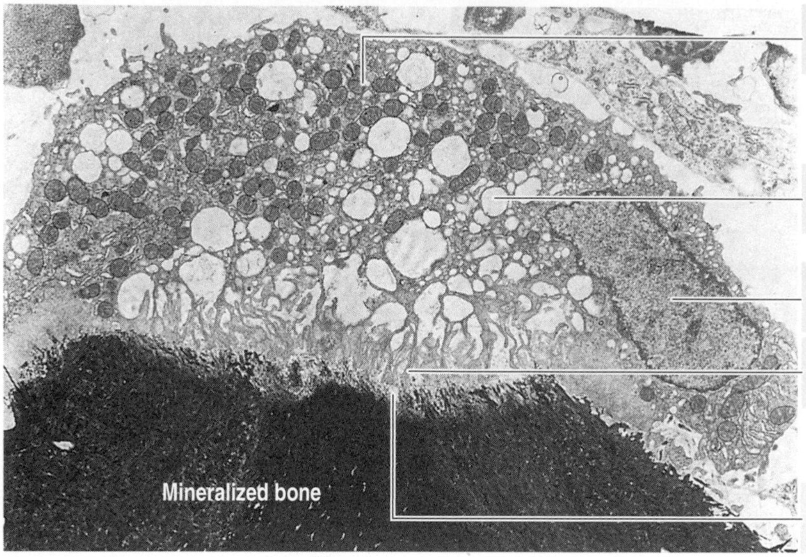
Mineralized bone
Mitochondria
Acidified vesicles
Nucleus
Ruffled border
Howship's lacuna or subosteoclastic compartment

The osteoclast is a highly polarized cell associated with a shallow concavity, **Howship's lacuna** or the **subosteoclastic compartment**.

The active surface facing the lacuna displays a **ruffled border**.

Osteoclasts are multinucleated cells and contain abundant mitochondria and acidified vesicles (containing electrogenic H^+-ATPase).

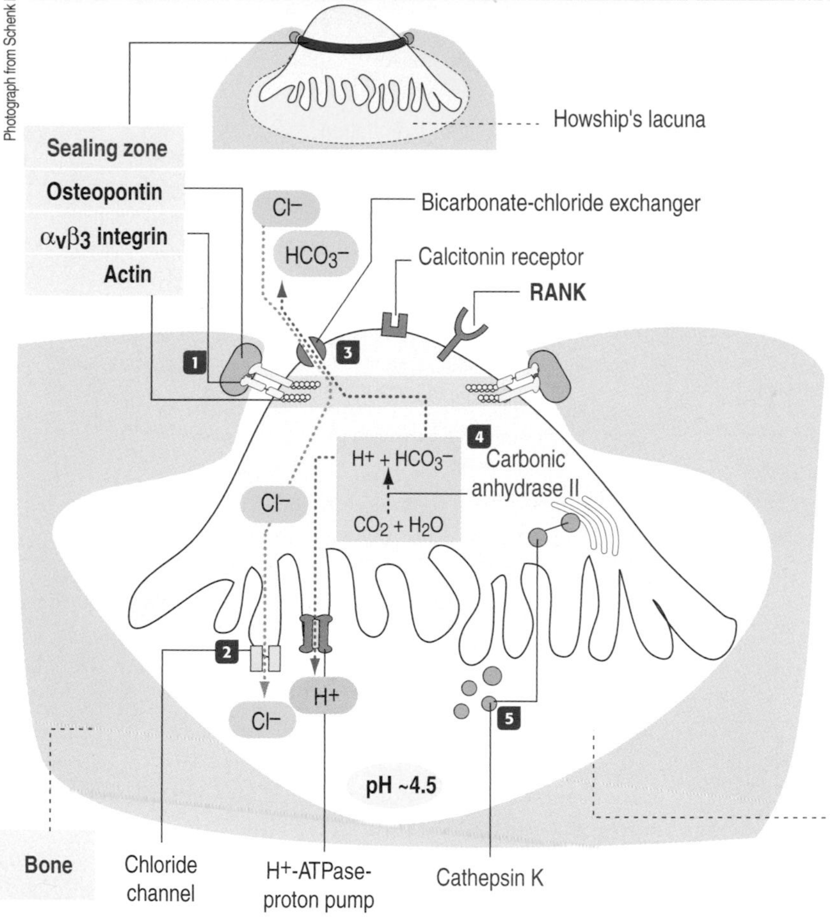
Howship's lacuna
Sealing zone
Osteopontin
$\alpha_v\beta_3$ integrin
Actin
Cl^-
HCO_3^-
Bicarbonate-chloride exchanger
Calcitonin receptor
RANK
1
3
4
$H^+ + HCO_3^-$
Carbonic anhydrase II
$CO_2 + H_2O$
Cl^-
2
H^+
Cl^-
5
pH ~4.5
Bone
Chloride channel
H^+-ATPase-proton pump
Cathepsin K
Howship's lacuna or subosteoclastic compartment

Osteoclast

1 Around the circumference of the ruffled border, where the the plasma membrane is closely applied to the bone, **actin filaments** accumulate to form a **sealing zone**, together with $\alpha_v\beta_3$ **integrin** and **osteopontin**.
2 A chloride channel prevents an excessive rise of intracellular pH.
3 Bicarbonate (HCO_3^-) is exchanged for chloride (Cl^-), which is then transported by the chloride channel (located in the ruffled membrane) to Howship's lacuna. A bicarbonate-chloride exchanger ensures the maintenance of cytoplasmic electroneutrality.
4 **Carbonic anhydrase II** generates protons (H^+) from CO_2 and H_2O. H^+ is released into Howship's lacuna by an **H^+-ATPase pump** to create an acidic environment (pH ~4.5) for solubilizing mineralized bone.
5 **Cathepsin K** is released into Howship's lacuna to degrade the exposed organic matrix (collagen and noncollagenous proteins) following solubilization of minerals by acidification.

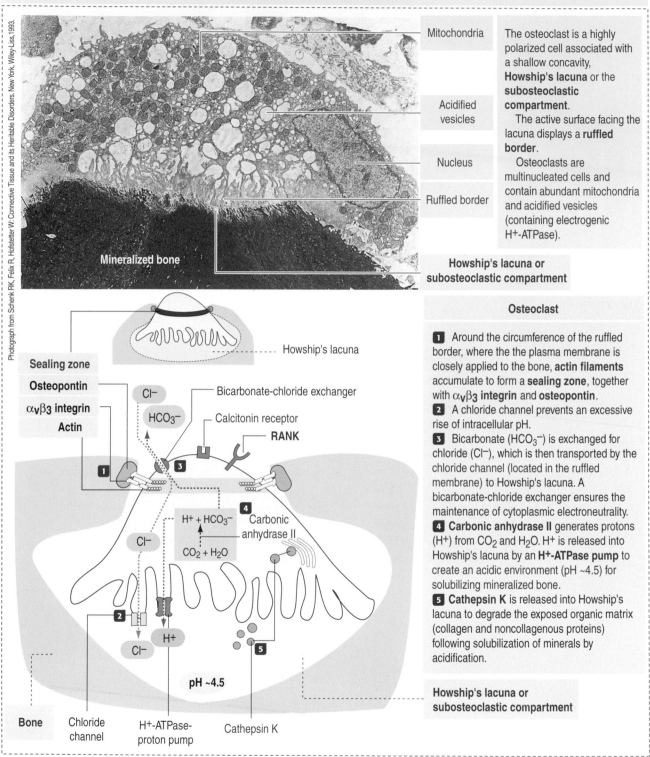

Photograph from Schenk RK, Felix R, Hofstetter W: Connective Tissue and its Heritable Disorders. New York, Wiley-Liss, 1993.

H^+-ATPase pumps required for the **acidification of the subosteoclastic compartment** for the subsequent **activation of the enzyme cathepsin K**. Cathepsin K breaks down the bone organic matrix following removal of the mineral component of bone. Figure 4-26 provides a step-by-step sequence of the activation of an osteoclast. We discuss in Chapter 15, Upper Digestive System, that the mechanism of production of HCl in the stomach is very similar to the acidification of Howship's lacuna.

Figure 4-26. Osteoclast differentiation

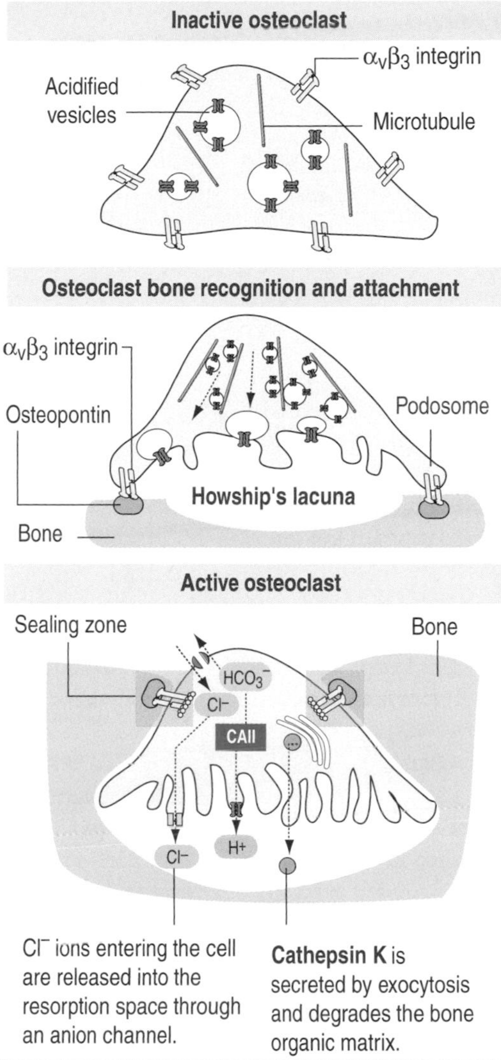
Inactive osteoclast
$\alpha_V\beta_3$ integrin
Acidified vesicles
Microtubule
Osteoclast bone recognition and attachment
$\alpha_V\beta_3$ integrin
Osteopontin
Podosome
Howship's lacuna
Bone
Active osteoclast
Sealing zone
Bone
HCO_3^-
Cl^-
CAII
Cl^-
H^+
Cl^- ions entering the cell are released into the resorption space through an anion channel.
Cathepsin K is secreted by exocytosis and degrades the bone organic matrix.

An inactive osteoclast (not attached to bone) contains **acidified vesicles with H^+-ATPase** on their membrane, microtubules, and a random distribution of $\alpha_V\beta_3$ integrin on the plasma membrane.

After attachment to bone, $\alpha_V\beta_3$ integrins concentrate on **podosomes**, sites contacting the bone matrix. Acidified vesicles associate to microtubules, and H^+-ATPases are inserted in the ruffling plasma membrane by vesicle exocytosis.

Bone degradation starts when the $\alpha_V\beta_3$ integrin-F-actin–osteopontin complex organizes the sealing zone resulting in the isolation of the resorption space from the extracellular space. Protons, generated by **carbonic anhydrase II (CAII)** activity, are transported through the H^+-ATPases present in the ruffled membrane and an acidic (~pH 4.5) environment mobilizes bone minerals. Intracellular equilibrium is maintained by Cl^-/HCO_3^- exchange.

The cell domain facing the lacuna has deep infoldings of the cell membrane, the **ruffled border**. When the cell is not active, the ruffled border disappears and the osteoclast enters into a resting phase. Around the circumference of the ruffled border—at the point where the cell membrane is closely applied to the bone just at the margins of the lacuna—**actin filaments** accumulate and participate, together with $\alpha_v\beta_3$ integrin, to form a **sealing zone**. The sealing zone seals off the bone resorption lacuna.

Osteoclasts are transiently active in response to a metabolic demand for the mobilization of calcium from bone into blood. Osteoclast activity is directly regulated by **calcitonin** (synthesized by neural crest derived parafollicular or **C cells** of the thyroid follicle), **vitamin D_3**, and regulatory molecules produced by osteoblasts and stromal cells of the bone marrow (see Osteoclastogenesis).

Osteoclastogenesis (osteoclast differentiation)

Osteoclastogenesis is triggered by two relevant molecules produced by the **osteoblast**: (1) **macrophage colony-stimulating factor (M-CSF)**, and (2) **nuclear factor kappa B (NF-κB) ligand (RANKL)**.

The osteoclast precursor, a member of the monocyte/macrophage family, responds to M-CSF, a secretory product of osteoblasts. M-CSF is required for the survival and proliferation of the osteoclast precursor (Figure 4-27). Its role was established by studies of the *op/op* mouse, which does not express M-CSF,

Figure 4-27. Osteoblasts regulate osteoclastogenesis

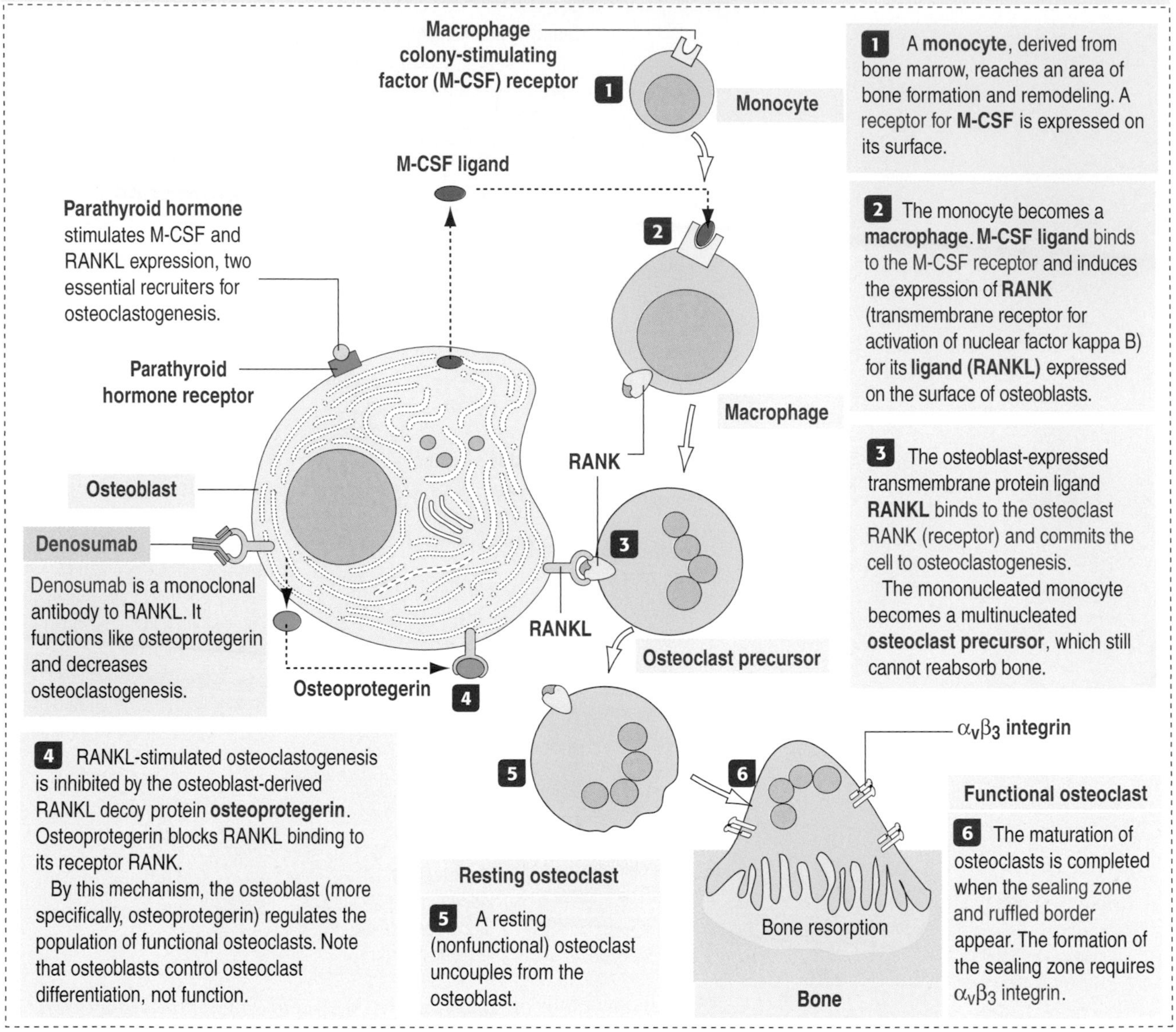
Macrophage colony-stimulating factor (M-CSF) receptor
1
Monocyte
1 A **monocyte**, derived from bone marrow, reaches an area of bone formation and remodeling. A receptor for **M-CSF** is expressed on its surface.
M-CSF ligand
Parathyroid hormone stimulates M-CSF and RANKL expression, two essential recruiters for osteoclastogenesis.
2
2 The monocyte becomes a **macrophage. M-CSF ligand** binds to the M-CSF receptor and induces the expression of **RANK** (transmembrane receptor for activation of nuclear factor kappa B) for its **ligand (RANKL)** expressed on the surface of osteoblasts.
Parathyroid hormone receptor
Macrophage
RANK
Osteoblast
3
Denosumab
3 The osteoblast-expressed transmembrane protein ligand **RANKL** binds to the osteoclast RANK (receptor) and commits the cell to osteoclastogenesis.
The mononucleated monocyte becomes a multinucleated **osteoclast precursor**, which still cannot reabsorb bone.
Denosumab is a monoclonal antibody to RANKL. It functions like osteoprotegerin and decreases osteoclastogenesis.
RANKL
Osteoclast precursor
Osteoprotegerin
4
$\alpha_v\beta_3$ integrin
4 RANKL-stimulated osteoclastogenesis is inhibited by the osteoblast-derived RANKL decoy protein **osteoprotegerin**. Osteoprotegerin blocks RANKL binding to its receptor RANK.
By this mechanism, the osteoblast (more specifically, osteoprotegerin) regulates the population of functional osteoclasts. Note that osteoblasts control osteoclast differentiation, not function.
5
6
Functional osteoclast
Resting osteoclast
5 A resting (nonfunctional) osteoclast uncouples from the osteoblast.
Bone resorption
Bone
6 The maturation of osteoclasts is completed when the sealing zone and ruffled border appear. The formation of the sealing zone requires $\alpha_v\beta_3$ integrin.

lacks osteoclasts, and has an increase in bone mass (**osteopetrosis;** Greek *osteon*, bone; *petra*, stone; *osis*, condition). In humans, **osteopetrosis is characterized by high-density bone due to absent osteoclastic activity**. In long bones, this condition leads to the **occlusion of marrow spaces** and to **anemia**.

Both **osteoblasts** and **stromal cells of the bone marrow** produce **RANKL**, a member of the **tumor necrosis factor** (TNF) **superfamily**. RANKL binds to **RANK receptor** present on the surface of differentiating osteoclasts. RANKL binding leads to RANK trimerization and the recruitment of an adaptor molecule called **TRAF6** (for TNF receptor–associated factor 6).

TRAF6 stimulates a downstream signaling cascade, including the nuclear relocation of two transcription factors: **NF-κB** and **NFATc1 (for nuclear factor–activated T cells c1)**. In the nucleus, these two transcription factors activate genes leading to osteoclast differentiation. We discuss in Chapter 3, Cell Signaling (Figure 3-8), that NF-κB is a critical transcription factor heterodimer activated in response to inflammatory or immunologic signaling.

TRAF6 also interacts with **c-Src** to stimulate a pathway leading to cytoskeletal reorganization and prevention of apoptosis. Figure 4-28 summarizes the relevant signaling steps following RANKL binding to RANK.

The interaction of the RANK receptor on osteoclast precursor cells with

RANKL, exposed on the surface of osteoblasts, determines cell-cell contact required for further maturation of the osteoclast precursor. Osteoblasts synthesize **osteoprotegerin**, a protein with high binding affinity for RANKL. Osteoprotegerin is a soluble "decoy" protein that binds to RANKL and prevents RANK-RANKL interaction. Consequently, **osteoprotegerin modulates the osteoclastogenic process.**

Parathyroid hormone stimulates the expression of osteoclastogenic RANKL. By this mechanism, the pool of RANKL increases relative to osteoprotegerin. An excess of parathyroid hormone enhances osteoclastogenesis (see Chapter 19, Endocrine System). Denosumab-induced inhibition of RANKL in hyperparathyroidism prevents bone loss caused by excessive production of parathyroid hormone.

We mentioned that a lack of M-CSF in the *op/op* mutant mouse results in **osteopetrosis**. For comparison, **osteosclerosis** is an increase in bone mass due to an **increase in osteoblastic activity**.

Clinical significance: Osteoporosis and osteomalacia

The realization that RANKL plays a major contribution in osteoclast development and in bone resorptive activity, stimulated the development of pharmaceutical

Figure 4-28. **RANK-RANKL signaling**

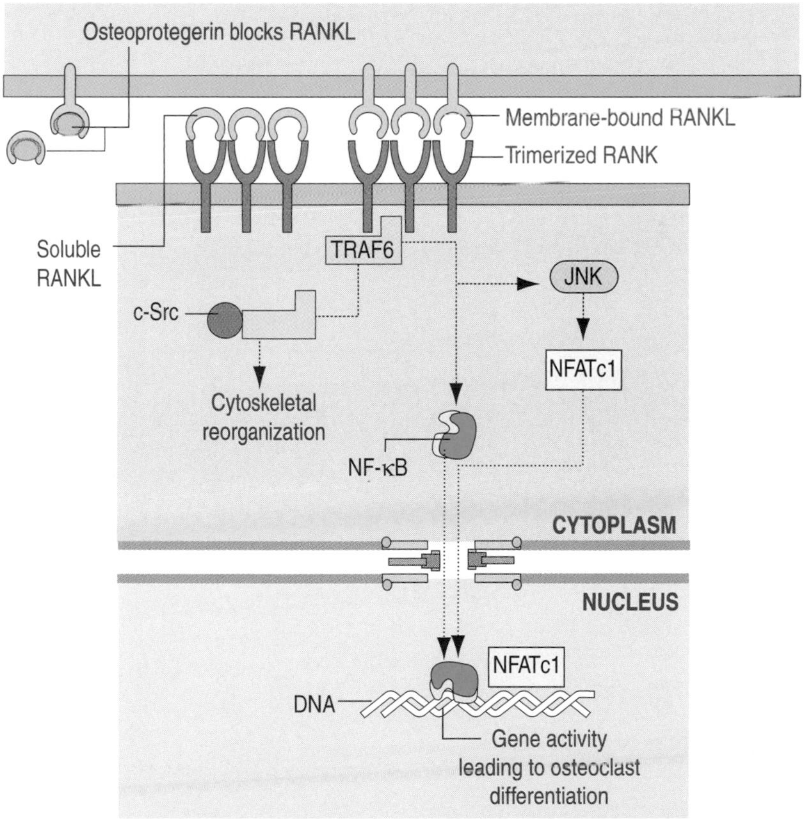

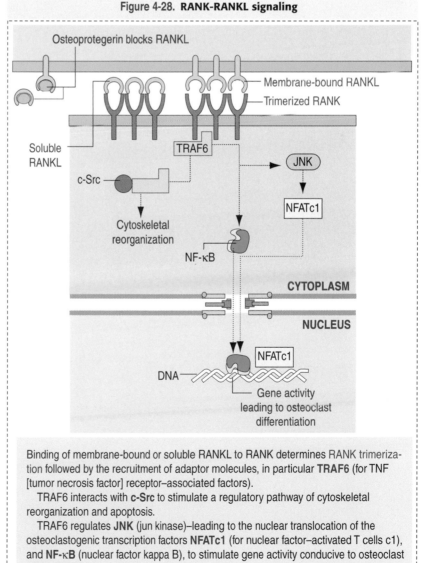

Binding of membrane-bound or soluble RANKL to RANK determines RANK trimerization followed by the recruitment of adaptor molecules, in particular **TRAF6** (for TNF [tumor necrosis factor] receptor–associated factors).

TRAF6 interacts with **c-Src** to stimulate a regulatory pathway of cytoskeletal reorganization and apoptosis.

TRAF6 regulates **JNK** (jun kinase)–leading to the nuclear translocation of the osteoclastogenic transcription factors **NFATc1** (for nuclear factor–activated T cells c1), and **NF-κB** (nuclear factor kappa B), to stimulate gene activity conducive to osteoclast differentiation.

agents to arrest skeletal disorders. **Osteoporosis** (Greek *osteon*, bone; *poros*, pore; *osis*, condition) is defined as the loss of bone mass leading to bone fragility and susceptibility to fractures.

The major factor in osteoporosis is the deficiency of the sex steroid **estrogen** that occurs in postmenopausal women. In this condition, the amount of reabsorbed old bone—due to an **increase in the number of osteoclasts**—exceeds the amount of formed new bone. This accelerated turnover state can be reversed by estrogen therapy and calcium and vitamin D supplementation. Osteoporosis and osteoporotic fractures are also observed in men.

Osteoporosis is asymptomatic until it produces skeletal deformity and bone fractures (typically in the spine, hip, and wrist). The **vertebral bones** are predominantly **trabecular bone** surrounded by a thin rim of compact bone. Therefore, they may be crushed or may wedge anteriorly, resulting in pain and in a reduction in height. Elderly persons with osteoporosis are unlikely to have a hip fracture unless they fall.

The diagnosis of osteoporosis is made radiologically or, preferentially, by measuring bone density by dual-energy x-ray absorptiometry (DEXA). DEXA measures photon absorption from an x-ray source to estimate the amount of bone mineral content.

A monoclonal antibody to RANKL, called **denosumab** (Amgen), functions like osteoprotegerin. The antibody has been administered subcutaneously every 3 months for 1 year in postmenopausal women with severe osteoporosis determined by low bone mineral density detected by DEXA. Denosumab mimics the function of osteoprotegerin and decreases bone resorption, as determined by measuring in urine and serum of bone-collagen degradation products and increased bone mineral density at 1 year. A concern with denosumab anti-RANKL treatment is the expression of RANKL-osteoprotegerin in cells of the immune system (dendritic cells and B and T cells).

Osteomalacia (Greek *osteon*, bone; *malakia*, softness) is a disease characterized by a progressive softening and bending of the bones. Softening occurs because of **a defect in the mineralization of the osteoid** due to lack of vitamin D or renal tubular dysfunction (see Chapter 14, Urinary System). In the young, a defect in **mineralization of cartilage** in the growth plate (see Chapter 5, Osteogenesis), causes a defect called **rickets (juvenile osteomalacia)**. Osteomalacia can result from a deficiency of vitamin D (for example, intestinal malabsorption) or heritable disorders of vitamin D activation (for example, **renal 1α-hydroxylase deficiency** in which **calciferol** is not converted to the active form of vitamin D, **calcitriol**; see vitamin D in Chapter 19, Endocrine System).

• Connective tissue provides support, or stroma, to the functional component, or parenchyma, of tissues. The functions of connective tissue include the storage of metabolites, immune and inflammatory responses, and tissue repair after injury.

Connective tissue consists of thee basic components: cells, fibers, and extracellular matrix (called ground substance). The proportion of these three components contributes to the classification of connective tissue.

Connective tissue can be classified into three major groups: (1) embryonic connective tissue, (2) adult connective tissue, and (3) special connective tissue (including adipose tissue, cartilage, bone, and hematopoietic tissue).

The embryonic connective tissue, or mesenchyme, consists predominantly of extracellular matrix. The umbilical cord contains this type of connective tissue, also called mucoid connective tissue or Wharton's jelly.

The adult connective tissue can be subclassified as loose or areolar connective tissue (more cells than fibers, found in the mesentery or lamina propria of mucosae) and dense connective tissue (more collagen fibers, arranged in bundles, than cells). The latter is subdivided into two categories: dense irregular connective tissue (with a random orientation of collagen bundles, found in the dermis of the skin) and dense regular connective tissue (with an orderly orientation of collagen bundles, found in tendon). A refinement of the adult connective tissue classification is based on which fibers predominate. Reticular connective tissue contains abundant reticular fibers (type III collagen). Elastic connective tissue, found in the form of sheets or laminae in the wall of the aorta, is rich in elastic fibers.

• There are two major classes of cells in the connective tissue: the resident fibroblasts, and the visiting macrophages, mast cells, and plasma cells.

The **fibroblast** synthesizes the precursor molecules of various types of collagens and elastin, and proteoglycans.

Collagen synthesis proceeds in an orderly sequence. Procollagen, the initial collagen precursor which contains hydroxyproline and hydroxylysine, is secreted by fibroblasts in the form of a triple helix flanked by nonhelical domains. Procollagen peptidase cleaves the nonhelical domains, and procollagen becomes tropocollagen. Tropocollagen molecules self-assemble in a staggered array in the presence of lysyl oxidase to form a cross-banded collagen fibril. Side-by-side linking of collagen fibrils, a process mediated by proteoglycans and a form of collagen with interrupted triple helices (called FACIT), results in the assembly of collagen fibers. What you see in the light microscope are bundles of collagen fibers.

Keep In mind that not only fibroblasts can produce collagens. Osteoblasts, chondroblasts, odontoblasts, and smooth muscle cells can also synthesize collagens. Even epithelial cells can synthesize type IV collagen. You have already seen that the basement membrane contains type IV collagen in the basal lamina and type III collagen in the reticular lamina.

Defects in the processing of procollagen and tropocollagen and the assembly of collagen fibrils give rise to variations of the Ehlers-Danlos syndrome, characterized by hyperelasticity of the skin and hypermobility of the joints.

Elastin, the precursor of elastic fibers, is also synthesized and processed sequentially. Fibroblasts or smooth muscle cells secrete desmosine- and isodesmosine-containing proelastin, which is partially cleaved to give rise to tropoelastin. These cells also produce fibrillin 1 and 2, and microfibril-associated glycoprotein (MAGP). Tropoelastin, fibrillins, and MAGP assemble into immature elastic fibers that aggregate to form bundles of mature elastic fibers.

A defect in fibrillin 1 affects the assembly of mature elastic fibers, a characteristic of Marfan syndrome.

Macrophages derive from monocytes produced in the bone marrow. A typical property of macrophages is phagocytosis. Their function in connective tissue is the turnover of fibers and extracellular matrix and, most important, the presentation of antigens to lymphocytes as an essential step of immune and inflammatory reactions.

Mast cells also originate in the bone marrow. They contain metachromatic granules, which stain with a color that is different from the color of the dye. The granules contain vasoactive mediators (histamine, heparin, and chemotactic mediators). Granules are released, by a process called degranulation, when a specific antigen (or allergen) dimerizes two adjacent IgE molecules anchored to FcεRI receptors and cytosolic calcium is released from intracellular storage sites. Leukotrienes are vasoactive agents not present in granules; they are metabolites of the plasma membrane–associated arachidonic acid. Like most vasoactive agents, they induce an increase in vascular permeability leading to edema.

Mast cells and basophils circulating in blood appear to derive from the same progenitor in the bone marrow.

Mast cells play a role in allergic hypersensitivity reactions associated with asthma, hay fever, and eczema.

Plasma cells derive from the differentiation of B lymphocytes (B cells). Three characteristics define the structure of a plasma cell: a well-developed rough endoplasmic reticulum, an extensive Golgi apparatus, and a prominent nucleolus. These features define the plasma cell as an actively protein-producing cell, whose main product are immunoglobulins.

The **extracellular matrix** is a combination of collagens, noncollagenous glycoproteins, and proteoglycans. Proteoglycan aggregates are the major components. Each proteoglycan consists of a core protein attached to a linear hyaluronan molecule by a linker protein. Attached to the core protein are numerous glycosaminoglycan chains (keratan sulfate, dermatan sulfate, and chondroitin sulfate). The extracellular matrix is maintained by a balance of matrix metalloproteinases and tissue inhibitors of metalloproteinases (TIMPs). Matrix metalloproteinases are zinc-dependent proteases, which include collagenases, stromelysins, gelatinases, and membrane-type matrix metalloproteinases.

• **Tumor invasion of the connective tissue.** Malignant cells that originated in a lining epithelium (carcinoma) or a glandular epithelium (adenocarcinoma) can break down the basement membrane and invade the underlying connective tissue. The first step leading to invasion is cessation in the expression of cadherins to weaken the cohesive nature of the epithelial tissue. The second step is the production of proteinases and cell adhesion molecules allowing the malignant cells to invade and attach to components of the connective tissue. The third step is the production by tumor cells of autocrine motility factors, to enable tumor cell motility; vascular permeability factors, to ensure a supply of nutrients; and angiogenic factors, to increase the vascular support of the growing tumors. Finally, tumor cells can produce chemokine molecules on their surface that facilitate their transendothelial migration to metastasize.

• **Adipose tissue** or fat is a special type of connective tissue. There are two types of adipose tissue: (1) white fat, the major reserve of long-term energy, and (2) brown fat, a thermogenic type of fat.

Mesenchymal cells give rise to preadipocytes. Preadipocytes, under control of insulin, bound to insulin-like growth factor-1 (IGF-1) receptor, synthesize lipoprotein lipase. Lipoprotein lipase is transferred to endothelial cells in the adjacent blood vessels to enable the passage of fatty acids and triglycerides into the adipocytes.

Fat can accumulate in a single lipid-strorage droplet (unilocular) or multiple small lipid droplets (multilocular). White fat is unilocular; brown fat is multilocular.

Fat can be mobilized by a lipolytic effect consisting in the activation of the enzyme lipase by a cAMP-mediated effect induced by epinephrine, glucagon, or ACTH. Fat deposits can increase by inhibiting lipase activity (antilipolytic effect) determined by insulin and prostaglandins.

Leptin, a peptide produced by adipocytes, regulates appetite, energy balance, and feeding. Leptin-deficient mice are obese and infertile, conditions that are reversible when leptin is administered to the mutants.

Adipocytes in brown fat contain abundant mitochondria. An important mitochondrial component is uncoupling protein-1 (UCP-1), a protein that allows the reentry of protons down their concentration gradient in the mitochondrial matrix, a process that results in the dissipation of energy in the form of heat (thermogenesis).

• **Cartilage** is another special type of connective tissue. Like adipocytes, chondroblasts derive from mesenchymal cells. Like a typical connective tissue member, cartilage consists of cells, fibers, and extracellular matrix. Chondroblasts and chondrocytes produce type II collagen (except in fibrocartilage, where chondrocytes produce type I collagen) and the proteoglycan aggrecan.

There are three major types of cartilages: (1) hyaline cartilage, (2) elastic cartilage, and (3) fibrocartilage.

Cartilage lacks blood vessels and is surrounded by the perichondrium (except in fibrocartilage and articular hyaline cartilage, which lack a perichondrium). The perichondrium consists of two layers: an outermost fibrous layer, consisting of elongated fibroblast-like cells, and the innermost chondrogenic cell layer.

Chondrogenesis (cartilage growth) takes place by two mechanisms: (1) interstitial growth (within the cartilage), and (2) appositional growth (at the perichondrial surface of the cartilage).

During interstitial growth, centers of chondrogenesis, consisting of chondroblasts located in lacunae and surrounded by a territorial matrix, divide by mitosis without leaving the lacunae and form isogenous groups. Isogenous groups are separated from each other by an interterritorial matrix. Interstitial growth is particularly prevalent during endochondral ossification.

During appositional growth, the cells of the perichondrial chondrogenic layer differentiate into chondroblasts following activation of the gene encoding the transcription factor Sox9. New layers are added to the surface of the cartilage by appositional growth.

A lack of Sox9 gene expression causes **campomelic dysplasia** consisting in bowing and angulation of long bones, hypoplasia of the pelvis and scapula, and abnormalities of the vertebral column.

• **Bone**. A mature long bone consists of a shaft or diaphysis, and two epiphyses at the endings of the diaphysis. A tapering metaphysis links each epiphysis to the diaphysis. During bone growth, a cartilaginous growth plate is present at the epiphysis-metaphysis interface. After growth, the growth plate is replaced by a residual growth line.

The diaphysis is surrounded by a cylinder of compact bone housing the bone marrow. The epiphyses consist of spongy or cancellous bone covered by a thin layer of compact bone. The periosteum covers the outer surface of the bone (except the articular surfaces and the tendon and ligament insertion sites). The endosteum lines the marrow cavity.

A cross section of a compact bone consists of the following components: (1) the periosteum, formed by an outer connective tissue layer pierced by periosteal blood vessels penetrating Volkmann's canals feeding each osteon or haversian system. An inner periosteal layer, attached to bone by Sharpey's fibers, is derived from the outer periosteal layer. (2) The outer circumferential lamellae. (3) Osteons or haversian systems, cylindrical structures parallel to the longitudinal axis of the bone. Blood vessels are present in the central canal, which is surrounded by concentric lamellae. Each lamella contains lacunae and radiating canaliculi occupied by osteocytes and their cell processes. Osteocyte cytoplasmic processes are connected to each other by gap junctions. A fluid containing ions is present in the lumen of the canaliculi. (4) The inner circumferential lamellae. (5) Spongy bone (trabecular or cancellous bone), consisting of lamellae lacking a central canal (lamellar bone but no haversian system), extending into the medullary cavity. (6) The endosteum, a lining of osteoprogenitor cells supported by reticular fibers. You can regard the endosteum as also the "capsule" of the bone marrow.

• The two major cell components of bone are the osteoblast and the osteoclast. Osteoblasts derive from mesenchyme-derived osteoprogenitor cells. Osteoclasts are monocyte-derived cells from the bone marrow.

The osteoblast is a typical protein-producing cell whose function is regulated by parathyroid hormone and IGF-1 (produced in liver following stimulation by growth hormone). Osteoblasts synthesize type I collagen, noncollagenous proteins, and proteoglycans. These are the components of the bone matrix or osteoid deposited during bone formation. In mature bone, the bone matrix consists of about 35% organic components and about 65% inorganic components (calcium phosphate with the crystalline characteristics of hydroxyapatite).

There are four noncollagenous proteins produced by osteoblasts that you should remember: macrophage-colony stimulating factor, RANKL, osteoprotegerin, and osteopontin. The first three play an essential role in osteoclastogenesis. Osteopontin contributes to the development of the sealing zone during osteoclast bone resorption activity.

Osteoblasts differentiate into osteocytes, which are trapped in lacunae in the bone lamellae. The differentiation process requires the participation of two transcription factors: Cbfa1/Runx2 and osterix. Cbfa1/Runx2-deficient mice have a skeleton consisting of cartilage and lack osteoclasts. In humans, **cleidocranial dysplasia**, characterized by hypoplastic clavicles and delayed ossification of sutures of certain skull bones, is associated with defective expression of the *Cbfa1/Runx2* gene.

The function of osteoclasts is regulated by calcitonin, produced by C cells located in the thyroid gland. Active osteoclasts, involved in bone resorption, are highly polarized cells. The free domain has a sealing zone, a tight belt consisting of $\alpha_v\beta_3$ integrin with its intracellular domain linked to F-actin and the extracellular domain attached to osteopontin on the bone surface. The domain associated to the subosteoclastic compartment (Howship's lacunae) displays a ruffled plasma membrane (ruffled border). The cytoplasm contains two relevant structures: mitochondria and acidified vesicles. The osteoclast is a multinucleated cell resulting from the fusion of several monocytes during osteoclastogenesis. You should be aware that the bone marrow contains megakaryocytes that may be confused with osteoclasts. Osteoclasts are intimately associated to bone and are multinucleated; megakaryocytes are surrounded by hematopoietic cells and their nucleus is multilobulated.

Howship's lacuna is the site where bone is removed by an osteoclast. Bone removal occurs in two phases: First, the mineral component is mobilized in an acidic environment (~pH 4.5); second, the organic component is degraded by cathepsin K.

Carbonic anhydrase II in the cytoplasm of the osteoclast

produces protons and bicarbonate from CO_2 and water. The acidified vesicles, with H^+-ATPase in their membranes, are inserted in the ruffling border. With the help of mitochondrial ATP, H^+ are released through the H^+-ATPase pump into Howship's lacuna and the pH becomes increasingly acidic.

Bicarbonate escapes the cell through a bicarbonate-chloride exchanger; chloride entering the osteoclast is released into the lacuna. Because of the significant H^+ transport, a parallel bicarbonate-chloride ion transport mechanism is required to maintain intracellular electroneutrality.

• Osteoclastogenesis. The osteoclast precursor is a member of the monocyte-macrophage lineage present in the adjacent bone marrow. Osteoblasts recruit monocytes and change them into osteoclasts, the cell in charge of bone remodeling and mobilization of calcium.

Osteoclastogenesis consists of several phases under strict control by the osteoblast: (1) macrophage colony-stimulating factor (M-CSF), produced by the osteoblast, binds to the M-CSF receptor on the monocyte surface and the monocyte becomes a macrophage. (2) The macrophage induces the expression of RANK, a transmembrane receptor, for the ligand RANKL produced by the osteoblast. (3) The RANK-RANKL interaction commits the macrophage to osteoclastogenesis. The macrophage becomes a multinucleated osteoclast precursor. (4) Osteoprotegerin, also produced by the osteoblasts, may bind to RANKL and prevent RANK-mediated association of the macrophage. This event can stop osteoclastogenesis (it does not stop osteoclast function). (5) The osteoclast precursor becomes a resting osteoclast waiting to attach to bone and become a functional osteoclast. (6) An osteoclast becomes functional when $\alpha_v\beta_3$ integrin binds to osteopontin and begins the formation of the sealing zone. Then, the H^+-ATPase-containing acidified vesicles are transported by motor proteins associated to microtubules to the ruffling border. The acidification of Howship's lacuna starts with the activation of carbonic anhydrase II.

The RANK-RANKL signaling pathway activates gene expression leading to osteoclast differentiation. RANKL binding trimerizes RANK, which then recruits TRAF6 to trigger jun kinase resulting in the nuclear translocation of NFATc1 and NF-κB.

5. OSTEOGENESIS

Bone formation (osteogenesis or ossification)

Bone develops by replacement of a preexisting connective tissue. The two processes of bone formation or osteogenesis observed in the embryo are: (1) **intramembranous bone formation**, in which bone tissue is laid down directly in primitive connective tissue or **mesenchyme** (Figures 5-1 and 5-2), and (2) **endochondral bone formation**, in which bone tissue replaces a preexisting **hyaline cartilage**, the template or anlage of the future bone (see Figures 5-3 to 5-5).

The mechanism of bone matrix deposition during intramembranous and endochondral ossification is essentially the same: **A primary trabecular network or primary spongiosa is first laid down and then transformed into mature bone.** But there is a difference: **In endochondral ossification, cartilage is replaced by bone matrix.**

Intramembranous bone formation

Membrane bones such as the flat bones of the skull develop by intramembranous

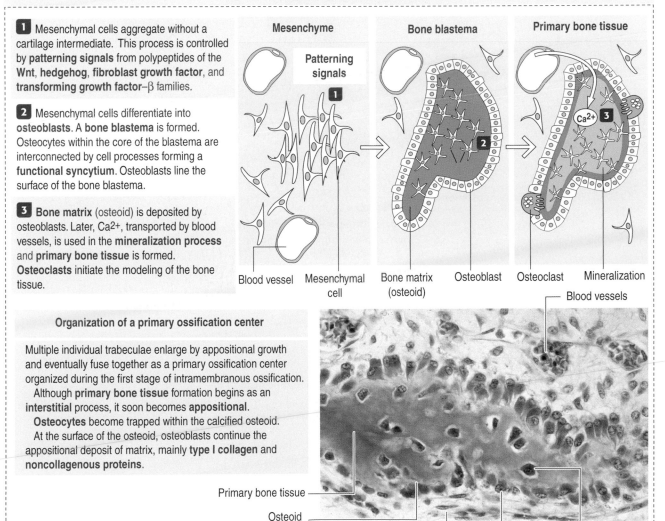

Figure 5-1. **Intramembranous ossification**

1 Mesenchymal cells aggregate without a cartilage intermediate. This process is controlled by **patterning signals** from polypeptides of the **Wnt**, **hedgehog**, **fibroblast growth factor**, and **transforming growth factor**–β families.

2 Mesenchymal cells differentiate into **osteoblasts**. A **bone blastema** is formed. Osteocytes within the core of the blastema are interconnected by cell processes forming a **functional syncytium**. Osteoblasts line the surface of the bone blastema.

3 **Bone matrix** (osteoid) is deposited by osteoblasts. Later, Ca^{2+}, transported by blood vessels, is used in the **mineralization process** and **primary bone tissue** is formed. **Osteoclasts** initiate the modeling of the bone tissue.

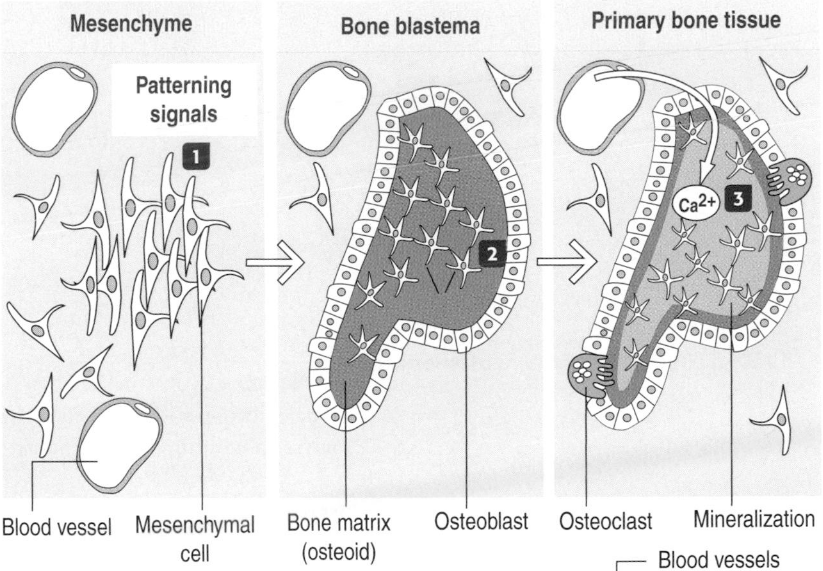

Mesenchyme
Bone blastema
Primary bone tissue
Patterning signals
1
2
3
Ca2+
Blood vessel
Mesenchymal cell
Bone matrix (osteoid)
Osteoblast
Osteoclast
Mineralization

Organization of a primary ossification center

Multiple individual trabeculae enlarge by appositional growth and eventually fuse together as a primary ossification center organized during the first stage of intramembranous ossification.

Although **primary bone tissue** formation begins as an **interstitial** process, it soon becomes **appositional**.

Osteocytes become trapped within the calcified osteoid.

At the surface of the osteoid, osteoblasts continue the appositional deposit of matrix, mainly **type I collagen** and **noncollagenous proteins**.

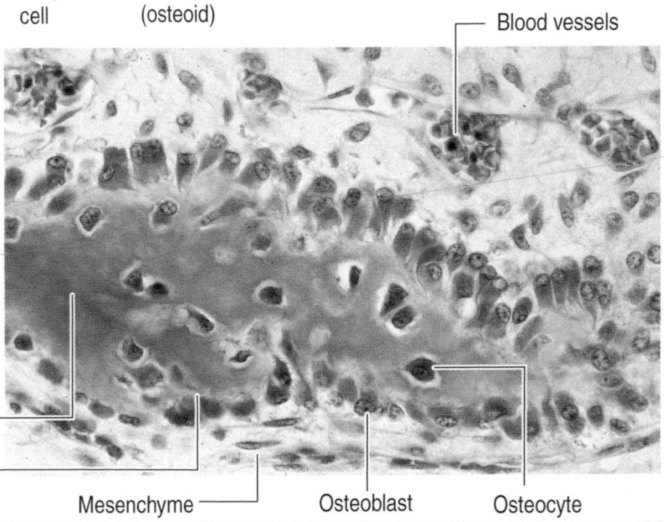

Blood vessels
Primary bone tissue
Osteoid
Mesenchyme
Osteoblast
Osteocyte

Figure 5-2. **Intramembranous ossification**

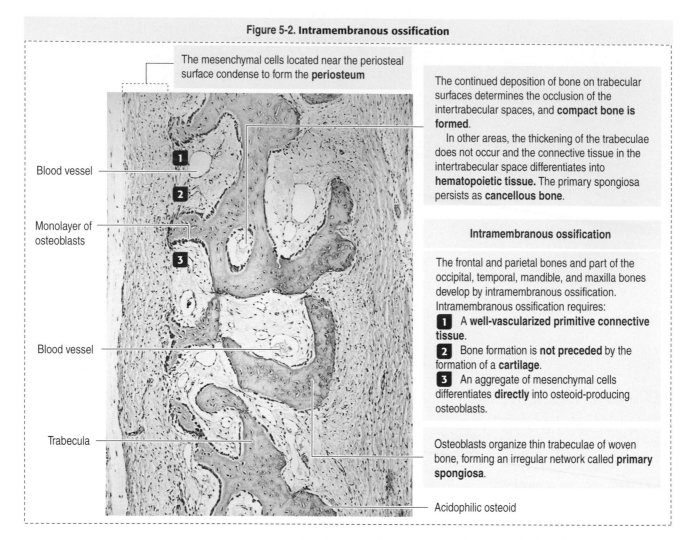

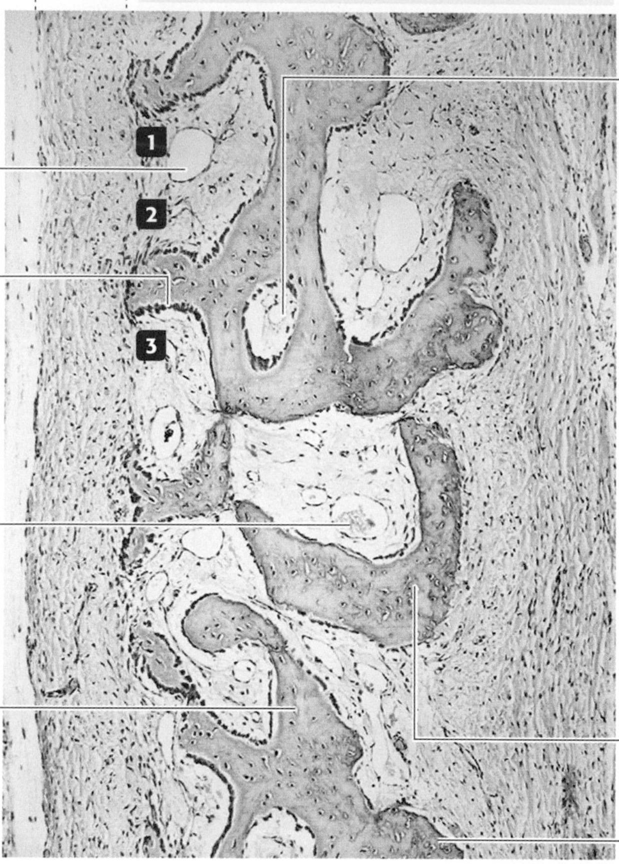
The mesenchymal cells located near the periosteal surface condense to form the **periosteum**
Blood vessel
Monolayer of osteoblasts
Blood vessel
Trabecula
1
2
3
The continued deposition of bone on trabecular surfaces determines the occlusion of the intertrabecular spaces, and **compact bone is formed**.
In other areas, the thickening of the trabeculae does not occur and the connective tissue in the intertrabecular space differentiates into **hematopoietic tissue.** The primary spongiosa persists as **cancellous bone**.
Intramembranous ossification
The frontal and parietal bones and part of the occipital, temporal, mandible, and maxilla bones develop by intramembranous ossification. Intramembranous ossification requires:
1 A **well-vascularized primitive connective tissue**.
2 Bone formation is **not preceded** by the formation of a **cartilage**.
3 An aggregate of mesenchymal cells differentiates **directly** into osteoid-producing osteoblasts.
Osteoblasts organize thin trabeculae of woven bone, forming an irregular network called **primary spongiosa**.
Acidophilic osteoid

ossification. Intramembranous ossification occurs in the following sequence (see Figure 5-1):

1. The embryonic mesenchyme changes into a highly vascularized connective tissue. Fibroblast-like mesenchymal cells, embedded in a gelatinous extracellular matrix containing collagen fibers, aggregate.

2. Mesenchymal cells acquire the typical columnar form of **osteoblasts** and begin to secrete **bone matrix** (see Box 5-A). Numerous ossification centers develop and eventually fuse, forming a network of anastomosing **trabeculae** resembling a sponge, the so-called **spongy bone** or **primary spongiosa**.

3. Because collagen fibers in the newly formed trabeculae are **randomly** oriented, the early intramembranous bone is described as **woven bone**—in contrast with **lamellar bone** formed later during bone remodeling.

4. Calcium phosphate is deposited in the bone matrix, which is laid down by **apposition. Interstitial bone growth does not occur.**

5. Bone matrix mineralization leads to two new developments (see Figure 5-2): the entrapment of osteoblasts as **osteocytes**, as trabeculae thicken, and the partial closing of the perivascular channels, which assume the new role of **hematopoiesis** by conversion of mesenchymal cells into blood-forming cells.

Osteocytes remain connected to each other by cytoplasmic processes enclosed within canaliculi, and new osteoblasts are generated from osteoprogenitor cells adjacent to the blood vessels.

The final developmental events include:

1. **The conversion of woven bone to lamellar bone.** In lamellar bone, the newly synthesized collagen fibers are aligned into **regular** bundles. Lamellae arranged in

Box 5-A | **From osteoblasts to osteocytes**

- Mesenchymal cells differentiate to osteoblasts when the transcription factors Cbfa1/Runx2 and osterix are expressed.
- The differentiation of osteoblasts to osteocytes also requires the expression of **Cbfa1/Runx2 and osterix.**
- The differentiation of mesenchymal cells to chondrocytes occurs when the gene encoding **Sox9** is expressed. During endochondral ossification (as we will see later), chondrocytes undergo considerable enlargement and become hypertrophic. The transition from chondrocyte to hypertrophic chondrocyte is stimulated by Cbfa1/Runx2 but inhibited by Sox9.
- Putting things together, Cbfa1/Runx2 has a role in both chondrocytic and osteoblastic differentiation. Osterix specifies the differentiation of osteoblasts to osteocytes. A lack of osterix gene expression affects osteoblastic differentiation but not chondrocyte maturation. An example is **cleidocranial dysplasia** with defects in both intramembranous and endochondral ossification.

concentric rings around a central blood vessel occupying the haversian canal form **osteons** or **haversian systems**. Membrane bones remain as spongy bone in the center, the **diploë**, enclosed by an outer and an inner layer of compact bone.

2. The condensation of the external and internal connective tissue layers to form the **periosteum** and **endosteum**, respectively, containing fusiform cells with osteoprogenitor cell potential.

At birth, bone development is not complete, and the bones of the skull are separated by spaces (**fontanelles**) housing osteogenic tissue. The bones of a young child contain both woven and lamellar bony matrix.

Endochondral ossification

Endochondral ossification is the process by which **skeletal cartilage templates** are replaced by bone. As you recall, intramembranous ossification is the process by which a **skeletal mesenchymal template** is replaced by bone without passing through the cartilage stage. Bones of the extremities, vertebral column, and pelvis derive from a hyaline cartilage template.

As in intramembranous ossification, a **primary ossification center** is formed during endochondral ossification (Figure 5-3). Unlike intramembranous ossification, this center of ossification derives from proliferated chondrocytes that have deposited an extracellular matrix containing type II collagen.

Shortly after, chondrocytes in the central region of the cartilage undergo maturation to hypertrophy and synthesize a matrix containing **type X collagen**, a marker for hypertrophic chondrocytes. **Angiogenic factors** secreted by hypertrophic chondrocytes (**vascular endothelial cell growth factor** [VEGF]) induce the formation of blood vessels from the perichondrium. Osteoprogenitor and hematopoietic cells arrive with the newly formed blood vessels.

These events result in the formation of the primary ossification center. Hypertrophic chondrocytes undergo apoptosis as **calcification of the matrix** in the middle of the shaft of the cartilage template takes place.

At the same time, the inner perichondrial cells exhibit their osteogenic potential, and a thin **periosteal collar** of bone is formed around the midpoint of the shaft,

Figure 5-3. Endochondral ossification: Primary ossification center

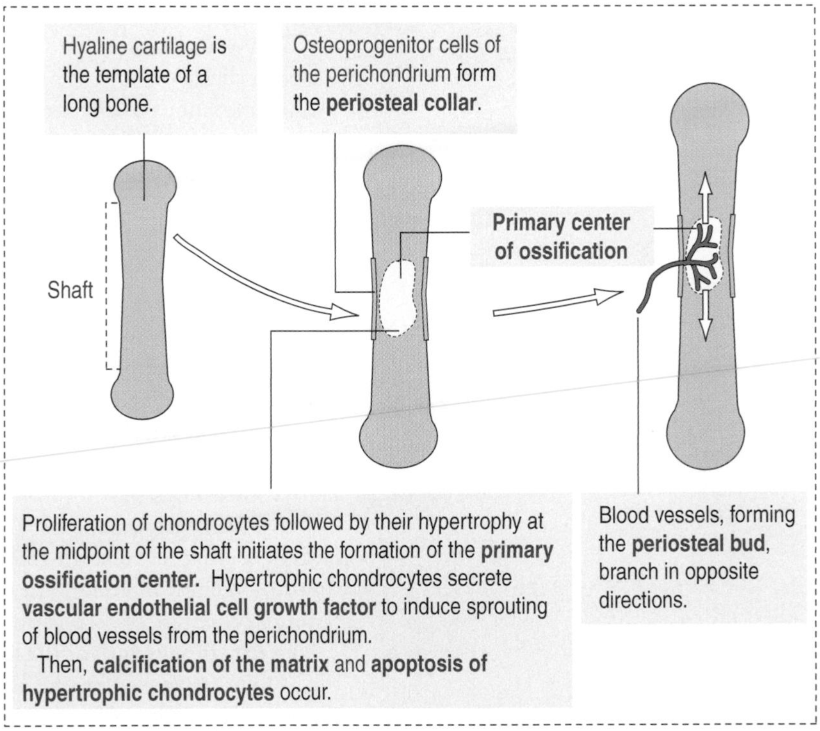

Hyaline cartilage is the template of a long bone.
Osteoprogenitor cells of the perichondrium form the **periosteal collar**.
Shaft
Primary center of ossification
Proliferation of chondrocytes followed by their hypertrophy at the midpoint of the shaft initiates the formation of the **primary ossification center.** Hypertrophic chondrocytes secrete **vascular endothelial cell growth factor** to induce sprouting of blood vessels from the perichondrium.
Then, **calcification of the matrix** and **apoptosis of hypertrophic chondrocytes** occur.
Blood vessels, forming the **periosteal bud**, branch in opposite directions.

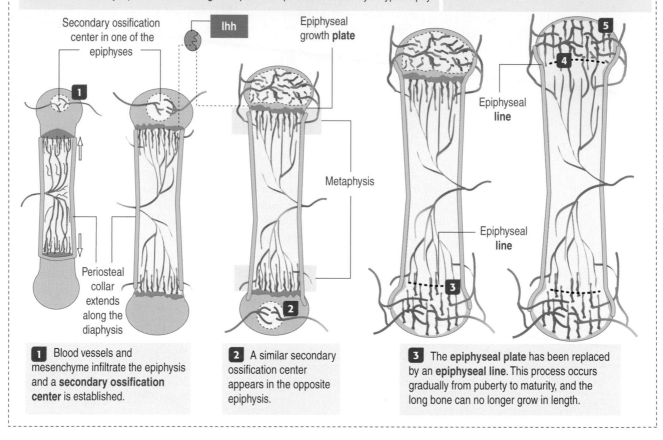

Figure 5-4. Endochondral ossification: Secondary ossification centers

The **metaphysis** is the portion of the diaphysis nearest to the epiphyses. The **epiphyseal cartilaginous growth plate** between the metaphysis and the epiphysis will eventually be replaced by bone. The bone at this site is particularly dense and is recognized as an **epiphyseal line**. **Indian hedgehog (Ihh)**, a member of the hedgehog protein family, stimulates chondrocyte proliferation in the growth plate and prevents chondrocyte hypertrophy.

4 Blood vessels from the diaphysis and epiphysis intercommunicate.
5 All the epiphyseal cartilage is replaced by bone, except for the **articular surface**.

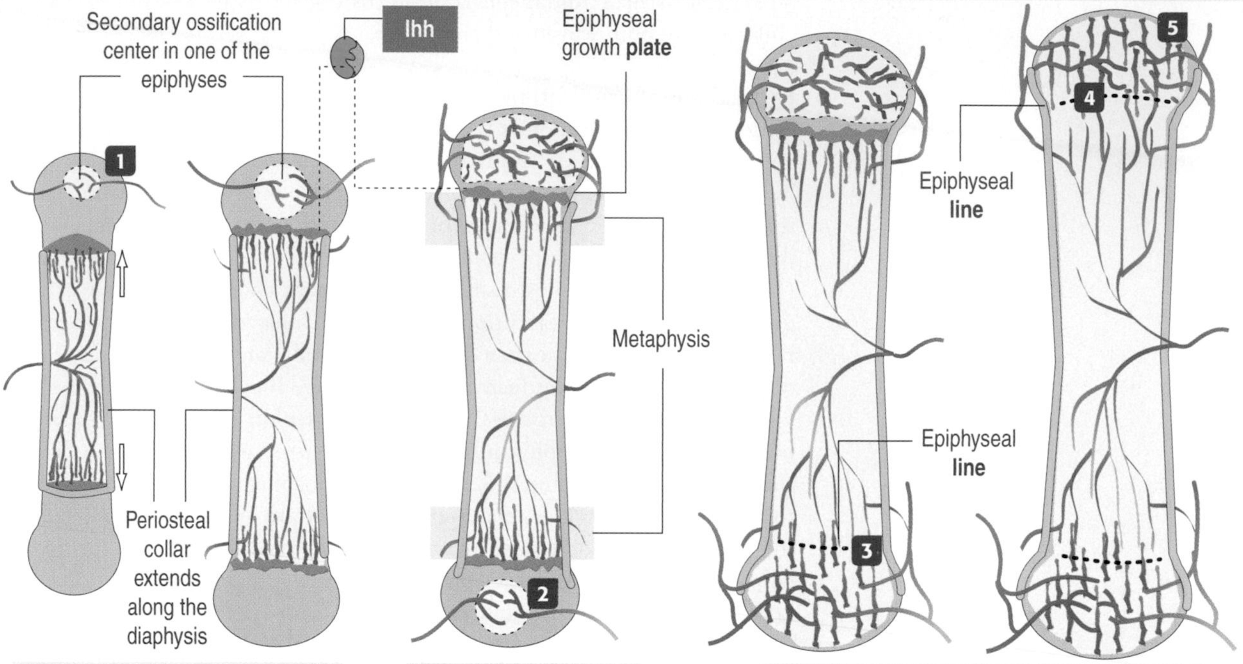

1 Blood vessels and mesenchyme infiltrate the epiphysis and a **secondary ossification center** is established.

2 A similar secondary ossification center appears in the opposite epiphysis.

3 The **epiphyseal plate** has been replaced by an **epiphyseal line**. This process occurs gradually from puberty to maturity, and the long bone can no longer grow in length.

the **diaphysis**. Consequently, the primary ossification center ends up located inside a cylinder of bone. **The periosteal collar formed under the periosteum by intramembranous ossification consists of woven bone**. As we will discuss later on, the periosteal collar is converted into compact bone.

The following sequence of events defines the next steps of endochondral ossification (Figure 5-4):

1. **Blood vessels** invade the space formerly occupied by the hypertrophic chondrocytes, and they branch and project toward either end of the center of ossification. Blind capillary ends extend into the cavities formed within the calcified cartilage.

2. **Osteoprogenitor cells** and hematopoietic stem cells reach the core of the calcified cartilage through the perivascular connective tissue surrounding the invading blood vessels. Then, osteoprogenitor cells differentiate into **osteoblasts** that aggregate on the surfaces of the calcified cartilage and begin to deposit **bone matrix (osteoid)**.

3. At this developmental step, a **primary center of ossification**—defined by both the **periosteal collar (intramembranous ossification type)** and the center of ossification in the interior of the cartilage template—is organized at the diaphysis. **Secondary centers of ossification** develop later in the **epiphyses**.

The **growth in length of the long bones** depends on the **interstitial growth** of the hyaline cartilage while the center of the cartilage is being replaced by bone at the equidistant zones of ossification.

Figure 5-5. Endochondral ossification: Four major zones

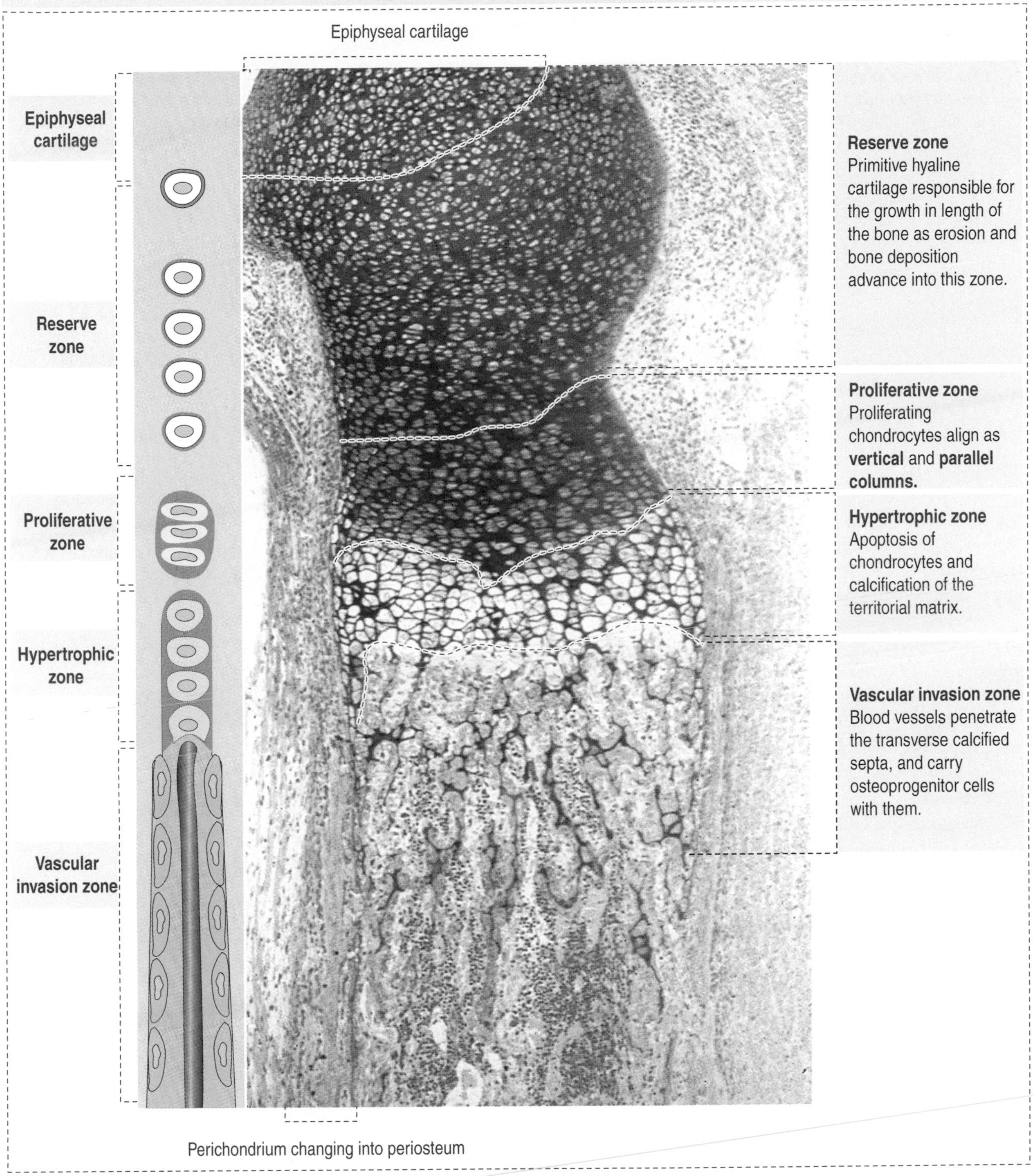
Epiphyseal cartilage
Epiphyseal cartilage
Reserve zone
Proliferative zone
Hypertrophic zone
Vascular invasion zone
Reserve zone
Primitive hyaline cartilage responsible for the growth in length of the bone as erosion and bone deposition advance into this zone.
Proliferative zone
Proliferating chondrocytes align as vertical and parallel columns.
Hypertrophic zone
Apoptosis of chondrocytes and calcification of the territorial matrix.
Vascular invasion zone
Blood vessels penetrate the transverse calcified septa, and carry osteoprogenitor cells with them.
Perichondrium changing into periosteum

Secondary centers of ossification and the epiphyseal growth plate

Up to this point, we have analyzed the development of **primary centers of ossification** in the **diaphysis** of long bones that occurs by the third month of fetal life.

After birth, **secondary centers of ossification** develop in the **epiphyses** (see Figure 5-4). As in the diaphysis, the space occupied by hypertrophic chondrocytes is invaded by blood vessels and osteoprogenitor cells from the perichondrium. Most of the hyaline cartilage of the epiphyses is replaced by the spongy bone, except for the **articular cartilage** and a thin disk, the **epiphyseal growth plate**,

Figure 5-6. **Endochondral ossification: Zones of proliferation, hypertrophy, and vascular invasion**

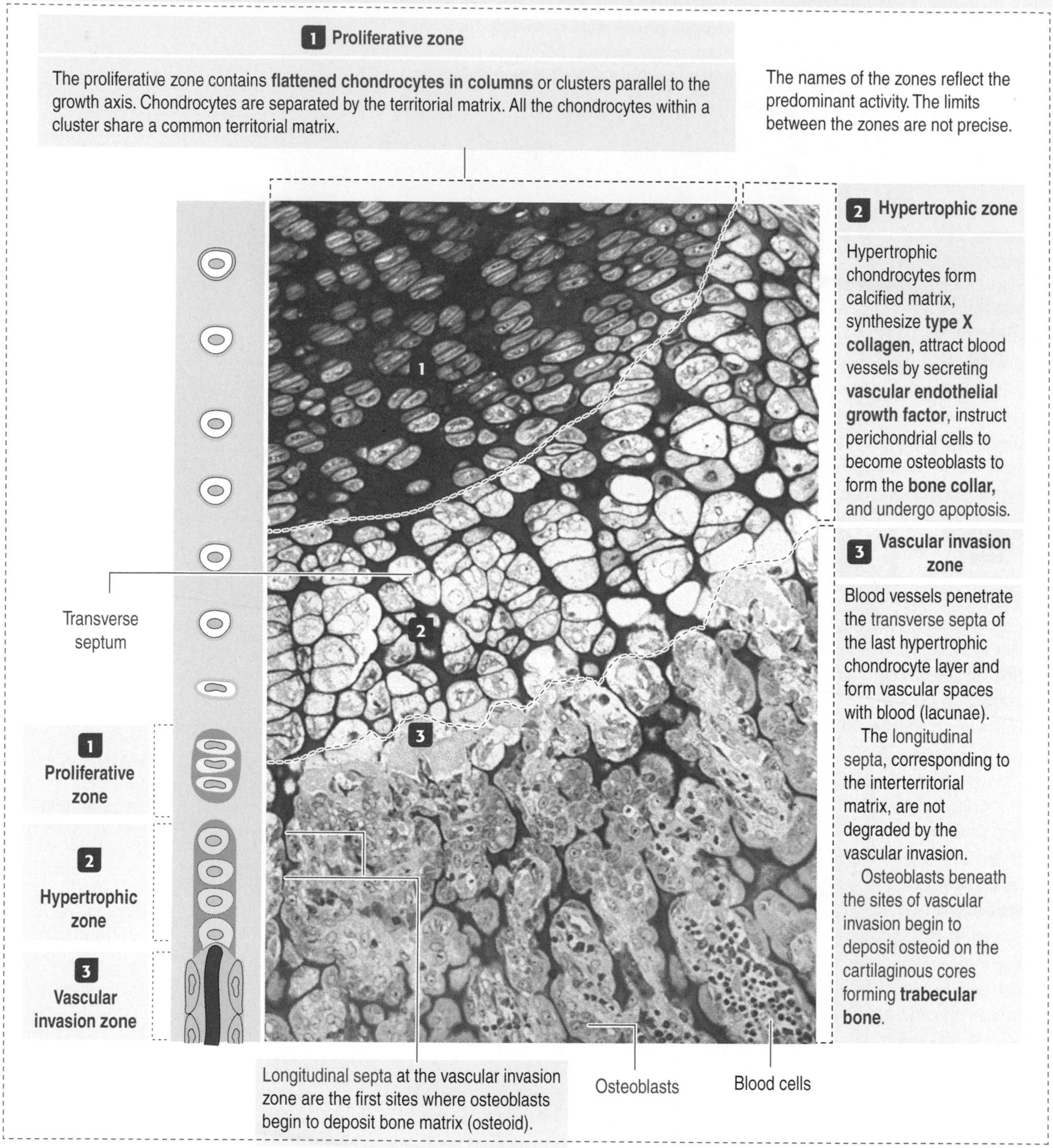

1 Proliferative zone
The proliferative zone contains **flattened chondrocytes in columns** or clusters parallel to the growth axis. Chondrocytes are separated by the territorial matrix. All the chondrocytes within a cluster share a common territorial matrix.
The names of the zones reflect the predominant activity. The limits between the zones are not precise.
2 Hypertrophic zone
Hypertrophic chondrocytes form calcified matrix, synthesize **type X collagen**, attract blood vessels by secreting **vascular endothelial growth factor**, instruct perichondrial cells to become osteoblasts to form the **bone collar,** and undergo apoptosis.
3 Vascular invasion zone
Blood vessels penetrate the transverse septa of the last hypertrophic chondrocyte layer and form vascular spaces with blood (lacunae).
The longitudinal septa, corresponding to the interterritorial matrix, are not degraded by the vascular invasion.
Osteoblasts beneath the sites of vascular invasion begin to deposit osteoid on the cartilaginous cores forming **trabecular bone**.
Transverse septum
1 Proliferative zone
2 Hypertrophic zone
3 Vascular invasion zone
1
2
3
Longitudinal septa at the vascular invasion zone are the first sites where osteoblasts begin to deposit bone matrix (osteoid).
Osteoblasts
Blood cells

located between the epiphyses and the diaphysis. The epiphyseal growth plate is responsible for subsequent growth in length of the bone.

Clinical significance: The epiphyseal growth plate and dwarfism

Indian hedgehog (**Ihh**), a member of the hedgehog family of proteins secreted by chondrocytes, **regulates chondrocyte proliferation of the growth plate in a paracrine fashion and delays chondrocyte hypertrophy** (see Figure 5-9). Ihh also regulates bone formation in the perichondrial collar. A lack of expression of Ihh protein in mutant mice results in dwarfism and lack of endochondral ossification. Essentially, **Ihh maintains the pool of proliferating chondrocytes in the growth**

Figure 5-7. Endochondral ossification: Zones of proliferation and hypertrophy

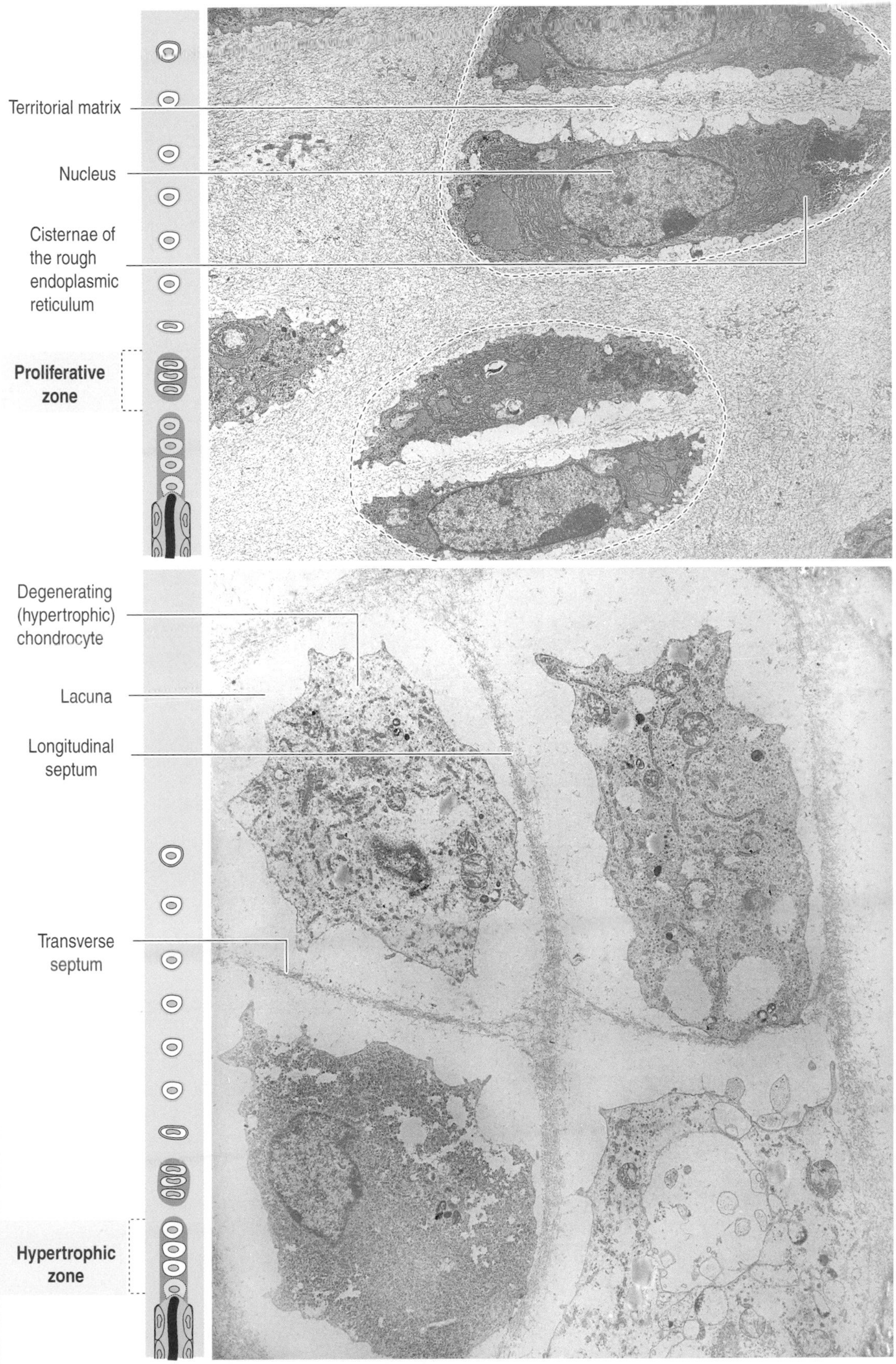

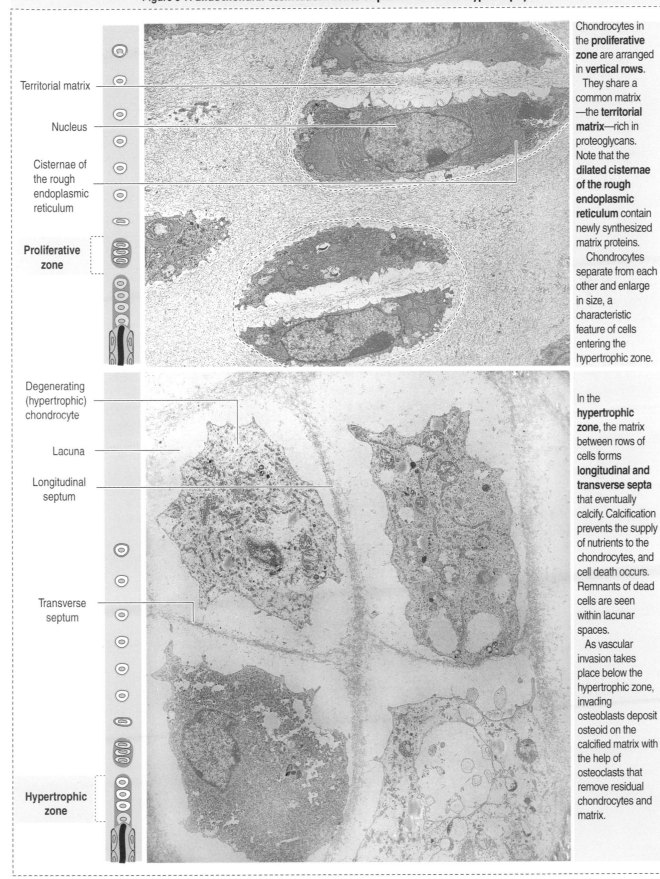

Territorial matrix
Nucleus
Cisternae of the rough endoplasmic reticulum
Proliferative zone
Degenerating (hypertrophic) chondrocyte
Lacuna
Longitudinal septum
Transverse septum
Hypertrophic zone

Chondrocytes in the **proliferative zone** are arranged in **vertical rows**.

They share a common matrix—the **territorial matrix**—rich in proteoglycans. Note that the **dilated cisternae of the rough endoplasmic reticulum** contain newly synthesized matrix proteins.

Chondrocytes separate from each other and enlarge in size, a characteristic feature of cells entering the hypertrophic zone.

In the **hypertrophic zone**, the matrix between rows of cells forms **longitudinal and transverse septa** that eventually calcify. Calcification prevents the supply of nutrients to the chondrocytes, and cell death occurs. Remnants of dead cells are seen within lacunar spaces.

As vascular invasion takes place below the hypertrophic zone, invading osteoblasts deposit osteoid on the calcified matrix with the help of osteoclasts that remove residual chondrocytes and matrix.

Figure 5-8. **Endochondral ossification: Zones of hypertrophy and vascular invasion**

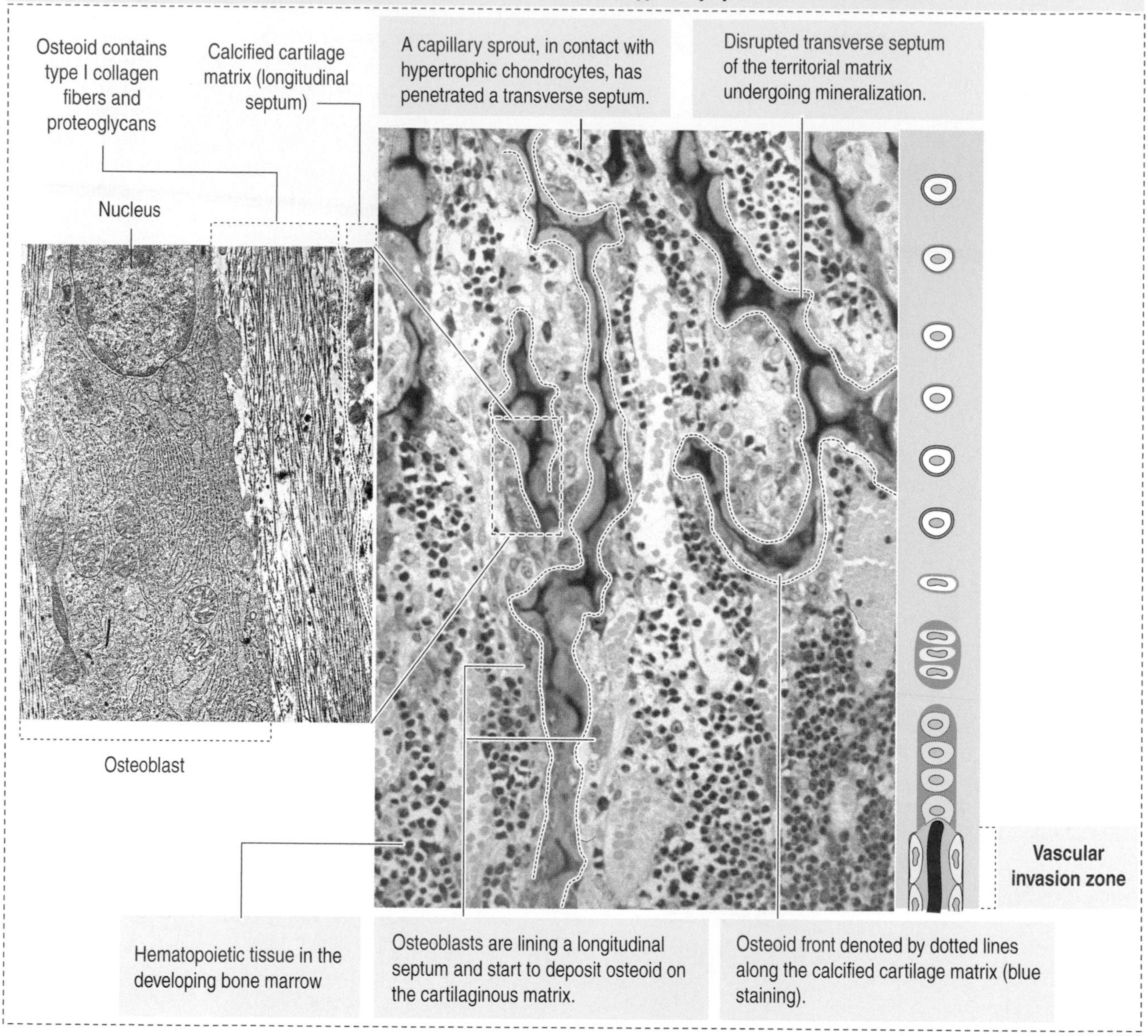

Osteoid contains type I collagen fibers and proteoglycans
Calcified cartilage matrix (longitudinal septum)
A capillary sprout, in contact with hypertrophic chondrocytes, has penetrated a transverse septum.
Disrupted transverse septum of the territorial matrix undergoing mineralization.
Nucleus
Osteoblast
Vascular invasion zone
Hematopoietic tissue in the developing bone marrow
Osteoblasts are lining a longitudinal septum and start to deposit osteoid on the cartilaginous matrix.
Osteoid front denoted by dotted lines along the calcified cartilage matrix (blue staining).

plate by delaying their hypertrophy. In addition, Ihh stimulates the expression of **parathyroid hormone–related peptide** (**PTH-RP**) in perichondrial chondrocytes adjacent to the articular surface. A feedback loop between Ihh and PTH-RP regulates the balance between proliferating and hypertrophic chondrocytes.

At the end of the growing period, the epiphyseal growth plate is gradually eliminated by a continuum established between the diaphysis and the epiphyses. No further growth in length of the bone is possible once the epiphyseal growth plate disappears at puberty.

Zones of endochondral ossification

As we have seen, the deposition of bone in the center of the diaphysis is preceded by an erosion process in the hyaline cartilage template (see Figure 5-4). This center of erosion, defined as the **primary ossification center**, extends in both directions of the template, in parallel with the formation of a bony collar.

The bony collar provides strength to the midsection of the diaphysis or shaft as the cartilage is weakened by the gradual removal of the cartilage before its replacement by bone.

The continuing process of cartilage erosion and bone deposition can be

Figure 5-9. Growth plates and bone growth in length

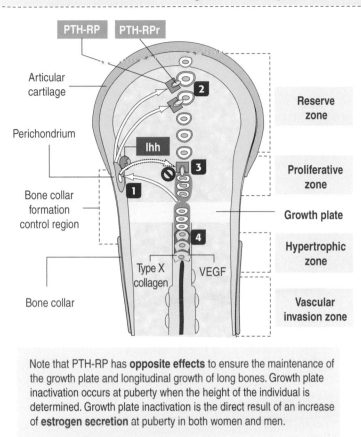

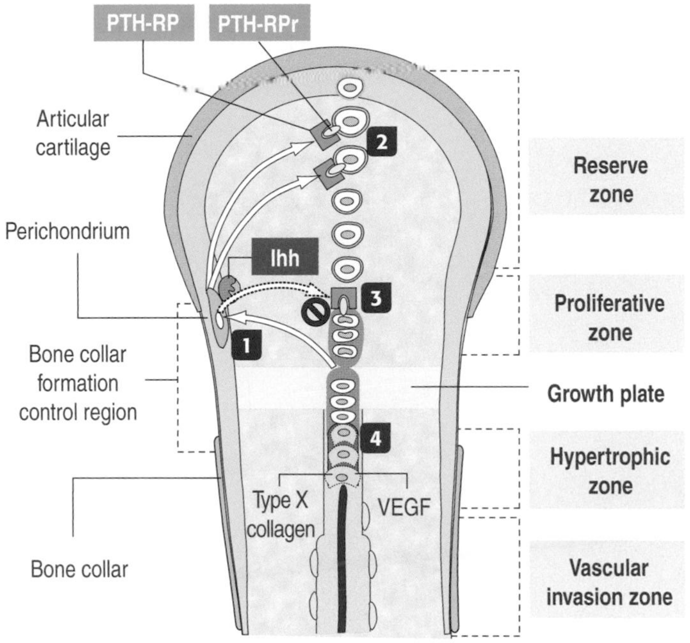
PTH-RP
PTH-RPr
Articular cartilage
Perichondrium
Ihh
Bone collar formation control region
Bone collar
Type X collagen
VEGF
1
2
3
4
Reserve zone
Proliferative zone
Growth plate
Hypertrophic zone
Vascular invasion zone

Note that PTH-RP has **opposite effects** to ensure the maintenance of the growth plate and longitudinal growth of long bones. Growth plate inactivation occurs at puberty when the height of the individual is determined. Growth plate inactivation is the direct result of an increase of **estrogen secretion** at puberty in both women and men.

Ihh is the vertebrate equivalent of a protein member of the fruit fly *Drosophila melanogaster* gene *hedgehog* involved in pattern determination of the limbs and trunks.

Growth of the epiphyseal growth plate cartilage

1 **Indian hedgehog (Ihh)** protein—secreted by chondrocytes of the proliferative zone—signals the synthesis and secretion of **parathyroid hormone–related protein (PTH-RP)** by cells of the chondrogenic layer of the perichondrium (epiphysis). Ihh has two functions: (1) regulation of the formation of the bone collar; (2) stimulation of PTH-RP secretion.

2 PTH-RP binds to its receptor (**PTH-RPr**) on the surface of chondrocytes of the reserve zone to **stimulate** their proliferation.

3 PTH-RP also binds to chondrocytes of the proliferative zone to **inhibit** their differentiation into hypertrophic chondrocytes.

4 Chondrocytes of the hypertrophic zone secrete **type X collagen**—a marker of differentiation—and **vascular endothelial growth factor (VEGF)**—an inducer of vascular invasion.

Clinical significance: Metaphyseal chondrodysplasia

Mutations of the genes encoding PTH-RP and PTH-RPr give rise to **Jansen's disease** or **metaphyseal chondrodysplasia**.

An excess of PTH-RP causes **hypercalcemia** and delay in maturation of proliferative chondrocytes into hypertrophic chondrocytes.

Circulating **parathyroid hormone cannot compensate for PTH-RP deficiencies** because the avascular nature of the cartilage makes parathyroid hormone circulating in blood relatively inaccessible to chondrocytes.

visualized histologically (Figure 5-5). **Four major zones** can be distinguished, starting at the end of the cartilage and approaching the zone of erosion:

1. The **reserve zone** is a site composed of primitive hyaline cartilage and is responsible for the growth in length of the bone as the erosion and bone deposition process advances. Essentially, chondrocytes are "running" as osteoclast-mediated erosion "**chases**" the chondrocytes of the reserve zone (see Figures 5-6 and 5-10).

2. The **proliferative zone** is characterized by active proliferation of chondrocytes aligning as cellular **stacks** parallel to the long axis of the cartilage template. This mitotically active zone represents the "running away" zone of the cartilage, a mechanism that eventually determines the elongation of the bone (Figures 5-6 and 5-7). We have already seen how **Ihh** and **PTH-RP** modulate the population of hypertrophic chondrocytes as a mechanism to ensure active growth plates until puberty (see Figure 5-9).

3. The **hypertrophic zone** is defined by both **chondrocyte apoptosis** and **calcification** of the territorial matrix surrounding the columns of previously proliferated chondrocytes (see Figures 5-6 and 5-7). Despite their "unhealthy" appearance, hypertrophic chondrocytes play an important role in bone growth. Hypertrophic chondrocytes have the following functional characteristics: They (1) direct the **mineralization of the surrounding cartilage matrix**, (2) **attract blood vessels through the secretion of vascular endothelial growth factor** (VEGF), (3) recruit **macrophages** (called **chondroclasts**) **to degrade the cartilage matrix**, (4) instruct **adjacent chondrocytes of the perichondrium to change into osteoblasts forming the bone collar**, (5) **produce type X collagen**, a marker of hypertrophic chondrocytes,

Figure 5-10. **Bone growth in length involves an osteoclastic "chase" and chondrocytic "run" sequence**

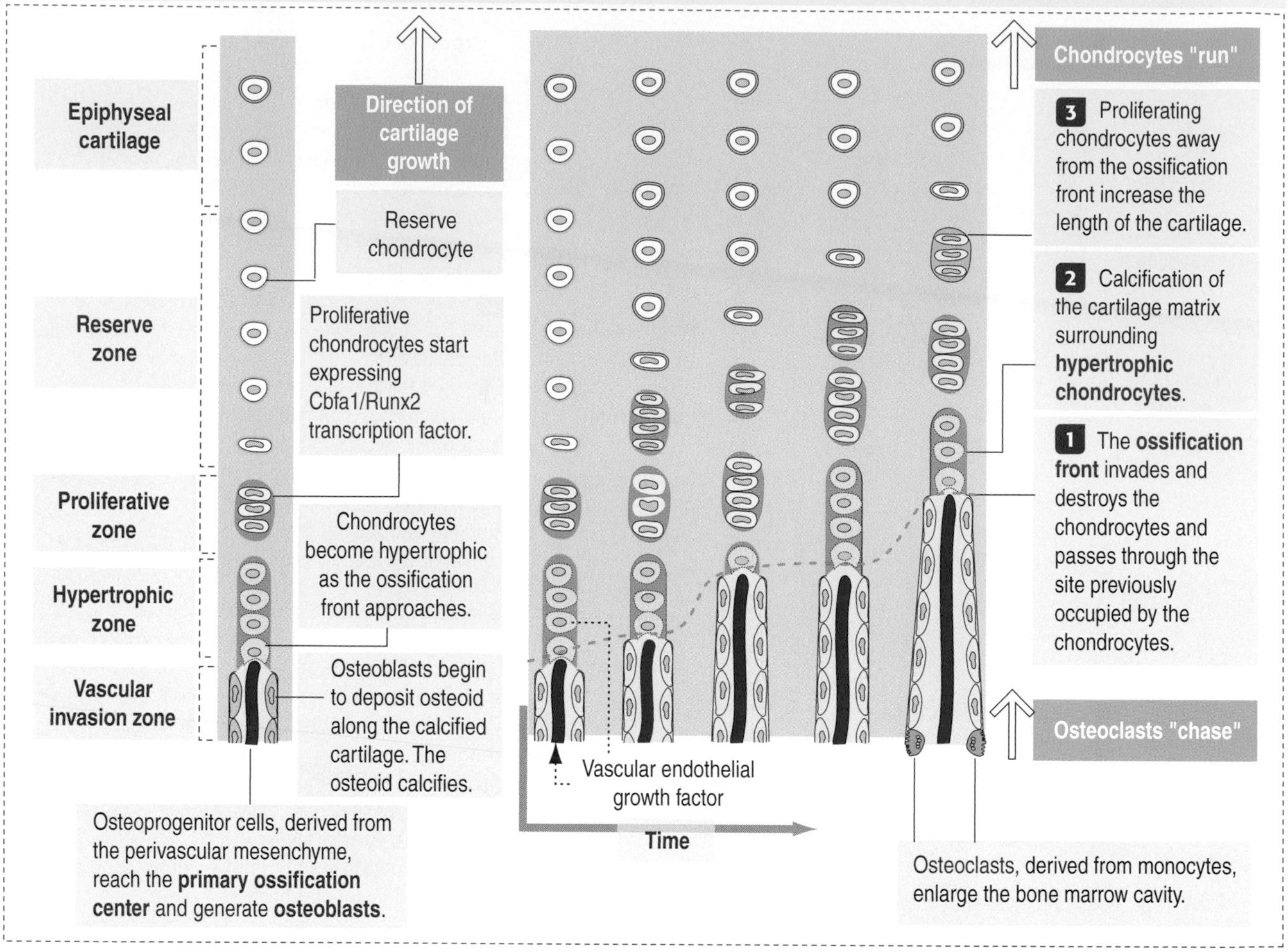

Epiphyseal cartilage
Reserve zone
Proliferative zone
Hypertrophic zone
Vascular invasion zone
Direction of cartilage growth
Reserve chondrocyte
Proliferative chondrocytes start expressing Cbfa1/Runx2 transcription factor.
Chondrocytes become hypertrophic as the ossification front approaches.
Osteoblasts begin to deposit osteoid along the calcified cartilage. The osteoid calcifies.
Osteoprogenitor cells, derived from the perivascular mesenchyme, reach the primary ossification center and generate osteoblasts.
Vascular endothelial growth factor
Time
Chondrocytes "run"
3 Proliferating chondrocytes away from the ossification front increase the length of the cartilage.
2 Calcification of the cartilage matrix surrounding hypertrophic chondrocytes.
1 The ossification front invades and destroys the chondrocytes and passes through the site previously occupied by the chondrocytes.
Osteoclasts "chase"
Osteoclasts, derived from monocytes, enlarge the bone marrow cavity.

and, when their task is accomplished, (6) they undergo **apoptosis**.

Chondrocytes in this zone are significantly enlarged (hypertrophic). As a result, the septa separating adjacent columns appear thinner due to a compression effect mediated by the hypertrophic chondrocytes. A provisional calcification begins in the **longitudinal septa. The** deepest layer, proximal to the vascular invasion zone, displays the blind end of capillary sprouts (Figure 5-8) derived from the developing bone marrow cavity occupied by hematopoietic cells (see Chapter 6, Blood and Hematopoiesis).

4. The **vascular invasion zone** is the site where blood vessels penetrate the transverse septa and carry migrating **osteoprogenitor cells** with them. Recall that hypertrophic chondrocytes secrete **VEGF** to stimulate angiogenesis in this zone (Figure 5-9).

Osteoprogenitor cells give rise to osteoblasts that begin lining the surfaces of the exposed cores of calcified cartilage (stained blue—basophilic—in the light microscopy photograph in Figure 5-8) and initiate the deposition of **osteoid** (stained pink—acidophilic—in Figure 5-8). The osteoid contains abundant type I collagen fibers embedded in the extracellular matrix.

The cartilage struts are gradually replaced by bone. The deposit of osteoid denotes the beginning of osteogenesis and results in the formation of **bone spicules** and, later, in **trabeculae**. As a consequence, **cancellous bone** appears in the midsection of the template.

As the ossification process advances toward the adjacent proliferative zones (a "chase" effect), the bone marrow cavity increases in size owing to loss of cartilage and erosion of newly formed bone spicules by osteoclasts (Figure 5-10).

The periosteal collar grows in length and thickness (by appositional growth) at the midsection of the shaft and compensates for the loss of endochondral bone, while also strengthening the gradually eroding cartilage template.

The reserve zone persists by continuous cell division and is responsible for a continued growth in length by the epiphyseal growth plate, which remains between the diaphysis and epiphysis of the bone. The **epiphyseal growth plate** becomes reduced to an **epiphyseal line** from puberty to maturity, and the long bone no longer grows in length.

After endochondral ossification, the general organization of a long bone is remodeled by combined **reabsorption** mediated by **osteoclasts** in certain areas and the deposition of new bone by osteoblasts in others. As a result, spongy bone is replaced by compact bone by a process in which osteoblasts produce overlapping layers of bone or **lamellae** on the surface of longitudinal cavities occupied by blood vessels. Consequently, a concentric arrangement of bone lamellae encircles a blood vessel entrapped within a canal to form a **primitive haversian system**.

Some variation exists in the literature concerning the classification of the zones of endochondral ossification. The reserve, proliferative, hypertrophic, and vascular invasion zones summarized earlier provide a simple way to guide you through the complexity of bone formation and the understanding of the mechanisms of bone repair.

Finally, it is important to stress that **local regulatory molecules** (bone morphogenetic proteins, hedgehog proteins, the RANK-RANKL signaling pathway, and fibroblast growth factors) and **blood circulating proteins** (insulin-like growth factor-1 [IGF-1], thyroid hormone, estrogens, androgens, vitamin D, retinoids, and glucocorticoids) control both bone development and remodeling throughout life. We will emphasize the specific function of these biological agents as we come across them. Their impact on skeletal biology and the therapeutic opportunities confronting an increasing number of genetic and degenerative diseases must be appreciated.

Growth in width of the diaphysis

As the bone grows in length, new layers of bone are added to the outer portions of the diaphysis by appositional growth. As a result, the thickness of the diaphysis increases. Simultaneous erosion of the inner wall of the diaphysis results in enlargement of the marrow cavity.

New bone in the form of haversian systems is added beneath the periosteum by its osteogenic layer. The surface of the diaphysis has **longitudinal ridges** with **grooves** between them. The periosteum contains blood vessels.

The following sequence is observed (Figure 5-11):

1. The ridges and grooves are lined by osteoblasts that proliferate and deposit osteoid. As a result, the ridges grow toward one another and enclose a periosteal vessel within a tunnel. Adjacent longitudinal periosteal capillaries within the tunnels are connected by transverse blood vessels. The latter become part of **Volkmann's canals. Unlike haversian canals, Volkmann's canals are not surrounded by concentric lamellae**.

2. Osteoblasts lining the tunnel deposit new lamellae and convert the tunnel into a haversian system, a central blood vessel surrounded by lamellae.

3. Appositional growth continuously adds lamellae under the periosteum in the cortical region of the diaphysis, which become the **outer circumferential lamellae**. This modeling and remodeling process occurs with the participation of osteoclasts that erode bone at the outer circumferential lamellae–osteon boundary. As a consequence, interstitial lamellae fill the spaces between the osteons and what remains of the outer circumferential lamellar system.

4. Osteoblasts lining the inner surface develop the **inner circumferential lamellae** by a similar mechanism described for the outer circumferential lamellae, except that the blood vessels enclosed in the tunnels are not periosteal but,

Figure 5-11. Periosteal bone growth

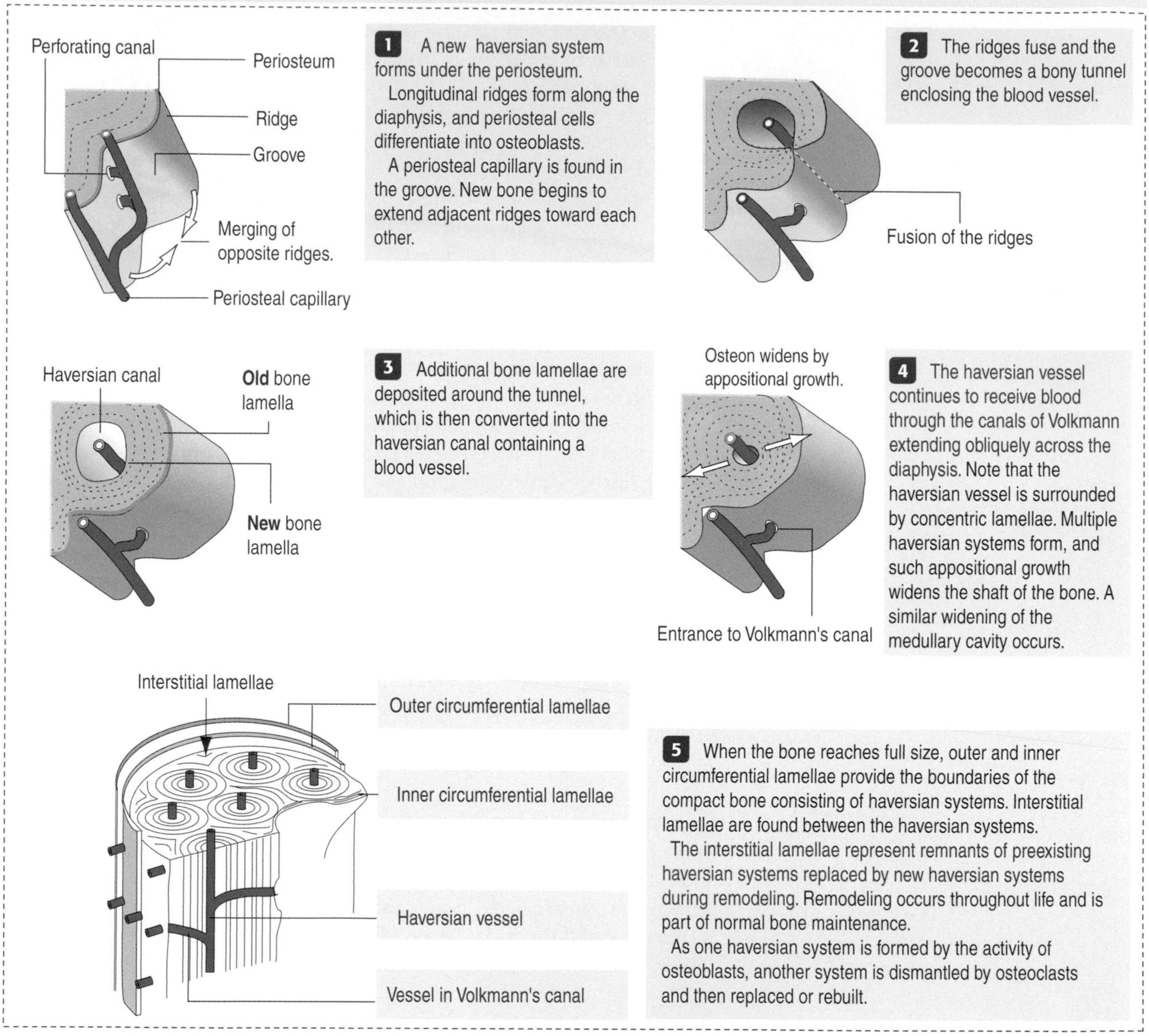

Perforating canal
Periosteum
Ridge
Groove
Merging of opposite ridges.
Periosteal capillary
1 A new haversian system forms under the periosteum.
Longitudinal ridges form along the diaphysis, and periosteal cells differentiate into osteoblasts.
A periosteal capillary is found in the groove. New bone begins to extend adjacent ridges toward each other.
2 The ridges fuse and the groove becomes a bony tunnel enclosing the blood vessel.
Fusion of the ridges
Haversian canal
Old bone lamella
New bone lamella
3 Additional bone lamellae are deposited around the tunnel, which is then converted into the haversian canal containing a blood vessel.
Osteon widens by appositional growth.
Entrance to Volkmann's canal
4 The haversian vessel continues to receive blood through the canals of Volkmann extending obliquely across the diaphysis. Note that the haversian vessel is surrounded by concentric lamellae. Multiple haversian systems form, and such appositional growth widens the shaft of the bone. A similar widening of the medullary cavity occurs.
Interstitial lamellae
Outer circumferential lamellae
Inner circumferential lamellae
Haversian vessel
Vessel in Volkmann's canal
5 When the bone reaches full size, outer and inner circumferential lamellae provide the boundaries of the compact bone consisting of haversian systems. Interstitial lamellae are found between the haversian systems.
The interstitial lamellae represent remnants of preexisting haversian systems replaced by new haversian systems during remodeling. Remodeling occurs throughout life and is part of normal bone maintenance.
As one haversian system is formed by the activity of osteoblasts, another system is dismantled by osteoclasts and then replaced or rebuilt.

instead, branches of the nutrient artery formed originally from a periosteal bud, as described earlier.

Bone remodeling

Bone remodeling consists in the replacement of newly formed and old bone by a resorption-production sequence with the participation of osteoclasts and osteoblasts. Bone remodeling is a continuous process throughout life and occurs at random locations. **The purpose of remodeling is to establish the optimum of bone strength by repairing microscopic damage (called microcracking) and to maintain calcium homeostasis.**

Under normal conditions, the same amount of resorbed bone is replaced by the same volume of new bone. If the volume of resorbed bone is not completely replaced by new bone, the tissue becomes weakened and a risk of spontaneous fractures arises.

There are two forms of bone remodeling: (1) **cortical bone remodeling**, and (2) **trabecular bone remodeling**.

Cortical bone remodeling is the resorption of an old haversian system followed by the organization of a new haversian system (Figure 5-12). Osteoclasts form a

Figure 5-12. **Bone remodeling**

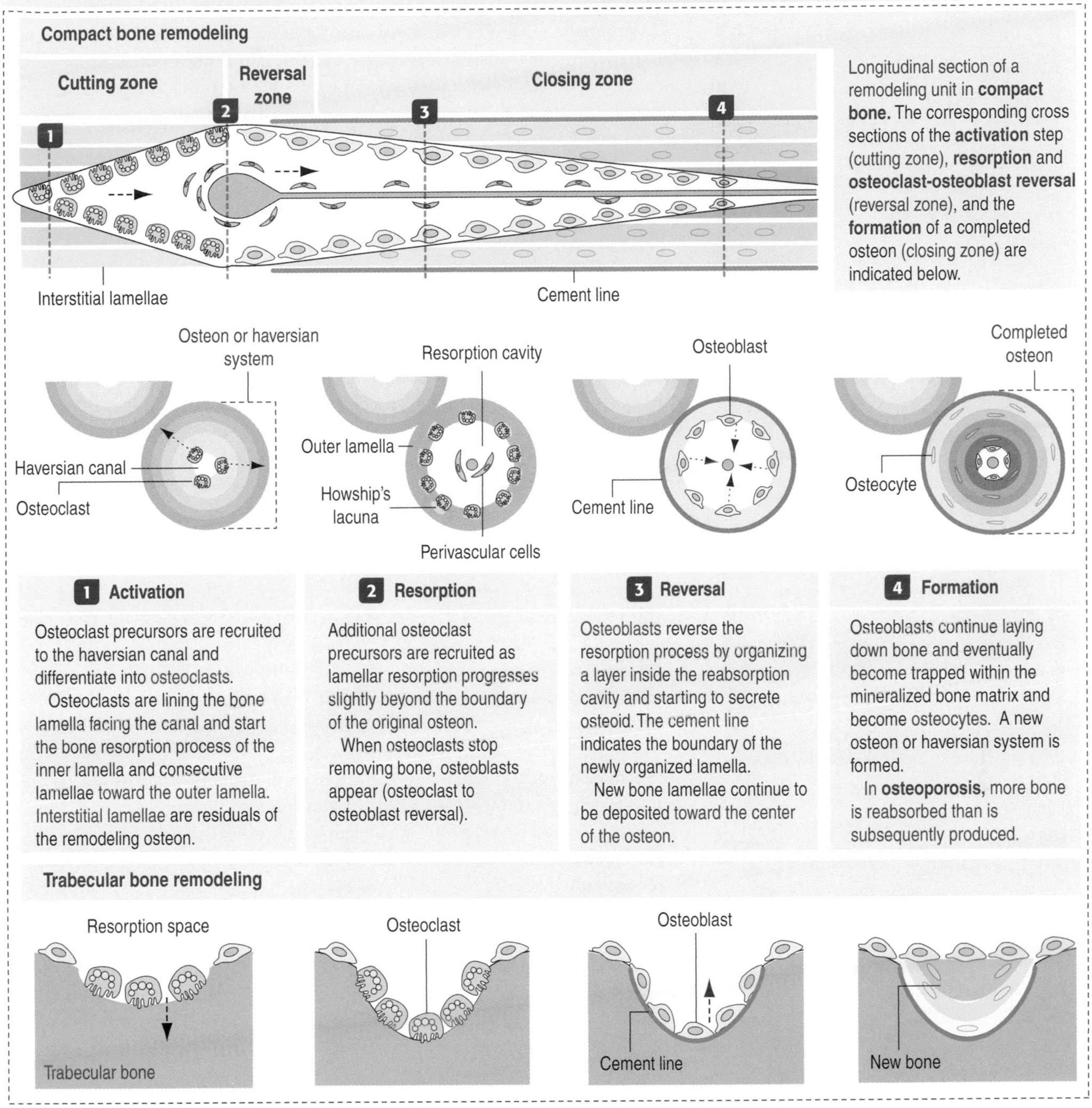

Compact bone remodeling
Cutting zone
Reversal zone
Closing zone
1
2
3
4
Interstitial lamellae
Cement line
Longitudinal section of a remodeling unit in **compact bone.** The corresponding cross sections of the **activation** step (cutting zone), **resorption** and **osteoclast-osteoblast reversal** (reversal zone), and the **formation** of a completed osteon (closing zone) are indicated below.
Osteon or haversian system
Haversian canal
Osteoclast
Resorption cavity
Outer lamella
Howship's lacuna
Perivascular cells
Osteoblast
Cement line
Completed osteon
Osteocyte
1 Activation
Osteoclast precursors are recruited to the haversian canal and differentiate into osteoclasts.
Osteoclasts are lining the bone lamella facing the canal and start the bone resorption process of the inner lamella and consecutive lamellae toward the outer lamella. Interstitial lamellae are residuals of the remodeling osteon.
2 Resorption
Additional osteoclast precursors are recruited as lamellar resorption progresses slightly beyond the boundary of the original osteon.
When osteoclasts stop removing bone, osteoblasts appear (osteoclast to osteoblast reversal).
3 Reversal
Osteoblasts reverse the resorption process by organizing a layer inside the reabsorption cavity and starting to secrete osteoid. The cement line indicates the boundary of the newly organized lamella.
New bone lamellae continue to be deposited toward the center of the osteon.
4 Formation
Osteoblasts continue laying down bone and eventually become trapped within the mineralized bone matrix and become osteocytes. A new osteon or haversian system is formed.
In **osteoporosis,** more bone is reabsorbed than is subsequently produced.
Trabecular bone remodeling
Resorption space
Trabecular bone
Osteoclast
Osteoblast
Cement line
New bone

centrifugal resorption tunnel (**cutting zone**) that is refilled centripetally by osteoblasts (**closing zone**). The **osteoclast-osteoblast reversal** occurs when the cutting zone has finished removing the outermost lamella of the osteon.

Note that: (1) the cutting zone is lined by osteoclasts and the closing zone by osteoblasts, (2) remnants of haversian lamellae surrounding the cutting zone become **interstitial lamellae**, filling the space between adjacent osteons, and (3) the haversian canal becomes narrow as new concentric lamellae, entrapping osteocytes in lacunae in the calcified bone matrix, are closing in.

A marker of the reversal zone is the **cement line**, the boundary of the newly formed bone lamella. Cement lines are not only a landmark of the initiation of lamellar remodeling. External forces acting on osteons may cause a damage called **microcracking.** A microcracking fracture can be neutralized by the cement line and by the alternating arrangement and orientation of mineralized collagen fibers

Figure 5-13. **Ectopic ossification**

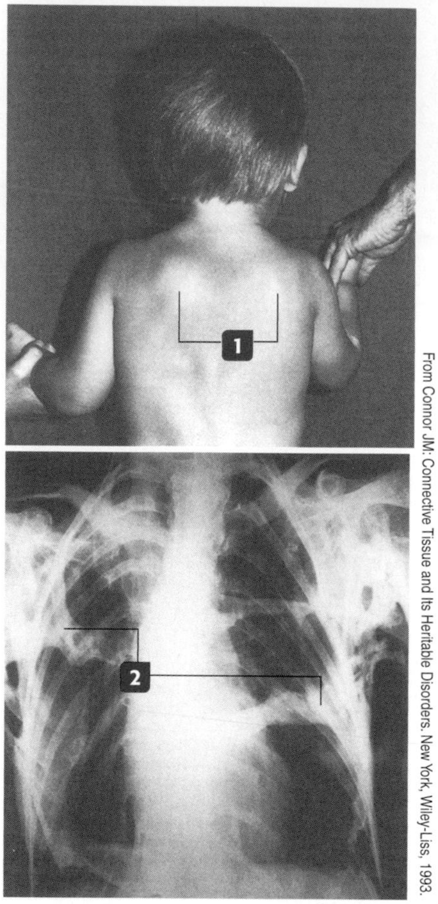

From Connor JM: Connective Tissue and Its Heritable Disorders. New York, Wiley-Liss, 1993.

Fibrodysplasia ossificans progressiva

1 Ectopic ossification is observed as lumps in the muscles of the neck and back. Lumps are first noted in children 1 to 3 years old.

2 Ectopic bone is visualized in radiographs after the initial appearance of ossifying lumps. Bone matures and develops a normal trabecular architecture.

in the lamellar bone. Examine once more Figure 4-20 in Chapter 4, Connective Tissue, to grasp this concept.

Microcracking, limited to a region of the osteon (for example, a damage to canaliculi which disrupts osteocyte cell-cell communication leading to cell death), can be repaired by the osteoclast-osteoblast remodeling process. When the architecture of the osteon is defective, microcracking becomes widespread and a complete bone fracture may occur.

Trabecular bone remodeling occurs on the bone surface (see Figure 5-12), in contrast to cortical bone remodeling, which occurs in a tunnel-like fashion. The trabecular endosteal surface is remodeled by this mechanism, whose steps are similar to cortical bone remodeling.

Clinical significance: Hereditary and degenerative bone disorders

Ossification includes **growth**, **modeling**, and **remodeling** of the bone, processes mediated by osteoblasts and osteoclasts under the control of local regulatory factors and blood-borne signaling molecules, including **parathyroid hormone** and **vitamin D_3**. A number of conditions can alter the skeleton by affecting cell-mediated bone remodeling or disturbing the mineralization of the extracellular matrix.

Rickets and **osteomalacia** are a group of bone diseases characterized by a **defect in the mineralization of the bone matrix** (osteoid), most often caused by a **lack of vitamin D_3**. Rickets is observed in children and produces skeletal deformities. Osteomalacia is observed in adults and is caused by poor mineralization of the bone matrix.

We have already stressed the importance of the RANK-RANKL signaling pathway as a pharmacologic target in the treatment of **osteoporosis** by controlling osteoclastogenesis.

Osteopetrosis ("stonelike bone") includes a group of hereditary diseases characterized by **abnormal osteoclast function**. The bone is abnormally brittle and breaks like a soft stone. The marrow canal is not developed, and most of the bone is woven because of absent remodeling.

We have already discussed a mutation in the ***colony-stimulating factor-1*** gene whose expression is required for the formation of osteoclasts (see Bone in Chapter 4, Connective Tissue). A clinical variant of osteopetrosis, also known as **marble bone disease**, or **Albers-Schönberg disease**, is caused by a deficiency in **carbonic anhydrase II**, required by osteoclasts to accumulate H^+ in Howship's resorption lacunae and acidify the environment for the activation of secretory cathepsin K enzyme.

Fibrodysplasia ossificans progressiva (FOP) is an inherited disorder of the connective tissue. The main clinical features are **skeletal malformations** and the **ossification of soft tissues** (muscles of the neck and back; Figure 5-13). Ectopic bone formation also occurs in ligaments, fasciae, aponeuroses, tendons, and joint capsules.

Patients with FOP have a mutation in the gene encoding **activin receptor type 1A (ACVR1)**, a receptor for bone morphogenetic protein. The mutation consists in the substitution of histidine for arginine at position 206 of the 509-amino-acids-long ACVR1. This single amino acid substitution results in the abnormal activation of ACVR1 leading to the transformation of connective tissue and muscle tissue into a secondary skeleton.

Joints

Bones are interconnected by articulations, or joints, that permit movement. **Synarthroses** are the joints that permit little or no movement (cranial bones, ribs, and the sternum). **Amphiarthroses** enable slight movement (intervertebral disks and bodies). **Diarthroses** permit free movement.

In a **diarthroidal joint**, a **capsule** links the ends of the bones. The capsule is lined by a **synovial membrane** that encloses the articular or synovial cavity. The

Figure 5-14. Joints and arthritis

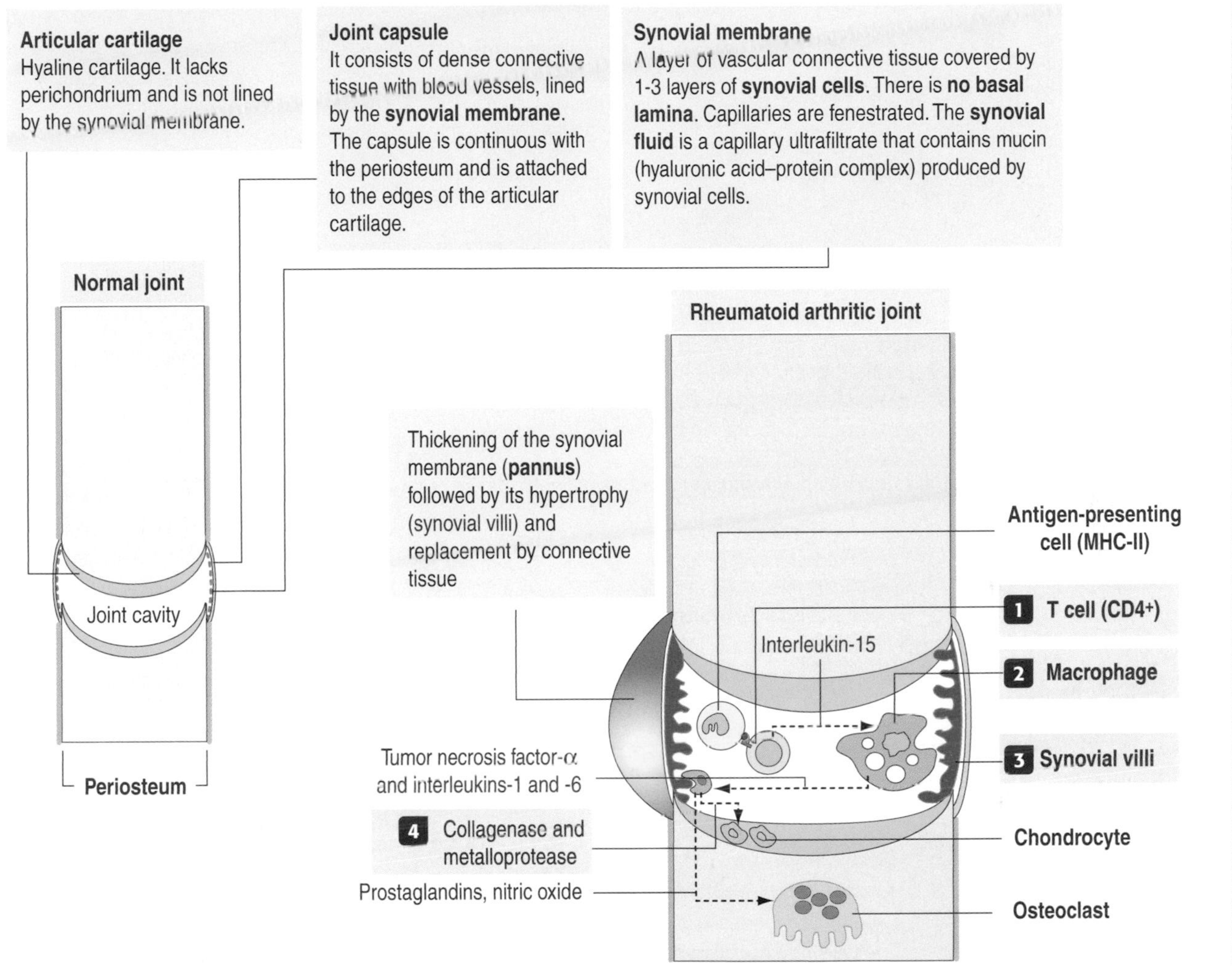
Articular cartilage
Hyaline cartilage. It lacks perichondrium and is not lined by the synovial membrane.
Joint capsule
It consists of dense connective tissue with blood vessels, lined by the synovial membrane. The capsule is continuous with the periosteum and is attached to the edges of the articular cartilage.
Synovial membrane
A layer of vascular connective tissue covered by 1-3 layers of synovial cells. There is no basal lamina. Capillaries are fenestrated. The synovial fluid is a capillary ultrafiltrate that contains mucin (hyaluronic acid–protein complex) produced by synovial cells.
Normal joint
Joint cavity
Periosteum
Rheumatoid arthritic joint
Thickening of the synovial membrane (pannus) followed by its hypertrophy (synovial villi) and replacement by connective tissue
Antigen-presenting cell (MHC-II)
1 T cell (CD4+)
Interleukin-15
2 Macrophage
3 Synovial villi
Tumor necrosis factor-α and interleukins-1 and -6
4 Collagenase and metalloprotease
Chondrocyte
Prostaglandins, nitric oxide
Osteoclast

Rheumatoid arthritis

Rheumatoid arthritis is a chronic inflammatory disease characterized by the presence of activated CD4+ T cells **1**, plasma cells, macrophages **2**, and **synovial cells** **3** changing the synovial membrane lining into villus-type inflammatory tissue called **pannus**. Within the pannus, cellular responses lead to release of collagenase and metalloproteases **4** and other effector molecules.

The initial cause of rheumatoid arthritis is a peptide antigen presented to T cells (CD4+) which, in turn, release **interleukin-15** to activate synovial macrophages normally present in the synovial membrane.

Synovial macrophages secrete **proinflammatory cytokines—tumor necrosis factor-α** and **interleukins-1** and **-6**—to induce the proliferation of synovial cells, which then release **collagenase**, **extracellular matrix metalloproteases**, **prostaglandins**, and **nitric oxide** targeted to the destruction of the **articular cartilage** and subjacent **bone tissue**. Both the chronic destruction of the articular cartilage and the hypertrophy of the synovial membrane are characteristic features of rheumatoid arthritis.

synovial cavity contains a **fluid** necessary for reducing the friction between the hyaline cartilage covering the opposing articular surfaces.

The articular cartilage is almost typical hyaline cartilage except that it **lacks a perichondrium** and has a unique collagen fiber organization in the form of overlapping arches. Collagen arcades sustain the mechanical stress on the joint surfaces.

The **joint capsule** consists of **two layers:** an outer layer of dense connective tissue with blood vessels and nerves, and an inner layer, called the **synovial membrane.** The inner surface of the synovial membrane is covered by one to two

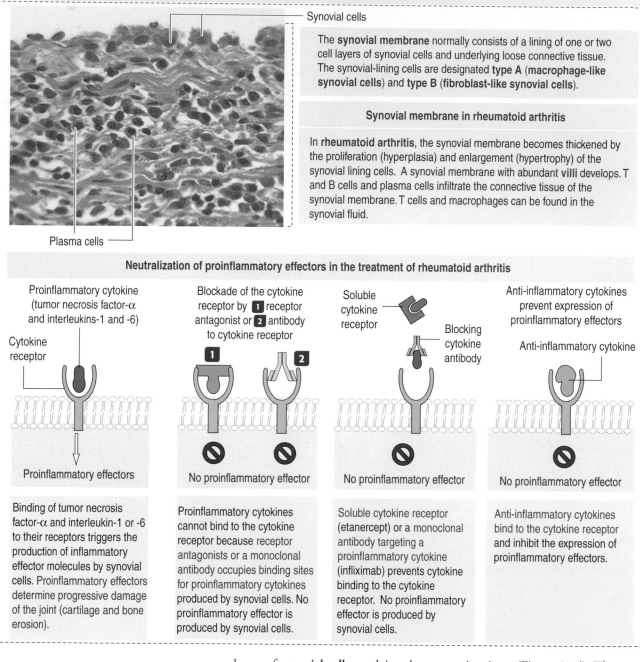

Figure 5-15. Synovial membrane in rheumatoid arthritis

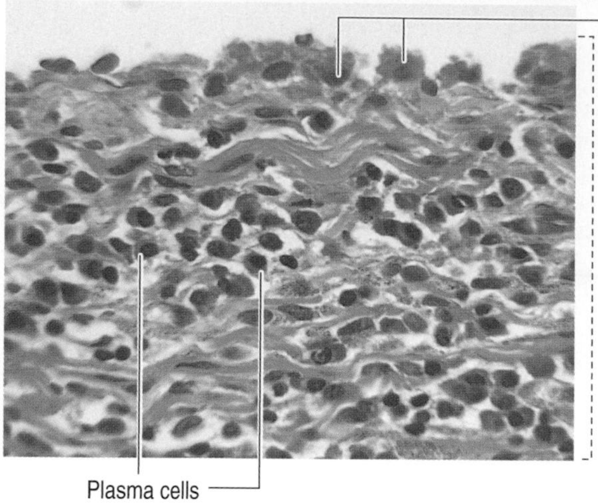

The **synovial membrane** normally consists of a lining of one or two cell layers of synovial cells and underlying loose connective tissue. The synovial-lining cells are designated **type A** (**macrophage-like synovial cells**) and **type B** (**fibroblast-like synovial cells**).

Synovial membrane in rheumatoid arthritis

In **rheumatoid arthritis**, the synovial membrane becomes thickened by the proliferation (hyperplasia) and enlargement (hypertrophy) of the synovial lining cells. A synovial membrane with abundant **villi** develops. T and B cells and plasma cells infiltrate the connective tissue of the synovial membrane. T cells and macrophages can be found in the synovial fluid.

Neutralization of proinflammatory effectors in the treatment of rheumatoid arthritis

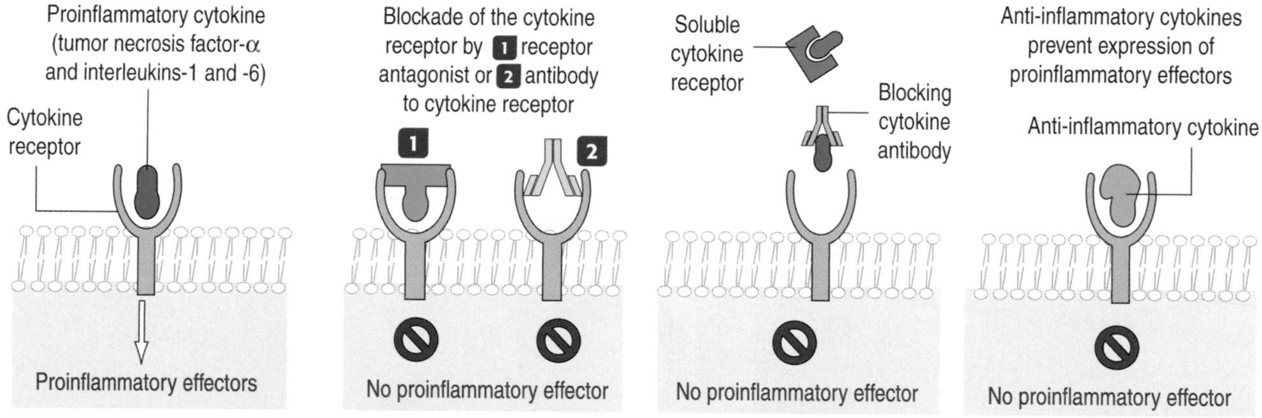

Binding of tumor necrosis factor-α and interleukin-1 or -6 to their receptors triggers the production of inflammatory effector molecules by synovial cells. Proinflammatory effectors determine progressive damage of the joint (cartilage and bone erosion).

Proinflammatory cytokines cannot bind to the cytokine receptor because receptor antagonists or a monoclonal antibody occupies binding sites for proinflammatory cytokines produced by synovial cells. No proinflammatory effector is produced by synovial cells.

Soluble cytokine receptor (etanercept) or a monoclonal antibody targeting a proinflammatory cytokine (infliximab) prevents cytokine binding to the cytokine receptor. No proinflammatory effector is produced by synovial cells.

Anti-inflammatory cytokines bind to the cytokine receptor and inhibit the expression of proinflammatory effectors.

layers of **synovial cells** overlying the connective tissue (Figure 5-14). There are two classes of synovial cells: (1) **type A macrophage-like synovial cells**, and (2) **type B fibroblast-like synovial cells.** There is no basal lamina separating synovial cells from the connective tissue. The connective tissue contains a rich network of **fenestrated capillaries**.

Synovial fluid is a combined product of the synovial cells and the ultrafiltrate of the capillaries. The fluid is rich in **hyaluronic acid**, **glycoproteins**, and **leukocytes.**

Clinical significance: Rheumatoid arthritis

Rheumatoid arthritis is a common chronic inflammatory and destructive disease of the joints that starts with a proliferative process of the synovial membrane, leading to the erosion of the articular cartilage and destruction of the subjacent bone.

The initial event is the activation of CD4$^+$ T cells by an undetermined antigen. Activated CD4$^+$ T cells stimulate the production of **tumor necrosis factor-α (TNF-α)**, **interleukin-2 (IL-2)** and **interleukin-6 (IL-6)**, and the secretion of **collagenase** and **metalloproteinases** by monocytes, macrophages, and fibroblast-like synovial cells. Activated CD4$^+$ T cells stimulate B cells to differentiate into **plasma cells** to produce immunoglobulins and **rheumatoid factor**.

TNF-α, IL-1, and IL-6 are key cytokines in driving inflammation in rheumatoid arthritis (Figure 5-14). TNF-α and IL-1 can be detected in synovial fluid of patients with rheumatoid arthritis. TNF-α and IL-1 stimulate fibroblast-like synovial cells, osteoclasts, and chondrocytes to release cartilage and bone-destroying matrix metalloproteinases.

The neutralization of proinflammatory cytokines by soluble receptors or monoclonal antibodies is currently used in the treatment of patients with rheumatoid arthritis. Figure 5-15 provides a summary of the major therapeutic strategies for suppressing inflammation and preventing joint damage.

Essential concepts | Osteogenesis

• There are two processes of osteogenesis (bone formation or ossification): (1) intramembranous bone formation, and (2) endochondral bone formation.

Both processes have a common aspect: the transformation of a primary trabecular network (also called primary spongiosa) into mature bone. However, they differ in the starting point: intramembranous bone formation consists in the transformation of a mesenchymal template into bone; endochondral ossification consists in the replacement of preexisting hyaline cartilage template into bone.

• **Intramembranous bone formation** is characteristic of skull flat bones. The following sequence is observed: (1) aggregates or mesenchymal condensations are formed in several sites, (2) mesenchymal cells differentiate into osteoblasts to form the bone blastema originated by interstitial growth, (3) bone matrix or osteoid, containing type I collagen and noncollagenous proteins, is deposited by osteoblasts, (4) blood-borne calcium is deposited in the osteoid, which becomes calcified (mineralized), (5) osteoblasts become enclosed in the mineralized matrix and differentiate into osteocytes, connected to each other by cellular processes forming a network, and (6) new osteoblasts appear along the surface of the primary bone tissue or primary ossification center, forming a trabecula. Several trabeculae enlarge by appositional growth and fuse together to form woven bone. Note that intramembranous bone formation starts as interstitial growth and continues by appositional growth.

The final steps include the conversion of woven bone in the outer and inner layers into compact or lamellar bone of haversian type (concentric lamellae around a space containing blood vessels). The center of the membranous bone remains as spongy bone, called diploë. The external and internal connective layers become the periosteum and endosteum, respectively.

• **Endochondral bone formation** is characteristic of long bones, vertebral column, and pelvis. The following sequence is observed: (1) chondrocytes in the center of the hyaline cartilage template become hypertrophic and start synthesizing type X collagen and vascular endothelial cell growth factor (VEGF), (2) blood vessels from the perichondrium invade the hypertrophic cartilage center, whose matrix becomes calcified; the primary ossification center is established, (3) the inner perichondrial cells form a thin periosteal collar at the midpoint of the shaft or diaphysis. The periosteal collar forms woven bone—by the intramembranous bone formation process—under the future periosteum, (4) blood vessels invade the space formerly occupied by hypertrophic chondrocytes and osteoprogenitor cells, and hematopoietic cells arrive through the perivascular tissue, and (5) osteoprogenitor cells differentiate into osteoblasts, which align along the calcified cartilage matrix and begin to deposit osteoid. The primary ossification center now consists of two components: the periosteal collar and the center of ossification in the interior of the cartilage template.

• Two steps will follow: (1) the growth in length of the future long bone, and (2) the development of secondary centers of ossification in the epiphyses.

The growth in length of the long bones depends on the interstitial growth of the hyaline cartilage while the center of the cartilage is being replaced by bone. The secondary centers of ossification consist in the replacement of hyaline cartilage by spongy bone, except the articular cartilage and a thin disk, the epiphyseal growth plate, in the metaphyses (linking the diaphysis to the epiphyses).

The growth plate retains the capacity of chondrogenesis and, after puberty, is replaced by the epiphyseal line. Chondrogenesis of the growth plate and the formation of the perichondrial collar are regulated by Indian hedgehog (Ihh) secretory protein in a paracrine manner.

Ihh, secreted by chondrocytes of the proliferative zone of the hyaline cartilage template close to the growth plate, stimulates the synthesis of parathyroid hormone-related peptide (PTH-RP) by cells of the chondrogenic layer of the perichondrium.

PTH-RP does two things: First, it binds to its receptor on the surface of chondrocytes of the reserve zone of the growth plate to stimulate cell proliferation; second, it binds to chondrocytes of the proliferative zone to prevent their hypertrophy. Essentially, PTH-RP keeps the developmental potential of the growth plate alive and going until the individual's programmed height has been accomplished.

• Endochondral bone formation consists of four major histologic zones: (1) The reserve zone, composed of hyaline cartilage "running away" from the "chasing" ossification front, the vascular invasion zone. (2) The proliferative zone, characterized by the active proliferation of chondrocytes, forming stacks of isogenous groups, also running away from the chasing vascular invasion zone. (3) The hypertrophic zone, the "facilitator" of the vascular invasion zone by producing VEGF, recruiting macrophage-like chondroclasts to destroy the calcified cartilage matrix, instructing the chondrogenic layers of the adjacent perichondrium to become osteoblast and form the bone collar, and producing type X collagen, an imprint of their hypertrophic nature. (4) The vascular invasion zone, the site where blood vessels sprout, penetrating the transverse calcified cartilage septa, bring osteoprogenitor cells and hematopoietic cells. A characteristic of this zone are the spicules, which will become trabeculae. A spicule consists of a core of longitudinal calcified cartilage septa coated by osteoid produced by osteoblasts lining the surface.

Woven or cancellous bone is formed and this type of primitive bone will change into a lamellar or primitive haversian system utilizing the blood vessel as the axial center for the concentric organization of lamellae. The latter process occurs with the help of osteoclasts. Recall that osteoblasts have two major tasks: to continue forming bone—until they become sequestered in the lacunae as osteocytes—and to direct osteoclastogenesis by the RANK-RANKL signaling pathway.

• Periosteal bone formation consists in the transformation of woven bone—produced by intramembranous bone formation—into compact lamellar bone forming now under the periosteum along the diaphysis. The task is to construct a strong cylindrical scaffold around the hollowing endochondral-forming bone and developing hematopoietic marrow.

The following components are observed: (1) longitudinal ridges of lamellar bone, (2) grooves between the ridges, and (3) a blood vessel occupying each groove. Ridges and grooves are lined by osteoblasts. The ridges advance toward one another and enclose the periosteal blood vessel within a tunnel. The longitudinal blood vessels will become the center of a haversian system or osteon; the supplying transverse blood vessels will occupy a tunnel called Volkmanns's canal. Keep in mind that the haversian system has concentric lamellae; the Volkmann's canal does not.

Appositional bone growth continues under the periosteum to form the outer circumferential lamellae. Osteoblasts lining the endosteum form the inner circumferential lamellae, also by appositional bone growth. A difference is that the blood vessels enclosed in the outer circumferential lamella are derived from branches of periosteal blood vessels and the inner circumferential lamellae are supplied by branches of the nutrient artery.

• Bone remodeling is a continuous and random process consisting in the replacement of newly formed bone and old bone by a resorption-production sequence with the cooperative participation of osteoblasts and osteoclasts.

There are two forms of bone remodeling: (1) cortical bone remodeling and (2) trabecular bone remodeling.

Cortical bone remodeling occurs in an old haversian system followed by the reorganization of a new one. Osteoclasts begin eroding the lamella facing the central canal until they reach the outermost lamella. This process is defined as a cutting cone: the apex of the cone initiates the osteoclast degradation process and the base of the cone concludes the degradation. Residual lamellae of the ongoing degradation process are pushed in between the existing intact osteons, forming the interstitial lamellae. The osteoclast-osteoblast reversal step indicates the beginning of the reconstruction process by osteoblasts progressing from the periphery to the central canal where a blood vessel is located. Again, do not forget that the RANK-RANKL signaling system coordinates the reversal step of bone remodeling. The starting point of the reconstruction is indicated by the cement line, a structure that absorbs microcracking created by load forces acting on bone.

Trabecular bone remodeling follows the same osteoclast resorption and osteoclast-osteoblast reversal sequence. A major difference is that this process occurs on the bone surface instead of in an osteon.

• **Osteopetrosis** includes a group of hereditary diseases characterized by abnormal or nonexisting osteoclast function. **Osteoporosis** is a degenerative bone disease in which the osteoclast-driven bone degradation process is not fully compensated by the same bone production volume by osteoblasts. **Rickets** is a defect in the mineralization of the bone matrix observed in children. **Osteomalacia** is the consequence of poor mineralization of the bone matrix observed in adults. **Fibrodysplasia ossificans progressiva** (FOP) is an inherited disorder of the connective tissue consisting in the aberrant ossification of muscle tissue and connective tissue and skeletal malformations. A mutation in the receptor ACVR1 (activin receptor type 1A) of bone morphogenetic protein leads to the unregulated activation of the receptor and the deposit of bone in nonskeletal tissues.

• Joints can be classified into synarthroses (which permit little or no movement), amphiarthroses (which enable slight movement), and diarthroses (which permit free movement). A diarthrodial joint consists of a vascularized outer layer of dense connective tissue capsule continuous with the periosteum. The capsule surrounds the joint and encloses the synovial cavity, containing fluid produced by the lining cells of the synovial membrane.

Rheumatoid arthritis is a chronic inflammatory and destructive disease of the joints. It starts by a proliferative process of the synovial membrane, followed by the erosion of the articular cartilage, and concludes with the destruction of the subjacent bone. The initial event is triggered by the activation of $CD4^+$ T cells by an undetermined antigen. $CD4^+$ T cells and antigen-presenting cells induce the villus-like proliferation of synovial cells (called pannus) and the production of tumor necrosis factor-α, interleukins, collagenases, and metalloproteinases (proinflammatory effectors), which continue triggering an inflammatory response by synovial cells. Proinflammatory effectors can be neutralized by the pharmacologic blocking of specific receptors.

6. BLOOD AND HEMATOPOIESIS

Blood

Blood is a specialized connective tissue consisting of **cells** and **plasma.** These components may be separated by centrifugation if blood is collected in the presence of anticoagulants. The sedimented erythrocytes or red blood cells (RBCs) constitute about **45%** of blood volume. This percentage of erythrocyte volume is the **hematocrit**. Sitting on top of the erythrocyte layer is the **buffy coat** layer, which contains **leukocytes** (white blood cells) and **platelets**. The translucent supernatant fraction above the packed RBCs consists of plasma. Normal adult blood volume measures **5** to **6** L.

Plasma

Plasma is the fluid component of blood (Figure 6-1). Plasma contains salts and organic compounds (including amino acids, lipids, vitamins, proteins, and hormones). In the absence of anticoagulants, the cellular elements of blood, together with plasma proteins (mostly **fibrinogen**), form a clot in the test tube. The fluid portion is called **serum**, which is essentially fibrinogen-free plasma.

Cellular elements of the blood: Red blood cells (erythrocytes)

RBCs, also called erythrocytes (Greek *erythros*, red; *kytos*, cell), are non-nucleated, biconcave-shaped cells measuring **7.8 μm** in diameter (unfixed). RBCs lack organelles and consist only of a plasma membrane, its underlying cytoskeleton (Figure 6-2), hemoglobin, and glycolytic enzymes.

RBCs (average number: **4 to 6 × 10^6 per mm^3**) circulate for **120 days**. Senescent RBCs are removed by phagocytosis or destroyed by **hemolysis** in the spleen. RBCs are replaced in the circulation by **reticulocytes**, which complete their hemoglobin synthesis and maturation 1 to 2 days after entering the circulation. Reticulocytes account for **1%** to **2%** of circulating RBCs. RBCs transport oxygen and carbon dioxide and are confined to the circulatory system.

Figure 6-1. **Blood: Plasma, serum, and cells**

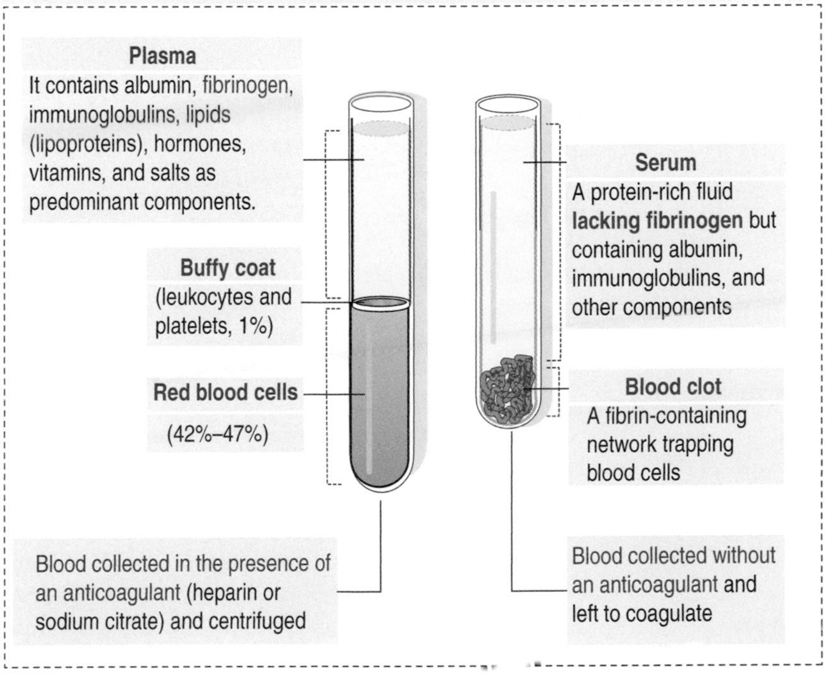

Plasma
It contains albumin, fibrinogen, immunoglobulins, lipids (lipoproteins), hormones, vitamins, and salts as predominant components.
Buffy coat
(leukocytes and platelets, 1%)
Red blood cells
(42%–47%)
Serum
A protein-rich fluid lacking fibrinogen but containing albumin, immunoglobulins, and other components
Blood clot
A fibrin-containing network trapping blood cells
Blood collected in the presence of an anticoagulant (heparin or sodium citrate) and centrifuged
Blood collected without an anticoagulant and left to coagulate

Figure 6-2. **Cell membrane of a red blood cell**

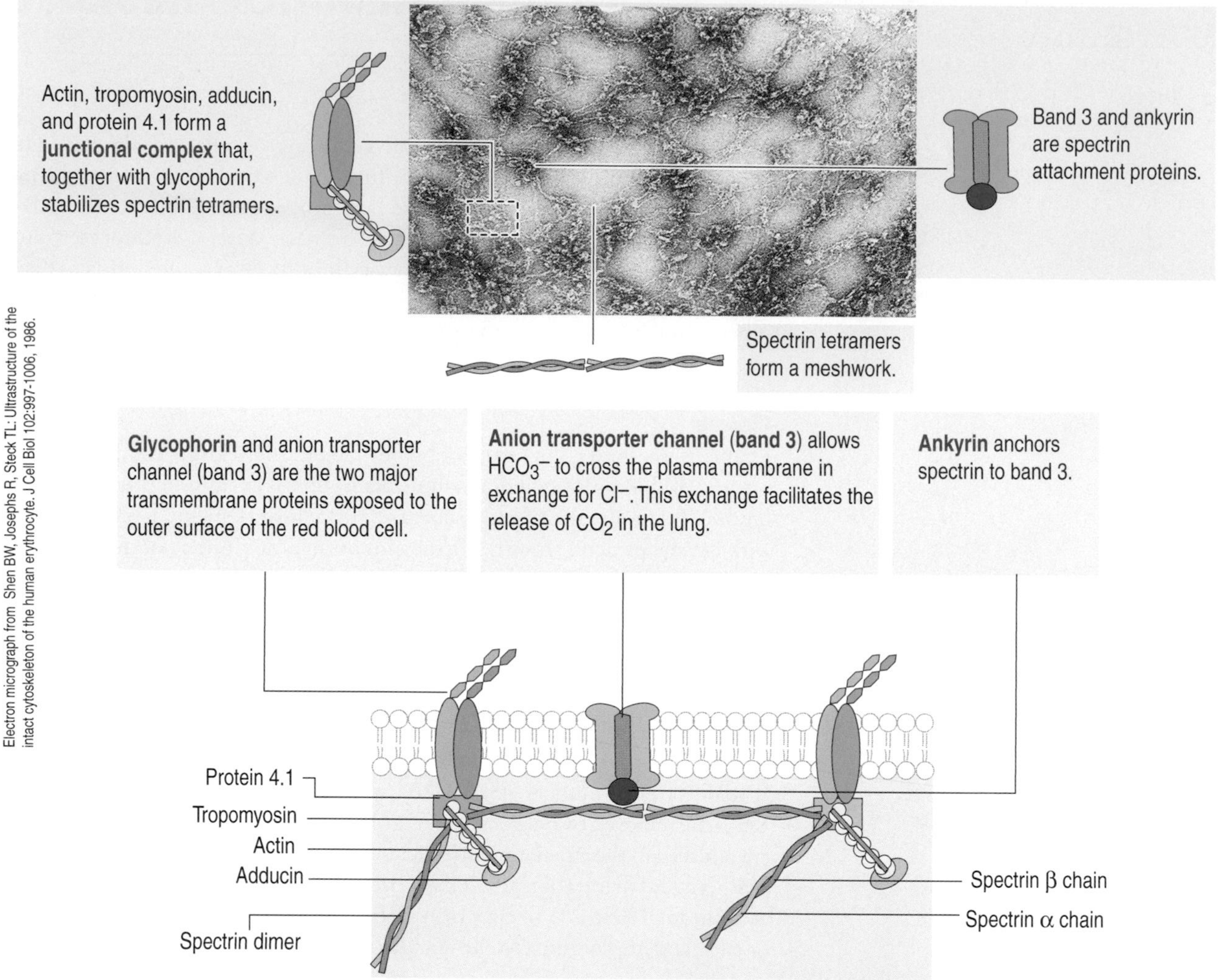

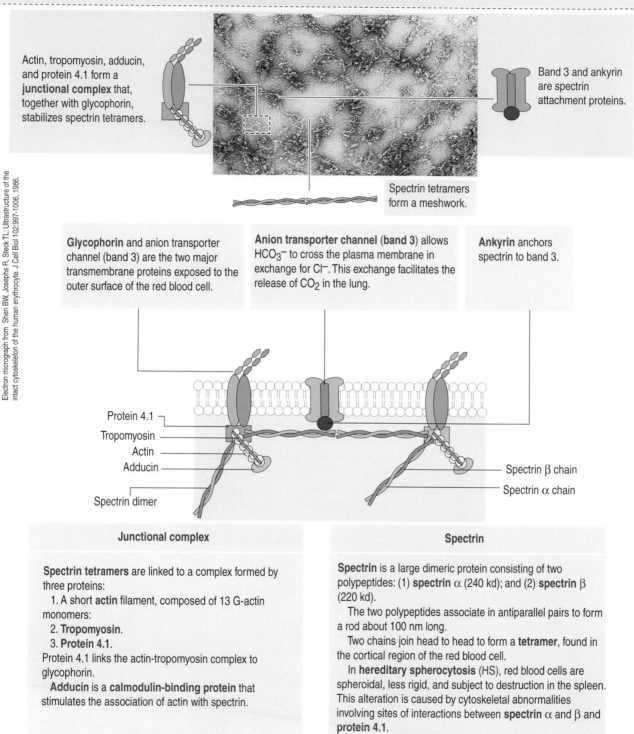

Actin, tropomyosin, adducin, and protein 4.1 form a **junctional complex** that, together with glycophorin, stabilizes spectrin tetramers.
Band 3 and ankyrin are spectrin attachment proteins.
Spectrin tetramers form a meshwork.
Glycophorin and anion transporter channel (band 3) are the two major transmembrane proteins exposed to the outer surface of the red blood cell.
Anion transporter channel (band 3) allows HCO_3^- to cross the plasma membrane in exchange for Cl^-. This exchange facilitates the release of CO_2 in the lung.
Ankyrin anchors spectrin to band 3.
Protein 4.1
Tropomyosin
Actin
Adducin
Spectrin dimer
Spectrin β chain
Spectrin α chain

Electron micrograph from Shen BW, Josephs R, Steck TL: Ultrastructure of the intact cytoskeleton of the human erythrocyte. J Cell Biol 102:997-1006, 1986.

Junctional complex

Spectrin tetramers are linked to a complex formed by three proteins:

1. A short **actin** filament, composed of 13 G-actin monomers:
2. **Tropomyosin.**
3. **Protein 4.1.**

Protein 4.1 links the actin-tropomyosin complex to glycophorin.

Adducin is a **calmodulin-binding protein** that stimulates the association of actin with spectrin.

Spectrin

Spectrin is a large dimeric protein consisting of two polypeptides: (1) **spectrin** α (240 kd); and (2) **spectrin** β (220 kd).

The two polypeptides associate in antiparallel pairs to form a rod about 100 nm long.

Two chains join head to head to form a **tetramer**, found in the cortical region of the red blood cell.

In **hereditary spherocytosis** (HS), red blood cells are spheroidal, less rigid, and subject to destruction in the spleen. This alteration is caused by cytoskeletal abnormalities involving sites of interactions between **spectrin** α and β and **protein 4.1**.

Clinical significance: Cytoskeletal and hemoglobin abnormalities

Elliptocytosis and **spherocytosis** are alterations in the shape of RBCs caused by defects in the cytoskeleton. **Elliptocytosis**, an autosomal dominant disorder characterized by the presence of oval-shaped RBCs, is caused by defective self-association of spectrin subunits, abnormal binding of spectrin to ankyrin, protein 4.1 defects, and abnormal glycophorin (see Figure 6-2). **Spherocytosis** is also an autosomal dominant condition involving a deficiency in **spectrin**. The common clinical features of elliptocytosis and spherocytosis are **anemia**, **jaundice**,

Figure 6-3. **Erythroblastosis fetalis: Hemolytic disease of the newborn**

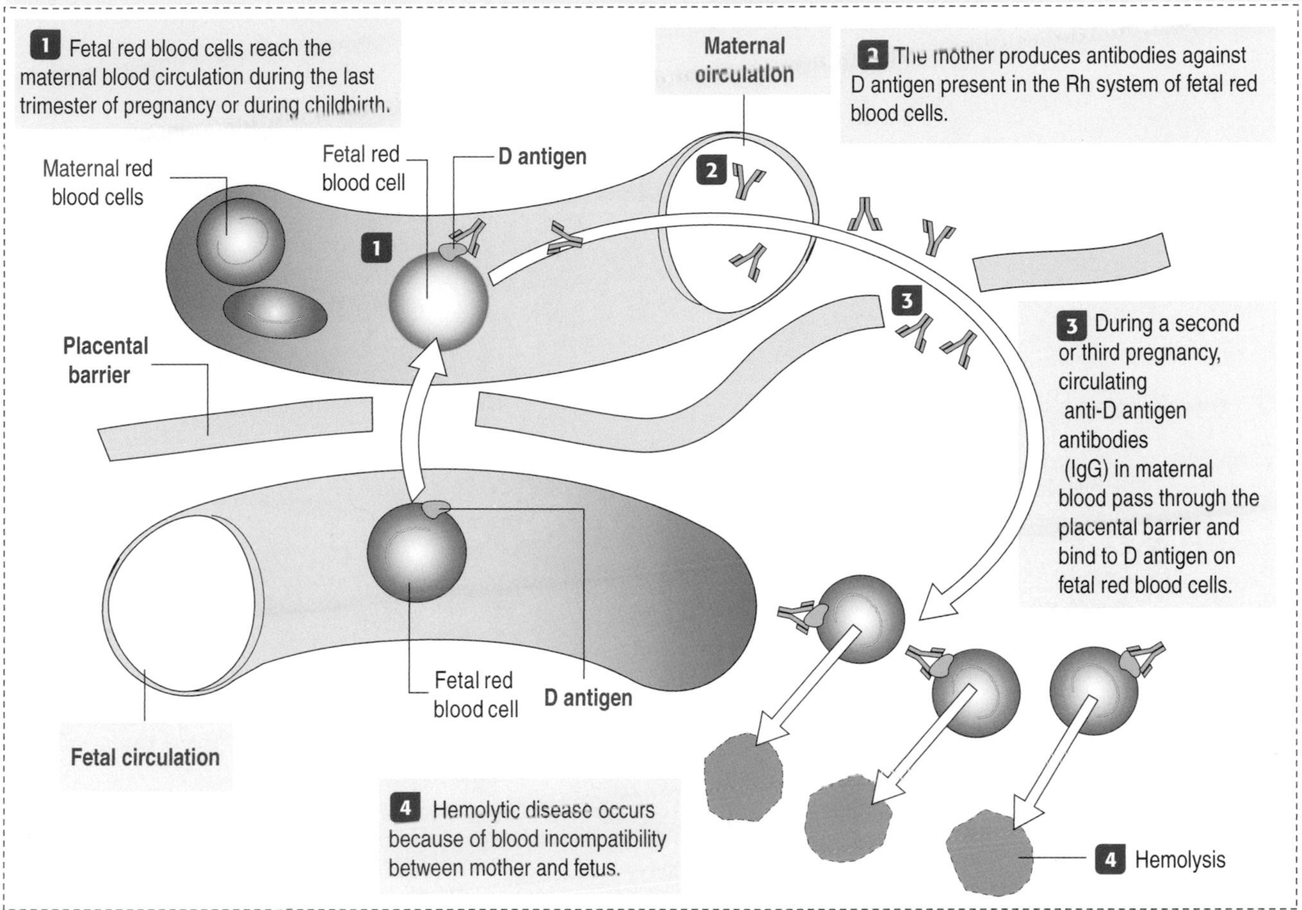
1 Fetal red blood cells reach the maternal blood circulation during the last trimester of pregnancy or during childbirth.
Maternal circulation
2 The mother produces antibodies against D antigen present in the Rh system of fetal red blood cells.
Maternal red blood cells
Fetal red blood cell
D antigen
1
2
3
Placental barrier
3 During a second or third pregnancy, circulating anti-D antigen antibodies (IgG) in maternal blood pass through the placental barrier and bind to D antigen on fetal red blood cells.
Fetal red blood cell
D antigen
Fetal circulation
4 Hemolytic disease occurs because of blood incompatibility between mother and fetus.
4 Hemolysis

and **splenomegaly** (enlargement of the spleen). **Splenectomy** is usually curative, since the spleen is the primary site responsible for the destruction of elliptocytes and spherocytes.

Hemoglobin genetic defects ($\alpha_2\beta S_2$) cause **sickle cell anemia** and **thalassemia** (Greek *thalassa*, sea; observed in populations along the Greek and Italian coasts). **Sickle cell anemia** results from a point mutation in which **glutamic acid** is replaced by **valine** at the sixth position in the β-globin chain. Defective hemoglobin (Hb S) tetramers aggregate and polymerize in deoxygenated RBCs, changing the biconcave disk shape into a rigid and less deformable sickle-shaped cell. Hb S leads to severe **chronic hemolytic anemia** and **obstruction of postcapillary venules** (see Spleen in Chapter 10, Immune-Lymphatic System).

Thalassemia syndromes are heritable anemias characterized by defective synthesis of either the α or β chains of the normal hemoglobin tetramer ($\alpha_2\beta_2$). The specific thalassemia syndromes are designated by the affected globin chain: **α-thalassemia** and **β-thalassemia. Thalassemia** syndromes are defined by anemia caused by defective synthesis of the hemoglobin molecule and hemolysis.

Box 6-A | **Hemolysis in erythroblastosis fetalis**

- The hemolytic process in erythroblastosis fetalis causes hemolytic anemia and jaundice.
- Hemolytic anemia causes hypoxic injury to the heart and liver leading to generalized edema (hydrops fetalis; Greek *hydrops*, edema).
- Jaundice causes damage to the central nervous system (German *kernicterus*, jaundice of brain nuclei).
- Hyperbilirubinemia is significant, and unconjugated bilirubin is taken up by the brain tissue.

Clinical significance: Erythroblastosis fetalis

Erythroblastosis fetalis is an antibody-induced hemolytic disease in the newborn that is caused by blood group incompatibility between mother and fetus (Figure 6-3 and Box 6-A). This incompatibility occurs when the fetus inherits RBC antigenic determinants that are foreign to the mother. ABO and Rh blood group antigens are of particular interest.

Essentially, the mother becomes sensitized to blood group antigens on **red blood cells**, which can reach maternal circulation during the last trimester of pregnancy (when the cytotrophoblast is no longer present as a barrier, as we

Figure 6-4. **Neutrophil**

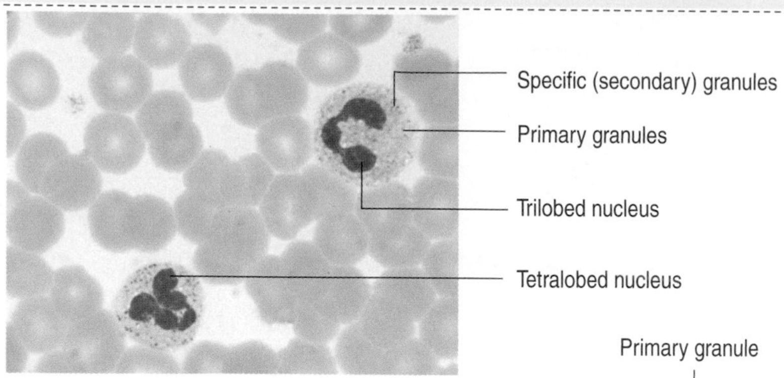

Neutrophils represent 50% to 70% of total leukocytes (the most abundant leukocyte in a normal blood smear). They measure 12 to 15 μm in diameter with a very pale pink cytoplasm (close in color to the erythrocyte).

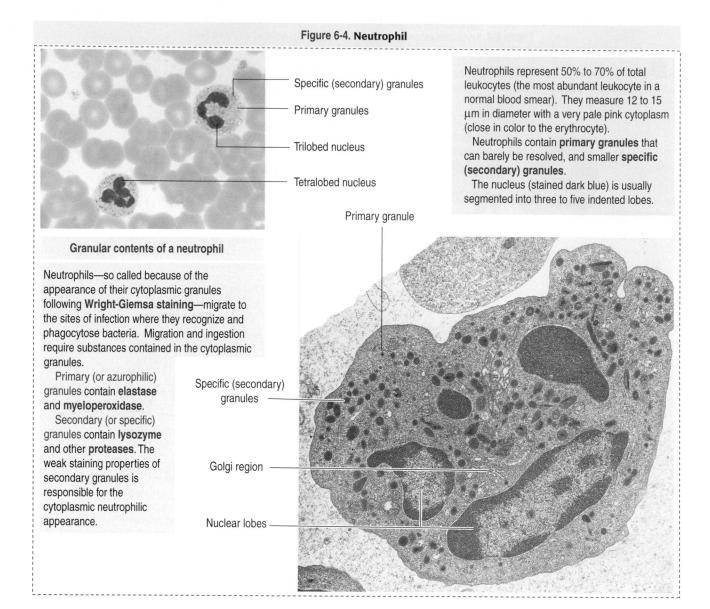

Neutrophils contain **primary granules** that can barely be resolved, and smaller **specific (secondary) granules**.

The nucleus (stained dark blue) is usually segmented into three to five indented lobes.

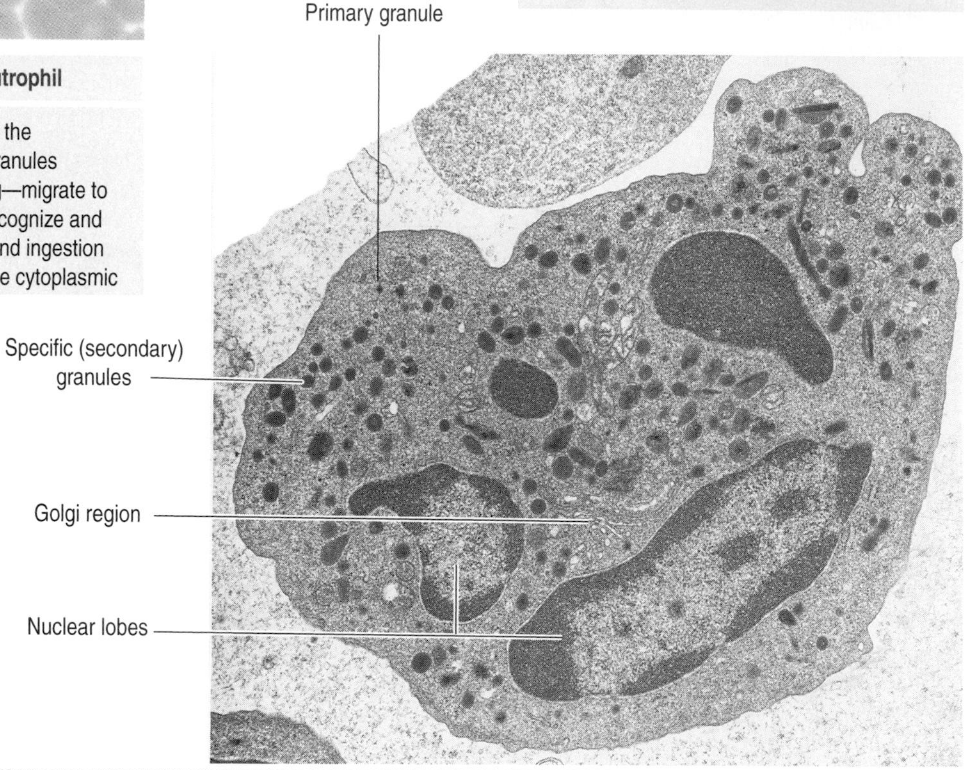

Granular contents of a neutrophil

Neutrophils—so called because of the appearance of their cytoplasmic granules following **Wright-Giemsa staining**—migrate to the sites of infection where they recognize and phagocytose bacteria. Migration and ingestion require substances contained in the cytoplasmic granules.

Primary (or azurophilic) granules contain **elastase** and **myeloperoxidase**.

Secondary (or specific) granules contain **lysozyme** and other **proteases**. The weak staining properties of secondary granules is responsible for the cytoplasmic neutrophilic appearance.

discussed in Chapter 23, Fertilization, Placentation, and Lactation) or during childbirth. Within the Rh system, **D antigen** is the major cause of Rh incompatibility. The initial exposure to the Rh antigen during the first pregnancy does not cause erythroblastosis fetalis because **immunoglobulin M (IgM)** is produced and IgMs cannot cross the placenta because of their large size.

Subsequent exposure to D antigen during the second or third pregnancy leads to a strong **immunoglobulin G (IgG)** response (IgGs can cross the placenta).

Rh-negative mothers are given anti-D globulin soon after the delivery of an Rh-positive baby. Anti-D antibodies mask the antigenic sites on the fetal RBCs that may have leaked into the maternal circulation during childbirth. This prevents long-lasting sensitization to Rh antigens.

Leukocytes

Leukocytes (**6 to 10 × 10^3 per mm^3**; see Box 6-B) are categorized as either **granulocytes (containing primary, and specific or secondary cytoplasmic granules,** Box 6-C) or **agranulocytes (containing only primary granules)**. In response to an appropriate stimulus, leukocytes may leave the bloodstream (**diapedesis**) and enter the connective tissue by the **homing** mechanism (see Figure 6-9).

Box 6-B | **Blood cells/μL or mm^3**

Erythrocytes	4-6 × 10^6	
Leukocytes	6000-10,000	
Neutrophils	5000	(60%-70%)
Eosinophils	150	(2%-4%)
Basophils	30	(0.5%)
Lymphocytes	2400	(28%)
Monocytes	350	(5%)
Platelets	300,000	

Figure 6-5. **Eosinophil**

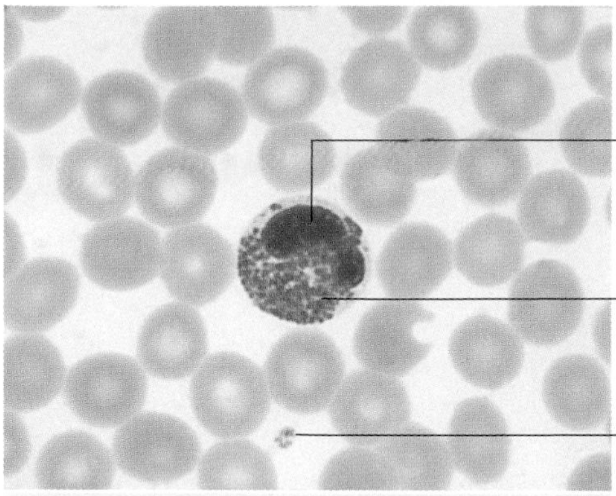

Eosinophils represent 1% to 5% of total leukocytes. They measure 12–15 μm in diameter.

Their cytoplasm contains large, refractile specific granules that appear bright red and are clearly discernible.

The nucleus of the eosinophil is typically bilobed.

Granular contents of an eosinophil

Eosinophil peroxidase
It binds to microorganisms and facilitates their killing by macrophages.

Major basic protein (MBP)
1. It is the predominant component of the crystalline center of the eosinophil granule.
2. It binds to and disrupts the membrane of parasites (binding is mediated by its Fc receptor).
3. It causes basophils to release histamine by a Ca^{2+}-dependent mechanism.

Eosinophil cationic protein
1. It neutralizes heparin.
2. Together with MBP, it causes the fragmentation of parasites.

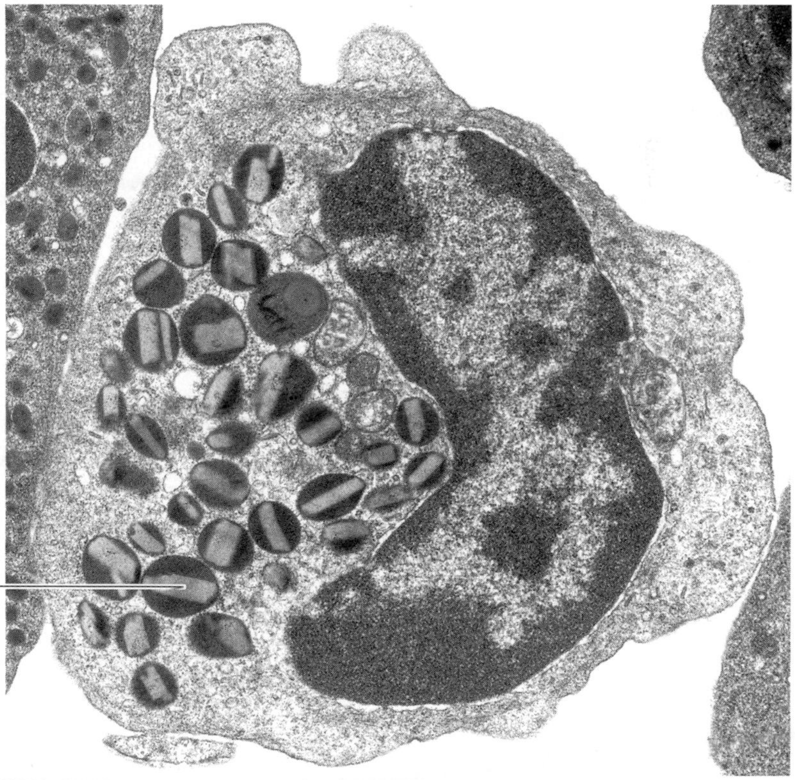

Box 6-C | **Primary and specific granules**

- Primary and specific (secondary) granules are membrane-bound lysosomes that contain enzymes.
- **Peroxidase is a marker enzyme of primary granules. The presence of alkaline phosphatase and a lack of peroxidase characterize the secondary granules.**
- Why are primary granules azurophilic with the Wright blood stain method? Because primary granules contain sulfated glycoproteins that presumably account for this deep-blue (azure) staining.

Granulocytes

These phagocytic cells have a **multilobed nucleus** and measure **12** to **15 μm** in diameter. Their average lifespan varies with cell type. Three types of granulocytes can be distinguished by their cytoplasmic granules:

1. **Neutrophils** (Figure 6-4). These cells have a lobulated nucleus. Their cytoplasm contains both secondary (specific) and primary granules (see Box 6-C). In stained smears, neutrophils appear very pale pink. Neutrophils, which constitute **60%** to **70%** of circulating leukocytes, have a lifespan of **6** to **7 hours** and may live for up to **4 days** in the connective tissue. After leaving the circulation through postcapillary venules, neutrophils act to eliminate opsonized bacteria or limit the extent of an inflammatory reaction in the connective tissue. The mechanism of bacterial opsonization is discussed in Chapter 10, Immune-Lymphatic System.

Enzymes contained in the primary granules (**elastase** and **myeloperoxidase**) and secondary granules (**lysozyme** and other **proteases**), specific receptors for **C5a** (produced by the complement system pathway, see Figure 10-10 in Chapter 10, Immune-Lymphatic System), and **L-selectin**, and **integrins** (with binding affinity to endothelial cell ligands such as **intercellular-adhesion molecules 1**

Figure 6-6. Basophil

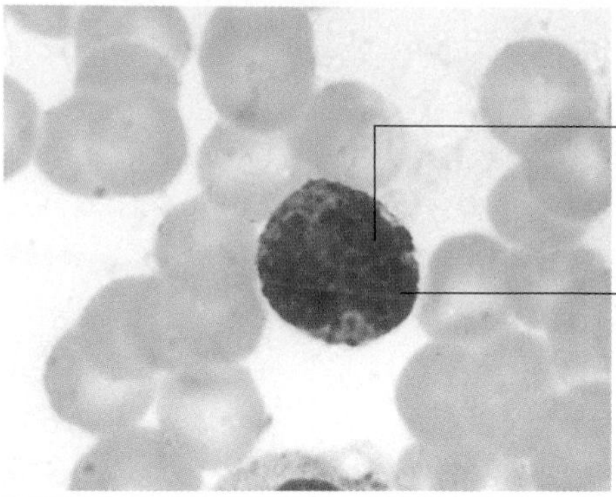

Basophils represent less than 1% of total leukocytes, so they may be difficult to find.

Their specific granules are large and stain dark blue or purple. Basophils also contain a few primary granules.

The nucleus, which is typically bilobed, is often obscured by the specific granules.

Granular contents of a basophil

Basophils contain large cytoplasmic granules with **sulfated** or **carboxylated acidic proteins** such as heparin. They stain dark blue with the **Wright-Giemsa stain**.

Basophils, similar to mast cells in the connective tissue, express on their surface **IgE receptors** and release histamine to mediate allergic reactions when activated by antigen binding.

An increase in the number of basophils (more than 150 basophils/μL) is called basophilia and is observed in acute hypersensitivity reactions, viral infections, and chronic inflammatory conditions, such as rheumatoid arthritis and ulcerative colitis.

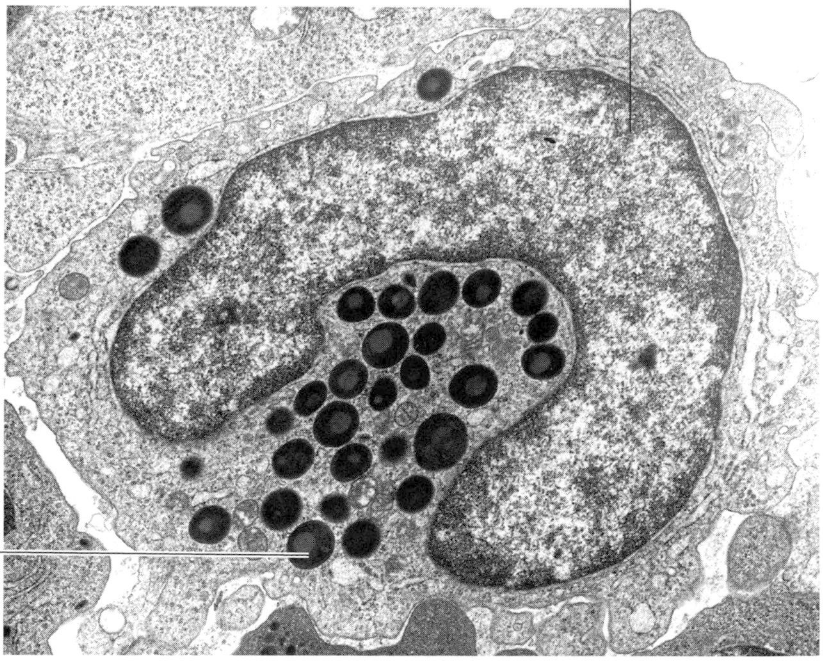

and 2 [**ICAM-1** and **ICAM-2**]) enable the antibacterial and homing function of neutrophils (see Figure 6-9).

2. **Eosinophils** (Figure 6-5). Like neutrophils, eosinophils have a characteristic bilobed nucleus. Their cytoplasm is filled with large, refractile granules that stain red in blood smears and tissue sections. Eosinophils constitute **2%** to **4%** of circulating leukocytes and may also leave the circulation and enter the connective tissue. These cells are the first line of defense against **parasites** and also participate in triggering **bronchial asthma** (see Chapter 13, Respiratory System).

3. **Basophils** (Figure 6-6). These granulocytes contain large, **metachromatic** cytoplasmic granules that often obscure the bilobed nucleus. Basophils represent only **1%** of circulating leukocytes. They may leave the circulation and enter the connective tissue, where they resemble **mast cells** (see Chapter 4, Connective Tissue, for additional differences between basophils and mast cells). Basophils play a role in immediate (**bronchial asthma**) and delayed hypersensitivity (**allergic skin reaction**) and in the propagation of the immune response.

Agranulocytes

Agranulocytes have a round or indented nucleus. They contain only lysosomal-type, **primary granules**. Agranulocytes include **lymphocytes** and **monocytes.**

Lymphocytes are either large (**3%** of lymphocytes; **9** to **12** μ**m**) or small (**97%** of lymphocytes; **6 to 8** μ**m** (Figure 6-7) cells. In either case, the nucleus is round

Figure 6-7. Lymphocyte

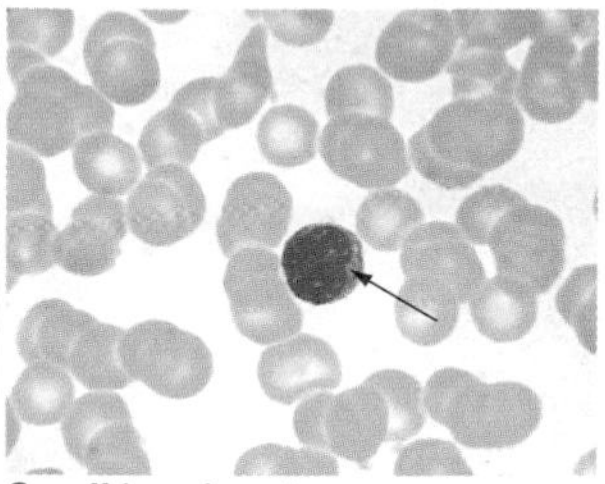

Small lymphocyte

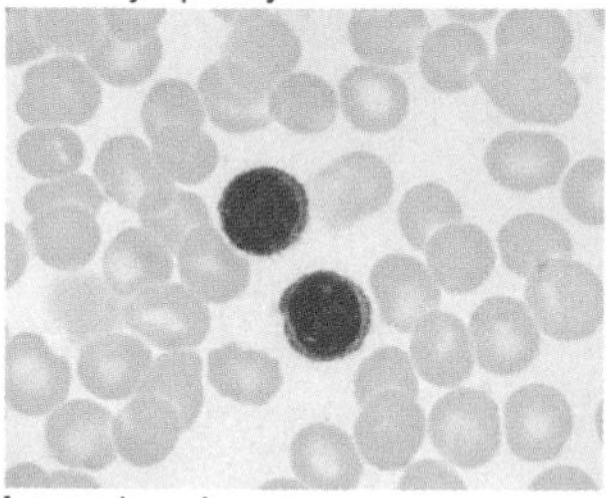

Large lymphocytes

Lymphocytes are relatively abundant, accounting for 20% to 40% of total leukocytes. In circulating blood, lymphocytes may range from approximately 7 to12 μm in diameter. However, the typical lymphocyte in a normal blood smear is small, about the size of a red blood cell.

The nucleus of a **small lymphocyte** is densely stained, with a round or slightly indented shape (*arrow*). The nucleus occupies most of the cell, reducing the cytoplasm to a thin basophilic rim.

Large lymphocytes have a round, slightly indented nucleus surrounded by a pale cytoplasm. Occasionally, a few primary granules (lysosomes) may be present.

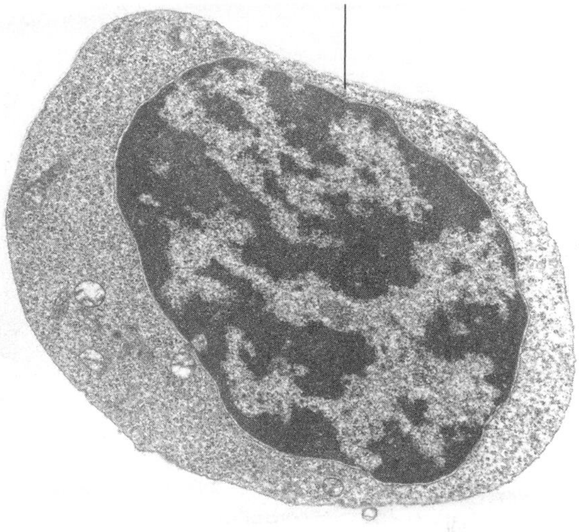

Small lymphocytes represent 97% of the population of circulating lymphocytes. Note that the nucleus is surrounded by a thin cytoplasmic rim. **Large lymphocytes** represent 3% of the population of circulating lymphocytes.

Lymphocytes are divided into two categories: **B lymphocytes**, produced in the bone marrow, and **T lymphocytes**, also produced in the bone marrow but that complete their maturation in the thymus.

A less abundant class is the **natural killer cell.**

During fetal development, the **yolk sac**, **liver**, and **spleen** are sites where lymphocytes originate. In postnatal life, the **bone marrow** and **thymus** are the **primary lymphoid organs** where lymphocytes develop before they are exposed to antigens.

Secondary lymphoid organs are the **lymph nodes**, the **spleen**, and lymphoid aggregates of the gastrointestinal and respiratory tracts.

and may be slightly indented. The cytoplasm is basophilic, often appearing as a thin rim around the nucleus (see Figure 6-7). A few primary granules may be present. Lymphocytes may live for a few days or several years.

Lymphocytes are divided into two categories: **B lymphocytes** (also called **B**

Figure 6-8. Monocyte

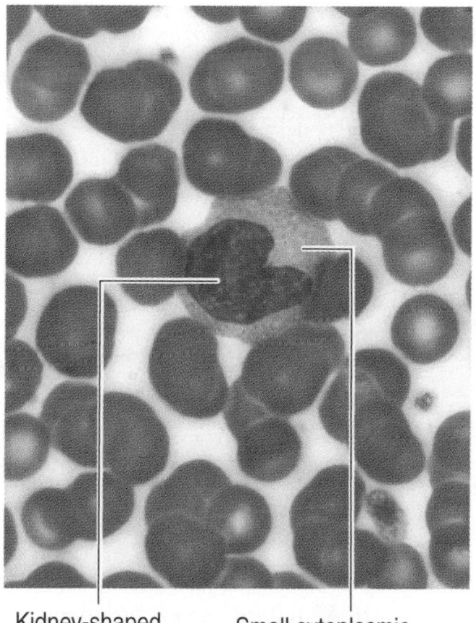

Monocytes (2% to 8% of total leukocytes) are the largest leukocytes, ranging in size from 15 to 20 μm.

The eccentrically placed nucleus is typically kidney-shaped and contains fine strands of chromatin.

The abundant cytoplasm stains pale gray-blue and is filled with small lysosomes that give a fine, granular appearance.

Monocytes travel briefly in the bloodstream (about 20 hours) and then enter the peripheral tissue where they are transformed into macrophages and survive a longer time. Macrophage-derived monocytes are more efficient phagocytic cells than neutrophils.

Figure 6-9. Homing and inflammation

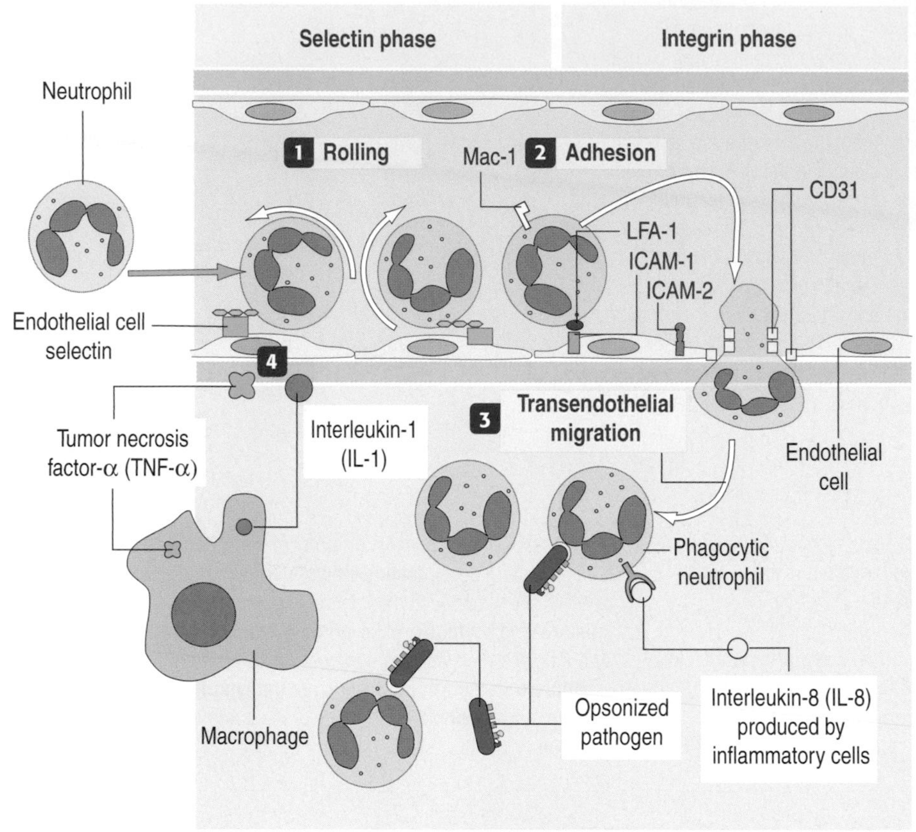
Selectin phase
Integrin phase
Neutrophil
1 Rolling
Mac-1
2 Adhesion
CD31
LFA-1
ICAM-1
ICAM-2
Endothelial cell selectin
4
Tumor necrosis factor-α (TNF-α)
Interleukin-1 (IL-1)
3 Transendothelial migration
Endothelial cell
Phagocytic neutrophil
Macrophage
Opsonized pathogen
Interleukin-8 (IL-8) produced by inflammatory cells

1 Rolling and attachment
Leukocytes (neutrophil in the diagram) establish reversible binding between selectins induced on the endothelial cell surface and carbohydrate ligands on the neutrophil surface. This binding is not strong and the cell keeps rolling.

2 Adhesion
A strong interaction occurs between the neutrophil and the endothelial cell. This interaction is mediated by intercellular adhesion molecules **ICAM-1** and **ICAM-2** on the endothelium and the **integrins LFA-1** (lymphocyte function–associated antigen 1) and **Mac-1** (macrophage-1). ICAM-1 is expressed in the presence of inflammation.

3 Transendothelial migration
T cells migrate across the endothelium along an **IL-8** concentration gradient produced by inflammatory cells. **CD31** contributes to diapedesis.

4 Activated macrophages secrete **TNF-α** and **IL-1** to stimulate the expression of selectins by endothelial cells.

cells) are produced and mature in bone marrow. Antigen-stimulated B cells differentiate into antibody-secreting **plasma cells. T lymphocytes** (also called **T cells**) are produced in bone marrow but complete their maturation in the **thymus.** Activated T cells participate in **cell-mediated immunity** (for additional details, see Chapter 10, Immune-Lymphatic System).

Monocytes (Figure 6-8) can measure **12** to **20** **μm** in diameter. Their nucleus is kidney-shaped or oval. Cytoplasmic granules are small and may not be resolved on light microscopy. Monocytes circulate in blood for **12** to **100 hours** and then enter the connective tissue. In the connective tissue, monocytes differentiate into macrophages, which are involved in bacterial phagocytosis, antigen presentation, and clean-up of dead cell debris. In bone, monocytes differentiate into **osteoclasts** under the control of osteoblasts (see Chapter 4, Connective Tissue).

Homing and inflammation

We have studied in Chapter 1, Epithelium (see Figure 1-11), the molecular principles of homing. We will expand the concept of homing by studying the mechanism of **migration of phagocytic neutrophils to the site of infection and inflammation** (Figure 6-9).

The first step is the binding of carbohydrate ligands on the surface of the neutrophil to an endothelial selectin (E selectin). This binding determines rolling adhesion of the neutrophil.

The second step is a stronger interaction of neutrophil **integrins LFA-1** (lymphocyte function–associated antigen 1) and **Mac-1** (macrophage-1) to **ICAM-1** and **ICAM-2** on the endothelial cell surface. ICAM-1 is induced by cytokine **tumor necrosis factor-**α, and **interleukin-1** (IL-1) is produced by activated macrophages present at the site of inflammation.

These molecular interactions determine (1) tight binding of the neutrophil, required for stopping rolling; (2) preparing the cell for squeezing between adjacent endothelial cells toward the chemoattractant **interleukin-8**, produced by inflammatory cells; and (3) **transendothelial migration**, or **diapedesis**, facilitated by the interaction of **CD31** molecules expressed on the surfaces of both the neutrophil and endothelial cell.

Clinical and pathologic significance of the homing process

Cell adhesion proteins play a significant role in immune surveillance, wound healing, tumor metastasis, and tissue morphogenesis. One of the main events in allergic inflammation is the recruitment of inflammatory cells into tissue sites where allergic reactions occur. To accomplish their migratory function, cell adhesion proteins on migratory cells bind to ligands found on the surface of other cells.

Two adhesion molecule deficiencies have been described, both characterized by a defect in wound healing, recurrent infections, and marked leukocytosis (increase in the number of leukocytes in blood).

Leukocyte adhesion deficiency I is caused by a defect in the β subunit of the integrin molecule. As a consequence, leukocytes are unable to leave blood vessels to enter the tissue by transendothelial migration. In these patients, inflammatory cell infiltrates are devoid of neutrophils.

In leukocyte adhesion deficiency II, the fucosyl-containing ligands for selectins are absent due to a congenital defect of endogenous fucose metabolism. As shown in Figure 6-9, selectin-carbohydrate interactions have a role in the rolling of leukocytes on an endothelial cell surface, a step required for the transendothelial migration of leukocytes into extravascular areas of inflammation.

Clinical significance: Mast cell–eosinophil interaction in asthma

We have already seen that both mast cells and eosinophils are immigrant cells of the connective tissue. These two cell types have a significant role in the pathogenesis of asthma.

Asthma, a condition in which extrinsic (allergens) or intrinsic (unknown) factors trigger variable air obstruction of the respiratory bronchi and bronchioles, provides a good example of mast cell–eosinophil interaction.

When **mast cells** degranulate and release chemical mediators, eosinophils and neutrophils are attracted from blood vessels into the connective tissue of the respiratory mucosa. **Eosinophils**, in turn, release additional mediators (leukotriene B_4 and others) to enhance bronchoconstriction and edema. The release of **eosinophil cationic protein** and **major basic protein** into the bronchial lumen damages the epithelial cell lining and disturbs mucociliary function (Figure 6-10).

Platelets

Platelets are small (**2 to 4 μm**) cytoplasmic fragments derived from the **megakaryocyte** (Figure 6-11) under the control of **thrombopoietin**, a 35- to 70-kd glycoprotein produced in the kidney and liver. Megakaryocytes develop cytoplasmic projections that become **proplatelets**, which fragment into platelets. This differentiation process takes 10 to 12 days. **Platelets bind and degrade thrombopoietin, a mechanism that regulates platelet production.**

The plasma membrane of a platelet invaginates to form a system of **cytoplasmic channels**, called the **open canalicular system**. The central region of the platelet, the **granulomere**, contains mitochondria, rough endoplasmic reticulum, the Golgi apparatus, and granules. The periphery of the platelet, the **hyalomere**, contains microtubules and microfilaments that regulate platelet shape and movement.

Clinical significance: Thrombocytopenia

About **300,000** platelets per microliter of blood circulate for **8** to **10** days. Platelets promote blood clotting and help to prevent blood loss from damaged vessels.

Figure 6-10. **Mast cell–eosinophil interaction in asthma**

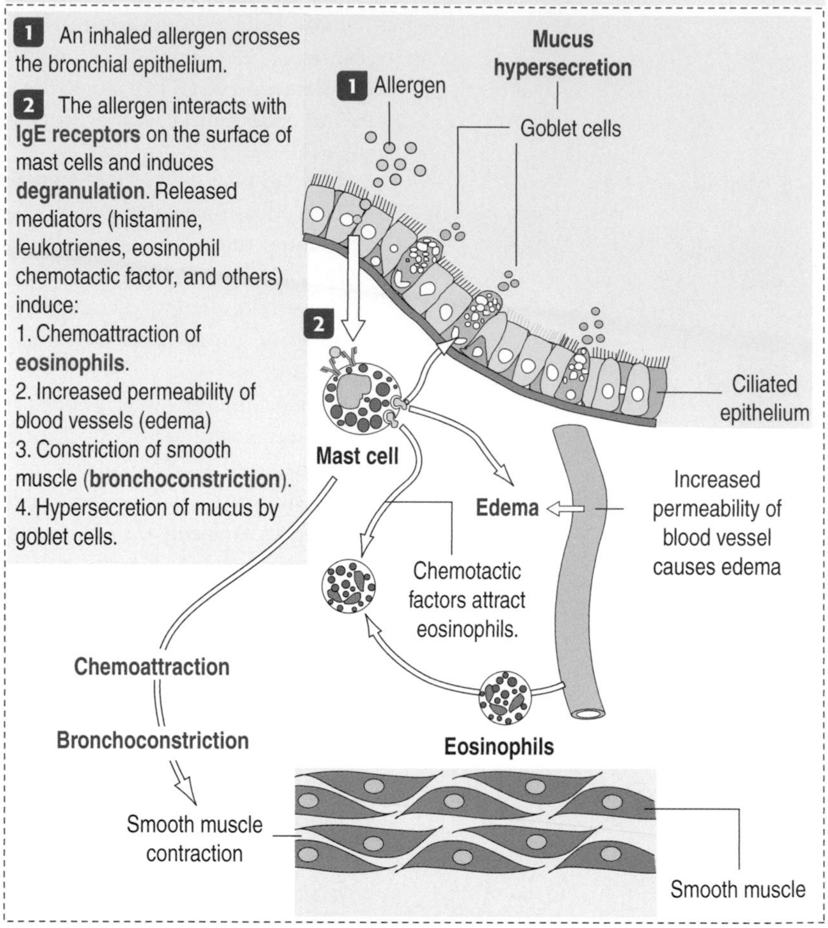
1 An inhaled allergen crosses the bronchial epithelium.
2 The allergen interacts with **IgE receptors** on the surface of mast cells and induces **degranulation**. Released mediators (histamine, leukotrienes, eosinophil chemotactic factor, and others) induce:
1. Chemoattraction of **eosinophils**.
2. Increased permeability of blood vessels (edema)
3. Constriction of smooth muscle (**bronchoconstriction**).
4. Hypersecretion of mucus by goblet cells.
Mucus hypersecretion
1 Allergen
Goblet cells
2
Ciliated epithelium
Mast cell
Edema
Increased permeability of blood vessel causes edema
Chemotactic factors attract eosinophils.
Chemoattraction
Bronchoconstriction
Eosinophils
Smooth muscle contraction
Smooth muscle

A reduction in the number of platelets in blood (**thrombocytopenia**) leads to increased susceptibility to bleeding. Thrombocytopenia is defined by a decrease in the number of platelets to less than 150,000/μL of blood. **Spontaneous bleeding** is observed with a platelet count of 20,000/μL. **Thrombocytosis** defines an increase in the number of platelets circulating in blood.

Thrombocytopenia can be caused by a **decrease in the production of platelets**, **an increase in the destruction of platelets** (determined by antibodies against platelets or megakaryocyte antigens [**autoimmune thrombocytopenic purpura, ITP**] or drugs—for example, penicillin, sulfonamides, and digoxin), and **aggregation of platelets in the microvasculature** (**thrombotic thrombocytopenic purpura**, [**TTP**]), probably a result of pathologic changes in endothelial cells producing procoagulant substances.

Deficiency of the **glycoprotein 1b–factor IX** complex, or **von Willebrand factor,** a protein associated with factor VIII, leads to two congenital bleeding disorders, **Bernard-Soulier syndrome** and **von Willebrand disease**, respectively (see Figures 6-11 to 6-13) (see Box 6-D). These two diseases are characterized by the inability of platelets to attach to vascular subendothelial surfaces. The **glycoprotein 1b–factor IX–von Willebrand factor complex is important for the aggregation of normal platelets when they are exposed to injured subendothelial tissues.**

Gray platelet syndrome, an autosomal dominant disease characterized by **macrothrombocytopenia** (thrombocytopenia with increased platelet volume), is due to a reduction in the content of alpha granules.

MYH9 (myosin heavy chain 9)-related disorders are also associated with macrothrombocytopenia. A defect in the *MYH9* gene, which encodes nonmuscle myosin heavy chain IIA, an isoform expressed in platelets and neutrophils, determines defective production of platelets during the formation of proplatelets.

Box 6-D | **Hemophilia**

- **Hemophilia** is a common hereditary disease associated with serious bleeding due to an inherited deficiency of **factor VIII** or **factor IX**.
- The genes for these blood coagulation factors lie on the X chromosome, and when mutated, they cause the X-linked recessive traits of **hemophilia A** and **B**. Hemophilia affects males, with females as carriers.
- A reduction in the amount or activity of **factor VIII**, a protein synthesized in the liver, causes **hemophilia A**. Deficiency in **factor IX** determines **hemophilia B**.
- Major trauma or surgery can determine severe bleeding in all hemophiliacs and, therefore, a correct diagnosis is critical. Plasma-derived or genetically engineered recombinant factors are available for the treatment of patients with hemophilia.
- **Von Willebrand disease**, the most frequent bleeding disorder, is also hereditary and related to a deficient or abnormal **von Willebrand factor**.

Figure 6-11. **Platelets**

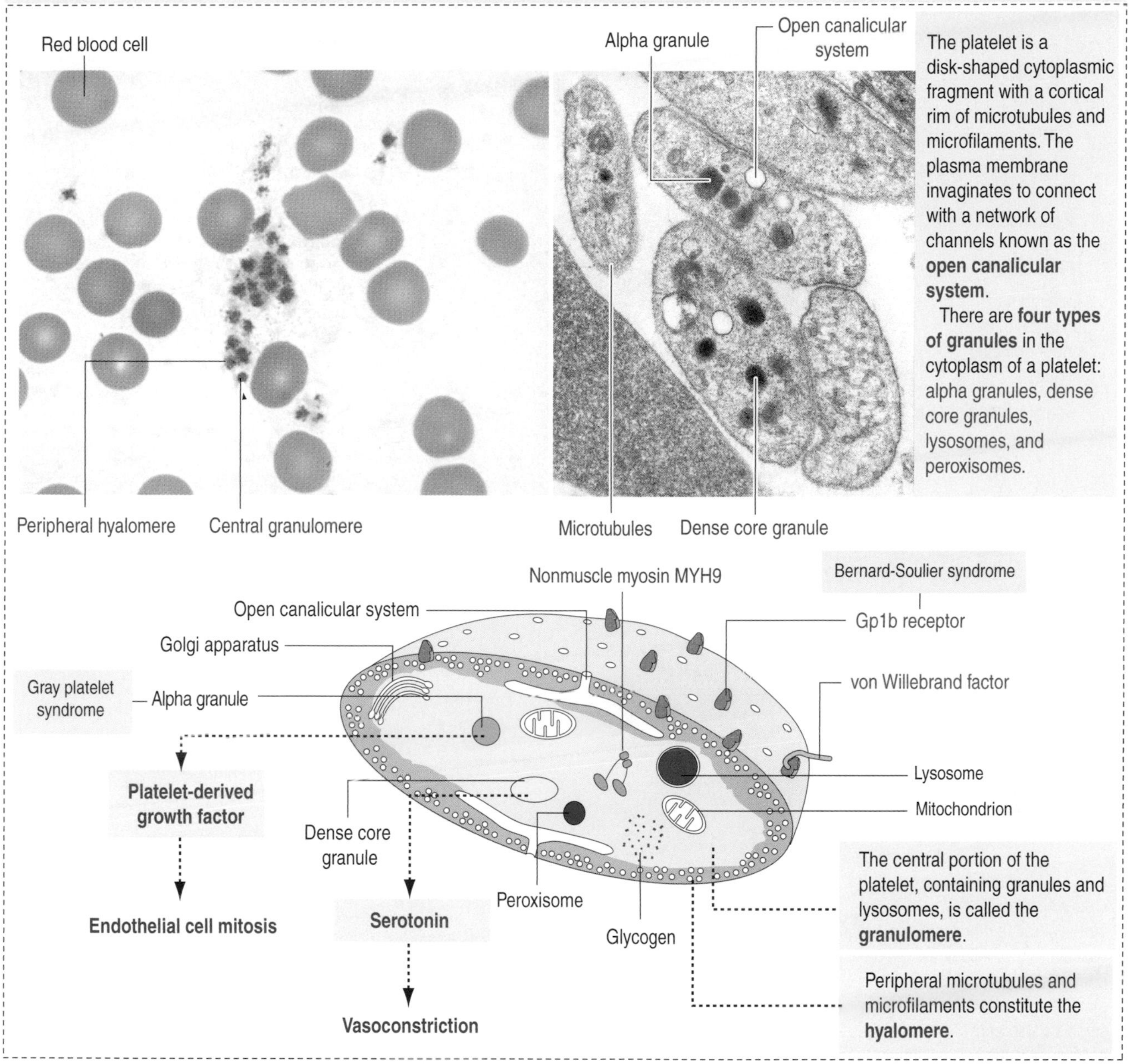

Red blood cell
Peripheral hyalomere
Central granulomere
Alpha granule
Open canalicular system
Microtubules
Dense core granule
The platelet is a disk-shaped cytoplasmic fragment with a cortical rim of microtubules and microfilaments. The plasma membrane invaginates to connect with a network of channels known as the **open canalicular system**.
There are **four types of granules** in the cytoplasm of a platelet: alpha granules, dense core granules, lysosomes, and peroxisomes.
Nonmuscle myosin MYH9
Bernard-Soulier syndrome
Gp1b receptor
Open canalicular system
Golgi apparatus
Gray platelet syndrome
Alpha granule
von Willebrand factor
Lysosome
Mitochondrion
Platelet-derived growth factor
Dense core granule
Endothelial cell mitosis
Serotonin
Peroxisome
Glycogen
Vasoconstriction
The central portion of the platelet, containing granules and lysosomes, is called the **granulomere**.
Peripheral microtubules and microfilaments constitute the **hyalomere**.

Clinical significance: Hemostasis and the blood clotting cascade

The blood clotting or coagulation cascade depends on the sequential activation of proenzymes to enzymes and the participation of endothelial cells and platelets to achieve **hemostasis** or arrest of bleeding. Hemostasis occurs when fibrin is formed to reinforce the platelet plug (Figure 6-12).

The blood clotting cascade has the following characteristics:

1. It is dependent on the presence of inactive precursor proteases (for example, factor XII) that are converted into active enzymes (for example, factor XIIa) by proteolysis.

2. It is composed of intrinsic and extrinsic pathways (see Figure 6-13).

3. The extrinsic and intrinsic pathways converge into the common pathway.

The **extrinsic pathway** is triggered by damage outside a blood vessel and is set in motion by the release of tissue factor. The **intrinsic pathway** is stimulated by damage to components of the blood and blood vessel wall. It is induced by contact of factor XII to subendothelial collagen. This contact results from damage to the wall of a blood vessel.

Figure 6-12. Blood clotting or hemostasis

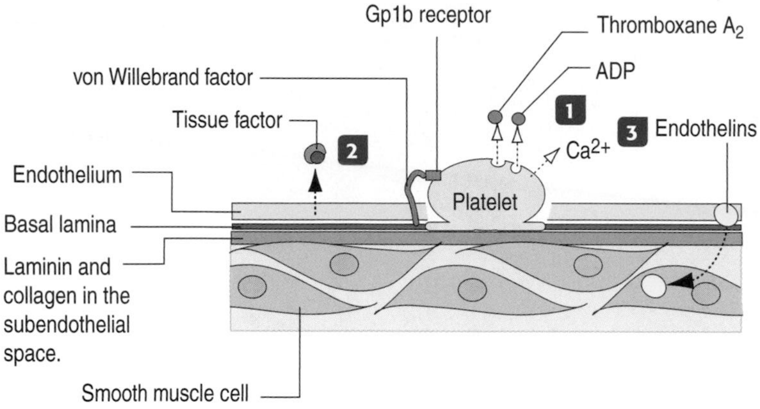

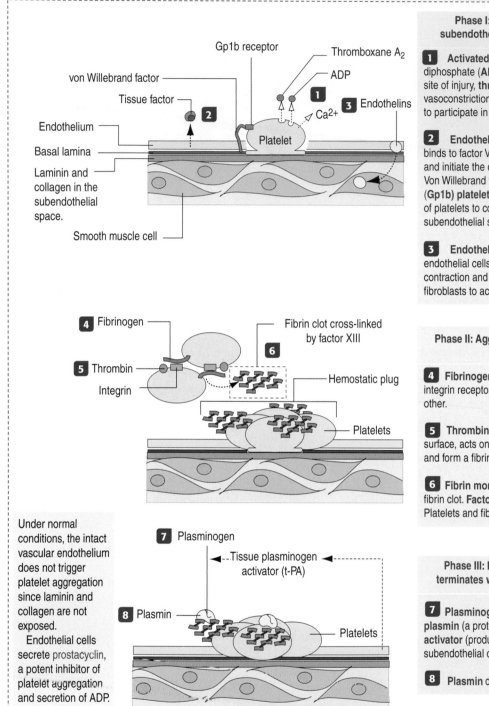

Phase I: Adhesion of platelets to the subendothelium of an injured blood vessel

1 **Activated platelets** release: adenosine diphosphate (**ADP**), to attract other platelets to the site of injury, **thromboxane A_2**, to cause vasoconstriction and platelet aggregation, and **Ca^{2+}**, to participate in clotting.

2 **Endothelial cells** release **tissue factor**, which binds to factor VIIa to convert factor X into factor Xa and initiate the common pathway of blood clotting. Von Willebrand factor binds to **glycoprotein 1b (Gp1b) platelet receptor** to facilitate the attachment of platelets to collagen and laminin in the subendothelial space.

3 **Endothelins**, peptide hormones secreted by endothelial cells, stimulate smooth muscle contraction and proliferation of endothelial cells and fibroblasts to accelerate the repair process.

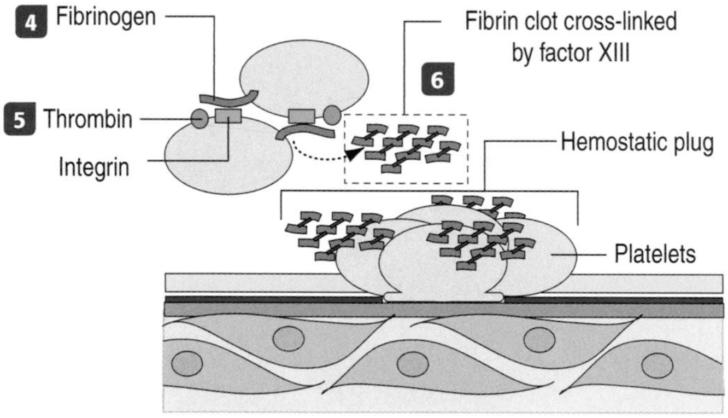

Phase II: Aggregation of platelets to form a hemostatic plug

4 **Fibrinogen** in plasma binds to activated integrin receptors, and platelets are bridged to each other.

5 **Thrombin**, bound to its receptor on the platelet surface, acts on **fibrinogen** to cleave fibrinopeptides and form a fibrin monomer.

6 **Fibrin monomers** aggregate to form a soft fibrin clot. **Factor XIII** cross-links fibrin monomers. Platelets and fibrin form a hemostatic plug.

Under normal conditions, the intact vascular endothelium does not trigger platelet aggregation since laminin and collagen are not exposed.
Endothelial cells secrete prostacyclin, a potent inhibitor of platelet aggregation and secretion of ADP.

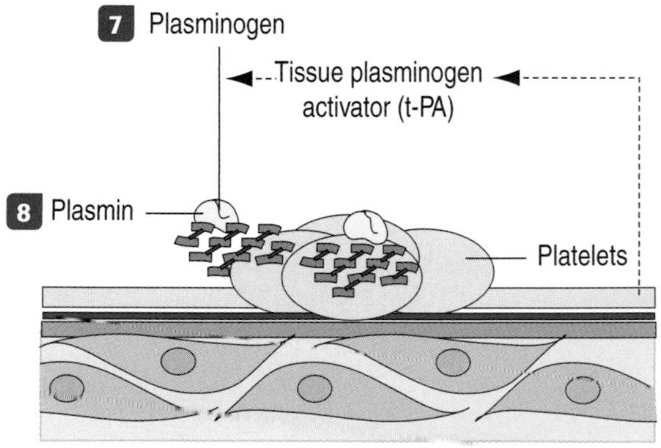

Phase III: Platelet procoagulation activity terminates with the removal of the fibrin clot

7 **Plasminogen** (a plasma protein) is converted to **plasmin** (a protease) by **tissue plasminogen activator** (produced by injured endothelial cells and subendothelial connective tissue).

8 **Plasmin** dissolves the fibrin clot.

Extrinsic and intrinsic pathways converge to a crucial step in which **fibrinogen is converted to fibrin**, which forms mesh that enables platelets to attach. The convergence starts with the activation of factor X to factor Xa, together with activated factor Va, resulting in the cleavage of **prothrombin** to **thrombin.** The initial hemostatic plug consists of a platelet scaffold for the conversion of prothrombin to thrombin, which changes fibrinogen into fibrin (see Figure 6-12).

Fibrinogen, produced by hepatocytes, consists of three polypeptide chains, which contain numerous negatively charged amino acids in the amino terminal. These characteristics allow fibrinogen to remain soluble in plasma. After cleavage,

Figure 6-13. **Phases of blood clotting**

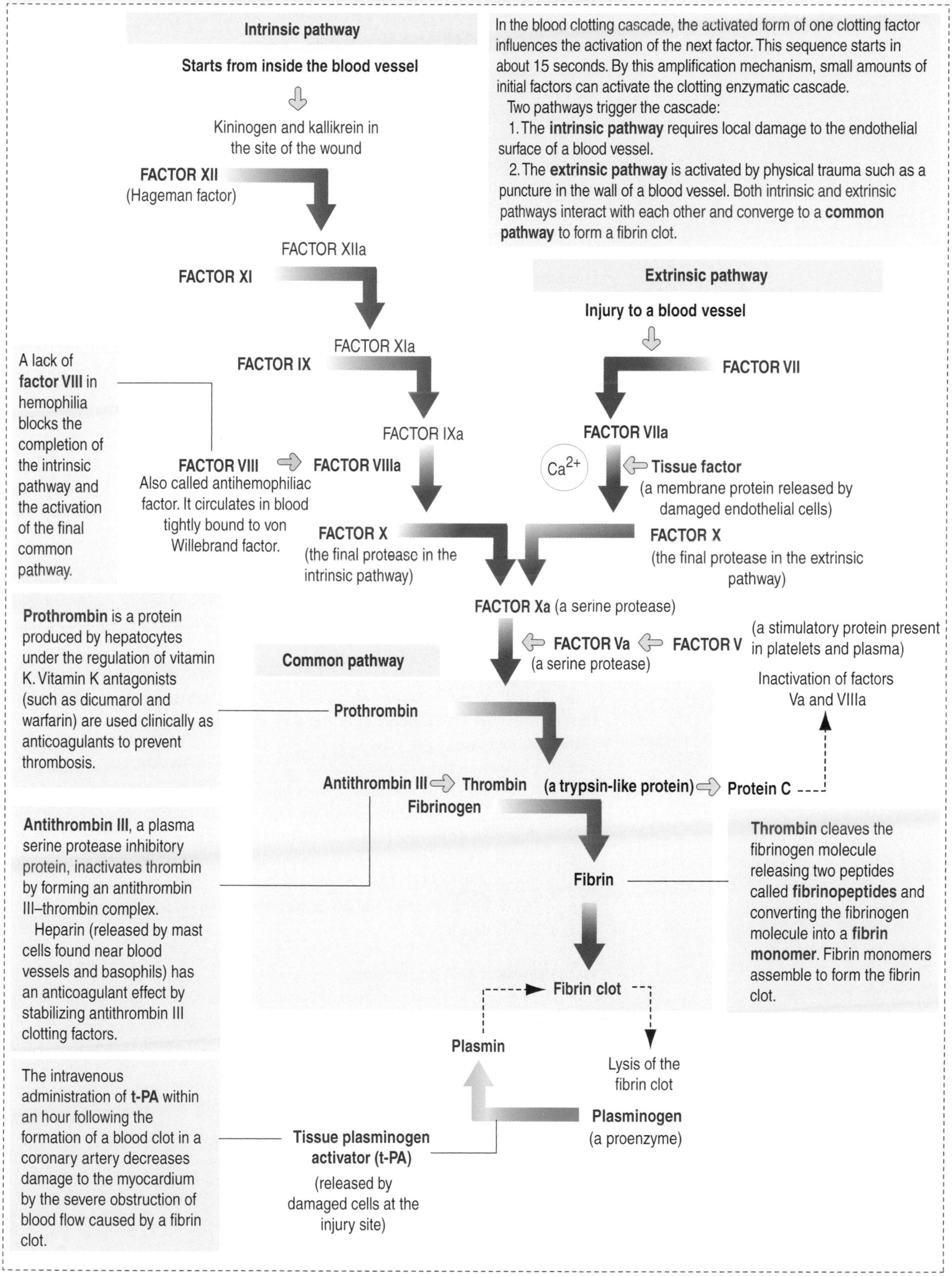

Intrinsic pathway
Starts from inside the blood vessel
Kininogen and kallikrein in the site of the wound
FACTOR XII (Hageman factor)
FACTOR XIIa
FACTOR XI
FACTOR XIa
FACTOR IX
FACTOR IXa
FACTOR VIII
FACTOR VIIIa
Also called antihemophiliac factor. It circulates in blood tightly bound to von Willebrand factor.
A lack of **factor VIII** in hemophilia blocks the completion of the intrinsic pathway and the activation of the final common pathway.
FACTOR X (the final protease in the intrinsic pathway)
In the blood clotting cascade, the activated form of one clotting factor influences the activation of the next factor. This sequence starts in about 15 seconds. By this amplification mechanism, small amounts of initial factors can activate the clotting enzymatic cascade.
Two pathways trigger the cascade:
1. The **intrinsic pathway** requires local damage to the endothelial surface of a blood vessel.
2. The **extrinsic pathway** is activated by physical trauma such as a puncture in the wall of a blood vessel. Both intrinsic and extrinsic pathways interact with each other and converge to a **common pathway** to form a fibrin clot.
Extrinsic pathway
Injury to a blood vessel
FACTOR VII
FACTOR VIIa
Ca^{2+}
Tissue factor (a membrane protein released by damaged endothelial cells)
FACTOR X (the final protease in the extrinsic pathway)
FACTOR Xa (a serine protease)
FACTOR Va (a serine protease)
FACTOR V (a stimulatory protein present in platelets and plasma)
Inactivation of factors Va and VIIIa
Common pathway
Prothrombin is a protein produced by hepatocytes under the regulation of vitamin K. Vitamin K antagonists (such as dicumarol and warfarin) are used clinically as anticoagulants to prevent thrombosis.
Prothrombin
Antithrombin III **Thrombin** **(a trypsin-like protein)** **Protein C**
Fibrinogen
Fibrin
Antithrombin III, a plasma serine protease inhibitory protein, inactivates thrombin by forming an antithrombin III–thrombin complex.
Heparin (released by mast cells found near blood vessels and basophils) has an anticoagulant effect by stabilizing antithrombin III clotting factors.
Thrombin cleaves the fibrinogen molecule releasing two peptides called **fibrinopeptides** and converting the fibrinogen molecule into a **fibrin monomer**. Fibrin monomers assemble to form the fibrin clot.
Fibrin clot
Plasmin
Lysis of the fibrin clot
Plasminogen (a proenzyme)
Tissue plasminogen activator (t-PA) (released by damaged cells at the injury site)
The intravenous administration of **t-PA** within an hour following the formation of a blood clot in a coronary artery decreases damage to the myocardium by the severe obstruction of blood flow caused by a fibrin clot.

the newly formed **fibrin** molecules aggregate forming a mesh. Fibrin, with the addition of **plasma fibronectin**, stabilizes the blood clot (Figure 6-13).

Hematopoiesis, the formation of blood cells

In the **fetus**, hematopoiesis (Greek *haima,* blood; *poiein,* to make) starts during the first trimester in islands of hematopoiesis found in the **yolk sac**. The islands develop from **hemangioblasts**, the progenitors of both hematopoietic and endothelial cells. Fetal hematopoiesis continues after the second trimester in the **liver** and then in the **spleen**. During the seventh month of intrauterine life, the **bone marrow** becomes the primary site of hematopoiesis, where it remains during adulthood. In the adult, an approximate volume of 1.7 L of marrow contains 10^{12} hematopoietic cells.

The bone marrow consists of two compartments: (1) the **marrow stromal compartment** and (2) the **hematopoietic cell compartment**.

The **marrow stromal compartment** is a framework of **adipose cells, fibroblasts, stromal cells, vascular endothelial cells, macrophages**, and **blood vessels** interspersed within trabecular bone (Figures 6-14 to 6-16). Endothelial cells, marrow fibroblasts, and stromal cells produce hematopoietic growth factors and cytokines that regulate the production of blood cells. Endothelial cells form a barrier that prevents immature hematopoietic cells from leaving the marrow and enables mature hematopoietic cells to enter the blood. Adipose cells provide a local source of energy as well as synthesize growth factors. Marrow macrophages remove apoptotic cells, residual nuclei from orthochromatic erythroblasts, and particles from entering the marrow. Osteoblasts and osteoclasts maintain and remodel the cancellous bone surrounding the marrow tissue.

The **hematopoietic cell compartment** is highly vascularized. It is supplied by the **central longitudinal artery**, derived from the **nutrient artery. Medullary capillary plexuses** and **periosteal capillary plexuses** are interconnected. **Medullary sinusoids** drain into the **central longitudinal vein** before leaving through the **nutrient vein** (see Figure 6-14).

Mature hematopoietic cells translocate from the site of growth through the sinusoid wall by active **transendothelial migration** across openings into the sinuses (see Figure 6-15) before entering the circulation through the central vein. Immature hematopoietic cells lack the capacity of transendothelial migration and are retained in the extravascular space by the vascular endothelial cells. The sinusoids of the marrow are lined by specialized endothelial cells with significant phagocytic activity and a capacity to produce growth factors that stimulate the proliferation and differentiation of hematopoietic cells.

The hematopoietic cell compartment consists of several cell types required for diverse physiologic needs. Hematopoietic cells occupy preferential sites in the bone marrow and have differing capacities for self-renewal, growth, differentiation, and maturation.

Hematopoietic cell populations

The bone marrow consists of three major populations (see Figure 6-16): (1) the **hematopoietic stem cells**, capable of **self-renewal**; (2) **committed precursor cells**, responsible for the generation of distinct cell lineages; and (3) **maturing cells**, resulting from the differentiation of the committed precursor cell population.

Hematopoietic stem cells can self-renew and produce two committed precursor cells: the **myeloid stem cell** and the **lymphoid stem cell**, that develop into distinct cell progenies. **Self-renewal** is an important property of hematopoietic stem cells. Self-renewal preserves the pool of stem cells and is critical for feeding common myeloid progenitor and common lymphoid progenitor into the differentiation or maturation pathway.

Hematopoietic stem cells are difficult to identify, mainly because they represent approximately 0.05% of total hematopoietic cells (about 10^6 to 10^7 stem cells). In

Figure 6-14. **Bone marrow: Structure and vascularization**

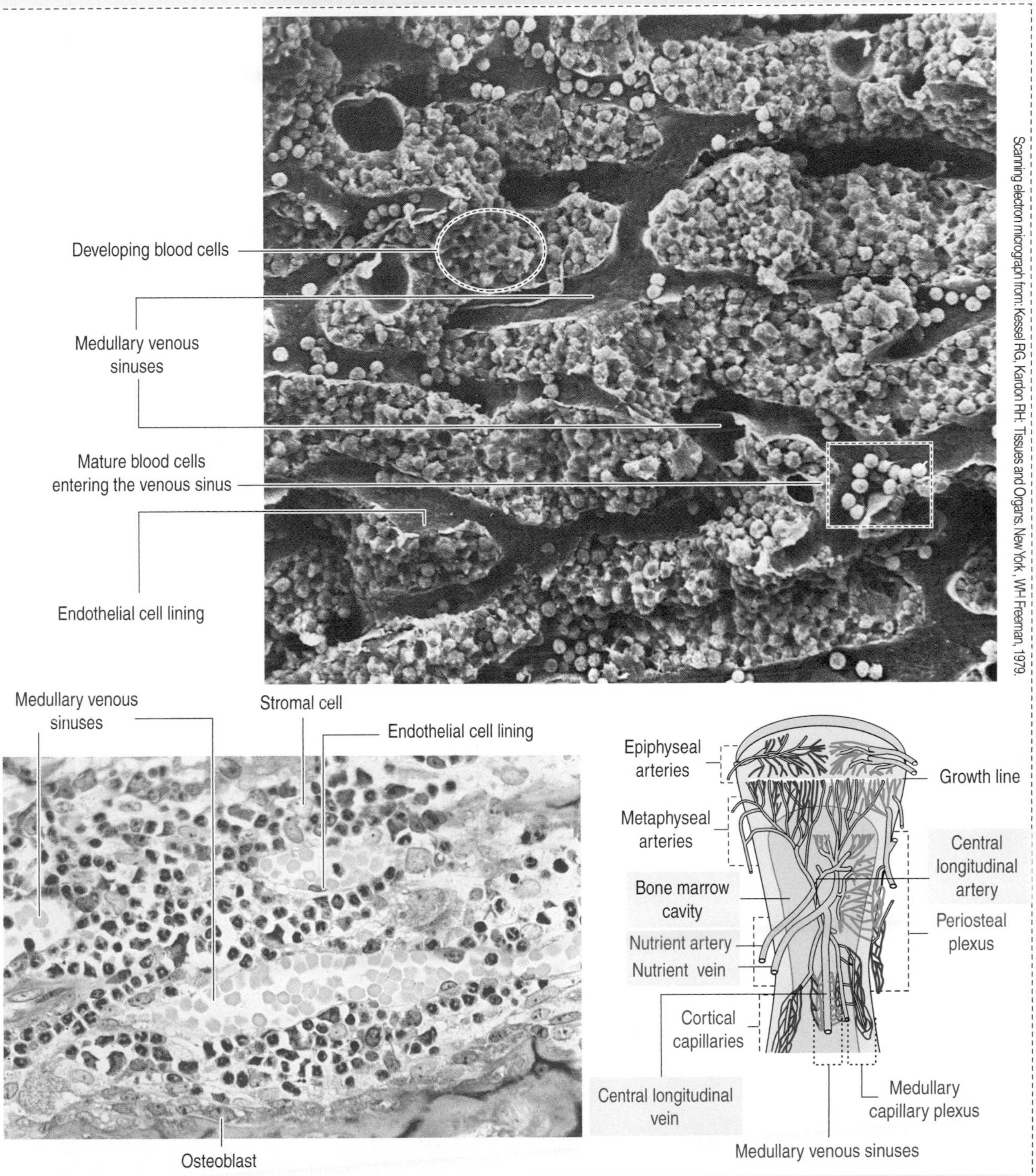

Developing blood cells
Medullary venous sinuses
Mature blood cells entering the venous sinus
Endothelial cell lining
Scanning electron micrograph from: Kessel RG, Kardon RH: Tissues and Organs. New York, WH Freeman, 1979.
Medullary venous sinuses
Stromal cell
Endothelial cell lining
Osteoblast
Epiphyseal arteries
Growth line
Metaphyseal arteries
Central longitudinal artery
Bone marrow cavity
Periosteal plexus
Nutrient artery
Nutrient vein
Cortical capillaries
Central longitudinal vein
Medullary capillary plexus
Medullary venous sinuses

The bone marrow can be **red** because of the presence of erythroid progenies, or **yellow**, because of adipose cells. Red and yellow marrow may be interchangeable in relation to the demands for hematopoiesis. In the adult, red bone marrow is found in the skull, clavicles, vertebrae, ribs, sternum, pelvis, and ends of the long bones of the limbs.

Blood vessels and nerves reach the bone marrow by piercing the bony shell. The **nutrient artery** enters the midshaft of a long bone and branches into the **central longitudinal artery**, which gives rise to a **medullary capillary plexus** continuous with the **medullary venous sinuses** and connected to cortical capillaries. Cortical capillaries and medullary capillaries extend into Volkmann's canals and haversian canals.

The venous sinuses empty into the **central longitudinal vein**. Periosteal blood vessels give rise to periosteal plexuses connected to medullary capillaries and medullary venous sinuses.

Figure 6-15. **Bone marrow: Structure**

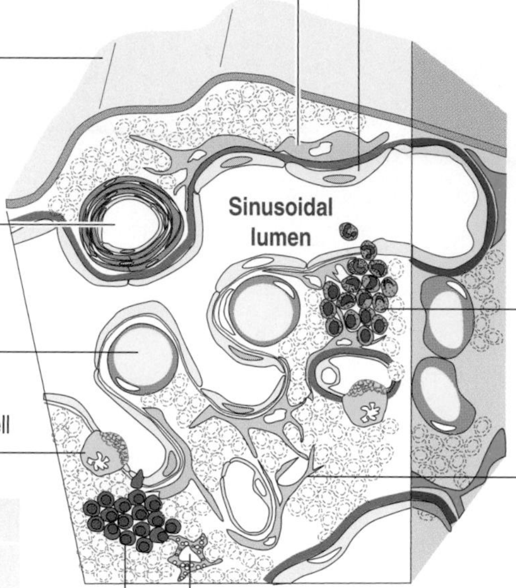

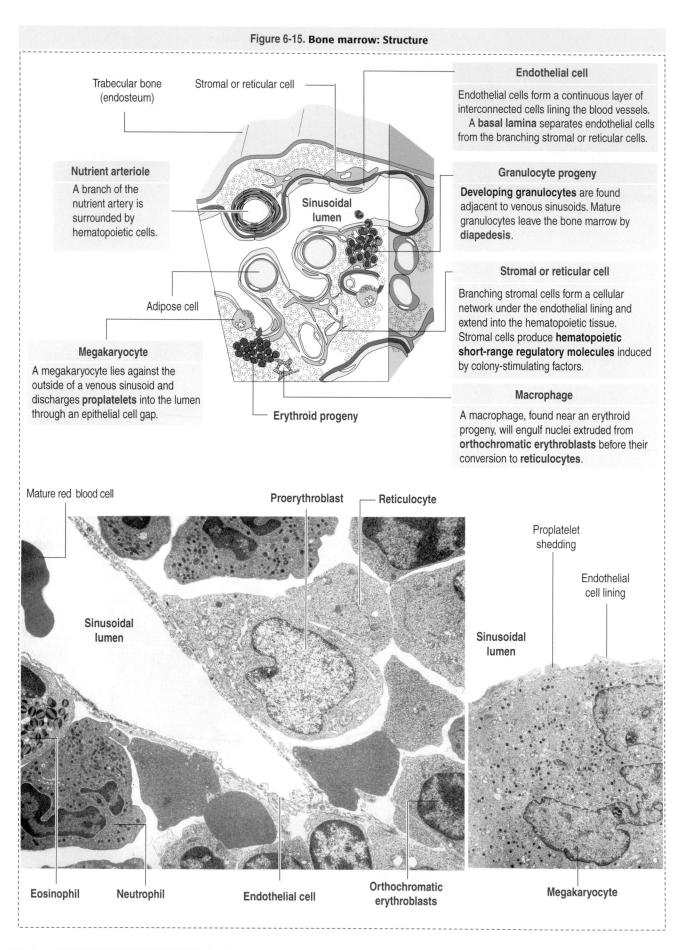

Trabecular bone (endosteum)
Stromal or reticular cell
Sinusoidal lumen
Adipose cell
Erythroid progeny

Endothelial cell

Endothelial cells form a continuous layer of interconnected cells lining the blood vessels.

A **basal lamina** separates endothelial cells from the branching stromal or reticular cells.

Nutrient arteriole

A branch of the nutrient artery is surrounded by hematopoietic cells.

Granulocyte progeny

Developing granulocytes are found adjacent to venous sinusoids. Mature granulocytes leave the bone marrow by **diapedesis**.

Stromal or reticular cell

Branching stromal cells form a cellular network under the endothelial lining and extend into the hematopoietic tissue. Stromal cells produce **hematopoietic short-range regulatory molecules** induced by colony-stimulating factors.

Megakaryocyte

A megakaryocyte lies against the outside of a venous sinusoid and discharges **proplatelets** into the lumen through an epithelial cell gap.

Macrophage

A macrophage, found near an erythroid progeny, will engulf nuclei extruded from **orthochromatic erythroblasts** before their conversion to **reticulocytes**.

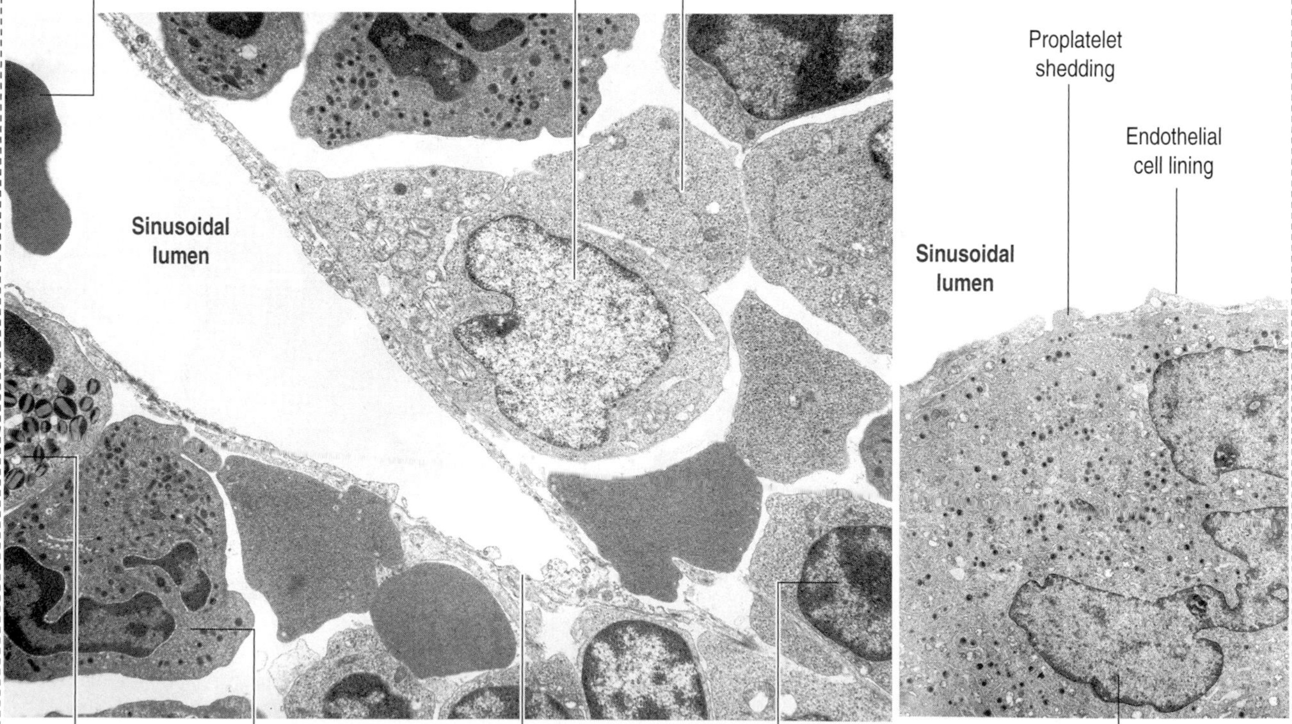

Mature red blood cell
Proerythroblast
Reticulocyte
Sinusoidal lumen
Proplatelet shedding
Endothelial cell lining
Sinusoidal lumen
Eosinophil
Neutrophil
Endothelial cell
Orthochromatic erythroblasts
Megakaryocyte

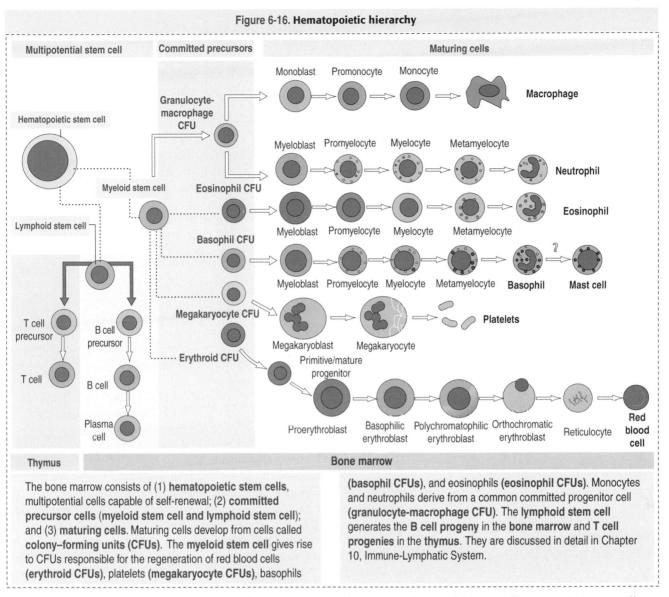

Figure 6-16. **Hematopoietic hierarchy**

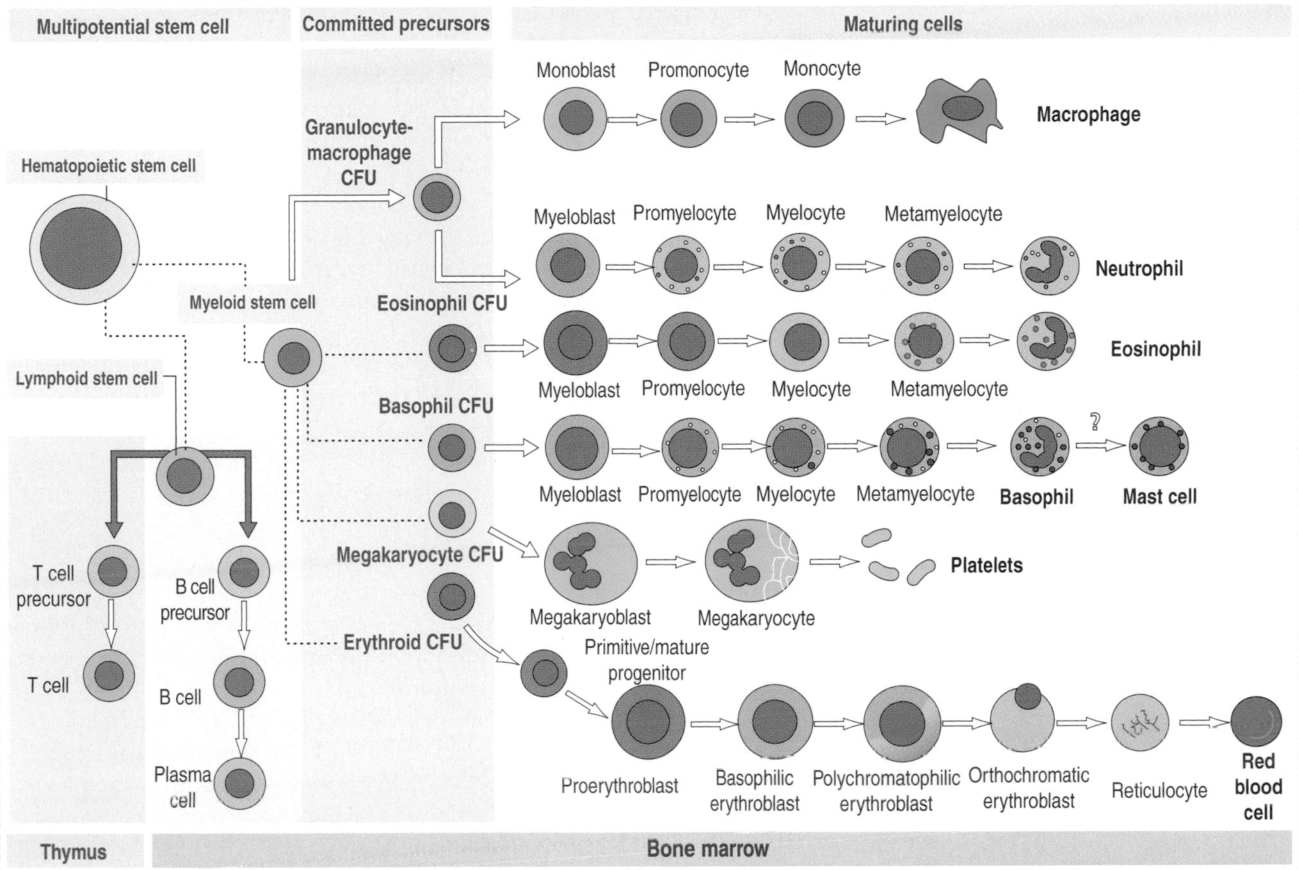

The bone marrow consists of (1) **hematopoietic stem cells**, multipotential cells capable of self-renewal; (2) **committed precursor cells (myeloid stem cell and lymphoid stem cell)**; and (3) **maturing cells**. Maturing cells develop from cells called **colony-forming units (CFUs)**. The **myeloid stem cell** gives rise to CFUs responsible for the regeneration of red blood cells **(erythroid CFUs)**, platelets **(megakaryocyte CFUs)**, basophils **(basophil CFUs)**, and eosinophils **(eosinophil CFUs)**. Monocytes and neutrophils derive from a common committed progenitor cell **(granulocyte-macrophage CFU)**. The **lymphoid stem cell** generates the **B cell progeny** in the **bone marrow** and **T cell progenies** in the **thymus**. They are discussed in detail in Chapter 10, Immune-Lymphatic System.

bone marrow transplantation, only 5% of the normal hematopoietic stem cells are needed to repopulate the entire bone marrow. **Hematopoietic stem cells cannot be identified by morphology, but they can be recognized by specific cell surface markers** (c-kit and Thy-1). $CD34^{+}$ committed precursor cell populations, also containing $CD34^{-}$ hematopoietic stem cells, are generally used for transplantation in the clinical treatment of malignant diseases with chemotherapeutic agents that deplete a certain group of committed precursor cells.

Myeloid and lymphoid stem cells are multipotential cells (see Figure 6-16). They are committed to the formation of cells of the blood and lymphoid organs. Five **colony-forming units** (**CFUs**) derive from the myeloid stem cell: the **erythroid** CFU, the **megakaryocyte** CFU, the **basophil** CFU, the **eosinophil** CFU, and the **granulocyte-macrophage** CFU. The erythroid CFU produces **red blood cells**. The megakaryocyte CFU generates **platelets**. The granulocyte-macrophage CFU produces both **monocytes** and **neutrophils**. Basophils and eosinophils derive from the basophil and eosinophil CFUs, respectively. The lymphoid stem cell gives rise to T cell and B cell precursors.

Clinical significance: Hematopoietic growth factors

Hematopoietic growth factors control the proliferative and maturational phases of hematopoiesis. In addition, they can extend the life span and function of a number of cells produced in the bone marrow. Several recombinant forms are available for clinical treatment of blood disorders.

Hematopoietic growth factors, also known as **hematopoietic cytokines**, are glycoproteins produced in the bone marrow by endothelial cells, stromal cells, fibroblasts, developing lymphocytes, and macrophages. Hematopoietic growth factors are also produced outside the bone marrow.

There are three major groups of hematopoietic growth factors: (1) **colony-stimulating factors**, (2) **erythropoietin** (Figure 6-17) and **thrombopoietin** (Greek *thrombos*, clot; *poietin*, to make), and (3) **cytokines** (primarily **interleukins**).

Colony-stimulating factors are so named because they are able to stimulate committed precursor cells to grow in vitro into cell clusters or colonies. Interleukins are produced by leukocytes (mainly lymphocytes) and affect other leukocytes (paracrine mechanism) or themselves (autocrine mechanism).

Hematopoietic cells express distinct patterns of **growth factor receptors** as they differentiate. Binding of the ligand to the receptor leads to a conformational change, activation of intracellular kinases, and the final induction of cell proliferation (see Chapter 3, Cell Signaling).

We discuss the role of specific hematopoietic growth factors when we analyze each cell lineage.

Erythroid lineage

Erythropoiesis includes the following sequence (Figure 6-18): **proerythroblast**, **basophilic erythroblast**, **polychromatophilic erythroblast**, **orthochromatic erythroblast**, **reticulocyte**, and **erythrocyte.**

The major regulator of erythropoiesis is **erythropoietin (EPO)** (see Figure 6-17), a glycoprotein produced primarily (90%) in the **kidney** (juxtatubular interstitial cells in the renal cortex) in response to **hypoxia** (a decrease in oxygen level in inspired air or tissues).

Renal juxtatubular interstitial cells sense oxygen levels through **oxygen-dependent prolyl hydroxylase**, a protein that hydroxylates the transcription factor **hypoxia-inducible factor 1α** (HIF-1α) to repress the activity of the *erythropoietin* gene. Under conditions of **low oxygen tension, the hydroxylase is inactive and nonhydroxylated** HIF-1α **can drive the production of erythropoietin.**

Erythropoietin stimulates the proliferation of erythroid progenitor cells by decreasing the levels of cell cycle inhibitors and increasing cyclins and the antiapoptotic protein $Bclx_L$. Erythropoietin is also produced by neurons and glial cells in the central nervous system and in the retina. The administration of erythropoietin exerts a protective effect on neurons after ischemia (stroke).

Erythropoietin production in **chronic renal diseases** is severely impaired. Recombinant erythropoietin can be administered intravenously or subcutaneously for the treatment of anemia caused by a decrease in the production of erythropoietin by the kidney. The effectiveness of erythropoietin treatment can be monitored by an **increase of reticulocytes in circulating blood.** Reticulocytes can be identified by the supravital stain of residual polyribosomes forming a reticular network (Figure 6-19).

Polychromatophilic erythroblasts are erythropoietin-independent, mitotically active, and specifically involved in the synthesis of hemoglobin. Derived orthochromatic erythroblasts, reticulocytes, and mature RBCs are postmitotic cells (not involved in mitosis).

Leukopoiesis

Leukopoiesis (Greek *leukos,* white; *poietin,* to make) results in the formation of cells belonging to the **granulocyte** and **agranulocyte** series. The **granulocyte lineage** (Figure 6-20) includes the **myeloblast**, **promyelocyte**, **myelocyte**, **metamyelocyte**, **band cell**, and **mature form**. The granulocyte-macrophage precursor gives rise to **neutrophils** and **monocytes**. The myeloid stem cell generates **eosinophil** and **basophil progenies. Agranulocytes** include **lymphocytes** and **monocytes**.

Figure 6-17. Erythropoietin

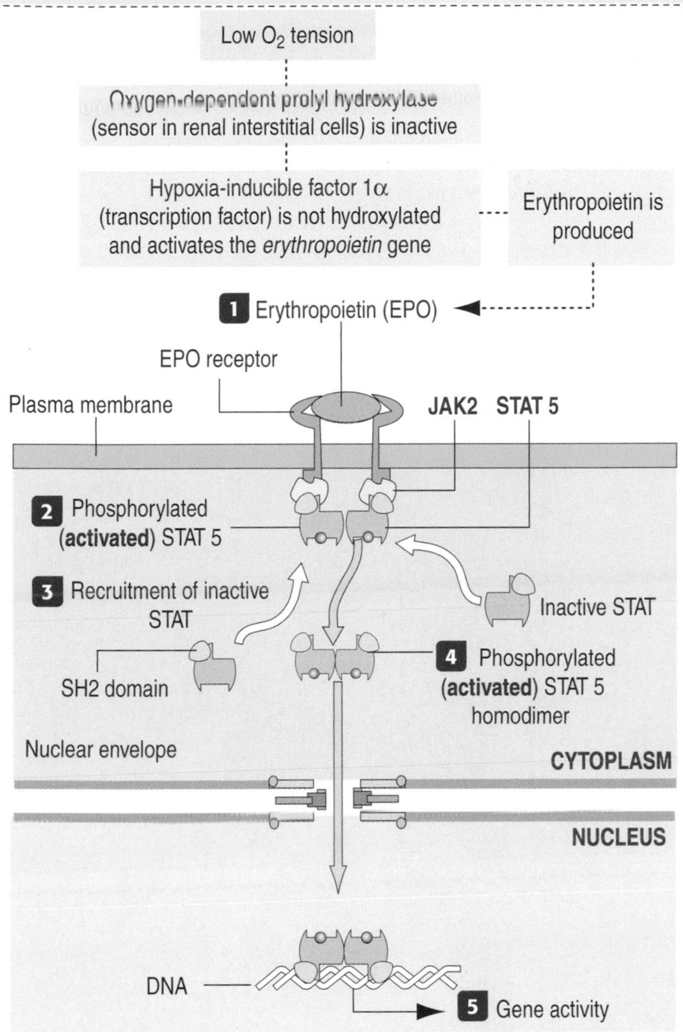

Low O_2 tension
Oxygen-dependent prolyl hydroxylase (sensor in renal interstitial cells) is inactive
Hypoxia-inducible factor 1α (transcription factor) is not hydroxylated and activates the *erythropoietin* gene
Erythropoietin is produced
1 Erythropoietin (EPO)
EPO receptor
Plasma membrane
JAK2
STAT 5
2 Phosphorylated (activated) STAT 5
3 Recruitment of inactive STAT
Inactive STAT
SH2 domain
4 Phosphorylated (activated) STAT 5 homodimer
Nuclear envelope
CYTOPLASM
NUCLEUS
DNA
5 Gene activity

Erythropoietin and the JAK-STAT signaling pathway

1 **Erythropoietin (EPO)**, produced by interstitial cells in the renal cortex, is transported to the bone marrow by the blood circulation.

2 In the bone marrow, EPO binds to the **dimerized erythropoietin receptor**, present in early stages of the **erythroid CFU progeny**, and induces binding of cytosolic **STAT 5** (signal transducers and activators of transcription 5) protein to **JAK2** (Janus kinase 2), a tyrosine kinase bound to the intracellular domain of the receptor.

3 The inactive (nonphosphorylated) form of STAT 5 contains an **SH2** (Src homology 2) domain. STAT 5 is recruited by JAK2 and binds to it through the SH2 domain. STAT 5 becomes active (phosphorylated) and homodimerizes.

4 The phosphorylated STAT 5 homodimer translocates into the nucleus.

5 After binding to DNA, the phosphorylated STAT 5 homodimer activates the transcription of specific genes required for erythropoiesis.

Granulocytes

Neutrophilic and macrophage cell lines share a common precursor cell: the granulocyte-macrophage CFU (see Figure 6-20). Eosinophils and basophils derive from independent eosinophil and basophil CFUs. Neutrophil, eosinophil, and basophil granulocytes follow a similar pattern of proliferation, differentiation, maturation, and storage in the bone marrow. Details of these processes are better recognized for neutrophils, the most abundant granulocyte in the bone marrow and blood. It takes 10 to 14 days for neutrophils to develop from early precursors, but this timing is accelerated in the presence of infections or by treatment with granulocyte colony-stimulating factor (CSF) or granulocyte-macrophage CSF (see below).

Myeloblasts, **promyelocytes**, and **myelocytes** are **mitotically dividing cells**; **metamyelocytes** and **band cells cannot divide** but continue to differentiate (see Figure 6-20). A typical feature of the maturation process of granulocytes is the appearance of **primary** (azurophilic) **granules** and **"specific"** or **secondary granules** in the cytoplasm (Figures 6-21 and 6-22).

Myeloblasts are undifferentiated cells lacking cytoplasmic granules. Promyelocytes and myelocytes display primary granules in cells of the neutrophil, eosinophil, and basophil series. **Secondary granules appear in myelocytes.** Primary granules do not transform into specific granules. Primary granules persist as such throughout the cell differentiation sequence (see Figure 6-22).

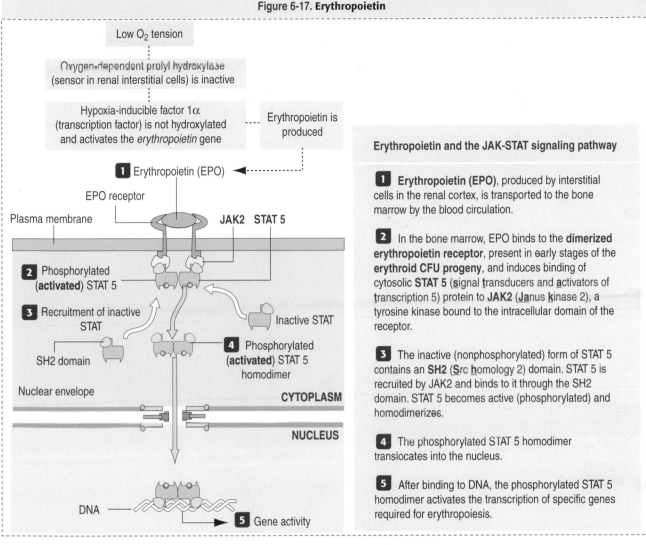

Eosinophils exhibit the same maturation sequence as neutrophils. Eosinophil-

Figure 6-18. Erythroid lineage

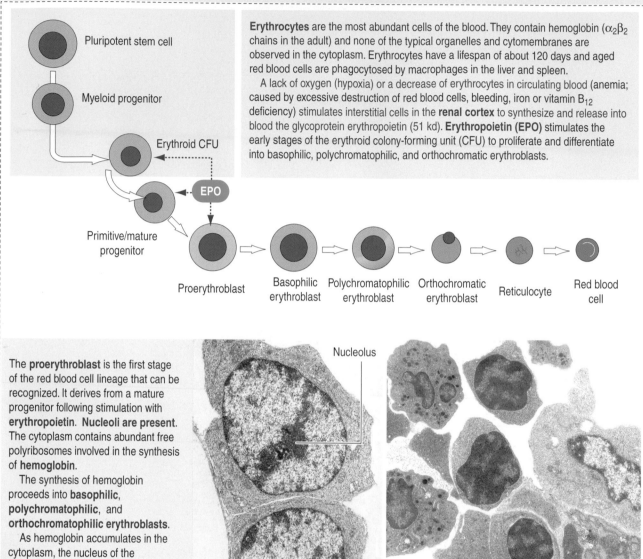

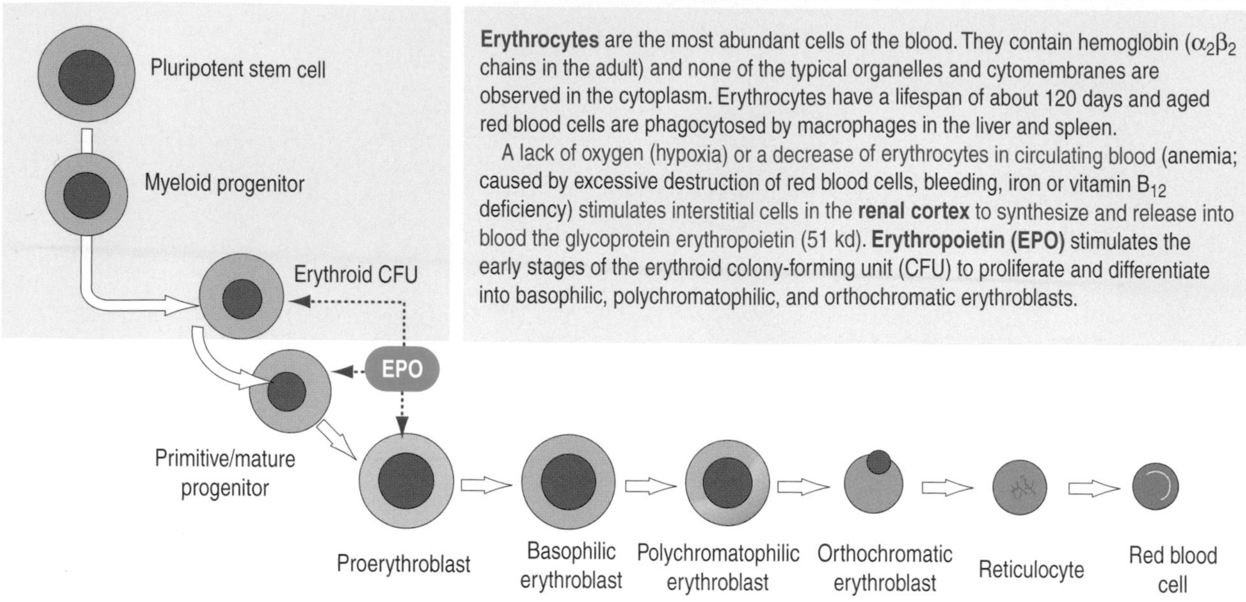

Erythrocytes are the most abundant cells of the blood. They contain hemoglobin ($\alpha_2\beta_2$ chains in the adult) and none of the typical organelles and cytomembranes are observed in the cytoplasm. Erythrocytes have a lifespan of about 120 days and aged red blood cells are phagocytosed by macrophages in the liver and spleen.

A lack of oxygen (hypoxia) or a decrease of erythrocytes in circulating blood (anemia; caused by excessive destruction of red blood cells, bleeding, iron or vitamin B_{12} deficiency) stimulates interstitial cells in the **renal cortex** to synthesize and release into blood the glycoprotein erythropoietin (51 kd). **Erythropoietin (EPO)** stimulates the early stages of the erythroid colony-forming unit (CFU) to proliferate and differentiate into basophilic, polychromatophilic, and orthochromatic erythroblasts.

The **proerythroblast** is the first stage of the red blood cell lineage that can be recognized. It derives from a mature progenitor following stimulation with **erythropoietin. Nucleoli are present.** The cytoplasm contains abundant free polyribosomes involved in the synthesis of **hemoglobin.**

The synthesis of hemoglobin proceeds into **basophilic, polychromatophilic**, and **orthochromatophilic erythroblasts.**

As hemoglobin accumulates in the cytoplasm, the nucleus of the differentiating erythroblasts is reduced in size, chromatin condenses, and free ribosomes decrease. The orthochromatophilic erythroblast displays maximum chromatin condensation.

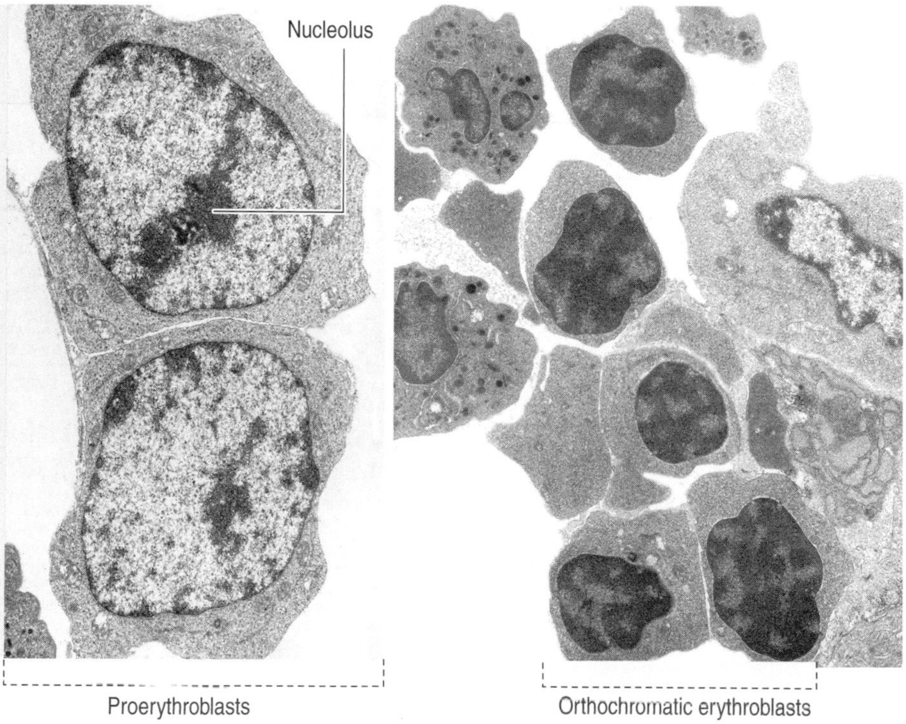

specific granules are larger than neutrophil granules and appear refractile under the light microscope. Eosinophilic granules contain **eosinophil peroxidase** (with antibacterial activity) and several cationic proteins (**major basic protein**, and **eosinophil cationic protein**, with antiparasitic activity).

Basophils are distinguished by their large, coarse, and darkly stained granules that fill the cytoplasm and often obscure the nucleus (Figure 6-23). The granules contain **peroxidase**, **heparin**, and **histamine** as well as **kallikrein**, a substance that attracts eosinophils.

We discuss in Chapter 4, Connective Tissue, that **mast cells** are structurally similar to basophils. However, mast cells are larger cells and are found in tissues,

Figure 6-19. Erythroid lineage

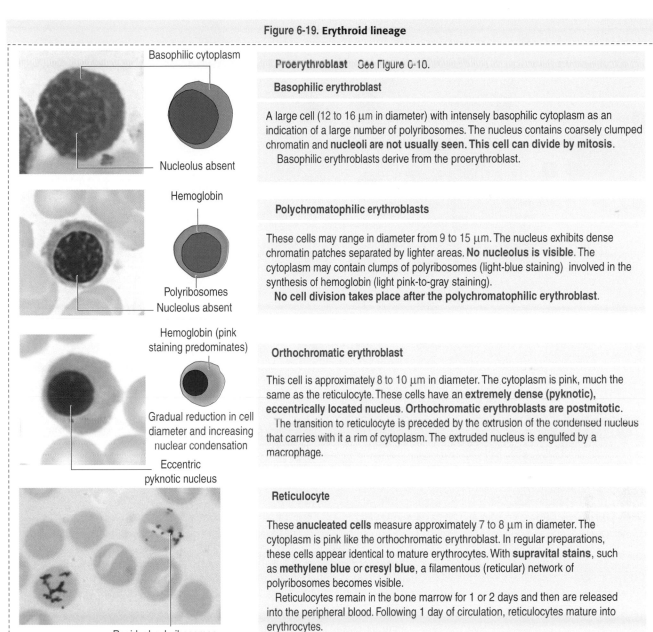

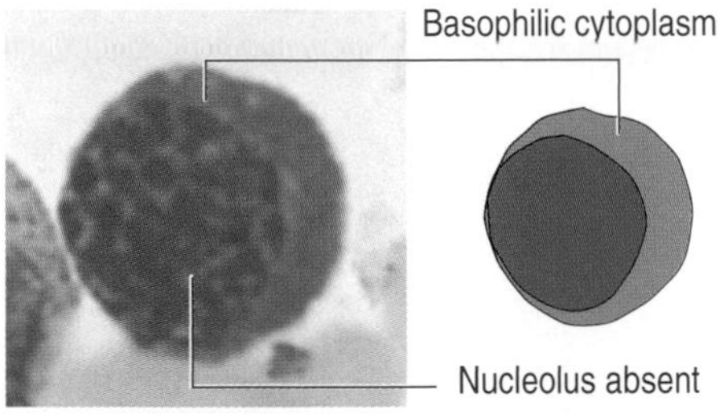
Basophilic cytoplasm
Nucleolus absent

Proerythroblast See Figure 6-18.

Basophilic erythroblast

A large cell (12 to 16 μm in diameter) with intensely basophilic cytoplasm as an indication of a large number of polyribosomes. The nucleus contains coarsely clumped chromatin and **nucleoli are not usually seen. This cell can divide by mitosis.**

Basophilic erythroblasts derive from the proerythroblast.

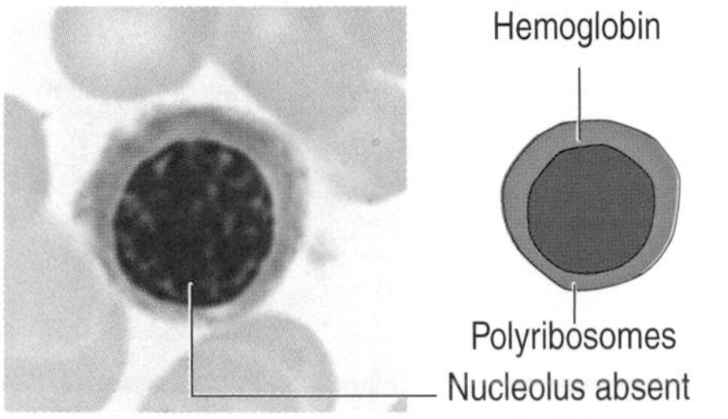
Hemoglobin
Polyribosomes
Nucleolus absent

Polychromatophilic erythroblasts

These cells may range in diameter from 9 to 15 μm. The nucleus exhibits dense chromatin patches separated by lighter areas. **No nucleolus is visible**. The cytoplasm may contain clumps of polyribosomes (light-blue staining) involved in the synthesis of hemoglobin (light pink-to-gray staining).

No cell division takes place after the polychromatophilic erythroblast.

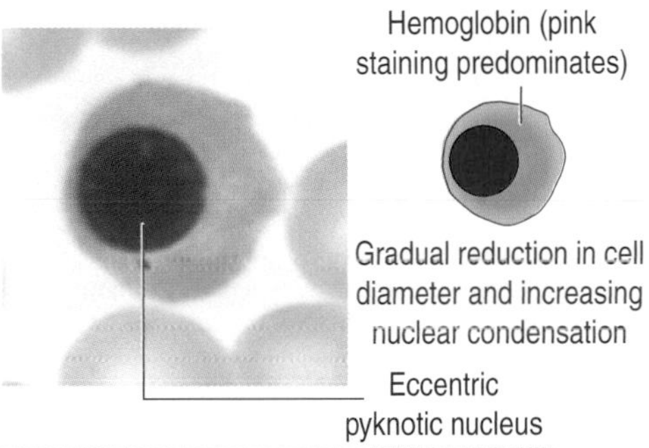
Hemoglobin (pink staining predominates)
Gradual reduction in cell diameter and increasing nuclear condensation
Eccentric pyknotic nucleus

Orthochromatic erythroblast

This cell is approximately 8 to 10 μm in diameter. The cytoplasm is pink, much the same as the reticulocyte. These cells have an **extremely dense (pyknotic), eccentrically located nucleus. Orthochromatic erythroblasts are postmitotic**.

The transition to reticulocyte is preceded by the extrusion of the condensed nucleus that carries with it a rim of cytoplasm. The extruded nucleus is engulfed by a macrophage.

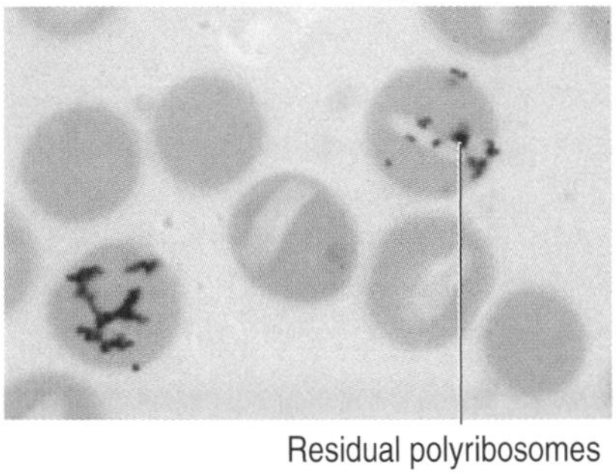
Residual polyribosomes

Reticulocyte

These **anucleated cells** measure approximately 7 to 8 μm in diameter. The cytoplasm is pink like the orthochromatic erythroblast. In regular preparations, these cells appear identical to mature erythrocytes. With **supravital stains**, such as **methylene blue** or **cresyl blue**, a filamentous (reticular) network of polyribosomes becomes visible.

Reticulocytes remain in the bone marrow for 1 or 2 days and then are released into the peripheral blood. Following 1 day of circulation, reticulocytes mature into erythrocytes.

close to blood vessels. A notable difference is that **mast cells contain serotonin and 5-hydroxytryptamine, which basophils do not contain**. In addition, mast cells discharge their granules into the extracellular space in contrast with basophils, which usually undergo diffuse internal degranulation.

Agranulocytes: Lymphocytes

Lymphocytes constitute a heterogeneous population of cells that differ from each other in terms of **origin**, **lifespan**, preferred sites of **localization within lymphoid organs**, **cell surface markers**, and **function**.

The pluripotent stem cell gives rise to all hematopoietic cells, including lymphocytes of the B and T cell lineage. **B cells mature in the bone marrow and then migrate to other lymphoid organs. T cells complete their maturation in the thymus and then migrate to specific lymphoid organs.**

A **lymphoblast** gives rise to a **prolymphocyte**, an intermediate stage that precedes the mature **lymphocyte. B and T lymphocytes are nonphagocytic cells. They are morphologically similar but functionally different**, as discussed in Chapter 10, Immune-Lymphatic System.

Figure 6-20. **Myeloid lineage**

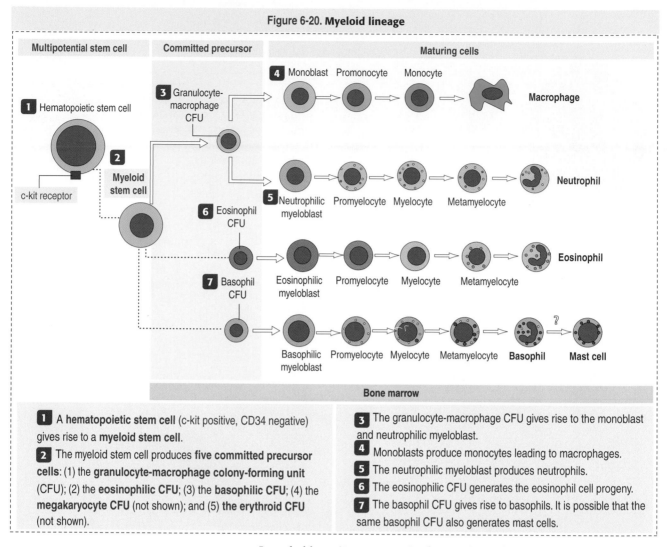

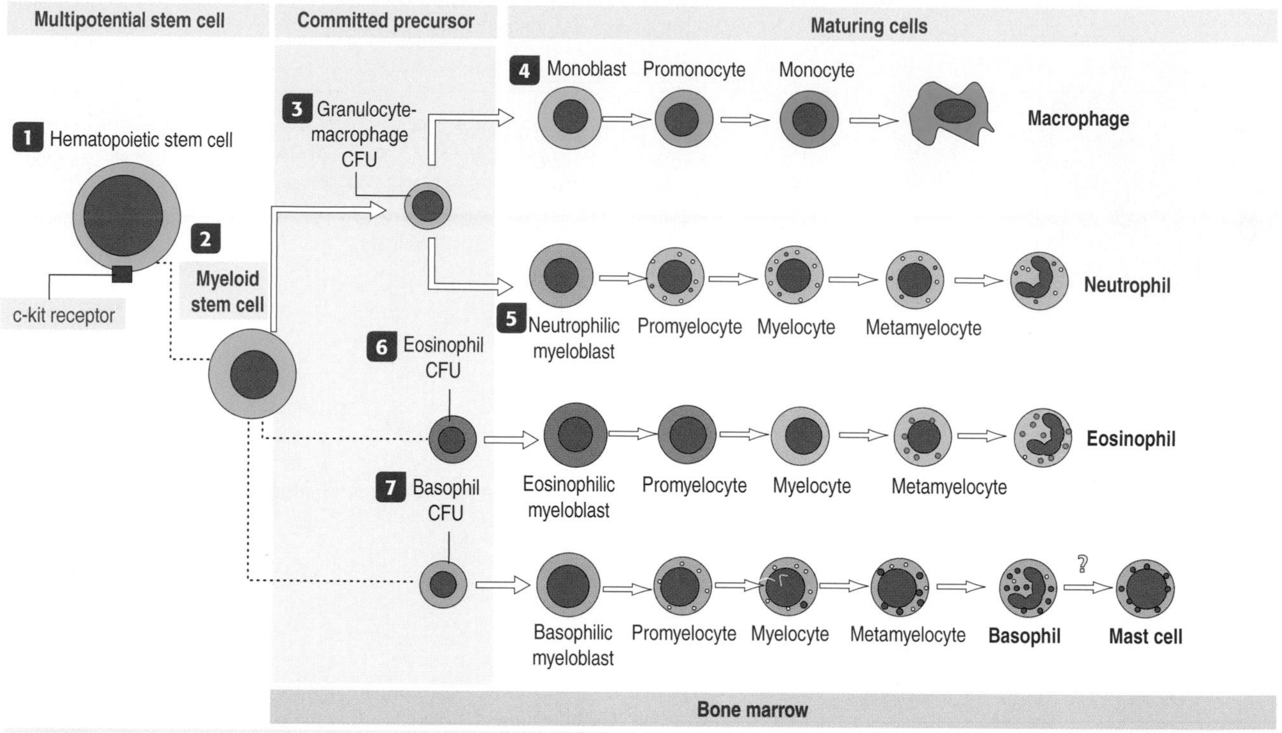

1 A **hematopoietic stem cell** (c-kit positive, CD34 negative) gives rise to a **myeloid stem cell.**

2 The myeloid stem cell produces **five committed precursor cells**: (1) the **granulocyte-macrophage colony-forming unit** (CFU); (2) the **eosinophilic CFU**; (3) the **basophilic CFU**; (4) the **megakaryocyte CFU** (not shown); and (5) **the erythroid CFU** (not shown).

3 The granulocyte-macrophage CFU gives rise to the monoblast and neutrophilic myeloblast.

4 Monoblasts produce monocytes leading to macrophages.

5 The neutrophilic myeloblast produces neutrophils.

6 The eosinophilic CFU generates the eosinophil cell progeny.

7 The basophil CFU gives rise to basophils. It is possible that the same basophil CFU also generates mast cells.

Lymphoblasts (8 to 12 μm in diameter) are the precursors of the lymphocytes. A lymphoblast has an uncondensed nucleus with a large nucleolus. The cytoplasm contains many polyribosomes and a few cisternae of the endoplasmic reticulum.

Lymphocytes (10 μm in diameter or less) contain a round or slightly indented condensed nucleus. The nucleolus is not visible. The cytoplasm is moderately basophilic and devoid of granules.

Monocytes

Monocytes derive from the **granulocyte-macrophage CFU.** We have already discussed that the granulocyte-macrophage CFU gives rise to the neutrophil lineage and the macrophage lineage. Under the influence of a specific CSF, each precursor cell establishes its own hierarchy: the granulocyte colony-stimulating factor (G-CSF) takes the granulocyte precursor cell into the **myeloblast** pathway; the granulocyte-macrophage colony-stimulating factor (GM-CSF) guides the monocyte precursor cell into the **monoblast** pathway, leading to the production of peripheral blood monocytes and tissue macrophages. Receptors for the macrophage-stimulating factor (M-CSF) are restricted to the monocyte lineage (see Osteoclastogenesis in Chapter 5, Osteogenesis).

Monoblasts (14 μm in diameter) are morphologically similar to myeloblasts. The monoblast is present in the bone marrow and is difficult to identify with certainty. The cytoplasm is basophilic and the nucleus is large and displays one or more nucleoli. The following cell in the series is the **promonocyte.**

Figure 6-21. **Myeloid lineage**

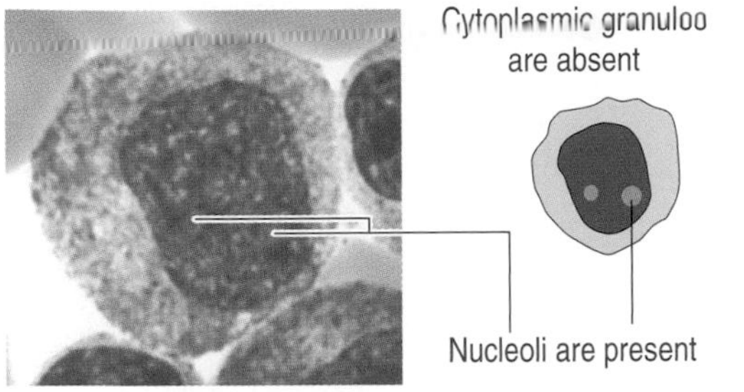

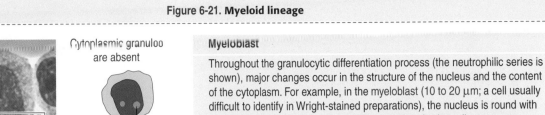

Cytoplasmic granules are absent
Nucleoli are present

Myeloblast

Throughout the granulocytic differentiation process (the neutrophilic series is shown), major changes occur in the structure of the nucleus and the content of the cytoplasm. For example, in the myeloblast (10 to 20 μm; a cell usually difficult to identify in Wright-stained preparations), the nucleus is round with uncondensed chromatin and a visible nucleolus. As the cell progresses through the subsequent stages of differentiation, the nucleus becomes indented, then segmented, and the chromatin increases its condensation. **The cytoplasm of the myeloblast is essentially granule-free.** Primary granules appear in the promyelocyte stage, while specific or secondary granules are synthesized by myelocytes.

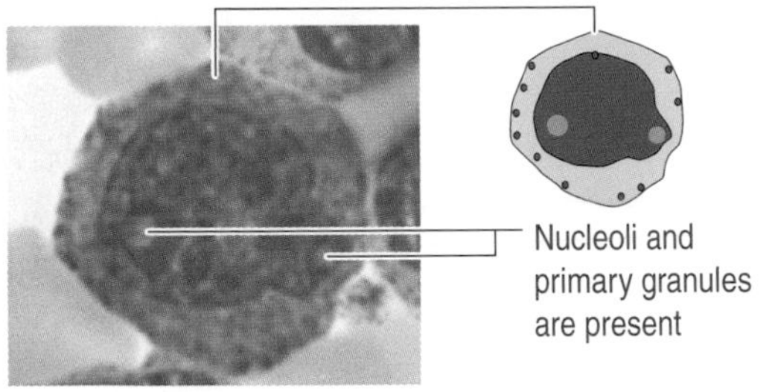

Nucleoli and primary granules are present

Promyelocyte

This cell measures approximately 15 to 20 μm in diameter. It has a large, round nucleus with uncondensed chromatin and one or more oval nucleoli. **The synthesis of primary granules, stained red or magenta, occurs exclusively at this stage.** The cytoplasm is basophilic due to the presence of abundant rough endoplasmic reticulum. **Promyelocytes give rise to neutrophilic, eosinophilic, or basophilic myelocytes.** It is not possible in conventional preparations to determine which type of granulocyte will be produced by a given promyelocyte.

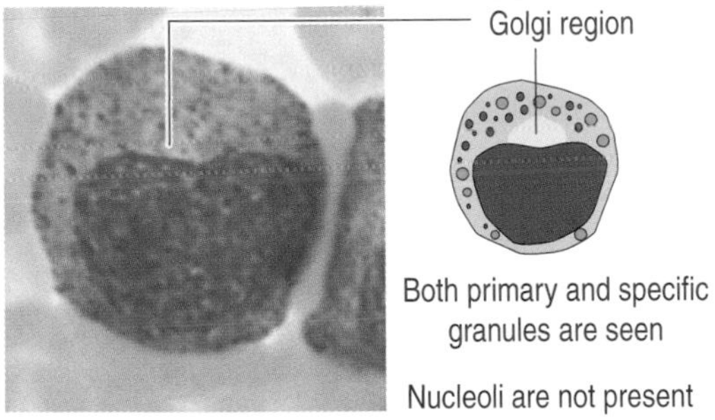

Golgi region
Both primary and specific granules are seen
Nucleoli are not present

Myelocyte

This cell, measuring 12 to 18 μm, has a round or oval nucleus that may be slightly indented; nucleoli are not present. **The basophilic cytoplasm contains primary granules produced in the promyelocyte stage as well as some specific granules, whose synthesis is detected in the myelocyte.** Consequently, the myelocyte cytoplasm begins to resemble that of the mature basophil, eosinophil, or neutrophil. The **myelocyte is the last stage capable of mitosis.** Myelocytes produce a large number of specific granules, but a finite number of primary granules (produced in the promyelocyte) are distributed among daughter myelocytes.

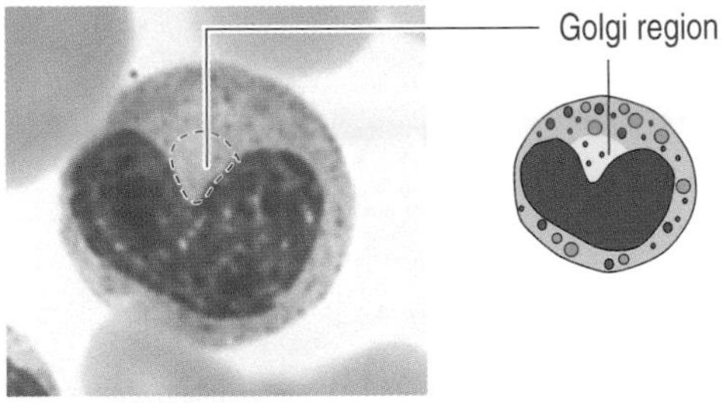

Golgi region

Metamyelocyte

This postmitotic cell measures 10 to 15 μm in diameter. The eccentric, bean-shaped nucleus now contains some condensed chromatin. The cytoplasm closely resembles that of the mature form. The specific granules outnumber the primary granules.

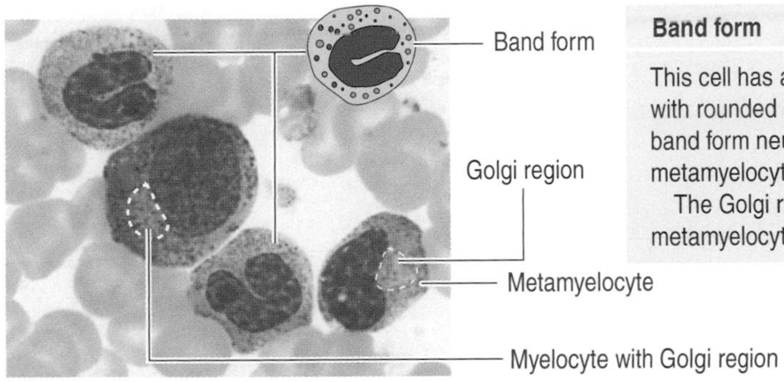

Band form
Golgi region
Metamyelocyte
Myelocyte with Golgi region

Band form

This cell has a diameter of about 9 to 15 μm. The nucleus is U-shaped with rounded ends. Its cytoplasm resembles that of the mature form. Two band form neutrophils are shown together with a myelocyte and a metamyelocyte neutrophil.

The Golgi region can be distinguished in the myelocyte and metamyelocyte.

Figure 6-22. Myeloid lineage: Cell types

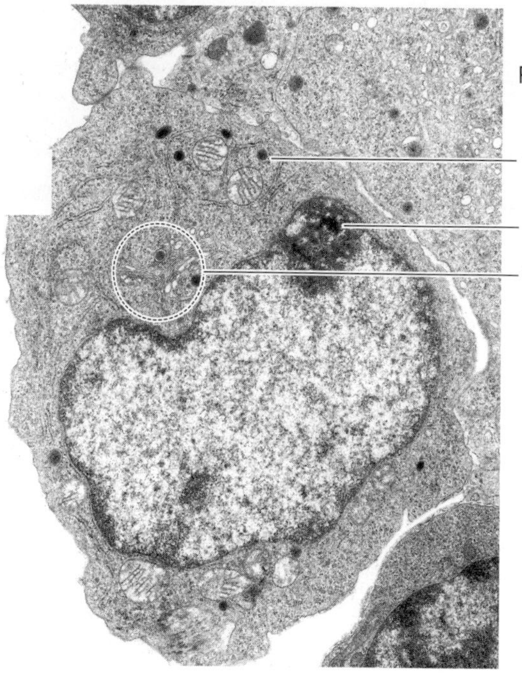

Early promyelocyte
A distinctive feature of promyelocytes is the **primary granules** (azurophilic in the neutrophilic lineage). **Several nucleolar masses** can be seen within an eccentric or central nucleus.

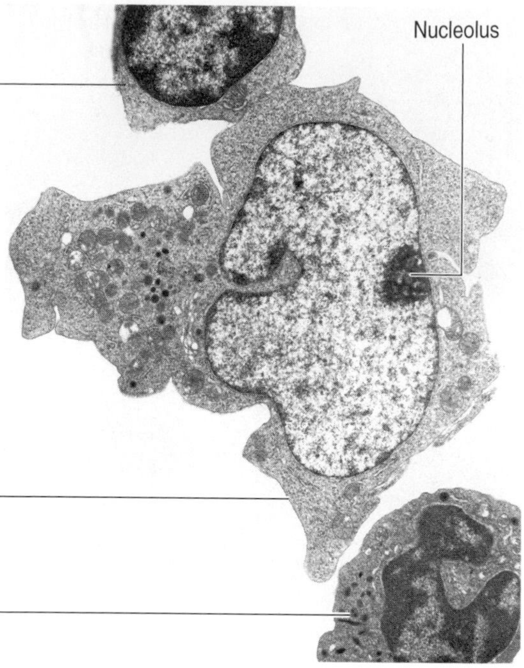

Promyelocyte
As promyelocytes advance in their development, **primary granules** become more abundant. Promyelocytes have a diameter of 15 to 20 μm, contrasting with the much smaller **band form** cell (9 to 15 μm) and polychromatophilic erythroblasts (12 to 15 μm) present in the field. A nucleolus is still visible.

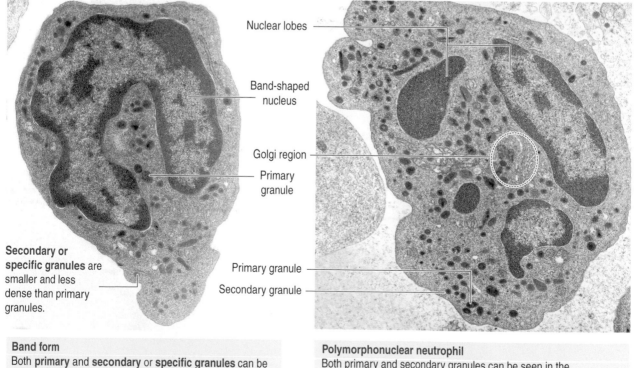

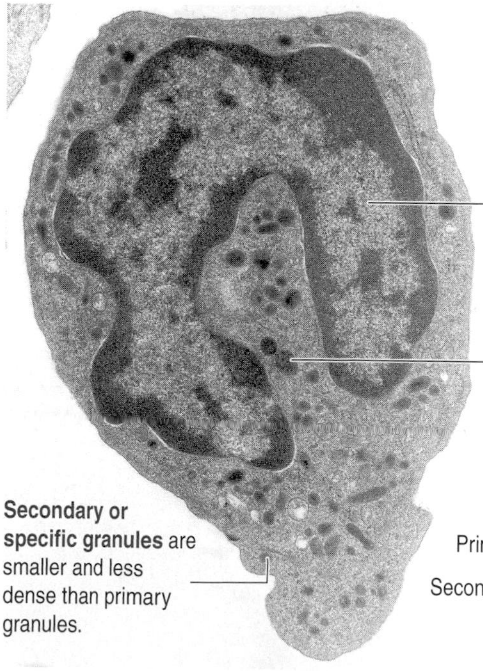

Band form
Both **primary** and **secondary** or **specific granules** can be seen in the cytoplasm of this **band form neutrophil**.

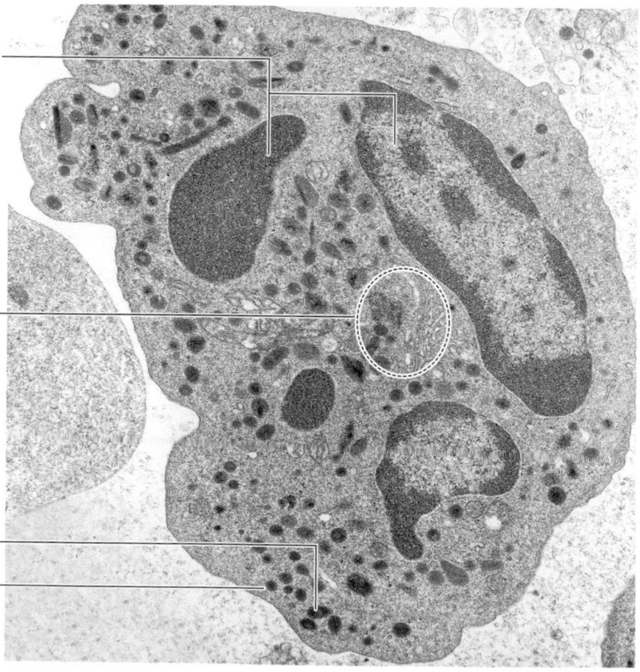

Polymorphonuclear neutrophil
Both primary and secondary granules can be seen in the cytoplasm of this cell displaying a **multilobulated nucleus**.

Figure 6-23. **Myeloid lineage: Basophil**

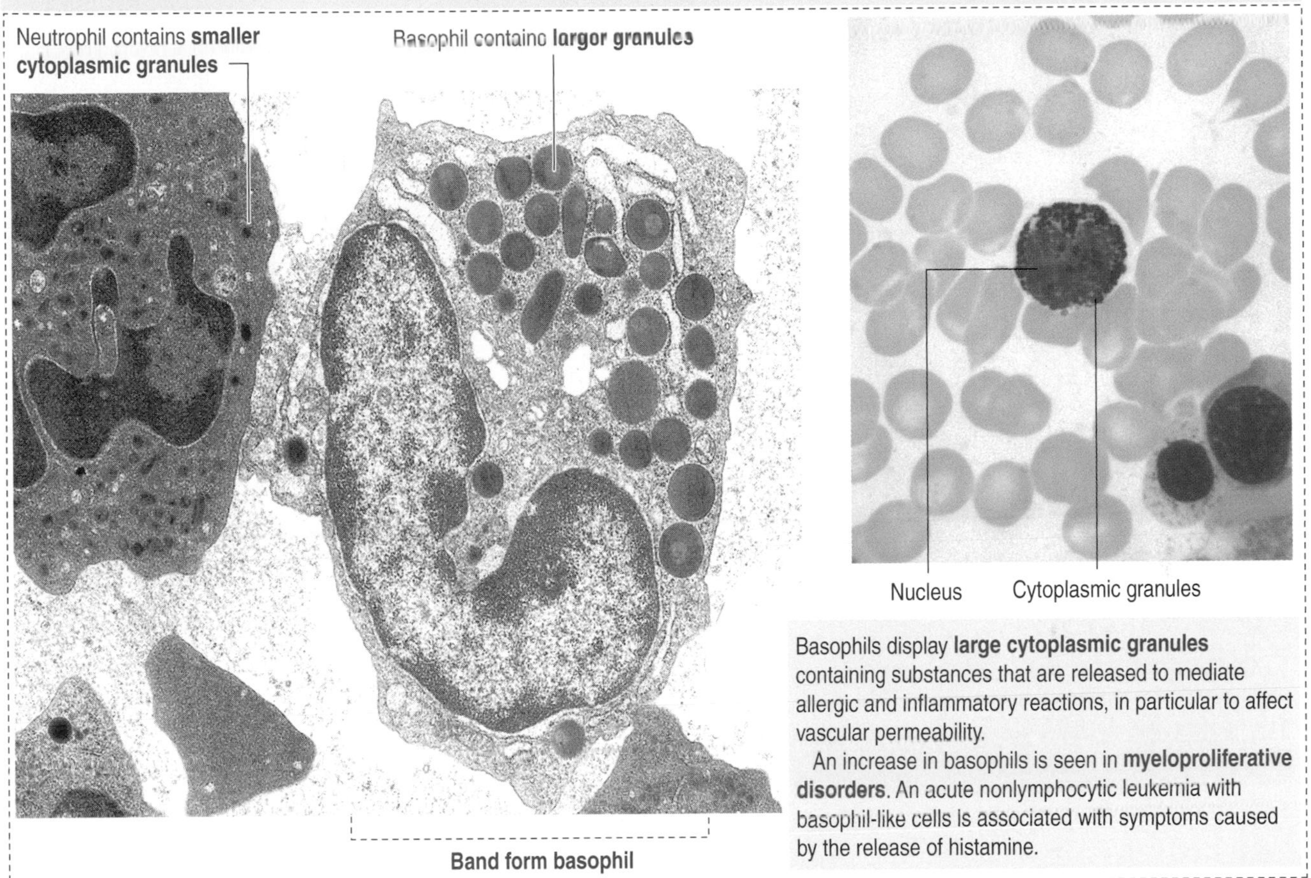

Neutrophil contains **smaller cytoplasmic granules**
Basophil contains **larger granules**
Nucleus
Cytoplasmic granules
Band form basophil

Basophils display **large cytoplasmic granules** containing substances that are released to mediate allergic and inflammatory reactions, in particular to affect vascular permeability.

An increase in basophils is seen in **myeloproliferative disorders**. An acute nonlymphocytic leukemia with basophil-like cells is associated with symptoms caused by the release of histamine.

Promonocytes (11 to 13 µm in diameter) contain a large nucleus with a slight indentation and uncondensed chromatin. A nucleolus may be visualized. The basophilic cytoplasm, due to polyribosomes, contains primary granules (lysosomes with **peroxidase**, **arylsulfatase**, and **acid phosphatase**). The primary granules are smaller and fewer than in promyelocytes. **Both monoblasts and promonocytes are mitotically active cells.**

Monocytes (12 to 20 µm in diameter) in the bone marrow and the blood have a large indented nucleus found in the central portion of the cytoplasm (Figure 6-24). Granules (**primary lysosomes**) and small vacuoles are typical features. Lysosomes lack peroxidase but contain other proteases and hydrolases. Monocytes are **motile** in response to chemotactic signals and attach to a surface.

Macrophages (15 to 80 µm in diameter) constitute a population of emigrated blood monocytes that differentiate in tissues (lung, spleen, liver, lymph node, peritoneum, gastrointestinal tract, and bone [osteoclasts]) in response to local conditions.

The structural and functional characteristics of tissue macrophages are discussed in Chapter 4, Connective Tissue. In Chapter 11, Integumentary System, we discuss the antigenic reactivity of monocyte-derived **Langerhans cells** in epidermis. In Chapter 17, Digestive Glands, we explore the important role of **Kupffer cells** in liver function, and in Chapter 10, Immune-Lymphatic System, we examine the phagocytic properties of macrophages in spleen.

Clinical significance: Colony-stimulating factors and interleukins

G-CSF is a glycoprotein produced by endothelial cells, fibroblasts, and macrophages in different parts of the body. The synthetic form of G-CSF (known as filgrastim or lenograstim) causes a dose-dependent increase of neutrophils in the blood. G-CSF is used for the treatment of **neutropenia** (neutrophil + Greek

Figure 6-24. Origin and fate of monocytes

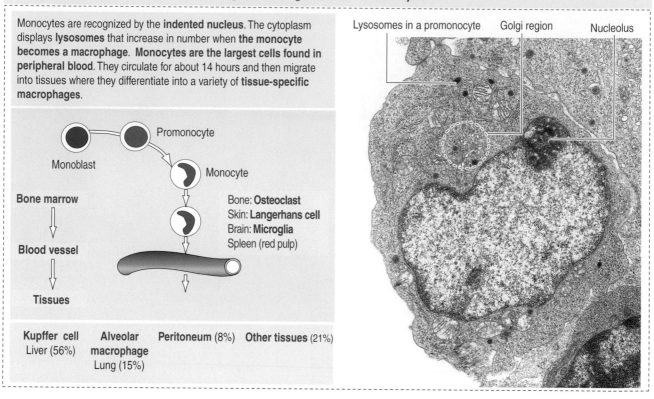

Monocytes are recognized by the **indented nucleus**. The cytoplasm displays **lysosomes** that increase in number when **the monocyte becomes a macrophage. Monocytes are the largest cells found in peripheral blood.** They circulate for about 14 hours and then migrate into tissues where they differentiate into a variety of **tissue-specific macrophages**.

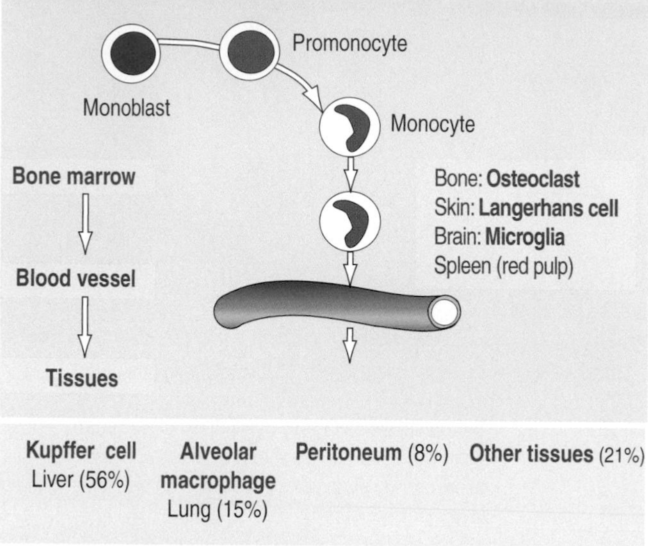

Promonocyte
Monoblast
Monocyte
Bone marrow
Blood vessel
Tissues
Bone: Osteoclast
Skin: Langerhans cell
Brain: Microglia
Spleen (red pulp)
Kupffer cell Liver (56%)
Alveolar macrophage Lung (15%)
Peritoneum (8%)
Other tissues (21%)

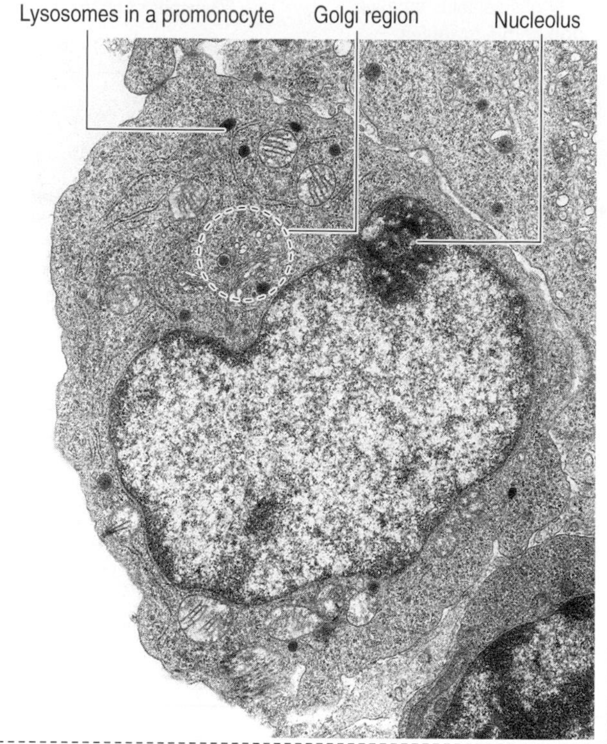

Lysosomes in a promonocyte
Golgi region
Nucleolus

penia, poverty; small numbers of neutrophils in circulating blood) after cancer chemotherapy, after bone marrow transplantation, to facilitate an increase of neutrophils, and in the treatment of chronic neutropenia.

GM-CSF is also a glycoprotein produced by endothelial cells, T cells, fibroblasts, and monocytes that stimulates the formation of neutrophils, eosinophils, basophils, monocytes, and dendritic cells (Figure 6-25). However, GM-CSF is less potent than G-CSF in increasing the levels of neutrophils during neutropenia. As is the case with G-CSF, a synthetic form of GM-CSF (sargramostim or molgramostim) is available for the treatment of neutropenia.

Interleukins have a relevant function in the formation and function of type B and T cells as we discuss in Chapter 10, Immune-Lymphatic System. IL-3 stimulates proliferation of hematopoietic stem cells and acts together with other growth factors, including stem cell factor, thrombopoietin, IL-1, IL-6, and Flt3 (fms-like tyrosine kinase 3) ligand (see Figure 6-25). IL-5 acts specifically on the eosinophil progeny.

Platelets and megakaryocytes

The precursor cell of the platelet (also called **thrombocyte**; Greek *thrombos,* clot) is the **megakaryoblast**, a cell derived from the **megakaryocyte CFU** (see Figure 6-16).

The megakaryoblast (15 to 50 μm in diameter) displays a single kidney-shaped nucleus with several nucleoli. The megakaryoblast enlarges to give rise to the **promegakaryocyte** (20 to 80 μm in diameter) with an irregularly shaped nucleus and a cytoplasm rich in azurophilic granules. The promegakaryocyte forms the mature megakaryocyte.

The **megakaryocyte** (35 to 160 μm in diameter; Figure 6-26) contains an irregularly **lobed nucleus produced by an endomitotic nuclear division process in which nuclear divisions occur without cell division (polyploid nucleus)**. Nucleoli are not detected.

The megakaryocyte can be mistaken for the osteoclast, another large cell in bone

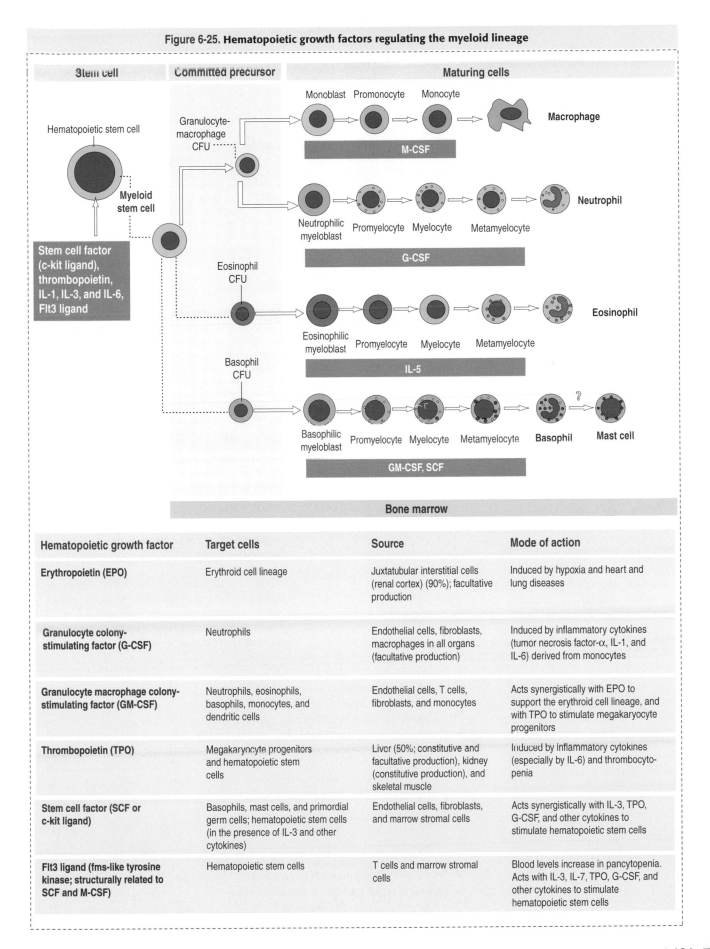

Figure 6-25. Hematopoietic growth factors regulating the myeloid lineage

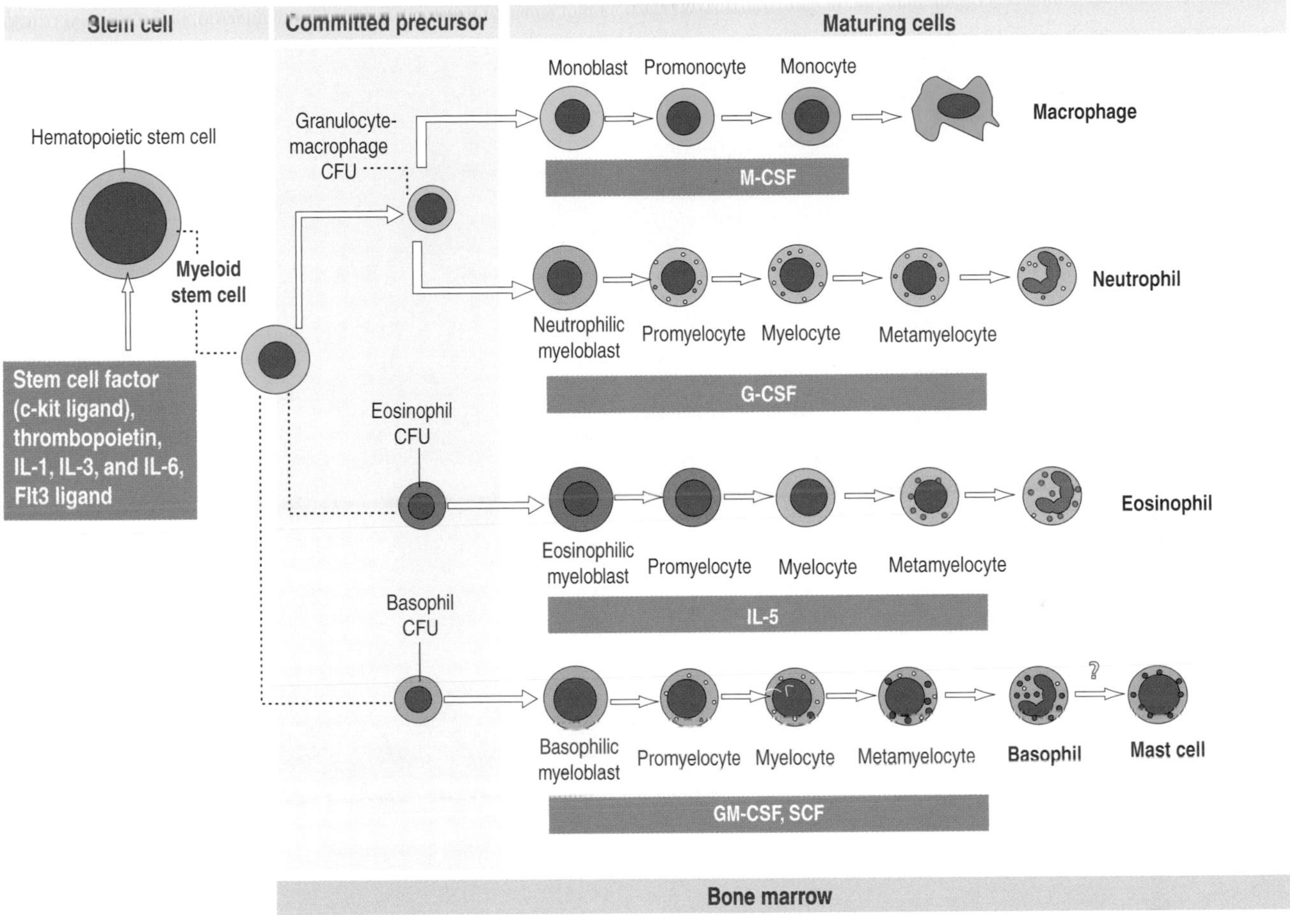

Hematopoietic growth factor	Target cells	Source	Mode of action
Erythropoietin (EPO)	Erythroid cell lineage	Juxtatubular interstitial cells (renal cortex) (90%); facultative production	Induced by hypoxia and heart and lung diseases
Granulocyte colony-stimulating factor (G-CSF)	Neutrophils	Endothelial cells, fibroblasts, macrophages in all organs (facultative production)	Induced by inflammatory cytokines (tumor necrosis factor-α, IL-1, and IL-6) derived from monocytes
Granulocyte macrophage colony-stimulating factor (GM-CSF)	Neutrophils, eosinophils, basophils, monocytes, and dendritic cells	Endothelial cells, T cells, fibroblasts, and monocytes	Acts synergistically with EPO to support the erythroid cell lineage, and with TPO to stimulate megakaryocyte progenitors
Thrombopoietin (TPO)	Megakaryocyte progenitors and hematopoietic stem cells	Liver (50%; constitutive and facultative production), kidney (constitutive production), and skeletal muscle	Induced by inflammatory cytokines (especially by IL-6) and thrombocytopenia
Stem cell factor (SCF or c-kit ligand)	Basophils, mast cells, and primordial germ cells; hematopoietic stem cells (in the presence of IL-3 and other cytokines)	Endothelial cells, fibroblasts, and marrow stromal cells	Acts synergistically with IL-3, TPO, G-CSF, and other cytokines to stimulate hematopoietic stem cells
Flt3 ligand (fms-like tyrosine kinase; structurally related to SCF and M-CSF)	Hematopoietic stem cells	T cells and marrow stromal cells	Blood levels increase in pancytopenia. Acts with IL-3, IL-7, TPO, G-CSF, and other cytokines to stimulate hematopoietic stem cells

Figure 6-26. **Megakaryocyte and the origin of platelets**

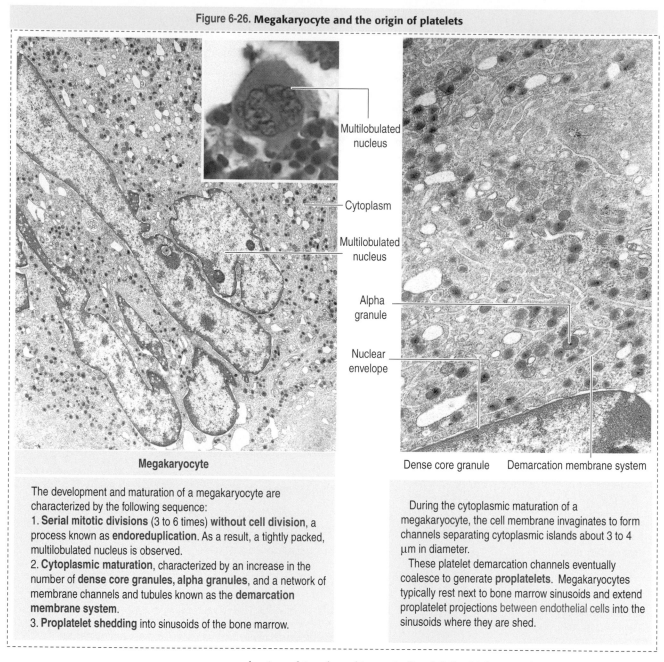

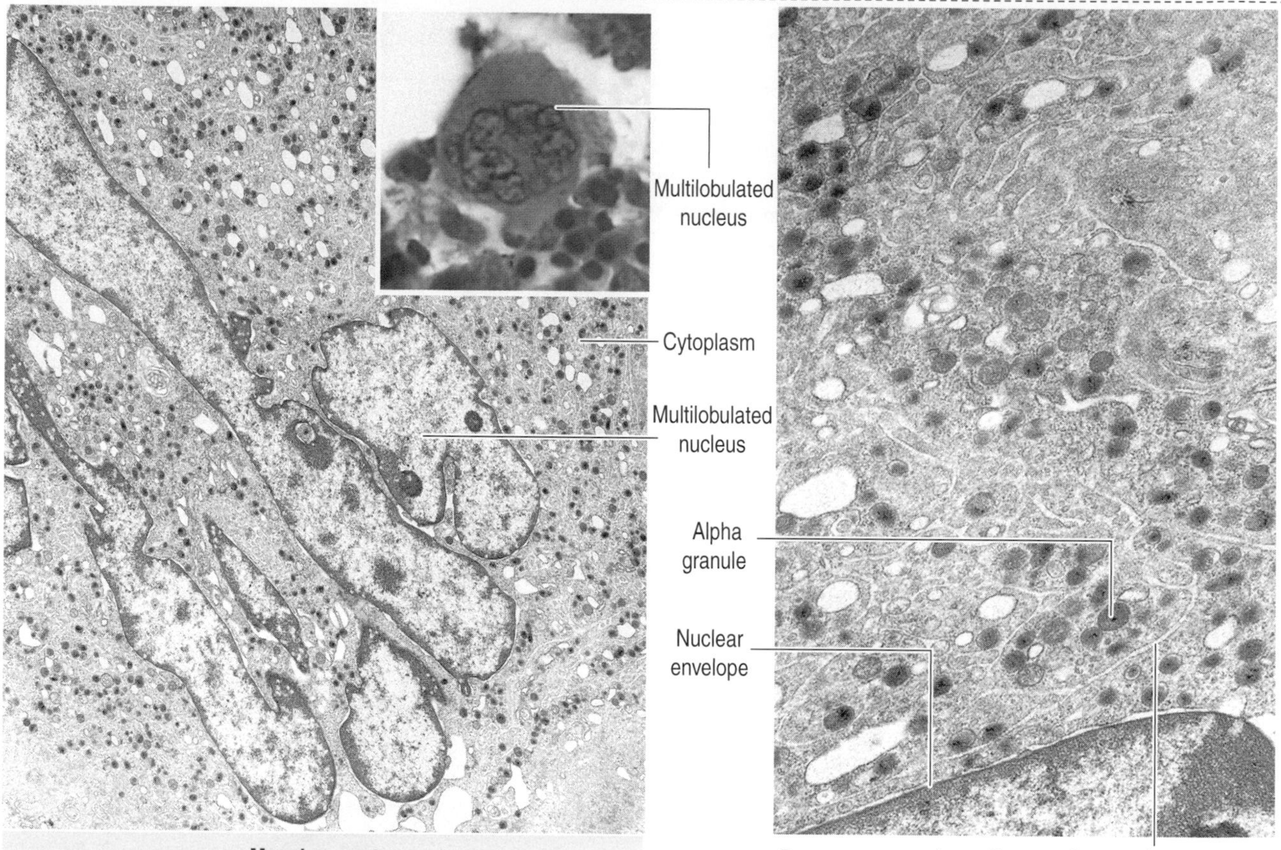
Multilobulated nucleus
Cytoplasm
Multilobulated nucleus
Alpha granule
Nuclear envelope
Megakaryocyte
Dense core granule
Demarcation membrane system

The development and maturation of a megakaryocyte are characterized by the following sequence:

1. **Serial mitotic divisions** (3 to 6 times) **without cell division**, a process known as **endoreduplication**. As a result, a tightly packed, multilobulated nucleus is observed.
2. **Cytoplasmic maturation**, characterized by an increase in the number of **dense core granules, alpha granules**, and a network of membrane channels and tubules known as the **demarcation membrane system**.
3. **Proplatelet shedding** into sinusoids of the bone marrow.

During the cytoplasmic maturation of a megakaryocyte, the cell membrane invaginates to form channels separating cytoplasmic islands about 3 to 4 μm in diameter.

These platelet demarcation channels eventually coalesce to generate **proplatelets**. Megakaryocytes typically rest next to bone marrow sinusoids and extend proplatelet projections between endothelial cells into the sinusoids where they are shed.

that is **multinucleated instead of multilobed**. The cytoplasm shows a **network of demarcation zones** formed by the invagination of the plasma membrane of the megakaryocyte. The coalescence of the demarcation membranes results in the formation of the plasma membrane of **proplatelets**, which fragment into platelets

Platelets play important roles in maintaining the integrity of blood vessels (see Figure 6-12). Keep in mind that platelet activation during hemostasis involves sequentially:

1. Platelet adhesion to the subendothelial matrix.
2. Platelet aggregation by binding to fibrinogen.
3. Platelet secretion of substances present in the granules, to recruit additional platelets.
4. Platelet procoagulant activity involving thrombin.

Clinical significance: Thrombopoietin

Thrombopoietin is produced in the **liver**, has a similar structure to erythropoietin, and stimulates the development of megakaryocytes from the megakaryocyte CFU

Figure 6-27. c-kit receptor

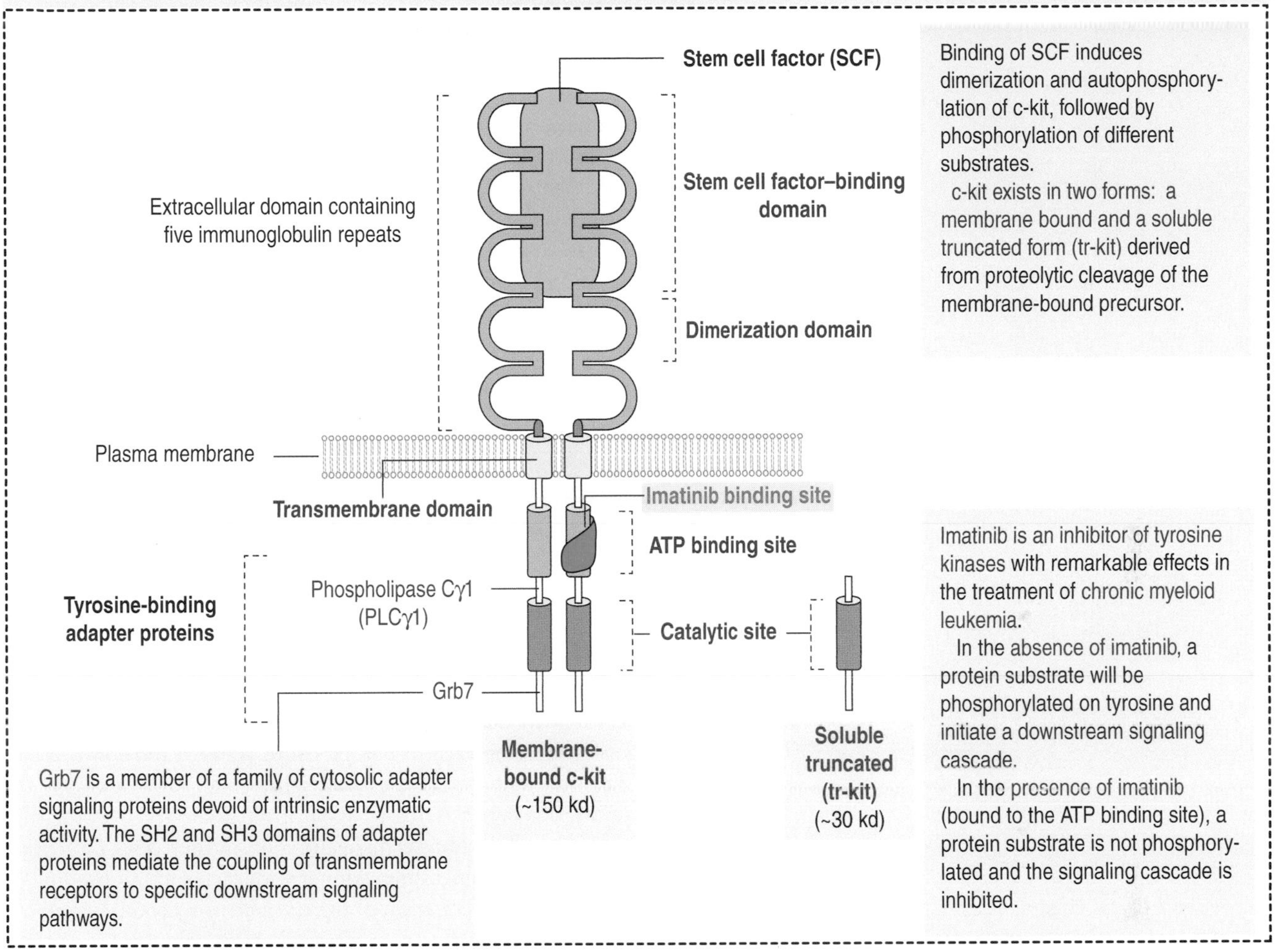
Stem cell factor (SCF)
Extracellular domain containing five immunoglobulin repeats
Stem cell factor–binding domain
Dimerization domain
Binding of SCF induces dimerization and autophosphorylation of c-kit, followed by phosphorylation of different substrates.
c-kit exists in two forms: a membrane bound and a soluble truncated form (tr-kit) derived from proteolytic cleavage of the membrane-bound precursor.
Plasma membrane
Transmembrane domain
Imatinib binding site
ATP binding site
Tyrosine-binding adapter proteins
Phospholipase Cγ1 (PLCγ1)
Catalytic site
Grb7
Imatinib is an inhibitor of tyrosine kinases with remarkable effects in the treatment of chronic myeloid leukemia.
In the absence of imatinib, a protein substrate will be phosphorylated on tyrosine and initiate a downstream signaling cascade.
In the presence of imatinib (bound to the ATP binding site), a protein substrate is not phosphorylated and the signaling cascade is inhibited.
Membrane-bound c-kit (~150 kd)
Soluble truncated (tr-kit) (~30 kd)
Grb7 is a member of a family of cytosolic adapter signaling proteins devoid of intrinsic enzymatic activity. The SH2 and SH3 domains of adapter proteins mediate the coupling of transmembrane receptors to specific downstream signaling pathways.

into platelets. Deficiencies in thrombopoietin cause **thrombocytopenia.** An excess of thrombopoietin causes **thrombocytosis.**

Platelets bind and degrade thrombopoietin, a process that autoregulates platelet production.

Clinical significance: Stem cell factor (also known as c-kit ligand)

Stem cell factor (SCF) is a ligand protein produced by fetal tissues and stromal cells of the bone marrow that binds to the stem cell factor receptor (c-kit receptor), a **tyrosine kinase.**

Stem cell factor exists in two forms: membrane-associated and soluble forms, the latter generated by proteolytic cleavage of the membrane-associated protein. The **c-kit receptor** has an **extracellular domain** consisting of five immunoglobulin motif repeats responsible for stem cell factor binding and dimerization (Figure 6-27). Binding of stem cell factor induces the dimerization of the c-kit receptor, followed by autophosphorylation. Autophosphorylated c-kit receptor is the docking site of specific signaling molecules.

The **intracellular domain** has an adenosine triphosphate (ATP) binding site and a catalytic site. The tyrosine kinase inhibitor **imatinib** binds to the ATP binding site and prevents the phosphorylation of substrates involved in the activation of downstream signaling. Imatinib shows remarkable results in the treatment of **chronic myeloid leukemia.**

The stem cell factor ligand by itself is a weak stimulator of hematopoiesis but makes hematopoietic stem cells responsive to other cytokines (see Figure 6-25). It does not induce the formation of cell colonies by itself. Flt3 (fms-like tyrosine kinase 3) ligand is closely related to c-kit receptor and stem cell factor. Similar to stem cell factor, Flt3 ligand acts on the pluripotent stem cell in synergy with thrombopoietin, stem cell factor, and interleukins.

The stem cell factor receptor is expressed by the c-kit **proto-oncogene.** A mutation in genes expressing the components of the stem cell factor receptor–ligand complex causes **anemia** and affects the **development of melanocytes in skin** and the **survival and proliferation of primordial germinal cells in the developing ovary and testis** (see Chapter 21, Sperm Transport and Maturation). Stem cell factor is potentially useful for the treatment of inherited and acquired disorders of hematopoiesis as well as in bone marrow transplantation.

In Chapter 4, Connective Tissue, we note that **mast cells** derive from a bone marrow precursor. The storage and release of histamine- and heparin-containing granules from mast cells are affected in mutants lacking stem cell factor.

Clinical significance: Transferrin and iron metabolites

In addition to erythropoietin, the formation of RBCs is highly dependent on **iron metabolism** and the water-soluble vitamins **folic acid** (folacin) and **vitamin B_{12}** (cobalamin).

Iron is involved in the transport of oxygen and carbon dioxide. Several iron-binding proteins store and transport iron, for example, **hemoglobin** in RBCs, and **myoglobin** in muscle tissue. Iron is coupled to **heme** (a molecule synthesized in the bone marrow, with one ferrous ion, Fe^{2+}, bound to a tetrapyrrolic ring) and **hematin** (with one ferric ion, Fe^{3+}, bound to a protein).

Transferrin, a serum protein produced in the liver, and **lactoferrin**, a protein present in maternal milk, are nonheme proteins involved in the **transport of iron** (Figure 6-28). Transferrin complexed to two Fe^{3+} ions is called **ferrotransferrin.** Transferrin devoid of iron is known as **apotransferrin.**

The iron-containing transferrin binds to a specific cell surface receptor that mediates the internalization of the transferrin ligand–transferrin receptor complex. The transferrin receptor is a transmembrane dimer with each subunit binding to a transferrin molecule. The internalization of the transferrin-receptor complex is dependent on receptor phosphorylation triggered by Ca^{2+}-calmodulin and the protein kinase C complex.

Inside the cell, iron is released within the acidic endosomal compartment and the **receptor-apotransferrin** (iron-free) complex returns to the cell surface where apotransferrin is released to be reutilized in blood plasma.

Ferritin, a major protein synthesized in the liver, is involved in the **storage of**

Figure 6-28. Uptake of iron by internalization of transferrin

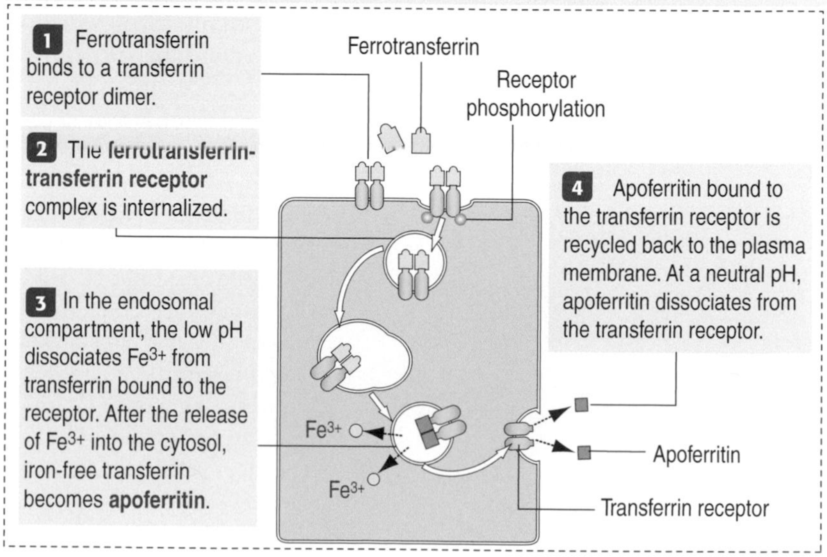

1 Ferrotransferrin binds to a transferrin receptor dimer.
2 The ferrotransferrin-transferrin receptor complex is internalized.
3 In the endosomal compartment, the low pH dissociates Fe3+ from transferrin bound to the receptor. After the release of Fe3+ into the cytosol, iron-free transferrin becomes apoferritin.
4 Apoferritin bound to the transferrin receptor is recycled back to the plasma membrane. At a neutral pH, apoferritin dissociates from the transferrin receptor.
Ferrotransferrin
Receptor phosphorylation
Fe3+
Fe3+
Apoferritin
Transferrin receptor

iron. A single ferritin molecule has the capacity to store up to 4500 iron ions. When the storage capacity of ferritin is exceeded, iron is deposited as **hemosiderin**. Ferritin with little iron is called **apoferritin**.

Patients with the heritable disorder **idiopathic hemochromatosis**, characterized by excessive iron absorption and tissue deposits, require periodic withdrawals of blood and the administration of **iron chelators** to facilitate the excretion of complexed iron in the urine. A **decrease in iron** by excessive menstrual flow or gastrointestinal bleeding determines a reduction in hemoglobin-containing iron. RBCs are smaller (**microcytic anemia**) and underpigmented (**hypochromic anemia**).

Folic acid regulates the **folate metabolism** leading to the increased availability of purines and deoxythymidine monophosphate (dTMP) required for DNA synthesis.

Vitamin B_{12} (known as **extrinsic factor**) binds to **intrinsic factor**, a protein produced by the parietal cells in the gastric glands. The vitamin B_{12}–intrinsic factor complex binds to specific receptor sites in the **ileum**, transported across enterocytes, and released in blood, where it binds to the transport protein *trans*-cobalaphilin III.

A decrease in vitamin B_{12}, due mainly to insufficient production of intrinsic factor or hydrochloric acid in the stomach, or both, can affect folate metabolism and folate uptake, thereby impairing DNA synthesis in bone marrow.

Vitamin B_{12} deficiency is rare because the liver stores up to a 6-year supply of vitamin B_{12}. Under deficiency conditions, the maturation of the erythroid cell progeny slows down, causing abnormally large RBCs (**megaloblasts**) with fragile cell membranes, resulting in the destruction of RBCs (**megaloblastic anemia**; see Box 6-E).

Box 6-E | Anemias

- **Anemia** is a reduction in the mass of circulating red blood cells. It is detected by analysis of peripheral blood (low hemoglobin, low red blood cell count, and low hematocrit). Anemia results in the lack of oxygen-carrying capacity, which is compensated for by a reduction in the affinity of hemoglobin for oxygen, an increase in cardiac output, and an attempt to increase red blood cell production. The most common cause of anemia is **iron deficiency** (low intake, chronic blood loss, or increased demand during pregnancy and lactation).
- Deficiency in **vitamin B_{12}** and **folic acid** causes **megaloblastic anemia**. This form of anemia is associated with the development of abnormally large red blood cell precursors (**megaloblasts**) that develop into large red blood cells (**macrocytes**). Vitamin B_{12} is normally absorbed in the small intestine after binding to **intrinsic factor**, a glycoprotein secreted by **gastric parietal cells**.

The lack of production of **intrinsic factor** (due to autoimmune atrophic gastritis, or after surgical gastrectomy) results in **pernicious anemia**.

Essential concepts | Blood and Hematopoiesis

- Blood is a specialized connective tissue consisting of plasma (an equivalent to extracellular matrix) and cells. Plasma contains proteins, salts, and organic compounds. Plasma contains fibrinogen; serum, the fluid after blood coagulation, is fibrinogen-free. The cellular elements of the blood are red blood cells (RBCs or erythrocytes) and leukocytes (white blood cells). Platelets are fragments of megakaryocytes.

- RBCs (4 to 6 × 10^6/mm^3; 7.8 μm in diameter) are non-nucleated cells containing hemoglobin, a heme protein involved in the transport of oxygen and carbon dioxide. The plasma membrane contains a cytoskeleton consisting of glycophorin and anion transporter channel (band 3), two transmembrane proteins. The protein ankyrin anchors spectrin, a spectin α–spectrin β dimeric protein, to band 3. Spectrin tetramers are linked to a complex of three proteins: F-actin, tropomyosin, and protein 4.1. Adducin is a calmodulin-binding protein that favors the association of F-actin to spectrin.

Elliptocytosis (caused by defective self-assembly of spectrin, abnormal binding of spectrin to ankyrin, and abnormal protein 4.1 and glycophorin) and **spherocytosis** (caused by spectrin deficiency) are alterations in the shape of RBCs. Anemia, jaundice, and splenomegaly are clinical features. **Sickle cell anemia** (glutamic acid replaced by valine in the β-globin chain) and **thalassemia** (defective globin α or β chains in hemoglobin) are caused by hemoglobin defects. **Chronic hemolytic anemia** is a clinical feature of the two conditions.

Erythroblastosis fetalis is an antibody-induced hemolytic disease in the newborn caused by Rh incompatibility between mother and fetus. The Rh-negative mother makes antibodies to D antigen present on the surface of fetal RBCs. During a second or third pregnancy, anti-D antigen antibodies cause hemolysis of fetal RBCs. Anemia and severe jaundice (which causes damage to the brain, a condition known as kernicterus) are clinical manifestations of the fetus.

- Leukocytes (6 to 10 × 10^3/mm^3) are classified as granulocytes (with primary, and specific or secondary cytoplasmic granules) and agranulocytes (containing only primary granules).

There are three types of granulocytes: (1) neutrophils (5 ×10^3/mm^3), (2) eosinophils (1.5 × 10^2/mm^3), and (3) basophils (0.3 × 10^2/mm^3).

Neutrophils (12 to 15 μm in diameter) have the following characteristics: (1) They contain primary granules (elastase and myeloperoxidase), and secondary granules (lysozyme and other proteases). (2) They enter a blood vessel by diapedesis and leave blood circulation by the mechanism of homing. (3) The nuclei are segmented (polymorphonucleated cell).

Eosinophils (12 to 15 μm in diameter) have the following features: (1) Cytoplasmic granules contain eosinophil peroxidase (binds to microorganisms to be phagocytosed by macrophages), major basic protein (MBP; a crystalline protein that disrupts the membrane of parasites), and eosinophilic cationic protein (works with MBP to fragment parasites). (2) They participate in allergic reactions. (3) They have a bilobed nucleus with refractile red cytoplasmic granules. Eosinophils and mast cells interact in **asthma**, a condition that causes obstruction of the small-caliber bronchi and bronchioles due to mucus hypersecretion and smooth muscle bronchial constriction.

Basophils (9 to12 μm in diameter) have the following features: (1) metachromatic coarse cytoplasmic granules and bilobed nucleus. (2) Similar to mast cells, basophils participate in allergic reactions. (3) They may leave blood circulation and enter the connective tissue.

There are two types of agranulocytes: lymphocytes and monocytes.

Lymphocytes are either large lymphocytes (9 to 12 μm in diameter) or small lymphocytes (6 to 8 μm in diameter). Lymphocytes are divided into two categories: B lymphocytes (or B cells; originate and differentiate in bone marrow), and T lymphocytes (or T cells; originate in bone marrow but differentiate in thymus).

Monocytes (12 to 20 μm in diameter). Monocytes circulate in blood for 12 to 100 hours before entering the connective tissue to become macrophages. Monocytes become osteoclasts in bone under the influence of osteoblasts.

• **Homing** is the mechanism by which neutrophils, lymphocytes, monocytes, and other cells circulating in blood leave a blood vessel to enter the connective tissue or a lymphoid organ or tissue. Homing occurs in two steps: (1) selectin-mediated attachment and rolling of a cell on the surface of an endothelial cell, and (2) integrin-mediated transendothelial migration of the cell. Homing plays a significant role in immune and inflammatory reactions, metastasis, and tissue morphogenesis. A defect in the integrin β subunit, the cause of **leukocyte adhesion deficiency I**, prevents migration of leukocytes and defects in wound healing and persistence of inflammation are seen. A defect in carbohydrate ligands for selectins, the cause of **leukocyte adhesion deficiency II**, results in chronic inflammation due to recurrent infections.

• Platelets (3×10^5/mm^3; 2 to 4 μm in diameter) are cytoplasmic fragment of mekagaryocytes, cells stimulated by thrombopoietin. Cytoplasmic projections, called proplatelets, enter blood circulation and fragment into platelets. A platelet has a central region, called a granulomere (containing alpha granules, lysosomes, mitochondria, and dense core granules), and a peripheral region, called a hyalomere (with microtubules and microfilaments and an open canalicular system). The surface of the platelet displays Gp1b receptor and von Willebrand factor (two molecules involved in blood clotting). Deficiency of these two proteins, and factors of the blood clotting cascade, causes **bleeding disorders** (Gp1b receptor–factor IX: **Bernard-Soulier syndrome**; von Willebrand factor–factor VIII: **von Willebrand disease**).

Thrombocytosis is an increase in circulating platelets. **Thrombocytopenia** is a reduction in the number of platelets (less than 1.5×10^5/mm^3) circulating in blood. **Autoimmune thrombocytopenic purpura** (ITP) is caused by antibodies targeting platelets or megakaryocytes, or drugs (penicillin, sulfonamides, and digoxin). **Thrombotic thrombocytopenic purpura** (TTP) is determined by pathologic changes in endothelial cells producing procoagulant substances. This condition leads to the aggregation of platelets in small blood vessels.

• Blood clotting or hemostasis. The process involves the conversion of proenzymes (designated factor X) to active enzymes (designated factor Xa) by proteolysis. It is characterized by an extrinsic pathway (initiated by damage outside a blood vessel), and an intrinsic pathway (initiated by damage inside a blood vessel, usually the wall of the vessel). Extrinsic and intrinsic pathways converge to a common pathway in which fibrinogen is converted to fibrin and platelets begin to attach to the fibrin mesh.

• Hematopoiesis is the formation of blood cells in the bone marrow (adult). The bone marrow consists of two compartments: (1) the marrow stromal compartment (the source of hematopoietic growth factors; it consists of adipose cells, fibroblasts, stromal cells, vascular endothelial cells, macrophages, and blood vessels), and (2) the hematopoietic cell compartment (the parenchyma; the site where erythroid, myeloid, lymphoid and megakaryoblast progenies develop).

Hematopoietic cell populations. The bone marrow consists of: (1) the hematopoietic stem cells, capable of self-renewal, (2) committed precursor cells (to produce distinct cell lineages), and (3) maturing cells (differentiating cells derived from committed precursor cells).

The hematopoietic stem cell gives rise to the myeloid stem cell and the lymphoid stem cell.

The myeloid stem cell generates five colony-forming units (CFU): (1) erythroid CFU, (2) megakaryocyte CFU, (3) basophil CFU, (4) eosinophil CFU, and (5) granulocyte-macrophage CFU. The granulocyte-macrophage CFU gives rise to neutrophils and monocytes.

The proliferation and maturation of the CFU is controlled by hematopoietic growth factors (called hematopoietic cytokines) produced by cells of the marrow stromal compartment and outside the bone marrow. There are three major groups of hematopoietic growth factors: (1) colony-stimulating factors (CSF), (2) erythropoietin (EPO), and (3) cytokines (mainly interleukins).

• Erythroid lineage. It consists of the following sequence: proerythroblast, basophilic erythroblast, polychromatophilic erythroblast, orthochromatic erythroblast, reticulocyte, and erythrocyte. EPO is the major regulator; it stimulates the erythroid CFU cell, derived cell (called mature or primitive progenitor), and proerythroblast. EPO is produced by interstitial cells of the renal cortex.

• Leukopoiesis is the development of cells of the granulocyte (neutrophil, basophil, and eosinophil) and agranulocyte (lymphocyte and monocyte) lineage. The granulocyte lineage consists of the following sequence: myeloblast, promyelocyte, myelocyte, metamyelocyte, band cell, and mature form.

A characteristic of granulocytes is the appearance in the cytoplasm of primary (azurophilic) granules (promyelocyte and myelocyte) followed by secondary or specific granules (from myelocyte on). Primary granules coexist with secondary or specific granules.

Agranulocytes. The lymphocyte lineage follows two routes: (1) B cells originate and mature in bone marrow. (2) T cells originate in bone marrow and mature in thymus. A lymphoblast gives rise to a prolymphocyte, which matures as a lymphocyte. B and T cells are morphologically similar but functionally different. The monocyte lineage derives from the granulocyte-macrophage CFU. A monoblast gives rise to a promonocyte; the final stage is monocyte, which differentiates in connective tissue into macrophage, and in bone differentiates into osteoclast.

Agranulocytes contain primary granules (lysosomes).

• CSF and interleukins. G-CSF stimulates the development of neutrophils. GM-CSF stimulates the formation of neutrophils, eosinophils, basophils, monocytes, and dendritic cells (present in lymphoid organs and lymphoid tissues). Interleukins have an important role in the development and function of the lymphoid lineage. Interleukins act synergistically with CSF, SCF, and Flt3 ligand to stimulate the development of the hematopoietic stem cells. Review additional details in Figure 6-25.

• Transferrin and iron metabolites, folic acid, and vitamin B_{12} are required, in addition to EPO, for the formation of RBCs. Iron, coupled to heme, is present in hemoglobin and myoglobin (muscle tissue).

Transferrin is produced in liver by hepatocytes. Transferrin complexed to two iron ions is called ferrotransferrin. Transferrin without iron ions is called apotransferrin. Ferritin is produced by hepatocytes to store iron. Apoferritin is ferritin with little iron.

Patients with **idiopathic hemochromatosis** absorb and deposit an excess of iron in tissues. A decrease in iron by excessive menstrual flow or gastrointestinal bleeding results in small RBCs (**microcytic anemia**).

Vitamin B_{12} (extrinsic factor) binds to intrinsic factor (produced by parietal cells in the stomach). The vitamin B_{12}–intrinsic factor complex binds to a specific receptor site in the ileum (small intestine), absorbed by enterocytes, and released into the bloodstream, where it binds to *trans*-cobalaphilin III, a transport protein. **Megaloblastic anemia** occurs when there is a deficiency of folate and vitamin B_{12}.

7. MUSCLE TISSUE

Muscle is one of the four basic tissues. There are three types of muscle: **skeletal**, **cardiac**, and **smooth**. All three types are composed of elongated cells, called **muscle cells**, **myofibers**, or **muscle fibers**, specialized for contraction. In all three types of muscle, energy from the hydrolysis of adenosine triphosphate (ATP) is transformed into mechanical energy.

Skeletal muscle

Muscle cells or fibers form a long multinucleated syncytium grouped in bundles surrounded by connective tissue sheaths and extending from the site of origin to their insertion (Figure 7-1). The **epimysium** is a dense connective tissue layer ensheathing the **entire muscle**. The **perimysium** derives from the epimysium and surrounds bundles or **fascicles** of muscle cells. The **endomysium** is a delicate layer of reticular fibers and extracellular matrix surrounding **each muscle cell**. Blood vessels and nerves use these connective tissue sheaths to reach the interior of the muscle. An extensive capillary network, flexible to adjust to contraction-relaxation changes, invests individual skeletal muscle cell.

The connective tissue sheaths blend and radiating-muscle fascicles interdigitate at each end of a muscle with regular dense connective tissue of the tendon to form a **myotendinous junction**. The tendon anchors into a bone through the periosteal Sharpey's fibers.

Characteristics of the skeletal muscle cell or fiber

Skeletal muscle cells are formed in the embryo by the fusion of myoblasts that produce a postmitotic, multinucleated **myotube**. The myotube matures into the long muscle cell with a diameter of 10 to 100 μm and a length up to several centimeters.

Figure 7-1. **General organization of the skeletal muscle**

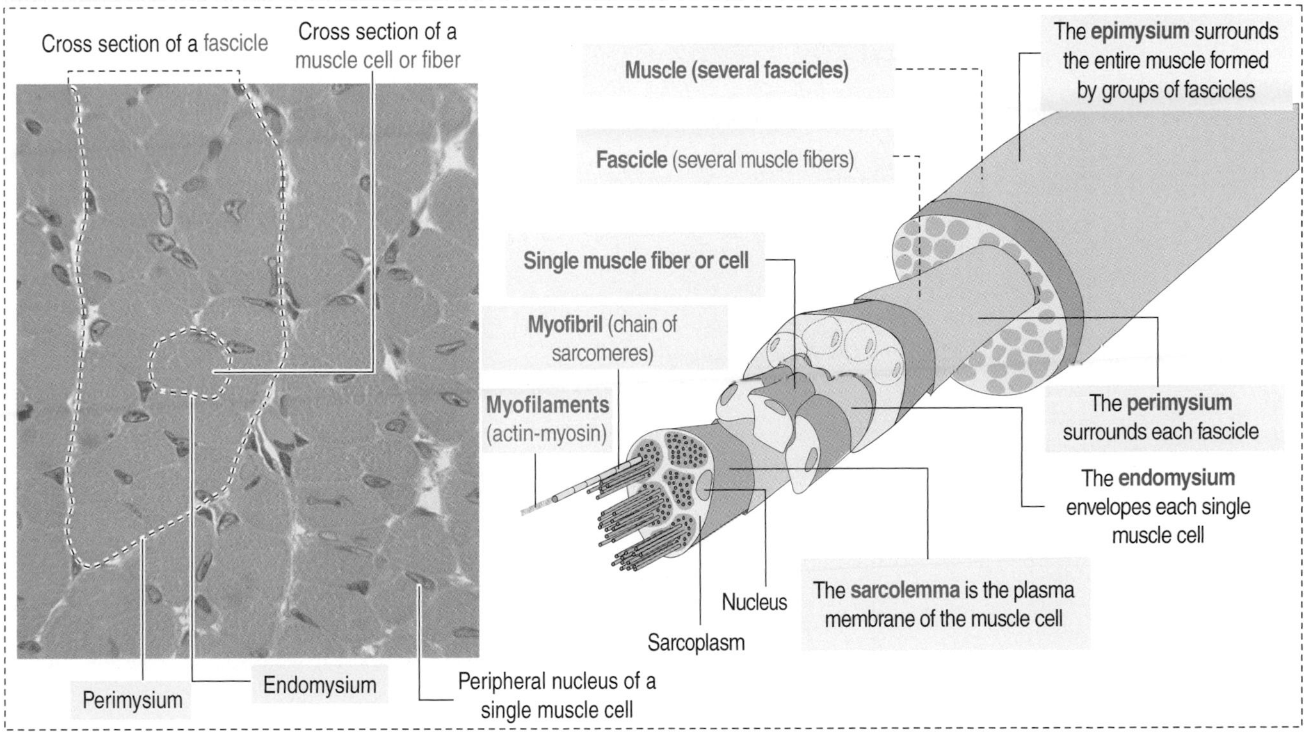

Cross section of a fascicle
Cross section of a muscle cell or fiber
Perimysium
Endomysium
Peripheral nucleus of a single muscle cell
Muscle (several fascicles)
Fascicle (several muscle fibers)
Single muscle fiber or cell
Myofibril (chain of sarcomeres)
Myofilaments (actin-myosin)
The epimysium surrounds the entire muscle formed by groups of fascicles
The perimysium surrounds each fascicle
The endomysium envelopes each single muscle cell
The sarcolemma is the plasma membrane of the muscle cell
Nucleus
Sarcoplasm

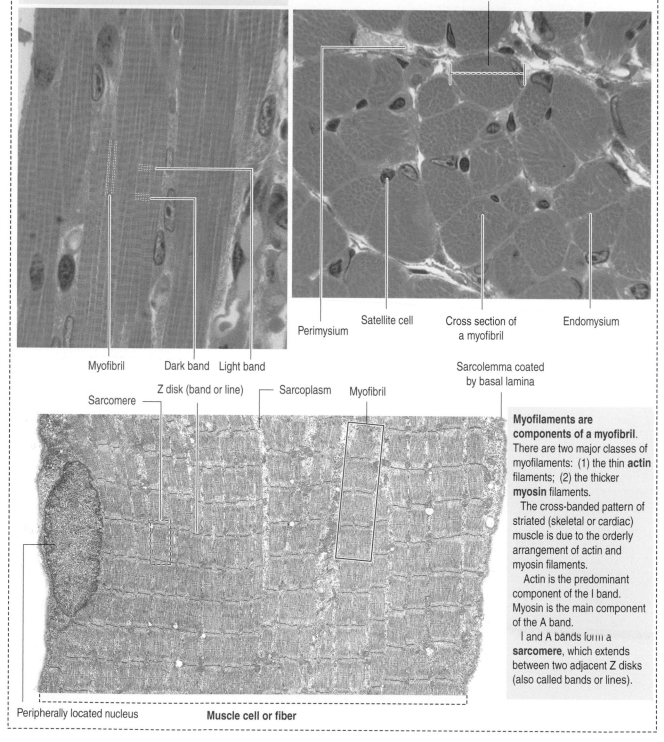

Figure 7-2. Skeletal muscle (striated)

The cytoplasm of the muscle cell or fiber contains an elaborate and regular arrangement of **myofibrils**, each organizing alternating short segments of differing refractive index: **dark A bands and light I bands**.

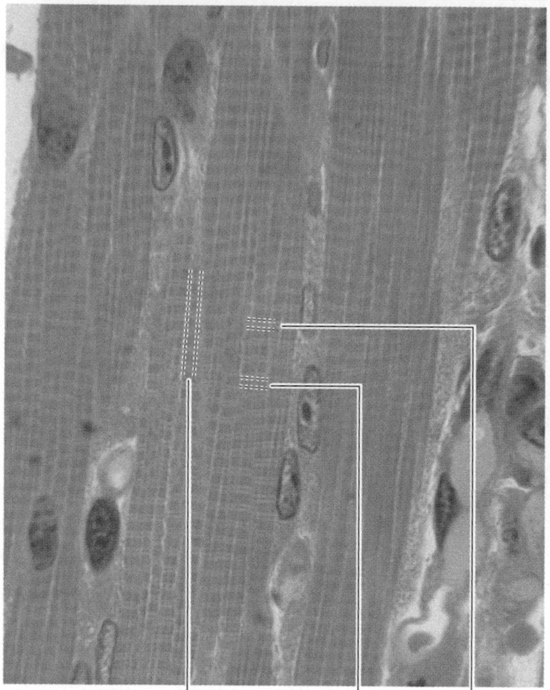

Myofibril
Dark band
Light band

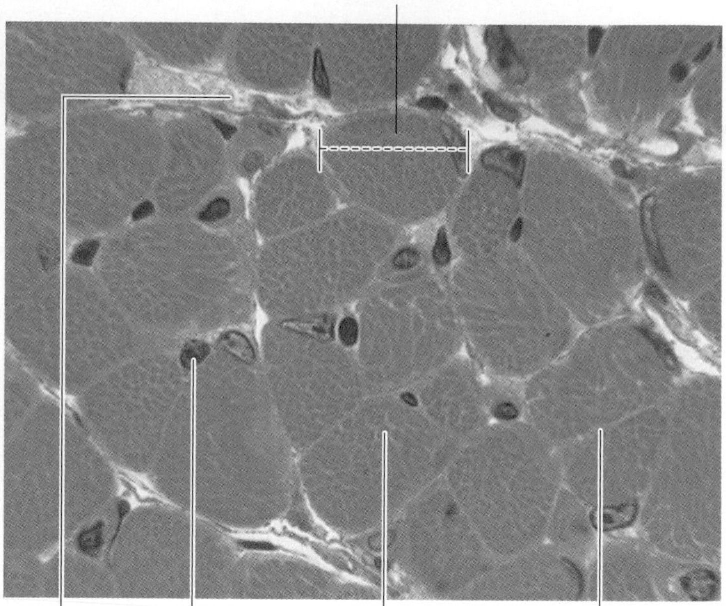

Cross section of a skeletal muscle cell with peripheral nucleus
Perimysium
Satellite cell
Cross section of a myofibril
Endomysium

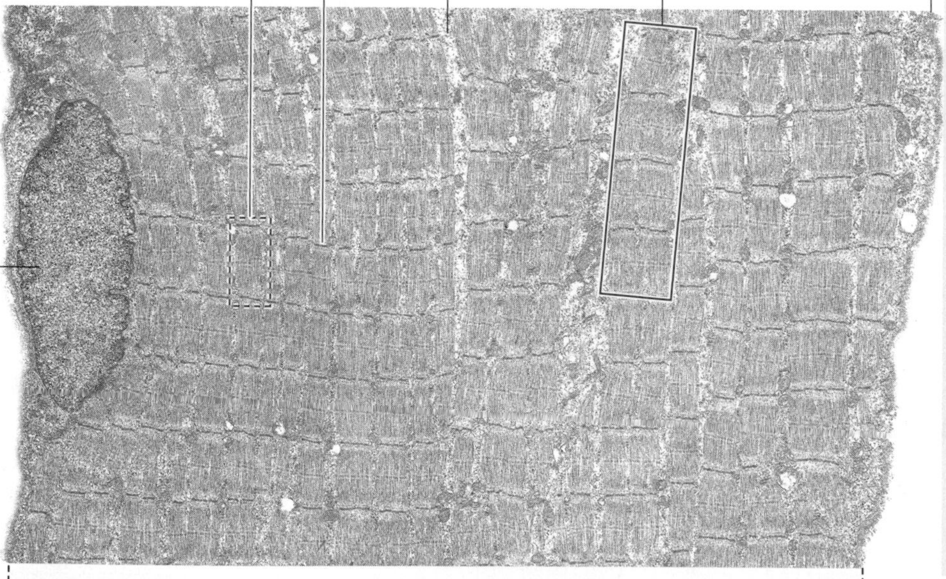

Sarcomere
Z disk (band or line)
Sarcoplasm
Myofibril
Sarcolemma coated by basal lamina
Peripherally located nucleus
Muscle cell or fiber

Myofilaments are components of a myofibril. There are two major classes of myofilaments: (1) the thin **actin** filaments; (2) the thicker **myosin** filaments.

The cross-banded pattern of striated (skeletal or cardiac) muscle is due to the orderly arrangement of actin and myosin filaments.

Actin is the predominant component of the I band. Myosin is the main component of the A band.

I and A bands form a **sarcomere**, which extends between two adjacent Z disks (also called bands or lines).

The plasma membrane (called the **sarcolemma**) of the muscle cell is surrounded by a **basal lamina** and **satellite cells** (Figure 7-2). We discuss the significance of satellite cells in muscle regeneration. The sarcolemma projects long, finger-like processes—called **transverse tubules** or **T tubules**—into the cytoplasm of the

Figure 7-3. Sarcomere

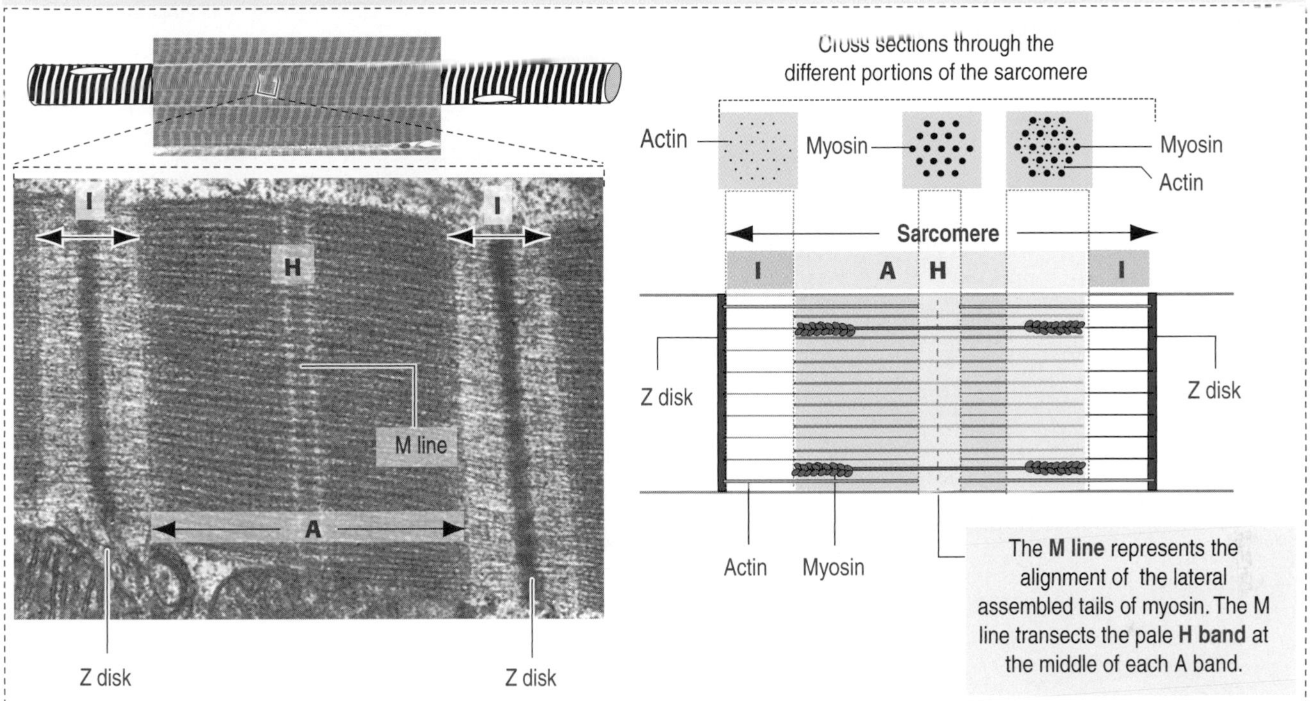

I
I
H
M line
A
Z disk
Z disk
Cross sections through the different portions of the sarcomere
Actin
Myosin
Myosin
Actin
Sarcomere
I
A
H
I
Z disk
Z disk
Actin
Myosin
The M line represents the alignment of the lateral assembled tails of myosin. The M line transects the pale H band at the middle of each A band.

cell—the **sarcoplasm**. T tubules make contact with membranous sacs or channels, the **sarcoplasmic reticulum**. The sarcoplasmic reticulum contains high concentrations of Ca^{2+}. The site of contact of the T tubule with the sarcoplasmic reticulum cisternae is called a **triad** because it consists of **two lateral sacs of the sarcoplasmic reticulum and a central T tubule**.

The many nuclei of the muscle fiber are located at the **periphery** of the cell, just under the sarcolemma.

About 80% of the sarcoplasm is occupied by myofibrils surrounded by **mitochondria** (called **sarcosomes**). Myofibrils are composed of two major filaments formed by contractile proteins: **thin filaments** contain **actin**, and **thick filaments** are composed of **myosin** (see Figure 7-2).

Depending on the type of muscle, mitochondria may be found parallel to the long axis of the myofibrils, or they may wrap around the zone of thick filaments. Thin filaments insert into each side of the Z disk (also called **band**, or **line**) and extend from the **Z disk** into the **A band**, where they alternate with thick filaments.

The myofibril is a repeat of sarcomere units

The **sarcomere** is the basic contractile unit of striated muscle (Figure 7-3). Sarcomere repeats are represented by **myofibrils** in the sarcoplasm of skeletal and cardiac muscle cells.

The arrangement of thick (myosin) and thin (actin) myofilaments of the sarcomere is largely responsible for the banding pattern observed under light and electron microscopy (see Figures 7-2 and 7-3). Actin and myosin interact and generate the contraction force. The Z disk forms a **transverse sarcomeric scaffold** to ensure the efficient transmission of the generated force.

Thin myofilaments measure 7 nm in width and 1 µm in length and form the **I band**. Thick filaments measure 15 nm in width and 1.5 µm in length and are found in the **A band**.

The A band is bisected by a light region called the **H band** (Figures 7-3 and 7-4). The major component of the H band is the enzyme **creatine kinase**, which catalyzes the formation of ATP from creatine phosphate and adenosine diphos-

Figure 7-4. **Skeletal muscle cell**

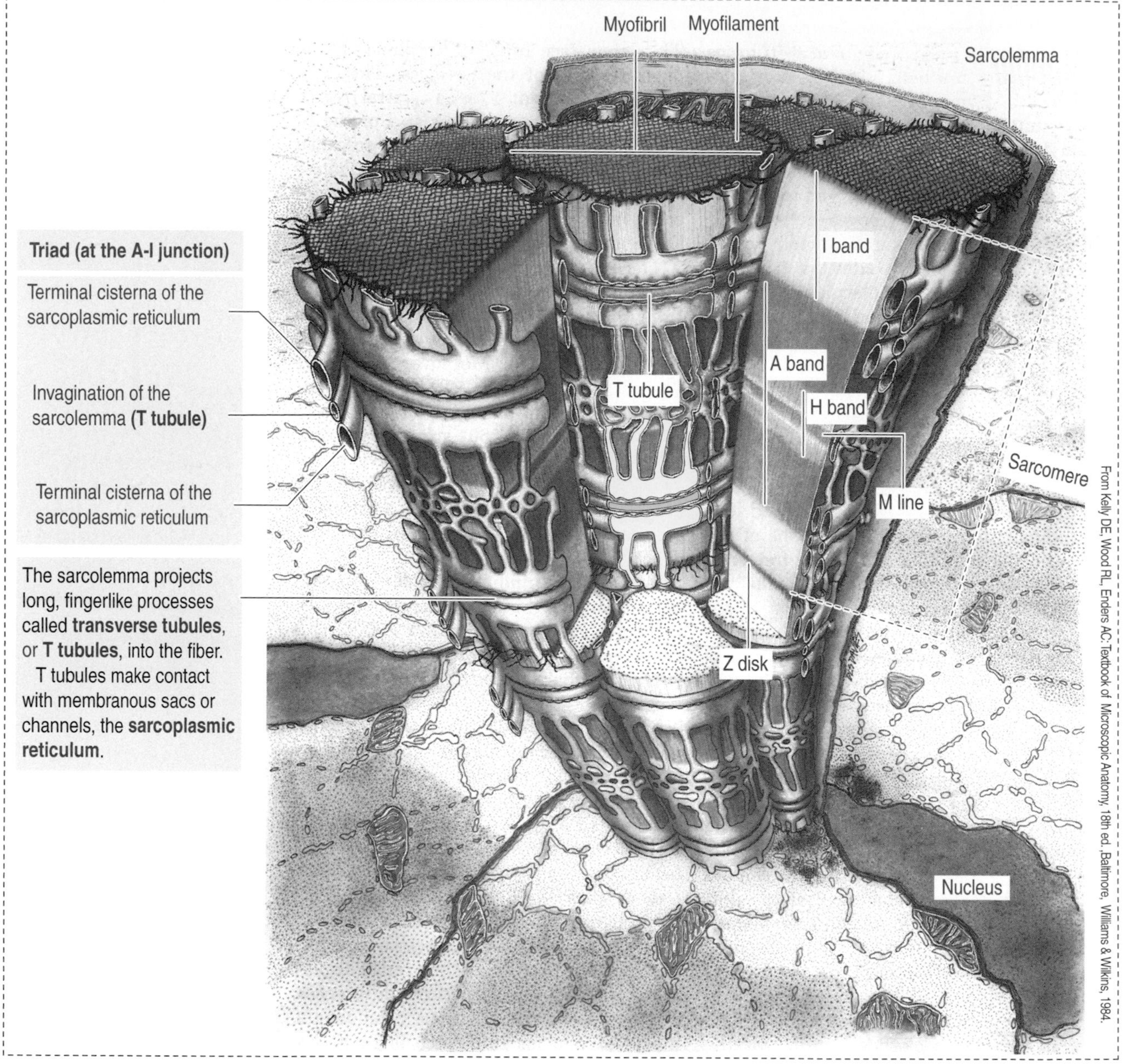
Myofibril
Myofilament
Sarcolemma
Triad (at the A-I junction)
Terminal cisterna of the sarcoplasmic reticulum
Invagination of the sarcolemma (T tubule)
Terminal cisterna of the sarcoplasmic reticulum
The sarcolemma projects long, fingerlike processes called transverse tubules, or T tubules, into the fiber.
T tubules make contact with membranous sacs or channels, the sarcoplasmic reticulum.
I band
A band
T tubule
H band
M line
Sarcomere
Z disk
Nucleus
From Kelly DE, Wood RL, Enders AC: Textbook of Microscopic Anatomy, 18th ed.,Baltimore, Williams & Wilkins, 1984.

phate (ADP). We discuss later how creatine phosphate maintains steady levels of ATP during prolonged muscle contraction.

Running through the midline of the H band is the **M line**. M-line striations correspond to a series of bridges and filaments linking the bare zone of thick filaments. Thin filaments insert into each side of the **Z disk**, whose components include **α-actinin**.

Components of the thin and thick filaments of the sarcomere

F-actin, the thin filament of the sarcomere, is double-stranded and twisted. F-actin is composed of globular monomers (**G-actin**; see Cytoskeleton in Chapter 1, Epithelium). G-actin monomers bind to each other in a head-to-tail fashion, giving the filament polarity, with barbed (plus) and pointed (minus) ends. The barbed end of actin filaments inserts into the Z disk.

Tropomyosin consists of two nearly identical α-helical polypeptides twisted around each other. Tropomyosin runs in the groove formed by F-actin strands. Each molecule of tropomyosin extends for the length of **seven actin monomers**

Figure 7-5. Troponin and tropomyosin

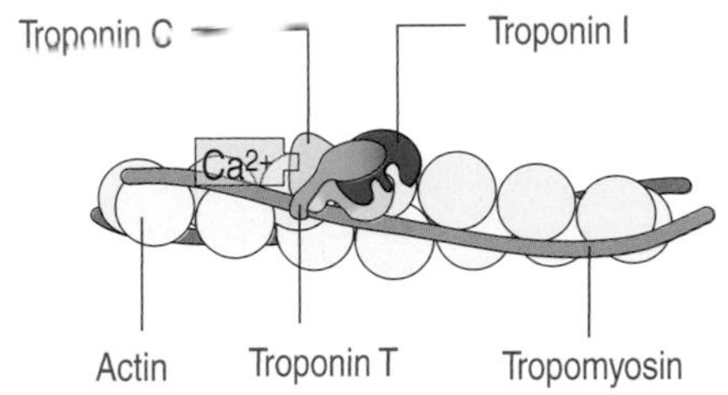

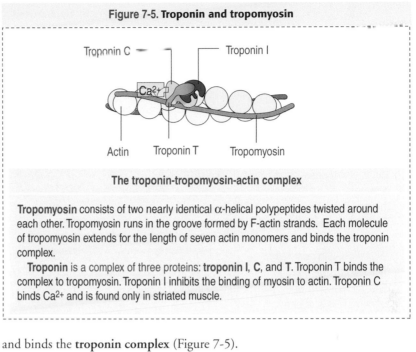

Troponin C
Troponin I
Ca2+
Actin
Troponin T
Tropomyosin

The troponin-tropomyosin-actin complex

Tropomyosin consists of two nearly identical α-helical polypeptides twisted around each other. Tropomyosin runs in the groove formed by F-actin strands. Each molecule of tropomyosin extends for the length of seven actin monomers and binds the troponin complex.

Troponin is a complex of three proteins: **troponin I, C**, and **T**. Troponin T binds the complex to tropomyosin. Troponin I inhibits the binding of myosin to actin. Troponin C binds Ca^{2+} and is found only in striated muscle.

and binds the **troponin complex** (Figure 7-5).

Troponin is a complex of three proteins: **troponin I, C,** and **T. Troponin T** binds the complex to tropomyosin. **Troponin I** inhibits the binding of myosin to actin. **Troponin C** binds Ca^{2+} and is found only in striated muscle.

Myosin, the major component of the thick filament, has adenosine triphosphatase (ATPase) activity (it hydrolyzes ATP) and binds to F-actin—the major component of the thin filament—in a reversible fashion.

Myosin consists of two identical **heavy chains** and two pairs of **light chains** (Figure 7-6; see Cytoskeleton in Chapter 1, Epithelium). At one end, each heavy chain forms a globular head. Two different light chains are bound to each head: the **essential light chain** and the **regulatory light chain**. The globular head has three distinct regions: (1) an actin-binding region; (2) an ATP-binding region; and (3) a light chain–binding region.

Figure 7-6. Myosin II

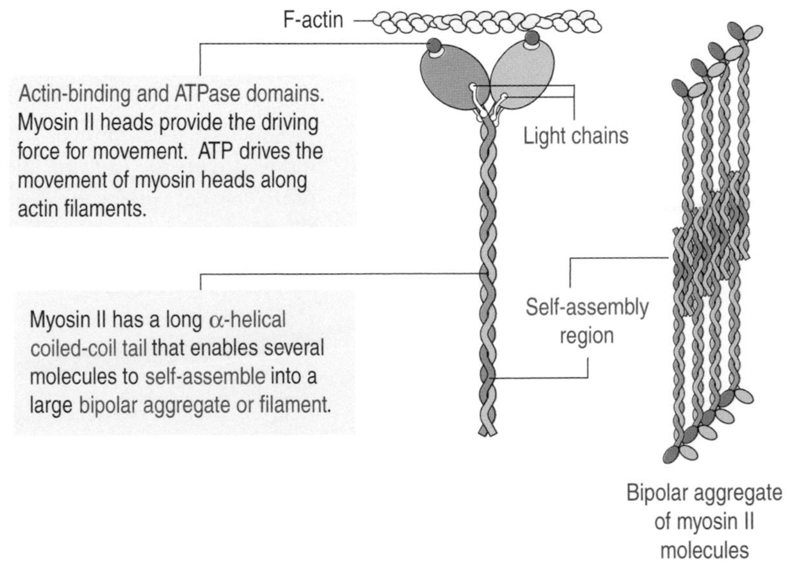

F-actin
Actin-binding and ATPase domains. Myosin II heads provide the driving force for movement. ATP drives the movement of myosin heads along actin filaments.
Light chains
Myosin II has a long α-helical coiled-coil tail that enables several molecules to self-assemble into a large bipolar aggregate or filament.
Self-assembly region
Bipolar aggregate of myosin II molecules

Figure 7-7. **Sarcomere: Nebulin and titin**

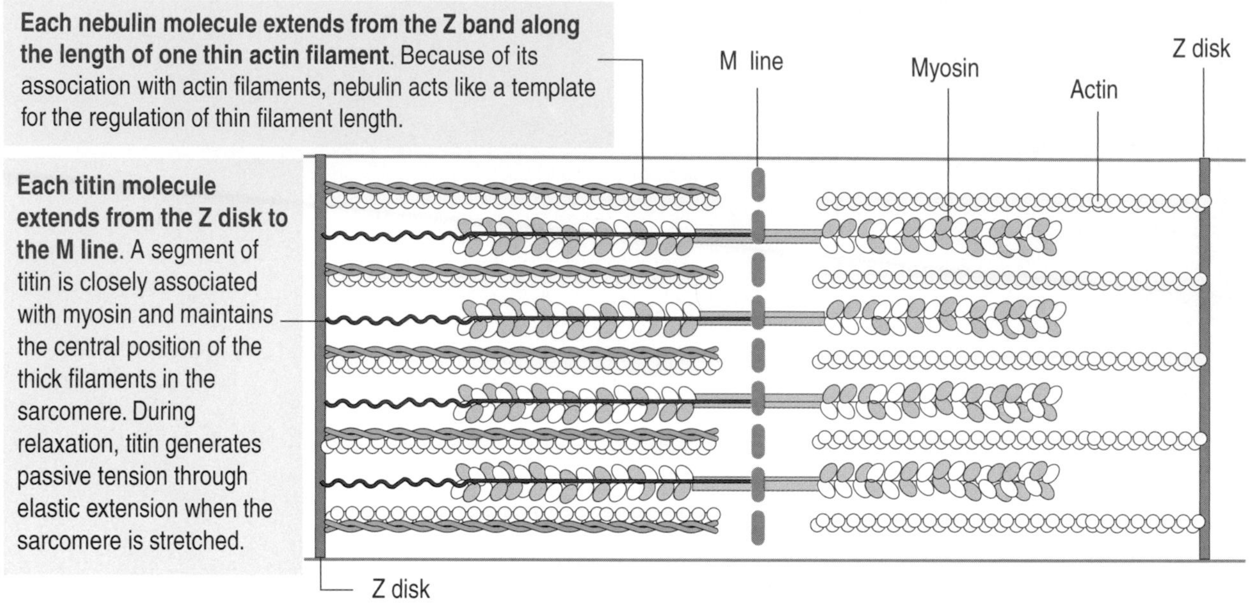
Each nebulin molecule extends from the Z band along the length of one thin actin filament. Because of its association with actin filaments, nebulin acts like a template for the regulation of thin filament length.
Each titin molecule extends from the Z disk to the M line. A segment of titin is closely associated with myosin and maintains the central position of the thick filaments in the sarcomere. During relaxation, titin generates passive tension through elastic extension when the sarcomere is stretched.
M line
Myosin
Actin
Z disk
Z disk

Nebulin (Figure 7-7) is associated with thin (actin) filaments; it inserts into the Z disk and acts as a template for determining the length of actin filaments.

Titin (Figure 7-7) is a very large protein with a molecular mass in the range of millions. Each molecule associates with thick (myosin) myofilaments and inserts into the Z disk, extending to the bare zone of the myosin filaments, close to the M line. Titin controls the assembly of the myosin myofilament by acting as a template. Titin has a role in sarcomere elasticity by forming a spring-like connection between the end of the thick myofilament and the Z disk.

Z disks are the insertion site of actin filaments of the sarcomere. A component of the Z disk, **α-actinin**, anchors the barbed end of actin filaments to the Z disk.

Desmin is a 55-kd protein that forms intermediate (10-nm) filaments. Desmin filaments encircle the Z disks of myofibrils and are linked to the Z disk and to each other by **plectin** filaments (Figure 7-8). Desmin filaments extend from the Z disk of one myofibril to the adjacent myofibril, forming a supportive latticework. Desmin filaments also extend from the sarcolemma to the nuclear envelope.

Desmin inserts into specialized sarcolemma-associated plaques, called **costameres.** Costameres, acting in concert with the dystrophin-associated protein complex, transduce contractile force from the Z disk to the basal lamina, maintain the structural integrity of the sarcolemma, and stabilize the position of myofibrils in the sarcoplasm.

The heat shock protein **αB-crystallin** protects desmin filaments from stress-induced damage. Desmin, plectin, and αB-crystallin form a mechanical stress protective network at the Z-disk level. Mutations in these three proteins lead to the destruction of myofibrils after repetitive mechanical stress.

Mechanism of muscle contraction

During muscle contraction, the muscle shortens about one third of its original length. The relevant aspects of muscle shortening are summarized in Figure 7-9 as follows:

1. The **length** of the thick and thin filaments **does not change** during muscle contraction (the length of the A band and the distance between the Z disk and the adjacent H band are constant).

2. The **length of the sarcomere decreases** because thick and thin filaments slide past each other (the size of the H band and I band decrease).

3. The force of contraction is generated by the process that moves one type of

Figure 7-8. **Cytoskeletal protective network of a skeletal muscle cell**

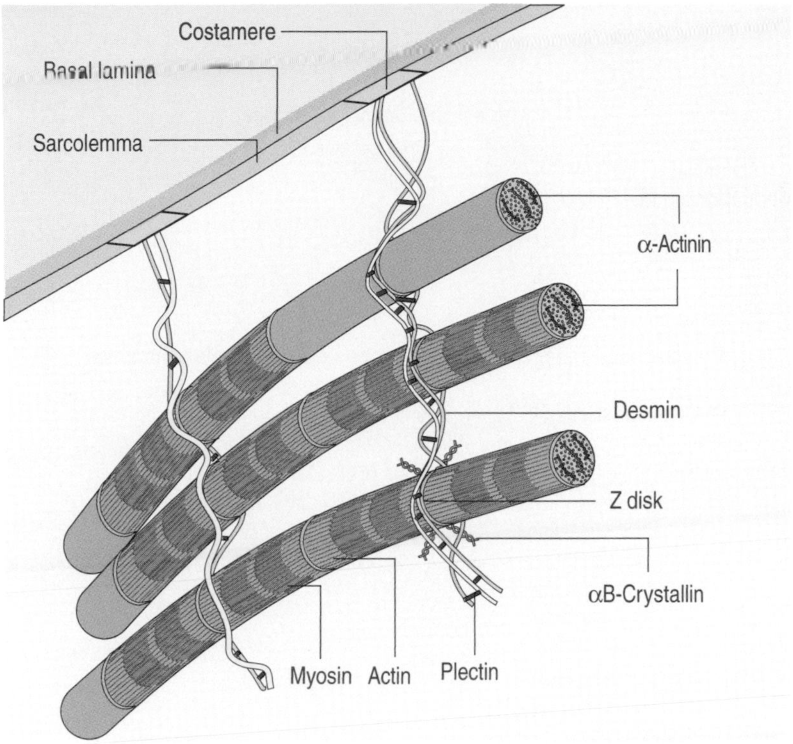
Costamere
Basal lamina
Sarcolemma
α-Actinin
Desmin
Z disk
αB-Crystallin
Myosin
Actin
Plectin

A mechanical stress protective network surrounds each myofibril at the Z disk.

Desmin, an intermediate filament extending from one myofibril to the other and anchored to the sarcolemma, encircles the Z disk of each sarcomere. Desmin inserts into specialized sarcolemma attachment regions known as **costameres**. Desmin filaments facilitate the coordinated contraction of individual myofibrils by holding adjacent myofibrils together and linking them to the sarcolemma.

Plectin links adjacent desmin filaments to each other.

αB-Crystallin, a heat shock protein associated with desmin, protects this intermediate filament from stress-induced damage.

α-Actinin anchors the barbed end of actin filaments to the Z disk.

filament past adjacent filaments of the other type.

Creatine phosphate, a backup energy source

Creatine phosphate is a backup mechanism to maintain steady levels of ATP during muscle contraction. Consequently, the concentration in muscle of free ATP during prolonged contraction does not change too much. Figure 7-10 provides a summary of the mechanism of regeneration of creatine phosphate, which takes place in mitochondria and diffuses to the myofibrils, where it replenishes ATP

Figure 7-9. **Sarcomere: Muscle contraction and relaxation**

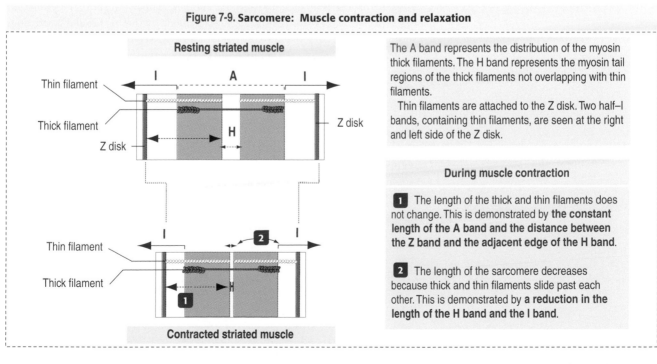

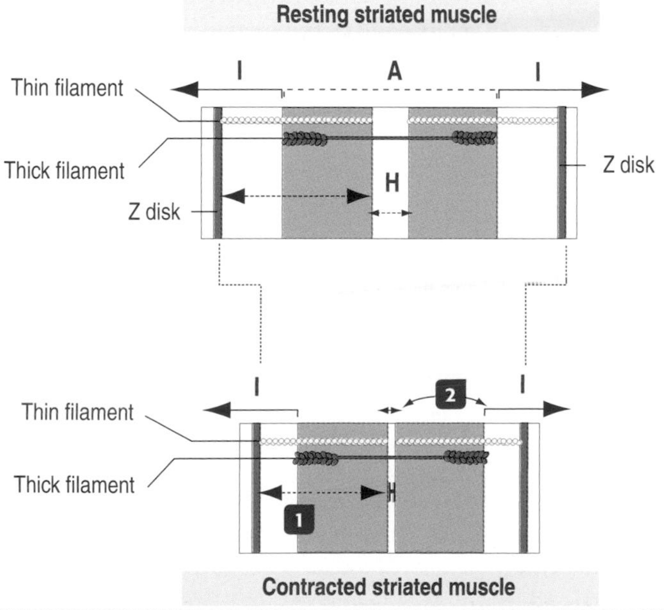
Resting striated muscle
Thin filament
Thick filament
Z disk
I
A
I
H
Z disk
Thin filament
Thick filament
I
2
I
1
Contracted striated muscle

The A band represents the distribution of the myosin thick filaments. The H band represents the myosin tail regions of the thick filaments not overlapping with thin filaments.

Thin filaments are attached to the Z disk. Two half–I bands, containing thin filaments, are seen at the right and left side of the Z disk.

During muscle contraction

1 The length of the thick and thin filaments does not change. This is demonstrated by **the constant length of the A band and the distance between the Z band and the adjacent edge of the H band.**

2 The length of the sarcomere decreases because thick and thin filaments slide past each other. This is demonstrated by **a reduction in the length of the H band and the I band.**

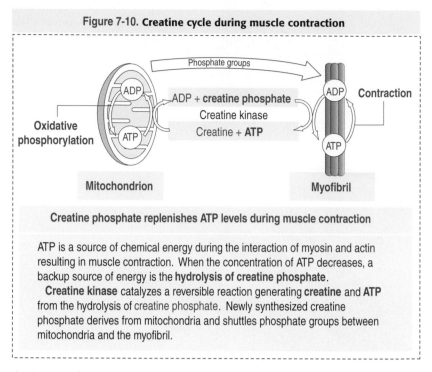

Figure 7-10. Creatine cycle during muscle contraction

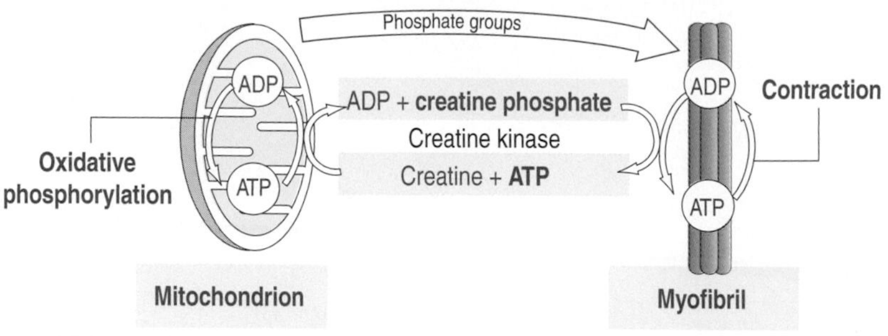
Phosphate groups
ADP
ADP + creatine phosphate
Creatine kinase
Creatine + ATP
ATP
Oxidative phosphorylation
ADP
Contraction
ATP
Mitochondrion
Myofibril

Creatine phosphate replenishes ATP levels during muscle contraction

ATP is a source of chemical energy during the interaction of myosin and actin resulting in muscle contraction. When the concentration of ATP decreases, a backup source of energy is the **hydrolysis of creatine phosphate**.

Creatine kinase catalyzes a reversible reaction generating **creatine** and **ATP** from the hydrolysis of creatine phosphate. Newly synthesized creatine phosphate derives from mitochondria and shuttles phosphate groups between mitochondria and the myofibril.

during muscle contraction.

A depolarization signal travels inside the muscle by T tubules

We discussed that the **triad** consists of a transverse T tubule flanked by sacs of the sarcoplasmic reticulum, and that the sarcoplasm of a skeletal muscle cell is packed with myofibrils (each consisting of a linear repeat of sarcomeres) with abundant mitochondria between them. How does a nerve impulse reach and deliver contractile signals to myofibrils located in the interior of the muscle cell?

An excitation-contraction signal is generated by **acetylcholine**, a chemical transmitter released from a nerve terminal in response to an **action potential**. Acetylcholine diffuses into a narrow gap, called the **neuromuscular junction**, between the muscle and a nerve terminal (Figure 7-11). The action potential spreads from the sarcolemma to the T tubules, which transport the excitation signal to the interior of the muscle cell. Remember that **T tubules** form rings around every sarcomere of every myofibril **at the A-I junction**.

We discuss later that the companions of the T tubule, the channels of the sarcoplasmic reticulum, contain calcium ions. Calcium ions are released inside the cytosol to activate muscle contraction when the action potential reaches the T tubule. This excitation-contraction sequence occurs in about 15 milliseconds.

Neuromuscular junction

The neuromuscular junction is a specialized structure formed by motor nerves associated with the target muscle and visible with the light microscope.

Once inside the skeletal muscle, the motor nerve gives rise to several branches. Each branch forms swellings called **presynaptic buttons** covered by **Schwann cells.** Each nerve branch **innervates a single muscle fiber.** The "parent" axon and all of the muscle fibers it innervates form a **motor unit**. Muscles that require fine control have few muscle fibers per motor unit. Very large muscles contain several hundred fibers per motor unit.

When myelinated axons reach the perimysium, they lose their myelin sheath but the presynaptic buttons remain covered with Schwann cell processes. A presynaptic button contains mitochondria and membrane-bound vesicles filled with the neurotransmitter **acetylcholine**. The neurotransmitter is released at dense areas on the cytoplasmic side of the axon membrane, called **active zones**.

Figure 7-11. Neuromuscular junction

Neuromuscular junction: The motor end plate

Motor axons branch at the muscle cell surface. Each branch forms **presynaptic buttons** covered by Schwann cells. Buttons lie over the **motor end plate** region, separated from the sarcolemma by the **synaptic cleft**. Each presynaptic button in the end plate is associated to a **primary synaptic cleft**, a depression of the muscle fiber formed by deep infoldings of the sarcolemma. **Junctional folds** (or secondary synaptic cleft) derive from the primary cleft. **Acetylcholine** receptors are found at the crest of the **junctional folds**. **Voltage-gated Na2+ channels** are found at the bottom of the junctional folds. The **basal lamina** contains **acetylcholinesterase**.

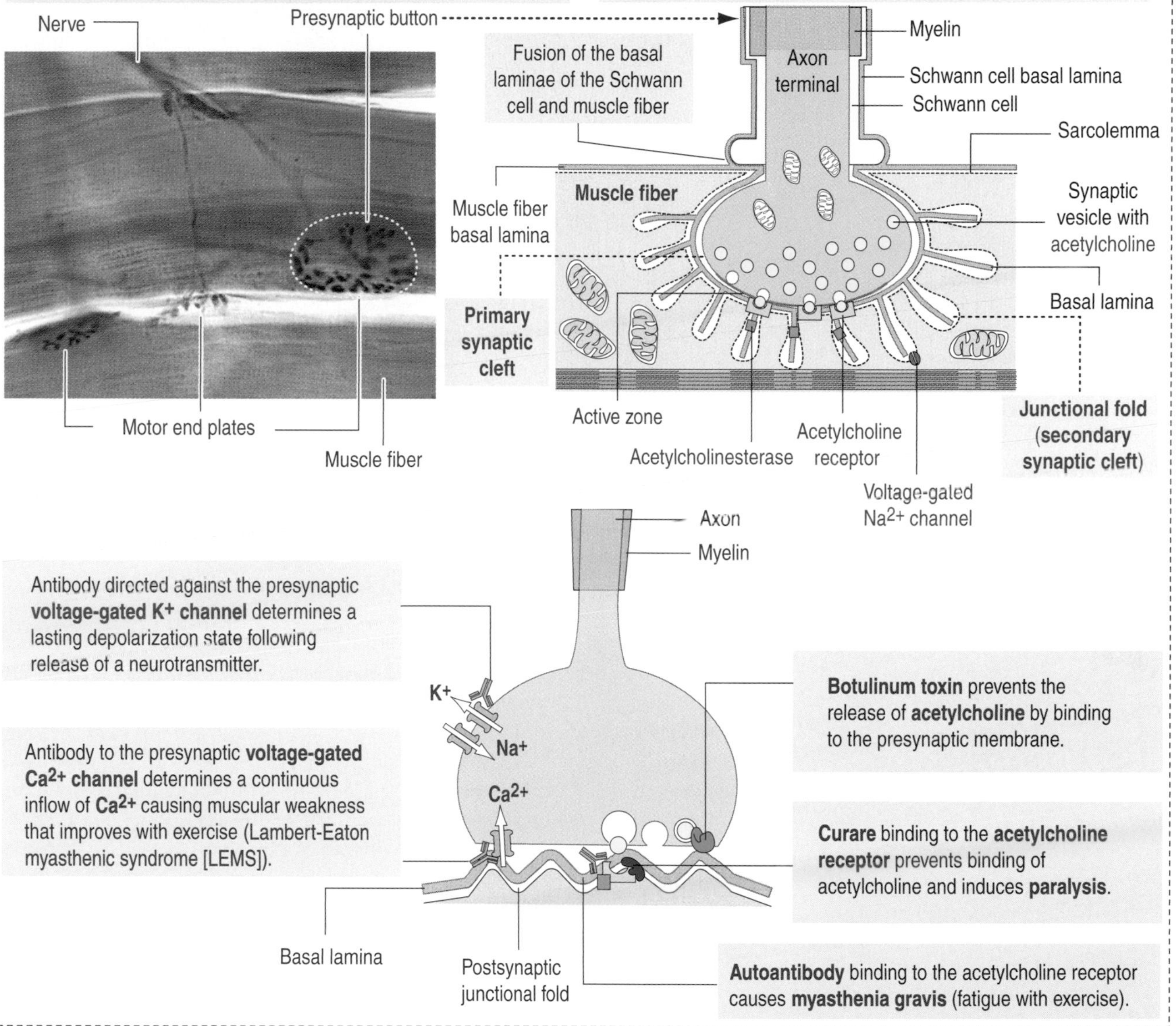

Nerve
Presynaptic button
Motor end plates
Muscle fiber
Myelin
Axon terminal
Fusion of the basal laminae of the Schwann cell and muscle fiber
Schwann cell basal lamina
Schwann cell
Sarcolemma
Muscle fiber
Muscle fiber basal lamina
Synaptic vesicle with acetylcholine
Basal lamina
Primary synaptic cleft
Junctional fold (secondary synaptic cleft)
Active zone
Acetylcholinesterase
Acetylcholine receptor
Voltage-gated Na2+ channel
Axon
Myelin
Antibody directed against the presynaptic voltage-gated K+ channel determines a lasting depolarization state following release of a neurotransmitter.
K+
Na+
Ca2+
Antibody to the presynaptic voltage-gated Ca2+ channel determines a continuous inflow of Ca2+ causing muscular weakness that improves with exercise (Lambert-Eaton myasthenic syndrome [LEMS]).
Botulinum toxin prevents the release of acetylcholine by binding to the presynaptic membrane.
Curare binding to the acetylcholine receptor prevents binding of acetylcholine and induces paralysis.
Basal lamina
Postsynaptic junctional fold
Autoantibody binding to the acetylcholine receptor causes myasthenia gravis (fatigue with exercise).

Synaptic buttons occupy a depression of the muscle fiber, called the **primary synaptic cleft**. In this region, the sarcolemma is thrown into deep **junctional folds (secondary synaptic clefts)**. **Acetylcholine receptors** are located at the crests of the folds and **voltage-gated Na^+ channels** are down into the folds (see Figure 7-11).

The basal lamina surrounding the muscle fiber extends into the synaptic cleft. The basal lamina contains **acetylcholinesterase**, which inactivates acetylcholine released from the presynaptic buttons into acetate and choline. The basal lamina covering the Schwann cell becomes continuous with the basal lamina of the muscle fiber.

Clinical significance: Disorders of neuromuscular transmission

Synaptic transmission at the neuromuscular junction can be affected by **curare**

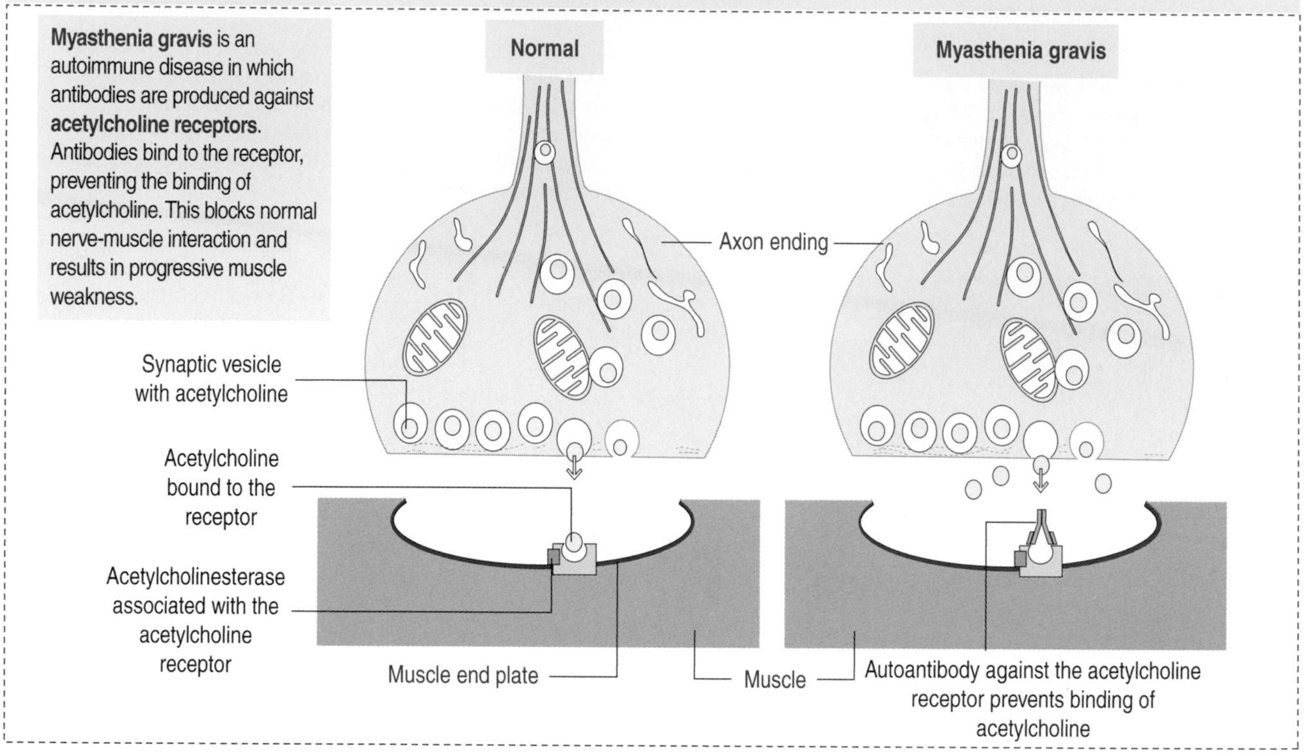
Myasthenia gravis is an autoimmune disease in which antibodies are produced against acetylcholine receptors. Antibodies bind to the receptor, preventing the binding of acetylcholine. This blocks normal nerve-muscle interaction and results in progressive muscle weakness.
Normal
Myasthenia gravis
Axon ending
Synaptic vesicle with acetylcholine
Acetylcholine bound to the receptor
Acetylcholinesterase associated with the acetylcholine receptor
Muscle end plate
Muscle
Autoantibody against the acetylcholine receptor prevents binding of acetylcholine
Figure 7-12. **Myasthenia gravis**

and **botulinum toxin** (see Figure 7-11).

Curare binds to the acetylcholine receptor and prevents binding of acetylcholine. Curare derivatives are used in surgical procedures in which muscle paralysis is necessary.

Botulinum toxin, an exotoxin from the bacterium *Clostridium botulinum*, prevents the release of acetylcholine at the presynaptic end. Muscle paralysis and dysfunction of the autonomous nervous system occur in cases of food poisoning mediated by botulinum toxin.

Myasthenia gravis is an autoimmune disease in which antibodies are produced against acetylcholine receptors (Figure 7-12). Autoantibodies bind to the receptor, preventing the binding of acetylcholine. This blocks normal nerve-muscle interaction and results in progressive muscle weakness.

Calcium controls muscle contraction

In the absence of Ca^{2+}, muscle is relaxed and the troponin-tropomyosin complex blocks the myosin binding site on the actin filament.

When a depolarization signal arrives, Ca^{2+} exits the terminal cisternae of the sarcoplasmic reticulum with the help of the **ryanodine-sensitive Ca^{2+} channel** (Figure 7-13). In the sarcomere, Ca^{2+} binds to troponin C and causes a change in configuration of the troponin-tropomyosin complex. As a result, the myosin-binding site on the actin filament is exposed. Myosin heads bind to the actin filament, and hydrolysis of ATP occurs. We have seen that steady levels of ATP rely on the mitochondrial supply of creatine phosphate and the availability of creatine kinase (see Figure 7-10).

Creatine kinase is an enzyme found in soluble form in the **sarcoplasm** and also is a component of the **M-line region** of the H band. Creatine kinase catalyzes the transfer of phosphate from creatine phosphate to ADP.

The energy of hydrolysis of ATP produces a change in the position of the myosin head, and the thin filaments are pulled past the thick filaments. Contraction results in the complete overlap of the A and I bands (see Figure 7-9). The contraction continues until Ca^{2+} is removed.

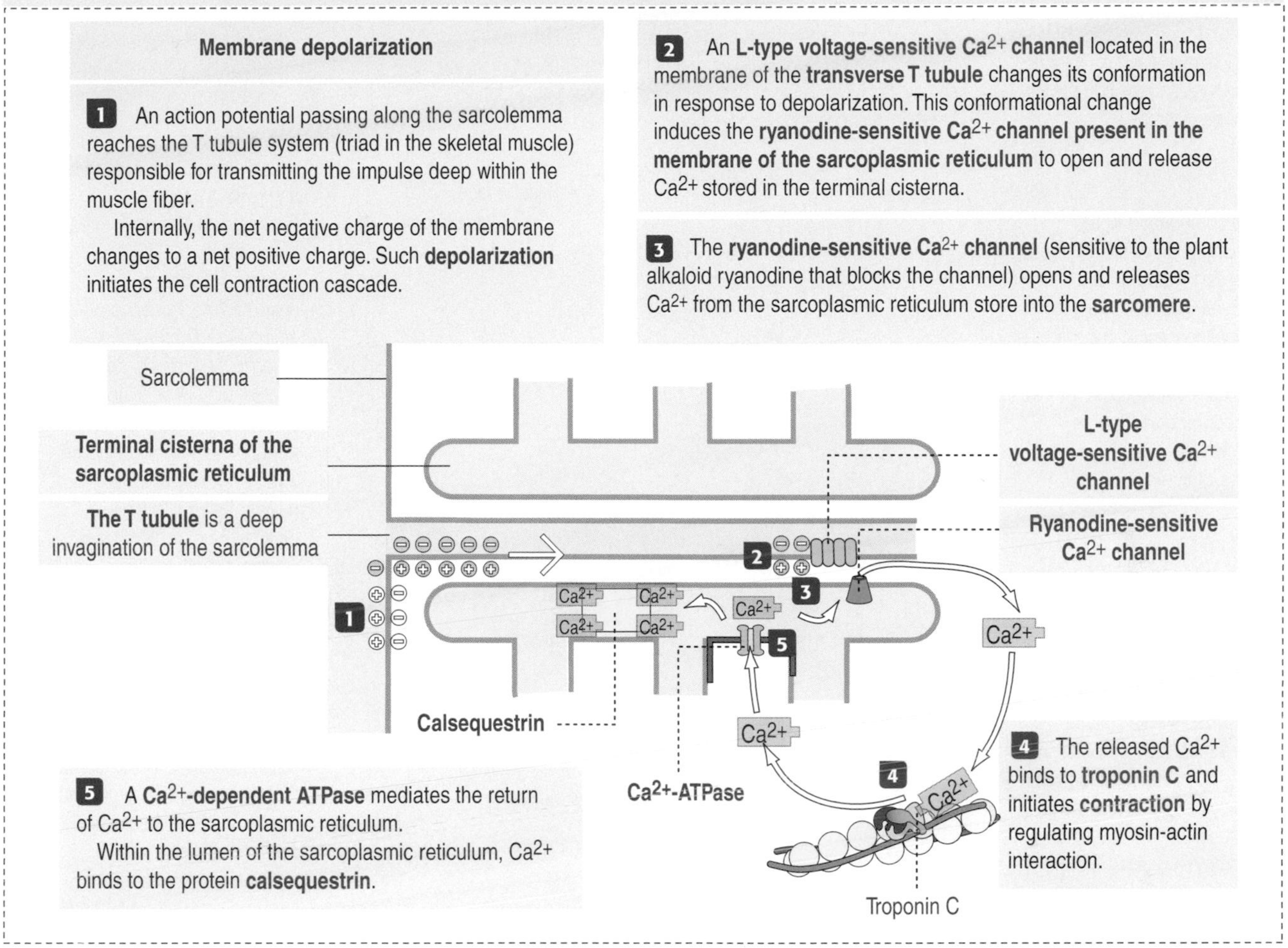
Membrane depolarization
1 An action potential passing along the sarcolemma reaches the T tubule system (triad in the skeletal muscle) responsible for transmitting the impulse deep within the muscle fiber.
Internally, the net negative charge of the membrane changes to a net positive charge. Such depolarization initiates the cell contraction cascade.
2 An L-type voltage-sensitive Ca2+ channel located in the membrane of the transverse T tubule changes its conformation in response to depolarization. This conformational change induces the ryanodine-sensitive Ca2+ channel present in the membrane of the sarcoplasmic reticulum to open and release Ca2+ stored in the terminal cisterna.
3 The ryanodine-sensitive Ca2+ channel (sensitive to the plant alkaloid ryanodine that blocks the channel) opens and releases Ca2+ from the sarcoplasmic reticulum store into the sarcomere.
Sarcolemma
Terminal cisterna of the sarcoplasmic reticulum
The T tubule is a deep invagination of the sarcolemma
L-type voltage-sensitive Ca2+ channel
Ryanodine-sensitive Ca2+ channel
Ca2+
Calsequestrin
Ca2+-ATPase
5 A Ca2+-dependent ATPase mediates the return of Ca2+ to the sarcoplasmic reticulum.
Within the lumen of the sarcoplasmic reticulum, Ca2+ binds to the protein calsequestrin.
4 The released Ca2+ binds to troponin C and initiates contraction by regulating myosin-actin interaction.
Troponin C

Figure 7-13. **Muscle contraction**

In summary, the sarcoplasmic reticulum, a network of smooth endoplasmic reticulum surrounding each myofibril (see Figure 7-4), stores Ca^{2+}. In response to depolarization signals, the sarcoplasmic reticulum releases Ca^{2+}. When membrane depolarization ends, Ca^{2+} is pumped back into the sarcoplasmic reticulum with the help of **Ca^{2+}-dependent ATPase**, and binds to the protein **calsequestrin** (see Figure 7-13). Contraction can no longer take place.

Clinical significance: Muscular dystrophies

Muscular dystrophies are a group of congenital muscular diseases characterized by muscle weakness, atrophy, elevation of serum levels of muscle enzymes, and destructive changes of muscle tissue (Figure 7-14).

Muscular dystrophies are caused by a deficiency in the **dystrophin-associated protein (DAP) complex**. The DAP complex consists of **dystrophin** and two subcomplexes: the **dystroglycan complex** (α and β subunits), and the **sarcoglycan complex** (α, β, γ, δ, ε, and ζ subunits; for simplicity, only four subunits are shown in Figure 7-14). Additional proteins include **syntrophins** (α, β1, β2, γ1, and γ2 subunits), **dystrobrevin**, and **sarcospan**. Dystrophin, syntrophins, and dystrobrevin are located in the sarcoplasm; dystroglycans, sarcoglycans, and sarcospan are transmembrane glycoproteins. Patients with a primary defect in dystroglycans and syntrophins have not been identified.

The most important muscle protein involved in muscular dystrophies is **dystrophin**, a 427-kd cytoskeletal protein associated to F-actin, dystroglycans, and syntrophins (see Figure 7-14). The absence of dystrophin determines the loss of components of the DAP complex. **The function of dystrophin is to reinforce and stabilize the sarcolemma during the stress of muscle contraction** by main-

Figure 7-14. **Muscular dystrophies**

A mutation in **laminin-2** (which consists of α, β, and γ chains), causes congenital muscle dystrophy.

The **dystroglycan complex links dystrophin to laminin-2.** Dystroglycan-α binds to the α chain of laminin-2 (called merosin) and dystroglycan-β binds to dystrophin. Patients with a primary defect in dystroglycans have not been identified.

The components of the **sarcoglycan complex** are specific for cardiac and skeletal muscle.

Defects in the components of the complex cause autosomal recessive **limb-girdle muscular dystrophies** (known as **sarcoglycanopathies**).

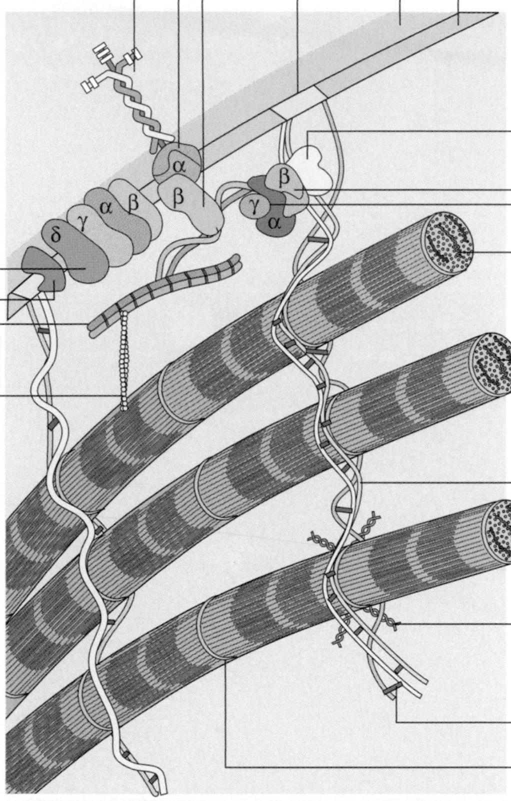

The **dystrophin-associated protein (DAP) complex** includes dystrophin and components of the dystroglycan complex and sarcoglycan complex.

Dystrophin reinforces and stabilizes the sarcolemma during the stress of muscle contraction by maintaining a link between the cytoskeleton and the extracellular matrix. When dystrophin is absent, the DAP complex is lost and the sarcolemma is disrupted, allowing unregulated calcium entry, which causes necrosis of the muscle fiber.

A deficiency in dystrophin is typical of **Duchenne's muscular dystrophy**, an X-linked recessive condition.

Structural muscle proteins associated with mutations causing myopathies

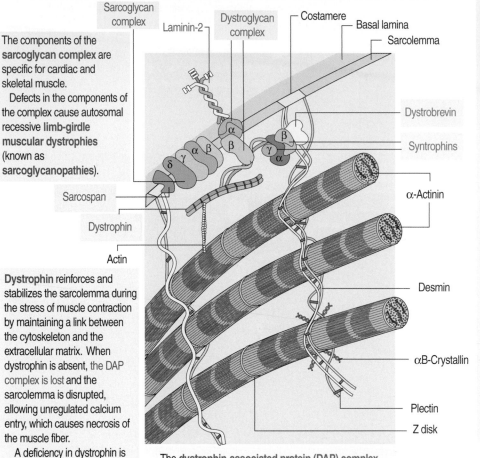

The **Z disk** is the insertion site of actin filaments of the sarcomere and plays a role in the transmission of tension through the myofibril.

Desmin filaments (intermediate filament protein) encircle the Z disks and are linked to them and to one another by **plectin** filaments. By this association, desmin: (1) **integrates mechanically the contractile action of adjacent myofibrils** and (2) **links the Z disk to the sarcolemma at costamere sites.**

The heat shock protein **αB-crystallin** protects desmin filaments from stress-dependent damage.

Note that **desmin, plectin, and αB-crystallin form a network around the Z disks,** thus protecting the integrity of the myofibrils during mechanical stress.

Mutations of desmin, plectin, and **αB-crystallin** cause fragility of the myofibrils and their destruction after continuous stress.

Cross section of a normal skeletal muscle fiber with the characteristic peripheral nucleus.

Degenerating skeletal muscle fiber in the early stages of Duchenne's muscular dystrophy.

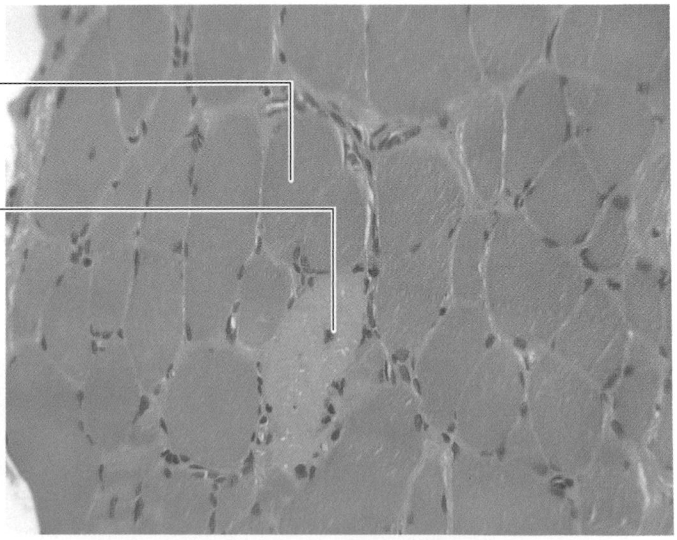

Muscular dystrophies are a heterogeneous group of congenital muscle diseases characterized by severe muscle weakness, and atrophy and destruction of muscle fibers.

The most important muscle protein involved in muscular dystrophies is **dystrophin.** The absence of dystrophin leads to a loss of the DAP complex (consisting of the subcomplexes **dystroglycan complex** and **sarcoglycan complex**).

Figure 7-15. Satellite cells and muscle regeneration

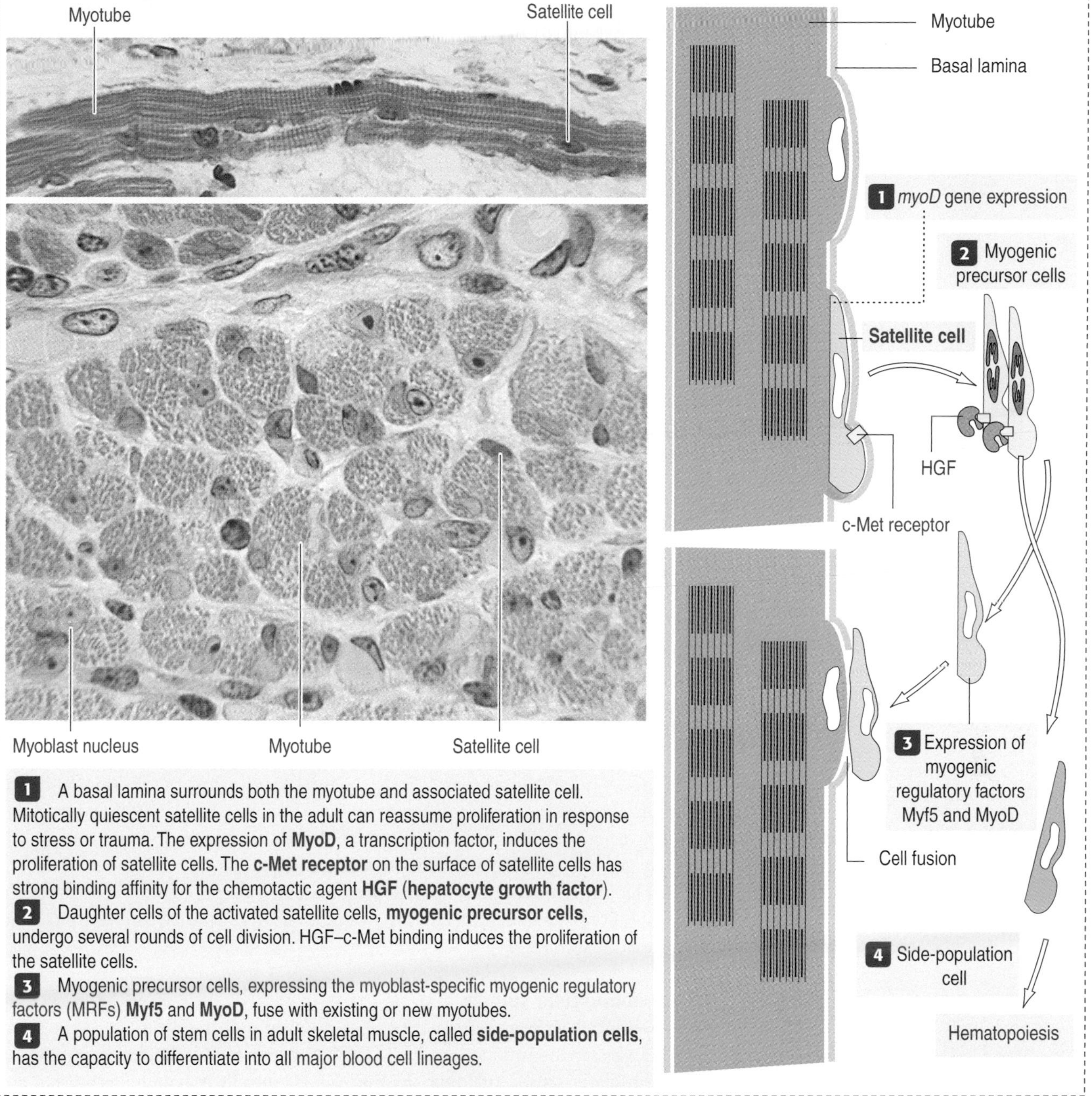

Myotube
Satellite cell
Myoblast nucleus
Myotube
Satellite cell
Myotube
Basal lamina
1 myoD gene expression
2 Myogenic precursor cells
Satellite cell
HGF
c-Met receptor
3 Expression of myogenic regulatory factors Myf5 and MyoD
Cell fusion
4 Side-population cell
Hematopoiesis

1 A basal lamina surrounds both the myotube and associated satellite cell. Mitotically quiescent satellite cells in the adult can reassume proliferation in response to stress or trauma. The expression of **MyoD**, a transcription factor, induces the proliferation of satellite cells. The **c-Met receptor** on the surface of satellite cells has strong binding affinity for the chemotactic agent **HGF** (**hepatocyte growth factor**).

2 Daughter cells of the activated satellite cells, **myogenic precursor cells**, undergo several rounds of cell division. HGF–c-Met binding induces the proliferation of the satellite cells.

3 Myogenic precursor cells, expressing the myoblast-specific myogenic regulatory factors (MRFs) **Myf5** and **MyoD**, fuse with existing or new myotubes.

4 A population of stem cells in adult skeletal muscle, called **side-population cells**, has the capacity to differentiate into all major blood cell lineages.

taining a mechanical link between the cytoskeleton and the extracellular matrix. Deficiencies of dystrophin are characteristic of **Duchenne's muscular dystrophy** (**DMD**). Most patients die young (in their late teens or early twenties) due to an involvement of the diaphragm and other respiratory muscles.

DMD is an X chromosome–linked recessive disorder caused by a mutation in the dystrophin gene. The disorder is detected in affected boys after they begin to walk. Progressive muscle weakness and wasting, sudden episodes of vomiting (caused by delayed gastric emptying), and abdominal pain are observed. A typical laboratory finding is **increased serum creatine kinase levels**.

Muscle biopsies reveal muscle destruction, **absence of dystrophin,** and a **substantial reduction of sarcoglycans,** and other components of the DAP complex, detected by immunohistochemistry.

Heterozygote female carriers may be asymptomatic or have mild muscle weakness, muscle cramps, and elevated serum **creatine kinase** levels. Women with these mutations may give birth to affected males or carrier females.

Sarcoglycanopathies in limb-girdle muscular dystrophies have mutations in the genes for α-, β-, γ-, and δ-sarcoglycan that cause defective assembly of the sarcoglycans, thus disrupting their interaction with the other dystroglycan complex proteins and the association of the sarcolemma with the extracellular matrix.

Clinical significance: Satellite cells and muscle regeneration

Muscle development involves the chain-like alignment and fusion of committed muscle cell precursors, the **myoblasts**, to form multinucleated **myotubes**.

Two crucial events occur during the commitment of the muscle cell precursor to myogenesis: (1) the cessation of proliferation of the precursor cell—determined by the upregulated expression of **myogenic regulatory factors** (**MRFs**), **Myf5** and **MyoD**, and the downregulation of **Pax**7, a transcription factor, and (2) the terminal differentiation of the muscle cell precursor—triggered by **myogenin** and **MRF4**.

Satellite cells are a cell population distinct from the myoblasts. They attach to the surface of the myotubes before a **basal lamina** surrounds the satellite cell and myotube (Figure 7-15). Satellite cells are of considerable significance in muscle maintenance, repair, and regeneration in the adult.

Satellite cells are mitotically **quiescent** in the adult, but can reassume **self-renewal** and **proliferation** in response to stress or trauma. **MyoD** expression induces the proliferation of satellite cells. The descendants of the activated satellite cells—called **myogenic precursor cells**—undergo multiple rounds of cell division before they can fuse with existing or new myofibers.

Quiescent satellite cells express a receptor on their surface encoded by the proto-oncogene **c-Met**. The c-Met receptor has strong binding affinity for the chemotactic agent **HGF** (hepatocyte growth factor). The HGF–c-Met complex upregulates a signaling cascade leading to proliferation of the satellite cells and the expression of Myf5 and MyoD.

In addition to satellite cells as progenitors of the myogenic cells in adult skeletal muscle, a population of stem cells in adult skeletal muscle—called **side-population cells**—has the capacity to differentiate into all major blood cell lineages as well as myogenic satellite cells. Side-population cells are present in bone marrow and may give rise to myogenic cells that can participate in muscle regeneration.

The pluripotent nature of satellite cells and side-population cells raises the possibility of stem cell therapy of a number of degenerative diseases, including muscular dystrophy.

Neuromuscular spindle

The central nervous system continuously monitors the position of the limbs and the state of contraction of the various muscles. Muscles have a specialized encapsulated sensor called the **neuromuscular spindle** that contains sensory and motor components (Figure 7-16).

A neuromuscular spindle consists of 2 to 14 specialized striated muscle fibers enclosed in a fusiform sheath or capsule of connective tissue. They are 5 to 10 mm long and therefore much shorter than the surrounding contractile muscle fibers.

The specialized muscle fibers in the interior of the neuromuscular spindle are called **intrafusal fibers** to distinguish them from the nonspecialized **extrafusal fibers** (Latin *extra*, outside; *fusus*, spindle), the regular skeletal muscle fibers.

There are two kinds of intrafusal fibers designated by their histologic appearance: (1) **nuclear bag fiber**, consisting of a central sensory (noncontractile) bag-like region, and (2) the **nuclear chain fiber**, so-called because its central portion contains a chain-like array of nuclei. The distal portion of both nuclear bag and nuclear chain fibers consists of striated muscle with contractile properties.

The neuromuscular spindle is innervated by two types of afferent axons making

Figure 7-16. Neuromuscular spindle

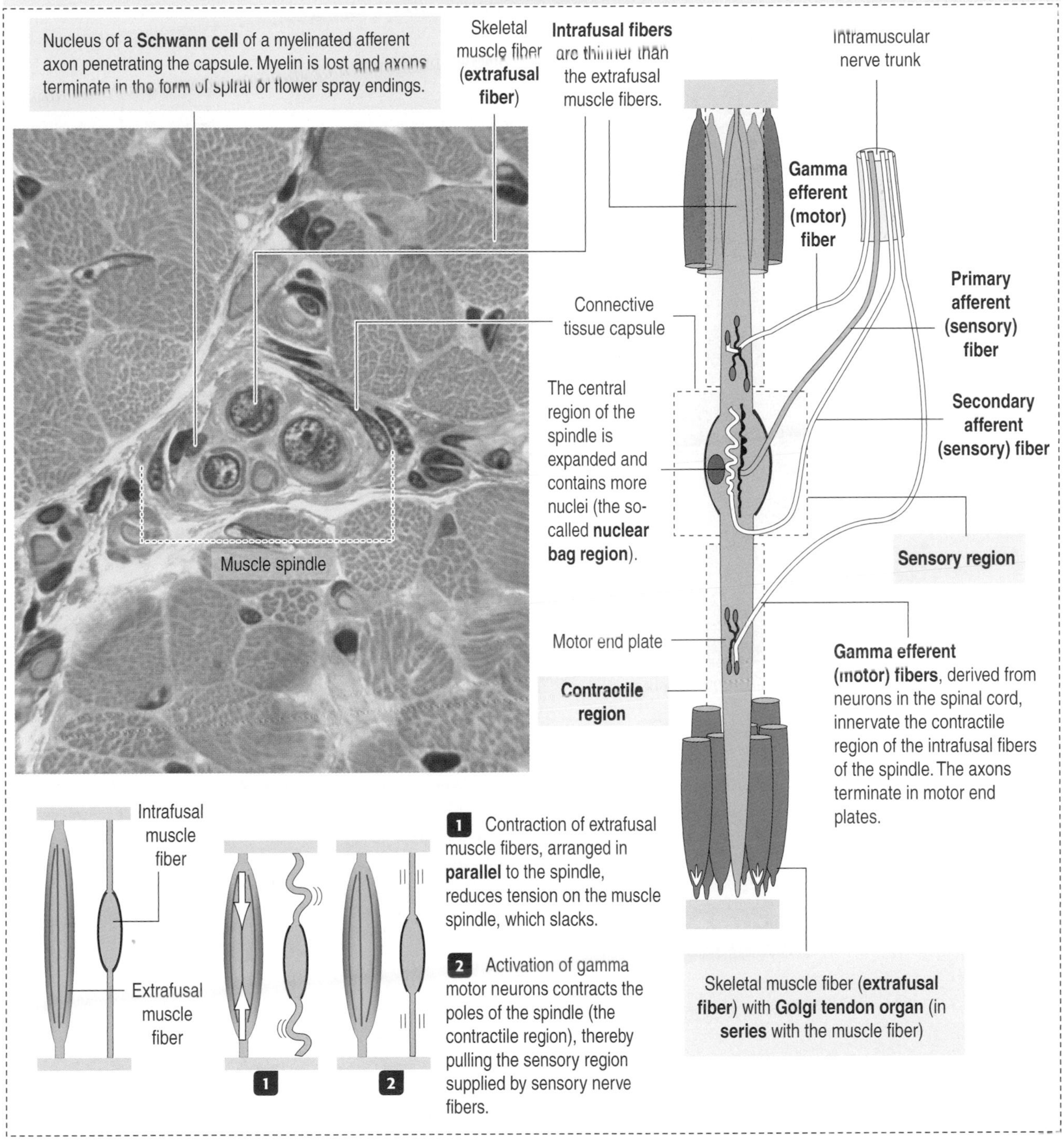

Nucleus of a **Schwann cell** of a myelinated afferent axon penetrating the capsule. Myelin is lost and axons terminate in the form of spiral or flower spray endings.
Skeletal muscle fiber (**extrafusal** fiber)
Intrafusal fibers are thinner than the extrafusal muscle fibers.
Intramuscular nerve trunk
Gamma efferent (motor) fiber
Connective tissue capsule
Primary afferent (sensory) fiber
Secondary afferent (sensory) fiber
The central region of the spindle is expanded and contains more nuclei (the so-called **nuclear bag region**).
Sensory region
Muscle spindle
Motor end plate
Contractile region
Gamma efferent (motor) fibers, derived from neurons in the spinal cord, innervate the contractile region of the intrafusal fibers of the spindle. The axons terminate in motor end plates.
Intrafusal muscle fiber
Extrafusal muscle fiber
1 Contraction of extrafusal muscle fibers, arranged in **parallel** to the spindle, reduces tension on the muscle spindle, which slacks.
2 Activation of gamma motor neurons contracts the poles of the spindle (the contractile region), thereby pulling the sensory region supplied by sensory nerve fibers.
Skeletal muscle fiber (**extrafusal fiber**) with **Golgi tendon organ** (in **series** with the muscle fiber)
1
2

contact with the central (receptor) region of the intrafusal fibers.

Two types of anterior motor neurons of the spinal cord give rise to motor nerve fibers: the large-diameter **alpha motor neurons** innervate the **extrafusal fibers** of muscles; the small-diameter **gamma motor neurons** innervate the **intrafusal fibers** in the spindle.

Sensory nerve endings are arranged around the central nuclear region and sense the degree of tension of the intrafusal fibers.

The intrafusal muscle fibers of the neuromuscular spindle are in **parallel** with the extrafusal muscle fibers. When the extrafusal muscle fibers contract (shorten), the neuromuscular spindle becomes slack. If the spindle remains slack, no further information about changes in **muscle length** can be transmitted to the spinal cord.

Figure 7-17. Cardiac muscle

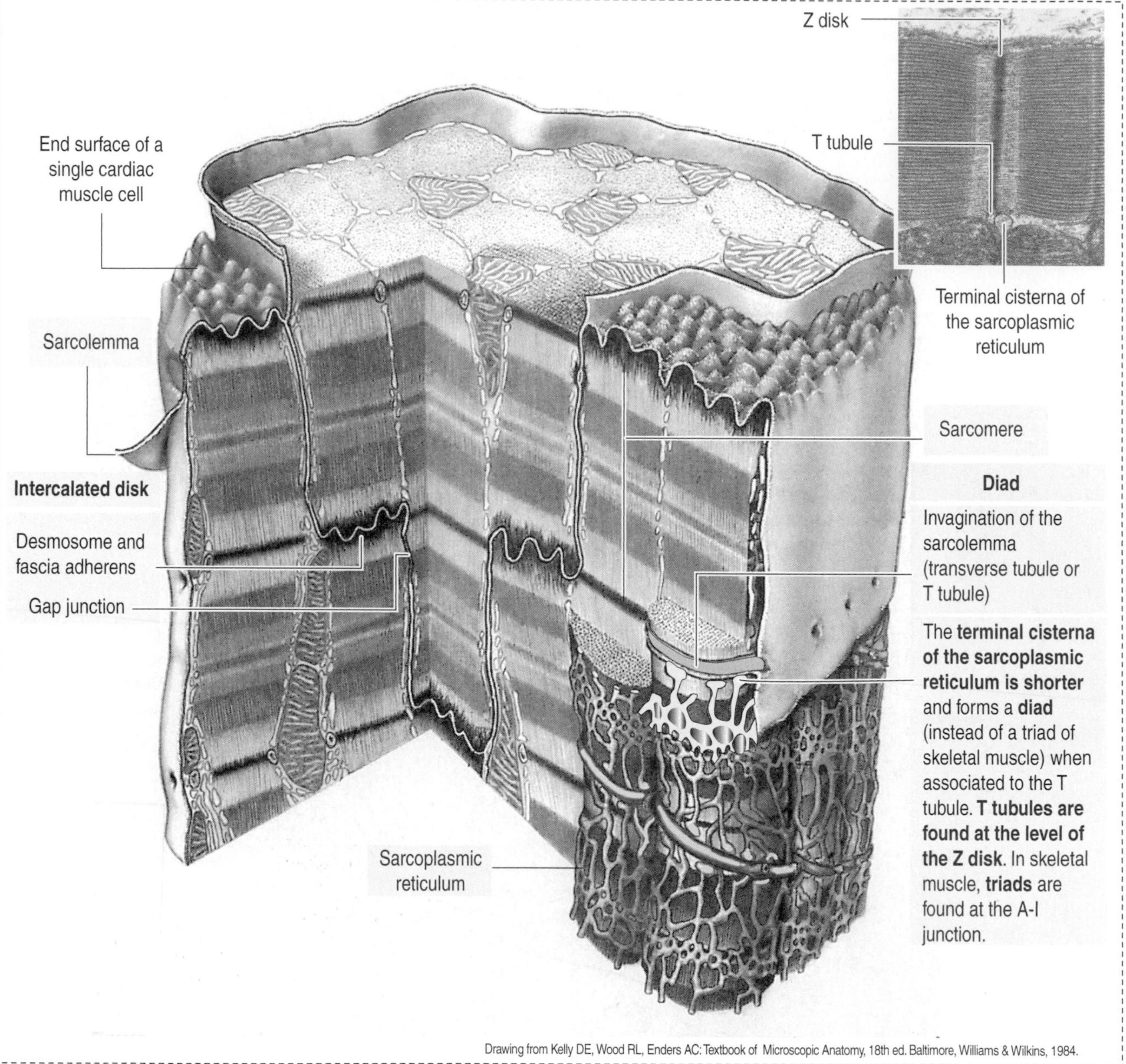

Z disk
T tubule
End surface of a single cardiac muscle cell
Sarcolemma
Intercalated disk
Desmosome and fascia adherens
Gap junction
Terminal cisterna of the sarcoplasmic reticulum
Sarcomere
Diad
Invagination of the sarcolemma (transverse tubule or T tubule)
The terminal cisterna of the sarcoplasmic reticulum is shorter and forms a diad (instead of a triad of skeletal muscle) when associated to the T tubule. T tubules are found at the level of the Z disk. In skeletal muscle, triads are found at the A-I junction.
Sarcoplasmic reticulum

Drawing from Kelly DE, Wood RL, Enders AC: Textbook of Microscopic Anatomy, 18th ed. Baltimore, Williams & Wilkins, 1984.

This situation is corrected by a feedback control mechanism by which the sensory region of the spindle activates gamma motor neurons, which contract the poles of the spindle (the contractile region). Consequently, the spindle stretches.

In addition to the neuromuscular spindle, **Golgi tendon organs**, located **in series** with the extrafusal muscle fibers, provide information about the **tension** or force of contraction of the skeletal muscle.

The neuromuscular spindle is an example of a **proprioceptor** (Latin, *proprius*, one's own; *capio*, to take), a structure that informs how the body is positioned and moves in space.

Types of skeletal muscle fibers

There are three types of skeletal muscle fibers: **red**, **white**, and **intermediate**. Most skeletal muscles contain a mixture of the three types of fibers. All myofibers in a given motor unit are of the same type.

Red fibers are found in **slow twitch** motor units. They are relatively small in diameter with abundant mitochondria. They are resistant to fatigue, and therefore are suited for prolonged muscular activity (for example, maintenance of posture).

White fibers are found in **fast twitch** motor units. They are relatively large, with fewer mitochondria than red fibers. They are rapidly contracting and generally responsible for movement (for example, extraocular muscle).

Intermediate fibers exhibit characteristics between red and white fibers. Human muscles often consist of a mixture of the three types.

Cardiac muscle

Cardiac cells (or **cardiocytes**) are branched cylinders, 85 to 100 μm long, approximately 1.5 μm in diameter (Figure 7-17), with a **single centrally located nucleus** (Figure 7-18).

The organization of contractile proteins is the same as found in skeletal muscle. However, the cytomembranes exhibit some differences:

1. T tubules **are found at the level of the Z disk**, and are substantially larger than those of skeletal muscle found at the A-I junction.
2. The sarcoplasmic reticulum is not as extensive as that of skeletal muscle.
3. **Diads**, rather than the triads seen in skeletal muscle are typical in cardiocytes (see Figure 7-17). A diad consists of a T tubule interacting with just one sarcoplasmic reticulum cisterna (instead of two, as in skeletal muscle).
4. **Mitochondria are more abundant in cardiac muscle** than in skeletal muscle and contain numerous cristae.

The cells are joined end-to-end by specialized junctional complexes called **intercalated disks**. Intercalated disks have a steplike arrangement, with **transverse portions** that run perpendicular to the long axis of the cell and longitudinal portions running in parallel to the myofibrils.

The transverse component is represented by the **Z disk** and consists of (1) **desmosomes**, which mechanically link cardiac cells, and (2) **fasciae adherentes,** which contain α-**actinin** and **vinculin** and provide an insertion site for the actin-containing thin filaments of the last sarcomere of each cardiocyte.

Gap junctions, restricted to the **longitudinal portion** of the intercalated disk, enable ionic communication between cells leading to synchronous muscle contraction.

The terminal fibers of the conducting system of the heart are specialized, glycogen-rich **Purkinje fibers**. Compared with the contractile fibers, Purkinje fibers are larger, paler-stained, and contain fewer myofibrils (see Chapter 12, Cardiovascular System, for additional details).

Clinical significance: Transport proteins on the sarcolemma of cardiocytes

The sarcolemma of the cardiocyte contains specific **transport proteins** (see Figure 7-18) controlling the release and reuptake of ions critical for systolic contractile function and diastolic relaxation.

Active transport of Ca^{2+} into the lumen of the sarcoplasmic reticulum by Ca^{2+}-dependent ATPase is controlled by **phospholamban**. The activity of phospholamban is regulated by phosphorylation. Changes in the amount and activity of phospholamban—regulated by **thyroid hormone**—may alter diastolic function during heart failure and thyroid disease. An increase in heart rate and cardiac output is observed in hyperthyroidism. We discuss the role of phospholamban in Graves' disease (hyperthyroidism) in Chapter 19, Endocrine System.

Additional transporters, including the **Na^{+}- Ca^{2+} exchanger** and **voltage-gated K^{+} channels**, regulate the intracellular levels of K^{+} and Na^{+}. **β-Adrenergic receptor** is also present in the sarcolemma.

Clinical significance: Myocardial infarction

Myocardial infarction is the consequence of a loss of blood supply to the myocardium caused by an obstruction of an atherosclerotic coronary artery. The clinical outcome depends on the anatomic region affected and the extent and duration

Figure 7-18. Cardiac muscle cell or cardiocyte

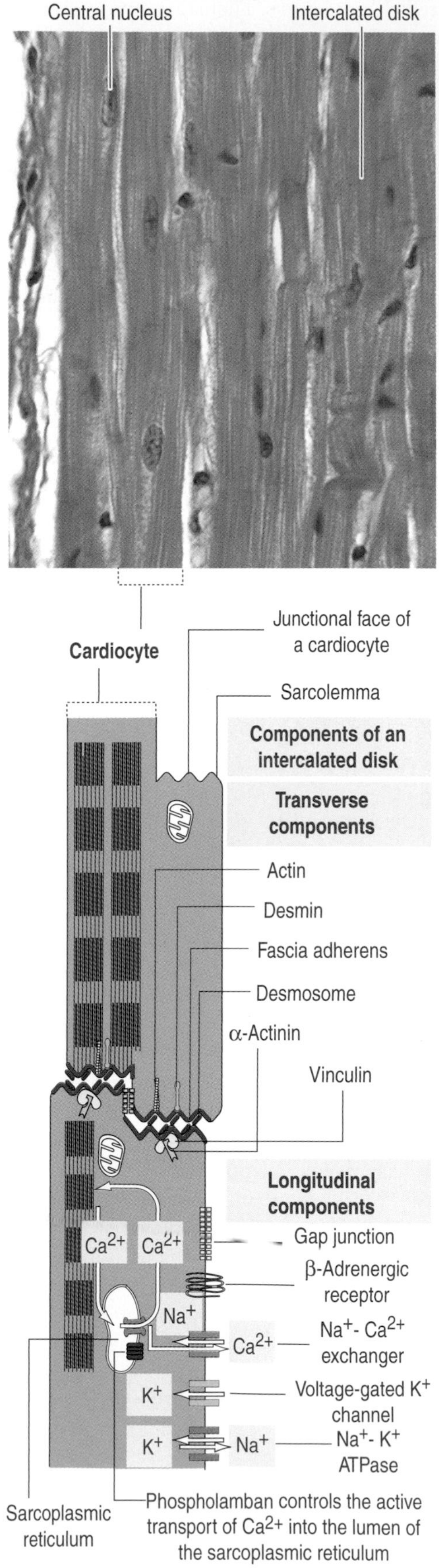

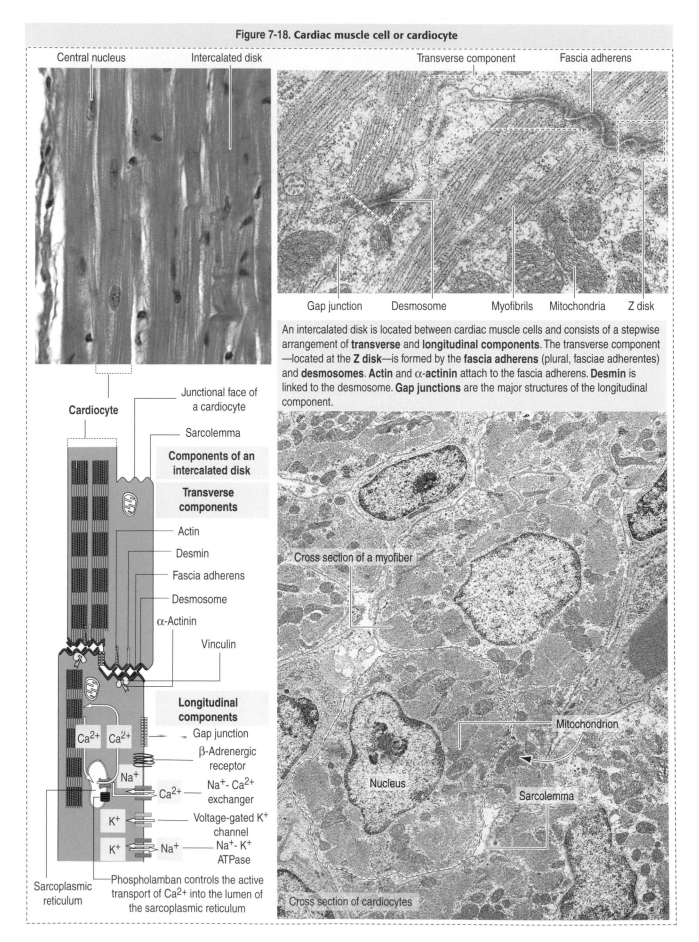

Central nucleus
Intercalated disk
Cardiocyte
Junctional face of a cardiocyte
Sarcolemma
Components of an intercalated disk
Transverse components
Actin
Desmin
Fascia adherens
Desmosome
α-Actinin
Vinculin
Longitudinal components
Gap junction
β-Adrenergic receptor
Ca2+
Ca2+
Na+
Ca2+
Na+- Ca2+ exchanger
K+
Voltage-gated K+ channel
K+
Na+
Na+- K+ ATPase
Sarcoplasmic reticulum
Phospholamban controls the active transport of Ca2+ into the lumen of the sarcoplasmic reticulum

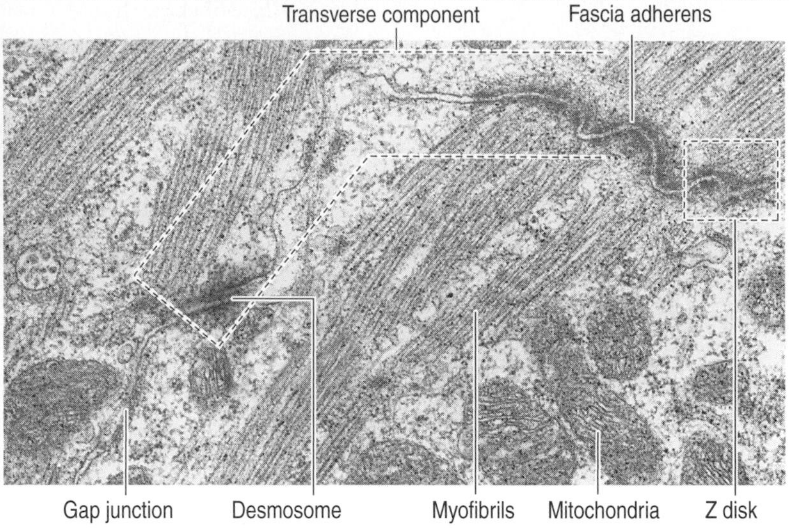

Transverse component
Fascia adherens
Gap junction
Desmosome
Myofibrils
Mitochondria
Z disk

An intercalated disk is located between cardiac muscle cells and consists of a stepwise arrangement of **transverse** and **longitudinal components**. The transverse component —located at the **Z disk**—is formed by the **fascia adherens** (plural, fasciae adherentes) and **desmosomes**. **Actin** and **α-actinin** attach to the fascia adherens. **Desmin** is linked to the desmosome. **Gap junctions** are the major structures of the longitudinal component.

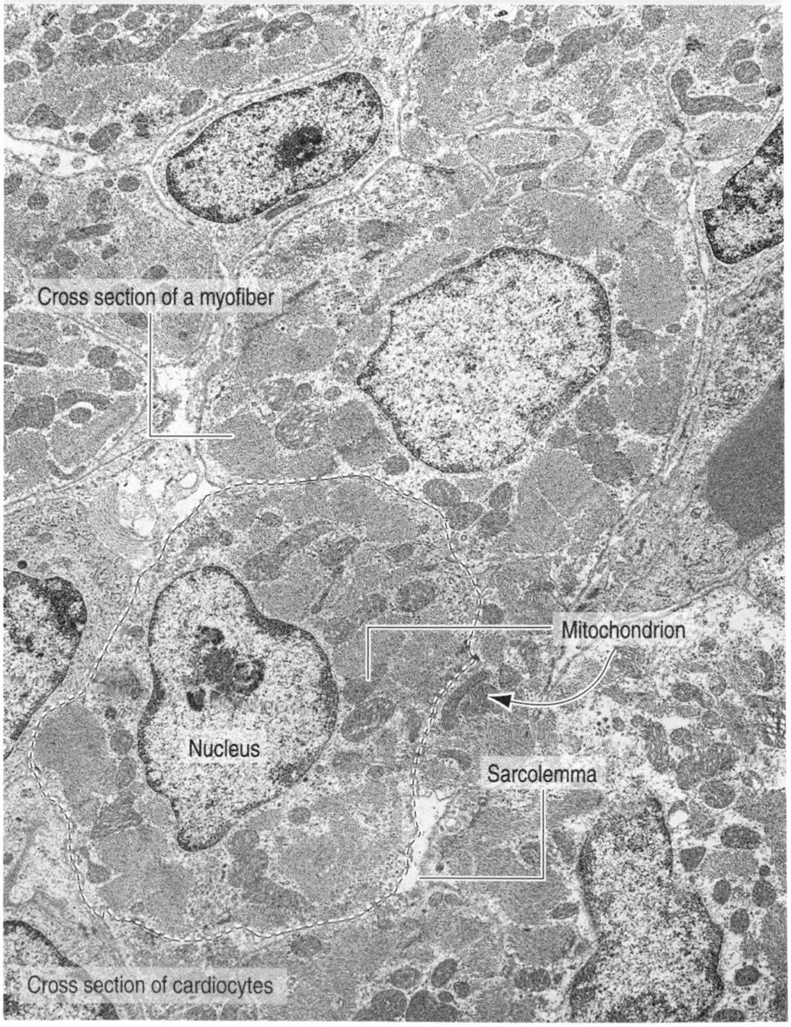

Cross section of a myofiber
Mitochondrion
Nucleus
Sarcolemma
Cross section of cardiocytes

Figure 7-19. **Myocardial infarction**

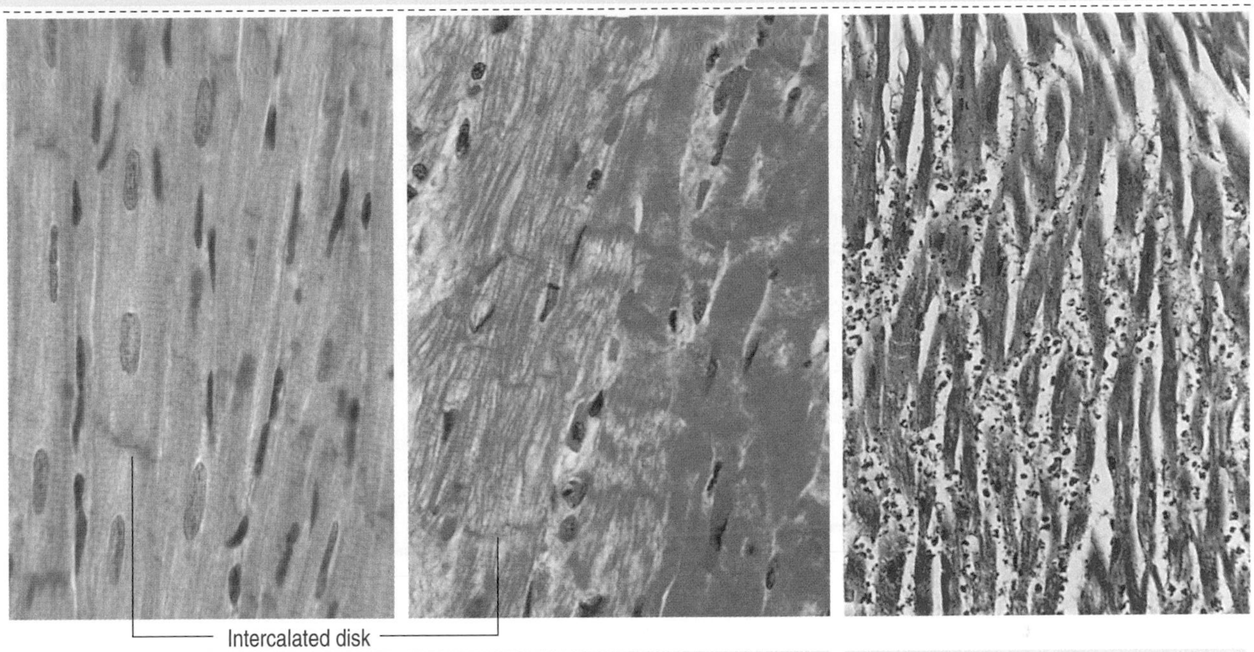

Micrographs left and center from Damjanov I, Linder J: Pathology. Mosby, 2000.

Normal cardiac tissue consists of branching and anastomosing striated cardiocytes with a central nucleus and intracellular contractile myofilaments. Intercalated disks join individual cardiocytes.

Myocardial ischemia caused by occlusion of the coronary artery results within the first **24 hours** in the necrosis of cardiocytes.

Cardiocytes display an eosinophilic cytoplasm lacking the characteristic intracellular striations detected in the adjacent unaffected cardiocytes. The nuclei are pyknotic (Greek, *pyknos*, dense, thick; *osis,* condition) and irregularly shaped. Lactic dehydrogenase-1 and creatine kinase MB*—released from dead cardiocytes—are detected in serum.

Serum levels of these enzymes remain elevated days after the myocardial infarction.

Three days later, the necrotic cardiocytes are surrounded by neutrophils.

After 3 weeks (not shown), capillaries, fibroblasts, macrophages, and lymphocytes are observed in the necrotic area. After 3 months, the infarcted region is replaced by scar tissue.

*Creatine kinase (CK) is composed of two dimers, M and B. CK-MM isoenzyme predominates in skeletal muscle and heart. CK-BB is present in brain, lung, and other tissues. CK-MB is characteristic of myocardium.

of disrupted blood flow.

Irreversible damage of cardiocytes occurs when the loss of blood supply lasts more than 20 minutes. If blood flow is restored in less than 20 minutes—an event known as **reperfusion**—cardiocyte cell viability is maintained. Timing is critical for implementing early therapy to reestablish blood flow by using thrombolytic agents. The histologic changes of myocardial infarction are summarized in Figure 7-19.

Creatine kinase, and its **MB isoenzyme** (CK-MB) are conventional markers of myocardial necrosis. A more sensitive marker is **cardiocyte-specific troponin** I not expressed in skeletal muscle. An increase of troponin I in serum of patients with acute coronary syndromes provides prognostic information on increased risk of death and enables treatment to decrease further myocardial necrosis.

Smooth muscle

Smooth muscle may be found as sheets or bundles in the walls of the gut, bile duct, ureters, urinary bladder, respiratory tract, uterus, and blood vessels.

Smooth muscle differs from skeletal and cardiac muscle: smooth muscle cells are **spindle-shaped, tapering cells** with a **central nucleus** (Figure 7-20). The perinuclear cytoplasm contains mitochondria, ribosomes, rough endoplasmic reticulum, a Golgi apparatus, a latticework of thick **myosin** filaments, thin actin filaments, and intermediate filaments composed of desmin and vimentin. **Actin**

Figure 7-20. Smooth muscle cell

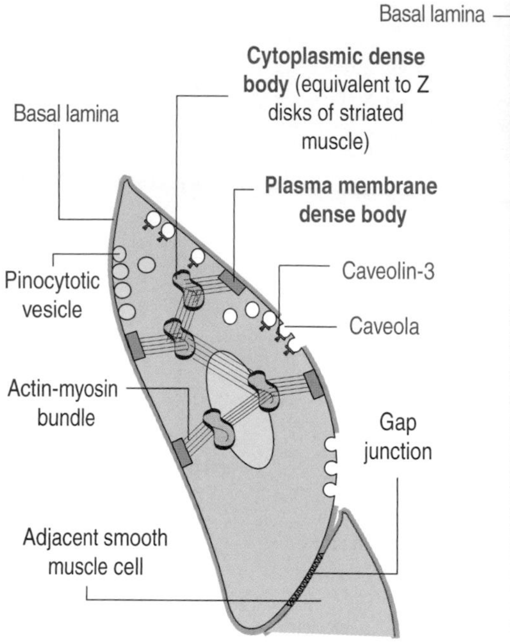

Basal lamina
Cytoplasmic dense body (equivalent to Z disks of striated muscle)
Basal lamina
Plasma membrane dense body
Pinocytotic vesicle
Caveolin-3
Caveola
Actin-myosin bundle
Gap junction
Adjacent smooth muscle cell

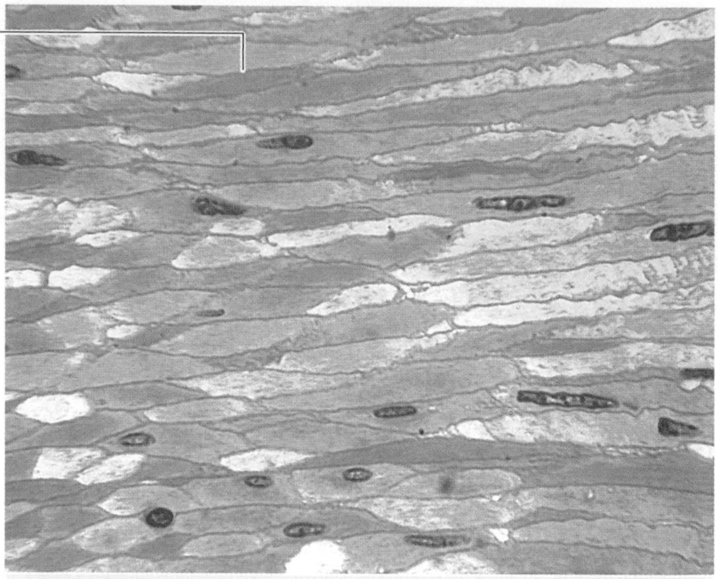

Longitudinal section of smooth muscle cells (muscularis of the stomach). A single oval nucleus is observed in the center of the cells. A **basal lamina** surrounds each smooth muscle cell.

Characteristics of smooth muscle

Smooth muscle is found in the walls of tubular organs, the walls of most **blood vessels**, the **iris** and **ciliary body** (eye), and **arrector pili muscle** (hair follicles), among other sites. It consists of fusiform individual cells or fibers with a **central nucleus**. Smooth cells in the walls of large blood vessels produce **elastin**.

Caveolae—depressions of the plasma membrane—are permanent structures involved in fluid and electrolyte transport (**pinocytosis**).

Caveolin-3, a protein encoded by a member of the caveolin gene family, is associated with **lipid rafts**. Complexes formed by caveolin-3 bound to **cholesterol** in a lipid raft invaginate and form caveolae. Caveolae detach from the plasma membrane to form **pinocytotic vesicles**.

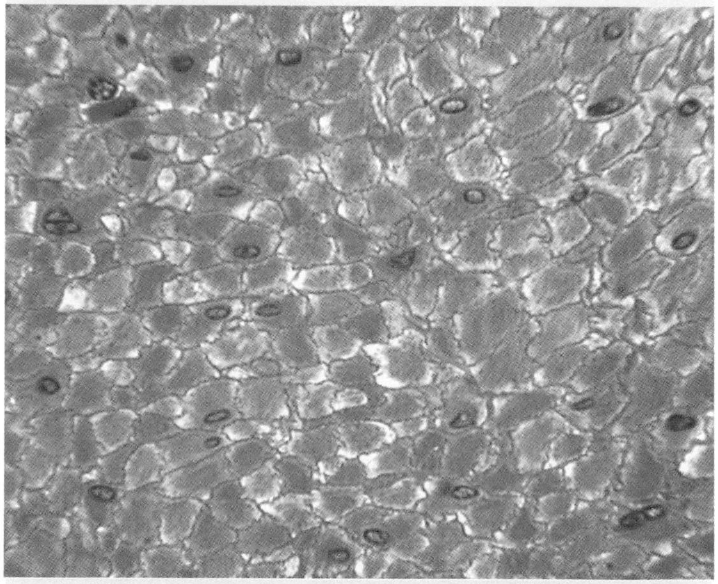

Cross section of smooth muscle cells. Depending on the section level, a central nucleus is observed in some of the muscle cells.

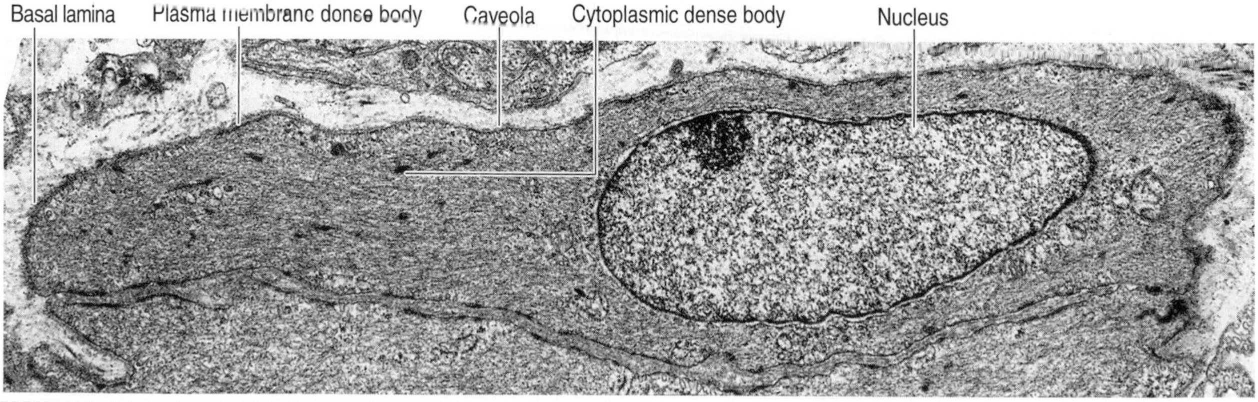

Basal lamina
Plasma membrane dense body
Caveola
Cytoplasmic dense body
Nucleus

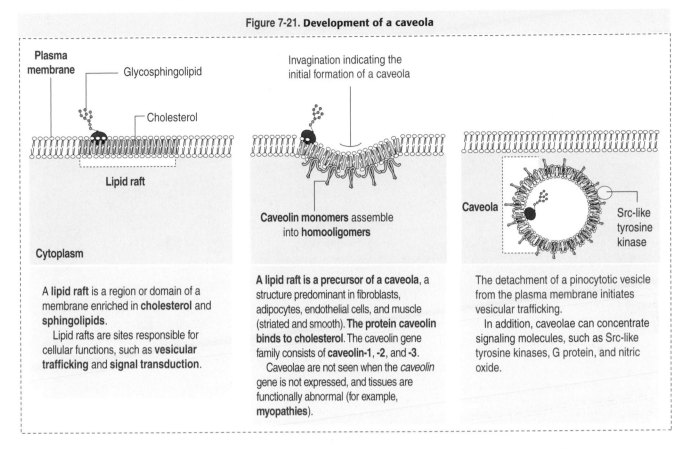

Figure 7-21. Development of a caveola

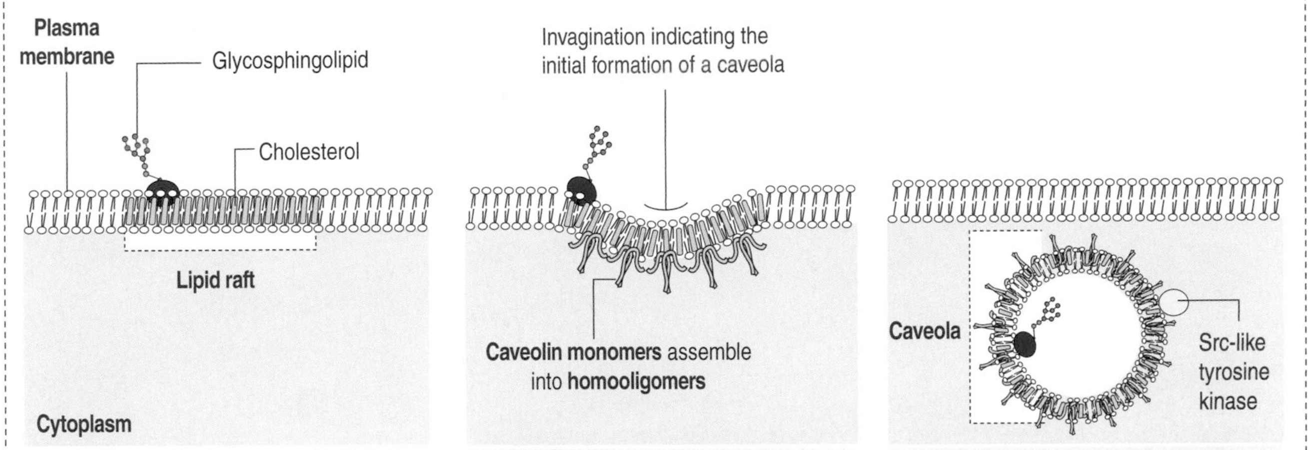
Plasma membrane
Glycosphingolipid
Cholesterol
Lipid raft
Cytoplasm
Invagination indicating the initial formation of a caveola
Caveolin monomers assemble into homooligomers
Caveola
Src-like tyrosine kinase

A **lipid raft** is a region or domain of a membrane enriched in **cholesterol** and **sphingolipids**.

Lipid rafts are sites responsible for cellular functions, such as **vesicular trafficking** and **signal transduction**.

A lipid raft is a precursor of a caveola, a structure predominant in fibroblasts, adipocytes, endothelial cells, and muscle (striated and smooth). **The protein caveolin binds to cholesterol**. The caveolin gene family consists of **caveolin-1**, **-2**, and **-3**.

Caveolae are not seen when the *caveolin* gene is not expressed, and tissues are functionally abnormal (for example, **myopathies**).

The detachment of a pinocytotic vesicle from the plasma membrane initiates vesicular trafficking.

In addition, caveolae can concentrate signaling molecules, such as Src-like tyrosine kinases, G protein, and nitric oxide.

and **intermediate filaments** insert into cytoplasmic and plasma membrane–associated structures rich in α-actinin, called **dense bodies**.

Invaginations of the plasma membrane, called **caveolae**, act as a primitive T tubule system, transmitting depolarization signals to the underdeveloped sarcoplasmic reticulum. The development of caveolae from **lipid rafts** and their diverse roles in several tissues are shown in Figure 7-21. Smooth muscle cells are linked to each other by gap junctions. Gap junctions permit synchronous contraction of the smooth muscle.

A **basal lamina** surrounds each muscle cell and serves to transmit forces produced by each cell.

Mechanism of smooth muscle contraction

Both the arrangement of the contractile proteins and the mechanism of contraction of smooth muscle differ from those of skeletal and cardiac muscle:

1. Actin and myosin filaments are not organized in sarcomeres as seen in cardiac and skeletal muscle.

2. **Smooth muscle cells do not contain troponin** but do contain tropomyosin, which binds to and stabilizes actin filaments.

3. Ca^{2+} ions that initiate contraction derive from outside the cell rather than from the sarcoplasmic reticulum.

4. **Myosin light-chain kinase,** instead of troponin, which is not present in smooth muscle cells, is responsible for the Ca^{2+} sensitivity of the contractile fibers in smooth muscle.

We have seen that the sliding of the myosin-actin complex in striated muscle is the basis for contraction (see Figure 7-9). In smooth muscle, actin filaments and associated myosin attach to cytoplasmic and plasma membrane **dense bodies,** representing the equivalent of the Z disk of striated muscle (see Figure 7–20). Dense bodies are attached to the plasma membrane through desmin and vimentin intermediate filaments. When the actin-myosin complex contracts, their attach-

Figure 7-22. Regulation of smooth muscle contraction

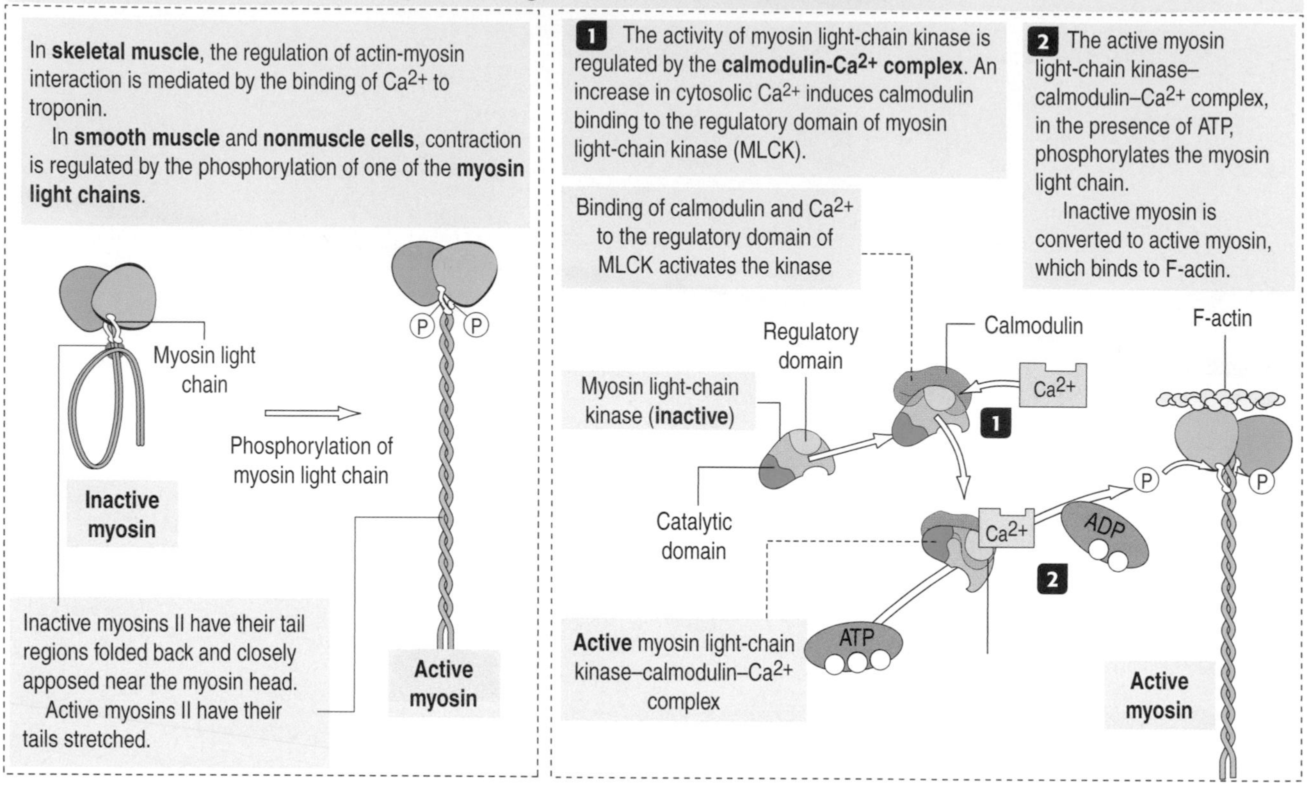

In **skeletal muscle**, the regulation of actin-myosin interaction is mediated by the binding of Ca^{2+} to troponin.
In **smooth muscle** and **nonmuscle cells**, contraction is regulated by the phosphorylation of one of the **myosin light chains**.
Myosin light chain
Phosphorylation of myosin light chain
P
P
Inactive myosin
Inactive myosins II have their tail regions folded back and closely apposed near the myosin head.
Active myosins II have their tails stretched.
Active myosin
1 The activity of myosin light-chain kinase is regulated by the **calmodulin-Ca^{2+} complex**. An increase in cytosolic Ca^{2+} induces calmodulin binding to the regulatory domain of myosin light-chain kinase (MLCK).
2 The active myosin light-chain kinase–calmodulin–Ca^{2+} complex, in the presence of ATP, phosphorylates the myosin light chain.
Inactive myosin is converted to active myosin, which binds to F-actin.
Binding of calmodulin and Ca^{2+} to the regulatory domain of MLCK activates the kinase
Regulatory domain
Calmodulin
F-actin
Myosin light-chain kinase (**inactive**)
Ca^{2+}
1
Catalytic domain
Ca^{2+}
ADP
2
ATP
Active myosin light-chain kinase–calmodulin–Ca^{2+} complex
Active myosin

ment to the dense bodies determines cell shortening.

Calcium-dependent phosphorylation of myosin regulatory light chains is responsible for the contraction of smooth muscle (Figure 7-22). We have already discussed this mechanism in Chapter 1, Epithelium, when we analyzed the role of different myosins in the cell.

Smooth muscle myosin is a **type II myosin**, consisting of two heavy chains and two pairs of light chains. The myosin molecule is folded when dephosphorylated.

When type II myosin phosphorylates, it unfolds and assembles into filaments, the actin binding site on the myosin head is exposed, and myosin can then bind to actin filaments to cause cell contraction.

Smooth muscle can be stimulated to contract by **nervous stimulation, hormonal stimulation**, or **stretch**. For example, intravenous **oxytocin** stimulates uterine muscle contractions during labor.

In response to an appropriate stimulus, there is an increase in cytoplasmic Ca^{2+}. Ca^{2+} binds to **calmodulin**. The Ca^{2+}-calmodulin complex activates **myosin light-chain kinase**, which catalyzes phosphorylation of the myosin light chain. When Ca^{2+} levels decrease, the myosin light chain is enzymatically dephosphorylated, and the muscle relaxes.

• There are three types of muscle: skeletal, cardiac, and smooth muscle.

Skeletal muscle is surrounded by the epimysium, a layer of dense connective tissue. The perimysium, derived from the epimysium, surrounds bundles or fascicles of muscle cells, also called muscle fibers. Each muscle fiber within a fascicle is surrounded by the endomysium, a thin layer of reticular fibers and extracellular matrix closely associated to a basal lamina enveloping each muscle cell.

Skeletal muscle cells are multinucleated cells, resulting from the fusion of myoblasts. Each skeletal muscle cell is surrounded by a plasma membrane (called sarcolemma). The sarcolemma is surrounded by a basal lamina and satellite cells. The sarcolemma projects long processes, called transverse tubules or T tubules, deep into the cytoplasm (called sarcoplasm). The sarcoplasm contains mitochondria (called sarcosomes). Each T tubule is flanked by sacs of the endoplasmic reticulum (called sarcoplasmic reticulum) forming a tripartite structure called a triad, found at the junction of the A band and I band. The nuclei are located at the periphery of the cell. An important component of the sarcoplasm is the myofibril.

A **myofibril** is a linear repeat of sarcomeres. Each sarcomere consists of two major cytoskeletal **myofilaments**: actin and myosin. Note the difference between myofibril and myofilament. The arrangement of these two myofilaments generates a banding pattern (or striation), characteristic of skeletal and cardiac muscle tissue. There is an A band (dark) and I band (light). The A band is at the center of the sarcomere; the Z disk bisects the I band. The A band is bisected by the H band, which contains creatine kinase. The M line runs through the midline of the H band.

A sarcomere is limited by two adjacent Z disks. Actin inserts into each side of the Z disk. Myosin myofilaments do not attach to the Z disk. Actin is associated with the tropomyosin-troponin complex (formed by troponin I, C, and T) and nebulin. Myosin (called myosin II) consists of two identical heavy chains (with a globular head) and two pairs of light chains. The globular heads have an actin-binding region, and ATP-binding region, and a light chain–binding region. Titin is associated with myosin.

Each Z disk is encircled by the intermediate filament desmin. Desmin filaments are linked to each other by plectin. The desmin-plectin complex forms a lattice with the opposite ends attached to costameres in the sarcolemma. This arrangement stabilizes the myofibrils in the sarcoplasm during muscle contraction.

• During muscle contraction, the length of myosin and actin myofilaments does not change. The length of the sarcomere decreases because actin and myosin slide past each other, represented by a reduction in the width of the I band and H band. ATP is an energy source for muscle contraction. Creatine phosphate (produced in sarcosomes) is a backup mechanism to maintain steady levels of ATP during muscle contraction. Creatine kinase catalyzes a reversible reaction generating creatine and ATP from the hydrolysis of creatine phosphate.

The neuromuscular junction is a specialized structure formed by a nerve associated with a target muscle. Inside the muscle, a motor nerve gives rise to numerous branches, each innervating a single muscle cell. The motor nerve and its innervating branches form a motor unit.

An excitation-contraction signal is produced by the release of acetylcholine from a presynaptic button into a primary synaptic cleft, an invagination on the surface of a muscle cell coated with basal lamina containing acetylcholinesterase. The primary synaptic cleft forms secondary synaptic clefts, also covered by basal lamina. Crests of the secondary synaptic clefts contain acetylcholine receptors.

An action potential depolarizes the sarcolemma, and the action potential travels inside the muscle cell along T tubules, which are in contact with channels of the sarcoplasmic reticulum containing calcium. Calcium ions are released, bind to troponin C, and initiate contraction by regulating myosin-actin interaction. When depolarization ends, calcium ions are pumped back into the sarcoplasmic reticulum channels and bind to calsequestrin.

Botulinum toxin binds to the presynaptic membrane of the nerve terminal and blocks the release of acetylcholine. **Curare** binds to the acetylcholine receptor, prevents binding of acetylcholine, and induces muscle paralysis. In **myasthenia gravis**, an autoimmune disease that produces fatigue with exercise, autoantibodies bind to the acetylcholine receptor and prevent binding of acetylcholine.

• **Muscular dystrophies** are a group of congenital muscular diseases characterized by muscle weakness, atrophy, serum levels increases of muscle enzymes, and destructive changes of muscle tissue.

The following protein complexes, some of them part of the dystrophin-associated protein (DAP) complex, are present in the sarcoplasm or in the sarcolemma adjacent to the sarcolemma. They provide mechanical stabilization during muscle contraction:

1. Dystroglycan complex consists of dystroglycan-α and dystroglycan-β. Dystroglycan-α binds to the α chain of laminin-2, and dystroglycan-β binds to dystrophin. No primary defects in the dystroglycan complex have been identified.

2. Sarcoglycan complex consists of six transmembrane subunits (α, β, γ, δ, ε, and ζ). **Sarcoglycanopathies** (for example, **limb-girdle muscular dystrophies**) are caused by defects in components of the sarcoglycan complex.

3. Dystrophin binds the dystroglycan complex to actin in the sarcoplasm. **Duchenne's muscular dystrophy**, an X-linked recessive condition, is caused by a deficiency in dystrophin. The absence of dystrophin results in the loss of syntrophins and other components of the DAP complex.

4. Dystrobrevin (α and β subunits), present in the sarcoplasm.

5. Syntrophins (α, β1, β2, γ1, and γ2 subunits) are found in the sarcoplasm and bind to dystrophin and dystrobrevin.

6. Sarcospan, a transmembrane protein.

• Satellite cells are closely associated to skeletal muscle cells and are covered by a basal lamina. In mature muscle, satellite cells are quiescent. Activated Satellite cells activated by trauma or mechanical stress can self-renew and proliferate. The expression of myogenic regulatory factors (for example, Myf5 and MyoD) activates satellite cells, which become myogenic precursor cells (to form muscle cells) or side-population cells (to differentiate into hematopoietic cells).

• The neuromuscular spindle is a specialized encapsulated sensor of the contraction of various muscles. It contains sensory and motor components and specialized muscle fibers called intrafusal fibers (designated nuclear bag fiber and nuclear chain fiber). Intrafusal fibers are in parallel with the striated extrafusal fibers. When extrafusal fibers contract, the neuromuscular spindle becomes slack. This information is transmitted to the spinal cord, which activates gamma motor neurons that stretch the spindle. In contrast to the neuromuscular spindle, the Golgi tendon organs are located in series with the extrafusal muscle fibers. They provide information about the force of contraction of the skeletal muscle.

• There are three major types of skeletal muscle fibers: red fibers (involved in maintenance of posture), white fibers (responsible for rapid contraction), and intermediate fibers (a combination of the characteristics of red and white fibers). Muscles contain a mixture of the three types of fibers.

• Cardiac muscle consists of branched cylindrical cells called cardiocytes. They contain a central nucleus and myofibrils in the cytoplasm. The organization of the sarcomere is similar to skeletal muscle. The following differences are observed:

(1) T tubules and short portions of the sarcoplasmic reticulum form diads (instead of triads). (2) Diads are found at the level of the Z disk (instead of the A-I band junction). (3) Mitochondria contain abundant cristae. (4) Cardiocytes are joined end-to-end by intercalated disks. (5) Intercalated disks display a steplike arrangement with a transverse portion (containing desmosomes and fasciae adherentes), and a longitudinal portion (where gap junctions are located).

A specialized type of cardiac fiber is the Purkinje fiber, a glycogen-rich cell with fewer myofibrils, involved in conductivity.

• Smooth muscle cells are found in the wall of the alimentary tube, urinary excretory passages, respiratory tract, uterus, and blood vessels.

Smooth muscle cells are spindle-shaped, tapering cells, with a central nucleus and surrounded by a basal lamina. We discussed the ability of smooth muscle cells to synthesize and secrete components of collagen and elastic fibers. The cytoplasm contains actin, myosin, and intermediate filaments.

A typical feature of muscle cells are caveolae, regarded as a primitive T tubule system. Caveolae develop from lipid rafts, a domain in the plasma membrane enriched in cholesterol and sphingolipids. The protein caveolin binds to cholesterol. Caveolae are not seen when the *caveolin* gene is not expressed. The detachment of caveolae forms pynocytotic vesicles, involved in vesicular trafficking and signaling.

• The contraction of smooth muscle cells differs from skeletal and cardiac muscle cells. Smooth muscle cells lack sarcomeres and troponin, and calcium ions initiate contraction from outside the cell, rather than from the sarcoplasmic reticulum.

Myosin light-chain kinase is responsible for the calcium sensitivity of the contractile actin-myosin component of smooth muscle. An equivalent to the Z disk of striated muscle are the dense bodies.

In response to a stimulus, an increase in cytoplasmic calcium binds to calmodulin. The calcium-calmodulin complex activates myosin light-chain kinase, which catalyzes phosphorylation of the myosin light chain and enables binding of activated myosin to actin.

8. NERVOUS TISSUE

General organization of the nervous system

Anatomically, the nervous system can be divided into (1) the **central nervous system (CNS)** (the brain, spinal cord, and neural parts of the eye) and (2) the **peripheral nervous system (PNS)** (peripheral ganglia, nerves, and nerve endings connecting ganglia with the CNS and receptors and effectors of the body). The CNS and PNS are morphologically and physiologically different, and these differences are significant in areas such as neuropharmacology.

The basic cell components of the CNS are **neurons** and **glia**. The PNS contains supporting cells called **satellite cells** and **Schwann cells**, analogous to the glial cells of the CNS.

We start the study of the nervous tissue by reviewing the highlights of the development of the nervous system.

Development of the nervous system

The CNS develops from the primitive ectoderm (Figure 8-1 and Box 8-A). A simple epithelial disk—the **neural plate**—rapidly rolls into a hollow cylinder—the **neural tube**. This process is known as **neurulation**. The neural tube differentiates into the very complex nervous system. During this process, a specialized portion of the neural plate —the **neural crest**— separates from both the neural tube and the overlying ectoderm. In later development, **the neural crest forms the neurons of the peripheral ganglia and other components of the PNS**. A defect in the closing of the neural tube causes different congenital malformations (see Box 8-B).

Neural crest cells remain separated from the neural tube and differentiate into (1) the sensory neurons of the dorsal root and cranial nerve ganglia and (2) the sympathetic and parasympathetic motor neurons of the autonomic ganglia.

Box 8-A | **Neural crest cells**

- The ectoderm germ cell layer gives rise to three major structures: (1) the **surface ectoderm**, primarily the epidermis of the skin (including hair, nails, and sebaceous glands), lens and cornea of the eye, anterior pituitary, and tooth enamel; (2) the **neural tube** (brain and spinal cord); (3) the **neural crest**.
- Cells of the neural crest migrate away from the neural tube and generate components of the peripheral nervous system (Schwann cells and the sympathetic and parasympathetic nervous system), the adrenal medulla, melanocytes of the skin, odontoblasts of the teeth, and neuroglial cells.

Figure 8-1. **Early stages of neural tube formation**

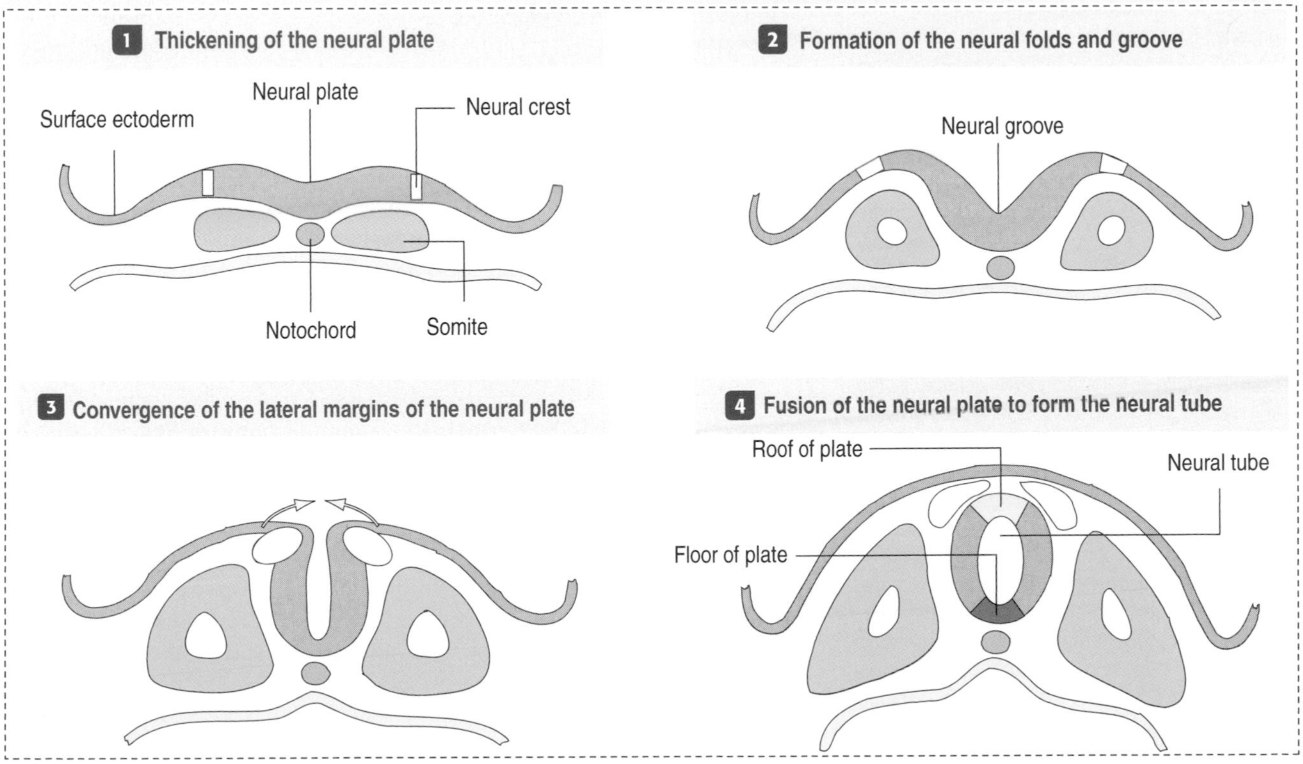

1 Thickening of the neural plate
Surface ectoderm
Neural plate
Neural crest
Notochord
Somite
2 Formation of the neural folds and groove
Neural groove
3 Convergence of the lateral margins of the neural plate
4 Fusion of the neural plate to form the neural tube
Roof of plate
Neural tube
Floor of plate

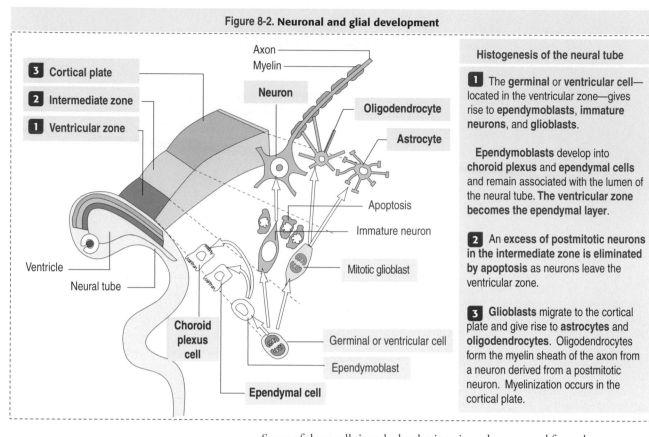

Figure 8-2. **Neuronal and glial development**

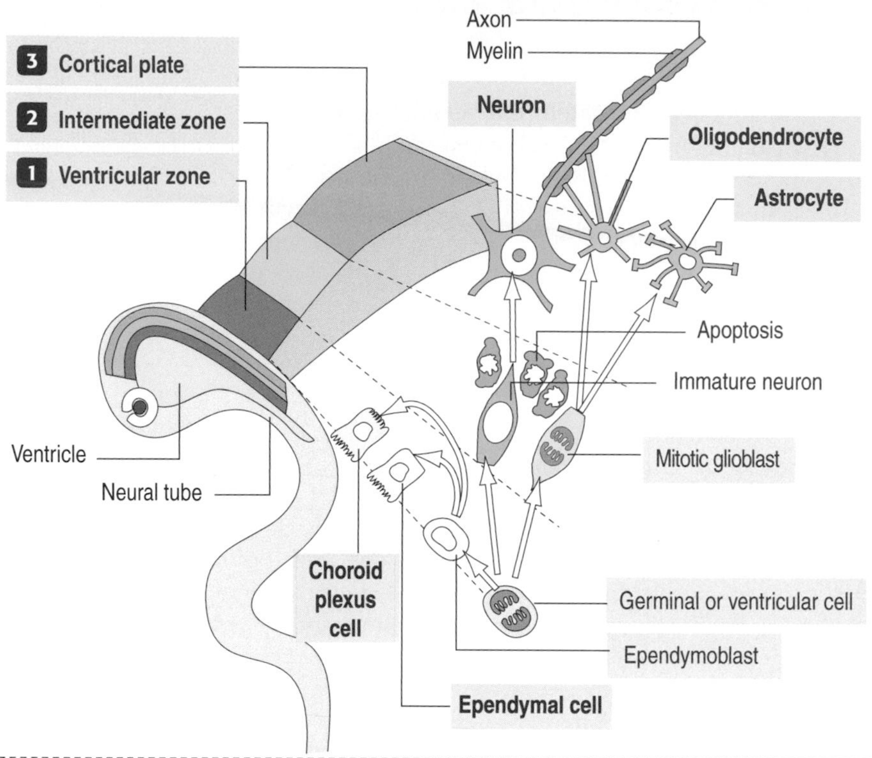

3 Cortical plate
2 Intermediate zone
1 Ventricular zone
Axon
Myelin
Neuron
Oligodendrocyte
Astrocyte
Apoptosis
Immature neuron
Mitotic glioblast
Ventricle
Neural tube
Choroid plexus cell
Germinal or ventricular cell
Ependymoblast
Ependymal cell
Histogenesis of the neural tube
1 The germinal or ventricular cell—located in the ventricular zone—gives rise to ependymoblasts, immature neurons, and glioblasts.
Ependymoblasts develop into choroid plexus and ependymal cells and remain associated with the lumen of the neural tube. The ventricular zone becomes the ependymal layer.
2 An excess of postmitotic neurons in the intermediate zone is eliminated by apoptosis as neurons leave the ventricular zone.
3 Glioblasts migrate to the cortical plate and give rise to astrocytes and oligodendrocytes. Oligodendrocytes form the myelin sheath of the axon from a neuron derived from a postmitotic neuron. Myelinization occurs in the cortical plate.

Box 8-B | **Neural tube defects**

- A defect in the closing of the neural tube causes different congenital malformations.

  Usually, skeletal (skull or vertebral column) defects occur along with malformations of the underlying brain and spinal cord. The latter results from an improper closure of the neural tube during neurulation. Congenital malformations associated with defective neurulation are designated **dysraphic defects**.
- **Spina bifida** is the most common of the spinal cord malformations caused by failure to close the **posterior** regions of the neural tube. The severity of spina bifida depends on the extent of spinal cord being exposed.
- The most severe example of a neural tube defect of the **anterior** region of the neural tube is **anencephaly**, a lethal condition defined by the absence of the brain and the surrounding bone, meninges, muscles, and skin.
- Failure to close the **entire** neural tube is called **craniorachischisis**.
- Closure of the neural tube in humans requires the expression of specific genes (***Pax3***, ***sonic hedgehog***, and ***openbrain***). Following closure, the neural tube separates from the surface ectoderm by a process mediated by cell-adhesion molecules **N-cadherin** and **neural cell adhesion molecule (N-CAM)**. The latter is a member of the immunoglobulin superfamily.

Some of these cells invade developing visceral organs and form the **parasympathetic** and **enteric ganglia** and the **chromaffin cells of the adrenal medulla.**

The Schwann cells and satellite cells of the dorsal root ganglia also develop from neural crest cells. Schwann cells ensheathe and myelinate the peripheral nerve fibers, and the satellite cells encapsulate the neuronal cell bodies in the dorsal root ganglia.

The early neural tube consists of a pseudostratified columnar epithelium formed by three zones (Figure 8-2): (1) the **ventricular zone**—the zone where progenitor cells give rise to most cells of the nervous tissue (except microglial cells); (2) the **intermediate zone**–where neurons migrate toward the cortical plate and where excess neurons are destroyed by apoptosis; and (3) the **cortical plate**—the future gray matter of the cerebral cortex.

In the ventricular zone, **germinal** or **ventricular cells** proliferate rapidly during early development to give rise to **ependymoblasts** (remaining in the ventricular zone) **and glioblasts** and **postmitotic neurons** (migrating to the intermediate zone).

Immature neurons leave the ventricular zone, migrate to the intermediate zone, lose their capacity to undergo cell division, and differentiate into functional neurons. During this differentiation process, a selection process—similar to that in the thymus for T cells (see Chapter 10, Immune-Lymphatic System)—results in either neuronal heterogeneity or death. Neurons that become postmitotic in the intermediate zone reach the outer layers of the cortical mantle and continue their differentiation.

Once the production of immature neurons is complete, the germinal or ventricular cells produce **glioblasts**, which differentiate into **astrocytes, oligodendrocytes,** and **ependymoblasts**. Ependymoblasts give rise to **ependymal cells**, lining the ventricular cavities of the CNS, and **choroid epithelial cells**, which are components of the choroid plexus.

Later, astrocytes develop vascular end-feet attached to blood vessels of the CNS. Coincident with vascularization is the differentiation of **microglia** from monocytes. Microglia respond to injury and become active phagocytic cells.

In later development, glioblasts give rise to **oligodendrocytes**, marking the beginning of **myelination** in the CNS. In contrast to neurons, glioblasts and derived glial cells retain the ability to undergo cell division.

The number of neurons in the human brain is in the range of 10^9 to 100^9. Up to 60% to 70% of these are present in the cerebral cortex. Most neurons are present at birth or shortly thereafter. As the brain continues to grow during the postnatal period, the number and complexity of interneuronal connections increase.

Cell types: Neurons and glia

Neuron

The functional unit of the nervous system is a highly specialized, excitable cell, the nerve cell or **neuron**. Neurons usually consist of three principal components (Figures 8-3 and 8-4): (1) **soma** or **cell body**, (2) **dendrites**, and (3) **axon**.

The soma contains the nucleus and its surrounding cytoplasm (also called **perikaryon**; Greek *peri*, around; *karyon*, nucleus).

The dendrites are processes that arise as multiple treelike branches of the soma, forming a **dendritic tree** collectively. The entire surface of the dendritic branches is covered by small protrusions called **dendritic spines**. Dendritic spines establish numerous axonal synaptic connections, as we will see later (see Figure 8-7).

Neurons have a **single axon** originating from the soma at the **axon hillock** and ending in a terminal arborization, the **telodendron**. Each terminal branch of the telodendron has an enlarged ending, the **synaptic terminal** or **synaptic bouton**.

Note that although dendrites and axons branch extensively, axons branch at their distal end (the telodendron), whereas dendrites are multiple extensions of the soma or cell body.

The surface membrane of the soma and the dendritic tree are specialized for the **reception** and **integration** of information, whereas the axon is specialized for the **transmission** of information in the form of an action potential or a nerve impulse.

Types of neurons

Different types of neurons can be identified on the basis of the **number** and **length** of **processes emerging from the soma** (Figure 8-5):

According to the **number of processes**, neurons can be classified as:

1. **Multipolar neurons**, which display **many processes** attached to a polygonal-shaped soma. The processes include a single axon and more than one dendrite. Multipolar neurons are the most abundant neurons in the nervous system. Pyramidal cells of the cerebral cortex and Purkinje cells and neurons of the cerebellar cortex are two typical examples.

2. **Bipolar neurons** have **two processes**. Bipolar neurons are typical of the visual, auditory, and vestibular system.

3. **Pseudounipolar neurons** have **only one short process** leaving the cell body and are localized in sensory ganglia of cranial and spinal nerves. Embryonically, pseudounipolar neurons derive from bipolar neuroblasts, and the two neuronal processes fuse during later development (hence the prefix **pseudo**).

Based on the **length of the axon relative to the dendritic tree**, multipolar neurons can be subclassified into (1) **Golgi type I** neurons, when the axon extends beyond the limits of the dendritic tree and (2) **Golgi type II** neurons, when an axon terminates in the immediate area of the cell body and does not extend beyond the limits of the dendritic tree. By definition, pyramidal cells and Purkinje cells can be regarded as Golgi type I neurons. Small **stellate cells** of the cerebral cortex are Golgi type II cells.

Designation of groups of neurons and axons

In the CNS, functionally and structurally related neurons form aggregates called **nuclei**. An area called the **neuropil** can be found within a **nucleus** and between the

Figure 8-3. **Components of a neuron**

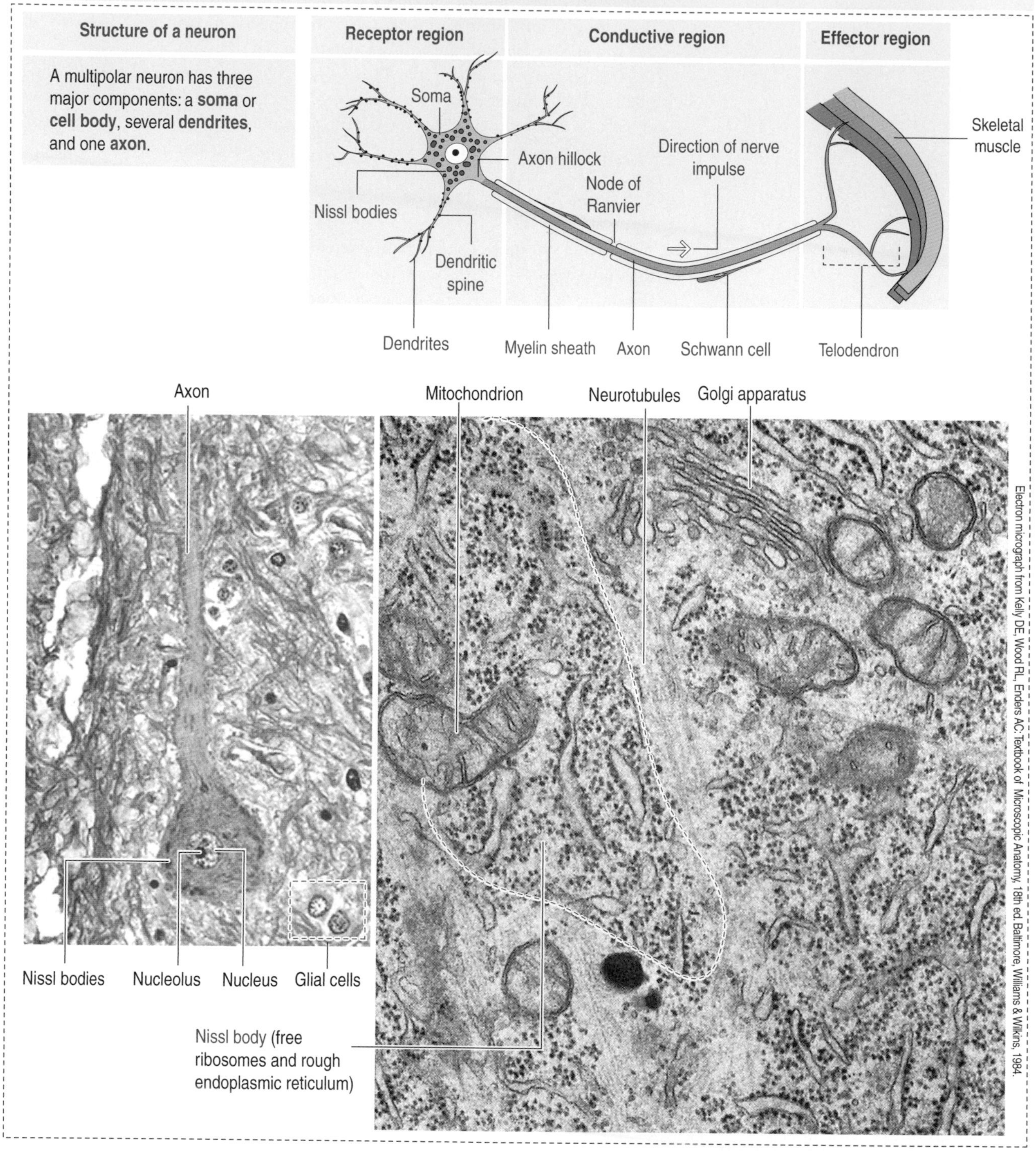
Structure of a neuron
A multipolar neuron has three major components: a **soma** or **cell body**, several **dendrites**, and one **axon**.
Receptor region
Conductive region
Effector region
Soma
Axon hillock
Direction of nerve impulse
Node of Ranvier
Nissl bodies
Dendritic spine
Skeletal muscle
Dendrites
Myelin sheath
Axon
Schwann cell
Telodendron
Axon
Mitochondrion
Neurotubules
Golgi apparatus
Nissl bodies
Nucleolus
Nucleus
Glial cells
Nissl body (free ribosomes and rough endoplasmic reticulum)

Electron micrograph from Kelly DE, Wood RL, Enders AC: Textbook of Microscopic Anatomy, 18th ed. Baltimore, Williams & Wilkins, 1984.

neuronal cell bodies. The term neuropil designates an area with packed dendrites, axonal branches with abundant synapses, and glial cells.

Clusters of neurons arranged in a layer form a **stratum** or **lamina** (cerebral cortex). When neurons form longitudinal groups, these groups are designated **columns**.

Bundles of axons in the CNS are called **tracts**, **fasciculi (bundles)**, or **lemnisci** (for example, the optic tract).

In the PNS, a cluster of neurons forms a **ganglion** (plural **ganglia**). A ganglion can be **sensory**—dorsal root ganglia and trigeminal ganglion—or **motor**—

Figure 8-4. Components of a neuron

Dendrites

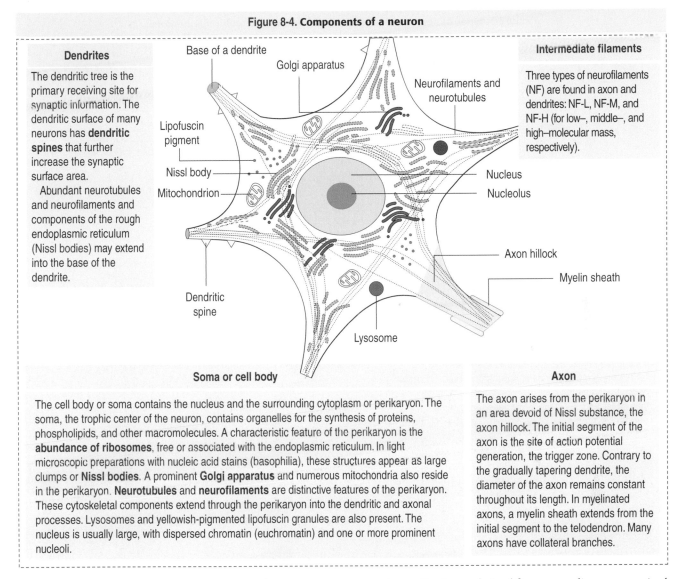

The dendritic tree is the primary receiving site for synaptic information. The dendritic surface of many neurons has **dendritic spines** that further increase the synaptic surface area.

Abundant neurotubules and neurofilaments and components of the rough endoplasmic reticulum (Nissl bodies) may extend into the base of the dendrite.

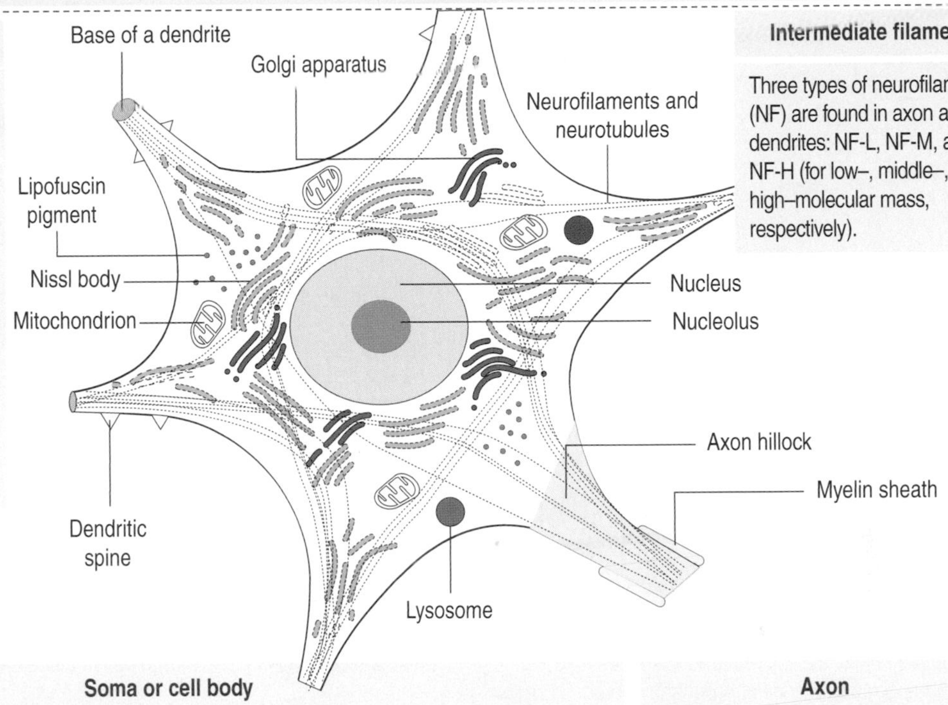

Base of a dendrite
Golgi apparatus
Neurofilaments and neurotubules
Lipofuscin pigment
Nissl body
Mitochondrion
Nucleus
Nucleolus
Axon hillock
Myelin sheath
Dendritic spine
Lysosome

Intermediate filaments

Three types of neurofilaments (NF) are found in axon and dendrites: NF-L, NF-M, and NF-H (for low–, middle–, and high–molecular mass, respectively).

Soma or cell body

The cell body or soma contains the nucleus and the surrounding cytoplasm or perikaryon. The soma, the trophic center of the neuron, contains organelles for the synthesis of proteins, phospholipids, and other macromolecules. A characteristic feature of the perikaryon is the **abundance of ribosomes**, free or associated with the endoplasmic reticulum. In light microscopic preparations with nucleic acid stains (basophilia), these structures appear as large clumps or **Nissl bodies**. A prominent **Golgi apparatus** and numerous mitochondria also reside in the perikaryon. **Neurotubules** and **neurofilaments** are distinctive features of the perikaryon. These cytoskeletal components extend through the perikaryon into the dendritic and axonal processes. Lysosomes and yellowish-pigmented lipofuscin granules are also present. The nucleus is usually large, with dispersed chromatin (euchromatin) and one or more prominent nucleoli.

Axon

The axon arises from the perikaryon in an area devoid of Nissl substance, the axon hillock. The initial segment of the axon is the site of action potential generation, the trigger zone. Contrary to the gradually tapering dendrite, the diameter of the axon remains constant throughout its length. In myelinated axons, a myelin sheath extends from the initial segment to the telodendron. Many axons have collateral branches.

visceromotor or autonomic ganglia. **Axons derived from a ganglion** are organized as **nerves**, **rami** (singular **ramus**), or **roots**.

Synaptic terminals and synapses

The **synaptic terminal** (Figure 8-6) is specialized for the transmission of a chemical message in response to an action potential. The **synapse** is the junction between the **presynaptic terminal** of an axon and a **postsynaptic membrane** receptor surface, generally a dendrite.

The prefixes **pre-** and **post-** refer to the direction of synaptic transmission: (1) **Presynaptic** refers to the transmitting side (usually axonal). (2) **Postsynaptic** identifies the receiving side (usually dendritic or somatic, sometimes axonal). The presynaptic and postsynaptic membranes are separated by a space: the **synaptic cleft**. A dense material coats the inner surface of these membranes: the **presynaptic and postsynaptic densities**.

Presynaptic terminals contain a large number of membrane-bound vesicles (40 to 100 nm in diameter), the **synaptic vesicles**. Synaptic vesicles originate in the neuronal soma and are transported by molecular motor proteins along the axon (**axonal transport**) (Figure 8-7). Each vesicle contains a **neurotransmitter**. Presynaptic terminals contain mitochondria, components of the smooth endoplasmic reticulum, microtubules, and a few neurofilaments.

Figure 8-5. Types of neurons: Bipolar, pseudounipolar, and multipolar neurons

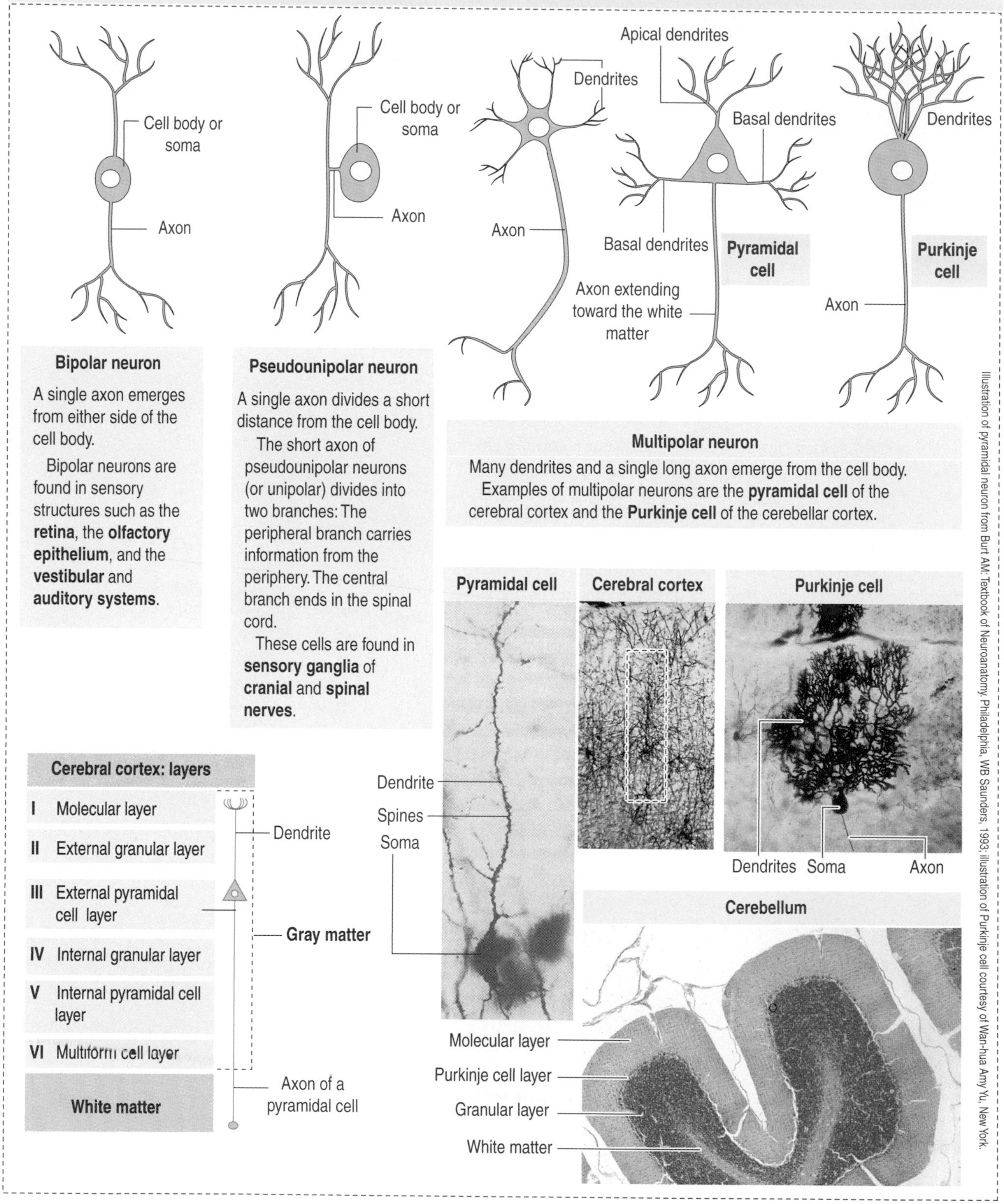

Cell body or soma
Axon
Bipolar neuron
A single axon emerges from either side of the cell body.
Bipolar neurons are found in sensory structures such as the **retina**, the **olfactory epithelium**, and the **vestibular** and **auditory systems**.
Cell body or soma
Axon
Pseudounipolar neuron
A single axon divides a short distance from the cell body.
The short axon of pseudounipolar neurons (or unipolar) divides into two branches: The peripheral branch carries information from the periphery. The central branch ends in the spinal cord.
These cells are found in **sensory ganglia** of **cranial** and **spinal nerves**.
Dendrites
Axon
Apical dendrites
Basal dendrites
Basal dendrites
Pyramidal cell
Axon extending toward the white matter
Dendrites
Purkinje cell
Axon
Multipolar neuron
Many dendrites and a single long axon emerge from the cell body.
Examples of multipolar neurons are the **pyramidal cell** of the cerebral cortex and the **Purkinje cell** of the cerebellar cortex.
Pyramidal cell
Cerebral cortex
Purkinje cell
Dendrite
Spines
Soma
Dendrites
Soma
Axon
Cerebellum
Molecular layer
Purkinje cell layer
Granular layer
White matter
Cerebral cortex: layers
I Molecular layer
II External granular layer
III External pyramidal cell layer
IV Internal granular layer
V Internal pyramidal cell layer
VI Multiform cell layer
White matter
Dendrite
Gray matter
Axon of a pyramidal cell
Illustration of pyramidal neuron from Burt AM: Textbook of Neuroanatomy. Philadelphia, WB Saunders, 1993; illustration of Purkinje cell courtesy of Wan-hua Amy Yu, New York.

Synapses are classified by their **location on the postsynaptic neuron** (Figure 8-8) as follows:

1. **Axospinous** synapses are axon terminals facing a dendritic spine.
2. **Axodendritic** synapses are axon terminals on the shaft of a dendrite.
3. **Axosomatic** synapses are axon terminals on the soma of a neuron.
4. **Axoaxonic** synapses are axon terminals ending on axon terminals.

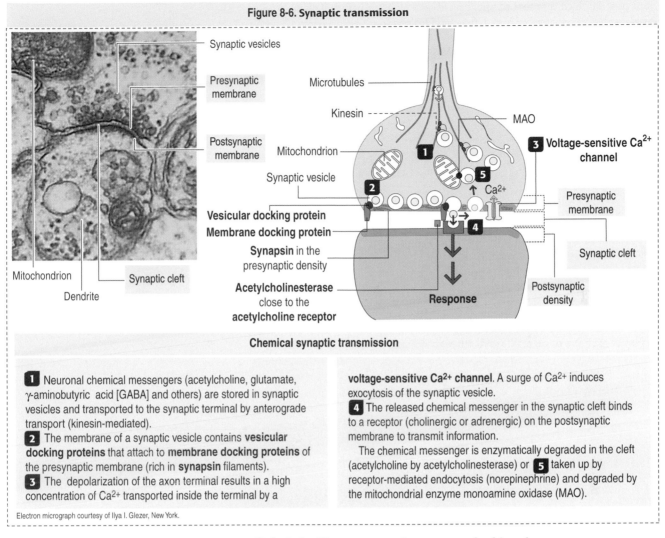

Figure 8-6. Synaptic transmission

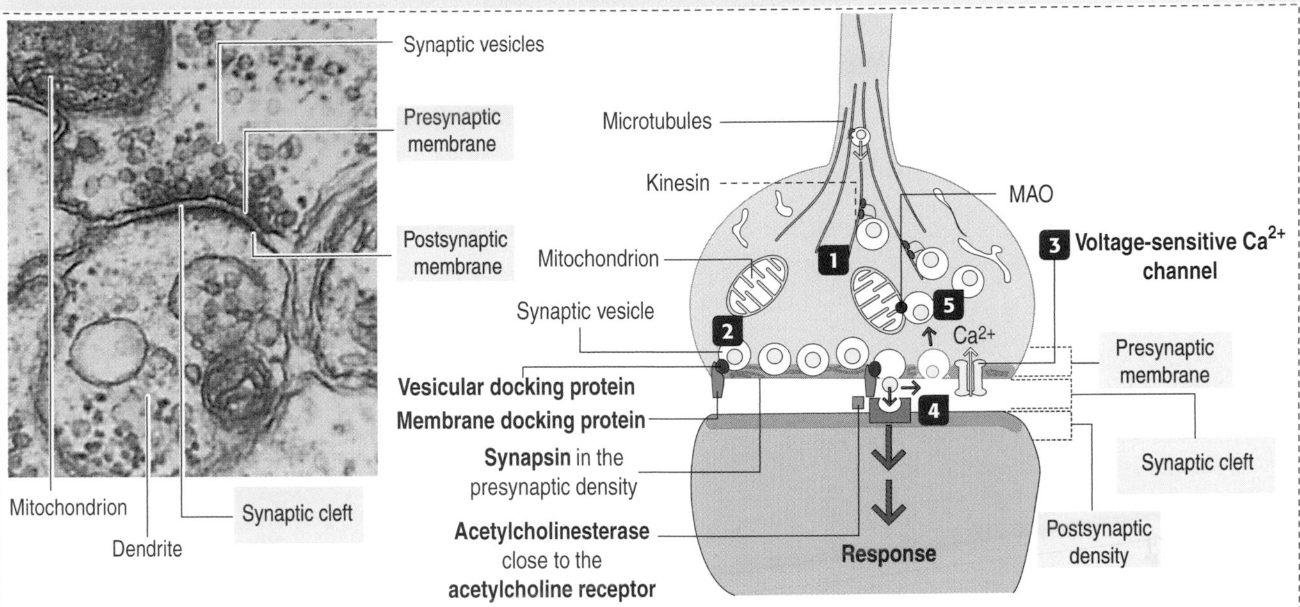

Synaptic vesicles
Presynaptic membrane
Postsynaptic membrane
Mitochondrion
Dendrite
Synaptic cleft
Microtubules
Kinesin
MAO
Mitochondrion
Synaptic vesicle
1
2
3 Voltage-sensitive Ca^{2+} channel
4
5
Ca^{2+}
Vesicular docking protein
Membrane docking protein
Synapsin in the presynaptic density
Acetylcholinesterase close to the acetylcholine receptor
Response
Presynaptic membrane
Synaptic cleft
Postsynaptic density

Chemical synaptic transmission

1 Neuronal chemical messengers (acetylcholine, glutamate, γ-aminobutyric acid [GABA] and others) are stored in synaptic vesicles and transported to the synaptic terminal by anterograde transport (kinesin-mediated).

2 The membrane of a synaptic vesicle contains **vesicular docking proteins** that attach to **membrane docking proteins** of the presynaptic membrane (rich in **synapsin** filaments).

3 The depolarization of the axon terminal results in a high concentration of Ca^{2+} transported inside the terminal by a **voltage-sensitive Ca^{2+} channel**. A surge of Ca^{2+} induces exocytosis of the synaptic vesicle.

4 The released chemical messenger in the synaptic cleft binds to a receptor (cholinergic or adrenergic) on the postsynaptic membrane to transmit information.

The chemical messenger is enzymatically degraded in the cleft (acetylcholine by acetylcholinesterase) or **5** taken up by receptor-mediated endocytosis (norepinephrine) and degraded by the mitochondrial enzyme monoamine oxidase (MAO).

Electron micrograph courtesy of Ilya I. Glezer, New York.

Clinical significance: Axonal transport of rabies virus

The role of the axonal cytoskeleton and motor proteins (kinesin and cytoplasmic dynein; see Figure 8-7) was discussed in the Cytoskeleton section of Chapter 1, Epithelium. We extend the discussion by emphasizing the bidirectional transport of molecules along the axon: **kinesin-mediated anterograde axonal transport** of neurotransmitters—from the cell body toward the axon terminals, and the **cytoplasmic dynein-mediated retrograde axonal transport** of growth factors and recycling of axon terminal components—from the axon terminals to the cell body (see Box 8-C).

Axonal transport is important in the pathogenesis of neurologic infectious diseases. For example, the **rabies virus** introduced by the bite of a rabid animal replicates in the muscle tissue from as short as 2 to 16 weeks or longer. After binding to the **acetylcholine receptor**, the viral particles are mobilized by **retrograde axonal transport** to the cell body of neurons supplying the affected muscle. The rabies virus continues to replicate within infected neurons and after the shedding of the virions by budding, they are internalized by the terminals of adjacent neurons. Further dissemination of the rabies virus occurs in the CNS. From the CNS, the rabies virus is transported by **anterograde axonal transport** by the peripheral nerves to the salivary glands. The virus enters the saliva to be transmitted by the bite. Painful **spasm of the throat muscles on swallowing** accounts for **hydrophobia** (aversion to swallowing water).

The retrograde axonal transport to the CNS of **tetanus toxin**—a protease produced by the vegetative spore form of *Clostridium tetani* bacteria after entering

Figure 8-7. **Axonal transport**

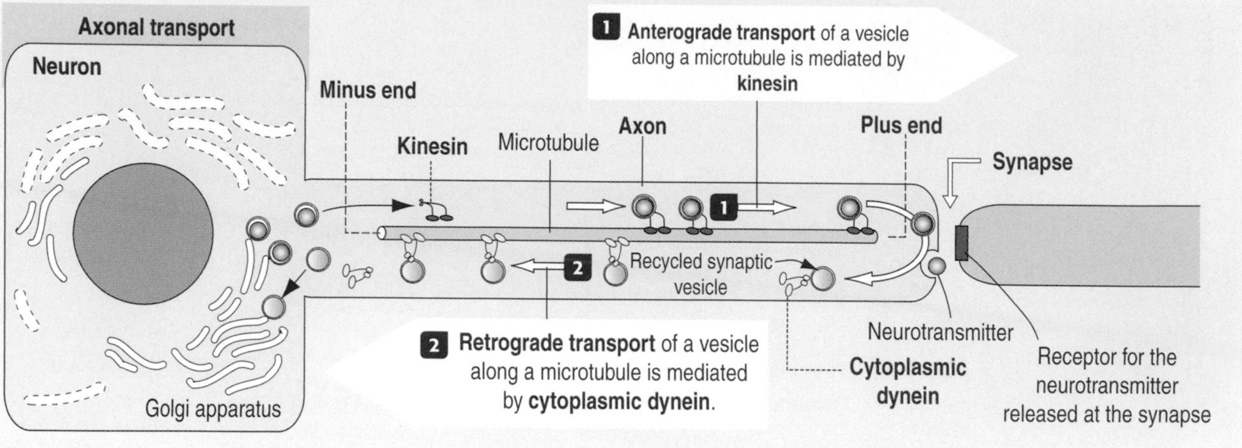

Axonal transport
Neuron
Minus end
Kinesin
Microtubule
Axon
Plus end
Synapse
1 Anterograde transport of a vesicle along a microtubule is mediated by kinesin
Recycled synaptic vesicle
Neurotransmitter
Receptor for the neurotransmitter released at the synapse
Cytoplasmic dynein
2 Retrograde transport of a vesicle along a microtubule is mediated by cytoplasmic dynein.
Golgi apparatus

at a wound site— blocks the release of inhibitory mediators at spinal synapses. Spasm contraction of the jaw muscles (known as **trismus**), exaggerated reflexes, and respiratory failure are characteristic clinical findings.

Glia, the "connective tissue" of the CNS

Glial cells (Greek *glia,* glue) are more numerous than neurons and retain the capacity to proliferate. Most brain tumors, benign or malignant, are of glial origin. When the CNS is injured, glial cells mobilize, clean up the debris, and seal off the local area, leaving behind a "glial scar" (gliosis), which interferes with neuronal regeneration.

Glial cells include (1) **astrocytes**, derived from the **neuroectoderm**; (2) **oligodendrocytes**, derived from the **neuroectoderm**; and (3) **microglia**, derived from the **mesoderm**.

Unlike neurons, glial cells do not propagate action potentials and their processes do not receive or transmit electrical signals. The **function of glial cells is to provide neurons with structural support and maintain local conditions for neuronal function.**

Astrocytes

Astrocytes are observed in the CNS and are divided into two categories: (1) **fibrous astrocytes**, and (2) **protoplasmic astrocytes**.

Fibrous astrocytes are found predominantly in **white matter** and have long thin processes with few branches. **Protoplasmic astrocytes** reside predominantly in **gray matter** and have shorter processes with many short branches. Astrocytic processes end in expansions called **end-feet** (Figure 8-9).

One of the distinctive features of astrocytes is the presence of a large number of **glial filaments** (**glial fibrillary acidic protein**, a class of intermediate filament studied in Chapter 1, Epithelium). Glial fibrillary acidic protein is a valuable marker for the identification of astrocytes by immunohistochemistry. Nuclei of astrocytes are large, ovoid, and lightly stained.

Most brain capillaries and the inner surface of the pia mater are completely surrounded by **astrocytic end-feet** (see Figure 8-9) forming the **glia limitans** (also called the glial limiting membrane). The close association of astrocytes and brain capillaries suggests a role in the regulation of brain metabolism.

Astrocytes surround neurons and neuronal processes in areas devoid of myelin sheaths and form the structural matrix for the nervous system.

Oligodendrocytes and Schwann cells: Myelinization

Oligodendrocytes are smaller than astrocytes and their nuclei are irregular and densely stained. The cytoplasm contains an extensive Golgi apparatus, many

Box 8-C | **Neurotransmitters**

- Incoming nerve impulses produce focal changes in the **resting membrane potential** of the neuron that spread along the membrane of dendrites and soma.
  Information is conducted along the processes as an electrical excitation (**depolarization**) generated across the cell membrane.
- As the resting membrane potential diminishes, a **threshold level** is reached, **voltage-gated Ca^{2+} channels** open, Ca^{2+} enters the cell, and at that point, the resting potential is reversed: the inside becomes positive with respect to the outside.
- In response to this reversal, the **Na^+ channel** closes and remains closed for the next 1 to 2 msec (the **refractory period**). Depolarization also causes the opening of **K^+ channels** through which K^+ leaves the cell, thus repolarizing the membrane.
- Neuron-to-neuron contacts or **synapses** are specialized for one-way transfer of excitation. Interneuronal communication occurs at a **synaptic junction**, the specialized communication site between the terminal of an axon of one neuron and the dendrite of another.
- When an action potential reaches the axon terminal, a chemical messenger or **neurotransmitter** is released to elicit an appropriate response.

Figure 8-8. Types of synapses

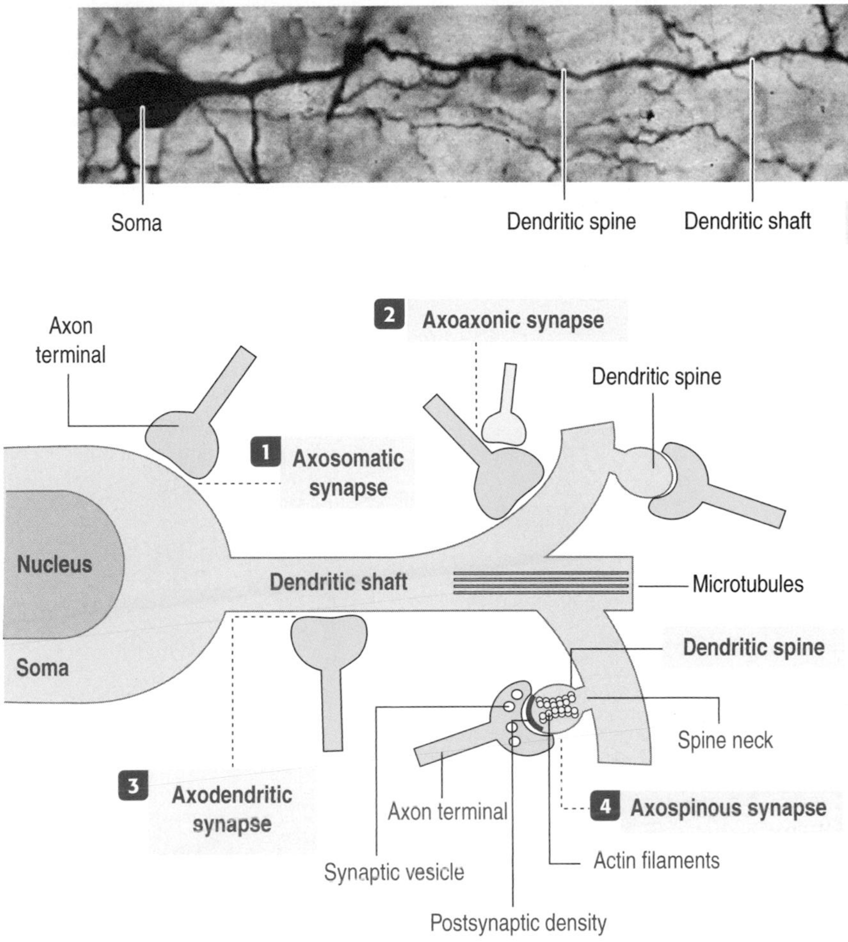

Types of synapses

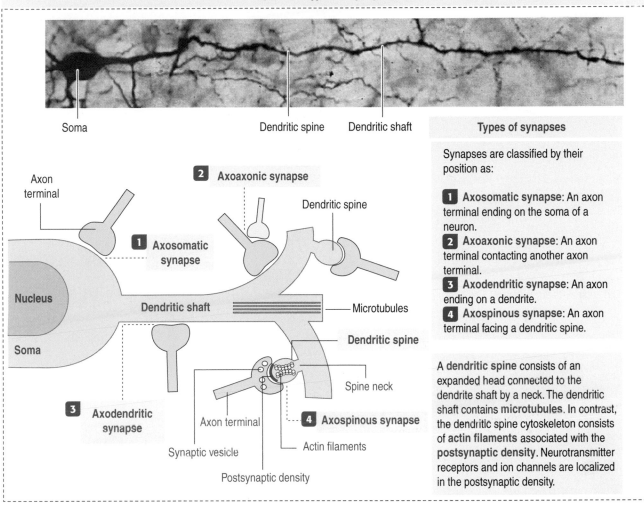

Synapses are classified by their position as:

1 Axosomatic synapse: An axon terminal ending on the soma of a neuron.
2 Axoaxonic synapse: An axon terminal contacting another axon terminal.
3 Axodendritic synapse: An axon ending on a dendrite.
4 Axospinous synapse: An axon terminal facing a dendritic spine.

A **dendritic spine** consists of an expanded head connected to the dendrite shaft by a neck. The dendritic shaft contains **microtubules**. In contrast, the dendritic spine cytoskeleton consists of **actin filaments** associated with the **postsynaptic density**. Neurotransmitter receptors and ion channels are localized in the postsynaptic density.

mitochondria, and a large number of microtubules. One function of oligodendrocytes is **axonal myelination**.

Processes of oligodendrocytes envelop axons and form a sheathlike covering (Figure 8-10). **The formation of this sheath is similar to that of Schwann cells in peripheral nerves.**

Myelin sheaths extend from the initial segments of axons to their terminal branches. The segments of myelin formed by individual oligodendrocyte processes are **internodes**. The periodic gaps between the internodes are the **nodes of Ranvier**.

A single oligodendrocyte has many processes and may form 40 to 50 internodes. The nodes of Ranvier are naked segments of axon between the internodal segments of myelin. This region contains a high concentration of voltage-gated sodium channels, essential for the **saltatory conduction** of the action potential. During saltatory conduction in the myelinated axons, the **action potential** "jumps" from one node to the next.

During the formation of the myelin sheath, a cytoplasmic process of the oligodendrocyte wraps around the axon and, after one full turn, the external surface of the glial membrane makes contact with itself, forming the **inner mesaxon** (Figure 8-11).

As the oligodendrocyte process continues to spiral around the axon, the external surfaces fuse to form the first **intraperiod line.** At the same time, the cytoplasm is squeezed off from the intracellular space (like toothpaste from a tube), and the cytoplasmic surfaces fuse to form the first **dense line**.

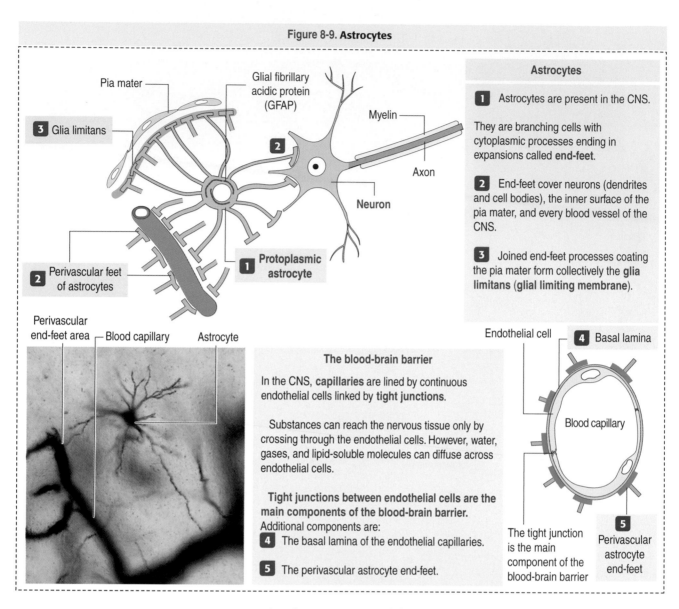

Figure 8-9. Astrocytes

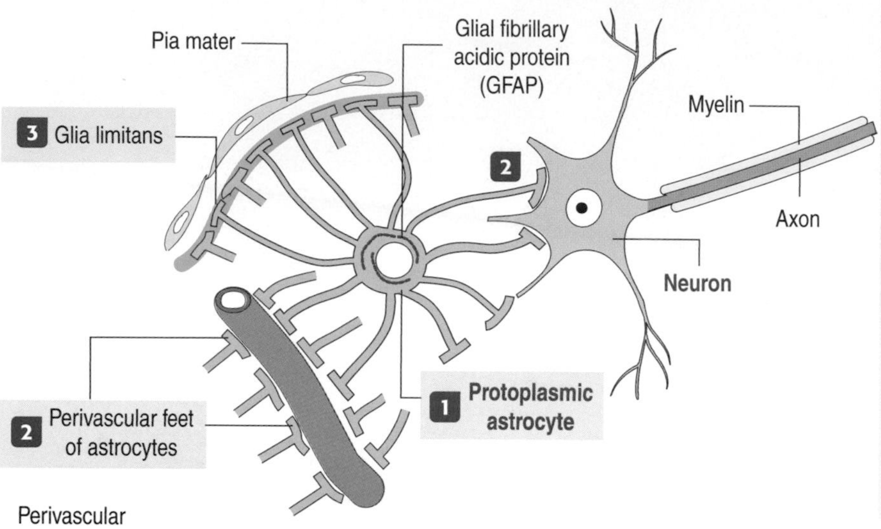

Pia mater
Glial fibrillary acidic protein (GFAP)
3 Glia limitans
2
Myelin
Axon
Neuron
2 Perivascular feet of astrocytes
1 Protoplasmic astrocyte

Astrocytes

1 Astrocytes are present in the CNS.

They are branching cells with cytoplasmic processes ending in expansions called **end-feet.**

2 End-feet cover neurons (dendrites and cell bodies), the inner surface of the pia mater, and every blood vessel of the CNS.

3 Joined end-feet processes coating the pia mater form collectively the **glia limitans (glial limiting membrane**).

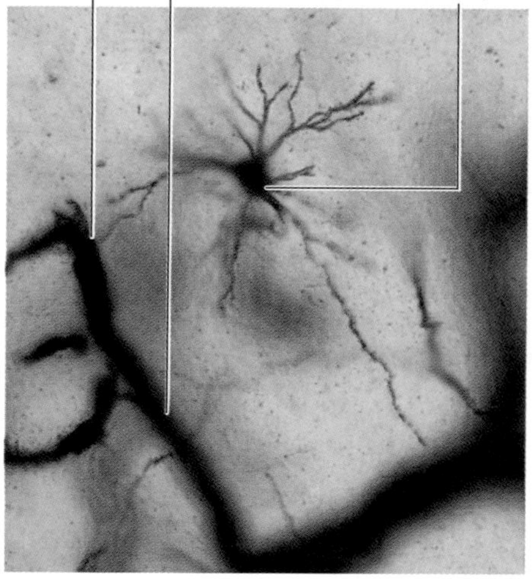

Perivascular end-feet area
Blood capillary
Astrocyte

The blood-brain barrier

In the CNS, **capillaries** are lined by continuous endothelial cells linked by **tight junctions.**

Substances can reach the nervous tissue only by crossing through the endothelial cells. However, water, gases, and lipid-soluble molecules can diffuse across endothelial cells.

Tight junctions between endothelial cells are the main components of the blood-brain barrier. Additional components are:

4 The basal lamina of the endothelial capillaries.

5 The perivascular astrocyte end-feet.

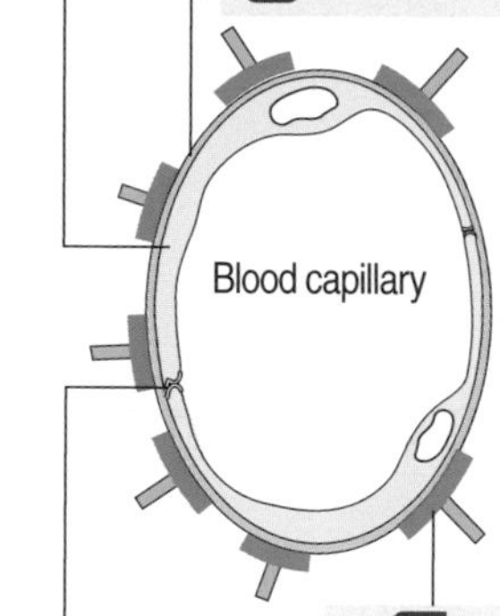

Endothelial cell
4 Basal lamina
Blood capillary
The tight junction is the main component of the blood-brain barrier
5 Perivascular astrocyte end-feet

Spiraling continues until the axon is invested with a number of wrappings. The alternate fusion of both the cytoplasmic and external surfaces of the membrane results in an interdigitated double spiral (see Figure 8-11), one of **intraperiod lines** (fused external surfaces with remnant extracellular space), and one of **major dense lines** (fused cytoplasmic surfaces).

The dense line terminates when the membrane surfaces separate to enclose the cytoplasm at the surface of the sheath (the **tongue**), and the intraperiod line terminates as the tongue turns away from the sheath. The **incisures of Schmidt-Lanterman** are seen in longitudinal sections of myelinated nerve fibers in the CNS and PNS. They correspond to areas of residual cytoplasm.

As the myelin sheath approaches the node of Ranvier region, an additional ring of cytoplasm separates the cytoplasmic surfaces of the cell membrane. These tongues make contact with the **axolemma**, or surface membrane of the axon, in the paranodal region. Axons branch to form collaterals at a node of Ranvier.

The apposed interdigitating processes of myelinating Schwann cells and the incisures of Schmidt-Lanterman are linked by **tight junctions**. They are called **autotypic tight junctions** because they link plasma membranes of the **same** cell. **Heterotypic tight junctions** are seen between the axolemma (surrounding the axon) and the Schwann cell paranodal cytoplasmic loops adjacent to the node of Ranvier.

Figure 8-10. Oligodendrocytes and nodes of Ranvier in the CNS and PNS

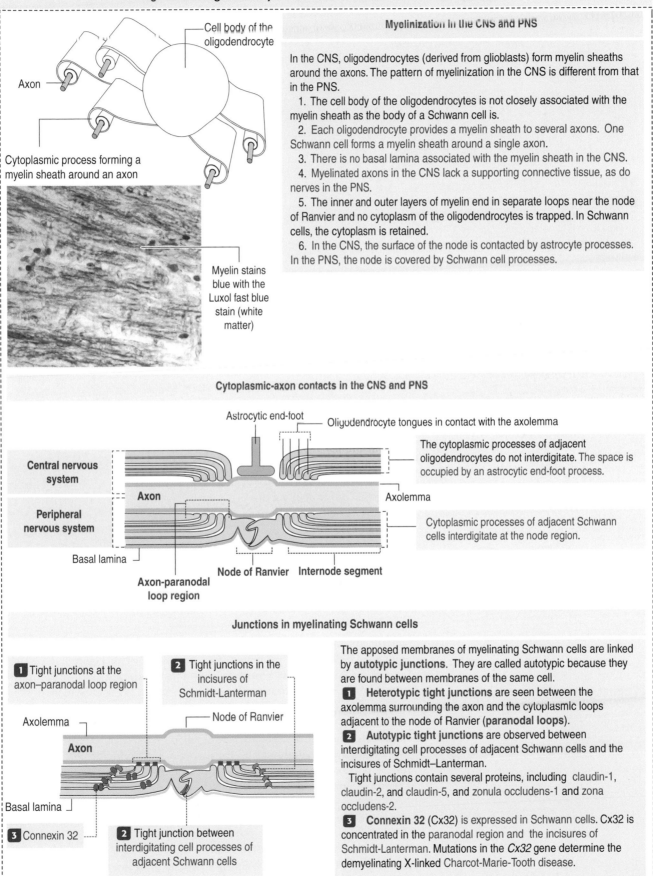

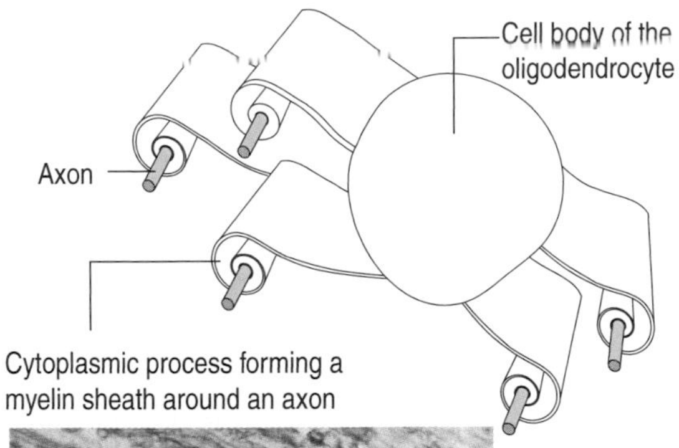

Cell body of the oligodendrocyte
Axon
Cytoplasmic process forming a myelin sheath around an axon

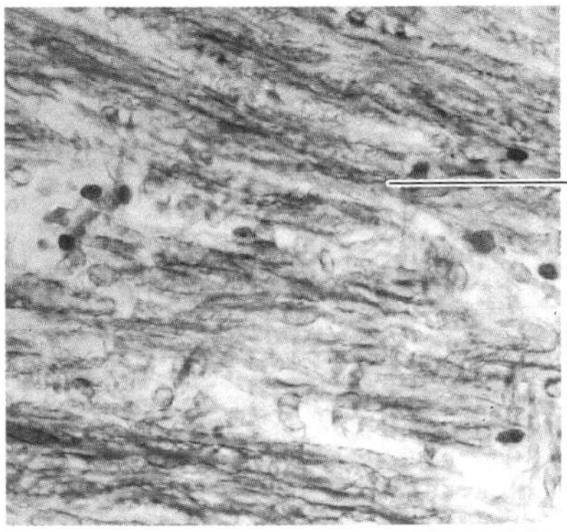

Myelin stains blue with the Luxol fast blue stain (white matter)

Myelinization in the CNS and PNS

In the CNS, oligodendrocytes (derived from glioblasts) form myelin sheaths around the axons. The pattern of myelinization in the CNS is different from that in the PNS.

1. The cell body of the oligodendrocytes is not closely associated with the myelin sheath as the body of a Schwann cell is.
2. Each oligodendrocyte provides a myelin sheath to several axons. One Schwann cell forms a myelin sheath around a single axon.
3. There is no basal lamina associated with the myelin sheath in the CNS.
4. Myelinated axons in the CNS lack a supporting connective tissue, as do nerves in the PNS.
5. The inner and outer layers of myelin end in separate loops near the node of Ranvier and no cytoplasm of the oligodendrocytes is trapped. In Schwann cells, the cytoplasm is retained.
6. In the CNS, the surface of the node is contacted by astrocyte processes. In the PNS, the node is covered by Schwann cell processes.

Cytoplasmic-axon contacts in the CNS and PNS

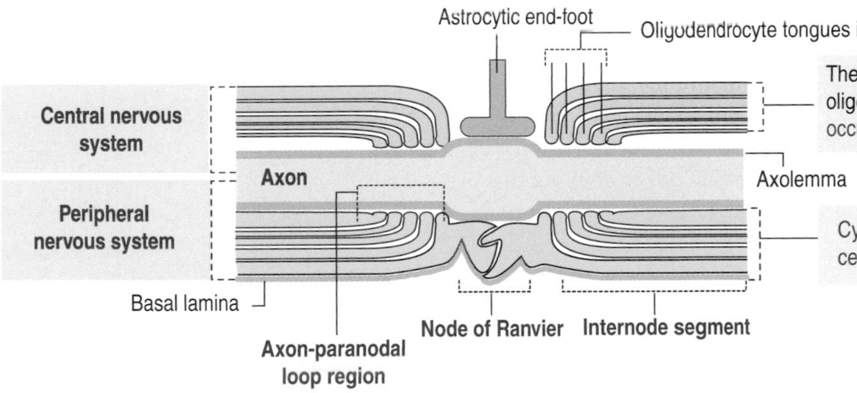

Astrocytic end-foot
Oligodendrocyte tongues in contact with the axolemma
Central nervous system
Axon
Axolemma
Peripheral nervous system
Basal lamina
Axon-paranodal loop region
Node of Ranvier
Internode segment

The cytoplasmic processes of adjacent oligodendrocytes do not interdigitate. The space is occupied by an astrocytic end-foot process.

Cytoplasmic processes of adjacent Schwann cells interdigitate at the node region.

Junctions in myelinating Schwann cells

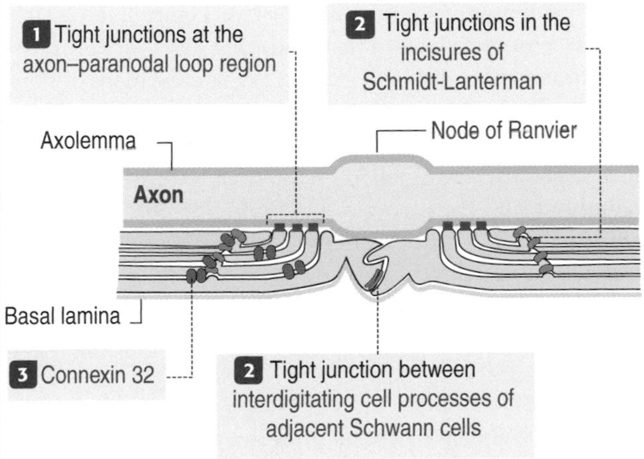

1 Tight junctions at the axon–paranodal loop region
2 Tight junctions in the incisures of Schmidt-Lanterman
Axolemma
Node of Ranvier
Axon
Basal lamina
3 Connexin 32
2 Tight junction between interdigitating cell processes of adjacent Schwann cells

The apposed membranes of myelinating Schwann cells are linked by **autotypic junctions**. They are called autotypic because they are found between membranes of the same cell.

1 **Heterotypic tight junctions** are seen between the axolemma surrounding the axon and the cytoplasmic loops adjacent to the node of Ranvier (**paranodal loops**).

2 **Autotypic tight junctions** are observed between interdigitating cell processes of adjacent Schwann cells and the incisures of Schmidt–Lanterman.

Tight junctions contain several proteins, including claudin-1, claudin-2, and claudin-5, and zonula occludens-1 and zona occludens-2.

3 **Connexin 32** (Cx32) is expressed in Schwann cells. Cx32 is concentrated in the paranodal region and the incisures of Schmidt-Lanterman. Mutations in the *Cx32* gene determine the demyelinating X-linked Charcot-Marie-Tooth disease.

Figure 8-11. **Myelinization**

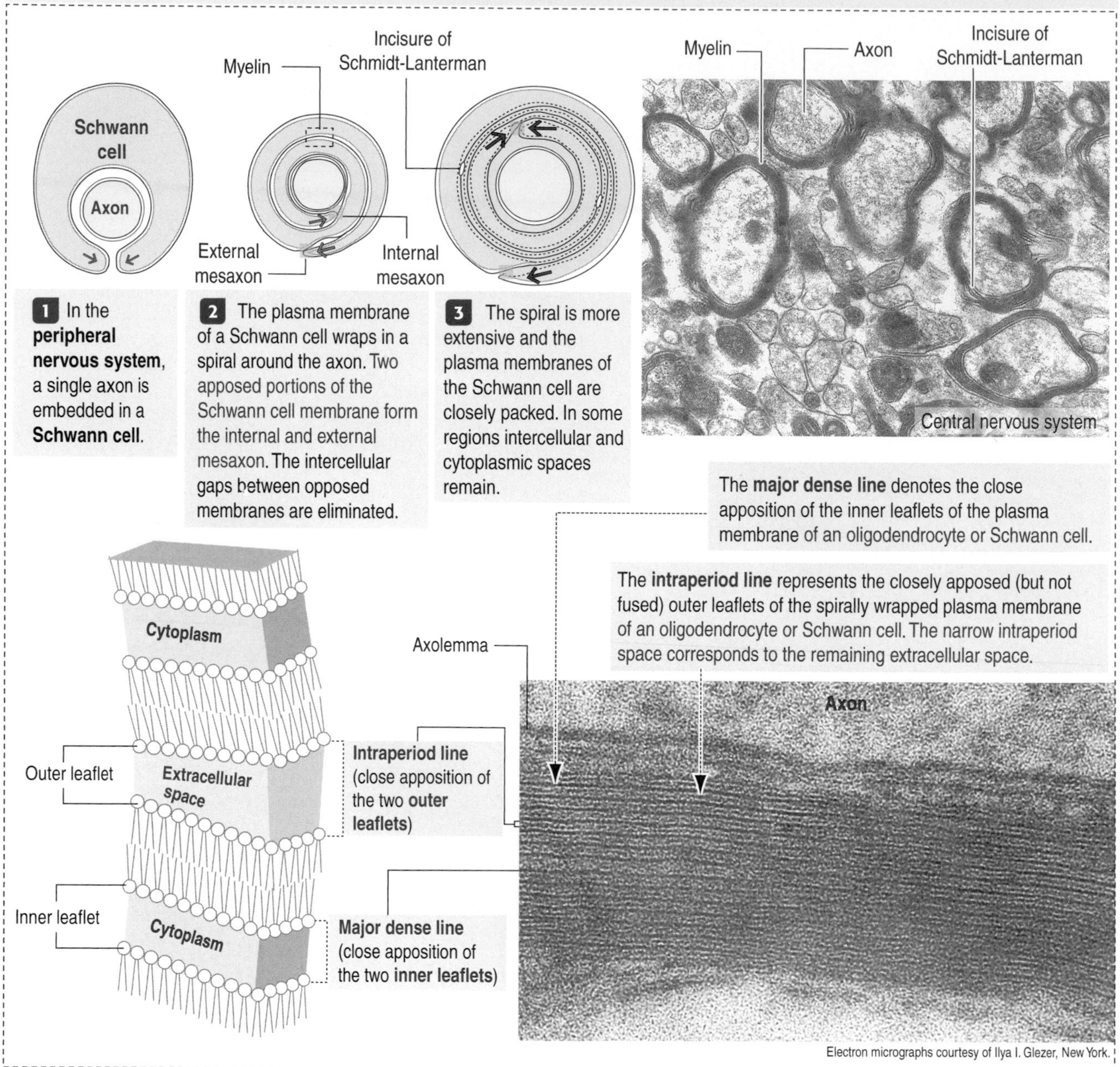

Schwann cell
Axon
Myelin
Incisure of Schmidt-Lanterman
External mesaxon
Internal mesaxon
1 In the **peripheral nervous system**, a single axon is embedded in a **Schwann cell**.
2 The plasma membrane of a Schwann cell wraps in a spiral around the axon. Two apposed portions of the Schwann cell membrane form the internal and external mesaxon. The intercellular gaps between opposed membranes are eliminated.
3 The spiral is more extensive and the plasma membranes of the Schwann cell are closely packed. In some regions intercellular and cytoplasmic spaces remain.
Myelin
Axon
Incisure of Schmidt-Lanterman
Central nervous system
The **major dense line** denotes the close apposition of the inner leaflets of the plasma membrane of an oligodendrocyte or Schwann cell.
The **intraperiod line** represents the closely apposed (but not fused) outer leaflets of the spirally wrapped plasma membrane of an oligodendrocyte or Schwann cell. The narrow intraperiod space corresponds to the remaining extracellular space.
Cytoplasm
Axolemma
Outer leaflet
Extracellular space
Intraperiod line (close apposition of the two **outer leaflets**)
Inner leaflet
Cytoplasm
Major dense line (close apposition of the two **inner leaflets**)
Axon
Electron micrographs courtesy of Ilya I. Glezer, New York.

Tight junctions contain **claudins** (claudin-1, claudin-2, and claudin-5) and **zonula occludens** (ZO) **proteins** (ZO-1 and ZO-2) (see Figure 8-10). Tight junctions (1) stabilize newly formed wraps of myelin during nerve development, (2) act as a selective permeability barrier, and (3) restrict the movement of lipids and proteins from specific membrane domains.

Connexin 32 (Cx32) is found in Schwann cells. Cx32 does not form gap junctions with other Schwann cells. Instead, Cx32 predominates in the paranodal membranes and incisures of Schmidt-Lanterman and forms intercellular channels linking portions of the same cell. Mutations in the *Cx32* gene causes **X-linked Charcot-Marie-Tooth disease**, a demyelinating disorder of the PNS characterized by the progressive loss of both motor and sensory functions of the distal legs (see Box 8-D).

Myelin: Protein and lipid components

Myelin in the CNS and PNS is similar in overall protein and lipid composition, except that myelin in the PNS contains more sphingomyelin and glycoproteins.

Figure 8-12. **Structure of myelin**

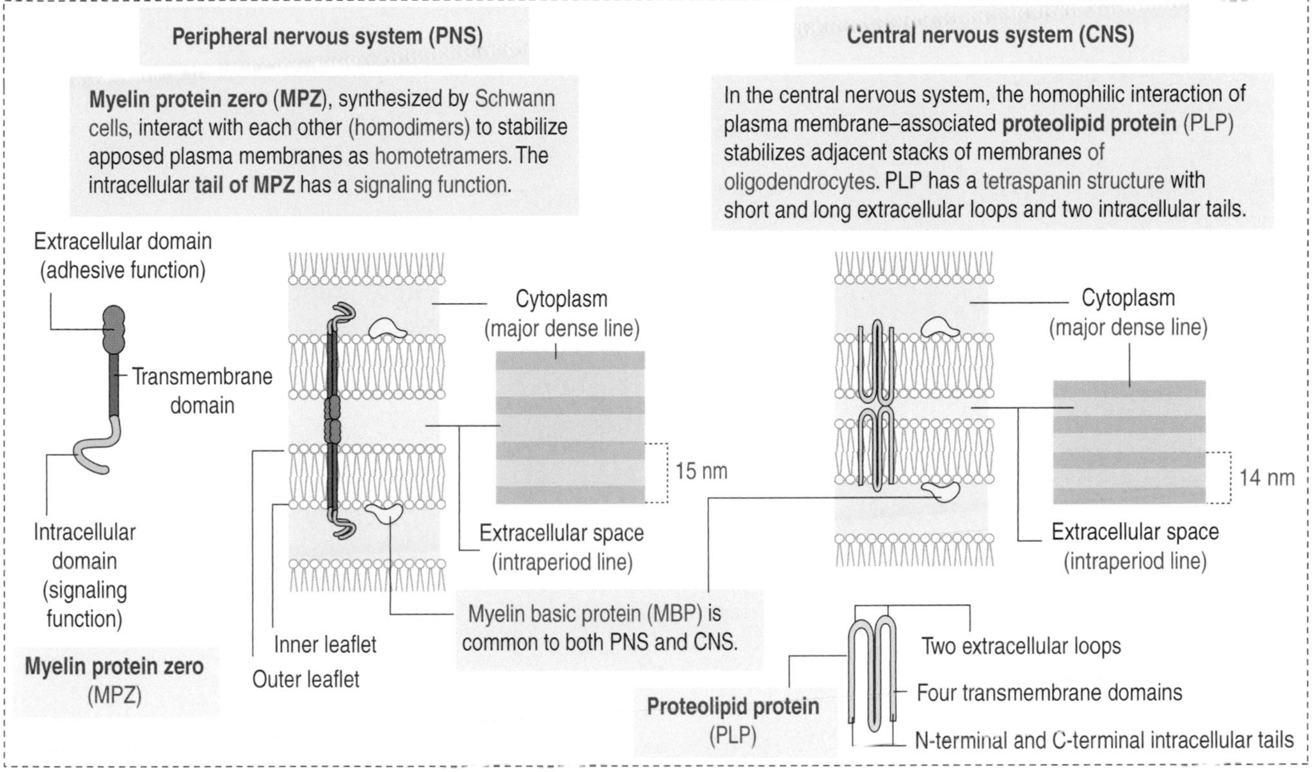

Peripheral nervous system (PNS)
Myelin protein zero (**MPZ**), synthesized by Schwann cells, interact with each other (homodimers) to stabilize apposed plasma membranes as homotetramers. The intracellular **tail of MPZ** has a signaling function.
Extracellular domain (adhesive function)
Transmembrane domain
Intracellular domain (signaling function)
Myelin protein zero (MPZ)
Inner leaflet
Outer leaflet
Cytoplasm (major dense line)
15 nm
Extracellular space (intraperiod line)
Myelin basic protein (MBP) is common to both PNS and CNS.
Central nervous system (CNS)
In the central nervous system, the homophilic interaction of plasma membrane–associated **proteolipid protein** (PLP) stabilizes adjacent stacks of membranes of oligodendrocytes. PLP has a tetraspanin structure with short and long extracellular loops and two intracellular tails.
Cytoplasm (major dense line)
14 nm
Extracellular space (intraperiod line)
Proteolipid protein (PLP)
Two extracellular loops
Four transmembrane domains
N-terminal and C-terminal intracellular tails

Three proteins are particularly relevant (Figure 8-12): **myelin basic protein (MBP)**, **proteolipid protein (PLP)**, and **myelin protein zero (MPZ)**.

MBP is a cytosolic plasma membrane–bound protein present in both the myelin of the PNS and CNS. PLP is a tetraspanin protein found only in the myelin of the CNS. PLP plays a significant role in neural development and is a structural component of myelin. A mutation of the *PLP* gene and its alternatively transcribed DM20 protein causes **Pelizaeus-Merzbacher disease**, an X-linked dysmyelinating neuropathty in which affected males have a reduction of white matter and a reduction in the number of oligodendrocytes. The most common characteristics of Pelizaeus-Merzbacher disease are flickering eyes, and physical and mental retardation.

The predominant protein in myelin of the PNS is **MPZ**, a functional equivalent to PLP in the CNS. The extracellular domain of two MPZ proteins extends into the extracellular space to establish homophilic interaction with a similar pair of MPZ molecules on an opposite membrane. The **homotetrameric** structure provides intermembrane adhesion essential for the compactation of myelin (see Figure 8-13). The intracellular domain of MPZ participates in a signaling cascade that regulates myelinogenesis. In the CNS, plasma membrane–associated PLPs interact with each other and have a similar stabilizing function.

Proteins of myelin are strong antigens with a role in autoimmune diseases such as **multiple sclerosis** in the CNS and **Guillain-Barré syndrome** in the PNS.

Some axons of the PNS are unmyelinated (Figure 8-13). A Schwann cell can accommodate several axons in individual cytoplasmic invaginations and no myelin is produced.

Clinical significance: Demyelinating diseases

The integrity of myelin, but not the axon, is disturbed in **demyelinating diseases** affecting the **survival of oligodendrocytes** or the **integrity of the myelin sheath.**

Demyelinating diseases can be (1) **immune-mediated**, (2) **inherited**, (3) **meta-**

Box 8-D | **Charcot-Marie-Tooth disease**

- Charcot-Marie-Tooth disease is a common and heterogeneous inherited disorder affecting the PNS. The disease is most often an autosomal dominant syndrome but is genetically heterogeneous.
- The most frequent form is Charcot-Marie-Tooth disease type I, a demyelinating polyneuropathy (with reduced nerve conduction velocity) caused by mutations affecting myelin components. Charcot-Marie-Tooth disease type 2 is an axonal polyneuropathy (with normal nerve conduction velocity) determined by defects in axonal transport (mutation of a kinesin), membrane trafficking, and protein synthesis.
- Myelin protein zero (MPZ) is a member of the immunoglobulin superfamily with a dual role: the compactation of myelin and cell signaling. Myelin in patients with mutations in the *MZP* gene is less compact because of a predominant defect in the extracellular domain of MZP, which is responsible for holding two membranes together. Mutations in the *MZP* gene causes the genetic and clinical variants of Charcot-Marie-Tooth disease type 1B and type 2.
- A duplication of the *peripheral myelin protein 22* (*PMP22*) gene causes Charcot-Marie-Tooth disease type 1A, the most common type of Charcot-Marie-Tooth disease.

Figure 8-13. Development of myelinated and unmyelinated nerves

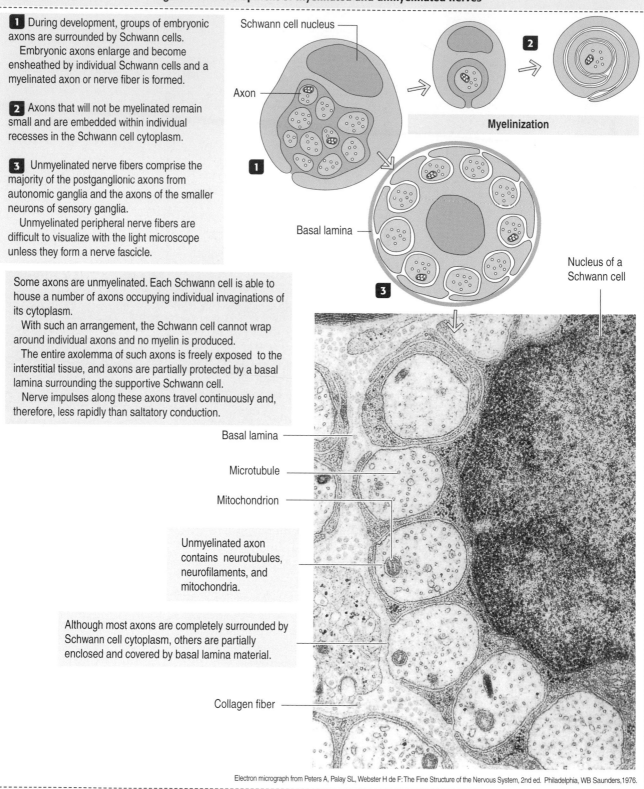

1 During development, groups of embryonic axons are surrounded by Schwann cells.
Embryonic axons enlarge and become ensheathed by individual Schwann cells and a myelinated axon or nerve fiber is formed.

2 Axons that will not be myelinated remain small and are embedded within individual recesses in the Schwann cell cytoplasm.

3 Unmyelinated nerve fibers comprise the majority of the postganglionic axons from autonomic ganglia and the axons of the smaller neurons of sensory ganglia.
Unmyelinated peripheral nerve fibers are difficult to visualize with the light microscope unless they form a nerve fascicle.

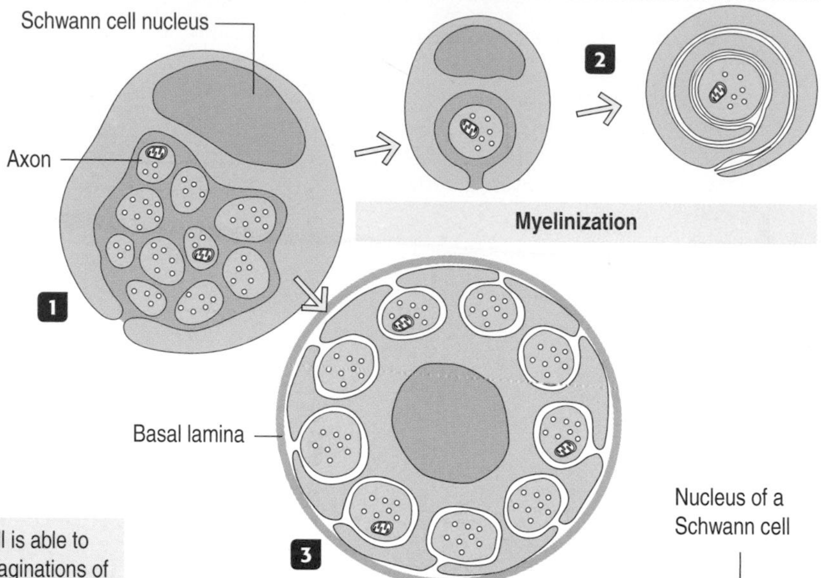

Schwann cell nucleus
Axon
1
2
Myelinization
Basal lamina
3

Some axons are unmyelinated. Each Schwann cell is able to house a number of axons occupying individual invaginations of its cytoplasm.
With such an arrangement, the Schwann cell cannot wrap around individual axons and no myelin is produced.
The entire axolemma of such axons is freely exposed to the interstitial tissue, and axons are partially protected by a basal lamina surrounding the supportive Schwann cell.
Nerve impulses along these axons travel continuously and, therefore, less rapidly than saltatory conduction.

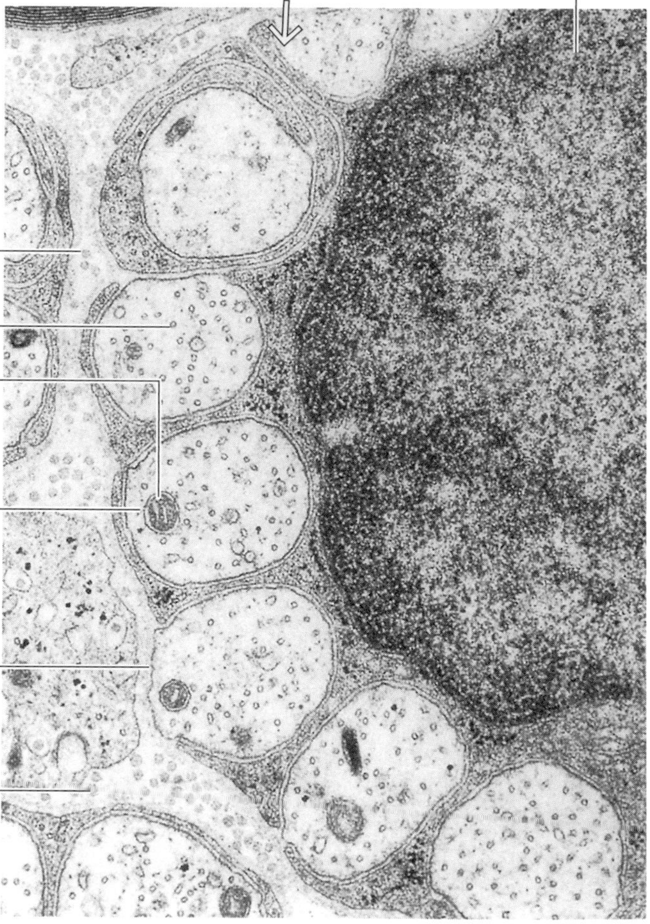

Nucleus of a Schwann cell
Basal lamina
Microtubule
Mitochondrion
Collagen fiber

Unmyelinated axon contains neurotubules, neurofilaments, and mitochondria.

Although most axons are completely surrounded by Schwann cell cytoplasm, others are partially enclosed and covered by basal lamina material.

Electron micrograph from Peters A, Palay SL, Webster H de F: The Fine Structure of the Nervous System, 2nd ed. Philadelphia, WB Saunders,1976.

bolic, and (4) **virus-induced**.

Immune-mediated demyelinating diseases include **multiple sclerosis** and **monophasic demyelinating diseases** (for example, **optic neuritis**).

Multiple sclerosis (Figure 8-14) is characterized by clinically recurrent or chronically progressive neurologic dysfunction caused by multiple areas of demyelination in the CNS, in particular the **brain**, **optic nerves**, and **spinal cord**.

Figure 8-14. **Pathogenesis of multiple sclerosis**

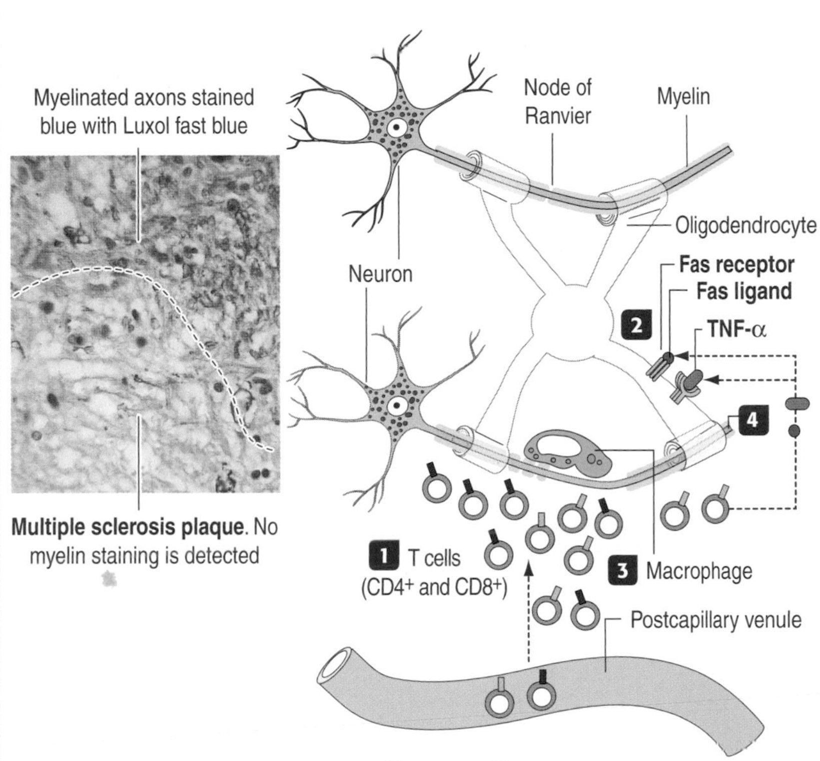
Myelinated axons stained blue with Luxol fast blue
Multiple sclerosis plaque. No myelin staining is detected
Node of Ranvier
Myelin
Oligodendrocyte
Neuron
Fas receptor
Fas ligand
TNF-α
2
4
1 T cells (CD4+ and CD8+)
3 Macrophage
Postcapillary venule

Multiple sclerosis

Multiple sclerosis is a demyelinating disorder characterized by episodes of neurologic dysfunction, separated in **time**, caused by lesions of the white matter, separated in **space.**

Two characteristic microscopic features are: (1) infiltration of inflammatory cells (T cells and macrophages) inside and around multiple sclerosis plaques; (2) plaques of astrocytic aggregates.

1 **CD8+ and CD4+ T cells**, recruited to multiple sclerosis lesions, **secrete cytokines** (interleukin-2, tumor necrosis factor-α [TNF-α], and interferon-γ).

2 T cells secrete **Fas ligand** that binds to **Fas receptor** on oligodendrocytes to induce their programmed cell death (apoptosis). TNF-α exerts a similar apoptotic effect.

3 Macrophages strip myelin off the axons. Macrophages contain myelin in phagocytic vacuoles.

4 Conduction in the demyelinated axon is blocked.

An immune-mediated origin of multiple sclerosis is supported by an increase of immunoglobulin G (IgG) in the cerebrospinal fluid (CSF), and abnormalities of T cell function. A characteristic pathologic finding is the **multiple sclerosis plaque,** a demyelination lesion of the white matter, where the primary target is the myelin sheath and oligodendrocytes.

An **inherited demyelination** disorder is **adrenoleukodystrophy,** in which **progressive demyelination** is associated with **dysfunction of the adrenal cortex.** The X-linked form of this disease is caused by a mutation of a gene encoding a membrane protein of **peroxisomes.** A defect in this gene leads to the accumulation of **very-long-chain fatty acids (VLCFAs)** in serum (discussed under Peroxisomes in Chapter 2, Epithelial Glands).

Metabolic demyelination disorders include **central pontine myelinolysis,** a syndrome in which neurologic dysfunction is observed following rapid correction of hyponatremia in individuals with alcohol abuse or malnutrition. A typical pathologic finding is the presence of **symmetrical demyelinated lesions in the central pons.**

Vitamin B_{12} deficiency results in demyelination of axons in the CNS (the spinal cord, in particular) and the PNS.

Virus-induced demyelination can be observed in **progressive multifocal encephalopathy** caused by an opportunistic viral infection of oligodendrocytes in patients with immunodeficiency.

Clinical significance: Neurodegenerative diseases

Degenerative processes of specific groups of neurons of the brain cause movement disorders, dementia syndromes, and autonomic perturbations. Neurodegenerative diseases include:

1. **Amyotrophic lateral sclerosis** (Figure 8-15) is a neurodegenerative disease characterized by progressive degeneration of motor neurons, starting with moderate weakness in one limb and progressing to severe paralysis (swallowing and respiratory disorders), leading to death in about 3 years. The term amyotrophic

Figure 8-15. Amyotrophic lateral sclerosis

Symmetrical loss of myelinated fibers in a section of spinal cord (crossed cerebrospinal tracts) from a patient with amyotrophic lateral sclerosis. The preparation was stained for myelin.

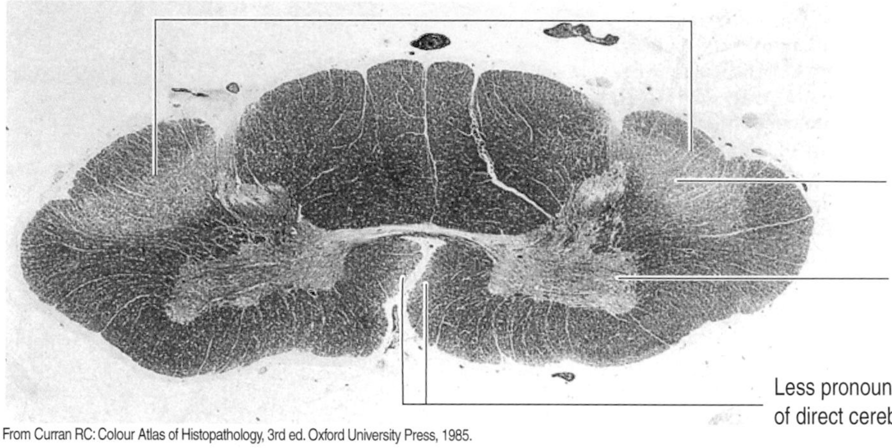
Demyelinization
Ventral horn
Less pronounced demyelinization of direct cerebrospinal tracts

From Curran RC: Colour Atlas of Histopathology, 3rd ed. Oxford University Press, 1985.

Amyotrophic lateral sclerosis (ALS; also known as **Lou Gherig's disease**) is a severe condition characterized by **progressive degeneration of motor neurons of the brainstem and spinal cord**.

Amyotrophic refers to **muscle atrophy**. Lateral sclerosis refers to the **hardness to palpation of the lateral columns of the spinal cord** in autopsy specimens. Lateral sclerosis is caused by an increased number of astrocytes (**astrocytic gliosis**) following the degeneration and loss of motor neurons.

ALS is a familial motor neuron disease in 5% to 10% of cases. The others are assumed to be sporadic. Mutations in the gene encoding **superoxide dismutase 1 (SOD1)** account for 20% of the cases of familial ALS. The remaining 80% are caused by mutations of other genes.

SOD1 is an enzyme that requires copper to catalyze the conversion of toxic superoxide radicals to hydrogen peroxide and oxygen. The toxic effects of mutant SOD1 result in the disorganization of intermediate filaments (NF-L, NF-M, and NF-H; see Figure 8-4), mitochondrial abnormalities, and apoptosis of motor neurons. Autoimmunity may have a role in the pathogenesis of ALS.

Patients with sporadic ALS have antibodies against voltage-gated Ca^{2+} channels, which may interfere with the regulation of intracellular Ca^{2+}, leading to the degeneration of motor neurons. However, immunotherapy has not been effective in patients with ALS.

The clinically apparent signs are overactive tendon reflexes, Hoffmann sign (digital reflex: flexion of the terminal phalanx of the thumb following nipping of the nail), Babinski sign (extension of the great toe and abduction of the other toes after plantar stimulation), and clonus (Greek *klonos*, a tumult; muscle contraction and relaxation of a muscle in rapid succession).

refers to muscle atrophy. Lateral sclerosis refers to the hardness to palpation of the lateral columns of the spinal cord. The cause is unknown. In a few familial cases, a mutation in the copper-zinc **superoxide dismutase** (***SOD1***) gene has been reported.

2. **Alzheimer's disease**, the most common neurodegenerative disease, a progressive cortical dementia affecting language, memory, and vision, as well as emotion or personality. Mutations in **presenilin-1** and -2, and in **β-amyloid precursor protein** (βAPP) genes are documented in familial forms of Alzheimer's disease. Figure 8-16 summarizes the major molecular events observed in the brains of patients with Alzheimer's disease, in particular the formation of **amyloid plaques**. Amyloid is the product of cleavage of βAPP by a series of proteases, the α-, β-, and γ-secretase. The γ-secretase is responsible for producing β-amyloid peptide, which forms insoluble toxic fibrils in the amyloid plaques. Alterations in the stabilizing function of **tau**, a microtubule-associated protein, result in the accumulation of twisted pairs of tau in neurons. Figure 8-7 stresses the role of microtubules in axonal transport, a function affected by abnormal tau.

Inheritance of one or more **apolipoprotein Eε4** alleles (**APOE locus**) is indicative of a susceptibility risk factor. The ε4 allele is associated with an earlier age of onset of the common form of Alzheimer's disease. The ε4/ε4 homozygotes, present in about 2% of the general population, have the greatest risk of developing the disease.

Figure 8-16. Alzheimer's disease

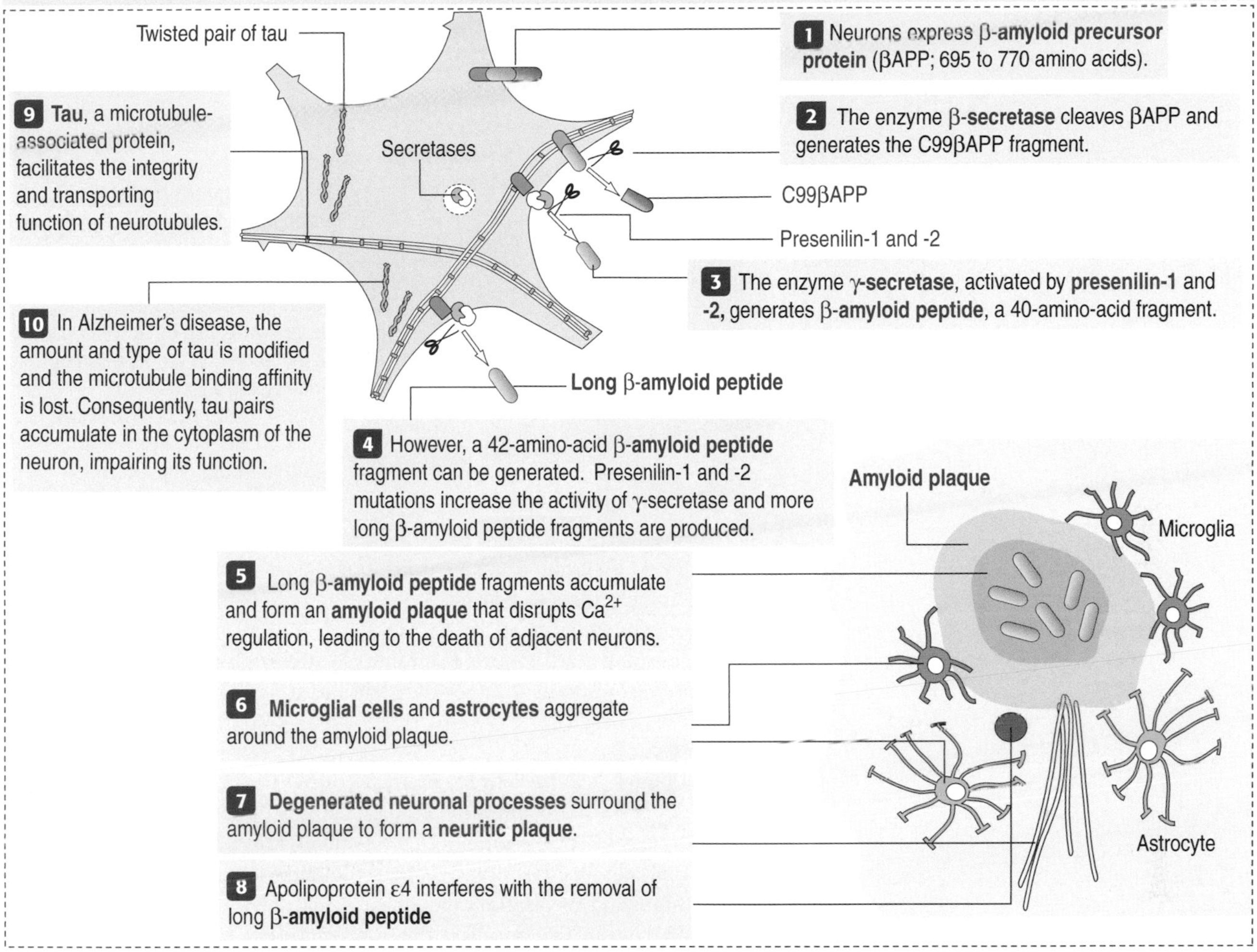

Twisted pair of tau
1 Neurons express β-amyloid precursor protein (βAPP; 695 to 770 amino acids).
9 Tau, a microtubule-associated protein, facilitates the integrity and transporting function of neurotubules.
Secretases
2 The enzyme β-secretase cleaves βAPP and generates the C99βAPP fragment.
C99βAPP
Presenilin-1 and -2
3 The enzyme γ-secretase, activated by presenilin-1 and -2, generates β-amyloid peptide, a 40-amino-acid fragment.
10 In Alzheimer's disease, the amount and type of tau is modified and the microtubule binding affinity is lost. Consequently, tau pairs accumulate in the cytoplasm of the neuron, impairing its function.
Long β-amyloid peptide
4 However, a 42-amino-acid β-amyloid peptide fragment can be generated. Presenilin-1 and -2 mutations increase the activity of γ-secretase and more long β-amyloid peptide fragments are produced.
Amyloid plaque
Microglia
5 Long β-amyloid peptide fragments accumulate and form an amyloid plaque that disrupts Ca2+ regulation, leading to the death of adjacent neurons.
6 Microglial cells and astrocytes aggregate around the amyloid plaque.
7 Degenerated neuronal processes surround the amyloid plaque to form a neuritic plaque.
Astrocyte
8 Apolipoprotein ε4 interferes with the removal of long β-amyloid peptide

No treatment is available for Alzheimer's disease. Symptomatic therapy is helpful during the early stages of dementia.

3. **Parkinson's disease**, the second most common neurodegenerative disease, is characterized clinically by **parkinsonism**, defined by resting tremor, slow voluntary movements (**hypokinetic disorders**), and movements with rigidity. This disease is pathologically defined by **a loss of dopaminergic neurons from the substantia nigra** and proteinaceous deposits in the cytoplasm of neurons (**Lewy bodies**) and threadlike inclusions in axons (**Lewy neurites**). The protein **α-synuclein** is present in Lewy bodies and axons. Although the cause of the disease is unknown, recent developments in understanding the functional organization of basal ganglia have led to the development of new pharmacologic and surgical (**thalamotomy** and **pallidotomy**) therapies.

Microglial cells

Microglial cells (Figure 8-17) have the following characteristics:

1. They are mesoderm-derived cells whose primary function is **phagocytosis**.
2. They are regarded as immune protectors of the brain and spinal cord.
3. They interact with neurons and astrocytes and migrate to the sites of dead neurons where they proliferate and phagocytose dead cells.
4. During histogenesis in the embryo, microglial cells discard an excess of nonviable neurons and glial cells, eliminated by apoptosis.

Substantial microglial activity has been observed in the brain of patients with **acquired immunodeficiency syndrome** (AIDS). **Human immunodeficiency virus**

Figure 8-17. **Microglial cells**

Microglial cells: Phagocytic cells of the CNS

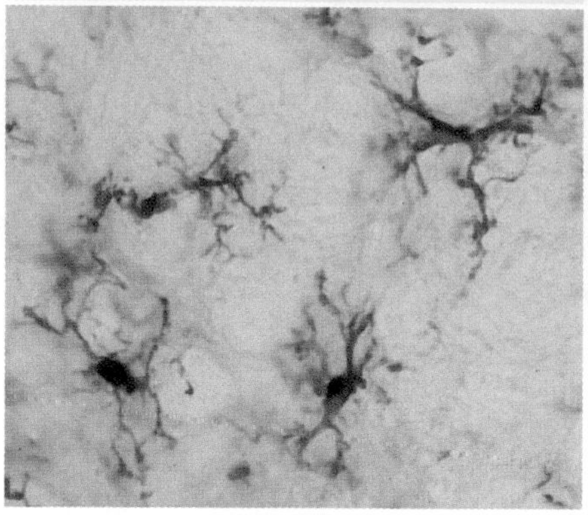

Immunocytochemical preparation courtesy of Wan-hua Amy Yu, New York.

Microglial cells, the resident macrophages of the CNS, are the primary cells to respond to injury to the brain (e.g., multiple sclerosis and trauma).

Microglial cells produce **chemoattractants** capable of **recruiting leukocytes across the blood-brain barrier to initiate neuroimmunologic diseases.**

Microglial cells and astrocytes interact with each other to modulate the initiation and progression of immune responses.

A lack of balance of this cell-cell interaction mechanism leads to CNS-directed **autoimmunity** and **inflammation**.

type 1 (HIV-1) does not attack neurons, but it does infect microglial cells that produce cytokines toxic to neurons.

The distinction between microglia, astrocytes, and oligodendrocytes is difficult in routine histologic techniques. Immunocytochemical and silver impregnation procedures are commonly used for the identification of glial cells.

Ependyma

Ependyma designates the **simple cuboidal epithelium** covering the surface of the ventricles of the brain and the central canal of the spinal cord. The ependyma consists of two cell types (Figure 8-18): (1) **ependymal cells** and (2) **tanycytes.**

Ependymal cells form a simple cuboidal epithelium, lining the ventricular cavities of the brain and the central canal of the spinal cord. These cells differentiate from **germinal** or **ventricular cells** of the embryonic neural tube (see Development of the Nervous System).

The apical domain of ependymal cells contains abundant **microvilli** and one or more cilia. **Desmosomes** link adjacent ependymal cells. The basal domain is in contact with **astrocytic processes.**

Tanycytes are specialized ependymal cells with basal processes extending between the astrocytic processes to form an end-foot on blood vessels.

Choroid plexus

During development, the ependymal cell layer comes in contact with the highly vascularized meninges, forming the **tela choroidea** in the roof of the third and fourth ventricles and along the choroid fissure of the lateral ventricles. These cells differentiate into secretory cells, which in combination with the meningeal blood vessels form the **choroid plexus.**

The cells of the choroid plexus are highly polarized (Figure 8-19). The **apical domain** contains microvilli, and **tight junctions** connect adjacent cells. The **basolateral domain** forms interdigitating folds, and the cell rests on a basal lamina.

Capillaries with fenestrated endothelial cells are located beneath the basal lamina. Macromolecules of the blood plasma can pass freely into the subepithelial space; however, they cannot pass directly into the CSF because of the elaborate interdigitations along the basolateral domain and the apical tight junctions.

Cerebrospinal fluid

The choroid plexuses of the lateral, third, and fourth ventricles produce CSF.

CSF flows from the fourth ventricle into the brain and spinal subarachnoid

Figure 8-18. **Ependyma and choroid plexus**

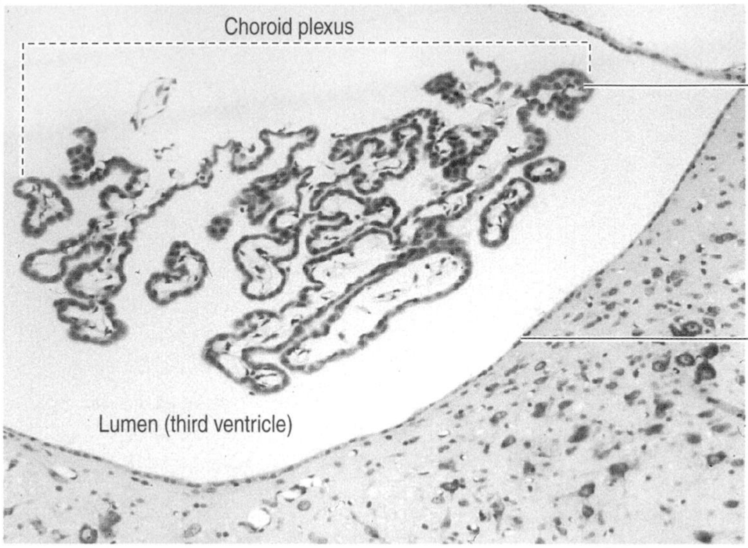
Choroid plexus
Lumen (third ventricle)

Choroid epithelium, formed by cuboidal cells linked by **tight junctions** with apical **microvilli**, infolding of the basal plasma membrane, and abundant mitochondria.

Choroidal epithelial cells produce cerebrospinal fluid.

Ependymal epithelium, formed by cuboidal cells linked by **desmosomes**, with apical microvilli and cilia and abundant mitochondria.

Tanycytes, specialized ependymal cells found in the third ventricle, have basal processes forming end-feet on blood vessels. **Tanycytes are linked to each other and to ependymal cells by tight junctions.**

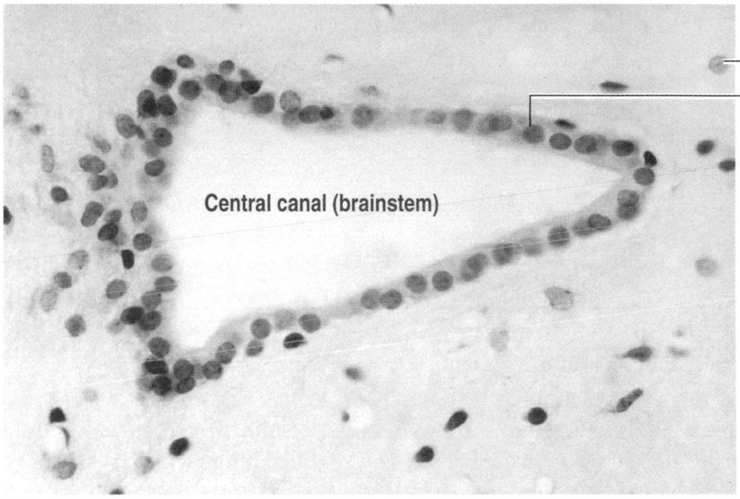
Glial cell
Central canal (brainstem)

The **central canal** is lined primarily by ependymal cells **(no tanycytes)**.

Preparations courtesy of Wan-hua Amy Yu, New York.

Ependyma

The brain ventricles and the central canal of the spinal cord are lined by a simple cuboidal epithelium, the **ependyma**.

The ependyma consists of two cell types:

1 **Ependymal cells**, with cilia and microvilli on the apical domain and abundant mitochondria. The basal domain is in contact with astrocytic processes. Ependymal cells are attached to each other by belt desmosomes.

2 **Tanycytes** (in the third ventricle) are specialized ependymal cells. Two different features are observed:
1. **Basal processes extend through the astrocytic processes layer to form end-feet on a blood vessel.**
2. **Tanycytes are attached to each other and to ependymal cells by tight junctions.**

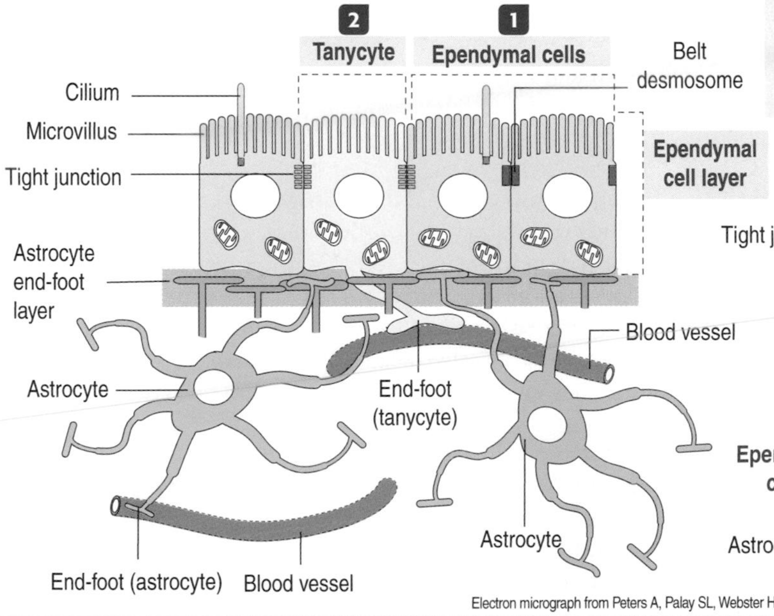
2
Tanycyte
1
Ependymal cells
Belt desmosome
Cilium
Microvillus
Tight junction
Ependymal cell layer
Astrocyte end-foot layer
Blood vessel
Astrocyte
End-foot (tanycyte)
Astrocyte
End-foot (astrocyte)
Blood vessel

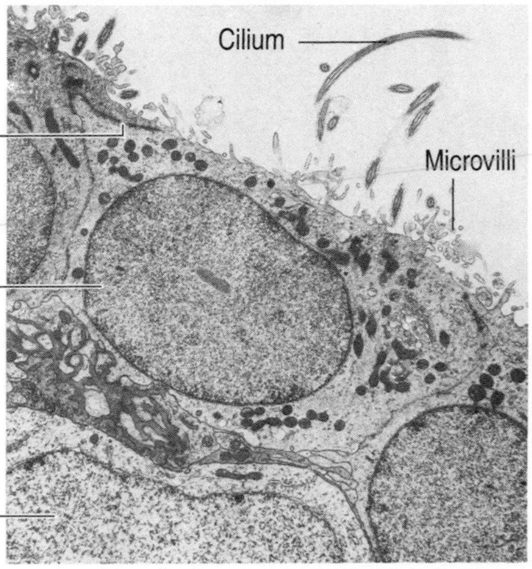
Cilium
Tight junction
Microvilli
Ependymal cells
Astrocyte

Electron micrograph from Peters A, Palay SL, Webster H de F: The Fine Structure of the Nervous System, 2nd ed. Philadelphia, WB Saunders, 1976.

Figure 8-19. **Choroid plexus**

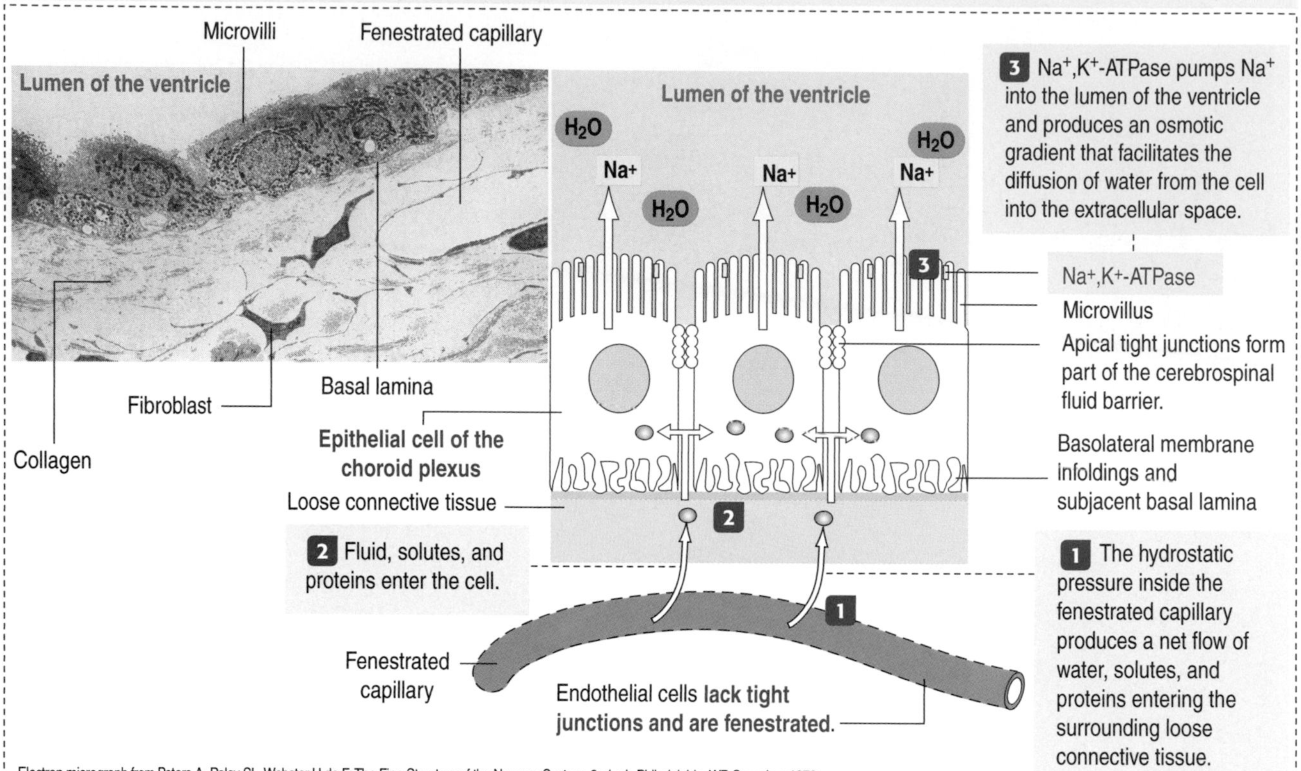

Microvilli
Fenestrated capillary
Lumen of the ventricle
Fibroblast
Basal lamina
Collagen
Epithelial cell of the choroid plexus
Loose connective tissue
2 Fluid, solutes, and proteins enter the cell.
Fenestrated capillary
Endothelial cells lack tight junctions and are fenestrated.
Lumen of the ventricle
H2O
Na+
3 Na+,K+-ATPase pumps Na+ into the lumen of the ventricle and produces an osmotic gradient that facilitates the diffusion of water from the cell into the extracellular space.
Na+,K+-ATPase
Microvillus
Apical tight junctions form part of the cerebrospinal fluid barrier.
Basolateral membrane infoldings and subjacent basal lamina
1 The hydrostatic pressure inside the fenestrated capillary produces a net flow of water, solutes, and proteins entering the surrounding loose connective tissue.

Electron micrograph from Peters A, Palay SL, Webster H de F: The Fine Structure of the Nervous System, 2nd ed. Philadelphia, WB Saunders, 1976.

space through median and lateral apertures. After entering the subarachnoid space, CSF flows outside the CNS into the blood, at the superior sagittal sinus (see Figure 8-18). The epithelium of the choroid plexus represents a barrier between the blood and the CSF. Several substances can leave the capillaries of the choroid plexus but cannot enter the CSF.

CSF protects and supports the brain and spinal cord from external forces applied to the skull or vertebral column (cushioning effect). In addition, the CSF allows the removal of metabolic wastes by continual drainage of the ventricular cavities and subarachnoid space. The volume of CSF varies with the intracranial blood volume. The free communication of CSF among compartments protects against pressure differences.

Lumbar puncture is a procedure to collect—with a needle inserted between the third and fourth and fourth and fifth lumbar vertebrae—a sample of CSF for biochemical analysis and pressure measurement. The total volume of CSF in an adult is 120 mL.

Clinical significance: Brain permeability barriers

The brain is supplied with blood from major arteries forming an anastomotic network around the base of the brain. From this region, arteries project into the subarachnoid space before entering the brain tissue.

In the brain, the perivascular space is surrounded by a basal lamina derived from both glial and endothelial cells: the **glia limitans**. Nonfenestrated endothelial cells, linked by tight junctions, prevent the diffusion of substances from the blood to the brain.

Tight junctions represent the structural basis of the blood-brain barrier. This barrier offers free passage to glucose and other selected molecules but excludes most substances, in particular potent drugs required for the treatment of an infection or tumor. If the blood-brain barrier breaks down, tissue fluid accumulates in the nervous tissue, a condition known as **cerebral edema**.

External to the capillary endothelial cell lining is a basal lamina and external

Figure 8-20. Brain permeability barriers

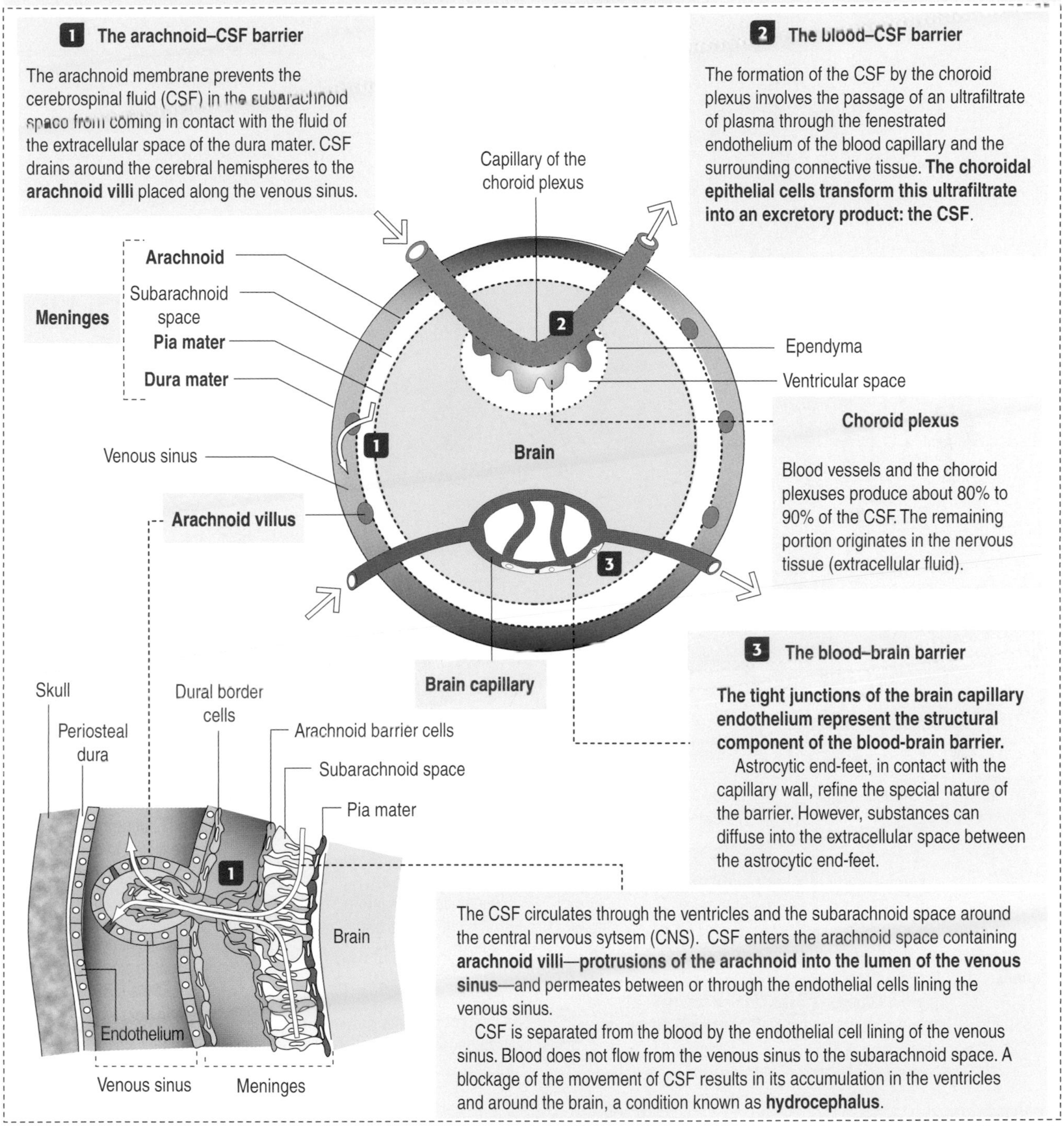
1 The arachnoid–CSF barrier
The arachnoid membrane prevents the cerebrospinal fluid (CSF) in the subarachnoid space from coming in contact with the fluid of the extracellular space of the dura mater. CSF drains around the cerebral hemispheres to the **arachnoid villi** placed along the venous sinus.
2 The blood–CSF barrier
The formation of the CSF by the choroid plexus involves the passage of an ultrafiltrate of plasma through the fenestrated endothelium of the blood capillary and the surrounding connective tissue. **The choroidal epithelial cells transform this ultrafiltrate into an excretory product: the CSF.**
Capillary of the choroid plexus
Meninges
Arachnoid
Subarachnoid space
Pia mater
Dura mater
Venous sinus
Arachnoid villus
Ependyma
Ventricular space
Brain
Choroid plexus
Blood vessels and the choroid plexuses produce about 80% to 90% of the CSF. The remaining portion originates in the nervous tissue (extracellular fluid).
Brain capillary
3 The blood–brain barrier
The tight junctions of the brain capillary endothelium represent the structural component of the blood-brain barrier.
Astrocytic end-feet, in contact with the capillary wall, refine the special nature of the barrier. However, substances can diffuse into the extracellular space between the astrocytic end-feet.
Skull
Periosteal dura
Dural border cells
Arachnoid barrier cells
Subarachnoid space
Pia mater
Brain
Endothelium
Venous sinus
Meninges
The CSF circulates through the ventricles and the subarachnoid space around the central nervous sytsem (CNS). CSF enters the arachnoid space containing **arachnoid villi—protrusions of the arachnoid into the lumen of the venous sinus**—and permeates between or through the endothelial cells lining the venous sinus.
CSF is separated from the blood by the endothelial cell lining of the venous sinus. Blood does not flow from the venous sinus to the subarachnoid space. A blockage of the movement of CSF results in its accumulation in the ventricles and around the brain, a condition known as **hydrocephalus**.

to this lamina are the end-feet of the astrocytes. Although the pericapillary end-feet of astrocytes are not part of the blood-brain barrier, they contribute to its maintenance by transporting fluid and ions from the perineuronal extracellular space to the blood vessels.

Figure 8-20 illustrates details of three brain permeability barriers: (1) the **arachnoid-CSF barrier**, represented by **arachnoid villi** distributed along the venous sinus, in particular the **arachnoid barrier cells** linked by tight junctions. Arachnoid villi transfer CSF to the venous system (superior sagittal sinus). Fluid in the subarachnoid space operates like a shock absorber, which prevents the mass of the brain from compressing nerve roots and blood vessels. (2) The **blood-CSF barrier**. It involves tight junctions in the choroidal epithelium, responsible for the production of the CSF. (3) The **blood-brain barrier**, represented by tight

Figure 8-21. Peripheral nerve

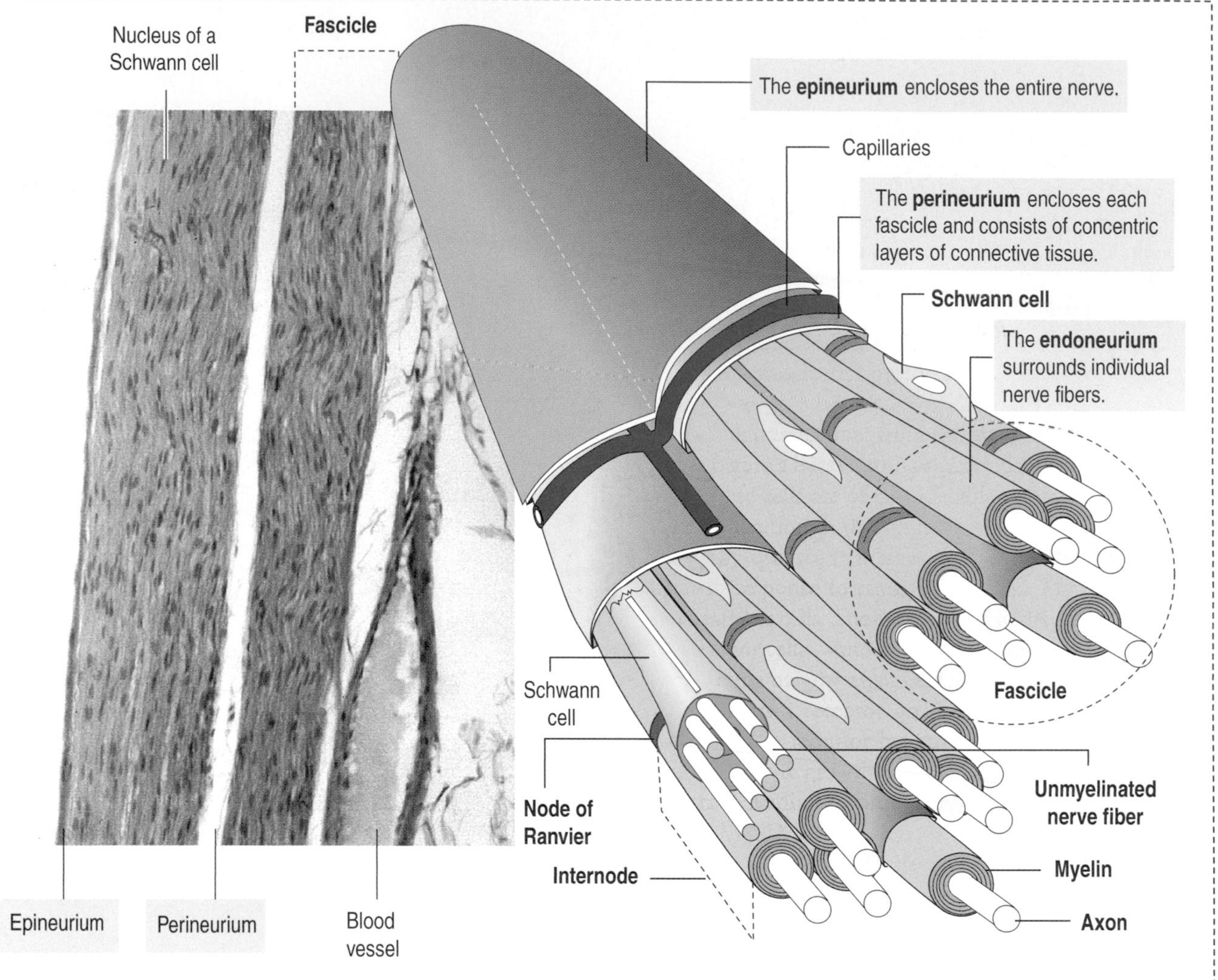

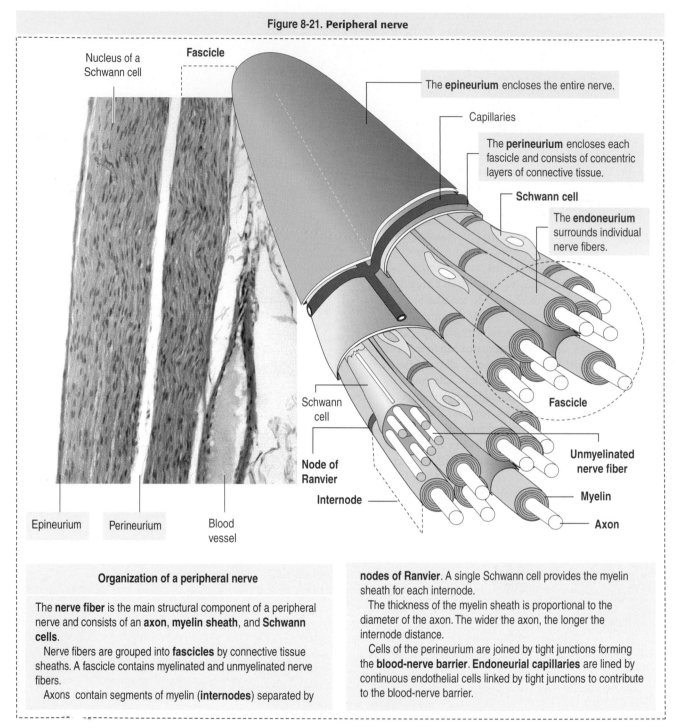

Nucleus of a Schwann cell
Fascicle
The epineurium encloses the entire nerve.
Capillaries
The perineurium encloses each fascicle and consists of concentric layers of connective tissue.
Schwann cell
The endoneurium surrounds individual nerve fibers.
Fascicle
Schwann cell
Node of Ranvier
Internode
Unmyelinated nerve fiber
Myelin
Axon
Epineurium
Perineurium
Blood vessel

Organization of a peripheral nerve

The **nerve fiber** is the main structural component of a peripheral nerve and consists of an **axon**, **myelin sheath**, and **Schwann cells**.

Nerve fibers are grouped into **fascicles** by connective tissue sheaths. A fascicle contains myelinated and unmyelinated nerve fibers.

Axons contain segments of myelin (**internodes**) separated by **nodes of Ranvier**. A single Schwann cell provides the myelin sheath for each internode.

The thickness of the myelin sheath is proportional to the diameter of the axon. The wider the axon, the longer the internode distance.

Cells of the perineurium are joined by tight junctions forming the **blood-nerve barrier**. **Endoneurial capillaries** are lined by continuous endothelial cells linked by tight junctions to contribute to the blood-nerve barrier.

junctions sealing the endothelial intercellular space.

Obstruction of CSF movement or defective absorption causes an accumulation of fluid in the ventricular spaces and around the brain. **Hydrocephalus** is a pathologic condition characterized by an increase in CSF volume and pressure, and enlargement of the ventricular space.

Peripheral nervous system

The PNS includes all neuronal elements outside the brain and spinal cord. The peripheral nerves are the **cranial** and **spinal nerves**.

The PNS contains two **supporting cell types:** (1) **Schwann cells**, analogous to the oligodendrocytes of the CNS and (2) the **satellite cells**, surrounding the cell bodies of neurons in sensory and autonomic ganglia. We discuss them later.

Figure 8-22. **Peripheral nerve**

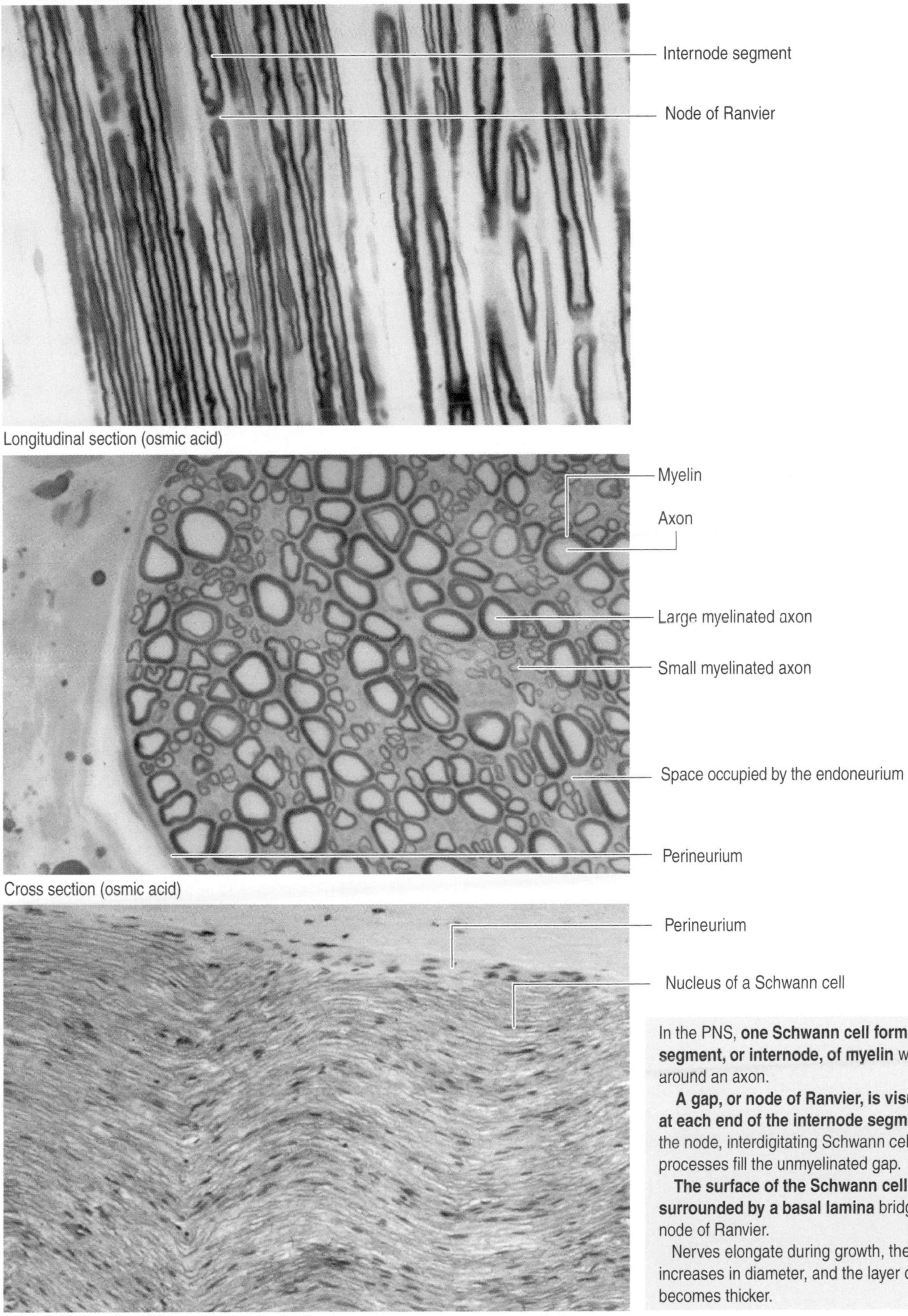

Internode segment
Node of Ranvier
Myelin
Axon
Large myelinated axon
Small myelinated axon
Space occupied by the endoneurium
Perineurium
Perineurium
Nucleus of a Schwann cell

Longitudinal section (osmic acid)

Cross section (osmic acid)

Longitudinal section (hematoxylin-eosin stain)

In the PNS, **one Schwann cell forms one segment, or internode, of myelin** wrapped around an axon.

A gap, or node of Ranvier, is visualized at each end of the internode segment. At the node, interdigitating Schwann cell processes fill the unmyelinated gap.

The surface of the Schwann cell is surrounded by a basal lamina bridging the node of Ranvier.

Nerves elongate during growth, the axon increases in diameter, and the layer of myelin becomes thicker.

Figure 8-23. Degeneration and regeneration of a peripheral nerve

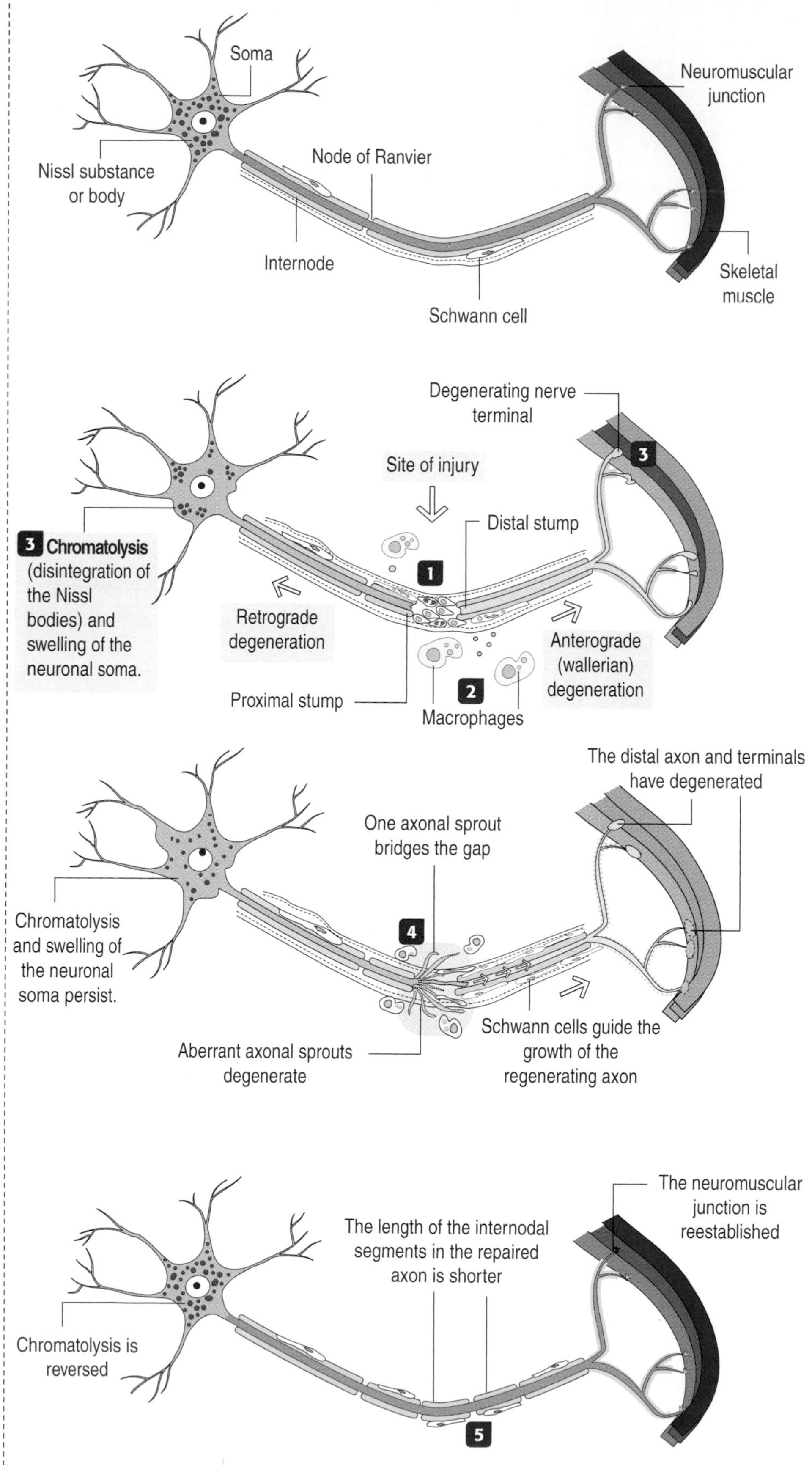

An intact motor neuron is shown with an axon ending in a neuromuscular junction. The axon is surrounded by a **myelin sheath** and a basal lamina—produced by Schwann cells—and the endoneurium.

The soma of the neuron contains abundant **Nissl bodies** (aggregates of ribosomes attached to the endoplasmic reticulum and free polyribosomes).

1 An injury damages the nerve fiber. Schwann cells undergo mitotic division and bridge the gap between the **proximal** and **distal** axonal stumps.
2 Schwann cells phagocytose myelin. Myelin droplets are extruded from Schwann cells and subsequently are phagocytosed by tissue macrophages.
3 **Chromatolysis** and degeneration of the axon terminals are seen. The distal and proximal segments of the axon degenerate (**anterograde** and **retrograde degeneration**, respectively).

4 The proximal axonal stump generates multiple **sprouts** advancing between Schwann cells. One sprout persists and grows distally (~1.5 mm per day) to reinnervate the muscle. The remaining sprouts degenerate.

In the CNS, degeneration of the axon and myelin is similar and microglial cells remove debris by phagocytosis.

The regeneration process starts but is aborted by the absence of endoneurium and lack of proliferation of oligodendrocytes.

5 Once the regenerated axon reaches the end organ (several months), Schwann cells start the production of myelin. **The internodal segments are shorter.**

The regenerated axon has a reduced diameter (80% of the original diameter) and, therefore, the conduction velocity of the nerve impulse is slower.

Individual nerve fibers of the PNS are ensheathed by **Schwann cells** (Figure 8-21). In **myelinated fibers**, individual Schwann cells wrap around the axon, forming a myelin sheath analogous to that of the oligodendrocytes of the CNS (see Figure 8-11). In **unmyelinated fibers**, a single Schwann cell envelops several axons (see Figure 8-13).

There are **two important differences between Schwann cells and oligodendrocytes:** (1) A single Schwann cell forms only one internodal segment of myelin, whereas a single oligodendrocyte may form 40 or 50. (2) Unmyelinated fibers in the PNS are embedded in Schwann cells, whereas those in the CNS are not ensheathed by oligodendrocytes but may have an investment of astrocytes.

Structure of a peripheral nerve

In addition to Schwann cells, peripheral nerves have three additional connective tissue coverings (see Figures 8-21 and 8-22): (1) the **epineurium**, (2) the **perineurium**, and (3) the **endoneurium**.

The epineurium is formed by type I collagen and fibroblasts and covers the entire nerve. Within the nerve, the perineurium segregates axons into **fascicles**. Several concentric layers of fibroblasts with two unusual characteristics form the perineurium: (1) A basal lamina surrounds the layers of fibroblasts. (2) Fibroblasts are joined to each other by tight junctions to form a protective barrier: the **blood-nerve barrier**.

The endoneurium surrounds individual axons and their associated Schwann cells. It consists of type III collagen fibrils and a few fibroblasts between individual nerve fibers. Additional components of the blood-nerve barrier are the endothelial cells of the **endoneurial capillaries**. Endoneurial capillaries derive from the vasa nervorum and are lined by continuous endothelial cells joined by tight junctions.

Clinical significance: Segmental demyelination and axonal degeneration

Diseases affecting Schwann cells lead to a loss of myelin, or **segmental demyelination**. Damage to the neuron and its axon leads to **axonal degeneration** (**wallerian degeneration**, first described by the English physiologist Augustus Volney Waller, 1816-1870).

Axonal degeneration (Figure 8-23) may be followed by **axonal regeneration**. Recall from our discussion in Chapter 7, Muscle Tissue, that the **motor unit** is the functional unit of the neuromuscular system. Therefore, segmental demyelination and axonal degeneration affect the motor unit and cause **muscle paralysis** and **atrophy**. Physiotherapy for the paralyzed muscles is necessary to prevent muscle degeneration before regenerating motor axons can reach the motor unit.

Segmental demyelination occurs when the function of the Schwann cell is abnormal or there is damage to the myelin sheath, for example, a crush nerve injury. If the nerve fiber is completely severed, the chances of recovery decrease unless a nerve segment is grafted. **The presence of the endoneurium is essential for the proliferation of Schwann cells.** Schwann cells guide an axonal sprout, derived from the proximal axonal stump, to reach the end organ (for example, a muscle).

Several sprouts can grow into the connective tissue and, together with proliferative Schwann cells, form a mass called an **amputation neuroma**. Amputation neuromas prevent regrowth of the axon after trauma and must be surgically removed to allow reinnervation of the peripheral end organ.

Axonal regeneration is a very slow process. It starts 2 weeks after injury and is completed, if successful, after several months. Schwann cells remyelinate the denuded portion of the axon, but the length of internodal myelin is shorter.

Axonal degeneration results from the primary destruction of the axon by metabolic or toxic damage and is followed by demyelination and degeneration of the neuronal cell body. This process is known as a "**dying back**" neuropathy.

Regeneration of nerve fibers in the CNS is not possible at present because of the following factors: (1) An endoneurium is not present. (2) Oligodendrocytes do not proliferate in contrast to Schwann cells, and a single oligodendrocyte serves a large number of axons. (3) Astrocytes deposit scar tissue (the astrocytic plaque).

Sensory ganglia

Sensory ganglia of the **posterior spinal nerve roots** and the **trunks of the trigeminal, facial, glossopharyngeal, and vagal cranial nerves** have a similar organization (Figure 8-24).

A connective tissue capsule, representing the continuation of the epineurium and perineurium, surrounds each ganglion. Neurons are **pseudounipolar** (unipolar), with a single **myelinated** process leaving each cell body. The short process bifurcates into a **peripheral** and a **central** branch. The peripheral branch reaches a peripheral sensory ending and terminates in dendrites. The central branch enters the CNS. The neuronal cell body is surrounded by a layer of flattened **satellite cells**, similar to Schwann cells and continuous with them as they enclose the peripheral and central process of each neuron.

A nerve impulse reaching the T-bifurcation junction bypasses the nerve cell body, traveling from the peripheral axon to the central axon.

Autonomic nervous system

The main divisions of the autonomic nervous system (ANS) are (1) the sympathetic nervous system, (2) the parasympathetic nervous system, and (3) the enteric nervous system. Neurons of the ANS derive from the neural crest and are situated in **ganglia** (a clustering of neurons acting as a transfer site for neuron stimulation), outside the CNS. The ANS consists of elements of the CNS and PNS; both the sympathetic and parasympathetic divisions contain ganglia.

Axons from neurons in the CNS (**preganglionic fibers**) extend to autonomic ganglia outside the CNS. Preganglionic fibers from a central neuron synapse with a second neuron within a ganglion. Nerve fibers derived from the second neuron are **postganglionic fibers**; they travel to a target organ or cell.

Sensory fibers, detecting pain from viscera, reach the CNS by either or both of the sympathetic and parasympathetic pathways. Their neurons are located in either the spinal ganglion (**dorsal root ganglion**) or the sensory ganglion of several cranial nerves.

The **enteric nervous system** consists of two interconnected plexuses—the **myenteric plexus of Auerbach** and the **submucosal plexus of Meissner**—within the walls of the alimentary tube. Each plexus consists of neurons and associated cells, and bundles of nerve fibers passing between plexuses. We discuss the enteric nervous system in Chapter 15, Upper Digestive Segment, and Chapter 16, Lower Digestive Segment.

Similar to the sensory ganglion, a layer of connective tissue continuous with the epineurium and perineurium of the peripheral nerve fiber (see Figure 8-24) surrounds each autonomic ganglion. The neurons of the autonomic ganglia are **multipolar. The dendrites are contacted by myelinated axons of preganglionic neurons (white rami)**. The **axons have a small diameter and are unmyelinated (grey rami)**. Each neuronal cell body is surrounded by Schwann cell–like **satellite cells.**

Neurohistochemistry

The nervous tissue has specialized features not observed in other basic tissues stained with routine staining methods such as hematoxylin-eosin. For example, **basic dyes** can demonstrate the cytoplasmic Nissl substance (ribonucleoproteins) in the cytoplasm of neurons (Figure 8-25).

Reduced silver methods produce dark deposits in various structures of neurons and glial cells. The **Golgi method** is particularly valuable for the study of dendrites. A variant of the Golgi method enables the identification of the cytomembranes

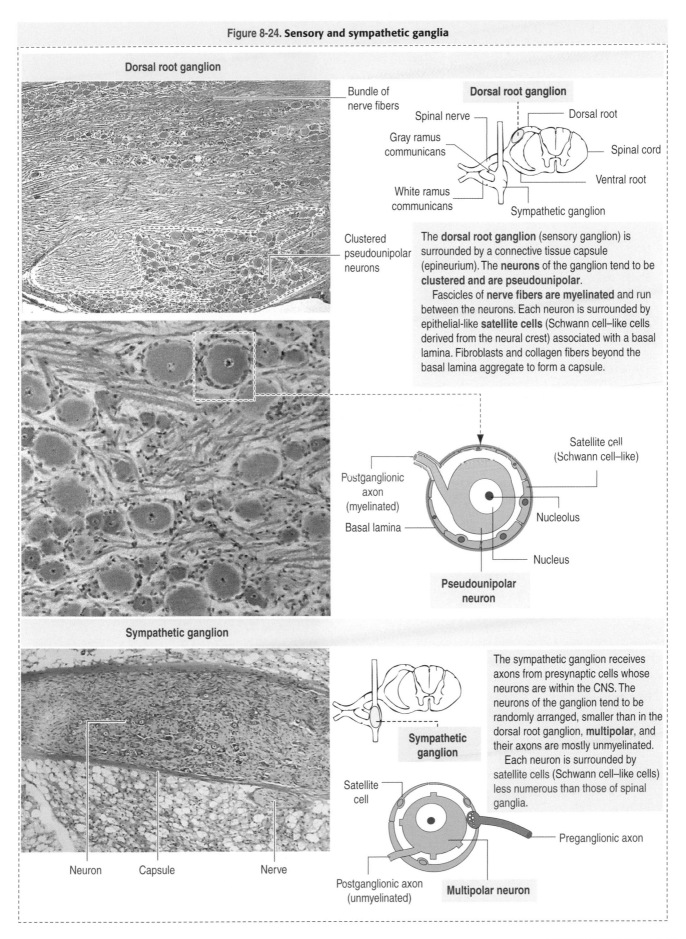

Figure 8-24. **Sensory and sympathetic ganglia**

Dorsal root ganglion

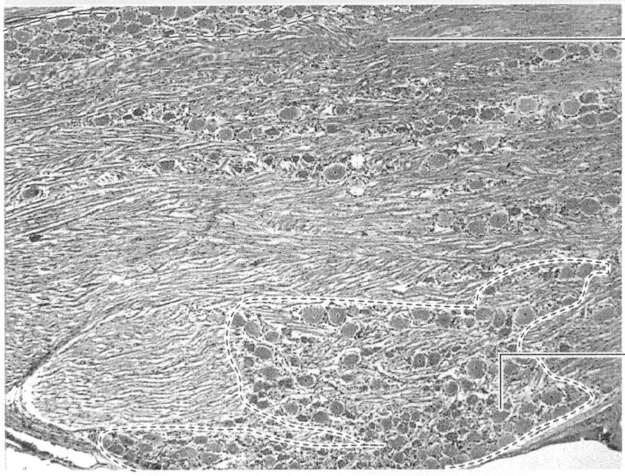
Bundle of nerve fibers
Clustered pseudounipolar neurons

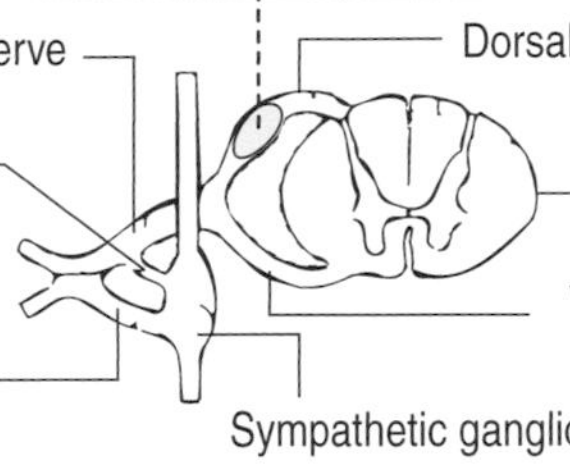
Dorsal root ganglion
Spinal nerve
Dorsal root
Gray ramus communicans
Spinal cord
Ventral root
White ramus communicans
Sympathetic ganglion

The **dorsal root ganglion** (sensory ganglion) is surrounded by a connective tissue capsule (epineurium). The **neurons** of the ganglion tend to be **clustered and are pseudounipolar**.

Fascicles of **nerve fibers are myelinated** and run between the neurons. Each neuron is surrounded by epithelial-like **satellite cells** (Schwann cell–like cells derived from the neural crest) associated with a basal lamina. Fibroblasts and collagen fibers beyond the basal lamina aggregate to form a capsule.

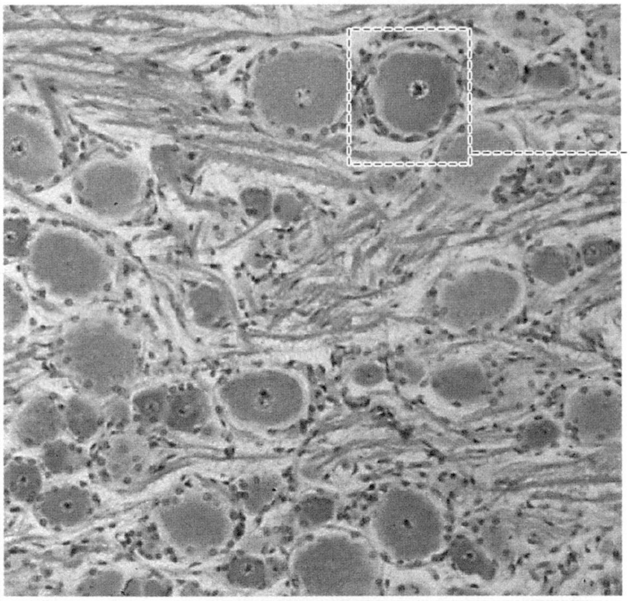

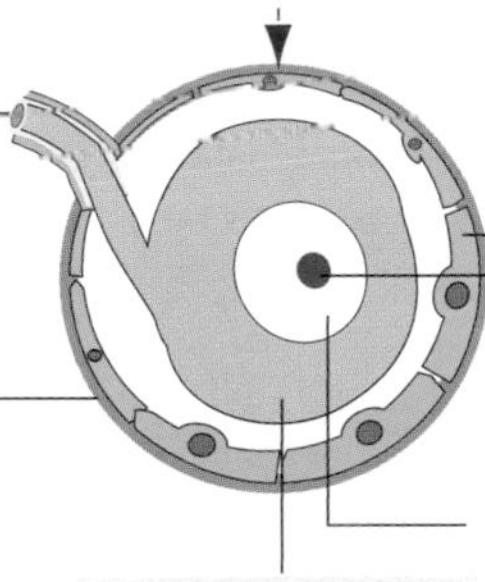
Satellite cell (Schwann cell–like)
Postganglionic axon (myelinated)
Nucleolus
Basal lamina
Nucleus
Pseudounipolar neuron

Sympathetic ganglion

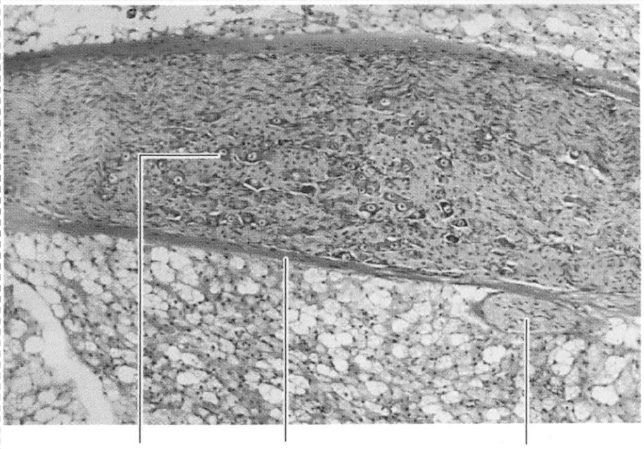
Neuron
Capsule
Nerve

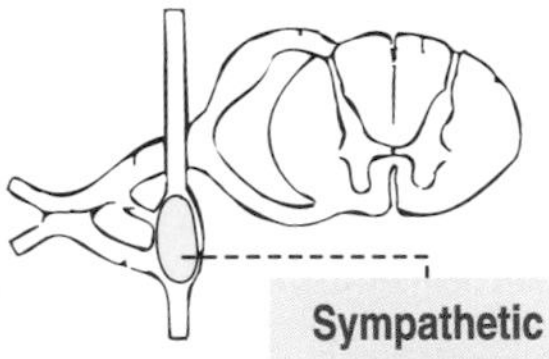
Sympathetic ganglion

The sympathetic ganglion receives axons from presynaptic cells whose neurons are within the CNS. The neurons of the ganglion tend to be randomly arranged, smaller than in the dorsal root ganglion, **multipolar**, and their axons are mostly unmyelinated.

Each neuron is surrounded by satellite cells (Schwann cell–like cells) less numerous than those of spinal ganglia.

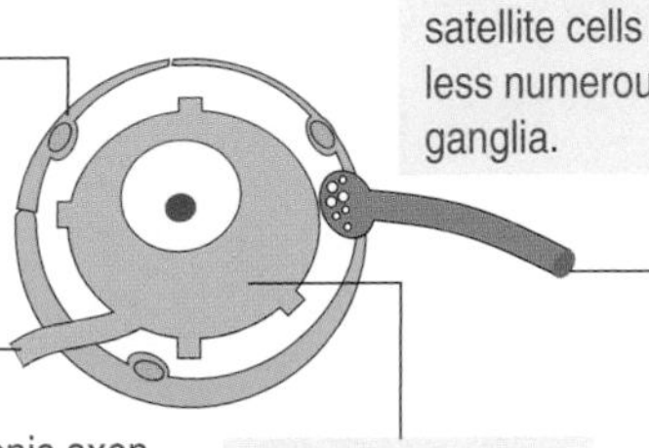
Satellite cell
Preganglionic axon
Postganglionic axon (unmyelinated)
Multipolar neuron

Figure 8-25. Neurohistochemistry

Methods	Reagents
Basic dyes	
Nissl	Basic dyes (methylene blue, cresyl violet, thionine, hematoxylin)
Metal impregnation methods	
Bielschowsky, Bodian, Cajal, Glees, Nauta	Reduced silver nitrate
Fink-Heimer, Nauta	Reduced silver nitrate
Golgi	Silver nitrate
Myelin stains	
Osmium tetroxide	Osmium tetroxide
Klüver-Barrera	Luxol fast blue, periodic acid–Schiff (PAS), and hematoxylin
Weigert-Pal	Iron-hematoxylin
Glial stains	
Cajal	Gold sublimate
Del Rio Hortega	Silver carbonate
Neurotransmitters	
Induced fluorescence Formaldehyde Glyoxylic acid	
Immunocytochemistry	**Specific antibodies** to neurotransmitters, synthesizing enzymes, and neuropeptides
Pathway tracing methods	
Anterograde transport	[^{3}H] **leucine** injected into the soma or perikaryon combined with autoradiography
Retrograde transport	**Horseradish peroxidase** injected near synaptic terminals; the marker is internalized and transported to the perikaryon

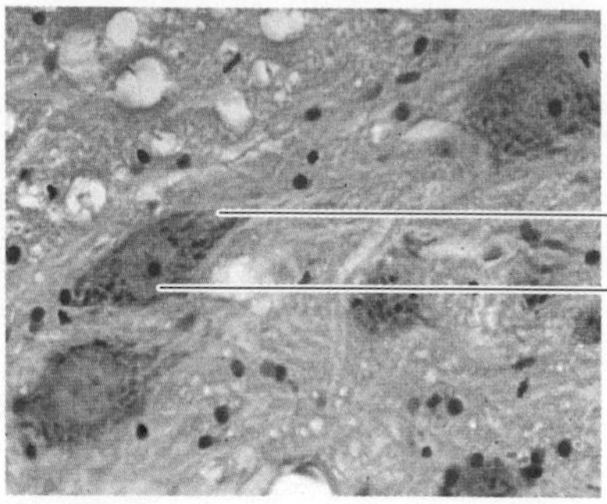

Nissl bodies
Nucleus and nucleolus

Nissl stain

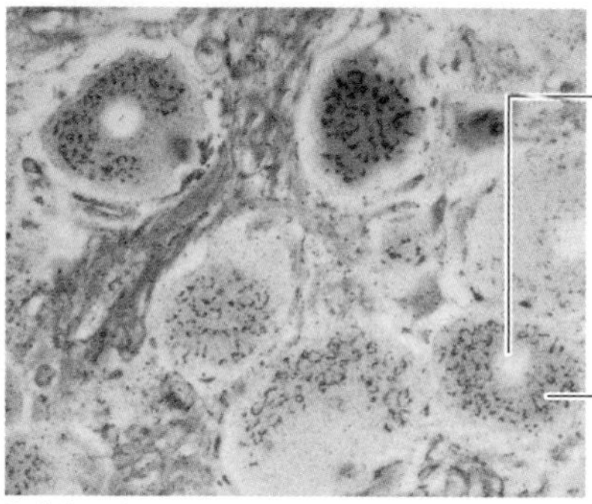

Nucleus
Golgi apparatus in a neuron of a peripheral ganglion. The nucleus is unstained.

Golgi stain

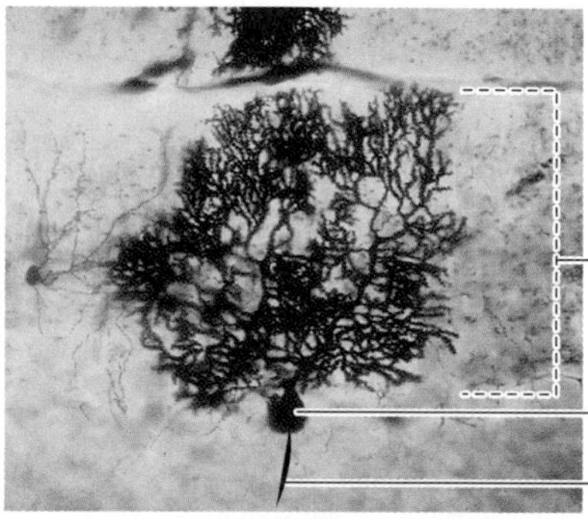

Dendrites
Soma
Axon

Silver impregnation (Purkinje cell)

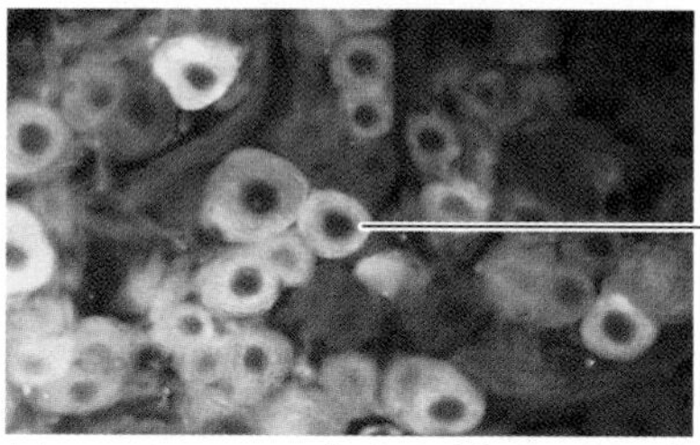

Neurons in the superior cervical ganglion contain catecholamines (green fluorescence).

Adrenergic neurons (induced fluorescence)

Purkinje cell (silver impregnation) courtesy of Wan-hua Amy Yu, New York. Adrenergic neurons (induced fluorescence) courtesy of Edward W. Gresik, New York.

and vesicles of the Golgi apparatus.

Myelin stains are based on the use of dyes with binding affinity for proteins bound to phospholipids. They are useful for the identification of tracts of fibers. Combined Nissl and myelin stains are used in neuropathology.

A tracer, such as horseradish peroxidase, injected into a neuron using a micropipet, has been used for anterograde transport studies. Similarly, tracers injected into nerve terminals can identify the putative neuron by its retrograde transport. Histochemical techniques are available for the localization of substances (for example, catecholamines, enzymes, and others) present in specific populations of neurons.

• The nervous system consists of a central nervous system (CNS) (brain, spinal cord, and the neural parts of the eye) and the peripheral nervous system (PNS) (peripheral ganglia, nerves, nerve endings linking ganglia with the CNS, and receptors and effectors of the body). The basic components of the CNS are neurons and glia (astrocytes and oligodendrocyte). The PNS includes Schwann cells (peripheral nerves) and satellite cells (ganglia).

• The CNS develops from the primitive ectoderm. A neural plate folds to form a hollow cylinder, the neural tube (a process known as neurulation). A region of the neural tube becomes the neural crest, which forms the neurons of peripheral ganglia and other components of the PNS. In addition, neural crest cells migrate along specific routes and differentiate into melanocytes, smooth muscle, and cartilaginous and skeletal components of the head. Some cells form the medulla of the adrenal gland; others organize the enteric nervous system of the alimentary tube.

Defects in the closing of the neural tube cause congenital malformation (for example, **spina bifida**, **anencephaly**, and **craniorachischisis**).

• The functional unit of the nervous system is the neuron. A neuron consists of a body (soma or perikaryon), multiple dendrites, and a single axon. Dendrites are covered by dendritic spines. The site of origin of the axon is called the axon hillock. The terminal portion of an axon has branches (called collectively telodendron); each branch has an enlarged synaptic ending or synaptic bouton. The body contains two important structures: Nissl body or substance (aggregates of polyribosomes and rough endoplasmic reticulum), and cytoskeletal components (neurofilaments and neurotubules), which extend into the dendritic and axonal processes. Nissl bodies stop at the axon hillock but extend into the base of the dendrites. Neurotubules play a significant role in anterograde and retrograde axonal transport of synaptic vesicles and other molecules, mediated by molecular motor proteins kinesin (anterograde transport) and cytoplasmic dynein (retrograde transport).

• Neurons can be classified as multipolar neurons (a single axon and multiple dendrites; for example, pyramidal cells of the cerebral cortex and Purkinje cells of the cerebellar cortex); bipolar neurons (with two processes; found in the sensory system); and pseudounipolar neurons (a single short process; localized in sensory ganglia of cranial and spinal nerves). Multipolar neurons can be subclassified as Golgi type I neurons (the axon extends beyond the limits of the dendritic tree; for example, pyramidal neurons and Purkinje neurons), and Golgi type II neurons (the axon terminates close to the body and does not extend beyond the limits of the dendritic tree; for example, stellate cells of the cerebral cortex).

• There is a specific nomenclature for groups of neurons and axons. A nucleus (plural nuclei) is an aggregate of neurons in the CNS. Neuropil designates the clustering of dendrites, axons, and glial cells within a nucleus and between neuronal bodies. A stratum or lamina is the aggregate of neurons in a layer. Bundles of axons in the CNS are called tracts, fasciculi (bundles), or lemnisci. A ganglion (plural ganglia) is a cluster of neurons in the PNS. A ganglion can be sensory (dorsal root ganglia and trigeminal ganglion) or motor (visceromotor or autonomic ganglia). Axons derived from a ganglion are organized as nerves, ramus (plural rami), or roots.

• A synapse is the junction between the presynaptic terminal of an axon (transmitting site) and the postsynaptic membrane (receiving site), usually of a dendrite, separated by a synaptic cleft. A presynaptic density (corresponding to specific protein—some of them associated to synaptic vesicles—and channels; the active site of a synaptic ending) and a postsynaptic density (receptors for neurotransmitters) are seen on the corresponding membranes.

Synapses can be axospinous (axon terminal facing a dendritic spine), axodendritic (axon terminal on the shaft of a dendrite), axosomatic (axon terminals on the soma of a neuron), and axoaxonic (axon terminal ending on an axon terminal).

• Glial cells include astrocytes (derived from the neuroectoderm), oligodendrocytes (derived from the neuroectoderm), and microglia (derived from the mesoderm). Astrocytes can be subdivided into fibrous astrocytes (predominant in white matter), and protoplasmic astrocytes (found mainly in gray matter). Astrocytes contain in their cytoplasm the intermediate filament protein glial fibrillary acidic protein. Brain capillaries and the inner surface of the pia are surrounded by the glia limitans, corresponding to astrocytic end-feet.

Oligodendrocytes are involved in axonal myelination within the CNS. Each oligodendrocyte provides myelin to several axons. The node of Ranvier (flanked by internode segments) is devoid of oligodendrocyte cytoplasm; the space is occupied by an astrocytic end-foot process.

Microglial cells are phagocytic cells and immunoprotect the brain and spinal cord.

• Myelin is a highly organized multilamellar structure formed by the plasma membrane of oligodendrocytes and Schwann cells. Myelin surrounds axons and facilitates conduction of a nerve impulse by providing insulation to axons and clustering Na^+ channels in the nodes of Ranvier. This arrangement enables the action potential to jump along nodes by a mechanism called saltatory conduction. Saltatory conduction decreases energy requirements for the transmission of a nerve impulse.

During myelinization, cytoplasmic processes of oligodendrocytes and Schwann cells wrap around the axon. Visualization of myelin by electron microscopy reveals two types of densities: the intraperiod line, representing the close apposition of the external surfaces of the plasma membrane with remnant extracellular space and the major dense line, corresponding to the apposition of the inner (cytoplasmic) surfaces of the plasma membrane. The incisures of Schmidt-Lanterman represent residual cytoplasm. The major dense line is slightly thinner in myelin of the CNS.

Proteins of myelin include myelin basic protein (MBP) present in myelin of the CNS and PNS, proteolipid protein (PLP) found in myelin of the CNS, and myelin protein zero (MPZ) the equivalent of PLP in the PNS. MPZ is responsible for maintaining myelin in a compact state. A mutation of the *PLP* gene and its alternatively transcribed protein DM20 causes **Pelizaeus-Merzbacher disease**, an X-linked neuropathy affecting males and characterized by a reduction in the white matter.

Proteins of myelin are strong antigens and have a role in the development of **multiple sclerosis** in the CNS and **Guillain-Barré syndrome** in the PNS.

Myelin is separated from the axon by the axolemma, the surface membrane of the axon. Tight junctions (represented by claudins and zonula occludens proteins) are found linking the plasma membranes of the same Schwann cell and adjacent Schwann cell at the level of the node of Ranvier. Gap junctions, containing connexin 32 (Cx32), are present in the region of the incisures of Schmidt-Lanterman. Mutations in the *Cx32* gene determine the **X-linked Charcot-Marie-Tooth disease**, a demyelinating disorder of the PNS.

• The ependyma lines the surface of the ventricles (brain) and central canal (spinal cord). It consists of two cell types: (1) ependymal cells, a simple cuboidal epithelium with apical microvilli, one or more cilia, linked by desmosomes, and a basal domain in contact with an astrocyte end-foot layer. (2) Tanycytes, a specialized ependymal cell with a basal cell process making contact with a blood vessel.

The choroid plexus produces cerebrospinal fluid (CSF). The plexus consists of epithelial cells linked by tight junctions and with apical microvilli containing Na^+,K^+-ATPase, which pumps Na^+ into the lumen of the ventricle. High Na^+ concentration in the ventricular lumen facilitates the diffusion of water by an osmotic gradient. The basal domain has numerous infoldings. Hydrostatic pressure inside the subjacent fenestrated capillaries produces a net flow of water, solutes, and proteins. The lining epithelium of the choroid plexus screens and excludes several substances from entering the CSF.

The CSF flows from the fourth ventricle into the brain and spinal subarachnoid space and exits the CNS at the superior sagittal sinus.

• Three brain permeability barriers exist: (1) The arachnoid-CSF barrier, consisting of the arachnoid membrane, which prevents the CSF from coming in contact with the extracellular space of the dura mater, and the arachnoid villi, which enable the CSF to permeate across arachnoid barrier cells and endothelial cells. (2) The blood-CSF barrier, with a role of the choroid epithelium in selecting protein and solutes that may reach the ventricular space. (3) The blood-brain barrier, represented by tight junctions sealing the interendothelial space. Astrocyte end-feet in contact with the capillary wall contribute to the barrier.

• The PNS consists of supporting cell types associated to axons extending from neuronal elements of the spinal cord and autonomic and sensory ganglia. Schwann cells are the equivalent of the oligodendrocytes of the CNS. Satellite cells surround the cell bodies of neurons in autonomic and sensory ganglia.

Schwann cells can provide a myelin sheath to a myelinated nerve fiber by forming only one internode segment of myelin (a single oligodendrocyte can form several internode segments). In contrast, several unmyelinated nerve fibers can be embedded in the cytoplasm of a single Schwann cell (in the CNS, unmyelinated nerves are ensheathed by astrocytes).

A peripheral nerve is covered by layers of connective tissue. The epineurium covers the entire nerve. The perineurium separates the nerve into fascicles, which are protected by the blood-nerve barrier consisting of fibroblasts and capillary endothelial cells linked by tight junctions. The endoneurium surrounds individual axons and their associated Schwann cells.

• Peripheral nerves can be injured (crush nerve injury) or diseases may affect the function of Schwann cells, leading to a loss of myelin (segmental demyelinization). A damage to a neuron and its axon causes axonal degeneration, also called wallerian degeneration. A characteristic of axonal degeneration, caused by toxic or metabolic damage, is chromatolysis, the dispersion of Nissl substance (polyribosomes and rough endoplasmic reticulum) in the neuronal soma, followed by demyelinization. Segmental demyelinization and axonal degeneration affect the motor unit and cause muscle paralysis. Axonal degeneration may be followed by axonal regeneration in the PNS. Axonal regeneration in the CNS is not feasible because the endoneurium is not present, oligodendrocytes—in contrast to Schwann cells—do not proliferate, and astrocytes deposit scar tissue (astrocytic plaque).

• **Neurodegenerative diseases**. (1) **Amyotrophic lateral sclerosis** is a motor neuron progressive disease starting with moderate weakness in one limb and progressing to severe paralysis. A mutation in the copper-zinc *superoxide dismutase* gene is frequently seen. (2) **Parkinson's disease**, the second most frequent after Alzheimer's disease, is caused by a loss of dopaminergic neurons from the substantia nigra. Resting tremor and movements with rigidity are typical clinical features. (3) **Alzheimer's disease**, the most frequent neurodegenerative disorder, is characterized by progressive cortical dementia affecting language and memory. A typical feature is the formation of amyloid plaques containing β-amyloid peptide.

• Sensory ganglia (dorsal root ganglia) are surrounded by a connective tissue capsule (epineurium). Neurons are clustered and are pseudounipolar. Nerve fascicles contain myelinated nerve fibers. Each neuron is surrounded by satellite cells supported by a basal lamina. Autonomic ganglia receive preganglionic axons from the CNS and give rise to postganglionic unmyelinated axons. Neurons are scattered and surrounded by satellite cells (less numerous than those of sensory ganglia).

9. SENSORY ORGANS: VISION AND HEARING

EYE

The eye can self-focus, adjust for light intensity, and convert light into electrical impulses interpreted by the brain. In humans, the eye is recessed in a bony orbit and is connected to the brain by the optic nerve. The eyeball protects and facilitates the function of the photoreceptive retina, the inner layer of the eyeball.

The eyeball consists of **three tunics** or **layers** which, from outside to inside, are (1) the **sclera** and the **cornea**, (2) the **uvea**, and (3) the **retina** (Figure 9-1).

Three distinct and interconnected chambers are found inside the eyeball: the **anterior chamber**, the **posterior chamber**, and the **vitreous cavity** (see Box 9-A). **Aqueous humor** circulates from the posterior to the anterior chamber. The **lens** is placed in front of the vitreous cavity, which contains **vitreous humor**. The **bony orbit**, the **eyelids**, the **conjunctiva**, and the **lacrimal apparatus** protect the eyeball.

The **ophthalmic artery**, a branch of the internal carotid artery, provides nutrients to the eye and the contents of the orbit. The **superior** and **inferior orbital veins** are the principal venous drainage of the eye. The veins empty into the **intracranial cavernous sinus**.

Development of the eye

A brief summary of the development of the eye is essential to the understanding of the relationship of the various layers in the eyeball. The components of the eye derive from (1) the surface **ectoderm** of the head; (2) the lateral **neuroectodermal** walls of the embryonic brain in the diencephalon region; and (3) the **mesenchyme**.

Lateral outpocketings of the right and left sides of the diencephalon give rise to

Box 9-A | Anatomy of the eye

- The eye consists of three chambers: (1) The **anterior chamber** is the space between the cornea and the anterior surface of the iris. (2) The **posterior chamber** extends from the posterior surface of the iris to the lens. (3) The **vitreous cavity** or **body** is posterior to the lens and is the largest compartment.
- The human eyeball is roughly spherical with a diameter of about 24 mm. The anterior pole of the eyeball is the center of the **cornea**.
- The posterior pole is located between the **optic disk** and the **fovea**, a shallow depression in the retina. The **anatomic axis** (also called the **optical axis**) is the line connecting the two poles. The **visual axis** joins the apparent center of the pupil and the center of the fovea and divides the eyeball into **nasal** and **temporal halves**.
- The eyeball is surrounded by a soft tissue cushion occupying the bony orbit of the skull. The soft tissue includes loose connective tissue, fat, muscles, blood and lymphatic vessels, nerves, and the lacrimal gland.
- The anterior surface of the eyeball is connected to the integument by the **conjunctiva**, which lines the inner surface of the lids and reflects over the eyeball to the edge of the cornea.

Figure 9-1. Anatomy of the eye

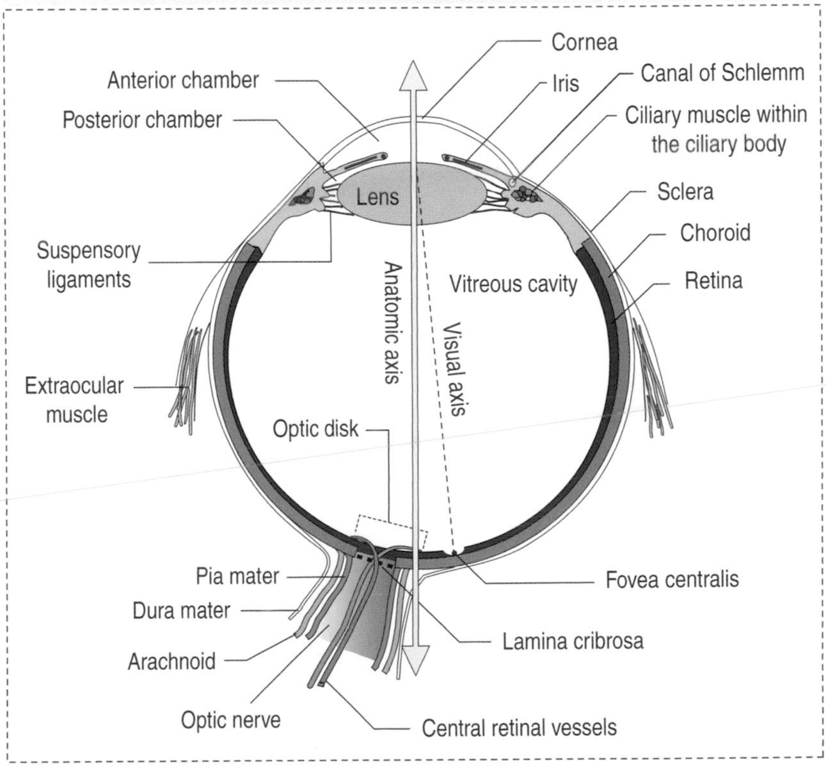

Cornea
Iris
Canal of Schlemm
Anterior chamber
Posterior chamber
Ciliary muscle within the ciliary body
Lens
Sclera
Choroid
Suspensory ligaments
Retina
Vitreous cavity
Anatomic axis
Visual axis
Extraocular muscle
Optic disk
Pia mater
Fovea centralis
Dura mater
Lamina cribrosa
Arachnoid
Optic nerve
Central retinal vessels

Figure 9-2. **Development of the eye**

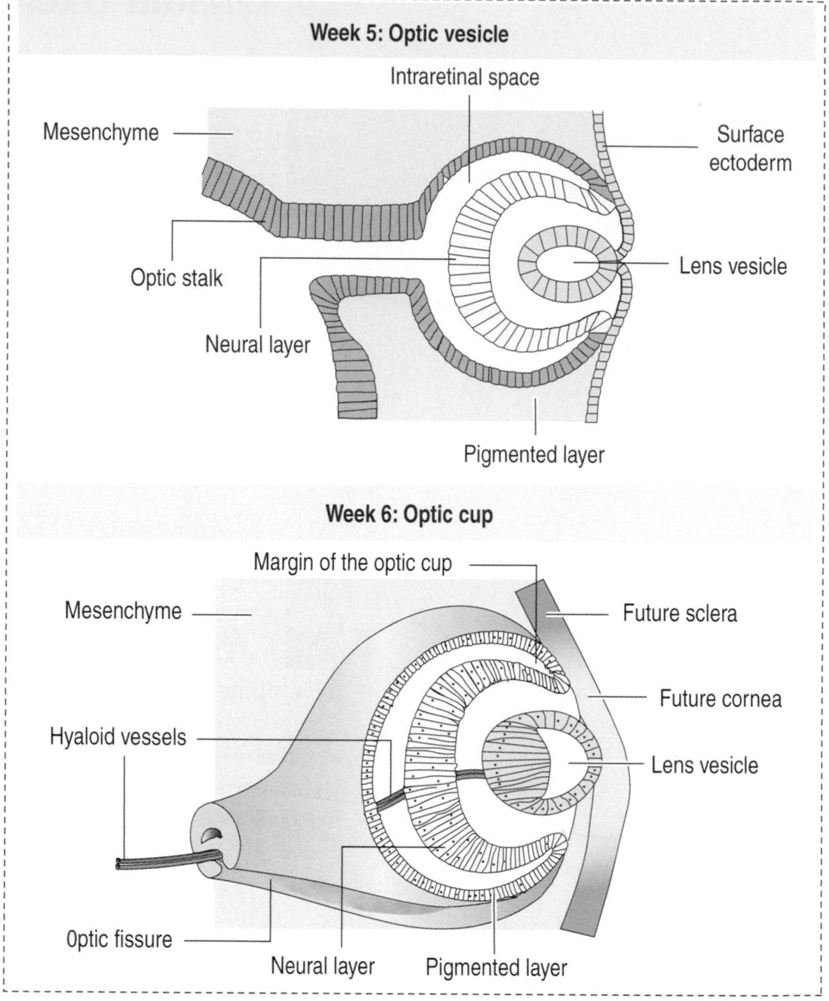
Week 5: Optic vesicle
Intraretinal space
Mesenchyme
Surface ectoderm
Optic stalk
Lens vesicle
Neural layer
Pigmented layer
Week 6: Optic cup
Margin of the optic cup
Mesenchyme
Future sclera
Future cornea
Hyaloid vessels
Lens vesicle
Optic fissure
Neural layer
Pigmented layer

two neuroepithelial **optic vesicles**, each remaining attached to the brain wall by a hollow **optic stalk** (Figure 9-2). The surface ectoderm of the head invaginates into the optical vesicle forming a **lens vesicle** that pinches off. Mesenchyme surrounds both the lens vesicle and the adjacent optic vesicle.

The optic vesicle invaginates and becomes a double-walled **optic cup** (see Figure 9-2). The **optic fissure** forms when the outer layer of the optic cup becomes the **pigmented epithelium**. Cells in the inner layer proliferate and stratify to form the **neural retina**. The mesenchyme extending into the invagination of the optic cup acquires a gelatinous consistency and becomes the **vitreous component** of the eye. The **lens vesicle** is kept in place by the free margins of the optic cup and the surrounding mesenchyme.

At the outer surface of the optic cup, the mesenchymal shell differentiates into the vascular **choroid coat** of the eye and the fibrous components of the **sclera** and **cornea** (Figure 9-3; see Box 9-B). Posterior to the lens, the vascular choroid coat forms the **ciliary body**, **ciliary muscle**, and **ciliary processes**. Anterior to the lens, the choroid coat forms the stroma of the **iris**. The ciliary processes secrete the **aqueous humor** that accumulates first in the **posterior chamber** (between iris and lens) and then passes into the anterior chamber (between lens and cornea) across the pupil. The aqueous humor leaves the anterior chamber by entering into the **canal of Schlemm**, a small vein (**sinus venosus of the sclera**) encircling the eye at the anterior edge of the choroid coat.

Around the rim of the optic cup, the inner and outer layers form the **posterior epithelium** of the **ciliary body** and **iris**. The sphincter and **dilator pupillae muscles**

Box 9-B | **Development of the cornea**

- The lens induces the differentiation of the overlying ectoderm. Cells of the mesenchyme secrete types I and II collagen, components of the primary stroma of the cornea.
- **Capillary endothelial cells** migrate into the primary stroma and produce hyaluronic acid, causing the stroma to swell.
- **Mesenchymal cells** in the surrounding space migrate into the stroma and secrete hyaluronidase. The stroma shrinks and the cornea acquires the correct shape and transparency.

Figure 9-3. **Development of the eye**

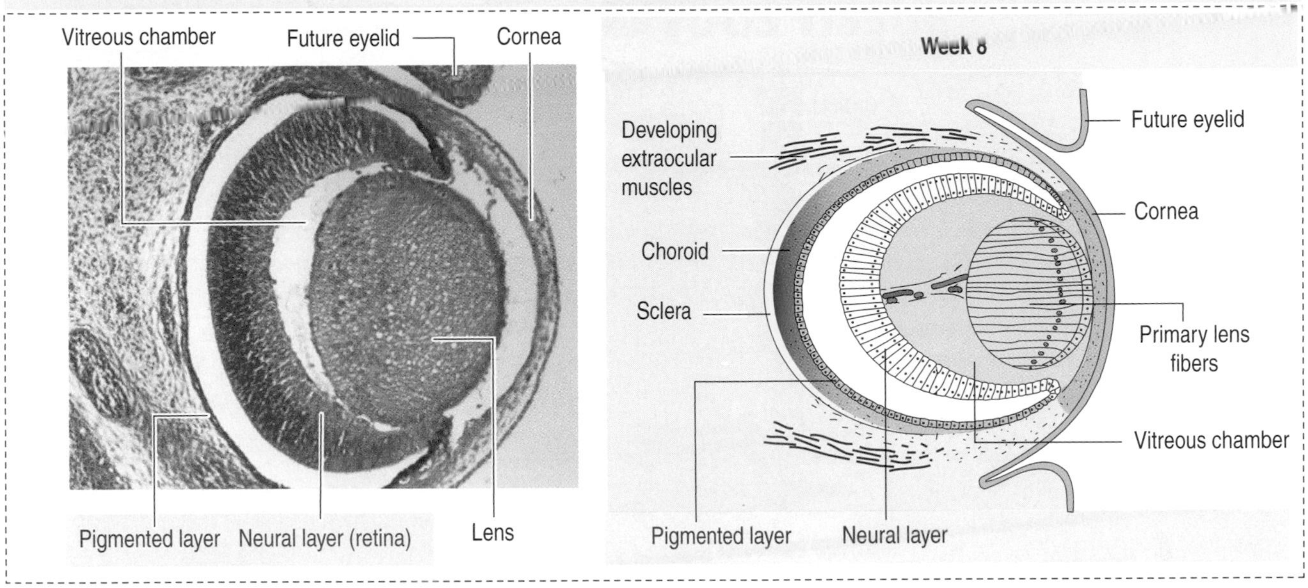

develop from the posterior epithelium.

The inner layer of the optic cup becomes the neural layer of the retina, which differentiates into **photosensory cells**, **bipolar neurons**, and **ganglionic neurons** (including interconnecting **horizontal** and **amacrine cells** and **glial Müller cells**). Axons from the ganglionic neurons form the nerve fiber layer of the retina, which converges on the optic stalk occupying the optic fissure as the **optic nerve**. The optic fissure becomes the escape route from the optic cup (except at its rim).

Outer tunic: Sclera and cornea

The sclera (Figure 9-4) is a 1.0- to 0.4-mm-thick layer of collagen and elastic fibers produced by fibroblasts. The inner side of the sclera faces the choroid, from which it is separated by a layer of loose connective tissue and an elastic tissue network known as the **suprachoroid lamina**. Tendons of the six extrinsic muscles of the eye are attached to the outer surface of the sclera.

Cornea

The cornea is 0.8 to 1.1-mm thick and has a smaller radius of curvature than the sclera. It is transparent, lacks blood vessels, and is extremely rich in nerve endings. The anterior surface of the cornea is always kept wet with a film of tears retained by microvilli of the apical epithelial cells. The cornea is one of the few organs that can be transplanted without a risk of being rejected by the host's immune system. This success can be attributed to the lack of corneal blood and lymphatic vessels.

The cornea is composed of five layers (Figure 9-5):

1. The **corneal epithelium**.
2. The **layer** or **membrane of Bowman**.
3. The **stroma** or **substantia propria**.
4. The **membrane of Descemet**.
5. The **corneal endothelium**.

The **corneal epithelium** is stratified squamous and consists of five to seven layers of cells. Cells of the outer surface have **microvilli** and all cells are connected to one another by desmosomes. The cytoplasm contains cytokeratin associated with desmosomes. The epithelium of the cornea is very sensitive, contains a large number of free nerve endings, and has a remarkable wound healing capacity. At the **limbus**, the corneoscleral junction, the corneal epithelium is continuous with that of the conjunctiva.

Figure 9-4. Three tunics of the eye

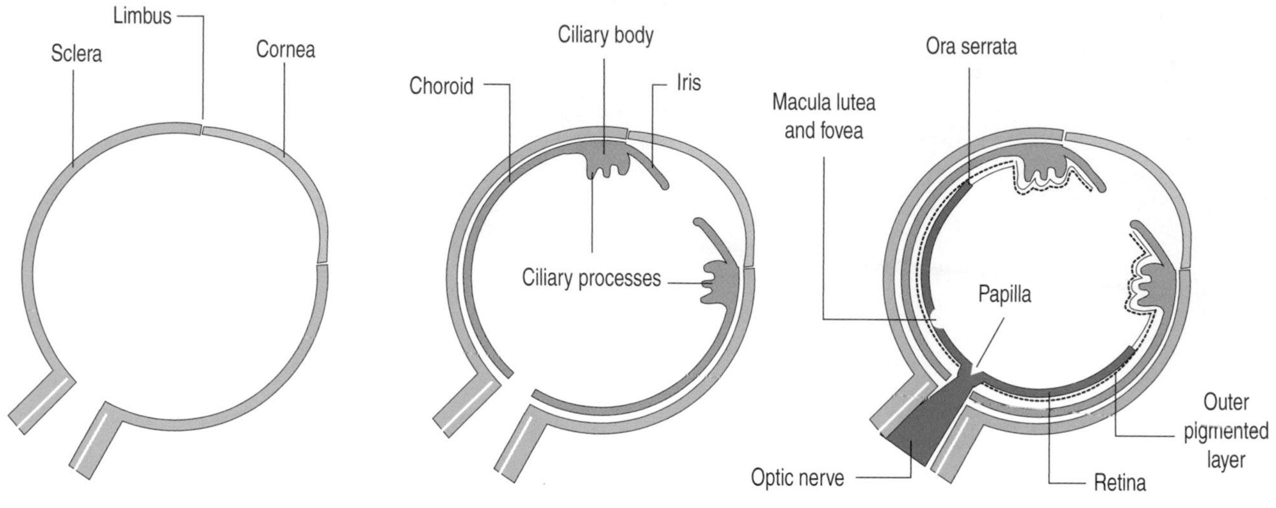
Limbus
Sclera
Cornea
Ciliary body
Choroid
Iris
Ciliary processes
Ora serrata
Macula lutea
and fovea
Papilla
Outer
pigmented
layer
Optic nerve
Retina

Outer tunic
Sclera and cornea

The cornea (Latin *corneus*, horny) is transparent. The rest of the wall of the eye, the **sclera** (Greek *scleros*, hard), is opaque and lined inside by the middle or vascular pigmented layer that absorbs light.

The **limbus** is the zone of transition of the epithelium of the conjunctiva with that of the cornea. The limbus is also the boundary of the transparent cornea with the opaque sclera.

The corneoscleral coat:

1. Protects the inner structures of the eye.
2. Together with the intraocular fluid pressure, it maintains the shape and consistency of the eyeball.

Middle tunic
Uvea

In the posterior two thirds of the eye, the vascular layer is called the choroid. In the anterior part of the eye the vascular layer thickens to form the **ciliary body**.

Ciliary processes extend inward from the ciliary body. The vascular layer continues as the iris, whose free edge outlines the **pupil**.

1. The vascular layer is **pigmented**, a property that light-proofs the inner surface of the eye and reduces reflection of the light.
2. Blood vessels travel through the middle layer.
3. Its anterior portion contains smooth muscle: the **muscle of the ciliary body** and the **dilator** and **constrictor of the iris**. The smooth muscle of the ciliary body regulates the tension of the **zonule** or **suspensory ligament** of the lens and, therefore, is an important element in the mechanism of **accommodation**.

Inner tunic
Retina

It consists of two layers: (1) an **outer pigmented layer** (pars pigmentosa) and (2) an **inner retinal layer** (pars nervosa or optica). The retina has a posterior two-thirds light-sensitive zone (pars optica) and an anterior one-third **light-nonsensitive zone** (pars ciliaris and iridica). The scalloped border between these two zones is called the **ora serrata** (Latin *ora*, edge; *serrata*, sawlike).

The retina contains **photoreceptor neurons** (cones and rods), **conducting neurons** (bipolar and ganglion cells), **association neurons** (horizontal and amacrine cells), and a **supporting neuroglial cell**, the Müller cell.

Each eye contains about 125 million rods and cones but only 1 million ganglion cells. The number of cones and rods varies over the surface of the retina. **Only cones are present in the fovea** (0.5 mm in diameter) where fine detail vision is best. Axons from the retinal ganglion cells pass across the surface of the retina, converge on the **papilla** or **optic disk**, and leave the eye through many openings of the sclera (the **lamina cribrosa**) to form the **optic nerve**.

Bowman's layer is 6 to 9 µm thick, consists of type I collagen fibrils, and lacks elastic fibers. This layer is transparent and does not have regenerative capacity. Bowman's layer is the anteriormost part of the corneal stroma, although differently organized. For this reason, it is designated "layer" instead of "membrane." Bowman's layer represents a protective barrier to trauma and bacterial invasion.

The highly transparent **stroma** or **substantia propria** represents about 90% of the thickness of the cornea. Bundles of **type I** and **V collagen** form thin layers regularly arranged in successive planes crossing at various angles and forming a **lattice** that is highly resistant to deformations and trauma. Fibers and layers are separated by an extracellular matrix rich in **proteoglycans** containing **chondroitin** and **keratan sulfate**.

Figure 9-5. **Cornea**

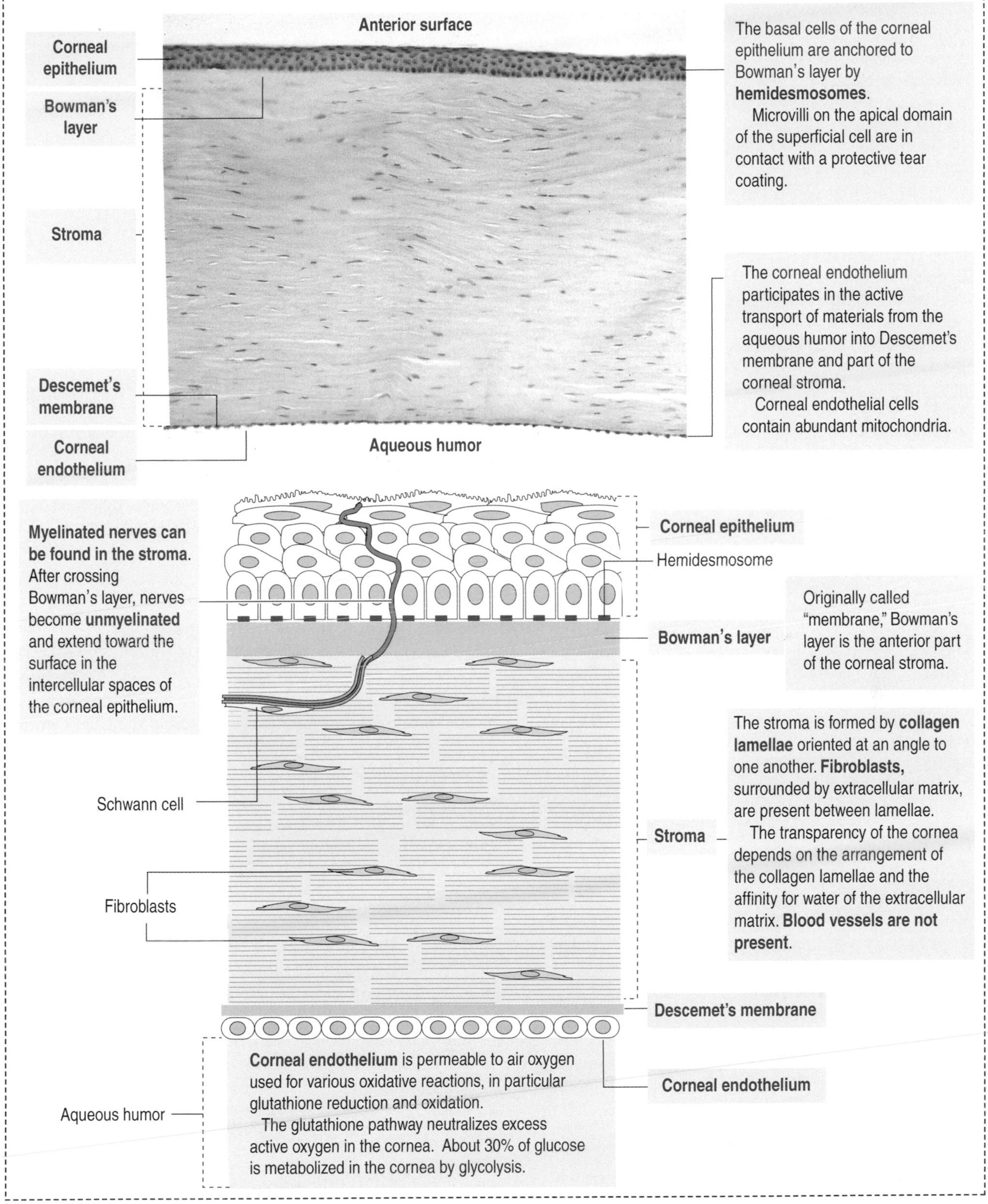
Anterior surface
Corneal epithelium
Bowman's layer
Stroma
Descemet's membrane
Corneal endothelium
Aqueous humor
The basal cells of the corneal epithelium are anchored to Bowman's layer by **hemidesmosomes**.
Microvilli on the apical domain of the superficial cell are in contact with a protective tear coating.
The corneal endothelium participates in the active transport of materials from the aqueous humor into Descemet's membrane and part of the corneal stroma.
Corneal endothelial cells contain abundant mitochondria.
Myelinated nerves can be found in the stroma. After crossing Bowman's layer, nerves become **unmyelinated** and extend toward the surface in the intercellular spaces of the corneal epithelium.
Corneal epithelium
Hemidesmosome
Originally called "membrane," Bowman's layer is the anterior part of the corneal stroma.
Bowman's layer
Schwann cell
Fibroblasts
Stroma
The stroma is formed by **collagen lamellae** oriented at an angle to one another. **Fibroblasts,** surrounded by extracellular matrix, are present between lamellae.
The transparency of the cornea depends on the arrangement of the collagen lamellae and the affinity for water of the extracellular matrix. **Blood vessels are not present.**
Descemet's membrane
Corneal endothelium
Aqueous humor
Corneal endothelium is permeable to air oxygen used for various oxidative reactions, in particular glutathione reduction and oxidation.
The glutathione pathway neutralizes excess active oxygen in the cornea. About 30% of glucose is metabolized in the cornea by glycolysis.

Nerves in transit to the corneal epithelium are found in the corneal stroma.

Descemet's membrane, one of the thickest basement membranes in the body (5 to 10 μm thick), is produced by the corneal endothelium and contains **type VII collagen**, which forms a hexagonal array of fibers.

The **corneal endothelium** lines the posterior surface of Descemet's membrane and faces the anterior chamber of the eye. It consists of a single layer of squamous epithelial cells, with impermeable intercellular spaces preventing influx of aqueous humor into the corneal stroma. The structural and functional integrity of the corneal endothelium is vital to the maintenance of corneal transparency (see Box 9-C).

Box 9-C | **Corneal transplantation**

- Corneal transplantation, also known as **penetrating keratoplasty**, is the most common form of tissue allotransplantation (Greek *allos*, other) with a rate of success over 90%.
- This success is related to various aspects of the cornea and the ocular microenvironment: (1) The expression of **major histocompatibility complex (MHC) class II** is negligible or absent in the normal cornea. (2) The **cornea secretes immunosuppressive factors** that inhibit T cell and complement activation (see Chapter 10, Immune-Lymphatic System). (3) Cells in the cornea express **Fas ligand**, which protects the eye from cell-mediated damage by eliminating apoptosis cells that can determine inflammatory damage (see Apoptosis in Chapter 3, Cell Signaling). (4) Corneal **Langerhans cells** (see Chapter 11, Integumentary System) and **antigen-presenting cells** are rare in the cornea. (5) The cornea is **avascular** and **lacks lymphatics**, thus preventing the arrival of immune elements.

Middle tunic: Uvea

The uvea forms the pigmented vascularized tunic of the eye and is divided into three regions: (1) the **choroid**, (2) the **ciliary body**, and (3) the **iris** (see Figure 9–7) (see Box 9-D).

The **choroid** consists of three layers (Figure 9-6):

1. **Bruch's membrane**, the innermost component of the choroid, consists of a network of collagen and elastic fibers and basal lamina material. Basal laminae derive from the pigmented epithelium of the retina and the endothelia of the underlying fenestrated capillaries.
2. The **choriocapillaris** contains fenestrated capillaries that supply oxygen and nutrients to the outer layers of the retina and the fovea.
3. The **choroidal stroma** consists of large arteries and veins surrounded by collagen and elastic fibers, fibroblasts, a few smooth muscle cells, neurons of the autonomic nervous system, and melanocytes.

The **ciliary body** (Figure 9-7) is anterior to the ora serrata and represents the ventral projection of both the choroid and the retina. It is made up of two components: (1) the **uveal portion** and (2) the **neuroepithelial portion.**

The **uveal portion** of the ciliary body includes:

1. The continuation of the outer layer of the choroid, known as the **supraciliaris.**
2. The **ciliary muscle**, a ring of smooth muscle tissue that, **when contracted, reduces the length of the circular suspensory ligaments of the lens**; this is known as the **ciliary zonule.**
3. A layer of **fenestrated capillaries** supplying blood to the ciliary muscle.

The **neuroepithelial portion** contributes the two layers of the **ciliary epithelium**:

1. An outer **pigmented epithelial layer**, continuous with the retinal pigmented epithelium. The pigmented epithelial layer is supported by a basal lamina continuous with Bruch's membrane.
2. An inner **nonpigmented epithelial layer**, which is continuous with the sensory retina.

Particular features of these two pigmented and nonpigmented epithelial cell layers are:

1. **The apical surfaces of the pigmented and nonpigmented cells face each other.**
2. The dual epithelium is smooth at its posterior end (pars plana) and folded at the anterior end (pars plicata) to form the **ciliary processes.**
3. The **aqueous humor** is secreted by epithelial cells of the ciliary processes supplied by fenestrated capillaries (Figure 9-8) .

The **iris** is a continuation of the ciliary body and is located in front of the lens. At this position, it forms a gate for the flow of aqueous humor between the anterior and posterior chambers of the eye and also controls the amount of light entering the eye.

The iris has two components: (1) the **anterior uveal** or **stromal** face and (2) the posterior **neuroepithelial** surface.

The **anterior** (outer) **uveal face** is of mesenchymal origin and has an irregular surface. It is formed by **fibroblasts** and pigmented **melanocytes** embedded in an extracellular matrix. The number of pigmented melanocytes determines the color of the iris. In albinos, the iris appears pink due to the abundant blood vessels.

Box 9-D | **Uveal tract**

- The **uveal tract** has significant clinical relevance. The uvea can be affected by several inflammatory processes known as **uveitis**, which can target the iris (**iritis**), the ciliary body (**cyclitis**), and the choroid (**choroiditis**).
- Uveal inflammation can be secondary to an **immune-mediated disease** or **infection** (for example, cytomegalovirus). An inflammatory exudate in choroiditis can lead to detachment of the retina. The inflammatory destruction of the choroid can cause degeneration of the photoreceptors whose nutrition depends on the integrity of the choroid.
- Melanocytes are abundant in the choroid and they can give rise to **ocular melanomas**, pigmented malignant tumors that can cause systemic metastasis.

Figure 9-6. Structure of the choroid

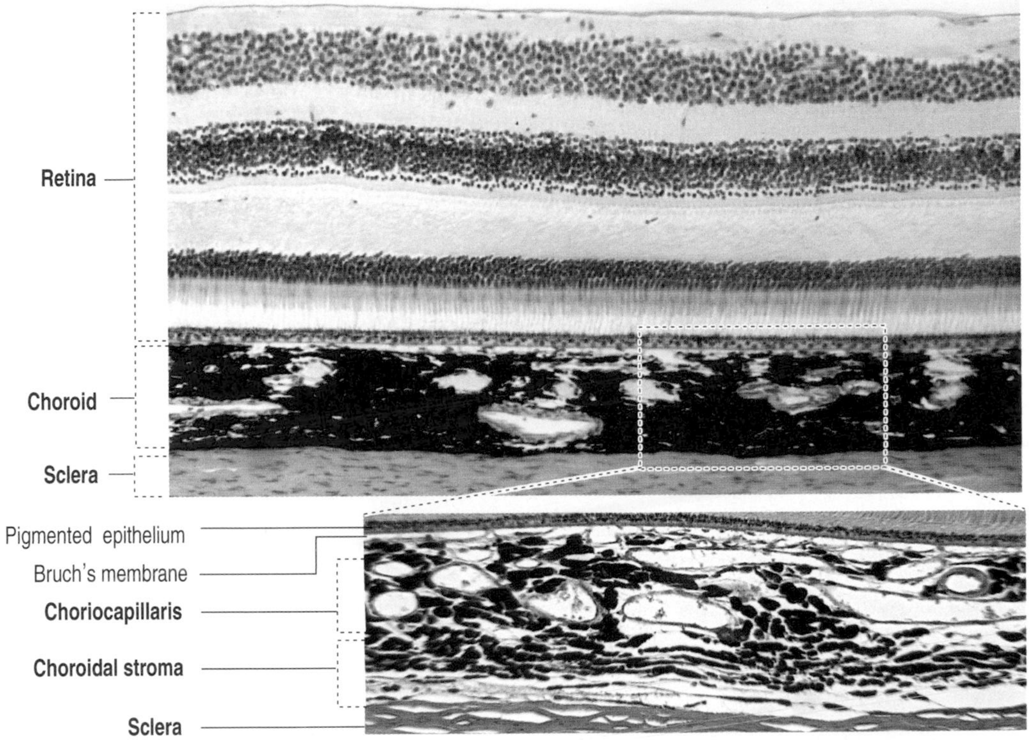

Retina
Choroid
Sclera
Pigmented epithelium
Bruch's membrane
Choriocapillaris
Choroidal stroma
Sclera

Bruch's membrane

Bruch's membrane is formed by:

1. The **basal lamina of the pigmented epithelium** of the retina.
2. Subjacent layers of **collagenous and elastic fibers**.
3. The **basal lamina of endothelial cells** of the underlying capillary network (choriocapillaris).

Choroidal stroma

The stroma contains collagen fibers, some smooth muscle cells, neurons of the autonomic nervous system, blood vessels (arteries and veins), and melanocytes.

Melanocytes are more numerous in heavily pigmented individuals than in persons with light pigment.

Choriocapillaris

Capillaries of the choriocapillaris connect with arteries (branches of the posterior ciliary arteries) and veins (vortex veins) in the choroidal stroma.

The choriocapillaris provides nutrients to the outer layers of the retina.

Drusen

The accumulation of **amyloid material** in the inner side of Bruch's membrane forms an inward bulging region called **drusen** (German *Drusen*, stony nodule).

A large drusen pushes away the photoreceptors from their blood supply. If the separation is too large, the pigmented epithelium and photoreceptors degenerate.

The earliest indication of **age-related macular degeneration** is the presence of drusen.

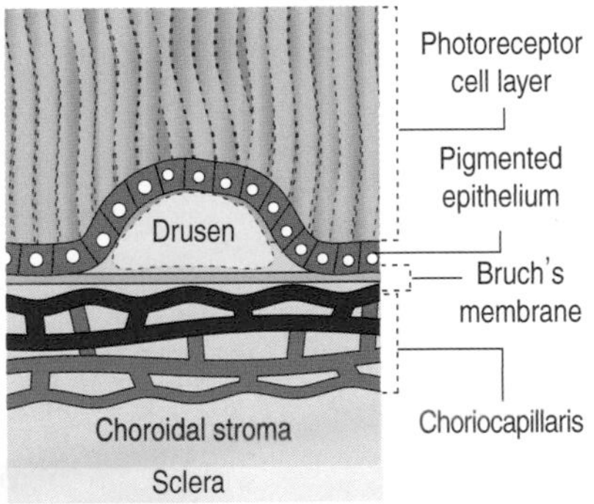

Photoreceptor cell layer
Pigmented epithelium
Drusen
Bruch's membrane
Choriocapillaris
Choroidal stroma
Sclera

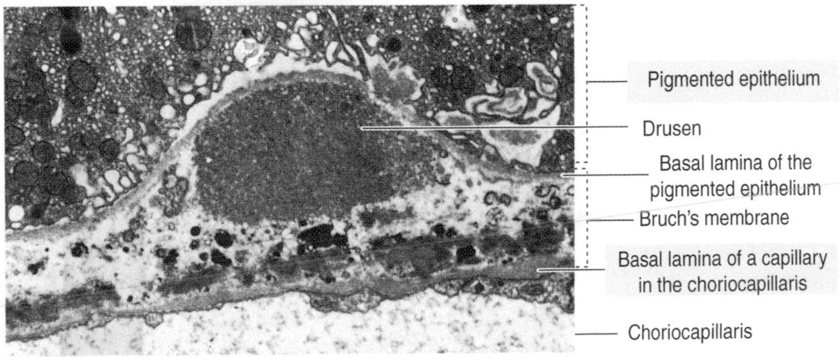

Pigmented epithelium
Drusen
Basal lamina of the pigmented epithelium
Bruch's membrane
Basal lamina of a capillary in the choriocapillaris
Choriocapillaris

Electron micrograph from Hogan MJ, Alvarado JA, Weddell JA: Histology of the Human Eye. Philadelphia, WB Saunders, 1971.

Blood vessels of the iris have a radial distribution and can adjust to changes in length in parallel to variations in the diameter of the pupil.

The **posterior** (inner) **neuroepithelial surface** consists of **two layers of pigmented epithelium**. The outer layer, a continuation of the pigmented layer of the ciliary epithelium, consists of **myoepithelial cells** that become the **dilator**

Figure 9-7. Ciliary body

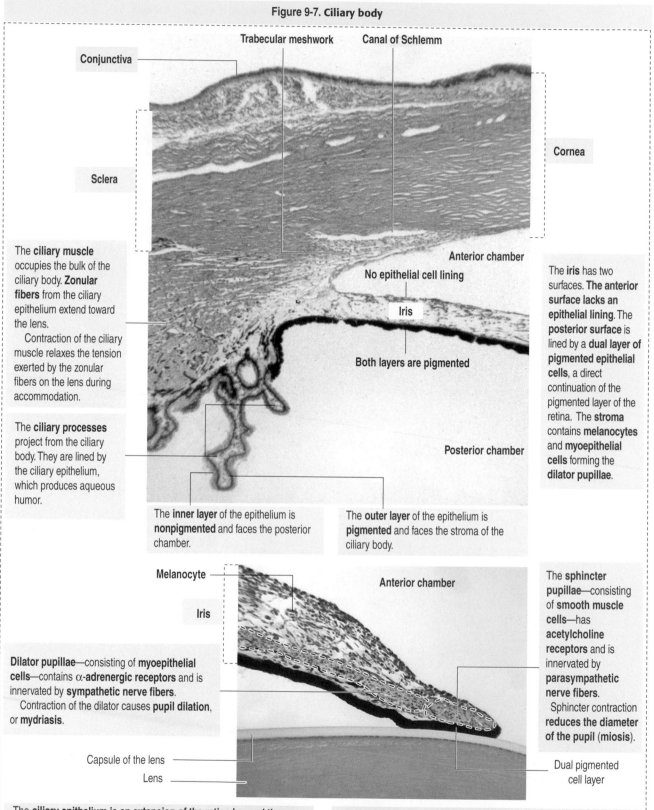

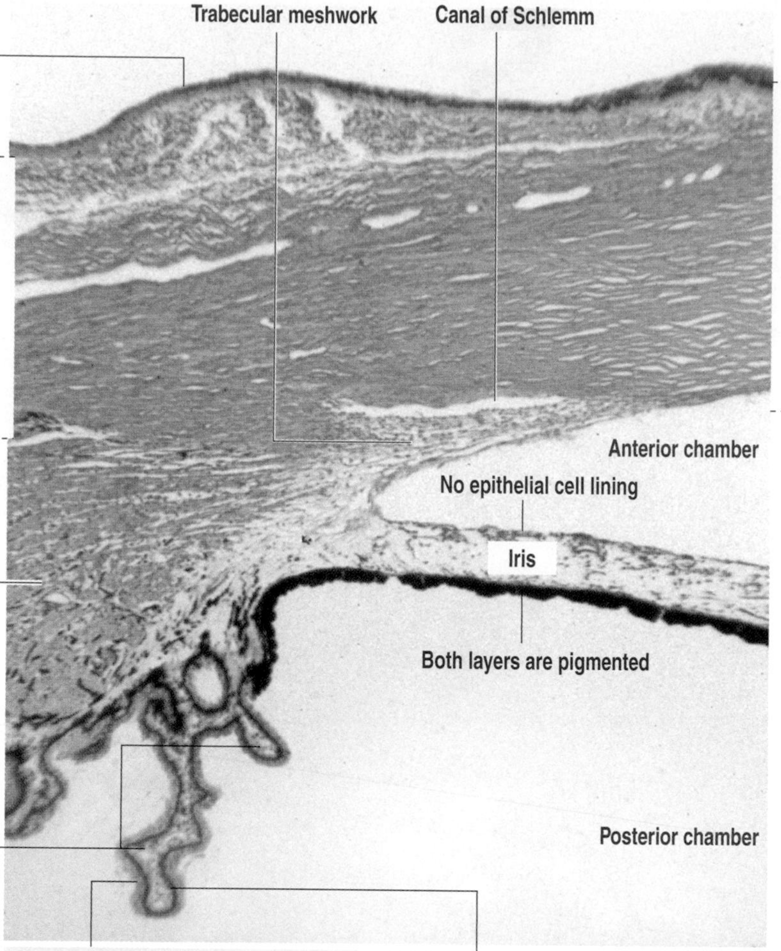

Trabecular meshwork
Canal of Schlemm
Conjunctiva
Sclera
Cornea
Anterior chamber
No epithelial cell lining
Iris
Both layers are pigmented
Posterior chamber

The **ciliary muscle** occupies the bulk of the ciliary body. **Zonular fibers** from the ciliary epithelium extend toward the lens.

Contraction of the ciliary muscle relaxes the tension exerted by the zonular fibers on the lens during accommodation.

The **ciliary processes** project from the ciliary body. They are lined by the ciliary epithelium, which produces aqueous humor.

The **inner layer** of the epithelium is **nonpigmented** and faces the posterior chamber.

The **outer layer** of the epithelium is **pigmented** and faces the stroma of the ciliary body.

The **iris** has two surfaces. **The anterior surface lacks an epithelial lining.** The **posterior surface** is lined by a **dual layer of pigmented epithelial cells**, a direct continuation of the pigmented layer of the retina. The **stroma** contains **melanocytes** and **myoepithelial cells** forming the **dilator pupillae**.

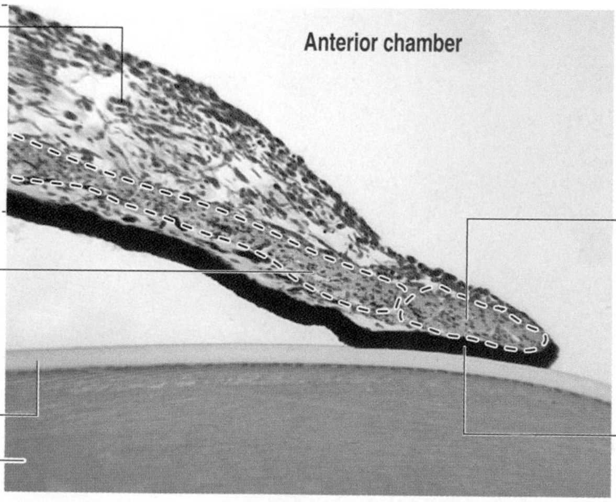

Melanocyte
Iris
Anterior chamber
Capsule of the lens
Lens
Dual pigmented cell layer

Dilator pupillae—consisting of **myoepithelial cells**—contains **α-adrenergic receptors** and is innervated by **sympathetic nerve fibers**.

Contraction of the dilator causes **pupil dilation**, or **mydriasis**.

The **sphincter pupillae**—consisting of **smooth muscle cells**—has **acetylcholine receptors** and is innervated by **parasympathetic nerve fibers**.

Sphincter contraction **reduces the diameter of the pupil (miosis)**.

The **ciliary epithelium is an extension of the retina beyond the ora serrata and covers the inner surface of the ciliary body**. It consists of two layers: an **inner layer of nonpigmented cells**—a direct continuation of the sensory retina—facing the posterior chamber, and **an outer layer of pigmented cells**—continuous with the retinal pigmented epithelium—in contact with the stroma of the ciliary body. As the ciliary epithelium approaches the base of the iris, the cells of the inner layer accumulate pigment granules and both layers are pigmented. **Aqueous humor is secreted by the epithelial cells of the ciliary processes** supplied by **fenestrated capillaries.** Zonular fibers, normally associated with the ciliary processes, are not seen in Figure 9-7 but are depicted in Figure 9-11.

Figure 9-8. Structure of the ciliary epithelium and secretion of aqueous humor

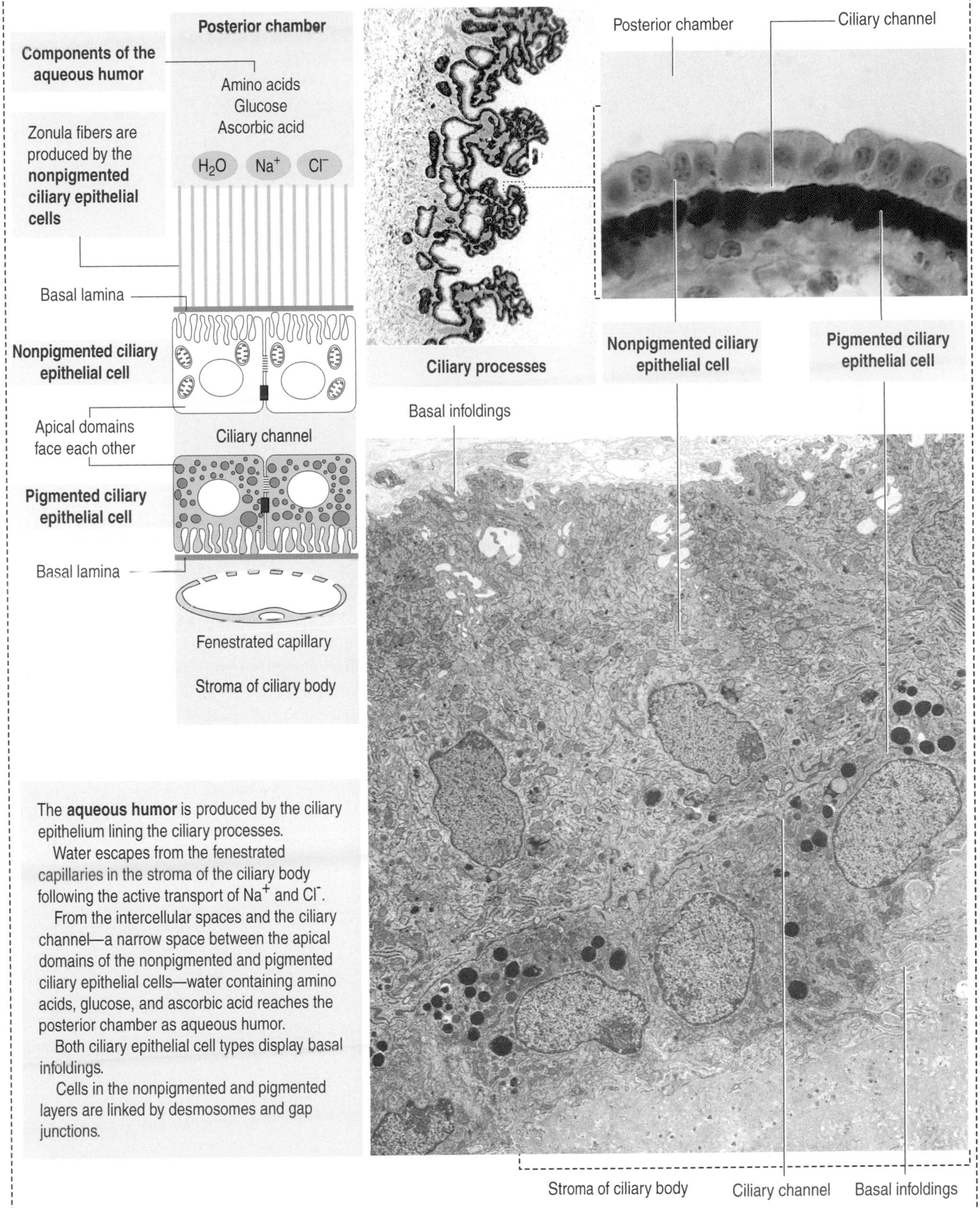

Posterior chamber
Components of the aqueous humor
Amino acids
Glucose
Ascorbic acid
Zonula fibers are produced by the **nonpigmented ciliary epithelial cells**
H_2O
Na^+
Cl^-
Basal lamina
Nonpigmented ciliary epithelial cell
Apical domains face each other
Ciliary channel
Pigmented ciliary epithelial cell
Basal lamina
Fenestrated capillary
Stroma of ciliary body
Ciliary processes
Posterior chamber
Ciliary channel
Nonpigmented ciliary epithelial cell
Pigmented ciliary epithelial cell
Basal infoldings
Stroma of ciliary body
Ciliary channel
Basal infoldings

The **aqueous humor** is produced by the ciliary epithelium lining the ciliary processes.

Water escapes from the fenestrated capillaries in the stroma of the ciliary body following the active transport of Na^+ and Cl^-.

From the intercellular spaces and the ciliary channel—a narrow space between the apical domains of the nonpigmented and pigmented ciliary epithelial cells—water containing amino acids, glucose, and ascorbic acid reaches the posterior chamber as aqueous humor.

Both ciliary epithelial cell types display basal infoldings.

Cells in the nonpigmented and pigmented layers are linked by desmosomes and gap junctions.

Electron micrograph from Hogan MJ, Alvarado JA, Weddell JA: Histology of the Human Eye. Philadelphia, WB Saunders,1971.

pupillae muscle. The **smooth muscle** of the **sphincter pupillae** is located in the iris stroma around the pupil.

Figure 9-9. **Path of aqueous humor**

1 The arrow indicates the pathway followed by **the aqueous humor produced by the epithelial lining of the ciliary processes**.

2 The aqueous fluid flows from the posterior chamber through the pupil into the anterior chamber. The **canal of Schlemm**, lined by an **endothelium**, does not communicate directly with the spaces of the trabecular meshwork. Instead, the fluid percolates through a thin endothelial lining and loose connective tissue.

3 **Aqueous veins** are collector channels draining the canal of Schlemm into the **episcleral veins**.

The drainage rate of aqueous humor is balanced by the rate of secretion. By this mechanism, the intraocular pressure is maintained constant (23 mm Hg).

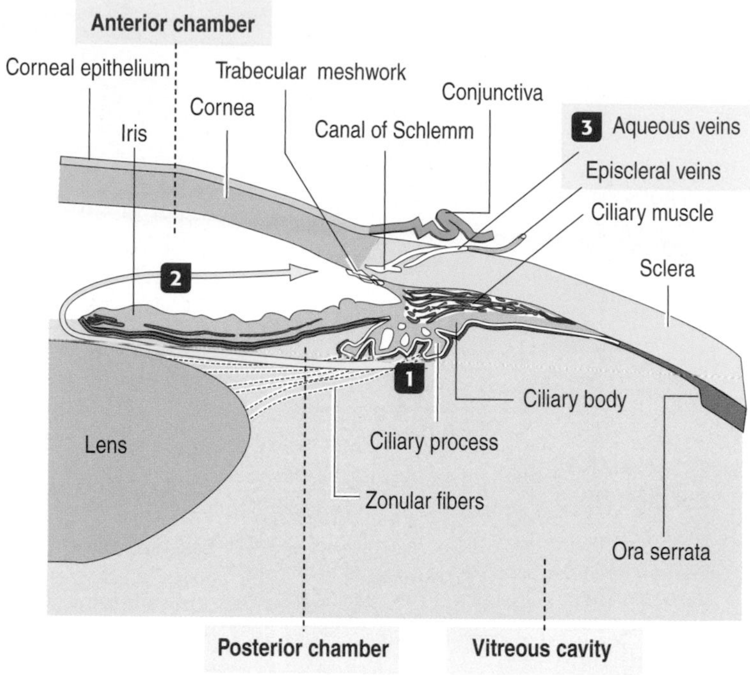

Three chambers of the eye

The eye contains three chambers (see Figure 9-1): (1) the **anterior chamber**, (2) the **posterior chamber**, and (3) the **vitreous cavity**.

The **anterior chamber** occupies the space between the **corneal endothelium** (anterior boundary) and the **anterior surface of the iris**, the **pupillary portion of the lens**, and the **base of the ciliary body** (posterior boundary). The circumferential angle of the anterior chamber is occupied by the **trabecular meshwork**, a drainage site for the aqueous humor into the **canal of Schlemm** (Figures 9-9 and 9-10).

The **posterior chamber** (see Figure 9-9) is limited anteriorly by the **posterior surface of the iris** and posteriorly by the **lens** and the **zonular fibers** (suspensory ligaments of the lens). The circumferential angle is occupied by the **ciliary processes**, the site of aqueous humor production.

The **vitreous cavity** is occupied by a transparent gel substance—the **vitreous humor**—and extends from the lens to the retina. The vitreous humor contains mostly water (99%), hyaluronic acid, and collagen fibers, both produced by **hyalocytes**.

Lens

The cornea, the three chambers of the eye, and the lens are three transparent structures through which light must pass to reach the retina.

The **lens** is a transparent, biconvex, elastic, and avascular structure (Figure 9-11). **Zonular fibers**, extending from the ciliary epithelium and inserting at the equatorial portion of the capsule, maintain the lens in place.

The lens consists of three components: (1) the **lens capsule**, (2) the **lens epithelium**, and (3) the **lens substance**, consisting of **cortical** and **nuclear lens cell fibers**.

The **lens capsule** is a thick and transparent basement membrane–like structure enclosing the lens. Beneath the anterior portion of the capsule is a single layer of **cuboidal epithelial cells** that extend posteriorly up to the equatorial region. There is no epithelial cell layer under the posterior surface of the capsule.

In the **cortical region of the lens**, elongated and concentrically arranged cells

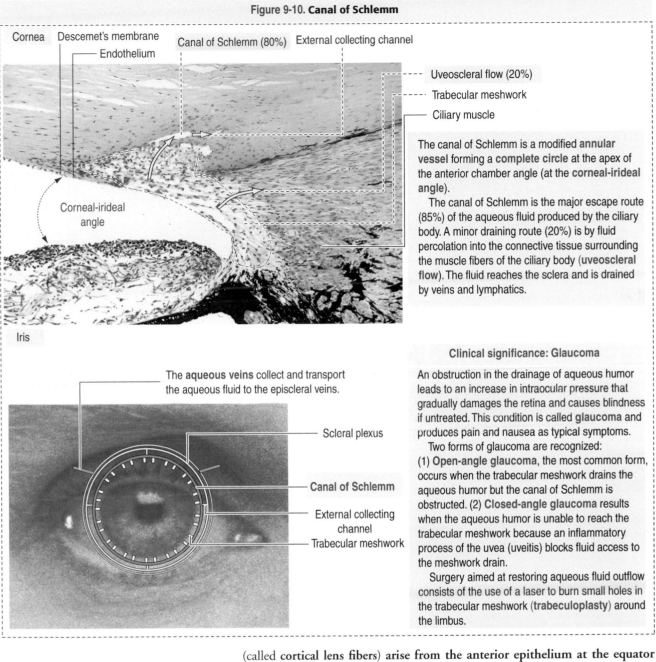

Figure 9-10. Canal of Schlemm

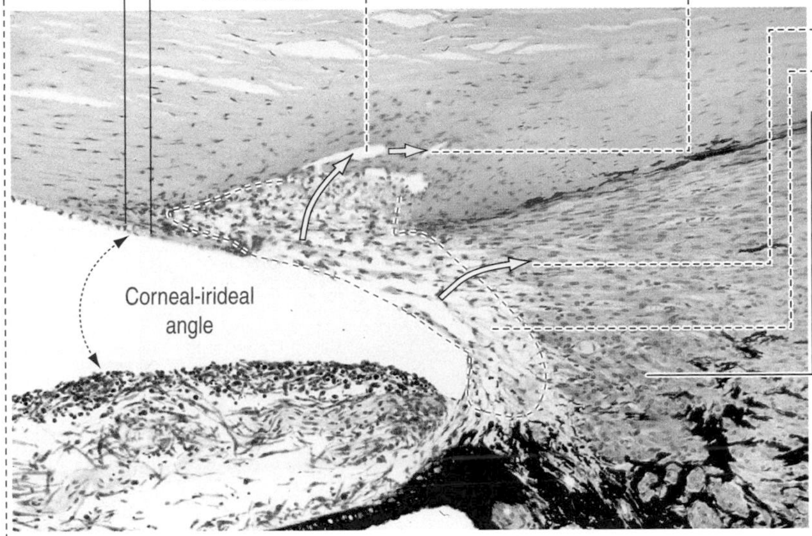

Cornea
Descemet's membrane
Endothelium
Canal of Schlemm (80%)
External collecting channel
Uveoscleral flow (20%)
Trabecular meshwork
Ciliary muscle
Corneal-irideal angle
Iris

The canal of Schlemm is a modified **annular vessel** forming a **complete circle** at the apex of the anterior chamber angle (at the **corneal-irideal angle**).

The canal of Schlemm is the major escape route (85%) of the aqueous fluid produced by the ciliary body. A minor draining route (20%) is by fluid percolation into the connective tissue surrounding the muscle fibers of the ciliary body (**uveoscleral flow**). The fluid reaches the sclera and is drained by veins and lymphatics.

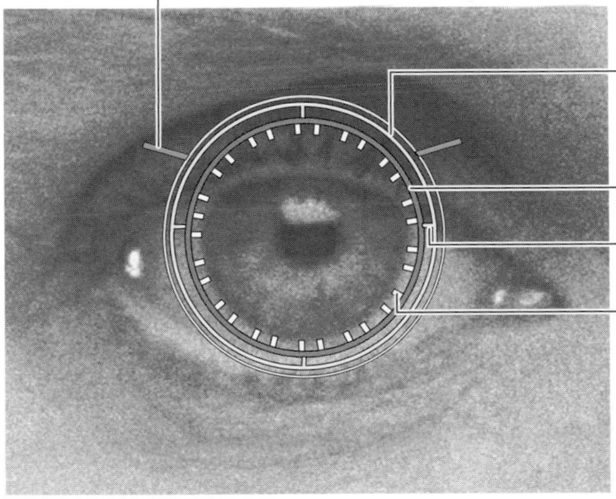

The **aqueous veins** collect and transport the aqueous fluid to the episcleral veins.
Scleral plexus
Canal of Schlemm
External collecting channel
Trabecular meshwork

Clinical significance: Glaucoma

An obstruction in the drainage of aqueous humor leads to an increase in intraocular pressure that gradually damages the retina and causes blindness if untreated. This condition is called **glaucoma** and produces pain and nausea as typical symptoms.

Two forms of glaucoma are recognized:
(1) **Open-angle glaucoma**, the most common form, occurs when the trabecular meshwork drains the aqueous humor but the canal of Schlemm is obstructed. (2) **Closed-angle glaucoma** results when the aqueous humor is unable to reach the trabecular meshwork because an inflammatory process of the uvea (uveitis) blocks fluid access to the meshwork drain.

Surgery aimed at restoring aqueous fluid outflow consists of the use of a laser to burn small holes in the trabecular meshwork (**trabeculoplasty**) around the limbus.

(called **cortical lens fibers**) **arise from the anterior epithelium at the equator region**. Cortical lens fibers contain a nucleus and organelles. The nucleus and organelles eventually disappear when the cortical lens fibers approach the center of the lens—**the nuclear lens fiber region**.

Lens cell differentiation consists of the appearance of unique cytoskeletal proteins: (1) **filensin**, an intermediate filament that contains attachment sites for crystallins and (2) lens-specific proteins called **crystallins** (α, β, and γ). Filensin and crystallins maintain the conformation and transparency of the lens fiber cell.

Lens cell fibers interdigitate at the medial **suture region**. At these contact sites, gap junctions and some spot desmosomes interlock the opposing cytoplasmic processes.

The inner cortical region and the core of the lens consist of older lens fibers lacking nuclei. About 80% of its available glucose is metabolized by the lens.

The lens is supported by the **suspensory ligament** (**zonular fibers**), formed by bundles of filaments linking the ciliary body to the equator of the lens. The ciliary body and zonular fibers play a role in accommodation.

Figure 9-11. Lens

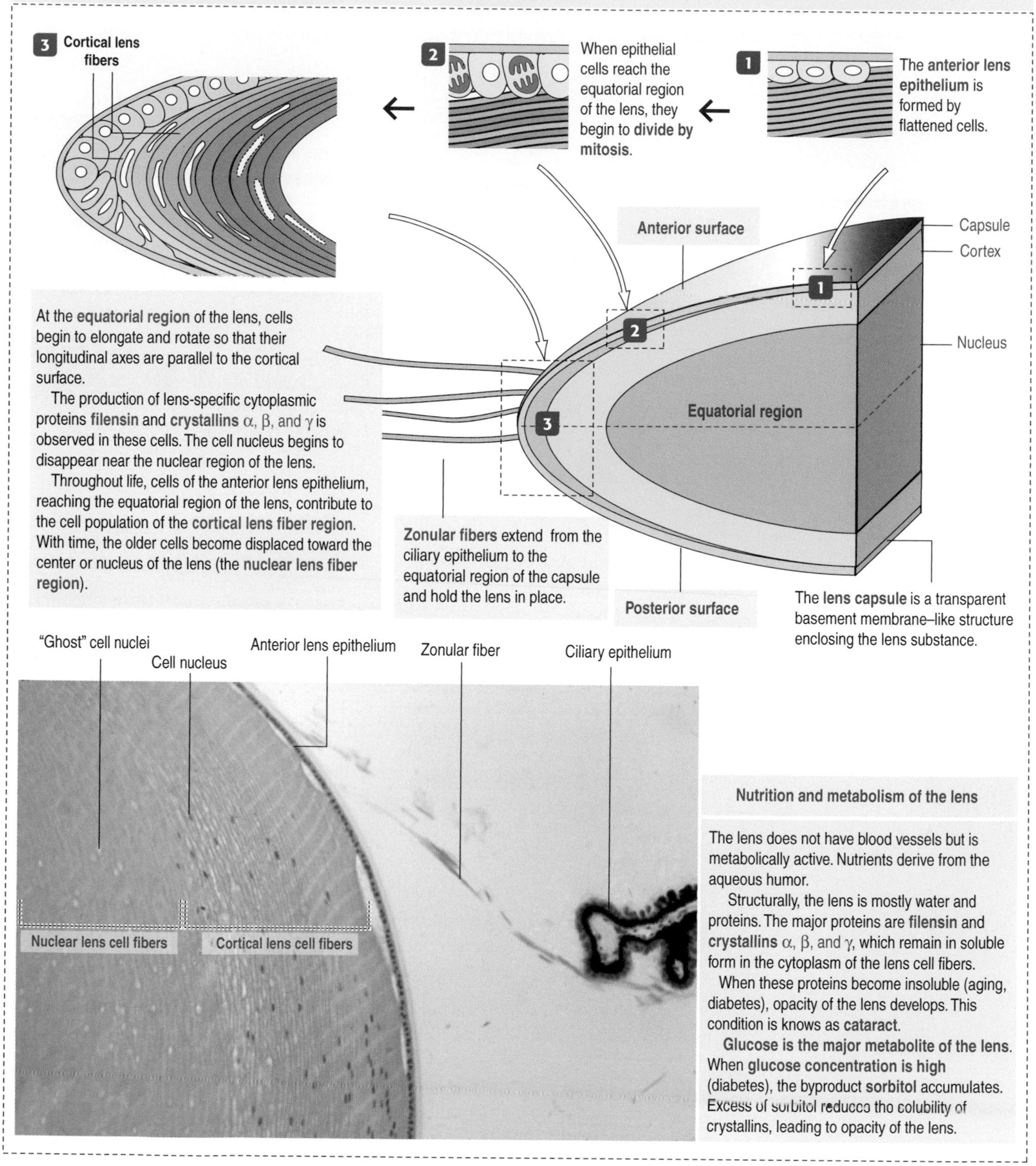

3 Cortical lens fibers
2 When epithelial cells reach the equatorial region of the lens, they begin to **divide by mitosis**.
1 The **anterior lens epithelium** is formed by flattened cells.
Anterior surface
Capsule
Cortex
Nucleus
Equatorial region
1
2
3
At the **equatorial region** of the lens, cells begin to elongate and rotate so that their longitudinal axes are parallel to the cortical surface.
The production of lens-specific cytoplasmic proteins **filensin** and **crystallins** α, β, and γ is observed in these cells. The cell nucleus begins to disappear near the nuclear region of the lens.
Throughout life, cells of the anterior lens epithelium, reaching the equatorial region of the lens, contribute to the cell population of the **cortical lens fiber region**. With time, the older cells become displaced toward the center or nucleus of the lens (the **nuclear lens fiber region**).
Zonular fibers extend from the ciliary epithelium to the equatorial region of the capsule and hold the lens in place.
Posterior surface
The **lens capsule** is a transparent basement membrane–like structure enclosing the lens substance.
"Ghost" cell nuclei
Cell nucleus
Anterior lens epithelium
Zonular fiber
Ciliary epithelium
Nuclear lens cell fibers
Cortical lens cell fibers
Nutrition and metabolism of the lens
The lens does not have blood vessels but is metabolically active. Nutrients derive from the aqueous humor.
Structurally, the lens is mostly water and proteins. The major proteins are **filensin** and **crystallins** α, β, and γ, which remain in soluble form in the cytoplasm of the lens cell fibers.
When these proteins become insoluble (aging, diabetes), opacity of the lens develops. This condition is knows as **cataract**.
Glucose is the major metabolite of the lens. When **glucose concentration is high** (diabetes), the byproduct **sorbitol** accumulates. Excess of sorbitol reduces the solubility of crystallins, leading to opacity of the lens.

Clinical significance: Cataracts

Cataracts are an opacity of the lens caused by a change in the solubility of lens proteins. This condition, observed during aging and diabetes, causes high light scattering by the aggregated filensin and crystallins and impairs accurate vision.

Accommodation

The sharpness of distant and close images focused on the retina depends on the **shape** of the lens (Figure 9-12). **Accommodation** defines the process by which the lens becomes **rounder** to focus the image of a **nearby object** on the retina and

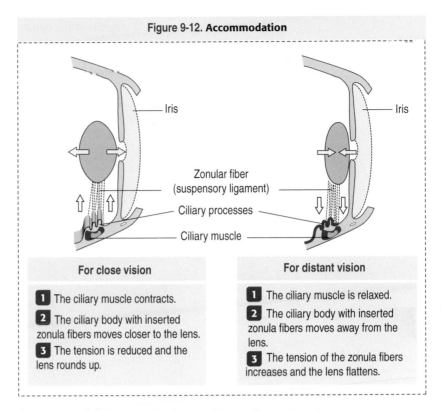

Figure 9-12. **Accommodation**

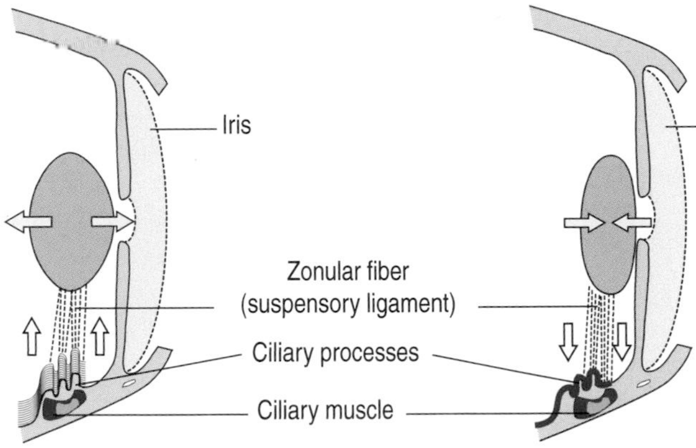

Iris
Iris
Zonular fiber
(suspensory ligament)
Ciliary processes
Ciliary muscle

For close vision

1 The ciliary muscle contracts.

2 The ciliary body with inserted zonula fibers moves closer to the lens.

3 The tension is reduced and the lens rounds up.

For distant vision

1 The ciliary muscle is relaxed.

2 The ciliary body with inserted zonula fibers moves away from the lens.

3 The tension of the zonula fibers increases and the lens flattens.

flattens when the image of a **distant object** is focused on the retina.

Accommodation determines that the distance between the center of the lens and the retina is equivalent to the focal distance needed for the formation of a sharp image on the retina.

Three components contribute to the accommodation process: (1) the **ciliary muscle**, (2) the **ciliary body**, and (3) the **suspensory ligaments**, inserted at the equatorial region of the lens capsule.

When the ciliary muscle **contracts**, the ciliary body moves toward the lens. Consequently, the tension of the suspensory ligaments is reduced, and the elastic capsule of the lens enables the lens to acquire a spherical shape. A rounded lens facilitates **close vision.**

When the ciliary muscle **relaxes**, the ciliary body keeps the tension of the suspensory ligaments that pull at the circumference of the lens. Thus, the lens remains flat to enable **distant vision**. This condition is known as **emmetropia** (Greek *emmetros*, in proper measure; *opia,* pertaining to the eye), or normal vision.

If the eyeball is too deep or the curvature of the lens is not flat enough, the image of a distant object forms in a plane **in front of the retina.** Distant objects are blurry because they are out of focus, but vision at close range is normal. This condition is called **myopia** (Greek *myein,* to shut), or **nearsightedness**.

If the eyeball is too shallow and the curvature of the lens is too flat, the distant image is formed at a plane **behind the retina.** Distant objects are well resolved but objects at a closer range are not. This condition is called **hyperopia** (Greek *hyper,* above), or **farsightedness.**

Older people become farsighted as the lens loses elasticity. This form of hyperopia is known as **presbyopia** (Greek *presbys*, old man).

Accommodation difficulties can be improved by the use of lenses. A diverging lens corrects myopia; a converging lens corrects hyperopia.

Inner layer: Retina

The retina consists of two regions (Figure 9-13): (1) the outer **nonsensory retinal pigmented epithelium**, and (2) the inner **sensory retina** (see Box 9-E).

The **nonsensory retinal pigmented epithelium** is a single layer of cuboidal cells

Figure 9-13. **Regions of the retina**

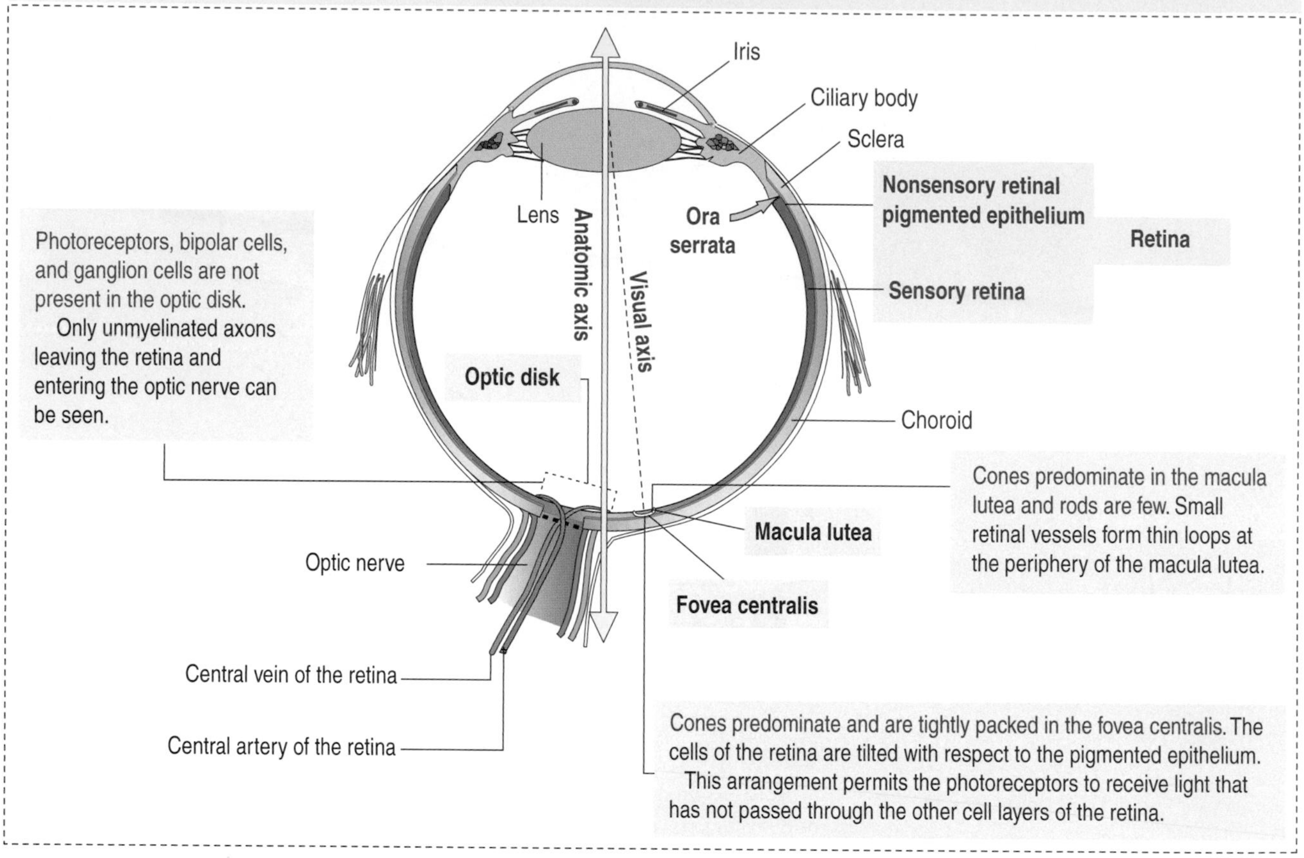
Iris
Ciliary body
Sclera
Nonsensory retinal pigmented epithelium
Retina
Sensory retina
Lens
Anatomic axis
Visual axis
Ora serrata
Photoreceptors, bipolar cells, and ganglion cells are not present in the optic disk.
Only unmyelinated axons leaving the retina and entering the optic nerve can be seen.
Optic disk
Choroid
Cones predominate in the macula lutea and rods are few. Small retinal vessels form thin loops at the periphery of the macula lutea.
Macula lutea
Optic nerve
Fovea centralis
Central vein of the retina
Central artery of the retina
Cones predominate and are tightly packed in the fovea centralis. The cells of the retina are tilted with respect to the pigmented epithelium.
This arrangement permits the photoreceptors to receive light that has not passed through the other cell layers of the retina.

extending from the edge of the **optic disk** to the **ora serrata**, where it continues as the pigmented layer of the ciliary epithelium.

The apical domain of the cuboidal nonsensory pigmented epithelium is sealed by **tight junctions** to form the **external retinal barrier** (Figure 9-14). Granules of **melanin** are present in the apical cytoplasm and apical cell processes. Melanin granules absorb excess light reaching the photoreceptors.

The apical surface contains **microvilli** that surround the outer segments of the photoreceptors (cones and rods). At this location, the sensory retina and the pigmented epithelium are attached to each other through an amorphous extracellular material, the **interphotoreceptor matrix** (Figure 9-15).

The inner **sensory retina** layer extends from the edge of the **optic disk** to the **ciliary epithelium**. The sensory retina has two clinically and anatomically important landmarks to remember: (1) the **fovea centralis**, a shallow depression of about 2.5 mm in diameter and (2) the **macula lutea**, a yellow rim surrounding the fovea centralis. **The fovea is the area of the retina where vision is the sharpest and is crossed by the visual axis.** We discuss these structures later.

Box 9-E | Highlights of the retina

- The retina derives from the neuroectoderm and represents an extension of the brain. The retina is a stratified layer of nervous cells formed by two layers: (1) the outer **retinal pigmented epithelium** and (2) the inner **sensory retina**.
- The **nonsensory retinal pigmented epithelium** is a **simple cuboidal epithelium** with **melanin** granules.
- The **sensory retina** spans from the margin of the **optic disk** posteriorly to the **ciliary epithelium** anteriorly.
- The optic disk includes the **optic papilla**, formed by protruding nerve fibers passing from the retina into the optic nerve. The optic papilla lacks photoreceptors and represents the **blind spot** of the retina.
- The **fovea centralis** is the area of sharpest vision.

Clinical significance: Detachment of the retina

A separation of the two layers by trauma, vascular disease, metabolic disorders, and aging results in the **detachment of the retina**. Retinal detachment affects the viability of the sensory retina and can be corrected by laser surgery.

The clinical significance of the detachment of the nonsensory retinal pigmented epithelium from the sensory retina is highlighted by the following functions of the pigmented epithelium:

1. The **transport of nutrients from the choroidal blood vessels to the outer layers of the sensory retina.**
2. The **removal of waste metabolic products from the sensory retina.**
3. **Active phagocytosis and recycling of photoreceptor disks shed from the**

Figure 9-14. Layers of the retina

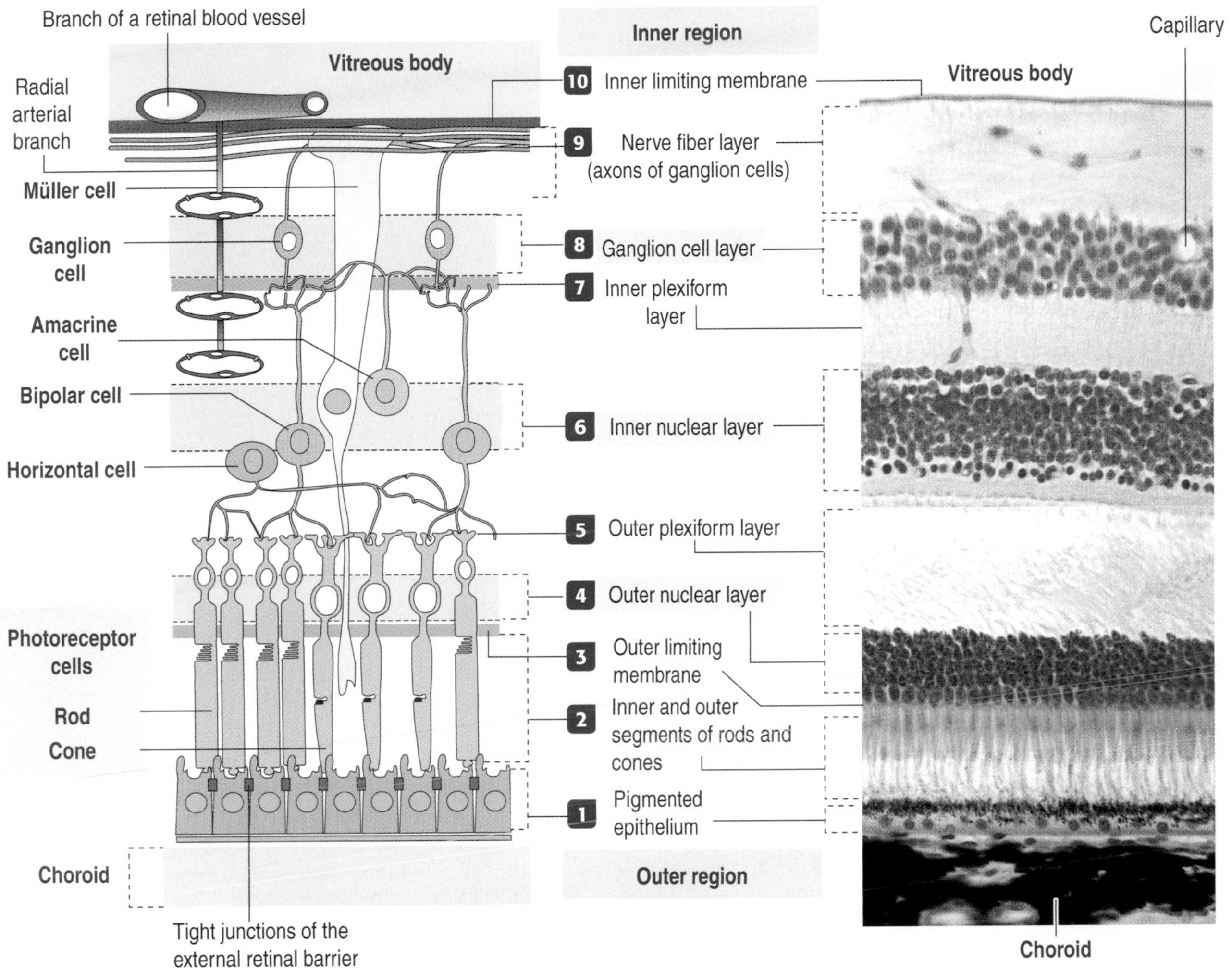

Branch of a retinal blood vessel
Vitreous body
Radial arterial branch
Müller cell
Ganglion cell
Amacrine cell
Bipolar cell
Horizontal cell
Photoreceptor cells
Rod
Cone
Choroid
Tight junctions of the external retinal barrier
Inner region
10 Inner limiting membrane
9 Nerve fiber layer (axons of ganglion cells)
8 Ganglion cell layer
7 Inner plexiform layer
6 Inner nuclear layer
5 Outer plexiform layer
4 Outer nuclear layer
3 Outer limiting membrane
2 Inner and outer segments of rods and cones
1 Pigmented epithelium
Outer region
Capillary
Vitreous body
Choroid

Light passes through several layers of the retina before activating the rod and cone photoreceptor cells. The layers of the retina observed in the photomicrograph are represented in the adjacent diagram. The synapses between the cells of each layer of the retina are also illustrated.

Radial branches from blood vessels (arteries and veins)—located on the retinal surface—are interconnected by **capillary beds** present in the inner layers of the retina. **Retinal capillary beds** are lined by **endothelial cells** linked by **tight junctions** creating an internal **blood-retinal barrier**. An **external retinal barrier** is formed by **tight junctions linking the cells of the pigmented epithelium**.

Note that the nuclei of rods and cones are present in the **outer nuclear layer**.

The axons of the cones and rods project into the **outer plexiform layer** and synapse with dendrites of the bipolar cells.

Nuclei of the bipolar cells contribute to the **inner nuclear layer**.

Axons of the bipolar cells synapse with dendrites of the ganglion cells in the **inner plexiform layer**.

Axons of the **ganglion cells** become part of the optic nerve.

Müller cells span most of the retina. The **inner limiting membrane** represents their basal lamina. Their nuclei form part of the inner nuclear layer.

The **outer limiting membrane** corresponds to junctional complexes (**zonula adherens**) between rods, cones, and Müller cells.

Horizontal cells synapse with several rods and cones.

Amacrine cells synapse with axons of bipolar cells and dendrites of ganglion cells.

outer segment of the cones and rods.

4. The **synthesis of basal lamina components of Bruch's membrane** to which the retinal pigmented epithelium is firmly attached.

5. It is essential for **the formation of the photopigment rhodopsin** because it regenerates the bleached photopigment by converting **all-*trans* retinol** into **retinal**, which is returned to the photoreceptor by **interstitial retinoid-binding protein (IRBP)**, a major protein in the interphotoreceptor matrix (see Figure 9-15).

Figure 9-15. Photoreceptors: Rod

The **modified cilium** connects the inner segment of the photoreceptor cell (the site of synthesis of proteins and other molecules) to the outer segment (containing a stack of disks). The **intraciliary transport** mechanism (see Cytoskeleton in Chapter 1, Epithelium) uses microtubule-based molecular motors (kinesins and cytoplasmic dyneins) to transport proteins, vesicles, and other materials from the inner segment to the outer segment. The modified cilium facilitates the delivery of molecules from a proximal site of synthesis to a distal site of assembly.

The plus/minus polarity of the microtubules enables an anterograde and retrograde transport mechanism through molecular motors.

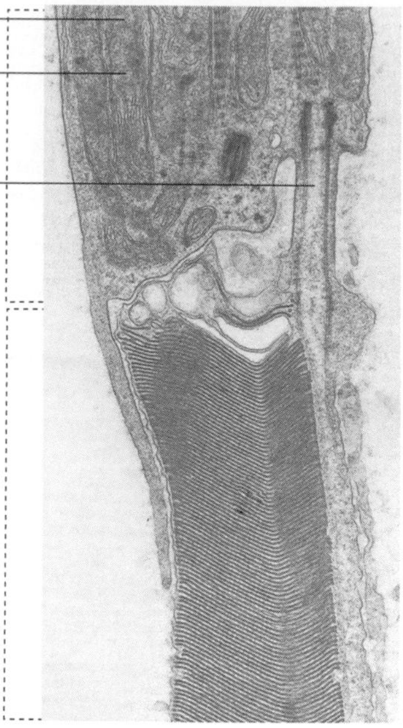

Mitochondria
Inner segment
Modified cilium
Outer segment

1 Interphotoreceptor matrix

A mixture of extracellular proteins—glycoproteins and glycosaminoglycans—link the outer segment of the photoreceptor cell to the pigmented epithelium by means of its viscosity.

A major protein of the matrix is **interstitial retinoid-binding protein (IRBP)**. IRBP transports **retinol** to the pigmented epithelium and returns **retinal** to the photoreceptor.

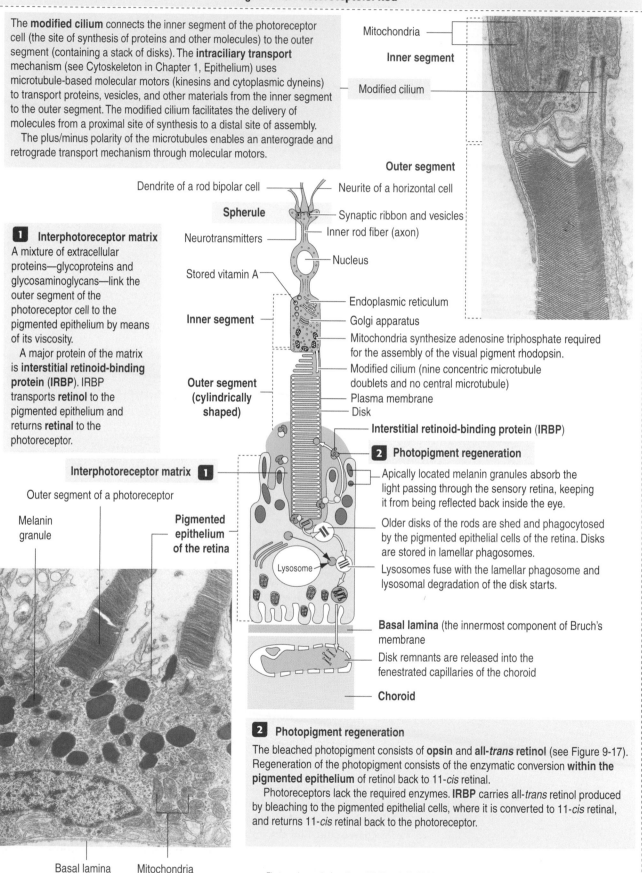

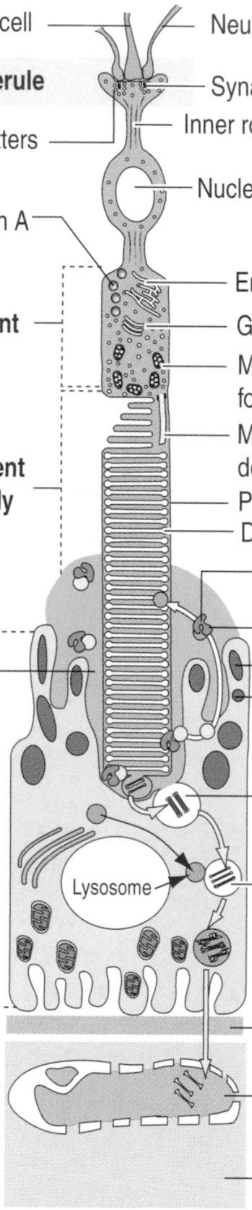

Dendrite of a rod bipolar cell
Neurite of a horizontal cell
Spherule
Synaptic ribbon and vesicles
Neurotransmitters
Inner rod fiber (axon)
Nucleus
Stored vitamin A
Endoplasmic reticulum
Inner segment
Golgi apparatus
Mitochondria synthesize adenosine triphosphate required for the assembly of the visual pigment rhodopsin.
Modified cilium (nine concentric microtubule doublets and no central microtubule)
Outer segment (cylindrically shaped)
Plasma membrane
Disk
Interstitial retinoid-binding protein (IRBP)
2 Photopigment regeneration
Interphotoreceptor matrix 1
Apically located melanin granules absorb the light passing through the sensory retina, keeping it from being reflected back inside the eye.
Pigmented epithelium of the retina
Older disks of the rods are shed and phagocytosed by the pigmented epithelial cells of the retina. Disks are stored in lamellar phagosomes.
Lysosome
Lysosomes fuse with the lamellar phagosome and lysosomal degradation of the disk starts.
Basal lamina (the innermost component of Bruch's membrane
Disk remnants are released into the fenestrated capillaries of the choroid
Choroid

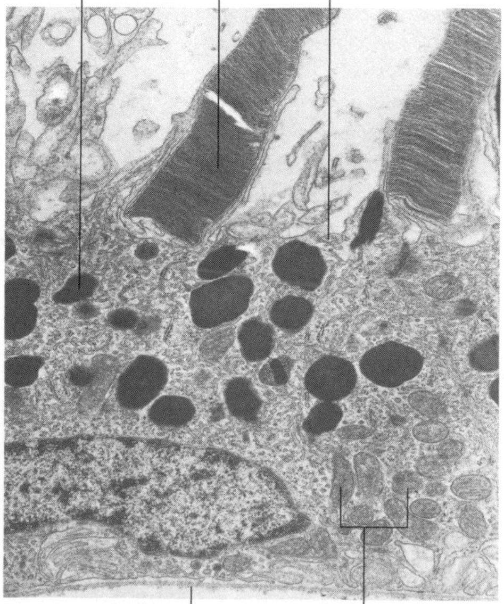

Outer segment of a photoreceptor
Melanin granule
Basal lamina
Mitochondria

2 Photopigment regeneration

The bleached photopigment consists of **opsin** and **all-*trans* retinol** (see Figure 9-17). Regeneration of the photopigment consists of the enzymatic conversion **within the pigmented epithelium** of retinol back to 11-*cis* retinal.

Photoreceptors lack the required enzymes. **IRBP** carries all-*trans* retinol produced by bleaching to the pigmented epithelial cells, where it is converted to 11-*cis* retinal, and returns 11-*cis* retinal back to the photoreceptor.

Electron micrographs from Hogan MJ, Alvarado JA, Weddell JA: Histology of the Human Eye. Philadelphia, WB Saunders, 1971.

Figure 9-16. Photoreceptors: Cone

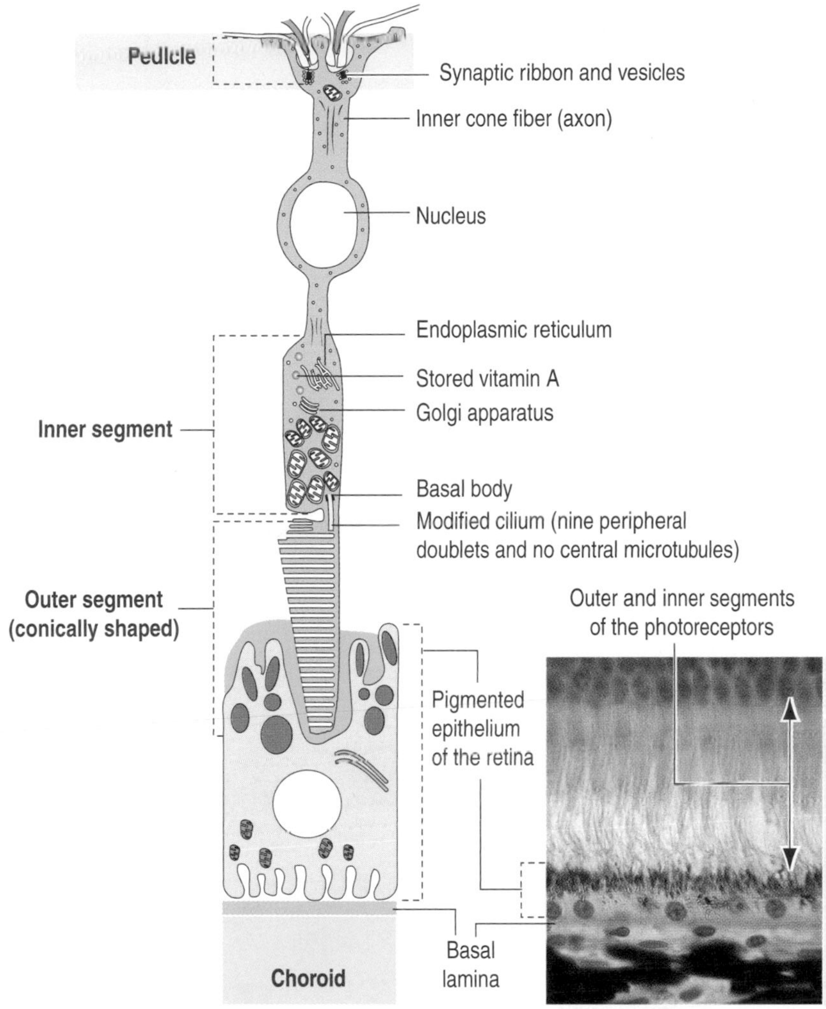

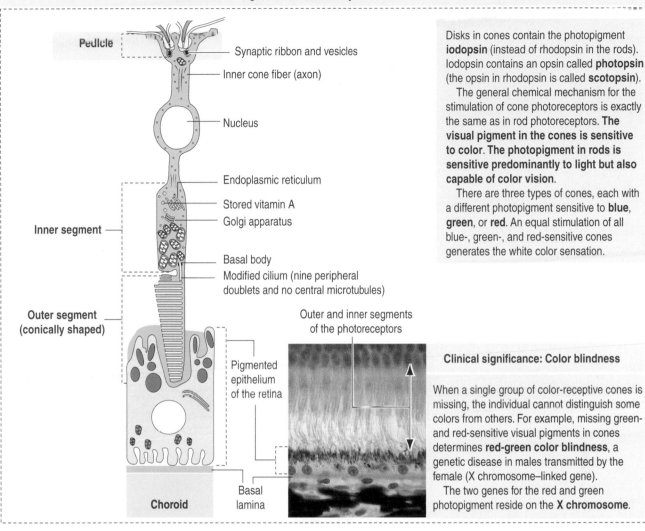

Pedicle
Synaptic ribbon and vesicles
Inner cone fiber (axon)
Nucleus
Endoplasmic reticulum
Stored vitamin A
Golgi apparatus
Inner segment
Basal body
Modified cilium (nine peripheral doublets and no central microtubules)
Outer segment (conically shaped)
Outer and inner segments of the photoreceptors
Pigmented epithelium of the retina
Basal lamina
Choroid

Disks in cones contain the photopigment **iodopsin** (instead of rhodopsin in the rods). Iodopsin contains an opsin called **photopsin** (the opsin in rhodopsin is called **scotopsin**).

The general chemical mechanism for the stimulation of cone photoreceptors is exactly the same as in rod photoreceptors. **The visual pigment in the cones is sensitive to color. The photopigment in rods is sensitive predominantly to light but also capable of color vision.**

There are three types of cones, each with a different photopigment sensitive to **blue**, **green**, or **red**. An equal stimulation of all blue-, green-, and red-sensitive cones generates the white color sensation.

Clinical significance: Color blindness

When a single group of color-receptive cones is missing, the individual cannot distinguish some colors from others. For example, missing green- and red-sensitive visual pigments in cones determines **red-green color blindness**, a genetic disease in males transmitted by the female (X chromosome–linked gene).

The two genes for the red and green photopigment reside on the **X chromosome**.

Cell layers of the retina

Four cell groups are found in the **sensory retina** (see Figure 9-14):

1. The **photoreceptor neurons—rods** and **cones**.
2. The **conducting neurons—bipolar** and **ganglion cells**.
3. The **association neurons—horizontal** and **amacrine cells**.
4. The **supporting neuroglial cells—Müller cells**.

Photoreceptor neurons: Rods and cones

Rods (see Figure 9-15) and cones (Figure 9-16) occupy specific regions in the sensory retina. Cones are predominant in the fovea centralis and perceive color and detail. Rods are concentrated at the periphery and function in peripheral and night vision.

Both rods and cones are elongated cells with specific structural and functional polarity. They consist of two major segments: an **outer segment** and an **inner segment**.

The outer segment contains stacks of flat **membranous disks** harboring a photopigment. The disks are infoldings of the plasma membrane that pinch off as they move away from the modified **cilium**, the outer-inner segment connecting region.

The various components of the disks are synthesized in the inner segment and are transported by molecular motors (kinesins and cytoplasmic dyneins) along microtubules toward the outer segment across the narrow cytoplasmic bridge

Figure 9-17. Visual pigment: Rhodopsin

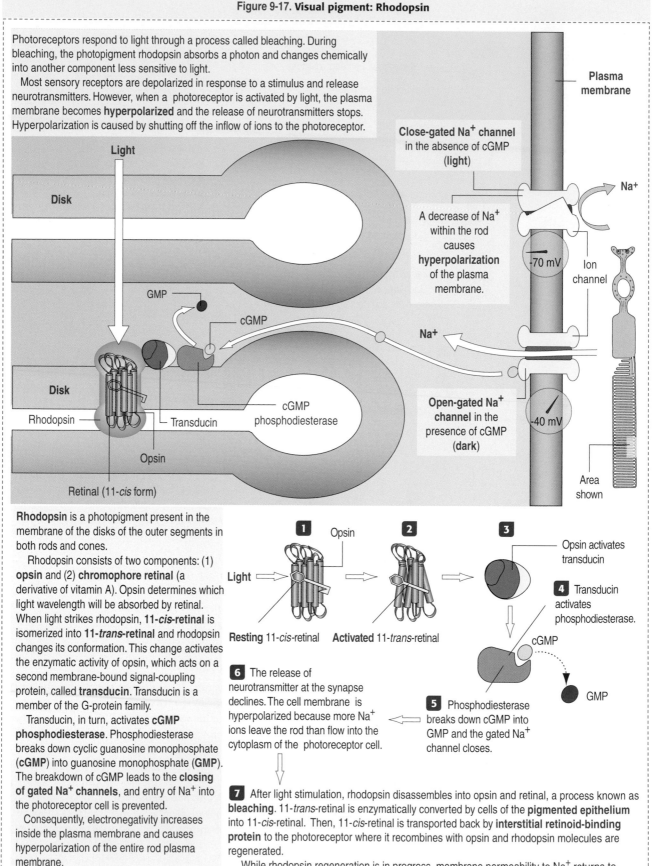

Photoreceptors respond to light through a process called bleaching. During bleaching, the photopigment rhodopsin absorbs a photon and changes chemically into another component less sensitive to light.

Most sensory receptors are depolarized in response to a stimulus and release neurotransmitters. However, when a photoreceptor is activated by light, the plasma membrane becomes **hyperpolarized** and the release of neurotransmitters stops. Hyperpolarization is caused by shutting off the inflow of ions to the photoreceptor.

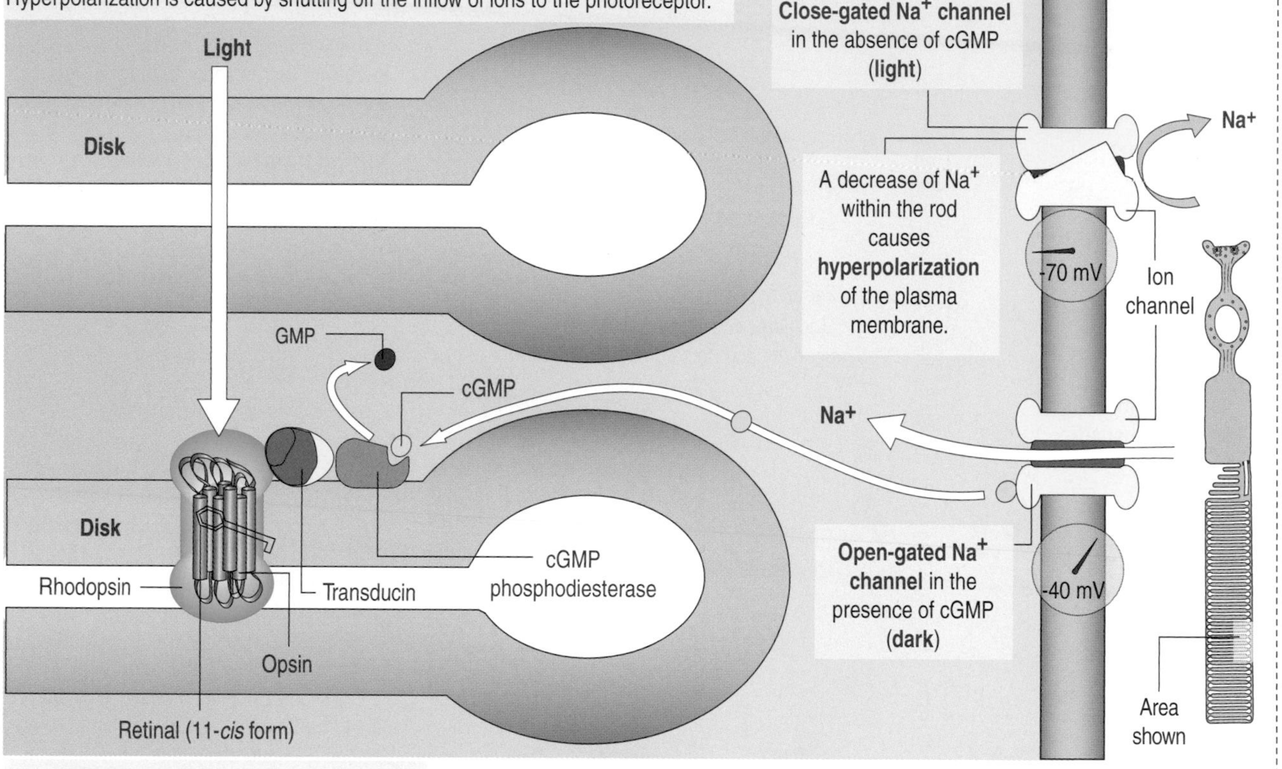

Plasma membrane
Close-gated Na^+ channel in the absence of cGMP (**light**)
Light
Na^+
Disk
A decrease of Na^+ within the rod causes **hyperpolarization** of the plasma membrane.
-70 mV
Ion channel
GMP
cGMP
Na^+
Disk
Rhodopsin
Transducin
cGMP phosphodiesterase
Open-gated Na^+ channel in the presence of cGMP (**dark**)
-40 mV
Opsin
Retinal (11-*cis* form)
Area shown

Rhodopsin is a photopigment present in the membrane of the disks of the outer segments in both rods and cones.

Rhodopsin consists of two components: (1) **opsin** and (2) **chromophore retinal** (a derivative of vitamin A). Opsin determines which light wavelength will be absorbed by retinal. When light strikes rhodopsin, **11-*cis*-retinal** is isomerized into **11-*trans*-retinal** and rhodopsin changes its conformation. This change activates the enzymatic activity of opsin, which acts on a second membrane-bound signal-coupling protein, called **transducin**. Transducin is a member of the G-protein family.

Transducin, in turn, activates **cGMP phosphodiesterase**. Phosphodiesterase breaks down cyclic guanosine monophosphate (**cGMP**) into guanosine monophosphate (**GMP**). The breakdown of cGMP leads to the **closing of gated Na^+ channels**, and entry of Na^+ into the photoreceptor cell is prevented.

Consequently, electronegativity increases inside the plasma membrane and causes hyperpolarization of the entire rod plasma membrane.

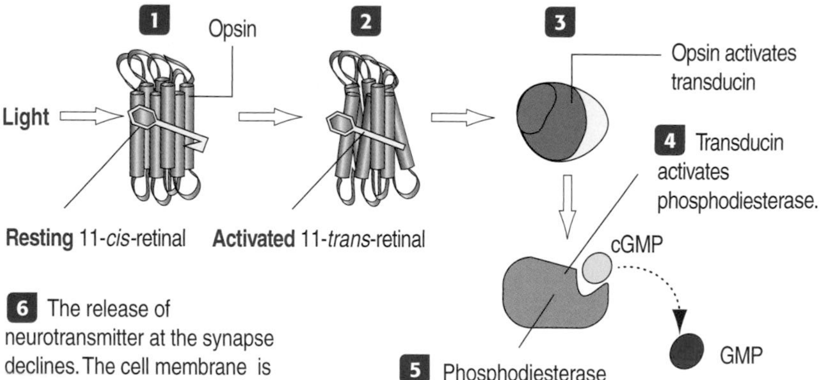

1
Opsin
2
3
Opsin activates transducin
Light
4 Transducin activates phosphodiesterase.
Resting 11-*cis*-retinal
Activated 11-*trans*-retinal
cGMP
GMP

5 Phosphodiesterase breaks down cGMP into GMP and the gated Na^+ channel closes.

6 The release of neurotransmitter at the synapse declines. The cell membrane is hyperpolarized because more Na^+ ions leave the rod than flow into the cytoplasm of the photoreceptor cell.

7 After light stimulation, rhodopsin disassembles into opsin and retinal, a process known as **bleaching**. 11-*trans*-retinal is enzymatically converted by cells of the **pigmented epithelium** into 11-*cis*-retinal. Then, 11-*cis*-retinal is transported back by **interstitial retinoid-binding protein** to the photoreceptor where it recombines with opsin and rhodopsin molecules are regenerated.

While rhodopsin regeneration is in progress, membrane permeability to Na^+ returns to normal as cGMP is also synthesized and opens the gated Na^+ channel.

Figure 9-18. **Rod spherules and cone pedicles**

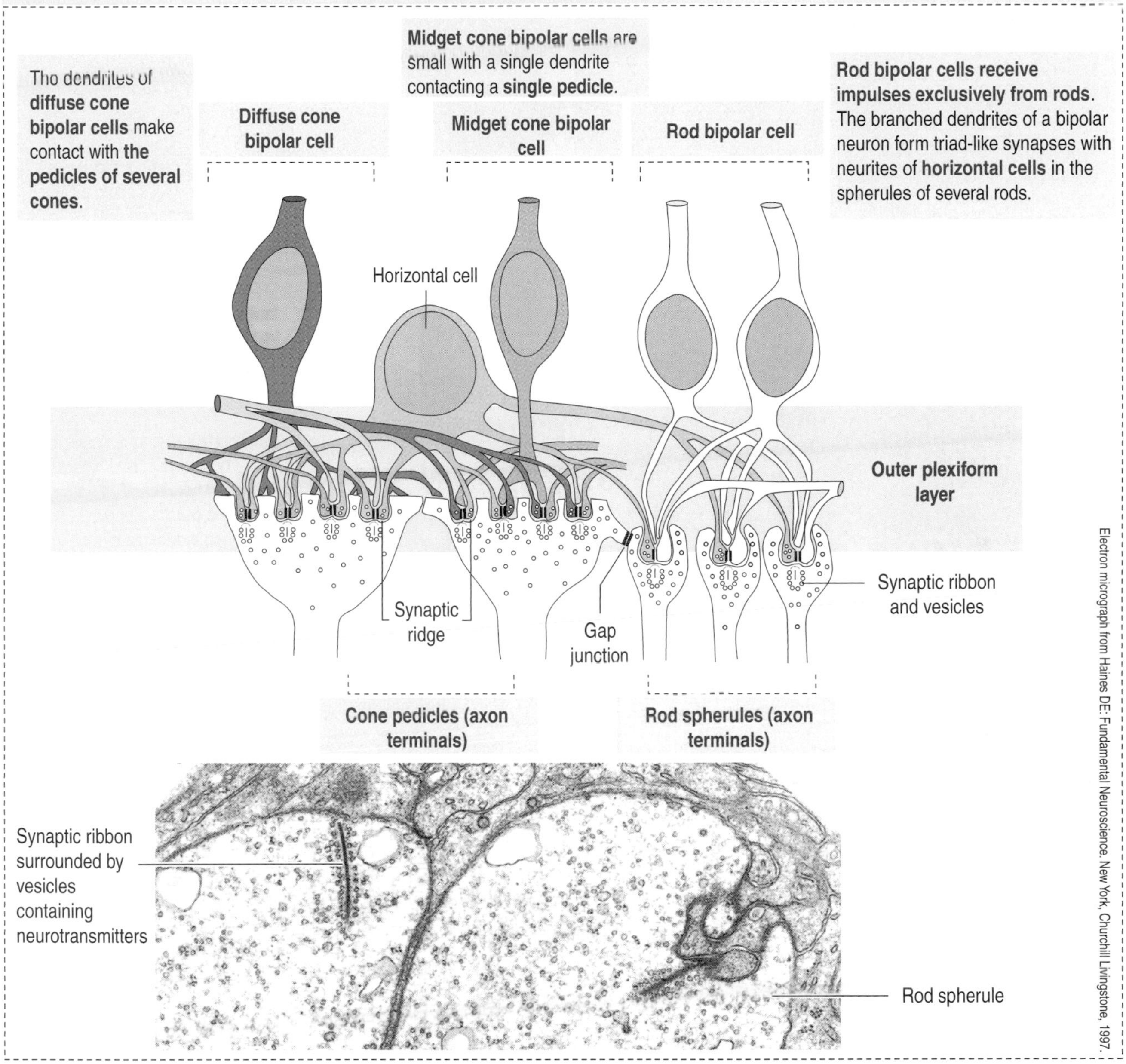

Midget cone bipolar cells are small with a single dendrite contacting a single pedicle.
The dendrites of diffuse cone bipolar cells make contact with the pedicles of several cones.
Diffuse cone bipolar cell
Midget cone bipolar cell
Rod bipolar cell
Rod bipolar cells receive impulses exclusively from rods. The branched dendrites of a bipolar neuron form triad-like synapses with neurites of horizontal cells in the spherules of several rods.
Horizontal cell
Outer plexiform layer
Synaptic ribbon and vesicles
Synaptic ridge
Gap junction
Cone pedicles (axon terminals)
Rod spherules (axon terminals)
Synaptic ribbon surrounded by vesicles containing neurotransmitters
Rod spherule
Electron micrograph from Haines DE: Fundamental Neuroscience. New York, Churchill Livingstone, 1997.

containing the modified cilium. We discuss in Chapter 1, Epithelium, details of the mechanism of **intraciliary transport**.

The production and turnover of the disks is continuous. New disks are added near the cilium. Older disks move apically toward the pigmented epithelium of the retina and once they reach the tip of the outer segment, they are phagocytosed by the cells of the pigmented epithelium. The duration of the disk recycling process is about 10 days.

The **inner segment** displays abundant mitochondria—involved in the synthesis of adenosine triphosphate (ATP), the Golgi apparatus, and rough and smooth endoplasmic reticulum. The modified cilium consists of **nine peripheral microtubule doublets** but **lacks the central pair** of microtubules. The terminal portion of the photoreceptors is equivalent to an axon forming synaptic contacts with cytoplasmic processes—**neurites**—of bipolar cells and horizontal cells.

There are three significant **differences between rods and cones**:

1. The **outer segment is cylindrical in the rods and conically shaped in the cones.**

Box 9-F | **Retinitis pigmentosa**

- Retinitis pigmentosa (RP) comprises a number of inherited defects of the retina causing blindness. The first indication of RP is night blindness caused by the degeneration of rod photoreceptor cells. Blood supply to the retina decreases and a pigment is observed on the retinal surface (hence the name retinitis pigmentosa).
- RP genes are located on the **X chromosome** and **chromosome 3**. The gene for the visual pigment **rhodopsin** also maps in the same chromosome 3 region. Mutations in the *rhodopsin* gene cause RP. **Peripherin**, a protein component of rods, is encoded by a gene of the RP family on **chromosome 6**.

Figure 9-19. **Conducting and integrating neurons**

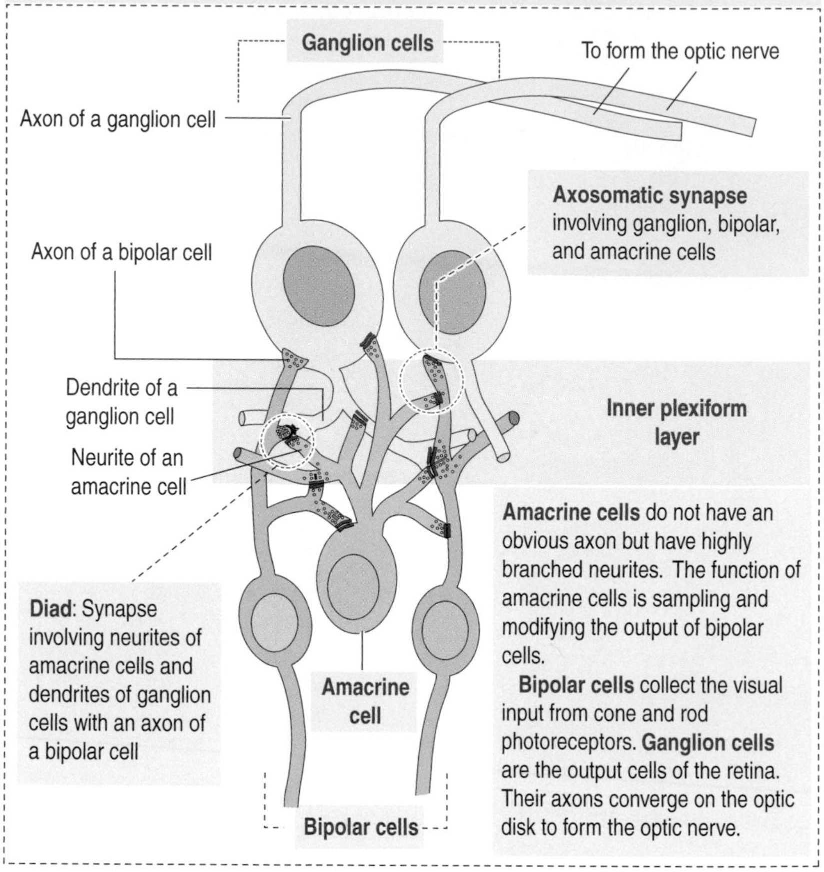
Ganglion cells
To form the optic nerve
Axon of a ganglion cell
Axosomatic synapse involving ganglion, bipolar, and amacrine cells
Axon of a bipolar cell
Dendrite of a ganglion cell
Inner plexiform layer
Neurite of an amacrine cell
Diad: Synapse involving neurites of amacrine cells and dendrites of ganglion cells with an axon of a bipolar cell
Amacrine cell
Bipolar cells

Amacrine cells do not have an obvious axon but have highly branched neurites. The function of amacrine cells is sampling and modifying the output of bipolar cells.

Bipolar cells collect the visual input from cone and rod photoreceptors. **Ganglion cells** are the output cells of the retina. Their axons converge on the optic disk to form the optic nerve.

2. The **rods** terminate in a small knob or **rod spherule**, which contacts dendrites of bipolar cells and neurites of horizontal cells. The **cones** end in a thicker **cone pedicle**. The cone pedicle also synapses with bipolar and horizontal cells. The synaptic ending of cones and rods—spherules and pedicles—contains a **synaptic ribbon** surrounded by **synaptic vesicles**.

3. Rods contain the photopigment **rhodopsin** (Figure 9-17). Cones contain a similar pigment called **iodopsin**. Rhodopsin operates during night vision. Iodopsin perceives detail and discriminates color (blue, green, and red). Both rhodopsin and iodopsin are transmembrane proteins bound to the prosthetic group **11-*cis*-retinal**. The protein lacking the prosthetic group is called **opsin**. See Box 9-F.

There are three different photopigments in cones with different light absorbance and sensitive to blue light (420 nm), green light (535 nm), and red light 565 nm), respectively. The isomerization of 11-*cis*-retinal to 11-*trans*-retinal is identical in rods and cones.

Conducting neurons: Bipolar and ganglion cells

Bipolar and ganglion cells conduct the impulse received by the photoreceptor cells.

Two major classes of bipolar cells can be distinguished (Figure 9-18):

1. **Rod bipolar cells**, linked to **rod spherules**.

2. **Cone bipolar cells**, linked to **cone pedicles**. Cone bipolar cells consist of two major classes: the **midget cone bipolar cell** and the **diffuse cone bipolar cell**.

Dendrites of the **diffuse cone bipolar cells** branch within the **outer plexiform layer** and contact several cone pedicles. On the opposite pole, the axon of a diffuse bipolar cell projects into the **inner plexiform layer** and contacts the dendrites of ganglion cells.

Midget cone bipolar cells synapse with a **single cone pedicle** and a single axon

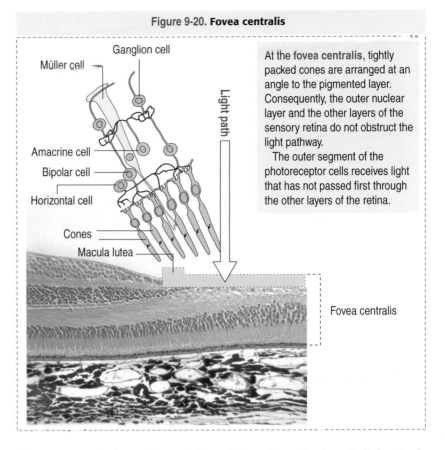

Figure 9-20. **Fovea centralis**

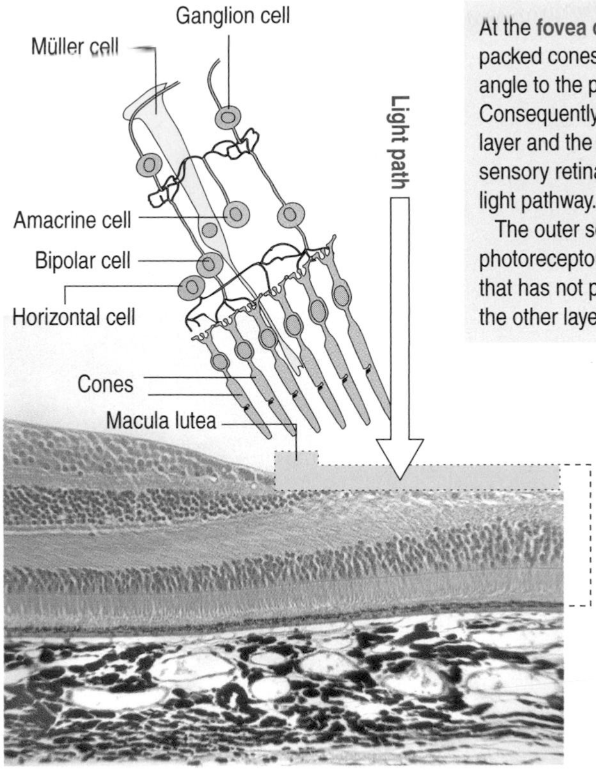
Ganglion cell
Müller cell
Light path
Amacrine cell
Bipolar cell
Horizontal cell
Cones
Macula lutea
Fovea centralis

At the **fovea centralis**, tightly packed cones are arranged at an angle to the pigmented layer. Consequently, the outer nuclear layer and the other layers of the sensory retina do not obstruct the light pathway.

The outer segment of the photoreceptor cells receives light that has not passed first through the other layers of the retina.

that contacts a **single ganglion cell**. Essentially, **midget bipolar cells link a single cone to an optic nerve fiber.** In contrast, **diffuse bipolar cells have wider input and output pathways.** The nuclei of the bipolar cells form part of the **inner nuclear layer** of the retina.

Ganglion cells extend their dendrites into the **inner plexiform layer**; the axons form part of the optic nerve. Two classes of ganglion cells exist: (1) **diffuse ganglion cells**, contacting several bipolar cells, and (2) **midget ganglion cells**, with their dendrites contacting a single midget bipolar cell. Note that midget ganglion cells receive impulses from cones only.

Association neurons: Horizontal and amacrine cells

Horizontal and amacrine cells do not have axons or dendrites, only **neuritic processes conducting in both directions.** The nuclei of the horizontal and amacrine cells contribute to the **inner nuclear layer.**

Horizontal cells give rise to **neurites** ending on **cone pedicles.** A single branching neurite synapses with **both rod spherules and cone pedicles** (see Figure 9-18). These neuritic synapses occur in the **outer plexiform layer** of the retina. This neurite and axonal distribution indicates that **horizontal cells integrate cones and rods of adjacent areas of the retina.**

Amacrine cells are found at the inner edge of the **inner nuclear layer.** They have a single neuritic process that branches to link the axonal terminals of the bipolar cells and the dendritic branches of the ganglion cells (Figure 9-19).

Supporting glial cells: Müller cells

The nuclei of Müller cells are located in the **inner nuclear layer.** The cytoplasmic processes extend to the **outer** and **inner limiting membrane.** The inner limiting membrane represents the basal lamina of the Müller cells and serves to separate the retina from the vitreous body.

The cytoplasmic processes of Müller cells fill the spaces between photorecep-

Figure 9-21. **Optic disk and fovea centralis**

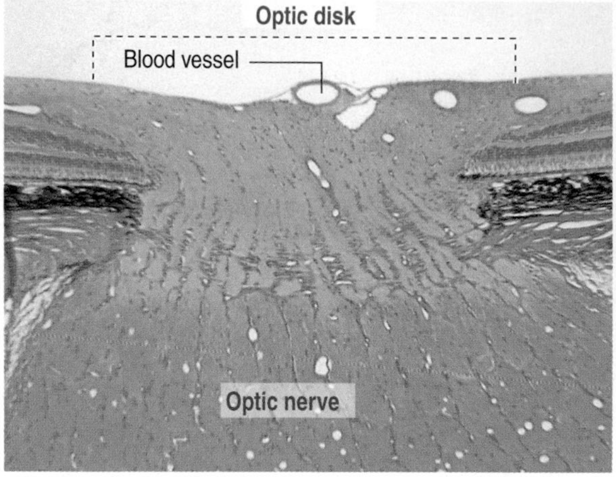

Optic disk
Blood vessel
Optic nerve

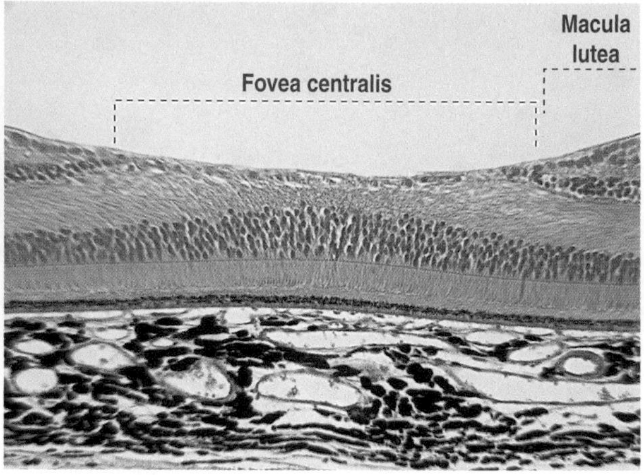

Macula lutea
Fovea centralis

The axons of the ganglion cells turn into the **optic nerve** at the **optic disk**, which lacks photoreceptors and corresponds to the **blind spot** of the retina.

The optic disk has a central depresion, the **optic cup**, that is pale in comparison to the surrounding nerve fibers. A loss of nerve fibers in glaucoma results in an increase in the optic cup area.

Retinal blood vessels can be visualized with an ophthalmoscope. When **intraocular pressure increases**, the disk of the optic nerve appears **concave**. The disk becomes swollen (**papilledema**) and the veins are dilated when intracranial pressure increases.

The **macula lutea**—yellow spot produced by **xanthophyll pigments** within retinal cells, which may absorb short wavelength light—provides for central vision. In its center, the **fovea** is for high quality vision. The rest of the retina is for peripheral vision. **Cones** are concentrated in the macula and are responsible for acute vision and color distinction. **Rods** are for vision in dim light and for movement detection.

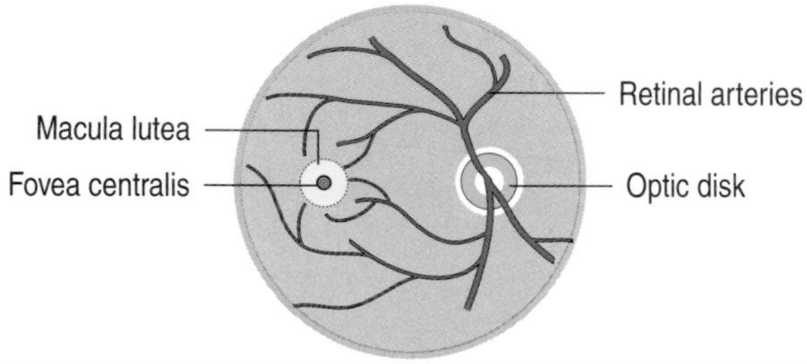

Retinal arteries
Macula lutea
Fovea centralis
Optic disk

tors and bipolar and ganglion cells. At the outer segment photoreceptor contact sites, a **zonula adherens** and **microvilli** extending from Müller cells stabilize the association between neuronal photoreceptors and glial Müller cells. This contact region is represented by the distinct boundary of the outer limiting membrane. In addition to glial Müller cells, microglial cells are present in all layers.

Areas of the retina with specific functions

The **fovea centralis**, surrounded by the **macula lutea** (Figures 9-20 and 9-21), is a specialized area of the retina for accurate vision under normal and dim illumination. The **optic disk**, which includes the **optic papilla**, is not suitable for vision.

The **fovea centralis** is located on the **temporal side** of the optic disk. **This area contains abundant cones but lacks rods and capillaries.** The cones synapse with the bipolar cells, both oriented **at an angle** around the margins of the fovea. This histologic feature enables free access of light to the photoreceptors. The **macula lutea** is characterized by a yellow pigment in the inner layers surrounding the shallow fovea.

The exit site from the retina of axons derived from ganglion cells is represented by the **optic disk**. The optic disk includes (1) the **optic papilla**, a protrusion formed by the axons entering the optic nerve and (2) the **lamina cribrosa** of the sclera, pierced by the axons of the optic nerve. Photoreceptors terminate at the edges of the optic disk, which represents the "blind spot" of the retina. **The central artery and vein of the retina pass through the optic disk.**

The eyelids, conjunctiva, and the lacrimal gland

The anterior portion of the eyeball is protected by the eyelids, the conjunctiva,

Figure 9-22. **Eyelid and its pathology**

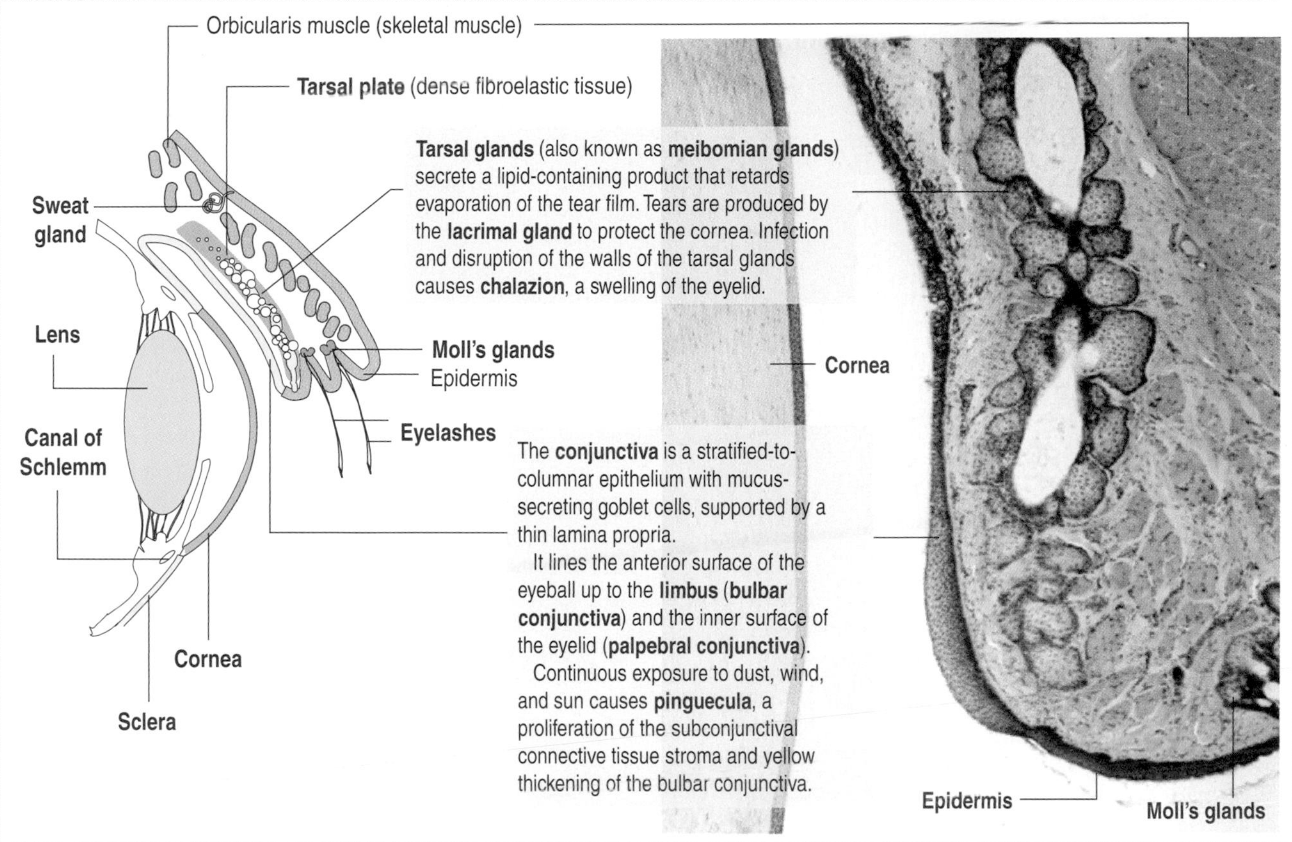

Orbicularis muscle (skeletal muscle)
Tarsal plate (dense fibroelastic tissue)
Tarsal glands (also known as **meibomian glands**) secrete a lipid-containing product that retards evaporation of the tear film. Tears are produced by the **lacrimal gland** to protect the cornea. Infection and disruption of the walls of the tarsal glands causes **chalazion**, a swelling of the eyelid.
Sweat gland
Lens
Canal of Schlemm
Cornea
Sclera
Moll's glands
Epidermis
Eyelashes
Cornea
The **conjunctiva** is a stratified-to-columnar epithelium with mucus-secreting goblet cells, supported by a thin lamina propria.
It lines the anterior surface of the eyeball up to the **limbus** (**bulbar conjunctiva**) and the inner surface of the eyelid (**palpebral conjunctiva**).
Continuous exposure to dust, wind, and sun causes **pinguecula**, a proliferation of the subconjunctival connective tissue stroma and yellow thickening of the bulbar conjunctiva.
Epidermis
Moll's glands

and the fluid produced by the lacrimal gland.

Each **eyelid** consists of two portions (Figure 9-22): (1) an outer **cutaneous portion** lined by a stratified squamous epidermis overlying a loose connective tissue dermis and skeletal muscle (**orbicularis oculi muscle**) and (2) an inner **conjunctival portion**, lined by a thin mucus membrane, the **conjunctiva**.

The cutaneous portion contains several skin appendages: (1) **sweat** and **se-**

Figure 9-23. **Lacrimal gland**

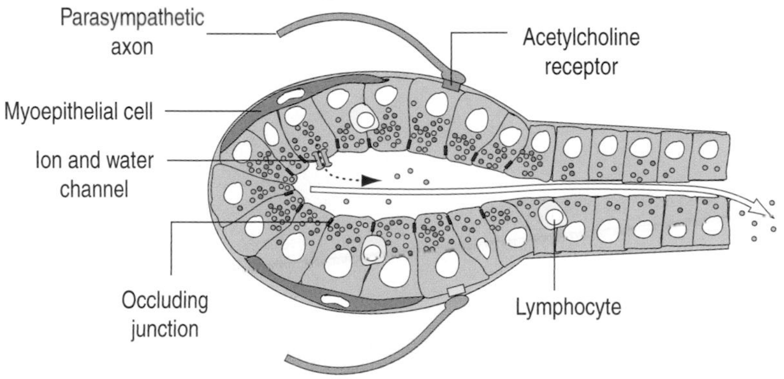

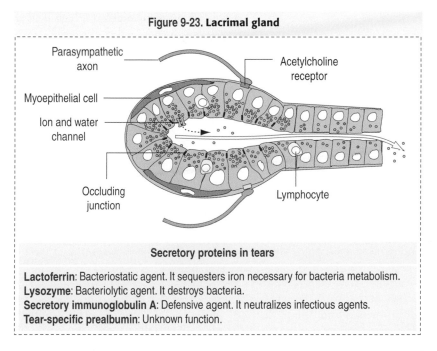

Parasympathetic axon
Acetylcholine receptor
Myoepithelial cell
Ion and water channel
Occluding junction
Lymphocyte

Secretory proteins in tears

Lactoferrin: Bacteriostatic agent. It sequesters iron necessary for bacteria metabolism.
Lysozyme: Bacteriolytic agent. It destroys bacteria.
Secretory immunoglobulin A: Defensive agent. It neutralizes infectious agents.
Tear-specific prealbumin: Unknown function.

baceous glands and (2) three to four rows of stiff hairs, the **eyelashes**, at the eyelid margins. Eyelashes are associated with modified sweat glands known as the **glands of Moll**.

Facing the conjunctival lining is the **tarsal plate**, a fibroelastic dense connective tissue containing large sebaceous **tarsal glands**, also known as **meibomian glands**. Each tarsal gland opens at the margin of the eyelid. The tarsal plate is responsible for the rigidity of the eyelids.

The junction between the cutaneous and conjunctival portions is demarcated clinically by the **sulcus**, a gray line located between the ducts of the meibomian glands and the eyelashes.

The **conjunctiva** is continuous with the skin lining and extends up to the periphery of the cornea. It consists of polygonal to columnar stratified epithelial cells with mucus-secreting goblet cells. At the corneal rim, the conjunctival epithelium becomes stratified squamous and is continuous with the corneal epithelium. A lamina propria with capillaries supports the lining epithelium.

The **lacrimal gland** produces a fluid, **tears**, that first accumulate in the conjunctival sac and then exit into the nasal cavity through a drainage duct (**nasolacrimal duct**). Tears evaporate in the nasal cavity but can produce a sniffy nose when excessive fluid is produced.

The lacrimal gland (Figure 9-23) is a **tubuloacinar serous gland** with **myoepithelial cells.** It is organized into separate lobes with 12 to 15 independent excretory ducts. Tears enter the excretory canaliculi through the **puncta** and reach the nasolacrimal sac and duct to eventually drain in the inferior meatus within the nasal cavity.

Lacrimal glands receive neural input from (1) **parasympathetic nerve fibers**, originating in the pterygopalatine ganglion; **acetycholine receptors** on glandular cells respond to acetylcholine released at the nerve terminals; and (2) **sympathetic nerve fibers**, arising from the superior cervical ganglion.

Blinking produces gentle compression of the lacrimal glands and the release of fluid. Tears keep the surface of the conjunctiva and cornea moist and rinse off dust particles. **Spreading of the mucus secreted by the conjunctival epithelial cells, the oily secretion derived from the tarsal glands, and the continuous blinking of the eyelids prevent rapid evaporation of the tear film**. Tears contain **lysozyme**, an antibacterial enzyme; **lactoferrin**; **secretory immunoglobulin A**; and **tear-specific prealbumin** (see Figure 9-23).

Excess production of tears occurs in response to chemical and physical irritants of the conjunctiva, high light intensity, and strong emotions. A disruption in the production of tears or damage to the eyelids results in the drying out of the cornea (**dry eye** or **keratoconjunctivitis sicca**), which is followed by ulceration, perforation, loss of aqueous humor, and blindness.

Clinical significance: Red eye

A red eye is the most frequent and relatively benign ocular alteration. In some cases, a red eye represents a vision-threatening condition.

A **subconjunctival hemorrhage** is the cause of acute ocular redness and can be produced by trauma, bleeding disorders, hypertension, and treatment with anticoagulants. No pain or vision impairment is associated with this disorder.

Conjunctivitis is the most common cause of red eye. The superficial blood vessels of the conjunctiva are dilated and cause edema of the conjunctiva with discharge. A purulent discharge indicates bacterial infection—predominantly gram-positive organisms. A watery discharge is observed in conjunctivitis caused by viral infection.

EAR

The ear consists of three components (Figure 9-24):

1. The **external ear**, which collects sound and directs it down the ear canal to

Figure 9-24. **General outline of the external, middle, and inner ear**

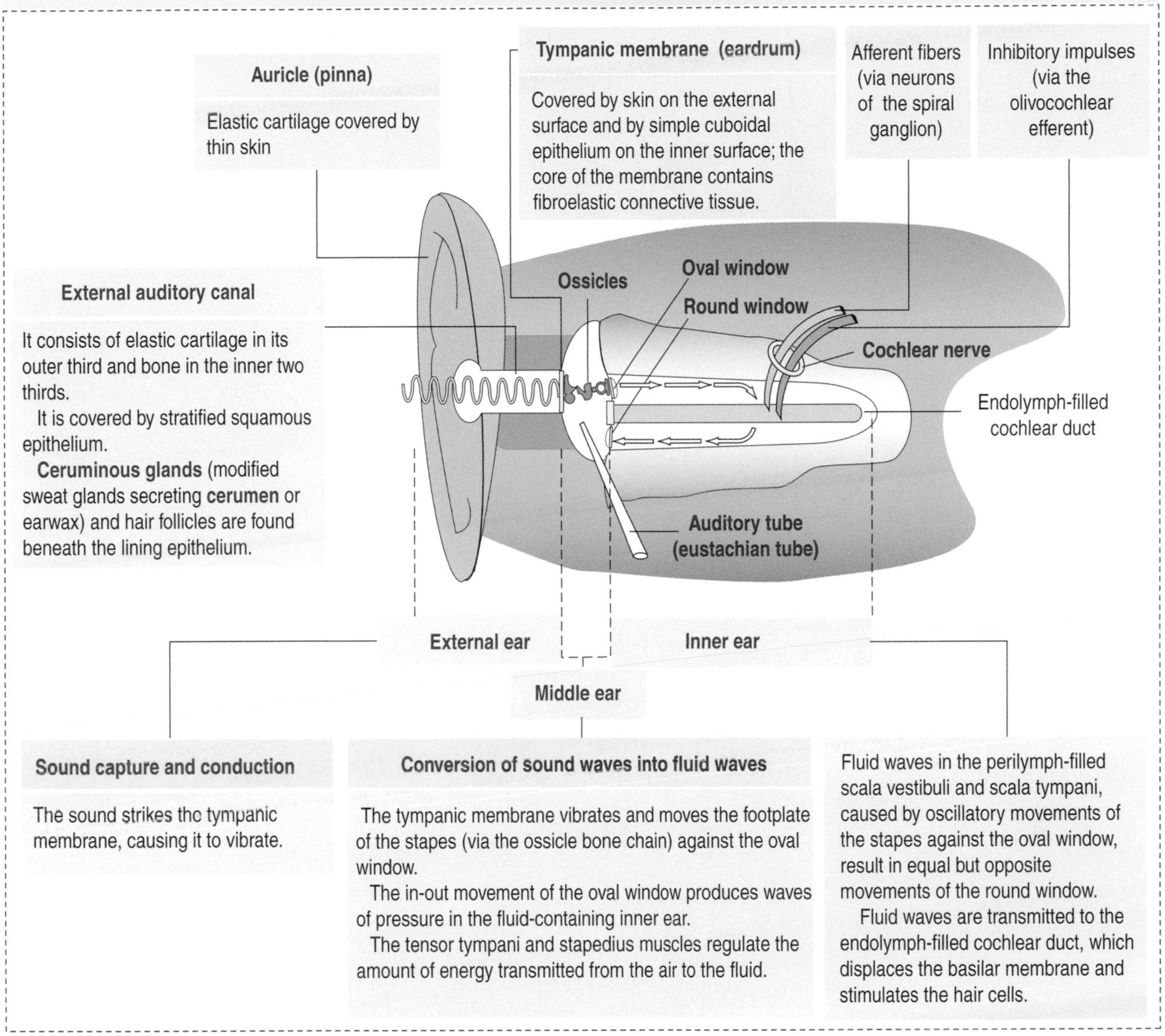

Auricle (pinna)
Elastic cartilage covered by thin skin
Tympanic membrane (eardrum)
Covered by skin on the external surface and by simple cuboidal epithelium on the inner surface; the core of the membrane contains fibroelastic connective tissue.
Afferent fibers (via neurons of the spiral ganglion)
Inhibitory impulses (via the olivocochlear efferent)
External auditory canal
It consists of elastic cartilage in its outer third and bone in the inner two thirds.
It is covered by stratified squamous epithelium.
Ceruminous glands (modified sweat glands secreting cerumen or earwax) and hair follicles are found beneath the lining epithelium.
Ossicles
Oval window
Round window
Cochlear nerve
Endolymph-filled cochlear duct
Auditory tube (eustachian tube)
External ear
Inner ear
Middle ear
Sound capture and conduction
The sound strikes the tympanic membrane, causing it to vibrate.
Conversion of sound waves into fluid waves
The tympanic membrane vibrates and moves the footplate of the stapes (via the ossicle bone chain) against the oval window.
The in-out movement of the oval window produces waves of pressure in the fluid-containing inner ear.
The tensor tympani and stapedius muscles regulate the amount of energy transmitted from the air to the fluid.
Fluid waves in the perilymph-filled scala vestibuli and scala tympani, caused by oscillatory movements of the stapes against the oval window, result in equal but opposite movements of the round window.
Fluid waves are transmitted to the endolymph-filled cochlear duct, which displaces the basilar membrane and stimulates the hair cells.

the tympanic membrane.

2. The **middle ear**, which converts sound pressure waves into mechanical motion of the tympanic membrane. The motion is in turn transmitted to the middle ear ossicles, which reduce the amplitude but increase the force of mechanical motion to overcome the resistance offered by the fluid-filled inner ear.

3. The **internal ear**, which houses the sensory organs for both hearing and balance, transmits mechanical vibrations to the fluid (the **endolymph**) contained in the **membranous labyrinth** and thereby converts these mechanical vibrations to electrical impulses on the same type of cell for sensory transduction: the **hair cell**.

The inner ear has two systems: (1) the **auditory system** for the perception of sound (hearing) and (2) the **vestibular system** for the perception of head and body motion (balance).

External ear

The first and second branchial arches, which include the arch ectoderm and mesoderm, are the major contributors to the embryologic origin of the external ear (Figure 9–25).

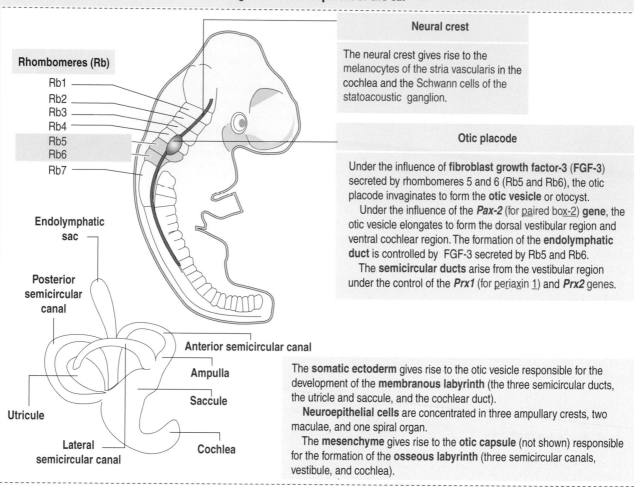

Figure 9-25. Development of the ear

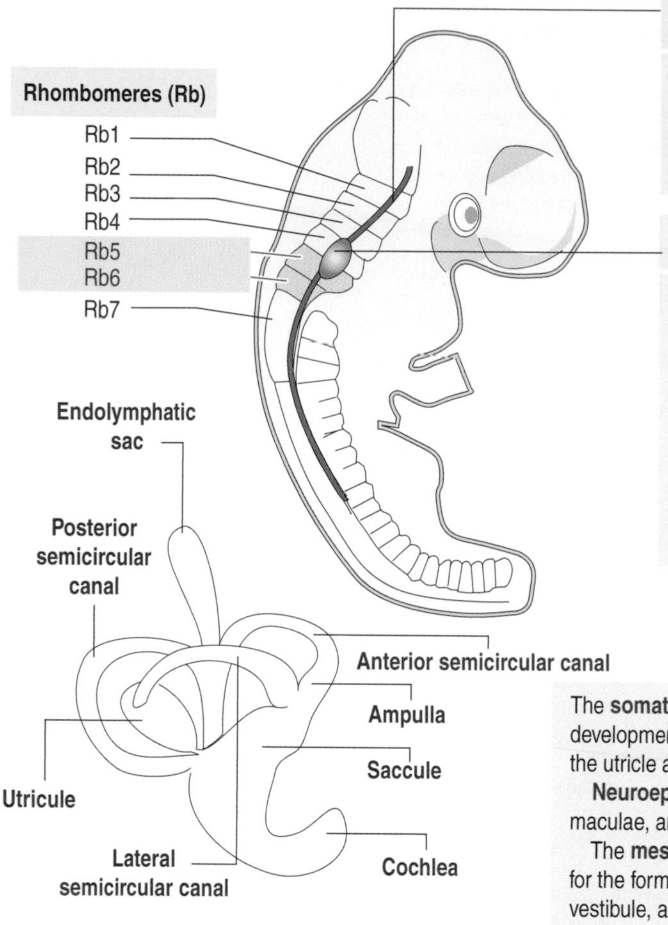

Rhombomeres (Rb)
Rb1
Rb2
Rb3
Rb4
Rb5
Rb6
Rb7
Endolymphatic sac
Posterior semicircular canal
Anterior semicircular canal
Ampulla
Saccule
Utricule
Lateral semicircular canal
Cochlea

Neural crest

The neural crest gives rise to the melanocytes of the stria vascularis in the cochlea and the Schwann cells of the statoacoustic ganglion.

Otic placode

Under the influence of **fibroblast growth factor-3 (FGF-3)** secreted by rhombomeres 5 and 6 (Rb5 and Rb6), the otic placode invaginates to form the **otic vesicle** or otocyst.

Under the influence of the ***Pax-2*** (for paired box-2) **gene**, the otic vesicle elongates to form the dorsal vestibular region and ventral cochlear region. The formation of the **endolymphatic duct** is controlled by FGF-3 secreted by Rb5 and Rb6.

The **semicircular ducts** arise from the vestibular region under the control of the ***Prx1*** (for periaxin 1) and ***Prx2*** genes.

The **somatic ectoderm** gives rise to the otic vesicle responsible for the development of the **membranous labyrinth** (the three semicircular ducts, the utricle and saccule, and the cochlear duct).

Neuroepithelial cells are concentrated in three ampullary crests, two maculae, and one spiral organ.

The **mesenchyme** gives rise to the **otic capsule** (not shown) responsible for the formation of the **osseous labyrinth** (three semicircular canals, vestibule, and cochlea).

The **auricle** (external ear or pinna) collects sound waves that are conducted across the **external acoustic meatus** to the **tympanic membrane.**

The **auricle** consists of a core of elastic cartilage surrounded by skin with hair follicles and sebaceous glands.

The **external acoustic meatus** is a passage extending from the auricle to the eardrum or **tympanic membrane**. The outer third of this passage is cartilage; the inner two thirds is part of the temporal bone. Skin lines the cartilage and the bone surfaces. A characteristic feature of this skin lining is the tubular coiled apocrine glands secreting a brown product called **cerumen.** Cerumen waterproofs the skin and protects the external acoustic meatus from exogenous agents such as insects.

Middle ear

The middle ear is formed by cells derived from the **neural crest** and **mesoderm** that initially migrated to the branchial arches (see Figure 9-25). Neural crest and mesodermic cells coalesce to form the components of the middle ear, lined by an **endodermal-derived epithelium** extending from the oral cavity (derived from the first pharyngeal pouch).

The middle ear, or **tympanic cavity**, is an air-filled space in the temporal bone interposed between the tympanic membrane and the structures contained in the inner ear. The main function of the middle ear is the transmission of sound from the tympanic membrane to the fluid-filled structures of the inner ear.

Sound transmission is carried out by the **auditory** or **bony ossicles** (**malleus, incus,** and **stapes**) organized in a chainlike fashion by interconnecting small liga-

Figure 9-26. Membranous labyrinth

Components of the membranous labyrinth

1 Two small sacs: the **utricle** and the **saccule**.
2 Three **semicircular ducts** open into the utricle. **Ampullae** are dilations connecting the ends of the semicircular ducts to the utricle.
3 Each ampulla contains the **crista ampullaris**. Sensory receptors in the crista ampullaris respond to the position of the head, generating nerve impulses necessary for correcting the position of the body.
4 The **cochlea**.

The sensory receptors of the membranous labyrinth are the **cristae ampullares** in the ampulla of each semicircular duct, the **macula utriculi** in the utricle, the **macula sacculi** in the saccule, and the **organ of Corti** in the cochlea.

The **ductulus reuniens** connects the saccule to the blind end of the cochlea proximal to the **cecum vestibulare**. The opposite blind end of the cochlea is the **cecum cupulare**.

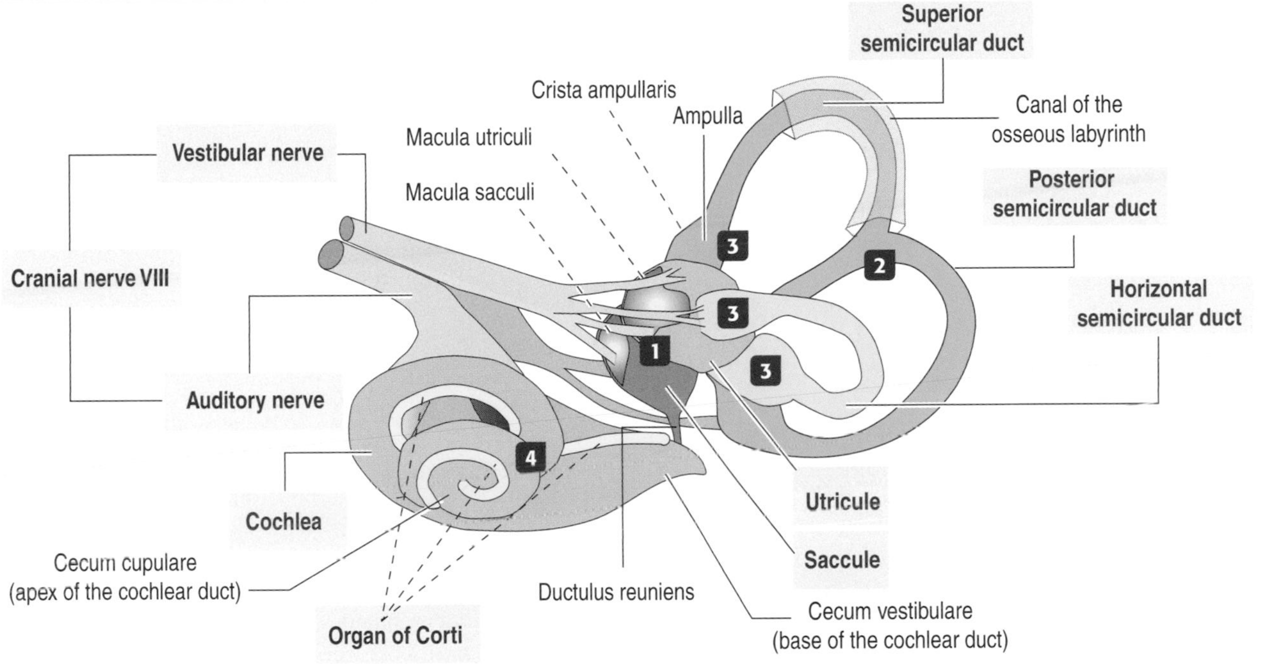

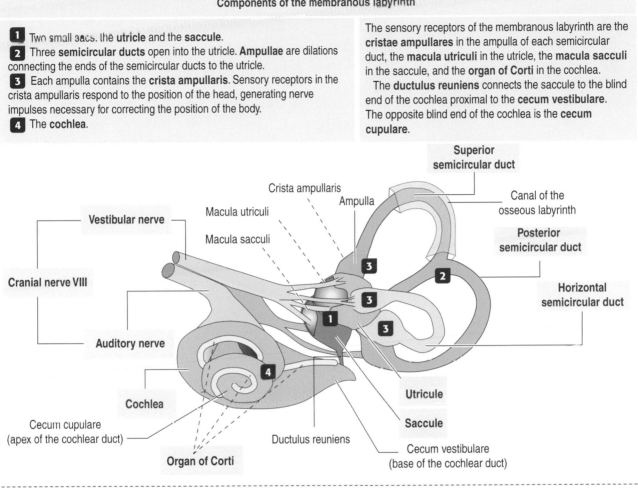

ments. In this chain, the arm of the malleus is attached to the **tympanic membrane** at one end; at the other end, the footplate of the stapes is applied to the **oval window** (fenestra vestibuli), an opening of the **bony labyrinth**. The **tensor tympani** (innervated by the trigeminal nerve [cranial nerve V]) and **stapedius muscles** (innervated by the facial nerve [cranial nerve VII]) keep the three auditory ossicles functionally linked.

The bony ossicles have two roles: (1) **they modulate the movement of the tympanic membrane**. (2) **They apply force to the oval window, thus amplifying the incoming sound waves. Otosclerosis** and **otitis media** affect the movements of the ossicles, conditions leading to hearing loss.

The **tympanic cavity** (also called the **tubotympanic recess** or **sulcus**) is lined by a squamous-to-cuboidal epithelium and lacks glands in the supporting connective tissue.

The **tympanic membrane** has an oval shape with a conical depression near the center caused by the attachment of the arm of the malleus. Two differently oriented layers of collagen fibers form the core of the membrane, and the two sides of the membrane are lined by a simple squamous-to-cuboidal epithelium.

The **auditory** or **eustachian tube** links the middle ear with the nasopharynx. Adjacent to the tympanic cavity, the tube is formed by the temporal bone. **Elastic cartilage** continues the bony portion of the tube, which then changes into **hyaline cartilage** near the nasopharynx opening. A ciliated epithelium with regional variations (low columnar-to-pseudostratified near the nasopharynx) and with mucus-secreting glands lines the bony and cartilaginous segments of the tube.

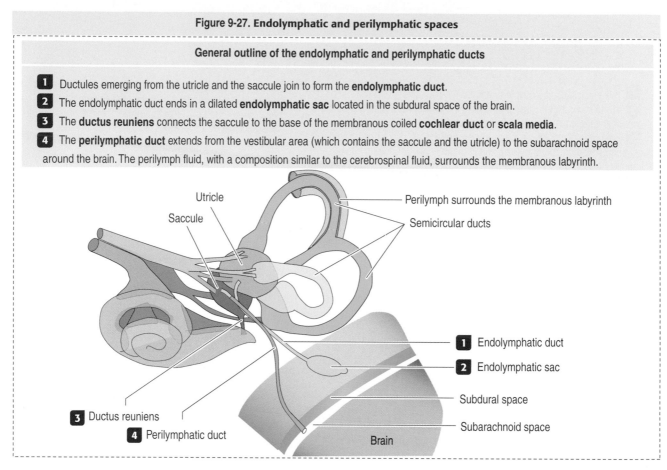

Figure 9-27. Endolymphatic and perilymphatic spaces

General outline of the endolymphatic and perilymphatic ducts

1 Ductules emerging from the utricle and the saccule join to form the **endolymphatic duct**.

2 The endolymphatic duct ends in a dilated **endolymphatic sac** located in the subdural space of the brain.

3 The **ductus reuniens** connects the saccule to the base of the membranous coiled **cochlear duct** or **scala media**.

4 The **perilymphatic duct** extends from the vestibular area (which contains the saccule and the utricle) to the subarachnoid space around the brain. The perilymph fluid, with a composition similar to the cerebrospinal fluid, surrounds the membranous labyrinth.

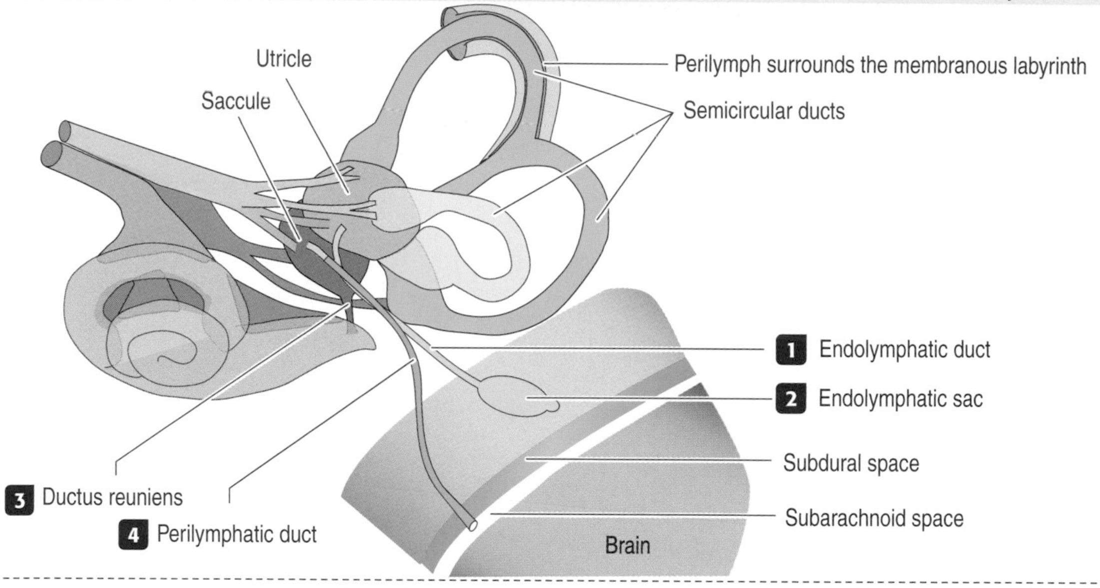

Utricle
Saccule
Perilymph surrounds the membranous labyrinth
Semicircular ducts
1 Endolymphatic duct
2 Endolymphatic sac
Subdural space
Subarachnoid space
3 Ductus reuniens
4 Perilymphatic duct
Brain

The **role of the auditory tube** is **to maintain a pressure balance between the tympanic cavity and the external environment.**

Defects in middle ear development include the absence of structural elements, such as the tympanic ring, which supports the tympanic membrane and the ossicles. The tympanic ring is derived from mesenchyme of the first pharyngeal arch (malleus and incus) and second pharyngeal arch (stapes), the middle ear muscles, and the tubotympanic recess.

Inner ear

Development of the inner ear

The inner ear and associated cranial ganglion neurons derive from an **otic placode** on the surface of the head. The placode invaginates and forms a hollow mass of cells called the **otic vesicle**, or **otocyst** (see Figure 9-25). Neural crest cells migrate out of the hindbrain and distribute around the otic vesicle. The otic vesicle elongates, forming the dorsal vestibular region and the ventral cochlear region under the influence of the ***Pax-2*** (for paired box-2) **gene**. Neither the cochlea nor the spiral ganglion form in the absence of *Pax-2*.

The endolymphatic duct derives from an invagination of the otocyst, regulated by **fibroblast growth factor-3**, secreted by cells in **rhombomeres** 5 and 6. A total of seven rhombomeres, called **neuromeres**, also provide signals for the development of the hindbrain. Two of the **semicircular ducts** derive from the vestibular region and develop under the control of the *Prx1* (for periaxin 1) and *Prx2* genes. Note that the auditory (cochlea) and vestibular portions (semicircular canals) are under separate genetic control (*Pax-2* and *Prx* genes, respectively).

Structure of the inner ear

The inner ear occupies the **osseous labyrinth** within the petrous portion of the temporal bone. The osseous labyrinth contains the **membranous labyrinth** (Figure

Figure 9-28. **Structure of the crista ampullaris**

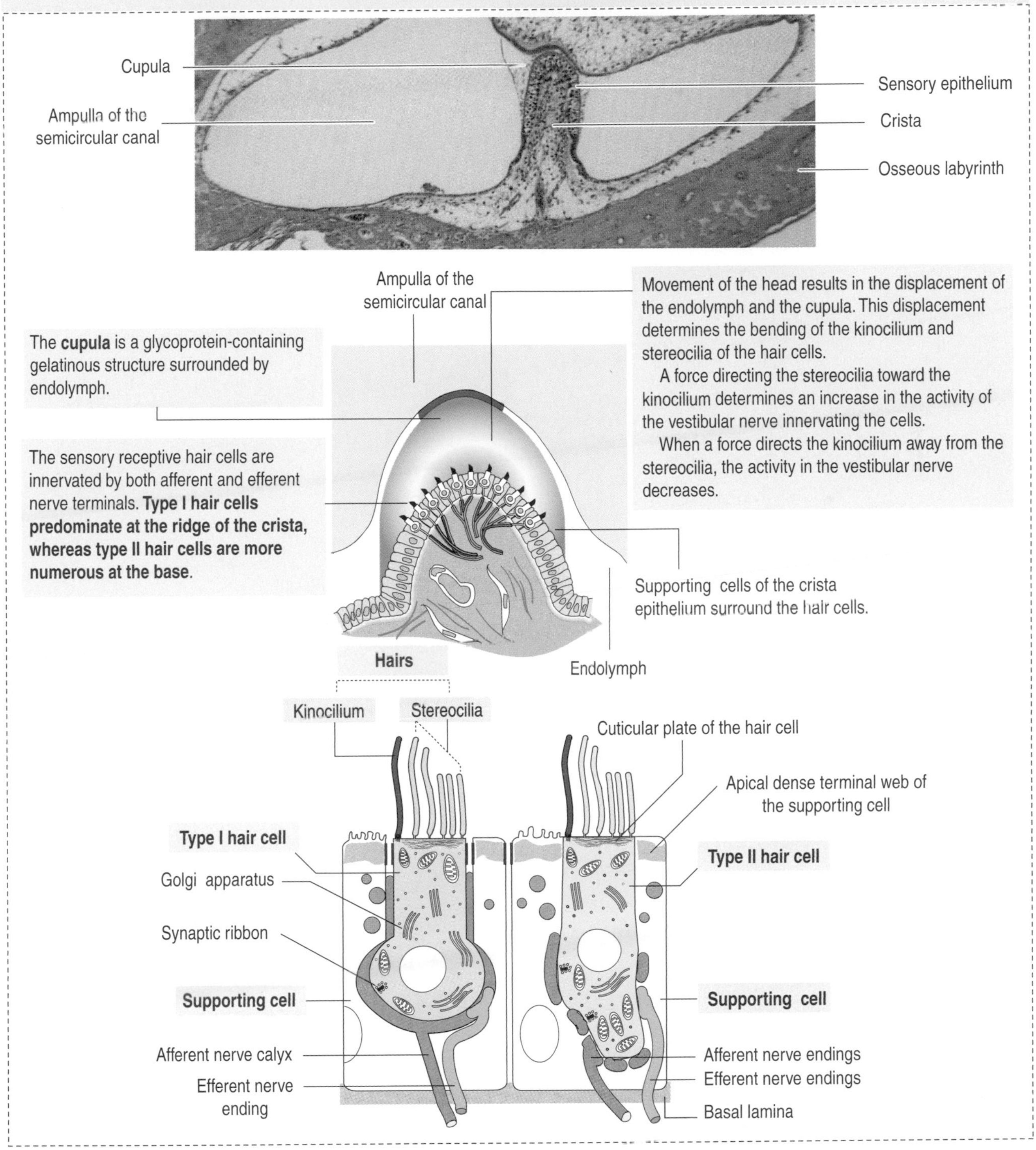
Cupula
Ampulla of the semicircular canal
Sensory epithelium
Crista
Osseous labyrinth
Ampulla of the semicircular canal
Movement of the head results in the displacement of the endolymph and the cupula. This displacement determines the bending of the kinocilium and stereocilia of the hair cells.
A force directing the stereocilia toward the kinocilium determines an increase in the activity of the vestibular nerve innervating the cells.
When a force directs the kinocilium away from the stereocilia, the activity in the vestibular nerve decreases.
The cupula is a glycoprotein-containing gelatinous structure surrounded by endolymph.
The sensory receptive hair cells are innervated by both afferent and efferent nerve terminals. Type I hair cells predominate at the ridge of the crista, whereas type II hair cells are more numerous at the base.
Supporting cells of the crista epithelium surround the hair cells.
Endolymph
Hairs
Kinocilium
Stereocilia
Cuticular plate of the hair cell
Apical dense terminal web of the supporting cell
Type I hair cell
Golgi apparatus
Synaptic ribbon
Supporting cell
Afferent nerve calyx
Efferent nerve ending
Type II hair cell
Supporting cell
Afferent nerve endings
Efferent nerve endings
Basal lamina

9-26), a structure that houses both the **vestibular** and **auditory systems.**

The **vestibular system** consists of two components: (1) two **sacs** (the **utricle** and **saccule**, also called **otolith organs**) and (2) **three semicircular canals** (superior, horizontal, and posterior) arising from the utricle.

The **auditory system** consists of the **cochlear duct**, lodged in a spiral bony canal anterior to the vestibular system.

The membranous labyrinth contains **endolymph**, a fluid with a high concentration of K^+ and a low concentration of Na^+. **Perilymph** (with a high Na^+ and low K^+ content) is present between the membranous labyrinth and the walls of

Figure 9-29. Structure of the macula of the saccule and utricle

The **maculae** are sensory receptor areas located in the wall of the **saccule** and **utricle**.
They are concerned with the detection of directional movement of the head. The position of the macula in the utricle is horizontal and it is vertical in the saccule.

A single layer of supportive cells associated with the basal lamina houses two types of sensory cells: **types I** and **II hair cells**. A long single kinocilium and 50 to 60 stereocilia project from the apical surface of the hair cells.

Otoliths contain calcium carbonate.
Changes in the position of the head cause a shift in the position of the otolithic membrane (including the otoliths) and endolymph.
This movement displaces the underlying kinocilium and stereocilia.

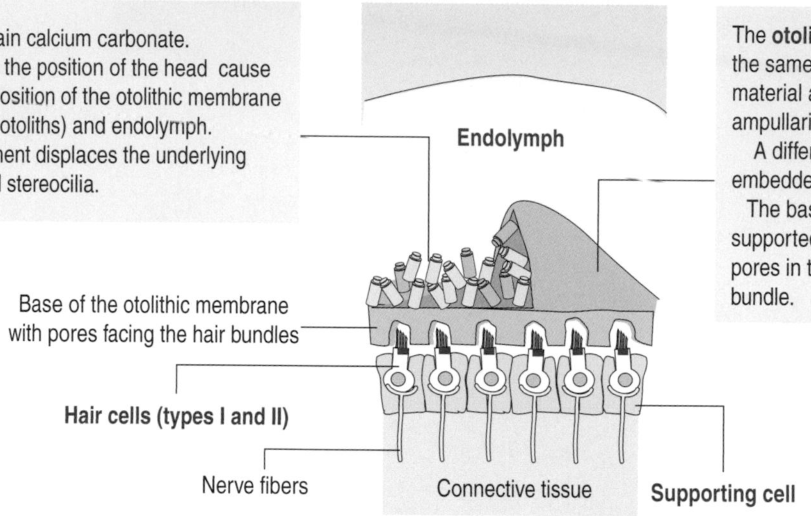

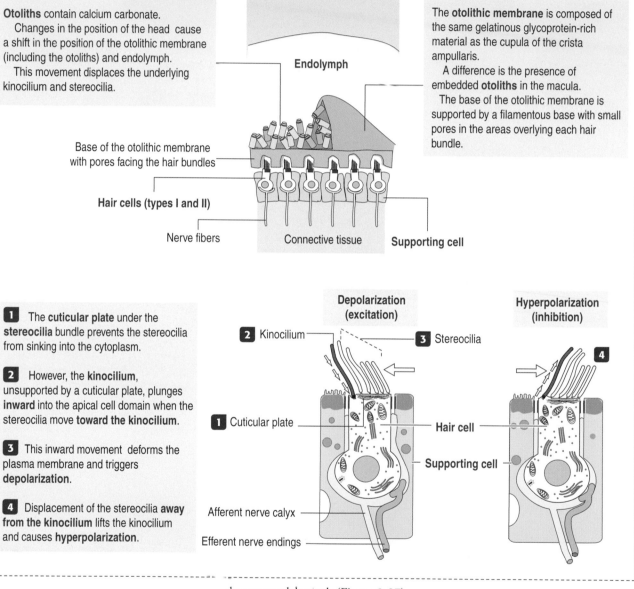

Endolymph
Base of the otolithic membrane with pores facing the hair bundles
Hair cells (types I and II)
Nerve fibers
Connective tissue
Supporting cell

The **otolithic membrane** is composed of the same gelatinous glycoprotein-rich material as the cupula of the crista ampullaris.
A difference is the presence of embedded **otoliths** in the macula.
The base of the otolithic membrane is supported by a filamentous base with small pores in the areas overlying each hair bundle.

1 The **cuticular plate** under the **stereocilia** bundle prevents the stereocilia from sinking into the cytoplasm.

2 However, the **kinocilium**, unsupported by a cuticular plate, plunges **inward** into the apical cell domain when the stereocilia move **toward the kinocilium**.

3 This inward movement deforms the plasma membrane and triggers **depolarization**.

4 Displacement of the stereocilia **away from the kinocilium** lifts the kinocilium and causes **hyperpolarization**.

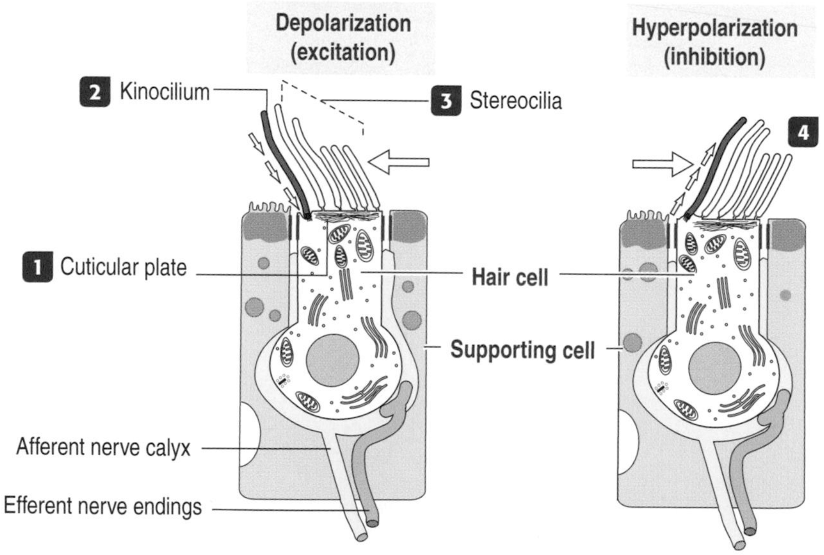

Depolarization (excitation)
Hyperpolarization (inhibition)
2 Kinocilium
3 Stereocilia
4
1 Cuticular plate
Hair cell
Supporting cell
Afferent nerve calyx
Efferent nerve endings

the osseous labyrinth (Figure 9-27).

Vestibular organ

The **semicircular canals** respond to **rotational movements** of the head and body (**angular accelerations**).

The **otolith organs** (saccule and utricle) respond to **translational movements** (**linear acceleration**).

Sensory cells in the vestibular organ are innervated by afferent fibers of the vestibular branch of the **vestibulocochlear nerve** (cranial nerve VIII). The **labyrinthine artery**, a branch of the anterior inferior cerebellar artery, supplies blood to the labyrinth. The **stylomastoid artery** supplies blood to the semicircular canals.

Figure 9-30. Organization of the macula

Sensory epithelium of the macula

This epithelium consists of **types I** and **II hair cells** embedded in **supporting cells** touching the basal lamina.

In vivo, kinocilia and stereocilia—extending from the surface of the hair cells—are coated by the **otolithic** (or statoconial) **membrane** containing **otoconia** (Greek "ear dust").

Otoconia are displaced by the endolymph during forward-backward and upward-downward movements of the head (**linear acceleration**).

The sensory epithelium of the macula in the otolithic organs (saccule and utricle) does not respond to head rotation.

The hair cells of the macula are **polarized**: The **kinocilium** is oriented with respect to an imaginary line called the **striola**, which divides the hair cells into two opposite fields.

In the utricule, the kinocilium faces the striola. In the saccule, the kinocilium faces away from the striola.

This orientation determines which population of hair cells will displace their hair bundles in response to a specific movement of the head.

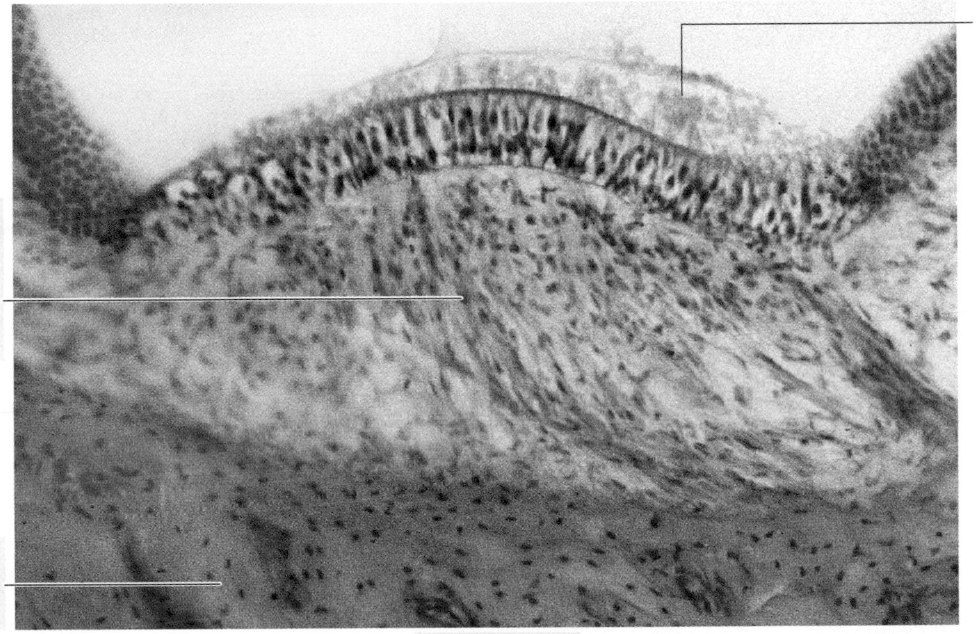

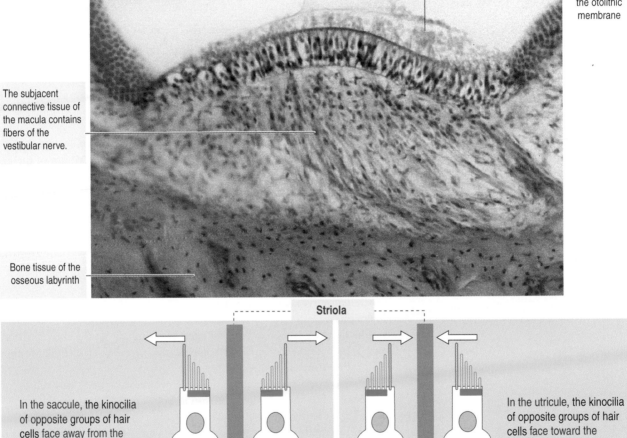

Remnant of the otolithic membrane
The subjacent connective tissue of the macula contains fibers of the vestibular nerve.
Bone tissue of the osseous labyrinth

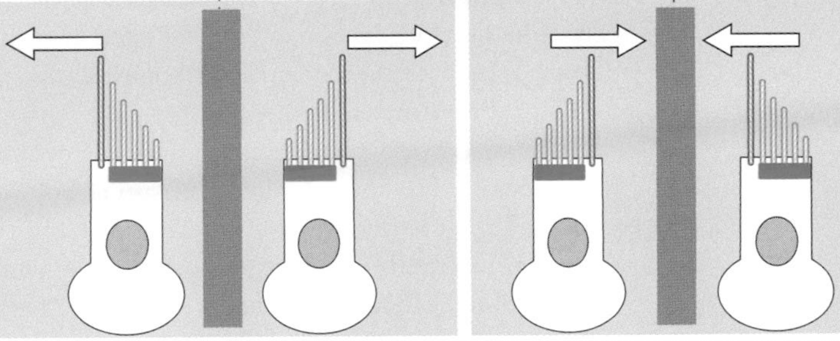

Striola
In the saccule, the kinocilia of opposite groups of hair cells face away from the striola.
In the utricule, the kinocilia of opposite groups of hair cells face toward the striola.

Semicircular canals

The semicircular ducts are contained within the osseous labyrinth. The three ducts are connected to the utricle. Ducts derived from the utricle and saccule join to form the **endolymphatic duct**. The endolymphatic duct ends in a small dilation called the **endolymphatic sac**, located between the layers of the meninges.

Small dilations —**ampullae**—are present at the semicircular duct–utricle connection sites. Each ampulla has a prominent ridge called the **crista ampullaris**.

The crista ampullaris (Figure 9-28) consists of a **sensory epithelium** covered by a gelatinous mass called the **cupula**.

The sensory epithelium consists of two cell types (see Figure 9-28): (1) the **hair cells** and (2) the **supporting cells**.

The basal surface of the supporting cells is attached to a basal lamina. In con-

Figure 9-31. **Topography of the cochlea**

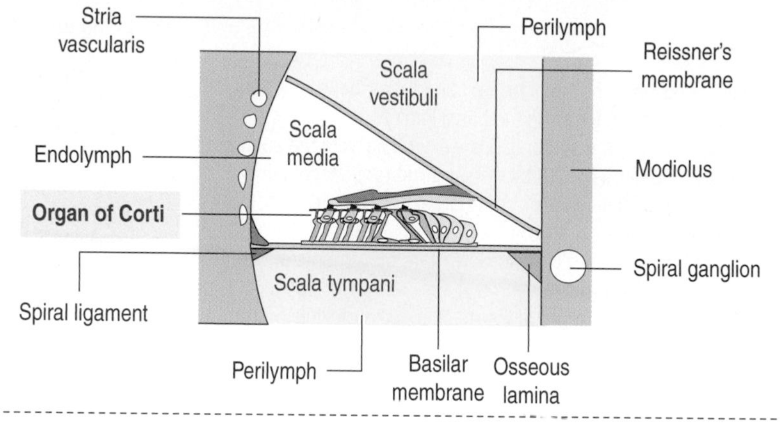

trast, the hair cells occupy a recess in the apical region of the supporting cells and do not reach the basal lamina. The apical domain of the hair cells contains 60 to 100 hairlike specialized **stereocilia** and a **single kinocilium**. Stereocilia are supported by an actin-containing **cuticular plate**. The free ends of both stereocilia and kinocilia are embedded in the **cupula**. The cupula attaches to the roof and walls of the ampulla and acts like a partition of the lumen of the ampulla (see Figure 9-28).

When the position of the cupula changes in response to movements of the endolymph, it causes displacement of the stereocilia and kinocilium of the hair cells (Figure 9-29). When stereocilia move **toward the kinocilium**, the plasma membrane of the hair cells **depolarizes** and the afferent nerve fibers are **stimulated (excitation)**. When stereocilia are **deflected away from the kinocilium**, the hair cell **hyperpolarizes** and afferent nerve fibers are **not stimulated (inhibition)**.

The cristae have two types of hair cells: (1) **type I hair cells** and (2) **type II hair cells**.

Both cell types are essentially similar in their internal structure, but differences exist in their shape and innervation:

1. **Afferent nerves**, with terminals containing the neurotransmitters **aspartate** and **glutamate**, enter the spaces separating the supporting cells and **form a calyx-like network** embracing the rounded basal domain of the type I hair cell. The cytoplasm displays **synaptic ribbons** and associated vesicles (similar to those found in the sensory retina).

2. The nerve endings in contact with the cylindrical type II hair cell do not form a basal calyx. Instead, **simple terminal boutons** can be visualized.

In addition to afferent nerves, both type I and type II hair cells receive **efferent nerve terminals** and have synaptic vesicles containing the neurotransmitter **acetylcholine**. Efferent nerve fibers control the sensitivity of the sensory receptor cells.

Supporting cells and hair cells are associated with each other by apical junctional complexes. Characteristic features of the supporting cells are an **apical dense terminal web** and the presence of **short microvilli**. Supporting cells lack stereocilia and kinocilia, two features typical of hair cells.

Clinical significance: Ménière's disease

Secretory cells in the membranous labyrinth and the endolymphatic sac maintain the ionic balance between endolymph and perilymph (see Figure 9-36). An **increase in the volume of endolymph** is the cause of **Ménière's disease**, which is characterized by vertigo (illusion of rotational movement in space), nausea, positional nystagmus (involuntary rhythmic oscillation of the eyes), vomiting, and ringing in the ears (**tinnitus**).

Figure 9-32. Cochlea

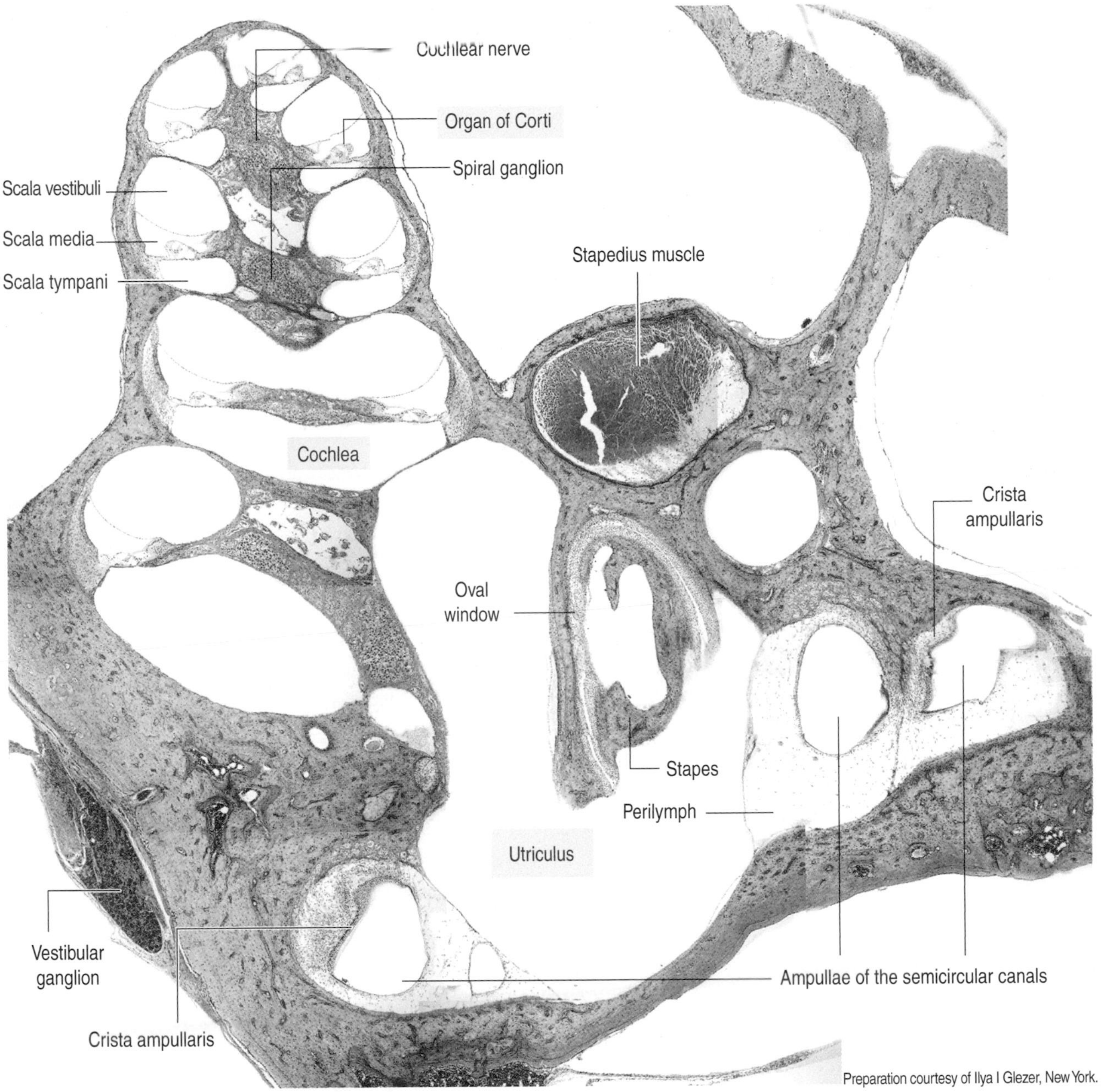

Cochlear nerve
Organ of Corti
Spiral ganglion
Scala vestibuli
Scala media
Scala tympani
Stapedius muscle
Cochlea
Crista ampullaris
Oval window
Stapes
Perilymph
Utriculus
Vestibular ganglion
Ampullae of the semicircular canals
Crista ampullaris

Preparation courtesy of Ilya I Glezer, New York.

The cochlea (Greek *kochlias*, spiral-shelled snail) is a spiral canal that winds more than two and a half times around a central bony axis, the **modiolus**. Within the bony modiolus is the **cochlear** (**spiral**) **ganglion**, spiraling around the inner side of the cochlea. The ganglion contains bipolar neurons: (1) The peripheral processes innervate the receptor cells. (2) The central processes enter the core of the modiolus, where they form the cochlear nerve (the cochlear division of cranial nerve VIII).

The membranous portion of the cochlea, the cochlear partition, contains the cochlear duct, or scala media. The cochlear partition spans the bony labyrinth dividing it into two separate canals: (1) the **scala vestibuli** and (2) the **scala tympani**.

The **vestibular membrane** (**Reissner's membrane**) and the **basilar membrane**, two membranes of the cochlear partition, separate the endolymph-filled cochlear duct from the perilymph-filled scala vestibuli and scala tympani. The lateral wall of the cochlear partition is the **stria vascularis**, a highly vascular tissue that covers a portion of the bony labyrinth and is responsible for the production and maintenance of the unique composition of the endolymph (K^+ homeostasis).

The cochlear duct does not extend to the apex or cupula of the cochlea but leaves a small opening of communication between the scala vestibuli and scala tympani at the apex, the **helicotrema** (see Figure 9-33). At the base of the cochlea, the stapes on the **oval window** and the membrane of the **round window** (not shown) separate the scala vestibuli and the scala tympani, respectively, from the middle ear cavity.

Figure 9-33. **Organ of Corti: The sound-transducing component of the inner ear**

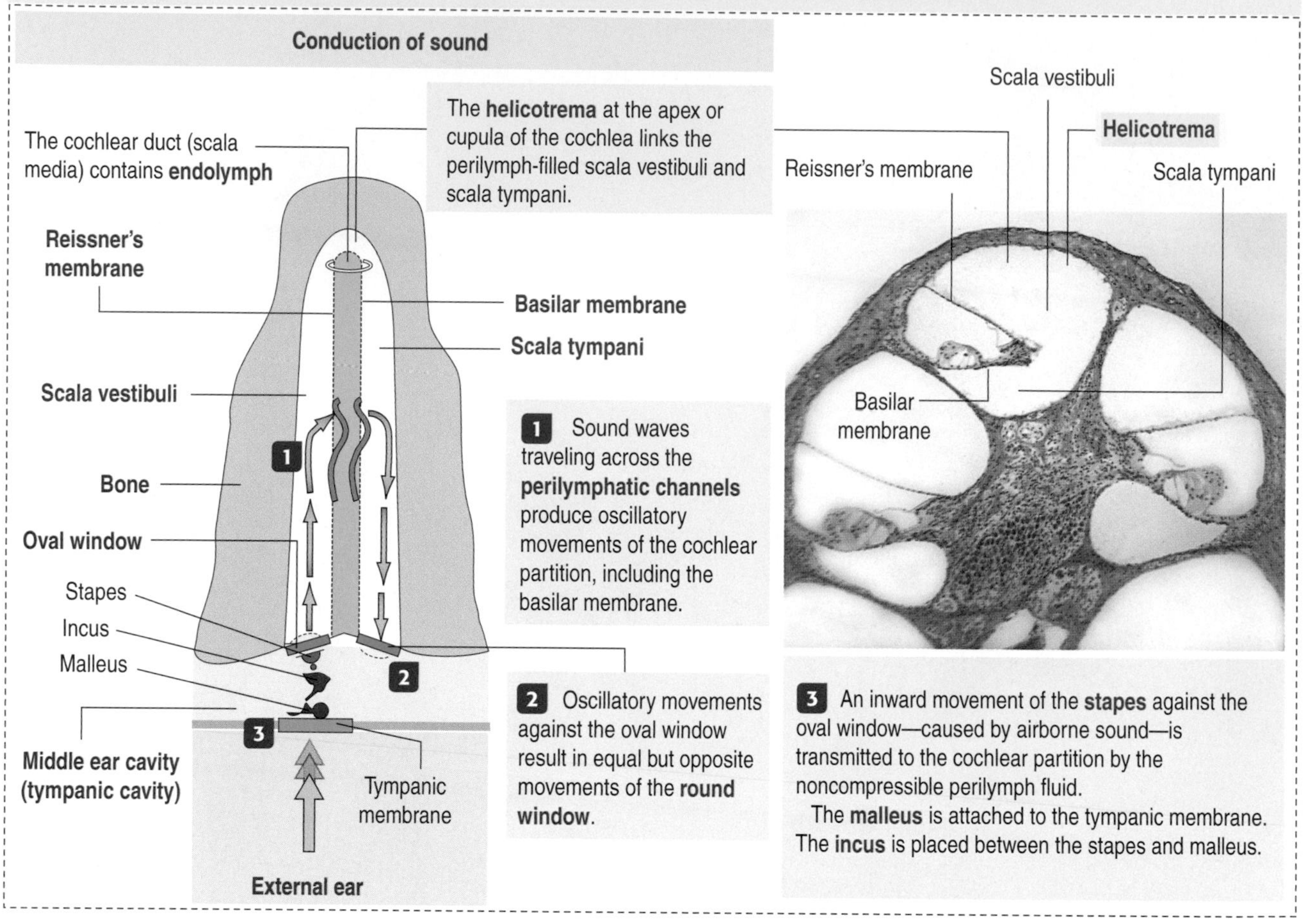

Conduction of sound
The cochlear duct (scala media) contains **endolymph**
The **helicotrema** at the apex or cupula of the cochlea links the perilymph-filled scala vestibuli and scala tympani.
Reissner's membrane
Basilar membrane
Scala tympani
Scala vestibuli
Bone
Oval window
Stapes
Incus
Malleus
Middle ear cavity (tympanic cavity)
Tympanic membrane
External ear
1 Sound waves traveling across the **perilymphatic channels** produce oscillatory movements of the cochlear partition, including the basilar membrane.
2 Oscillatory movements against the oval window result in equal but opposite movements of the **round window**.
Scala vestibuli
Helicotrema
Reissner's membrane
Scala tympani
Basilar membrane
3 An inward movement of the **stapes** against the oval window—caused by airborne sound—is transmitted to the cochlear partition by the noncompressible perilymph fluid.
The **malleus** is attached to the tympanic membrane. The **incus** is placed between the stapes and malleus.

Otolithic organs

The utricle and saccule display a sensory epithelium called a **macula** (Figure 9-30). Like the sensory epithelium of the crista ampullaris in the semicircular canals, the macula contains hair cells and supporting cells. The macula is covered by a gelatinous substance containing calcium carbonate–protein complexes forming small crystals called **otoliths** (see Figure 9-29). Otoliths are not present in the cupula overlying the hairs of the crista ampullaris. Small ductules derived from the utricle and saccule join to form the **endolymphatic duct** ending in the **endolymphatic sac**. The **ductus reuniens** links the saccule to the base of the membranous cochlear duct.

Cochlea

The cochlear duct is a membranous coiled duct inserted in the bony cochlea. It consists of an **apex** and a **base**. The coiled duct makes about two and two-thirds turns with a total length of 34 mm.

The cochlea has **three spiraling chambers** (Figures 9-31 to 9-33):

1. The **cochlear duct** (also called the **scala media**) represents the central chamber and contains endolymph.

2. Above the cochlear duct is the **scala vestibuli**, starting at the oval window.

3. Below the cochlear duct is the **scala tympani**, ending at the **round window**.

The scalae vestibuli and tympani are filled with perilymph and communicate at the **helicotrema** (see Figure 9-33).

In cross section, the boundaries of the scala media are the **basilar membrane** at the bottom, the **vestibular** or **Reissner's membrane** above, and the **stria vascularis** externally. The cells and capillaries of the stria vascularis produce endolymph. The

Figure 9-34. Organ of Corti

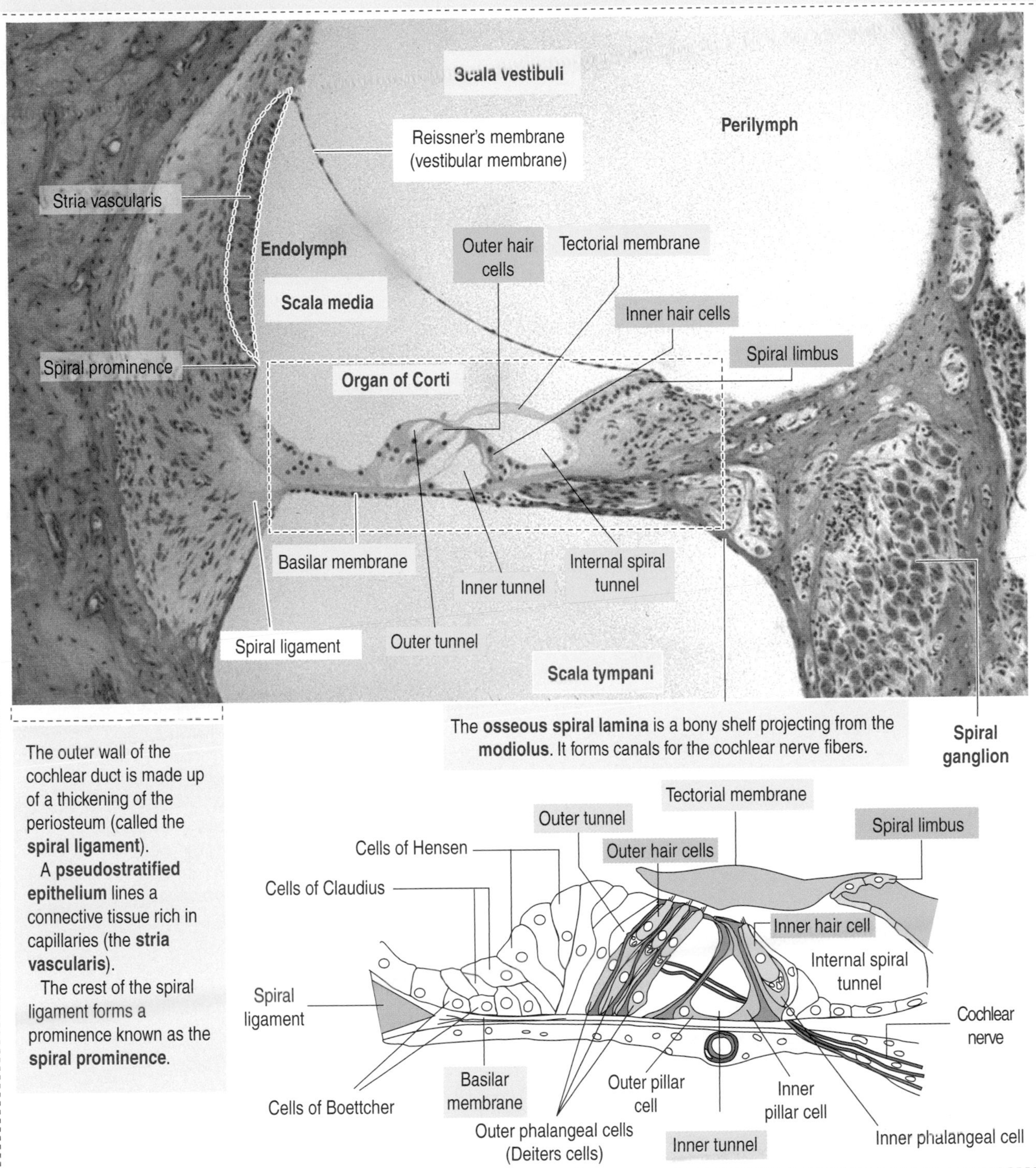

Scala vestibuli
Reissner's membrane (vestibular membrane)
Perilymph
Stria vascularis
Endolymph
Outer hair cells
Tectorial membrane
Scala media
Inner hair cells
Spiral limbus
Spiral prominence
Organ of Corti
Basilar membrane
Internal spiral tunnel
Inner tunnel
Spiral ligament
Outer tunnel
Scala tympani
Spiral ganglion
Tectorial membrane
Outer tunnel
Spiral limbus
Cells of Hensen
Outer hair cells
Cells of Claudius
Inner hair cell
Internal spiral tunnel
Spiral ligament
Cochlear nerve
Basilar membrane
Outer pillar cell
Inner pillar cell
Cells of Boettcher
Outer phalangeal cells (Deiters cells)
Inner tunnel
Inner phalangeal cell

The **osseous spiral lamina** is a bony shelf projecting from the **modiolus**. It forms canals for the cochlear nerve fibers.

The outer wall of the cochlear duct is made up of a thickening of the periosteum (called the **spiral ligament**).

A **pseudostratified epithelium** lines a connective tissue rich in capillaries (the **stria vascularis**).

The crest of the spiral ligament forms a prominence known as the **spiral prominence**.

spiraling bony core of the cochlea is the **modiolus**. On the inner side, the spiral osseous lamina projects outward from the modiolus to join the basilar membrane. On the external side, the basilar membrane is continuous with the **spiral ligament.** The scala vestibuli meets the scala tympani at an opening at the apex of the cochlea. This connecting site is called the **helicotrema**.

The **organ of Corti** (Figure 9-34) is the sensory epithelium of the cochlea. It is formed by (1) **inner** and **outer hair cells**; (2) **supporting cells**; (3) the **tectorial membrane**, extending from the **spiral limbus**; and (4) the **inner tunnel**, limited by the **outer** and **inner pillar cells**, separating inner from outer hair cells.

Figure 9-35. Organ of Corti

Structure of the organ of Corti

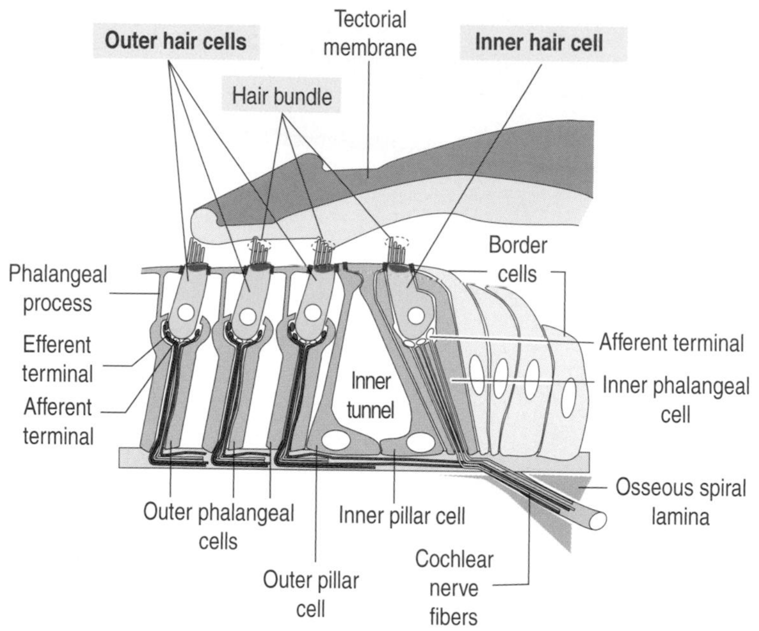

The **organ of Corti** is located in the scala media and extends the full length of the basilar membrane. Hair cells are the sensory receptors of the organ of Corti.

Two classes of hair cells with distinct functions are present in the human cochlea: (1) the **inner hair cell** and (2) the **outer hair cells**. **Only outer hair cells are in direct contact with the tectorial membrane**.

Both have hairs, bundles of stereocilia projecting from their apical surfaces. From the base to the apex of the cochlear duct, inner hair cells are arranged in a single row and outer hair cells in three to four rows.

Hair cells are kept in position by two supporting epithelial cell types: (1) the **pillar cells** and (2) the **phalangeal cells**.

Outer phalangeal cells (**Deiters cells**) surround the lower third of the outer hair cells and the nerve terminals around the base of the hair cell. A phalangeal process projects toward the apical surface of the hair cell and flattens into a plate. The **inner phalangeal cells** lack the phalangeal process and extensively surround the inner hair cell and its nerve terminal.

The **tectorial membrane** extends above the hair cells from the inner side of the organ of Corti.

Hair bundle, an array of stereocilia arranged in a staircase

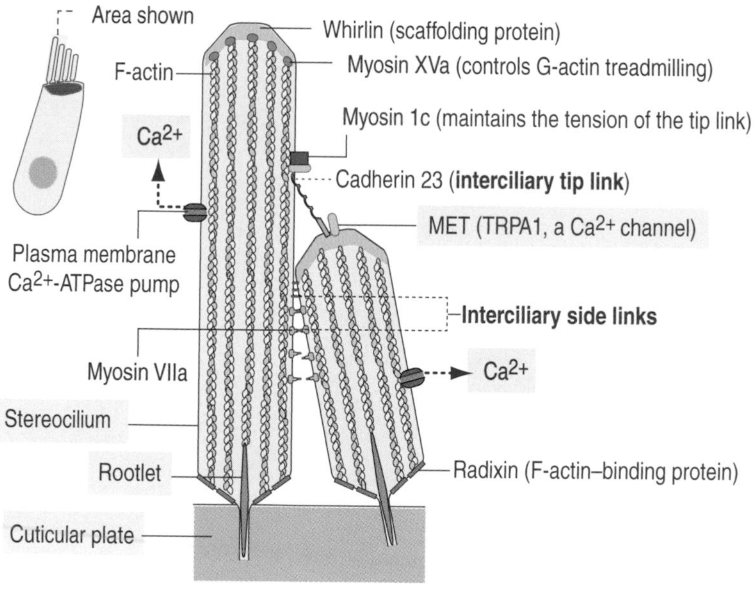

Deflections of the hair bundle are caused by sound vibrations initiated in each eardrum, conducted through the three ossicles in the middle ear, and transmitted within the cochlea as pressure waves. The end result is the displacement of the basilar membrane to elicit an electrical response in hair cells.

Sound-induced motion of the basilar membrane deflects the hair bundles of the hair cells to activate mechanoelectrical transduction (MET) ion channels represented by transient receptor potential channel A1 (TRPA1) linked by an interciliary tip link (for example, Ca^{2+}-dependent cadherin 23). The tension of the tip link is maintained by myosin 1c. Force applied to the interciliary tip link appears to activate TRPA1, which becomes permeable to Ca^{2+}. Plasma membrane Ca^{2+}-ATPase pumps are present. Side links (for example, myosin VIIa) stabilize the cohesion of adjacent hair bundles.

Each hair bundle consists of an F-actin core capped by the scaffolding protein whirlin and associated myosin XVa. G-actin is added at the tip of the stereocilia.

A **single line** of inner hair cells extends from the base to the apex of the cochlea (see Figures 9-34 and 9-35). The outer hair cells are arranged in **three parallel rows**, also extending from the base to the apex of the cochlea. A **hair bundle**, formed by 50 to 150 **stereocilia** in a long-to-short gradient arrangement, extends from the apical domain of each hair cell. **No kinocilium is present in the hair bundle of the cochlea.**

Each member of the hair bundle consists of a core of actin filaments. The tip of the actin bundle is the site where actin monomers are added under control of **myosin XVa** in association with the protein **whirlin**. Defects in myosin Va and

Figure 9-36. Functions of the organ of Corti

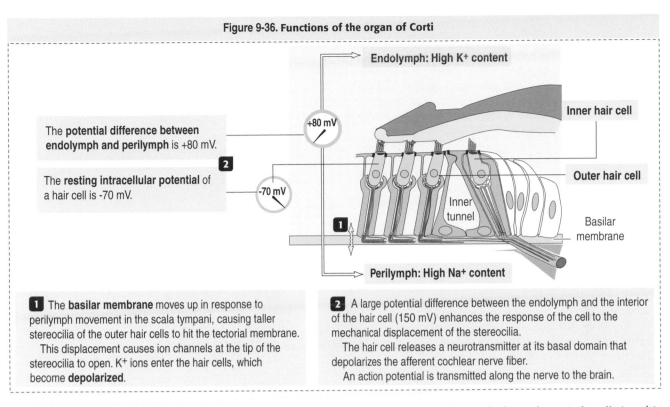

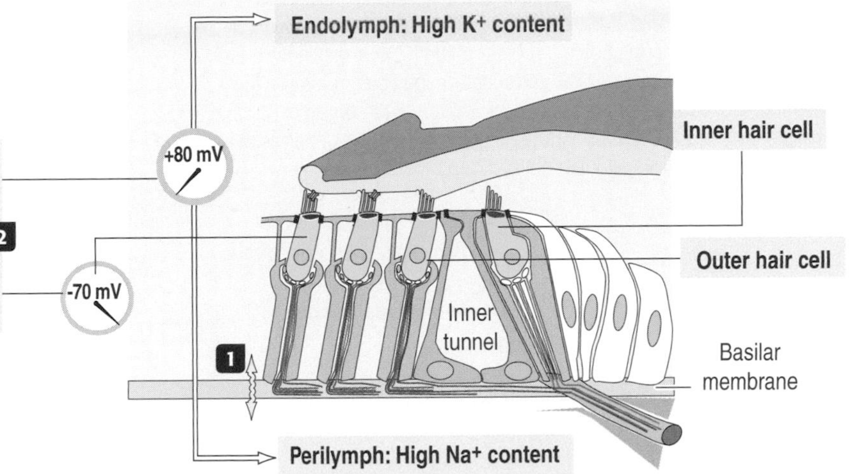
Endolymph: High K+ content
Inner hair cell
The potential difference between endolymph and perilymph is +80 mV.
+80 mV
2
The resting intracellular potential of a hair cell is -70 mV.
-70 mV
Outer hair cell
Inner tunnel
1
Basilar membrane
Perilymph: High Na+ content

1 The **basilar membrane** moves up in response to perilymph movement in the scala tympani, causing taller stereocilia of the outer hair cells to hit the tectorial membrane.

This displacement causes ion channels at the tip of the stereocilia to open. K^+ ions enter the hair cells, which become **depolarized**.

2 A large potential difference between the endolymph and the interior of the hair cell (150 mV) enhances the response of the cell to the mechanical displacement of the stereocilia.

The hair cell releases a neurotransmitter at its basal domain that depolarizes the afferent cochlear nerve fiber.

An action potential is transmitted along the nerve to the brain.

whirlin cause abnormally short stereocilia. At the base, the actin bundle is stabilized by the protein **radixin** (see Figure 9-35). Stereocilia within a hair bundle are interconnected by extracellular filaments (**interciliary links**). **Side links** (**myosin VIIa** and associated proteins) connect stereocilia along their shafts. **Tip links** (**cadherin 23**) extend from the tip of a stereocilium to the side of the taller adjacent stereocilium. The tension of the tip link is controlled by **myosin 1c**. Defects in interciliary links result in **Usher's syndrome**, characterized by disorganization of hair bundles leading to sensorineural deafness of cochlear origin combined with retinitis pigmentosa (loss of vision).

Interciliary links regulate the opening and closing of **mechanoelectrical transduction** (MET) **ion channels**, permeable to Ca^{2+}. Deflection of the hair bundle toward the taller stereocilia side opens the MET channels; displacements in the opposite direction close these channels. Interciliary links ensure a uniform response of MET channels. MET Ca^{2+} channels are essential for the conversion of a sound stimulus to an equivalent electrical signal and frequency tuning.

The **tectorial membrane** contains **α-** and **β-tectorin** proteins and extends outward over the sensory epithelium, from the spiral limbus of the osseous spiral lamina. The tectorial membrane is in close contact with the taller stereocilia of the hair bundle. When the basilar membrane and organ of Corti are displaced, stereocilia hit the tectorial membrane and **depolarization** of the hair cells occurs (Figure 9-36).

The **spiral ganglion** is housed in the modiolus. Processes of the bipolar sensory neurons of the spiral ganglion extend into the osseous spiral lamina, lose their myelin, pierce the basilar membrane, and synapse on the basal domain of the inner and outer hair cells.

There are two types of bipolar sensory neurons in the spiral ganglion: (1) **type I cells** (90% to 95%) whose fibers contact inner hair cells and (2) **type II cells** (5% to 10%) that synapse with outer hair cells.

The neuronal processes of type I and II cells form the cochlear branch of the vestibulocochlear nerve. Olivocochlear efferent fibers run along the basilar membrane to contact the inner and outer hair cells. Neurons of the auditory and vestibular ganglia fail to develop when the ***neurogenin 1* gene** is deleted.

Figure 9-37. **Deafness and balance**

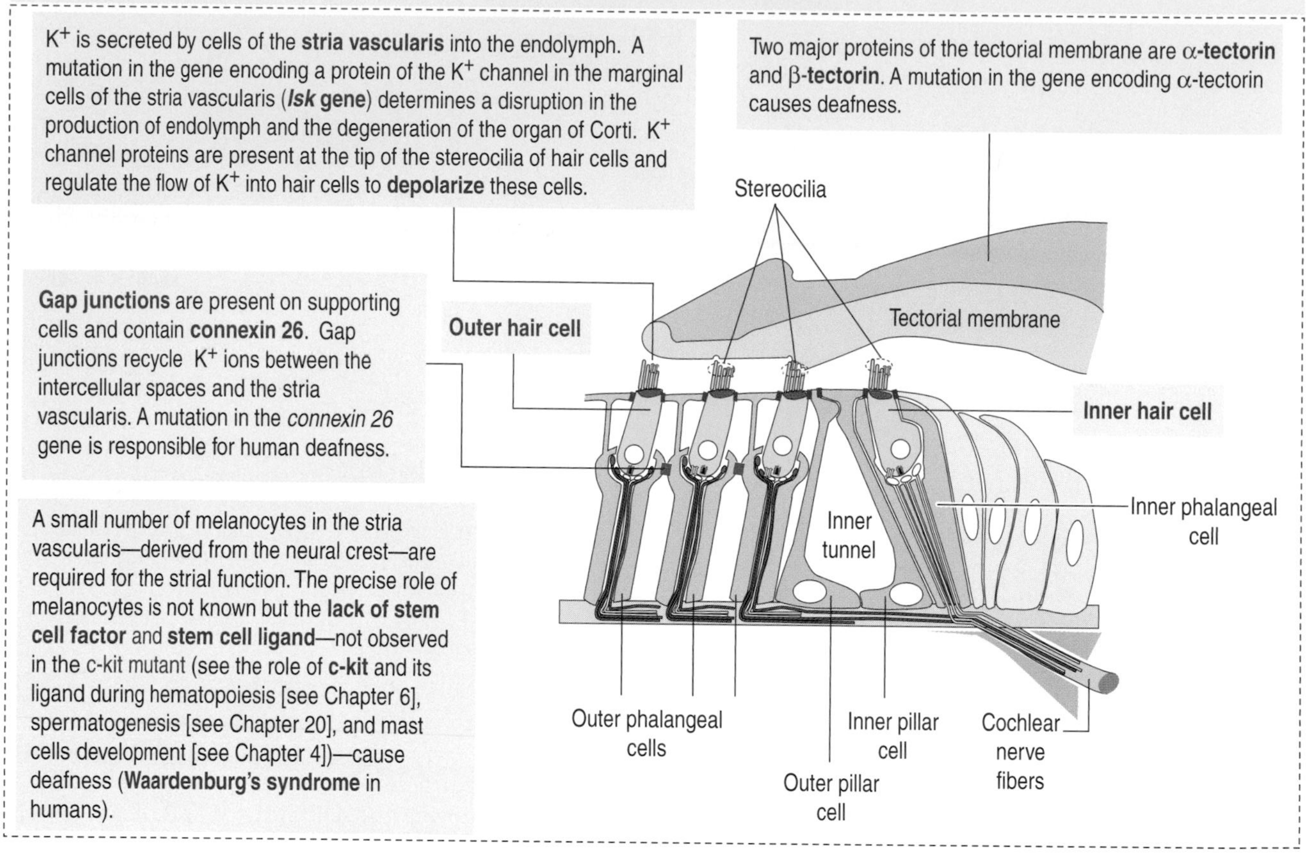

K^+ is secreted by cells of the **stria vascularis** into the endolymph. A mutation in the gene encoding a protein of the K^+ channel in the marginal cells of the stria vascularis (***Isk* gene**) determines a disruption in the production of endolymph and the degeneration of the organ of Corti. K^+ channel proteins are present at the tip of the stereocilia of hair cells and regulate the flow of K^+ into hair cells to **depolarize** these cells.
Two major proteins of the tectorial membrane are **α-tectorin** and **β-tectorin**. A mutation in the gene encoding α-tectorin causes deafness.
Stereocilia
Tectorial membrane
Gap junctions are present on supporting cells and contain **connexin 26**. Gap junctions recycle K^+ ions between the intercellular spaces and the stria vascularis. A mutation in the *connexin 26* gene is responsible for human deafness.
Outer hair cell
Inner hair cell
A small number of melanocytes in the stria vascularis—derived from the neural crest—are required for the strial function. The precise role of melanocytes is not known but the **lack of stem cell factor** and **stem cell ligand**—not observed in the c-kit mutant (see the role of **c-kit** and its ligand during hematopoiesis [see Chapter 6], spermatogenesis [see Chapter 20], and mast cells development [see Chapter 4])—cause deafness (**Waardenburg's syndrome** in humans).
Inner tunnel
Inner phalangeal cell
Outer phalangeal cells
Inner pillar cell
Cochlear nerve fibers
Outer pillar cell

Hearing process

Two factors play a significant role during the hearing process (see Figure 9-36):

(1) The high concentration of K^+ in the endolymph and the high concentration of Na^+ in the perilymph determine an electrical potential difference. The ion concentration is regulated by the absorptive and secretory activity of the stria vascularis. (2) Fluid movement in the scala tympani induces the movement of the basilar membrane causing the taller stereocilia to be displaced by the tectorial membrane.

As a result, ion channels at the stereocilia tip open driving K^+ into the cell, which then becomes depolarized. Upon depolarization, an **influx of Ca^{2+}** to the basal region of the hair cells determines the release of neurotransmitters at the hair cell–cochlear nerve fiber synapse and generation of a stimulus. Note the presence of **ribbon synapses** at the base of the hair cells. Changes in electrical potential between the perilymph and the hair cells occur in response to the magnitude of sound.

Clinical significance: Deafness and balance

Cytoskeletal components in the apical domain of hair cells are relatively abundant. Hair cells convert mechanical input, determined by the deflection of apical bundles of stereocilia embedded in the tectorial membrane and the otolithic membrane of the cupula, into an electromechanical input leading to synaptic transmission.

In the absence of the transcription factor **Pou4f3** (for POU domain, transcription factor 4, class 3), hair cells express specific markers (including unconventional **myosin VI** and **VIIa**), and both hair cells and spiral ganglion neurons degenerate.

The tectorial membrane and otolith membrane contain two proteins: **α-tectorin** and **β-tectorin**. When the ***α-tectorin*** encoding gene is mutated, deafness occurs (Figure 9-37).

A mutation in the gene for **connexin 26**, a component of gap junctions on the surface of supporting cells, is responsible for deafness because the recycling of endolymph K^+ from the intercellular spaces to the stria vascularis is disrupted. Connexin 26 is not present in hair cells.

There are several mouse mutants with a decrease in neural crest–derived melanocytes in the stria vascularis. Although the particular role of melanocytes in the stria vascularis is not known, a mutation in the **c-*kit* gene** (encoding the stem cell factor receptor and its ligand; see Chapter 6, Blood and Hematopoiesis, for a discussion of the c-*kit* gene) affects the function of the stria vascularis and the mice are deaf.

Waardenburg's syndrome in humans is an autosomal dominant type of congenital deafness associated with pigment abnormalities, such as partial albinism, and abnormal development of the vestibulocochlear ganglion. Recall that melanocytes have a common origin in the neural crest and are migratory cells.

Essential concepts | Sensory Organs: Vision and Hearing

• Eye

The eyeball consists of three tunics (from outside to inside): (2) Sclera and cornea, (2) uvea, and (3) retina. The interconnected chambers are inside the eye: (1) the anterior chamber (between the corneal endothelium and the anterior surface of the iris), (2) the posterior chamber (between the posterior surface of the iris and the lens and associated with zonular fibers or suspensory ligaments of the lens), and (3) the vitreous cavity (from the lens to the retina).

Aqueous humor (produced by the ciliary body) circulates from the posterior to the anterior chambers. Aqueous humor is drained from the trabecular meshwork into the canal of Schlemm located at the corneal-irideal angle.

The eyeball is protected by the bony orbit, the eyelids, conjunctiva, and the lacrimal apparatus. The ophthalmic artery (a branch of the internal carotid artery) provides nutrients to the eye and the orbit contents.

• The components of the eye derive from three different sites: (1) the surface ectoderm of the head, (2) the lateral neuroectodermal walls of the embryonic brain (diencephalon region), and (3) the mesenchyme. Each optic vesicle, an outpocketing on the right and left side of the diencephalon, becomes a two-layered optic cup. The outer layer becomes the pigmented epithelium; the inner neural layer becomes the retina. The surface of the ectoderm invaginates into the optical vesicle forming the future lens. The outer surface of the optic cup differentiates into the vascular choroid coat (which gives rise to the ciliary body, ciliary muscle, and ciliary processes), the sclera, and the cornea. The mesenchyme, extending into the invagination of the optic cup, forms the vitreous component of the eye.

• Outer tunic: sclera and cornea. The sclera is a thick layer of collagen and elastic fibers produced by fibroblasts. The cornea is a transparent, avascular, and innervated tissue. It consists of five layers: (1) a stratified corneal epithelium exposed to the environment, (2) a supporting membrane or layer of Bowman, (3) a regularly oriented corneal stroma, (4) the membrane of Descemet, and (5) the corneal endothelium (a simple squamous epithelium in contact with aqueous humor).

Middle tunic: uvea. The uvea consists of three regions: (1) choroid, (2) ciliary body, and (3) iris.

The choroid consists of three layers: (1) Bruch's membrane (formed by the basal lamina of the pigmented epithelium of the retina, the basal lamina of fenestrated capillaries corresponding to the choriocapillaris, and connective tissue in between, the site of deposits of amyloid material called drusen), (2) choriocapillaris (the source of nutrients to the outer layers of the retina), and (3) the choroid stroma (containing melanocytes, blood vessels, and neurons of the autonomic nervous system).

The ciliary body, anterior to the ora serrata, consists of two portions: (1) the uveal portion (the supraciliaris portion of the choroid; the ciliary muscle, which controls the curvature of the lens by modifying the length of the suspensory ligaments; and fenestrated capillaries). (2) The neuroepithelial portion (which contributes two cell layers to the ciliary epithelium: a pigmented cell layer and a nonpigmented cell layer, continuous with the sensory retina; the apical surfaces of these two layers face each other and secrete aqueous humor).

The iris is a continuation of the ciliary body. It has an anterior surface without epithelial lining (melanocytes and fibroblasts), and a posterior surface lined by a dual layer of pigmented cells. The stroma contains myoepithelial cells (dilator pupillae muscle) and smooth muscle cells (sphincter pupillae).

The lens is a biconvex, transparent, elastic, and avascular structure kept in place by zonular fibers (extending from the ciliary epithelium and inserting at the equatorial region of the lens capsule). The lens consists of (1) a capsule, (2) an epithelium, and (3) a lens substance (consisting of cortical and nuclear lens fibers). Filensin and crystallins (α, β, and γ) are intermediate filament proteins found in the lens. **Cataracts**, an opacity of the lens, is caused by a change in the solubility of these proteins.

Accommodation is the process by which the lens becomes rounder (to focus the image of a nearby object on the retina) and flattens (when the image of a distant object is focused on the retina).

Accommodation involves the participation of the ciliary muscle, the ciliary body, and the suspensory ligaments. When the ciliary muscle contracts, the tension of the ligaments is reduced (because the ciliary body moves closer to the lens), and the lens acquires a spherical shape (close vision). When the ciliary muscle relaxes, the tension of the ligaments increases (the ciliary body moves away from the lens), and the lens becomes flat (distant vision).

Emmetropia is normal vision. **Myopia** (or nearsightedness) occurs when the eyeball is too deep or the curvature of the lens is not flat enough for distant vision; the image of a distant object forms in front of the retina. **Hyperopia** (or farsightedness) is when the eyeball is too shallow and the curvature of the lens is too flat; the image of a distant object forms behind the retina. Older people become farsighted as the lens loses elasticity, a condition known as **presbyopia**.

Inner tunic: retina. The retina consists of two regions: (1) the outer nonsensory retinal pigmented epithelium (a single layer of pigmented cuboidal cells extending from the optic disk to the ora serrata) and (2) the inner sensory retina (extending from the optic disk to the ciliary epithelium).

The separation of these two layers, resulting from trauma, vascular disease, metabolic disorders, and aging, results in **detachment of the retina**. The pigmented epithelium of the retina is essential for the transport of nutrients from the choroidal blood vesssels to the outer layers of the retina, the removal of waste metabolic products from the sensory retina, the phagocytosis and recycling of photoreceptor disks, and the recycling of the photobleached pigment rhodopsin. The basal lamina of the pigmented epithelium is a component of Bruch's membrane.

The sensory retina consists of four cell groups: (1) photorecepor neurons (rods and cones), (2) conducting neurons (bipolar and ganglion cells), (3) association neurons (horizontal and amacrine cells), and (4) supporting neuroglia Müller cells. Cells are distributed in 10 layers summarized in Figure 9-14. There are three distinct nuclear regions: (1) the outer nuclear layer corresponds to the nuclei of the photoreceptors; (2) the inner nuclear layer corresponds to the nuclei of bipolar cells, horizontal and amacrine cells, and Müller cells; and (3) the ganglion layer contains the nuclei of the ganglion cells. The plexiform and limiting membranes represent sites of contacts among the retinal cells.

Photoreceptor cells (rods and cones) are elongated and consist of two segments: an outer segment, which contains flat membranous disks and an inner segment, the site of synthesis of various cell components. A modified cilium connects the outer and inner segments. It also provides microtubules for molecular motor proteins (kinesins and cytoplasmic dyneins) to deliver materials to the disk assembly site by the mechanism of intraciliary transport. The differences between rods and cones are the following: (1) the outer segment of the rod is cylindrical; in cones it is conical. (2) Rods terminate in a spherule; cones end in a pedicle. Both endings interact with bipolar and horizontal cells. (3) Rods contain the photopigment rhodopsin (night vision); cones contain a similar pigment, iodopsin (color vision).

Bipolar and ganglion cells are connecting neurons receiving impulses from photoreceptor cells.

Horizontal and amacrine cells do not have axons or dendrites, only neuritic processes conducting in both directions.

Müller cells are columnar cells that occupy the spaces between photoreceptor and bipolar and ganglion cells. Müller cells contact the outer segment of the photoreceptors, establishing zonulae adherentes and microvilli, corresponding to the outer limiting membrane. The inner limiting membrane represents the basal lamina of Müller cells.

The fovea centralis, surrounded by the macula lutea, is a specialized area for accurate vision. The optic disk (the exit site of axons derived from ganglion cells and the passage site of blood vessels), including the optic papilla, is not suitable for vision (the blind spot of the retina).

• The eyelids consist of two portions: (1) the outer cutaneous portion and (2) the inner conjunctival portion. The cutaneous portion contains sweat and sebaceous glands, and eyelashes associated with glands of Moll. The tarsal plate (fibroelastic connective tissue) faces the conjunctival lining. Large sebaceous glands, called tarsal glands or meibomian glands, open at the margin of the eyelids. The conjunctiva (polygonal to columnar stratified epithelial lining with mucus-secreting cells) is continuous with the skin and ends at the margin of the cornea, where it becomes stratified squamous epithelium and is continuous with the corneal epithelium.

The lacrimal gland is a tubuloacinar serous gland with myoepithelial cells. Blinking produces compression of the lacrimal glands and the release of fluid (tears).

• Ear

The ear consists of three portions: (1) external ear, (2) middle ear, and (3) inner ear.

The external ear consists of the auricle (external ear), which collects sound waves that are conducted across the external acoustic meatus to the tympanic membrane.

The middle ear (or tympanic cavity) is an air-filled space in the temporal bone that contains the auditory or bony ossicles (malleus, incus, and stapes). The arm of the malleus is attached to the tympanic membrane at one end; the footplate of the stapes is applied to the oval window, an opening of the bony labyrinth. Bony ossicles modulate the movement of the tympanic membrane and apply force to the oval window (to amplify the incoming sound waves). **Otitis media** and **otosclerosis** affect the movement of the ossicles and can lead to hearing loss. The auditory or eustachian tube (elastic cartilage changing to hyaline catilage) links the middle ear to the nasopharynx. It maintains a pressure balance between the tympanic cavity and the external environment.

The inner ear occupies the osseous labyrinth, which contains the membranous labyrinth. The membranous labyrinth houses the vestibular and auditory systems. The membranous labyrinth contains endolymph (high concentration of K^+ and low concentration of Na^+). Perilymph (high concentration of Na^+ and low concentration of K^+) is present between the osseous labyrinth and the membranous labyrinth.

The vestibular system consists of two sacs (utricle and saccule), and three semicircular canals (superior, horizontal, and posterior) arising from the utricle. Ampullae are present at the semicircular canal–utricle connection site.

The endolymphatic duct derives from the utricle and saccule and fuses into a single duct, which terminates in a small dilation, the endolymphatic sac, located between the layers of the meninges. An increase in the volume of endolymph causes **Ménière's disease**, characterized by vertigo, nausea, positional nystagmus, vomiting, and tinnitus (ringing in the ears).

The ampulla has a crista, an elevation covered by sensory epithelium consisting of type I and II hair cells and supporting cells, topped by the cupula, a gelatinous substance surrounded by endolymph. Semicircular canals respond to rotational movements of the head and body (angular acceleration).

Hair cells have an apical domain containing 60 to 100 stereocilia (supported by an actin-containing cuticular plate) and a single kinocilium. The free ends of the stereocilia and kinocilium are embedded in the cupula.

The maculae of the utricle and saccule respond to translational movements (linear acceleration). Maculae consist of a sensory epithelium (type I and II hair cells and supporting cells) topped by the otolithic membrane, a gelatinous substance similar to cristae, except for the presence of otoliths containing calcium carbonate.

The auditory system consists of the cochlea, a coiled duct. The cochlea has three spiraling chambers: (1) the cochlear duct (called scala media), (2) the scala vesibuli, starting at the oval window, and (3) the scala tympani, ending at the round window. The scala vestibuli and scala tympani contain perilymph and communicate at the helicotrema. Review Figures 9-31 and 9-33.

The organ of Corti is the sensory epithelium of the cochlea. It contains hair cells and supporting cells. Instead of a cupula found in the crista and macula, the sensory epithelium of the cochlea is in contact with the tectorial membrane. The organ of Corti consists of two groups of hair cells: inner and outer hair cells, separated from each other by the inner tunnel, limited by outer and inner pillar cells. Additional cell types can be reviewed in Figure 9-34.

The modiolus, the spiraling bony axis of the cochlea, houses the spiral ganglion.

Deafness occurs when α-tectorin is defective in the tectorial membrane, connexin 26 is not present in gap junctions linking cochlear supporting cells, and the vestibulocochlear ganglion is not developed (Waardenburg's syndrome).

10. IMMUNE-LYMPHATIC SYSTEM

Organization of the immune-lymphatic system

The lymphatic system includes **primary** and **secondary lymphoid organs.**

The primary lymphoid organs produce the cell components of the immune system. They are (1) the **bone marrow** (Figure 10-1) and (2) the **thymus.**

The secondary lymphoid organs are the sites where immune responses occur. They include (1) the **lymph nodes**, (2) the **spleen**, (3) the **tonsils**, and (4) aggregates of lymphocytes and antigen-presenting cells in the **lung** (bronchial-associated lymphoid tissue [BALT] and the mucosa of the **digestive tract** (gut-associated lymphoid tissue [GALT] including **Peyer's patches**).

The main function of the **lymphoid organs**, as components of the immune system, is to protect the body against invading **pathogens** or **antigens** (bacteria, viruses, and parasites). The basis for this defense mechanism, or **immune response**, is the ability to distinguish **self** from **nonself.** Because pathogens can enter the body at any point, the lymphatic system is widely distributed.

The **two key cell components of the immune system** are **lymphocytes** and

Figure 10-1. **Lineage origin of the lymphoid progeny within the context of hematopoiesis**

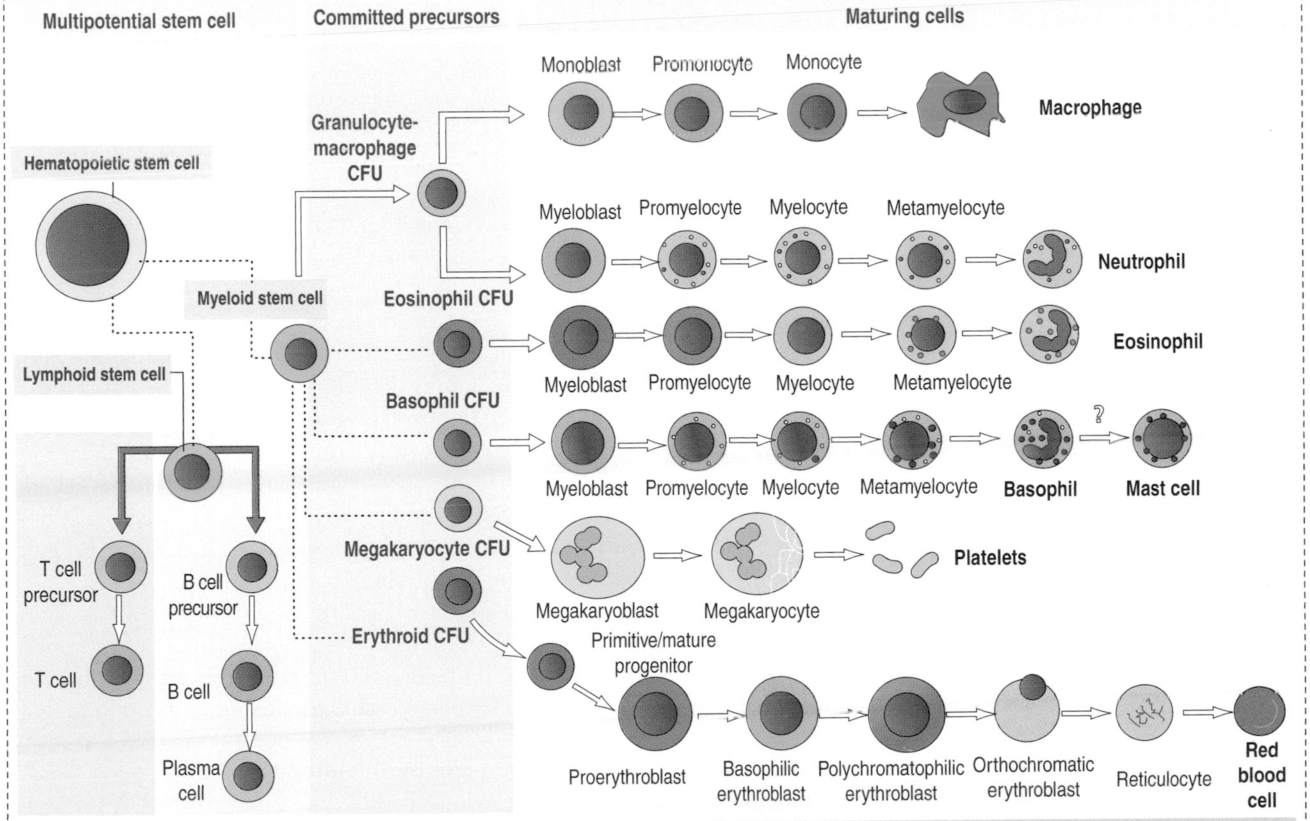

The cells of the immune system arise from the hematopoietic stem cell in the bone marrow. We discuss in Chapter 6, Blood and Hematopoiesis, that hematopoietic stem cells divide to produce two specialized stem cells: **lymphoid stem cell**, which generates B and T lymphocytes, and a **myeloid stem cell**, which gives rise to leukocytes, erythrocytes, megakaryocytes, and macrophages.

B lymphocytes (B cells) differentiate in the bone marrow, When activated outside the bone marrow, B cells differentiate into antibody-secreting **plasma cells. T lymphocytes** (T cells) differentiate in the **thymus** into cells that can activate other cells of the immune system (helper cells) or kill bacteria- or virus-infected cells (cytolytic or cytotoxic cells). **CFU**: colony-forming unit.

Table 10-1 Cells participating in immune reactions

Lymphocytes	
B cells	Respond to cell-free and plasma membrane–bound antigens
T cells Helper T cells Cytolytic T cells (CTLs)	Respond to cell-bound antigens
Natural killer cells	Cell population lacking T cell receptor (TCR) and CD4 and CD8 coreceptors
Accessory cells	
Macrophages	Monocyte-derived cells
Dendritic cells	Monocyte-derived cells (e.g., Langerhans cells of the epidermis)
Follicular dendritic cells	Found in lymphatic nodules
Effector cells	
Macrophages, CTLs, neutrophils	

accessory cells (Table 10-1). Lymphocytes include two major cell groups: (1) **B cells**, responding to cell-free and cell-bound antigens; and (2) **T cells**, subdivided into two categories: **helper T cells** and **cytolytic** or **cytotoxic T cells**. T cells respond to cell-bound antigens presented by specific molecules.

After leaving the two **primary** organs (bone marrow and thymus), mature B and T cells circulate in the blood until they reach one of the various **secondary lymphoid organs** (lymph nodes, spleen, and tonsils).

B and T cells can leave the bloodstream through specialized venules called **high endothelial venules**, so called because they are lined by tall endothelial cells instead of the typical squamous endothelial cell type. In this chapter we review the mechanism of cell homing within the context of **inflammation**.

The accessory cells include two monocyte-derived cell types: **macrophages** and **dendritic cells.** An example of a dendritic cell is the **Langerhans cell** found in the epidermis of the skin. A third type, the **follicular dendritic cell**, is present in lymphatic nodules of the lymph nodes. Follicular dendritic cells differ from ordinary dendritic cells in that they do not derive from a bone marrow precursor.

Before we start our discussion of the origin, differentiation, and interaction of lymphocytes and accessory cells, we will define the characteristics of the immune system. Then, we will be able to integrate the structural aspects of each major lymphatic organ with the specific characteristics of the immune responses.

Innate (natural) and adaptive (acquired) immunity

Immunity in general is the reaction of cells and tissues to foreign (nonself) substances or **pathogens** such as microorganisms, parasites, proteins, and polysaccharides (Table 10-2).

Innate or **natural immunity** is the simplest mechanism of protection, does not require previous exposure to a pathogen, and has rapid responsiveness. A consequence of an initial exposure to a pathogen is adaptive or acquired immunity. The contributors to innate immunity are an epithelial surface or barrier, neutrophils and macrophages with phagocytic properties, natural killer cells (which we analyze later), and a number of proteins, including cytokines and components

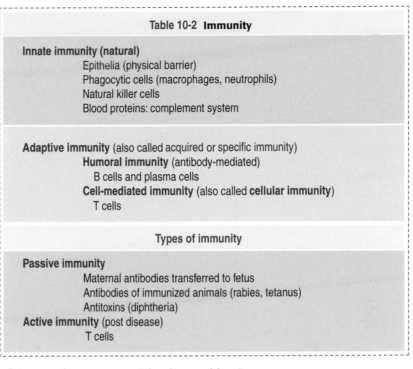

Table 10-2 **Immunity**	
Innate immunity (natural)	
	Epithelia (physical barrier)
	Phagocytic cells (macrophages, neutrophils)
	Natural killer cells
	Blood proteins: complement system
Adaptive immunity (also called acquired or specific immunity)	
	Humoral immunity (antibody-mediated)
	B cells and plasma cells
	Cell-mediated immunity (also called **cellular immunity**)
	T cells
Types of immunity	
Passive immunity	
	Maternal antibodies transferred to fetus
	Antibodies of immunized animals (rabies, tetanus)
	Antitoxins (diphtheria)
Active immunity (post disease)	
	T cells

of the complement system (also discussed later).

Adaptive or **acquired immunity** develops when an individual is exposed to an infectious pathogen. Lymphocytes and cytokines are directly involved in generating an adaptive or acquired immune response against a pathogen or antigen. To achieve an immune response, adaptive immunity relies on an effector mechanism with the participation of **effector cells**, also utilized by innate immunity: macrophages, neutrophils, and killer cells. Essentially, adaptive immunity is the perfection of innate immunity.

Adaptive immunity involves two types of responses to an antigen (pathogen): The first response is mediated by **antibodies** produced by plasma cells, the final differentiation product of B cells as we have seen in Chapter 4, Connective Tissue. This response is known as **humoral immunity** and operates against antigens located outside a cell or bound to its surface. When antibodies bind to an antigen or toxins produced by a pathogen, they can facilitate the phagocytic action of macrophages or recruit leukocytes and mast cells to take advantage of their cytokines and mediators, respectively, and strengthen a response. Humoral immunity results in persistent antibody production and production of memory cells.

The second type of response **requires the uptake of a pathogen by a phagocyte**. An intracellular pathogen is not accessible to antibodies and requires a cell-mediated response, or **cell-mediated immunity**. T cells, B cells, and antigen-presenting cells are the key players in cell-mediated immunity.

A consequence of adaptive or acquired immunity is the protection of the individual when a second encounter with the pathogen occurs. This protection is specific against the same pathogen and, therefore, adaptive or acquired immunity is also called **specific immunity**.

Active immunity is the form of immunity resulting from exposure to a pathogen. **Passive immunity** is a temporary form of immunity conferred by serum or lymphocytes transferred from an immunized individual to another individual who has not been exposed or cannot respond to a pathogen. The transfer of maternal antibodies to the fetus is a form of passive immunity that protects newborns from infections until they can develop active immunity.

Properties of adaptive or acquired immunity

Both humoral and cell-mediated immunity developed against foreign pathogens

Figure 10-2. **Development of B cells in bone marrow**

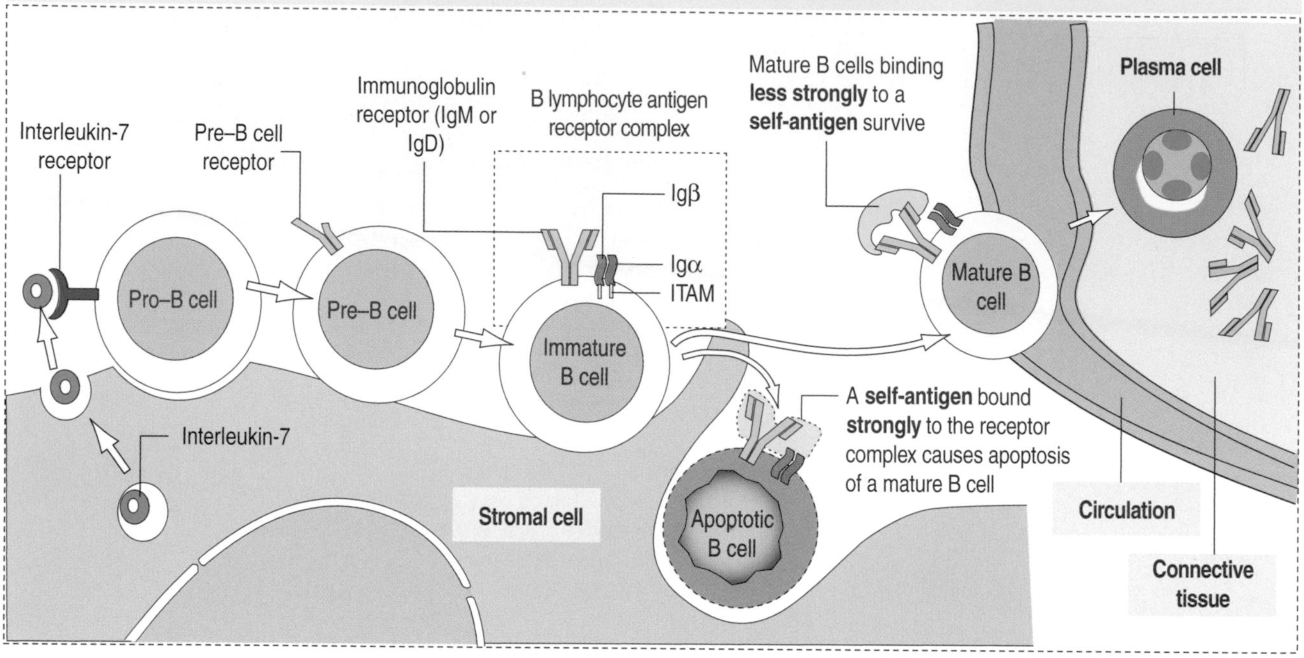

have the following characteristics:

1. **Specificity**: Specific domains of an antigen are recognized by individual lymphocytes. We will see later how cell membrane receptors on lymphocytes can distinguish and respond to subtle variations in the structure of antigens.

2. **Diversity**: Lymphocytes utilize molecular mechanisms to modify their antigen receptors in such a way that they can recognize and respond to a large number and types of antigenic domains.

3. **Memory**: The exposure of lymphocytes to an antigen results in two events: their antigen-specific clonal expansion by mitosis, as well as the generation of reserve **memory cells**. Memory cells can react more rapidly and efficiently when exposed again to the same antigen.

4. **Self-limitation**: An immune response is stimulated by a specific antigen. When the antigen is neutralized or disappears, the response ceases.

5. **Tolerance**: An immune response pursues the removal of a non-self antigen while being "tolerant" to self-antigens. Tolerance is achieved by a selection mechanism that eliminates lymphocytes expressing receptors specific for self-antigens. A failure of self-tolerance (and specificity) leads to a group of disorders called **autoimmune diseases**.

Development of B cells

Figure 10-1 illustrates the concept that the bone marrow is the site of origin of B and T lymphocytes from a lymphoid stem cell. In Chapter 6, Blood and Hematopoiesis, we discuss developmental aspects of the myeloid and erythroid lineages from a hematopoietic stem cell. The same hematopoietic stem cell gives rise to a **lymphoid stem cell** that generates precursors for B cells, T cells, and natural killer cells. **B cells mature in the bone marrow**, whereas **the thymus is the site of maturation of T cells.**

Stem B cells in the bone marrow proliferate and mature in contact with bone marrow **stromal cells** under the influence of **interleukin**-7 (IL-7) (Figure 10-2). During maturation, on their surface B cells express **immunoglobulins M** (IgM) or **D** (IgD) interacting with two additional proteins linked to each other, **immunoglobulins** α (**Ig**α) and β (**Ig**β). The cell surface IgM or IgD, together with the conjoined **Ig**α and **Ig**β, form the **B cell antigen receptor complex**. The intracellular domains of Igα and Igβ contain a tyrosine-rich domain called

Box 10-A | CD antigens

- Cell surface molecules recognized by monoclonal antibodies are called **antigens.** These antigens are **markers** that enable the identification and characterization of cell populations. A surface marker that identifies a member of a group of cells, has a defined structure, and is also recognized in other members of the group by a monoclonal antibody is called a **cluster of differentiation (CD)**.
- A **helper T cell**, which expresses the **CD4** marker, can be differentiated from a **killer T cell**, which does not contain CD4 but expresses the **CD8** marker.
- CD markers permit the classification of T cells that participate in inflammatory and immune reactions. **CD antigens promote cell-cell interaction and adhesion as well as signaling leading to T cell activation.**

immunoreceptor tyrosine-based activation motif (ITAM).

Binding of an antigen to the B cell antigen receptor complex induces the phosphorylation of tyrosine in the ITAM, which, in turn, activates transcription factors that drive the expression of genes required for further development of B cells.

Self-antigens present in the bone marrow test the antigen-binding specificity of IgM or IgD on B cell surfaces. This is a required testing step before B cells can continue their maturation, enter peripheral lymphoid tissues, and interact with foreign (non-self) antigens. **Self-antigens** binding **strongly** to two or more IgM or IgD receptor molecules on B cells induce **apoptosis. Self-antigens** with a **weaker binding affinity** for the B cell antigen receptor complex enable the survival and maturation of these B cells when ITAMs of IgM- or IgD-associated Igα and Igβ transduce signaling events, resulting in further differentiation of B cells and the entrance of mature B cells into the circulation.

Major histocompatibility complex and human leukocyte antigens

The presentation of antigens to T cells is carried out by specialized proteins encoded by genes in the major histocompatibility locus and present on the surface of antigen-presenting cells. Antigen-presenting cells survey the body, find and internalize antigens by phagocytosis, break them down into antigenic peptide fragments, and bind them to **major histocompatibility complex** (MHC) molecules (Figure 10-3) so that the **antigen peptide fragment–MHC complex** can be exposed later on the surface of the cells. The *MHC* gene locus expresses gene products responsible for the rejection of grafted tissue between two genetically incompatible hosts.

There are two types of mouse MHC gene products: **class I MHC** and **class II MHC.** The class I MHC molecule consists of two polypeptide chains: an **α chain**, consisting of three domains (α_1, α_2 and α_3) encoded by the *MHC* gene locus, and **β_2-microglobulin**, not encoded by the *MHC* gene locus. Antigens are housed in a cleft formed by the α_1 and α_2 domains. CD8, a coreceptor on the surface of cytolytic T cells, binds to the α_3 domain of class I MHC. See Box 10-A.

Class II MHC consists of two polypeptide chains, an α chain and a β chain. Both chains are encoded by the *MHC* gene locus. The α_1 and β_1 domains form an antigen-binding cleft. CD4, a coreceptor on the surface of helper T cells, binds to the β_2 domain of class II MHC.

All nucleated cells express class I MHC molecules. Class II MHC molecules are restricted mainly to antigen-presenting cells (dendritic cells, macrophages, and B cells), epithelial reticular cells of the thymus, and endothelial cells.

The MHC-equivalent molecules in the human are designated **human leukocyte antigens (HLAs)**. HLA molecules are structurally and functionally homologous to mouse MHC molecules and the gene locus (3500 kilobases in length) is present on human chromosome 5 (β_2-microglobulin is encoded by a gene on chromosome 15).

The **class I MHC locus encodes** three major proteins in the human: **HLA-A, HLA-B**, and **HLA-C.** The **class II MHC locus encodes HLA-DR** (R for antigenically related), **HLA-DQ**, and **HLA-DP** (Q and P preceding R in the alphabet).

T cell receptor complex

In addition to MHC molecules, subsets of T cells have cell surface receptors that enable each of them to recognize a different antigen peptide–MHC combination. Antigen recognition involves stable antigen-presenting cell–T cell adhesiveness followed by an activating signaling cascade by T cells.

The receptor that recognizes specific antigenic peptides presented by class I and class II MHC molecules is the **T cell receptor (TCR)**. TCR acts together with accessory cell surface molecules, called **coreceptors**, to stabilize the binding of antigen-presenting cells to T cells.

The TCR consists of two disulfide-linked transmembrane polypeptide chains:

Figure 10-3. **Structure of the T cell receptor and class I and II major histocompatibility complex (MHC)**

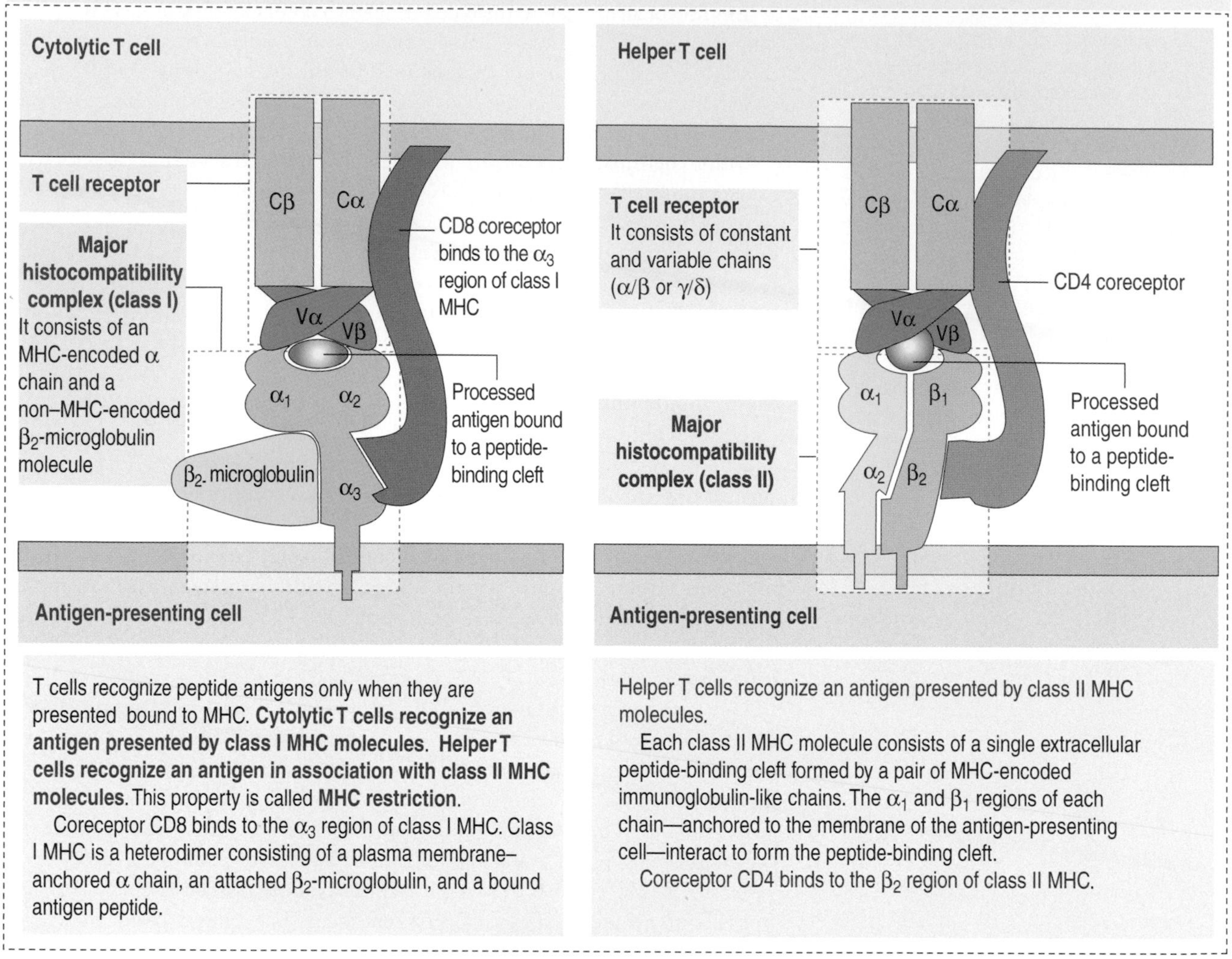
Cytolytic T cell
T cell receptor
Major histocompatibility complex (class I)
It consists of an MHC-encoded α chain and a non–MHC-encoded β2-microglobulin molecule
Cβ
Cα
Vα
Vβ
α1
α2
α3
β2- microglobulin
CD8 coreceptor binds to the α3 region of class I MHC
Processed antigen bound to a peptide-binding cleft
Antigen-presenting cell
Helper T cell
T cell receptor
It consists of constant and variable chains (α/β or γ/δ)
Major histocompatibility complex (class II)
β1
β2
CD4 coreceptor
Processed antigen bound to a peptide-binding cleft
Antigen-presenting cell
T cells recognize peptide antigens only when they are presented bound to MHC. Cytolytic T cells recognize an antigen presented by class I MHC molecules. Helper T cells recognize an antigen in association with class II MHC molecules. This property is called MHC restriction.
Coreceptor CD8 binds to the α3 region of class I MHC. Class I MHC is a heterodimer consisting of a plasma membrane–anchored α chain, an attached β2-microglobulin, and a bound antigen peptide.
Helper T cells recognize an antigen presented by class II MHC molecules.
Each class II MHC molecule consists of a single extracellular peptide-binding cleft formed by a pair of MHC-encoded immunoglobulin-like chains. The α1 and β1 regions of each chain—anchored to the membrane of the antigen-presenting cell—interact to form the peptide-binding cleft.
Coreceptor CD4 binds to the β2 region of class II MHC.

the α **chain** and the β **chain** (see Figure 10-3). A limited number of T cells have a TCR composed of γ and δ chains. Each α and β chain consists of a **variable** (Vα and Vβ) domain and a **constant** (Cα and Cβ) domain. When compared with the immunoglobulin molecule, the Vα and Vβ domains are structurally and functionally similar to the antigen-binding fragment (Fab) of immunoglobulins.

The TCR molecule is associated with two proteins, CD3 and ζ (not shown in Figure 10-3), forming the **TCR complex**. CD3 and ζ have a signaling role and are present in all T cells. CD3 contains the ITAM cytoplasmic domain previously mentioned as part of the B cell antigen receptor complex and involved in signaling functions.

CD4 and CD8 coreceptors

CD4 and CD8 are T cell surface proteins interacting selectively with class II MHC and class I MHC molecules, respectively. When the TCR recognizes an antigen bound to the cleft of MHC, CD4 or CD8 coreceptors cooperate in the activation of T cell function (see Figure 10-3).

CD4 and CD8 are members of the immunoglobulin (Ig) superfamily. In Chapter 1, Epithelium, we discuss the function and structure of cell adhesion molecules belonging to the Ig superfamily.

Members of the Ig superfamily have a variable number of extracellular Ig-like domains. The two terminal Ig-like domains of CD4 bind to the β_2 domain of the class II MHC (see Figure 10-3). The single Ig-like domain of CD8 binds to the α_3 domain of the class I MHC. Thus, **CD4$^+$ helper T cells recognize**

Figure 10-4. **General features of helper and cytolytic T cells**

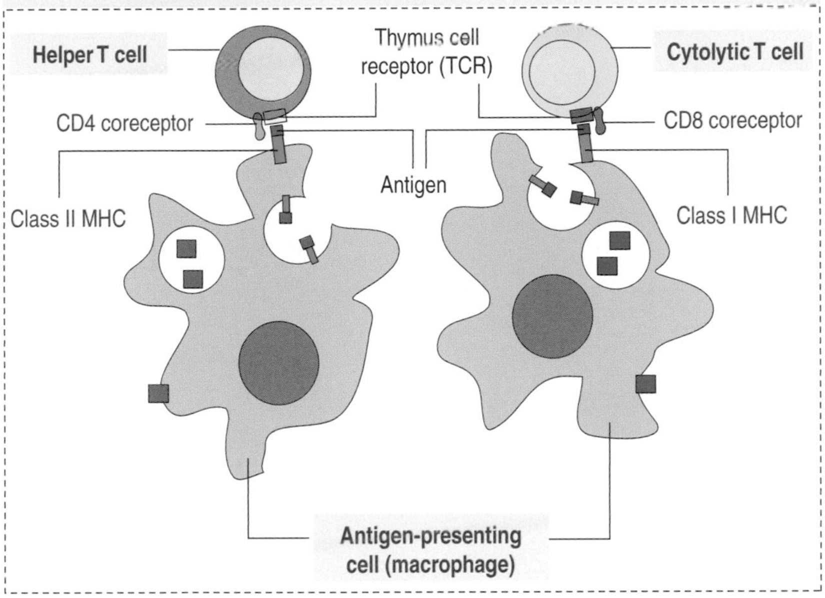
Helper T cell
Thymus cell
receptor (TCR)
Cytolytic T cell
CD4 coreceptor
CD8 coreceptor
Antigen
Class II MHC
Class I MHC
Antigen-presenting
cell (macrophage)

antigens associated with class II MHC, and **CD8$^+$ cytolytic T cells (cytolytic thymus-derived lymphocytes [CTL]) respond to antigens presented by class I MHC** (Figure 10-4).

MHC molecules and adaptive immune responses

T cells are **MHC-restricted.** T cells are able to react against a **foreign** antigen fragment bound to their **own** (**self**-) MCH molecules and contribute to **adaptive immune responses.** T cells should **not respond** to self-antigen peptide fragments bound to self-MHC molecules.This lack of response is called **self-tolerance.** Developing T cells express unique TCRs generated by random rearrangement of a variety of gene segments. These randomly produced TCRs provide the diversity required to identify numerous foreign peptides.

During their maturation in the thymus, T cells are selected to be **self-MHC–restricted** and **self-tolerant.** This selective process, known as **positive selection** (see Figure 10-5), occurs only when self-MCH–restricted T cells are selected. **Negative selection** takes place when T cells **do not bind to any MHC** or bind to the **body's tissue-specific antigens (self-molecules).** We discuss later how a portfolio of self-antigens expressed in the thymus permits the elimination of autoreactive T cells by apoptosis. Only those **T cells that can recognize foreign peptides and self-MHC survive,** leave the thymus, and migrate into the secondary lymphoid organs.

The clonal selection process occurs in the thymus (Figure 10-5). The cortex of the thymus contains branching and interconnected **thymic cortical epithelial cells** involved in the **positive selection of T cells.** The medulla of the thymus houses **thymic medullary epithelial cells** involved in the **negative selection of potentially autoreactive T cells.** Contact between MHC molecules on the thymic epithelial cell surfaces and TCRs of developing T cells is an important feature in positive selection.

T cells developing in the thymus express specific cell surface molecules

Two major events take place in the thymus during T cell maturation (see Figure 10-5): (1) a rearrangement of the gene-encoding protein components of the **TCR** and (2) the transient coexistence of TCR-associated **coreceptors CD4 and CD8.**

When precursor cells—derived from the bone marrow—enter the **cortex** of the thymus, they lack surface molecules typical of mature T cells. Because **they still**

Figure 10-5. Maturation of T cells involves changes in cell surface molecules

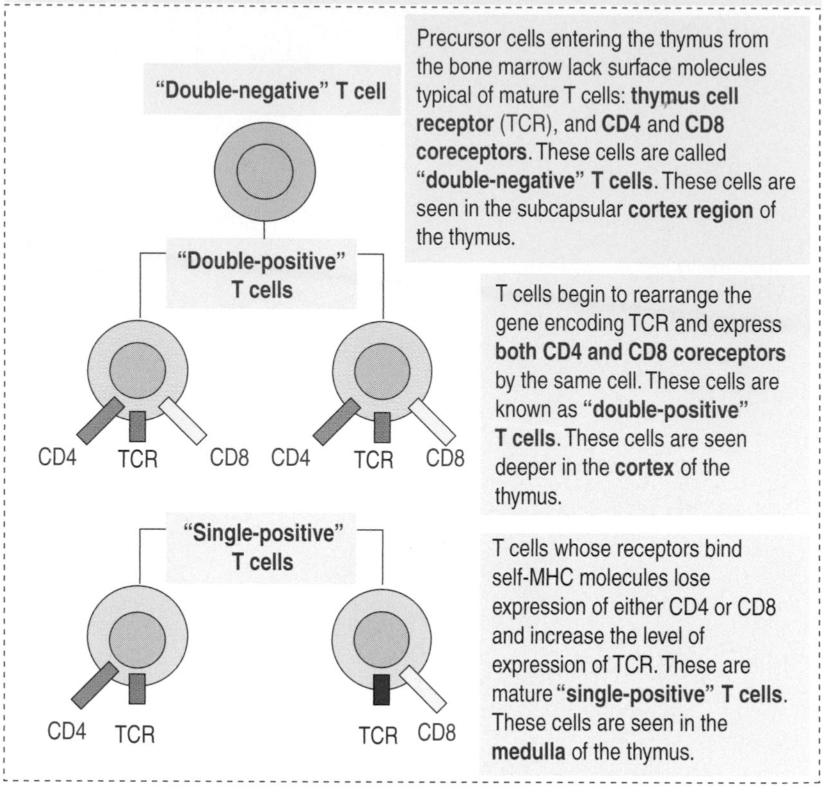
"Double-negative" T cell
Precursor cells entering the thymus from the bone marrow lack surface molecules typical of mature T cells: **thymus cell receptor** (TCR), and **CD4** and **CD8 coreceptors**. These cells are called **"double-negative" T cells**. These cells are seen in the subcapsular **cortex region** of the thymus.
"Double-positive" T cells
CD4
TCR
CD8
CD4
TCR
CD8
T cells begin to rearrange the gene encoding TCR and express **both CD4 and CD8 coreceptors** by the same cell. These cells are known as **"double-positive" T cells**. These cells are seen deeper in the **cortex** of the thymus.
"Single-positive" T cells
CD4
TCR
TCR
CD8
T cells whose receptors bind self-MHC molecules lose expression of either CD4 or CD8 and increase the level of expression of TCR. These are mature **"single-positive" T cells**. These cells are seen in the **medulla** of the thymus.

do not express CD4 and CD8, they are called "double-negative" T cells.

After interacting with thymic **epithelial cells**, double-negative T cells proliferate, differentiate, and express the first T cell–specific molecules: TCR and coreceptors CD4 and CD8.

TCR consists of two pairs of subunits: **αβ chains** or **γδ chains** (see Figure 10-3). Each chain can vary in sequence from one T cell to another. This variation is determined by the random combination of gene segments and has a bearing on which foreign antigen T cells can recognize.

Maturation of T cells proceeds through a stage where **both CD4 and CD8 coreceptors and low levels of TCR are expressed by the same cell**. These cells are known as **"double-positive" T cells.** Double-positive T cells **can** or **cannot** recognize self-MHC. Those cells that can recognize self-MHC eventually mature and express one of the two coreceptor molecules (CD4 or CD8) and become **"single-positive" T cells.** Double-positive cells that cannot recognize self-MHC fail positive selection and are discarded.

T cell–mediated immunity

When T cells complete their development in the thymus, they enter the bloodstream and migrate to the peripheral lymphoid organs in search of an antigen on the surface of an **antigen-presenting cell.**

Helper T cells contain both the **TCR** and **CD4 coreceptor**. Helper T cells recognize **class II MHC** on antigen-presenting cells.

There are **two distinct subtypes of helper T cells** derived from the same $CD4^+$ T cell precursor: **TH1** and **TH2** cells.

Immune responses controlled by TH2 cells are observed in patients with **helminthic** (Greek *helmins*, worm) **intestinal parasites.** TH2 cells produce interleukin-4 (IL-4) and interleukin-13 (IL-13), among other cytokines, and determine the production of immunoglobulin E by plasma cells to activate the responses of mast cells, basophils, and eosinophils. The activation of macrophage responses is minimal in TH2-driven immune responses.

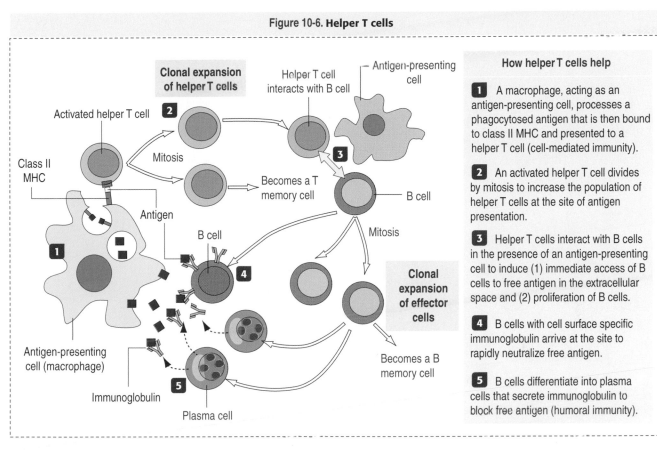

Figure 10-6. **Helper T cells**

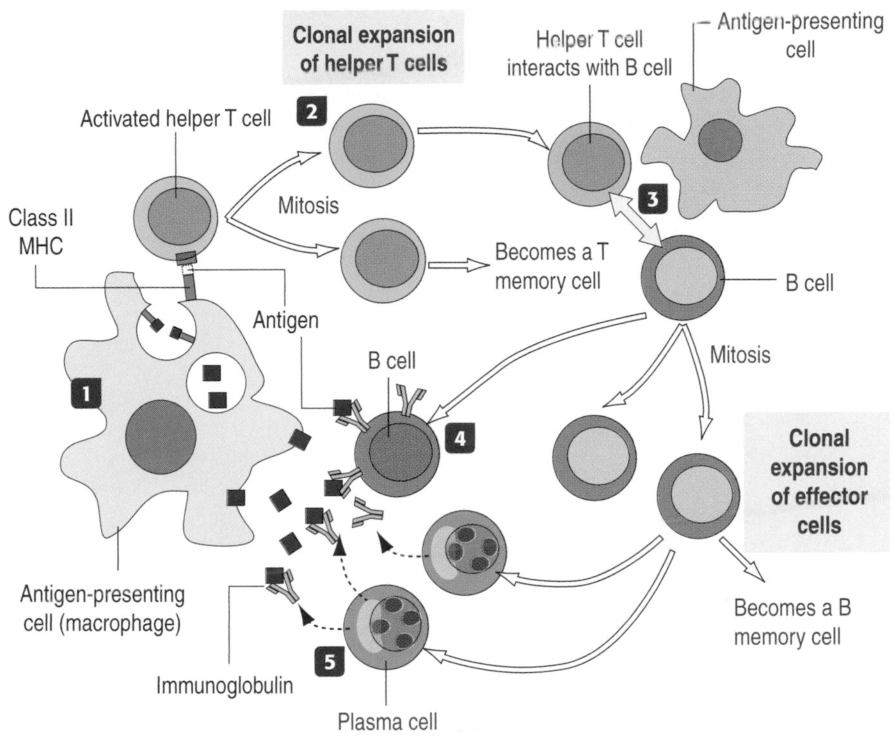
Clonal expansion of helper T cells
Helper T cell interacts with B cell
Antigen-presenting cell
Activated helper T cell
2
Mitosis
3
Class II MHC
Becomes a T memory cell
B cell
Antigen
B cell
Mitosis
1
4
Clonal expansion of effector cells
Antigen-presenting cell (macrophage)
Becomes a B memory cell
Immunoglobulin
5
Plasma cell

How helper T cells help

1 A macrophage, acting as an antigen-presenting cell, processes a phagocytosed antigen that is then bound to class II MHC and presented to a helper T cell (cell-mediated immunity).

2 An activated helper T cell divides by mitosis to increase the population of helper T cells at the site of antigen presentation.

3 Helper T cells interact with B cells in the presence of an antigen-presenting cell to induce (1) immediate access of B cells to free antigen in the extracellular space and (2) proliferation of B cells.

4 B cells with cell surface specific immunoglobulin arrive at the site to rapidly neutralize free antigen.

5 B cells differentiate into plasma cells that secrete immunoglobulin to block free antigen (humoral immunity).

By contrast, TH1 cells participate in the regulation of immune responses caused by **intracellular pathogens** (viruses causing infections, certain bacteria, or single-cell parasites) with the significant participation of macrophages. TH1 cells produce interferon-γ, which can suppress the activity of TH2 cells.

Cytolytic or **killer T cells** display both the **TCR** and **CD8 coreceptor**. CTLs recognize **class I MHC** on antigen-presenting cells. We will return to the clinical significance of helper and cytolytic T cells when we discuss their involvement in the pathology of human immunodeficiency virus-type 1 (HIV-1) infection, allergy, and cancer immunotherapy.

How do helper T cells help?

Helper T cells are activated when they recognize the antigen peptide–class II MHC complex (Figure 10-6).

In the presence of cells with antigen peptide bound to class II MHC, helper T cells proliferate by mitosis and secrete **cytokines**, also called **interleukins**. These chemical signals, in turn, attract B cells, which also have receptor molecules of single specificity on their surface (**immunoglobulin receptor**). **Unlike helper T cells, B cells can recognize free antigen peptides without MHC molecules.**

When activated by interleukins produced by the proliferating helper T cells, B cells also divide and differentiate into **plasma cells secreting immunoglobulins**, a soluble form of their receptors. Secreted immunoglobulins diffuse freely, bind to antigen peptides to neutralize them, or trigger their destruction by enzymes or macrophages.

Plasma cells synthesize **only one class of immunoglobulin** (several thousand immunoglobulin molecules per second; lifetime of a plasma cell is from 10 to 20 days). Five classes of immunoglobulins are recognized in humans: **IgG, IgA, IgM, IgE**, and **IgD**.

Some T and B cells become **memory cells**, ready to eliminate the same antigen if it recurs in the future. The **secondary immune response** (reencounter with

Figure 10-7. **Cytolytic T cells**

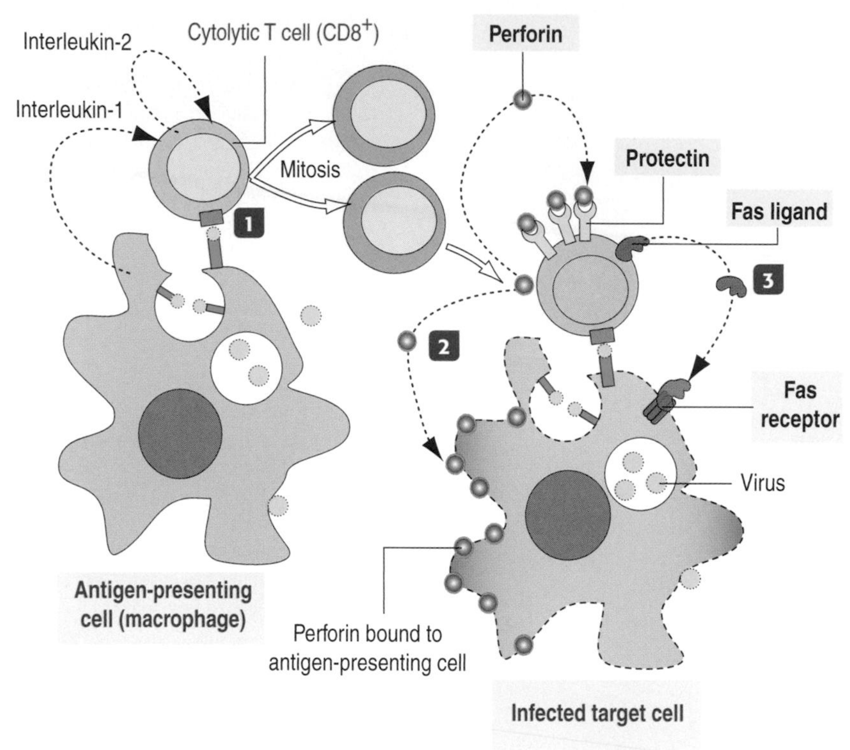

How cytolytic T cells kill

1 A cytolytic T cell binds to an antigen-presenting cell and is activated by interleukin-1 produced by the antigen-presenting cell (paracrine mechanism), and by interleukin-2, produced by the cytolytic T cell (autocrine mechanism). The cytolytic T cell divides by mitosis to increase the cell population.

2 In the presence of an antigen-presenting cell containing a pathogen antigen (a virus), cytolytic T cells release **perforin** to kill the infected macrophage. The cytolytic T cell protects itself with **protectin**, a cell surface molecule that binds perforin. However, the infected antigen-presenting cell lacks protectin and is vulnerable to the action of perforin. Perforin alters cell permeability to ions and the antigen-presenting cell is destroyed.

3 **Fas ligand**, released by the cytolytic T cell, destroys by **apoptosis** the target cell by binding to its **Fas receptor**.

the same antigen that triggered their production) is more rapid and of greater magnitude. Memory cells recirculate for many years and provide a surveillance system directed against foreign antigens.

How do cytolytic T cells kill?

Another function of helper T cells is **to secrete cytokines to stimulate the proliferation of cytolytic T cells** that recognize the antigen peptide–class I MHC complex on the surface of antigen-presenting cells.

The subset of CTLs initiates a **target cell destruction** process (Figure 10-7) by (1) attaching firmly to the antigen-presenting cell with the help of integrins and cell adhesion molecules (CAMs) on the cell surface of the target cell and (2) inducing cell membrane damage by the release of pore-forming proteins (called **perforins**). These pores facilitate the unregulated entry of various lytic substances, water, and salts. The CTL protects itself by a membrane protein, **protectin**, that inactivates perforin, blocking its insertion into the CTL membrane.

CTLs can also destroy target cells by the **Fas-Fas ligand mechanism** seen during **apoptosis** (see Chapter 3, Cell Signaling). When the CTL receptor recognizes an antigen on the surface of a target cell, Fas ligand is induced in the CTL. The interaction of Fas ligand with the trimerized Fas receptor on the target cell surface (see Figure 10-7) triggers the apoptotic cascade by activation of procaspases into caspases that determine cell death.

Players in the immune responses: Regulatory and effector cells

B cells can differentiate into immunoglobulin-secreting plasma cells. Plasma cells are **effector cells**. T cells differentiate into **regulatory**, **suppressor**, and **effector T cells**.

Regulatory T cells include **helper T cells**, which cooperate with B cells to stimulate the proliferation and differentiation of B cells into immunoglobulin-secreting plasma cells and the cytolytic activation of killer T cells.

Figure 10-8. Natural killer T cells

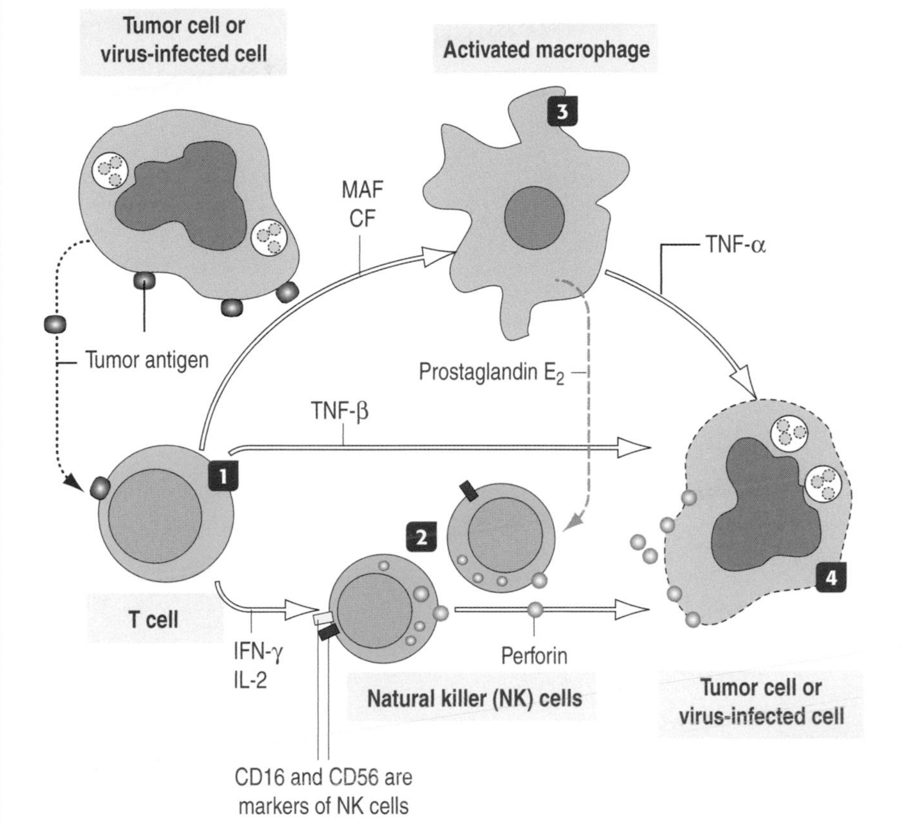

How natural killer cells kill

1 T cells are activated by tumor antigens that induce them to release cytokines, such as **interleukin-2** (IL-2), **interferon-γ** (IFN-γ), **macrophage-activating factor** (MAF), **chemotactic factor** (CF), and **tumor necrosis factor-β** (TNF-β).

2 Natural killer (NK) cells represent a population of naturally occurring cells cytotoxic to tumor cells or virus-infected cells. IL-2 stimulates the proliferation of NK cells. IFN-γ activates NK cells, which destroy tumor cells by the release of perforin. NK cells are not activated by direct action of an antigen and lack T cell receptor.

3 Macrophages are attracted to the tumor site and are activated by MAF and CF. Activated macrophages inhibit tumor cell proliferation or kill tumor cells by releasing **tumor necrosis factor-α** (TNF-α). **Prostaglandin E_2** downregulates NK cell activity.

4 Tumor cells or virus-infected cells are directly destroyed by TNF-β (produced by T cells activated by the tumor antigen), TNF-α (produced by macrophages), and **perforin** (released by activated NK cells).

Suppressor T cells, acting on helper T cells to moderate or inhibit their activities, also modulate the differentiation of B cells into plasma cells. There are two subsets of T cells (TH1 and TH2) that produce different cytokines with distinct functions. TH1 cells produce interferon-γ, whereas TH2 cells produce IL-4 and IL-13. Interferon-γ, produced by TH1 cells, stimulates the differentiation of TH1 cells but suppresses the proliferation of TH2 cells. Furthermore, TH2-derived IL-4 suppresses the activation of TH1 cells.

Effector T cells include **cytolytic** or **killer T cells** and **natural killer cells**. CTLs can lyse cells that bear antigens for which they are specific. Cell killing is caused by the release of perforin or Fas ligand as already discussed.

Natural killer cells (Figure 10-8) destroy virus-infected and tumor cells, but this activity **does not depend on antigen activation**. Natural killer cells can destroy antibody-coated target cells by a mechanism called **antibody-dependent cell-mediated cytotoxicity** (ADCC). Natural killer cells do not belong to the T or B cell types (they do not express TCR) and have **CD16** and **CD56 receptors**.

Patients deficient in natural killer cells are susceptible to the early phases of **herpesvirus infection**.

Clinical significance: Acquired immunodeficiency syndrome

The **acquired immunodeficiency syndrome** (AIDS) is caused by HIV-1 and is characterized by significant immunosuppression associated with opportunistic infections, malignancies, and degeneration of the central nervous system.

HIV infects macrophages, dendritic cells, and predominantly CD4-bearing

Figure 10-9. Immune system and HIV infection

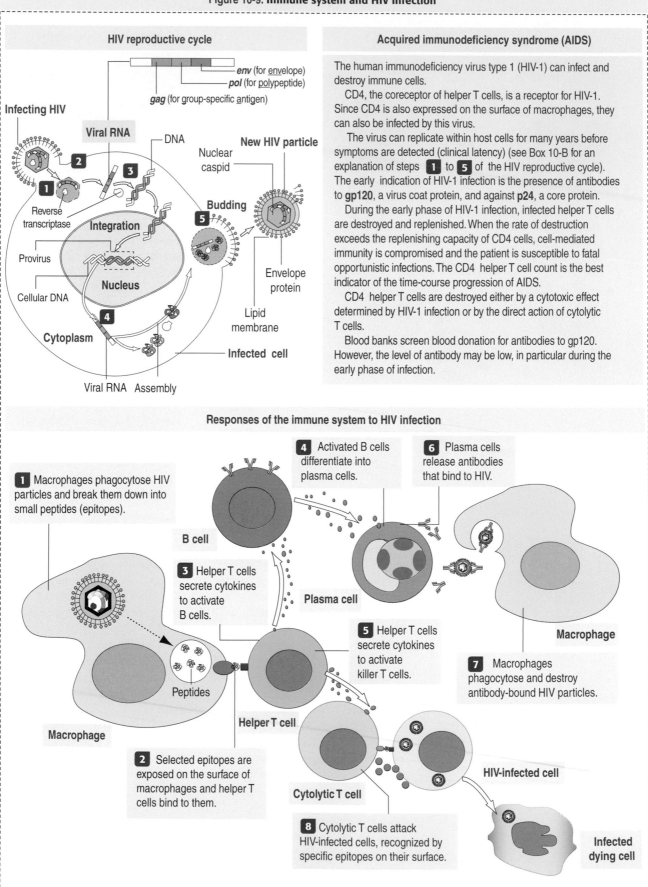

HIV reproductive cycle

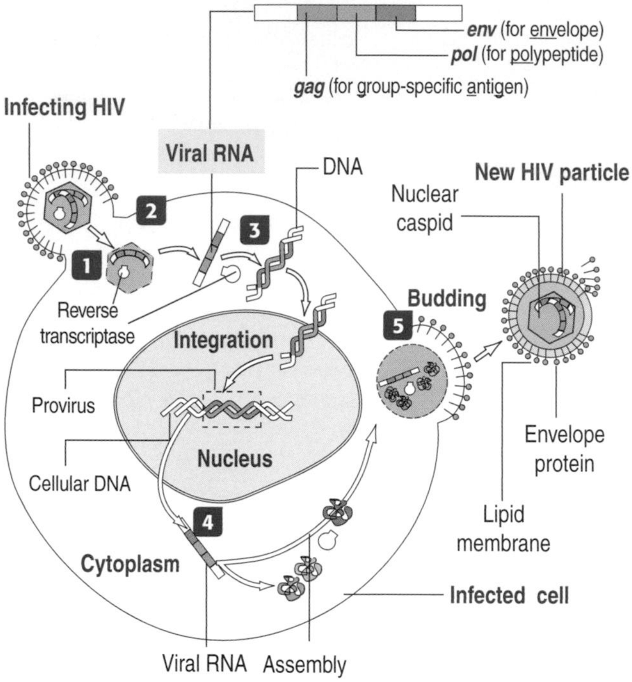

env (for envelope)
pol (for polypeptide)
gag (for group-specific antigen)
Infecting HIV
Viral RNA
DNA
New HIV particle
Nuclear caspid
Budding
Reverse transcriptase
Integration
Provirus
Nucleus
Cellular DNA
Cytoplasm
Envelope protein
Lipid membrane
Infected cell
Viral RNA
Assembly

Acquired immunodeficiency syndrome (AIDS)

The human immunodeficiency virus type 1 (HIV-1) can infect and destroy immune cells.

CD4, the coreceptor of helper T cells, is a receptor for HIV-1. Since CD4 is also expressed on the surface of macrophages, they can also be infected by this virus.

The virus can replicate within host cells for many years before symptoms are detected (clinical latency) (see Box 10-B for an explanation of steps 1 to 5 of the HIV reproductive cycle). The early indication of HIV-1 infection is the presence of antibodies to **gp120**, a virus coat protein, and against **p24**, a core protein.

During the early phase of HIV-1 infection, infected helper T cells are destroyed and replenished. When the rate of destruction exceeds the replenishing capacity of CD4 cells, cell-mediated immunity is compromised and the patient is susceptible to fatal opportunistic infections. The CD4 helper T cell count is the best indicator of the time-course progression of AIDS.

CD4 helper T cells are destroyed either by a cytotoxic effect determined by HIV-1 infection or by the direct action of cytolytic T cells.

Blood banks screen blood donation for antibodies to gp120. However, the level of antibody may be low, in particular during the early phase of infection.

Responses of the immune system to HIV infection

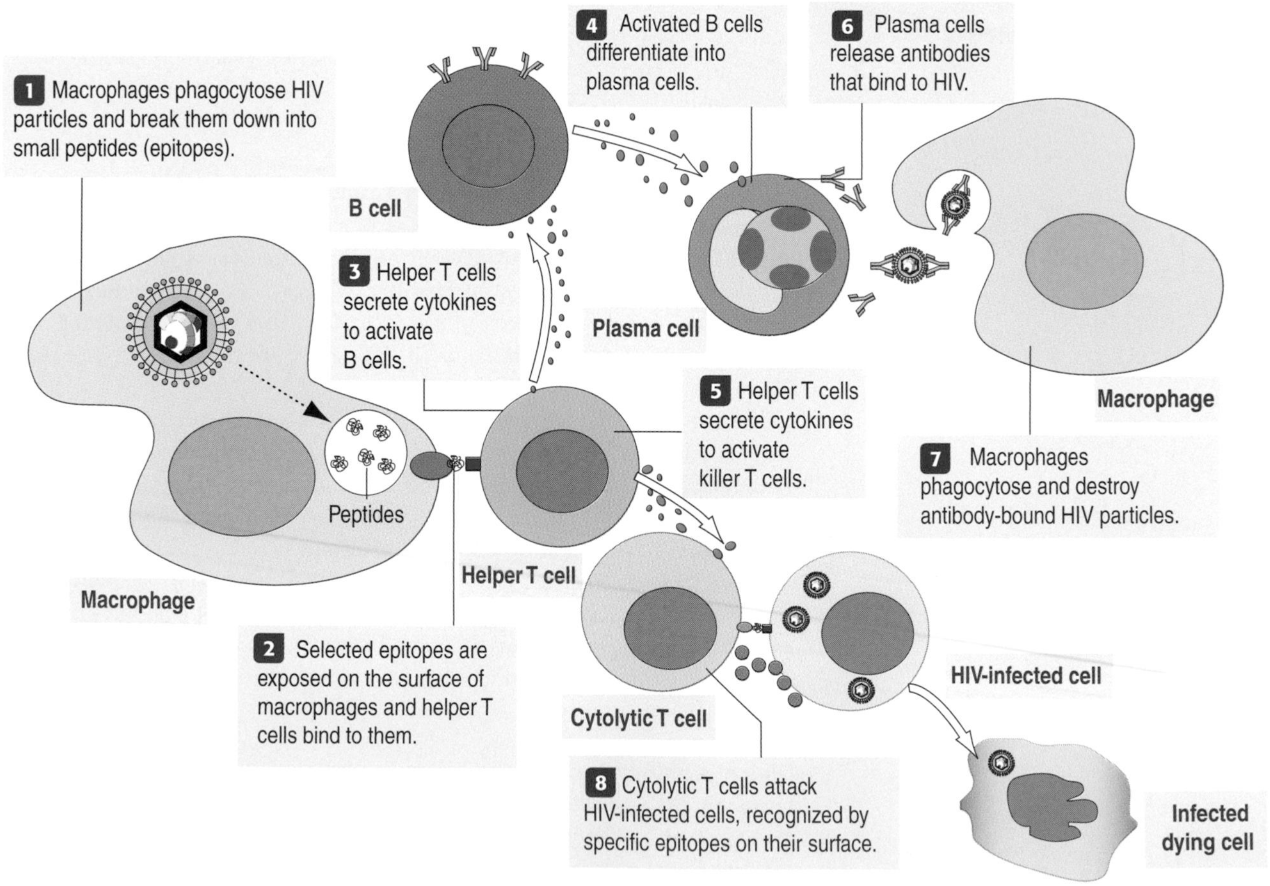

1 Macrophages phagocytose HIV particles and break them down into small peptides (epitopes).
B cell
4 Activated B cells differentiate into plasma cells.
6 Plasma cells release antibodies that bind to HIV.
3 Helper T cells secrete cytokines to activate B cells.
Plasma cell
5 Helper T cells secrete cytokines to activate killer T cells.
Macrophage
7 Macrophages phagocytose and destroy antibody-bound HIV particles.
Peptides
Helper T cell
Macrophage
2 Selected epitopes are exposed on the surface of macrophages and helper T cells bind to them.
HIV-infected cell
Cytolytic T cell
8 Cytolytic T cells attack HIV-infected cells, recognized by specific epitopes on their surface.
Infected dying cell

Box 10-B | **HIV reproductive cycle**

1. The life cycle of a retrovirus begins when the virus binds and enters a cell and introduces its genetic material (RNA) and proteins into the cytoplasm.
2. The genome of a typical retrovirus includes three coding regions: **gag**, **pol**, and **env**, specifying, respectively, proteins of the viral core, the enzyme **reverse transcriptase**, and constituents of the viral coat.
3. In the cytoplasm, reverse transcriptase converts viral RNA into DNA which is then inserted into cellular DNA. This process is called **integration**.
4. The provirus DNA directs the synthesis of viral proteins and RNA.
5. The proteins enclose the RNA, forming viral particles that bud from the cell.

helper T cells. HIV is a member of the lentivirus family of animal retroviruses and causes long-term latent cellular infection. HIV includes two types, designated HIV-1 and HIV-2. HIV-1 is the cause of AIDS. The genome of the infectious HIV consists of two strands of RNA enclosed within a core of viral proteins and surrounded by a lipid envelope derived from the infected cell. The lipid envelope contains viral proteins designated gp41 and gp120, encoded by the *env* viral sequence. The glycoprotein gp120 has binding affinity for CD4 and a coreceptor. HIV particles are present in blood, semen, and other body fluids. Transmission is by sexual contact or needle injection.

Figure 10-9 presents a summary of the cellular events associated with HIV infection. Box 10-B summarizes the steps of the HIV reproductive cycle. A relevant event of HIV infection is the destruction of $CD4^+$ helper T cells responsible for the initiation of immune responses, leading to the elimination of HIV infection. **Cytolytic T cells** (that attach to virus-infected cells) and **B cells** (that give rise to antibody-producing plasma cells) represent an adaptive response to HIV infection. Antibodies to HIV antigens are detected within 6 to 9 weeks after infection.

Clinical significance: Allergy

Allergy refers to immune responses characterized by the participation of **IgE** bound to a special receptor, designated **FcεRI**. When an antigen or **allergen** binds to two adjacent IgE molecules, it induces aggregation of the IgE molecules and associated FcεRI receptors. This event results in a signaling cascade that leads to the release of mediators and cytokines (Figure 10-10).

Note that two subtypes of helper T cell, TH1 and TH2, trigger distinct responses when activated by specific antigens.

Complement system

The main function of the complement system is to enable the **direct destruction of pathogens or target cells by phagocytes** (macrophages and neutrophils) by a mechanism known as **opsonization** (Greek *opsonein*, to buy provisions) **by producing proteolytic enzyme complexes** (Figure 10-11).

Complement provides a rapid and efficient mechanism for eliminating pathogens to prevent tissue injury or chronic infection. Host tissues have cell surface–anchored regulatory proteins, which can inhibit complement activation and prevent unintended damage.

The complement system consists of about 20 plasma proteins, synthesized mainly in the liver, that "complement," or enhance, a tissue response to pathogens. Several components of this system are **proenzymes** converted to active enzymes.

Activation of the complement cascade can be triggered by (1) antibodies bound to a pathogen (**classical pathway**); (2) binding of mannose-binding lectin to a bacterial carbohydrate moiety (**lectin pathway**); and (3) by spontaneous activation of C3, a proenzyme of the complement sequence (**alternative pathway**).

The critical molecule of the complement cascade is **C1**, a hexamer, called **C1q**, with binding affinity to the **Fc region** of an immunoglobulin. C1q is also associated with two molecules, **C1r** and **C1s**.

When the globular domains of C1q bind to the Fc regions of immunoglobulins already bound to the surface of a pathogen, C1r is activated and converts C1s into a serine protease. **Activation of C1s marks the initiation of the complement activation cascade**.

The second step is the cleavage of complement protein C4 by C1s. Two fragments are produced: (1) the small fragment C4a is discarded; and (2) the large fragment C4b binds to the pathogen surface.

The third step occurs when complement protein **C2** is cleaved by C1s into C2a (discarded) and C2b. C2b binds to the already bound C4b, forming the **complex C4b-2b**, also called **C3 convertase**, on the surface of a pathogen.

The fourth step takes place when complement protein **C3** is cleaved by C3

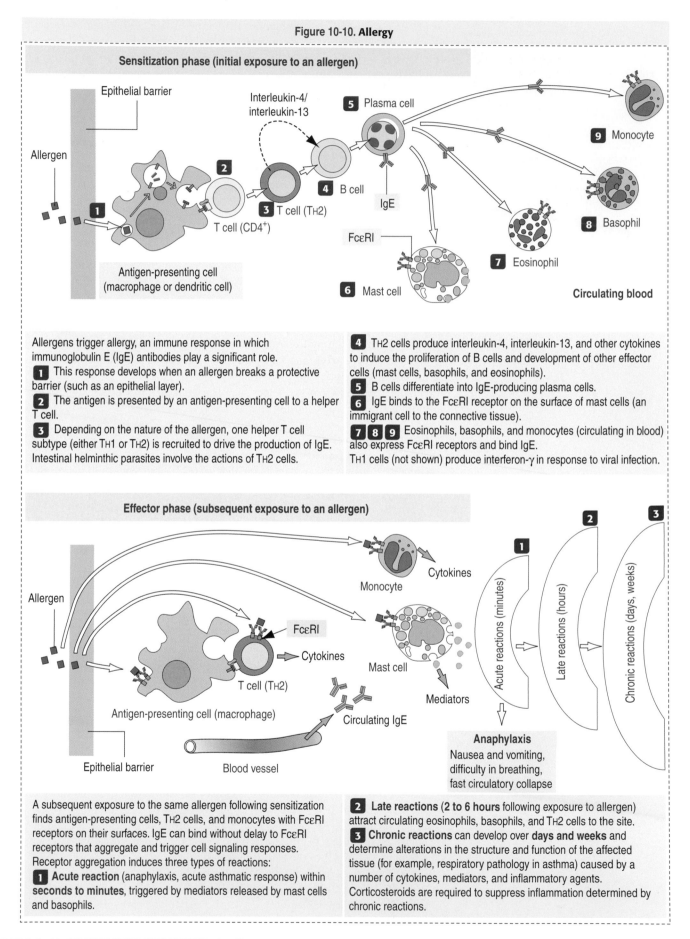

Figure 10-10. **Allergy**

Sensitization phase (initial exposure to an allergen)

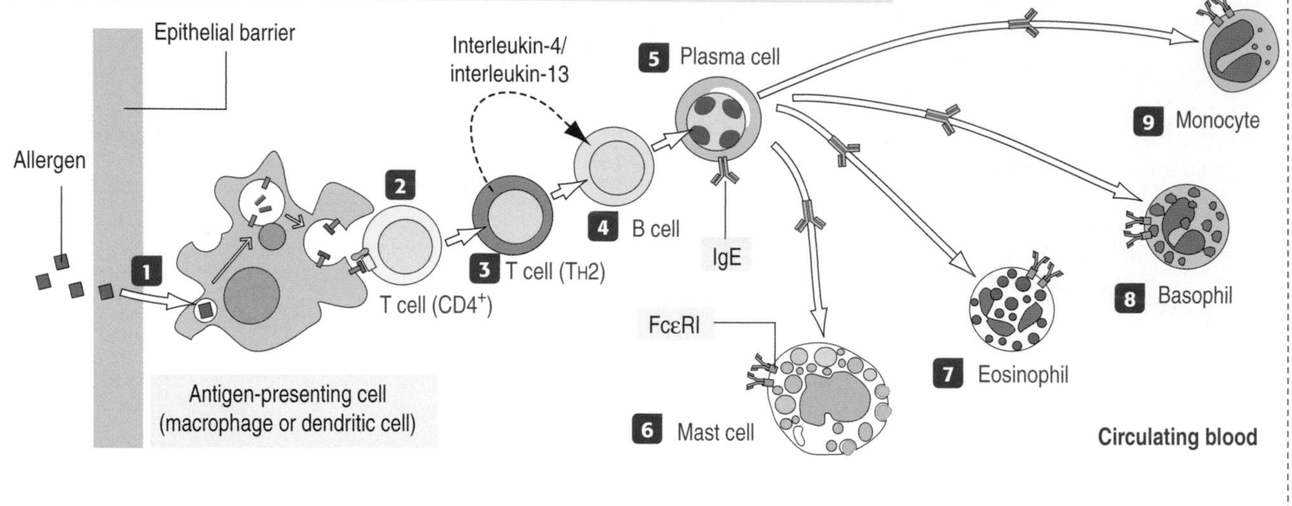
Epithelial barrier
Allergen
1
Antigen-presenting cell
(macrophage or dendritic cell)
2
T cell (CD4+)
Interleukin-4/
interleukin-13
3 T cell (TH2)
4 B cell
5 Plasma cell
IgE
FcεRI
6 Mast cell
7 Eosinophil
8 Basophil
9 Monocyte
Circulating blood

Allergens trigger allergy, an immune response in which immunoglobulin E (IgE) antibodies play a significant role.

1 This response develops when an allergen breaks a protective barrier (such as an epithelial layer).

2 The antigen is presented by an antigen-presenting cell to a helper T cell.

3 Depending on the nature of the allergen, one helper T cell subtype (either TH1 or TH2) is recruited to drive the production of IgE. Intestinal helminthic parasites involve the actions of TH2 cells.

4 TH2 cells produce interleukin-4, interleukin-13, and other cytokines to induce the proliferation of B cells and development of other effector cells (mast cells, basophils, and eosinophils).

5 B cells differentiate into IgE-producing plasma cells.

6 IgE binds to the FcεRI receptor on the surface of mast cells (an immigrant cell to the connective tissue).

7 8 9 Eosinophils, basophils, and monocytes (circulating in blood) also express FcεRI receptors and bind IgE.

TH1 cells (not shown) produce interferon-γ in response to viral infection.

Effector phase (subsequent exposure to an allergen)

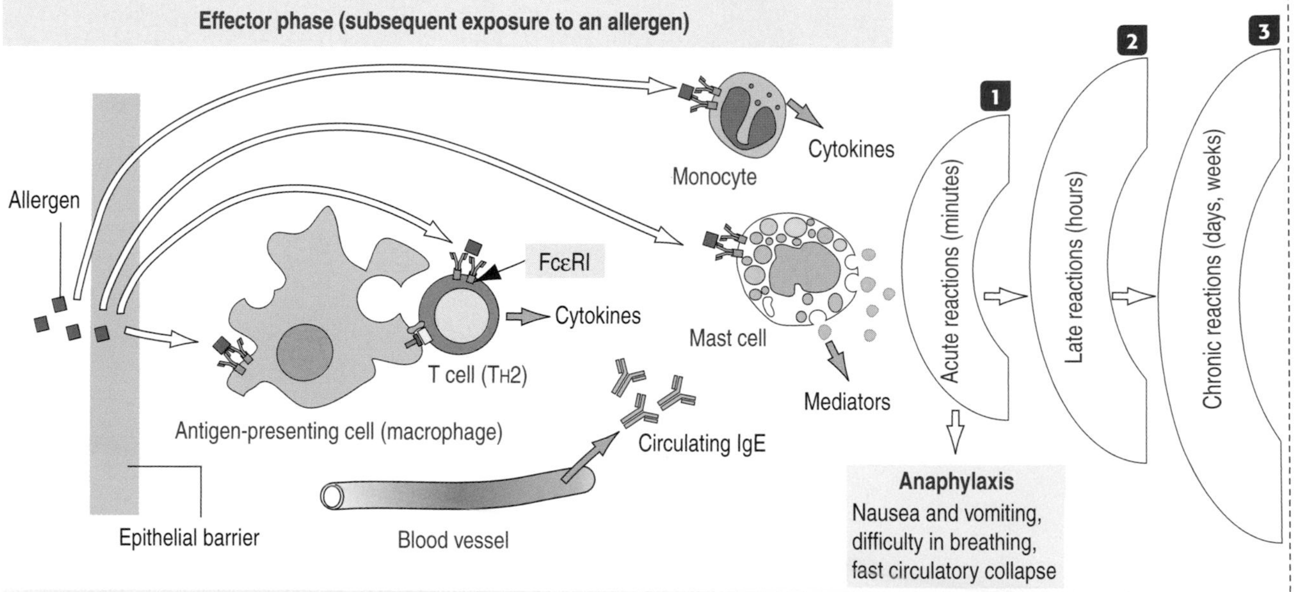
Allergen
Epithelial barrier
Antigen-presenting cell (macrophage)
FcεRI
Cytokines
T cell (TH2)
Blood vessel
Circulating IgE
Monocyte
Cytokines
Mast cell
Mediators
1
Acute reactions (minutes)
2
Late reactions (hours)
3
Chronic reactions (days, weeks)
Anaphylaxis
Nausea and vomiting,
difficulty in breathing,
fast circulatory collapse

A subsequent exposure to the same allergen following sensitization finds antigen-presenting cells, TH2 cells, and monocytes with FcεRI receptors on their surfaces. IgE can bind without delay to FcεRI receptors that aggregate and trigger cell signaling responses. Receptor aggregation induces three types of reactions:

1 **Acute reaction** (anaphylaxis, acute asthmatic response) within **seconds to minutes**, triggered by mediators released by mast cells and basophils.

2 **Late reactions** (**2 to 6 hours** following exposure to allergen) attract circulating eosinophils, basophils, and TH2 cells to the site.

3 **Chronic reactions** can develop over **days and weeks** and determine alterations in the structure and function of the affected tissue (for example, respiratory pathology in asthma) caused by a number of cytokines, mediators, and inflammatory agents. Corticosteroids are required to suppress inflammation determined by chronic reactions.

Figure 10-11. Complement system

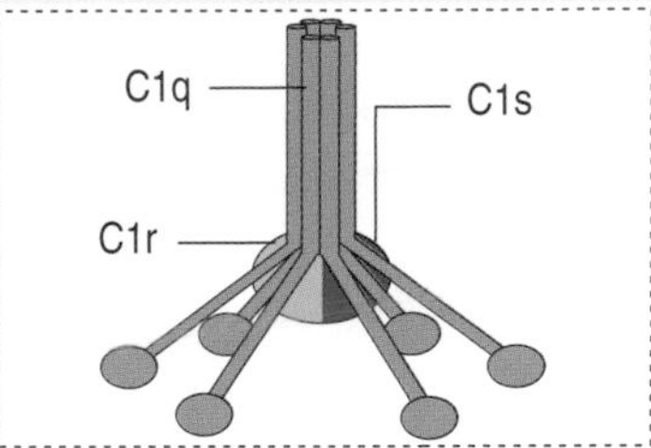

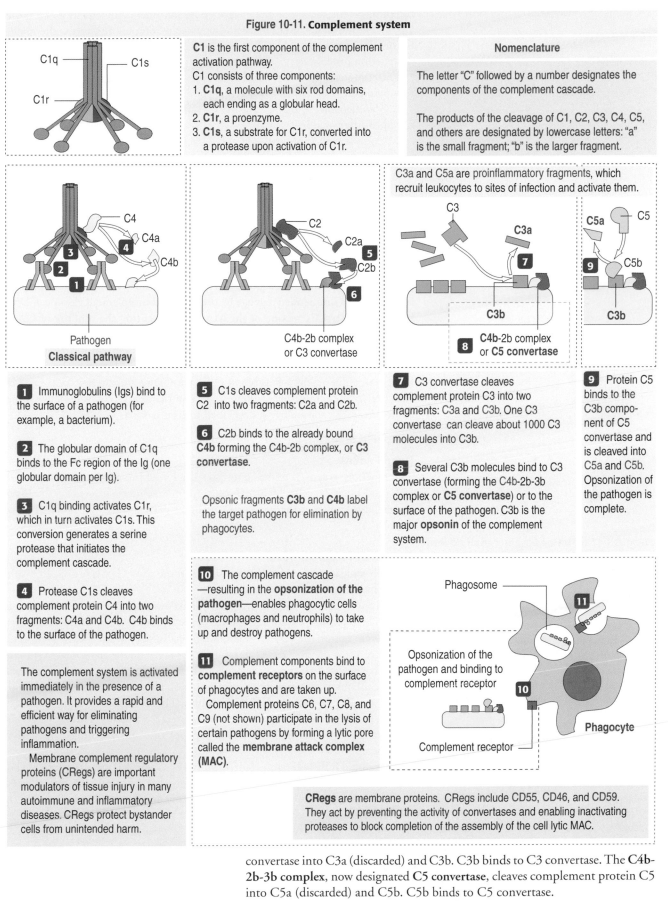

C1 is the first component of the complement activation pathway.
C1 consists of three components:
1. **C1q**, a molecule with six rod domains, each ending as a globular head.
2. **C1r**, a proenzyme.
3. **C1s**, a substrate for C1r, converted into a protease upon activation of C1r.

Nomenclature

The letter "C" followed by a number designates the components of the complement cascade.

The products of the cleavage of C1, C2, C3, C4, C5, and others are designated by lowercase letters: "a" is the small fragment; "b" is the larger fragment.

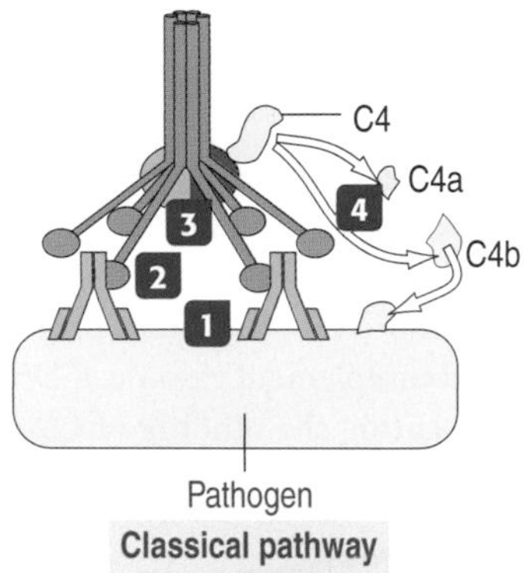

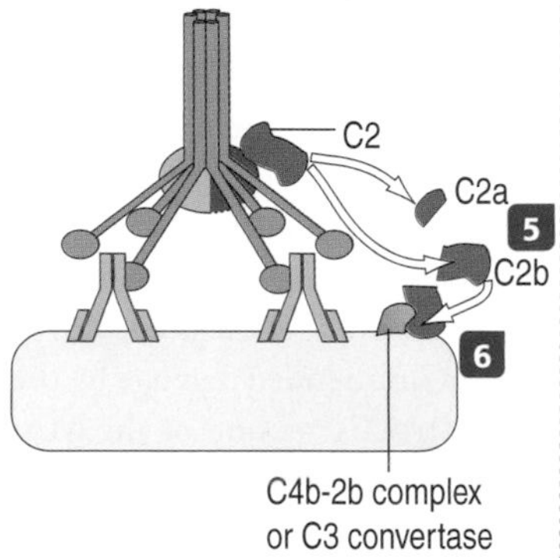

C3a and C5a are proinflammatory fragments, which recruit leukocytes to sites of infection and activate them.

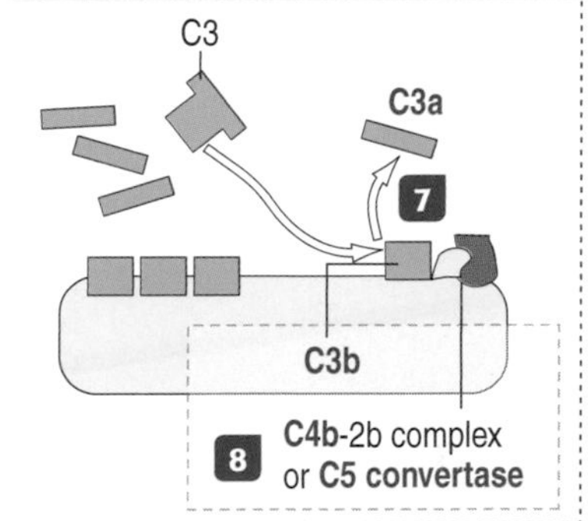

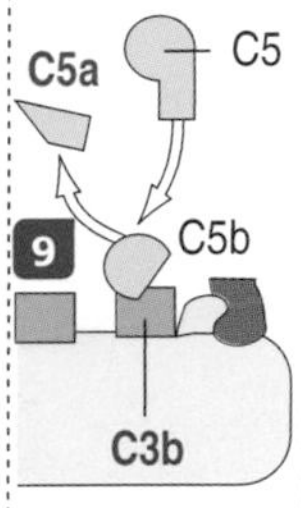

1 Immunoglobulins (Igs) bind to the surface of a pathogen (for example, a bacterium).

2 The globular domain of C1q binds to the Fc region of the Ig (one globular domain per Ig).

3 C1q binding activates C1r, which in turn activates C1s. This conversion generates a serine protease that initiates the complement cascade.

4 Protease C1s cleaves complement protein C4 into two fragments: C4a and C4b. C4b binds to the surface of the pathogen.

5 C1s cleaves complement protein C2 into two fragments: C2a and C2b.

6 C2b binds to the already bound **C4b** forming the C4b-2b complex, or **C3 convertase**.

Opsonic fragments **C3b** and **C4b** label the target pathogen for elimination by phagocytes.

7 C3 convertase cleaves complement protein C3 into two fragments: C3a and C3b. One C3 convertase can cleave about 1000 C3 molecules into C3b.

8 Several C3b molecules bind to C3 convertase (forming the C4b-2b-3b complex or **C5 convertase**) or to the surface of the pathogen. C3b is the major **opsonin** of the complement system.

9 Protein C5 binds to the C3b component of C5 convertase and is cleaved into C5a and C5b. Opsonization of the pathogen is complete.

The complement system is activated immediately in the presence of a pathogen. It provides a rapid and efficient way for eliminating pathogens and triggering inflammation.

Membrane complement regulatory proteins (CRegs) are important modulators of tissue injury in many autoimmune and inflammatory diseases. CRegs protect bystander cells from unintended harm.

10 The complement cascade—resulting in the **opsonization of the pathogen**—enables phagocytic cells (macrophages and neutrophils) to take up and destroy pathogens.

11 Complement components bind to **complement receptors** on the surface of phagocytes and are taken up.

Complement proteins C6, C7, C8, and C9 (not shown) participate in the lysis of certain pathogens by forming a lytic pore called the **membrane attack complex (MAC)**.

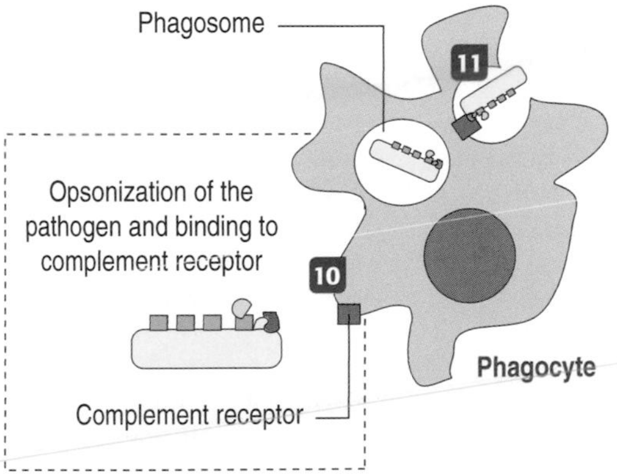

CRegs are membrane proteins. CRegs include CD55, CD46, and CD59. They act by preventing the activity of convertases and enabling inactivating proteases to block completion of the assembly of the cell lytic MAC.

convertase into C3a (discarded) and C3b. C3b binds to C3 convertase. The **C4b-2b-3b complex**, now designated **C5 convertase**, cleaves complement protein C5 into C5a (discarded) and C5b. C5b binds to C5 convertase.

The last steps consist in the binding of the opsonized pathogen to complement receptors on the surface of the phagocyte. Additional complement proteins are C6, C7, C8, and C9. CD9 binds to the protein complex and forms the **membrane attack complex** (MAC), a cytolytic pore that directly initiates the cell destruction process.

The complement system has the following specific characteristics important to remember:

1. Complement fragments C3a and C5a, produced by the enzymatic cascade, have **proinflammatory** activity.
2. Complement fragment C3a and C5a recruit leukocytes to the infection site, which become activated and activate other cells.
3. Other fragments (C3b and C4b), mark targets for destruction by phagocytes.
4. Destruction of a pathogen is mediated by the final assembly of the **MAC**, a **transmembrane cytolytic pore**.
5. **Complement regulators** (**CRegs**; for example, **CD55**, **CD46**, and **CD59**) regulate the production of complement fragments, accelerate the decay of the already produced fragments, and block the final cytolytic action of the MAC by preventing its assembly. **CRegs are cell surface–anchored proteins that protect host cells from unintended damage by the activated complement cascade. CD59 blocks the destructive action of the MAC by preventing the binding of C9 to C8. CD59** also modulates the activity of T cells.
6. **Paroxysmal nocturnal hemoglobinuria** (PNH) determines episodes of hemolysis represented by dark urine and anemia, stomach and back pain, and formation of blood clots. **Red blood cells lack CD59** and are susceptible to destruction by the complement system. Therapeutic means to prevent or arrest the complement cascade are being developed to treat patients with PNH.

Lymphoid organs

Lymph nodes

The function of lymph nodes is to filter the lymph, maintain and produce B cells, and house T cells. Helper T cells are preferentially located in the **deep cortex** (also known as the **paracortex** or **inner cortex**) of lymph nodes (Figure 10-12).

Structure of a lymph node

A lymph node is surrounded by a capsule, and the parenchyma is divided into a **cortex** and a **medulla**.

The **capsule** consists of dense irregular connective tissue surrounded by adipose tissue. The capsule at the convex surface of the lymph node is pierced by numerous **afferent lymphatic vessels**. Afferent lymphatic vessels have **valves** to prevent the reflux of lymph entering a lymph node.

The **cortex** has two zones: the **outer cortex** and the **inner cortex**. The outer cortex contains **B cell–rich lymphoid follicles**. The deep cortex houses **CD4$^+$ helper T cells** and **high endothelial venules**. The deep cortex is a paracortical zone in which mainly CD4$^+$ helper T cells interact with B cells to induce their proliferation and differentiation when exposed to a specific antigen (adaptive immune response).

A **lymphoid follicle** (Figure 10-13) consists of a **mantle** (facing the cortex) and a **germinal center** containing mainly proliferating B cells or **lymphoblasts**, resident **follicular dendritic cells** (**FDCs**), migrating **dendritic cells** (see Box 10-C), **macrophages,** and supporting **reticular cells**, which produce reticular fibers (type III collagen). A **primary lymphoid follicle** lacks a mantle and germinal center. A **secondary lymphoid follicle** has a mantle and a germinal center. The mantle and germinal center **develop in response to antigen stimulation**.

FDCs are branched (hence the name **dendritic**) cells forming a network within the lymphoid follicle. In contrast to migrating dendritic cells, which derive from bone marrow and interact with T cells, resident FDCs do not derive from a bone

Box 10-C | **Dendritic cells and lymph nodes**

- Terminal afferent lymphatic vessels, transporting lymph to the lymph nodes, derive from collecting lymphatic vessels.
- Terminal afferent lymphatic vessels penetrate the connective tissue cortex of a lymph node and empty their content in the subcapsular sinus.
- The flow of lymph into lymph nodes is regulated by smooth muscle cells present in the wall of collecting lymphatic vessels (intrinsic pumping activity) and by movements in the surrounding tissue (passive extrinsic activity).
- Collecting lymphatic vessels have valves that allow unidirectional flow of lymph and cells (for example, dendritic cells and leukocytes) from lymph node to lymph node. Valves prevent the backflow of lymph processed in the preceding lymph node.
- Dendritic cells are highly mobile. They are distributed as sentinels in the periphery to monitor the presence of foreign antigens. They relocate to secondary lymphoid organs, lymph nodes in particular, to interact with memory T cells present in the deep cortex. An example is the Langerhans cell present in epidermis.

Figure 10-12. Lymph node

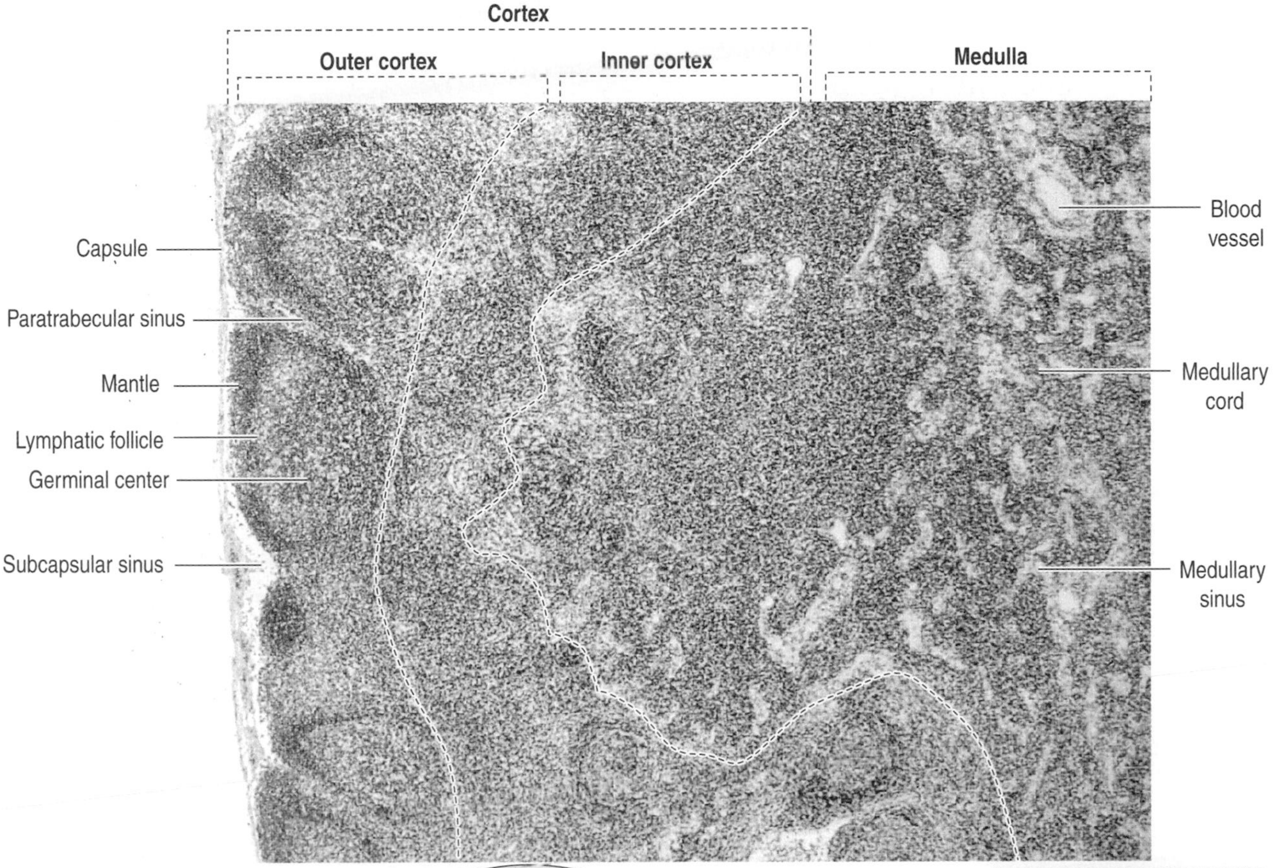

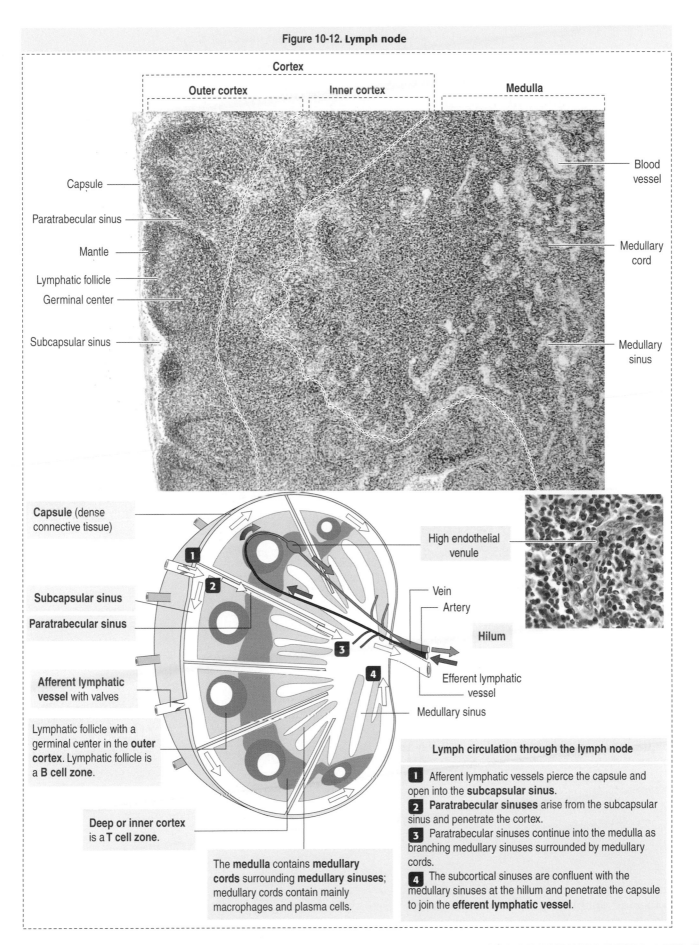

Cortex
Outer cortex
Inner cortex
Medulla
Capsule
Paratrabecular sinus
Mantle
Lymphatic follicle
Germinal center
Subcapsular sinus
Blood vessel
Medullary cord
Medullary sinus

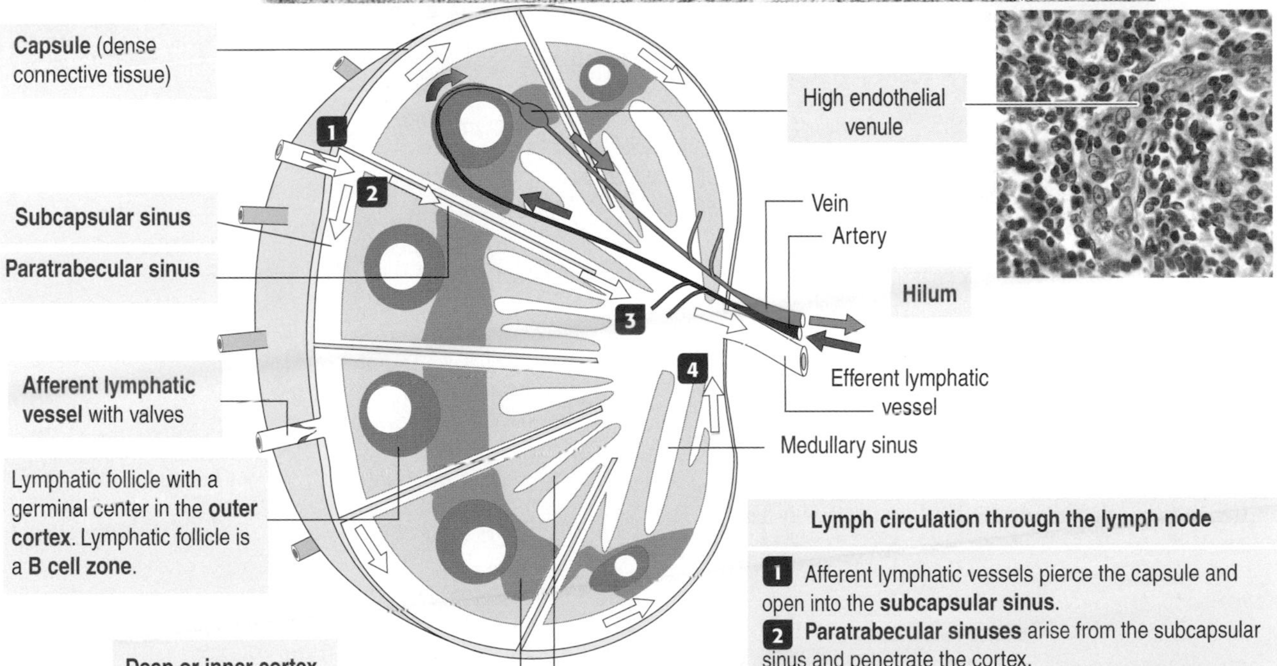

Capsule (dense connective tissue)
Subcapsular sinus
Paratrabecular sinus
Afferent lymphatic vessel with valves
Lymphatic follicle with a germinal center in the **outer cortex**. Lymphatic follicle is a **B cell zone**.
High endothelial venule
Vein
Artery
Hilum
Efferent lymphatic vessel
Medullary sinus
1
2
3
4
Deep or inner cortex is a **T cell zone.**
The **medulla** contains **medullary cords** surrounding **medullary sinuses**; medullary cords contain mainly macrophages and plasma cells.

Lymph circulation through the lymph node

1 Afferent lymphatic vessels pierce the capsule and open into the **subcapsular sinus.**

2 **Paratrabecular sinuses** arise from the subcapsular sinus and penetrate the cortex.

3 Paratrabecular sinuses continue into the medulla as branching medullary sinuses surrounded by medullary cords.

4 The subcortical sinuses are confluent with the medullary sinuses at the hillum and penetrate the capsule to join the **efferent lymphatic vessel**.

Figure 10-13. Lymphatic follicle

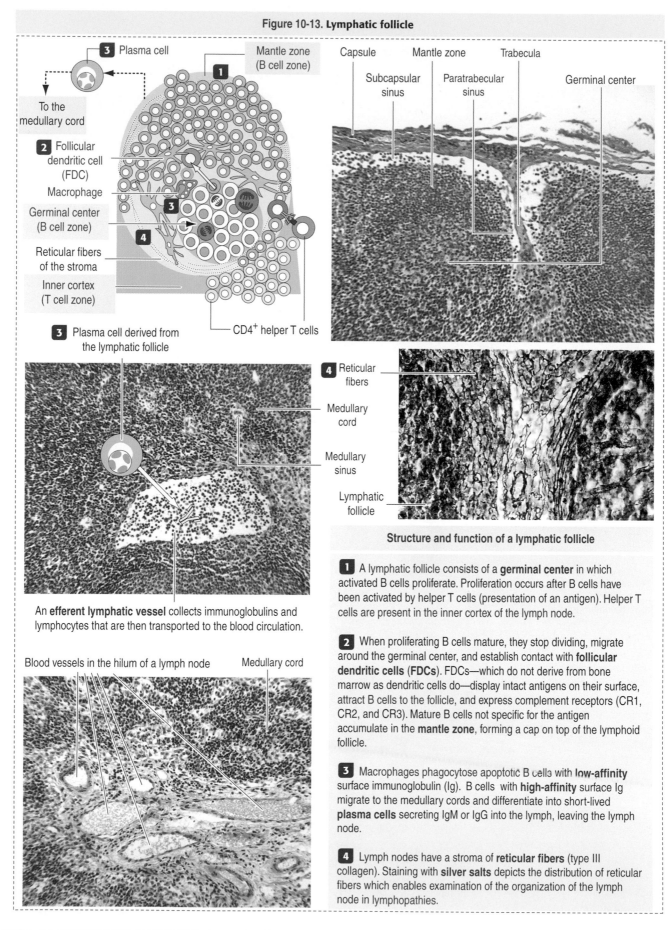

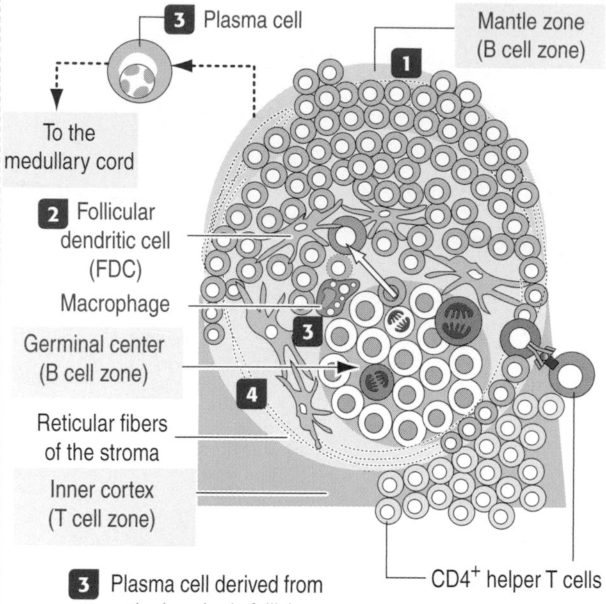

3 Plasma cell
Mantle zone
(B cell zone)
1
To the
medullary cord
2 Follicular
dendritic cell
(FDC)
Macrophage
3
Germinal center
(B cell zone)
4
Reticular fibers
of the stroma
Inner cortex
(T cell zone)
CD4+ helper T cells

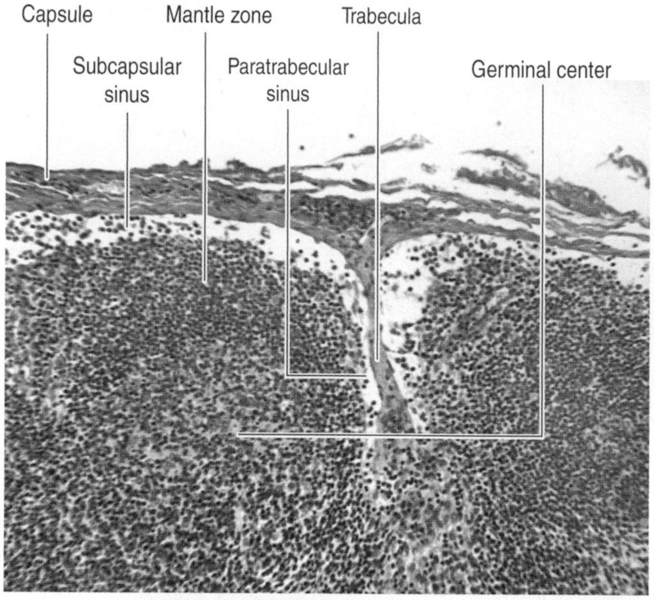

Capsule
Mantle zone
Trabecula
Subcapsular
sinus
Paratrabecular
sinus
Germinal center

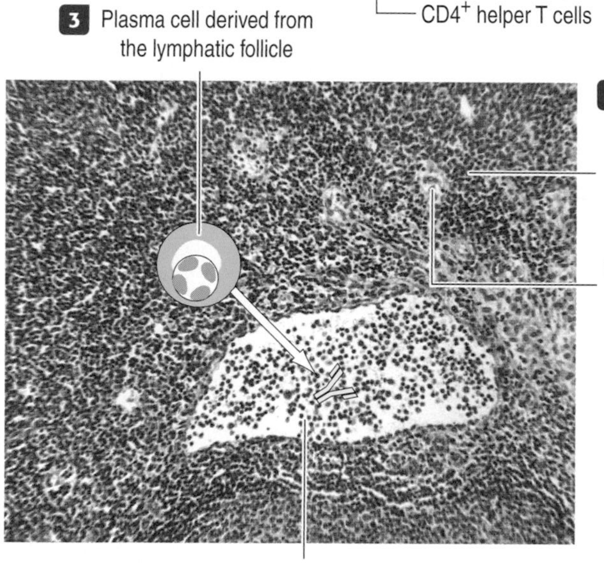

3 Plasma cell derived from
the lymphatic follicle
Medullary
cord
Medullary
sinus

An **efferent lymphatic vessel** collects immunoglobulins and lymphocytes that are then transported to the blood circulation.

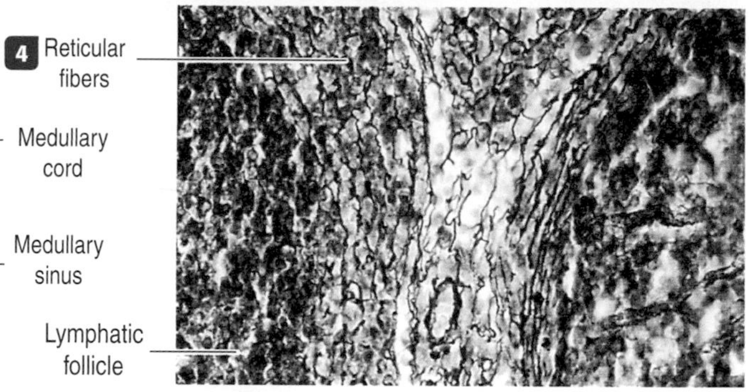

4 Reticular
fibers
Lymphatic
follicle

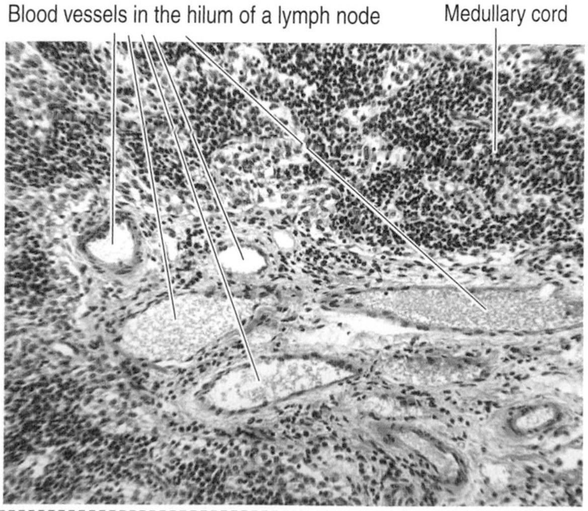

Blood vessels in the hilum of a lymph node
Medullary cord

Structure and function of a lymphatic follicle

1 A lymphatic follicle consists of a **germinal center** in which activated B cells proliferate. Proliferation occurs after B cells have been activated by helper T cells (presentation of an antigen). Helper T cells are present in the inner cortex of the lymph node.

2 When proliferating B cells mature, they stop dividing, migrate around the germinal center, and establish contact with **follicular dendritic cells** (**FDCs**). FDCs—which do not derive from bone marrow as dendritic cells do—display intact antigens on their surface, attract B cells to the follicle, and express complement receptors (CR1, CR2, and CR3). Mature B cells not specific for the antigen accumulate in the **mantle zone**, forming a cap on top of the lymphoid follicle.

3 Macrophages phagocytose apoptotic B cells with **low-affinity** surface immunoglobulin (Ig). B cells with **high-affinity** surface Ig migrate to the medullary cords and differentiate into short-lived **plasma cells** secreting IgM or IgG into the lymph, leaving the lymph node.

4 Lymph nodes have a stroma of **reticular fibers** (type III collagen). Staining with **silver salts** depicts the distribution of reticular fibers which enables examination of the organization of the lymph node in lymphopathies.

Figure 10-14. Development of the thymus

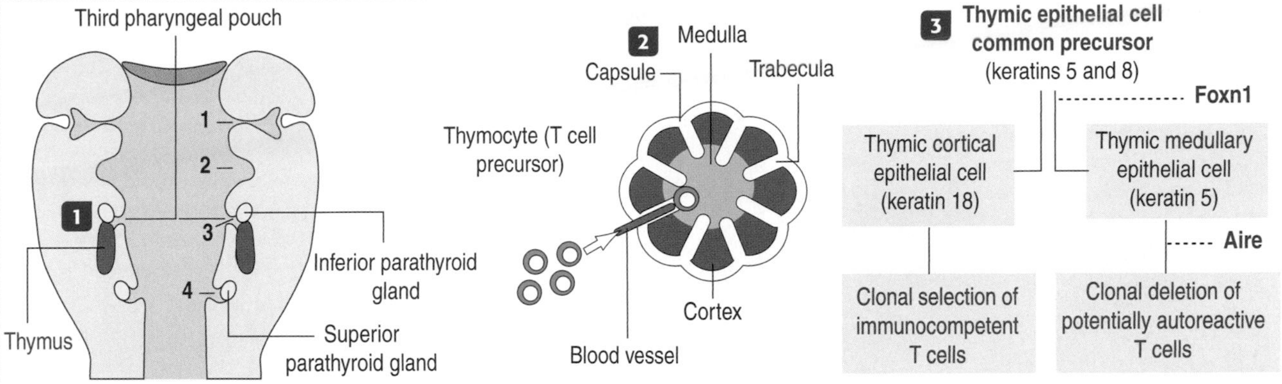

Third pharyngeal pouch
1
2
3
4
1
Thymus
Inferior parathyroid gland
Superior parathyroid gland
2
Medulla
Capsule
Trabecula
Thymocyte (T cell precursor)
Cortex
Blood vessel
3
Thymic epithelial cell common precursor
(keratins 5 and 8)
Foxn1
Thymic cortical epithelial cell (keratin 18)
Thymic medullary epithelial cell (keratin 5)
Aire
Clonal selection of immunocompetent T cells
Clonal deletion of potentially autoreactive T cells

1 The thymus rudiments originate from the caudal region of the endodermic **third pharyngeal pouch** on each side, proliferate, migrate to the thorax, and become connected by connective tissue.

Parathyroid gland tissue, developing from the same pouch, migrates with the thymus and becomes the inferior parathyroid glands. The superior parathyroid glands originate from the fourth pharyngeal pouch. The numbers 1 to 4 indicate the pharyngeal pouches.

2 A **capsule** forms from the neural crest mesenchyme. Capsule-derived trabeculae extending into the future corticomedullary region of the thymus divide the thymus into **incomplete lobules.**

By 14 weeks, thymocyte precursors arrive from bone marrow through blood vessels, after interconnected **thymic epithelial cells** form a three-dimensional network and **macrophages** are present. By 17 weeks, the thymus is beginning to produce T cells.

3 Thymic epithelial cells play important functions in clonal selection and clonal deletion of differentiating T cells:

1. A common precursor (keratins 5 and 18) gives rise to thymic cortical (keratin 18) and medullary (keratin 5) epithelial cells.
2. Thymic epithelial cells express two essential transcription factors: **Foxn1** (for forkedhead box N1), and **aire** (for autoimmune regulator). **Foxn1** is essential for the differentiation of thymic epithelial cells. **Aire** promotes the expression of a portfolio of tissue-specific cell proteins by thymic **medullary** epithelial cells, which normally do not express these proteins. These proteins permit the identification and disposal of autoreactive T cells. A mutation of the aire gene in humans causes autoimmune polyendocrinopathy–candidiasis–ectodermal dystrophy (APECED).

marrow cell precursor. FDCs are observed at the edge of the germinal centers, interacting with mature B cells. FDCs trap antigens bound to immunoglobulins or complement proteins on their surface for recognition by B cells. **The interaction of mature B cells with FDCs** (displaying an antigen that complements a **high-affinity surface immunoglobulin**) **rescues the B cell from apoptosis. Only B cells with low-affinity surface immunoglobulin are induced to apoptosis. Macrophages** in the lymphoid follicle phagocytose apoptotic B cells.

Lymphatic sinuses are spaces lined by endothelial cells under the capsule (**subcapsular sinus**) and along trabeculae of connective tissue derived from the capsule and entering the cortex (**paratrabecular sinus**). Highly phagocytic macrophages are distributed along the subcapsular and paratrabecular sinuses to remove particulate matter present in the percolating lymph. Lymph entering the paratrabecular sinus through the subcapsular sinus percolates to the medullary sinuses and exits through a single efferent lymphatic vessel. Lymph in the subcapsular sinus can bypass the paratrabecular and medullary sinuses and exit through the efferent lymphatic vessel.

High endothelial venules (**HEVs**) (see Figure 10-12), located in the deep cortex, are the sites of entry of most B and T cells into the lymph node (by the lymphocyte homing mechanism). HEVs are specialized venules present in several lymphatic tissues, including **Peyer's patches** in the small intestine and the cortex of the **thymus**.

The **medulla** is surrounded by the cortex, except at the region of the **hilum** (see

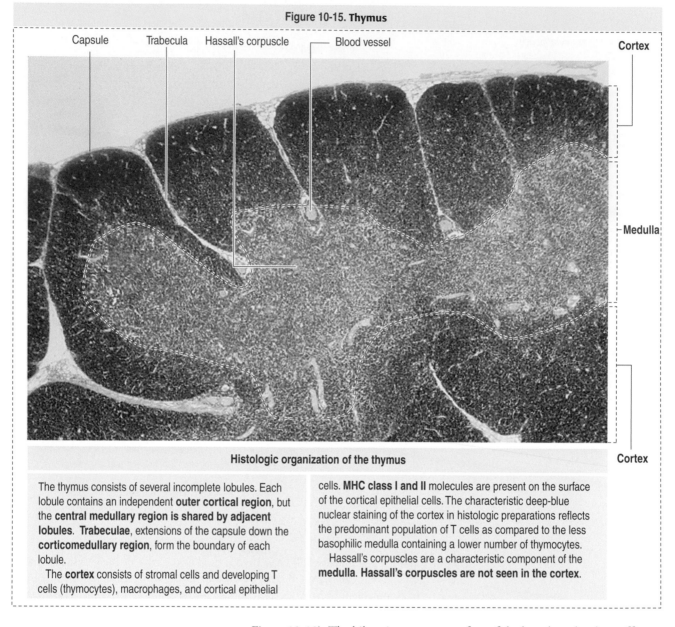

Figure 10-15. Thymus

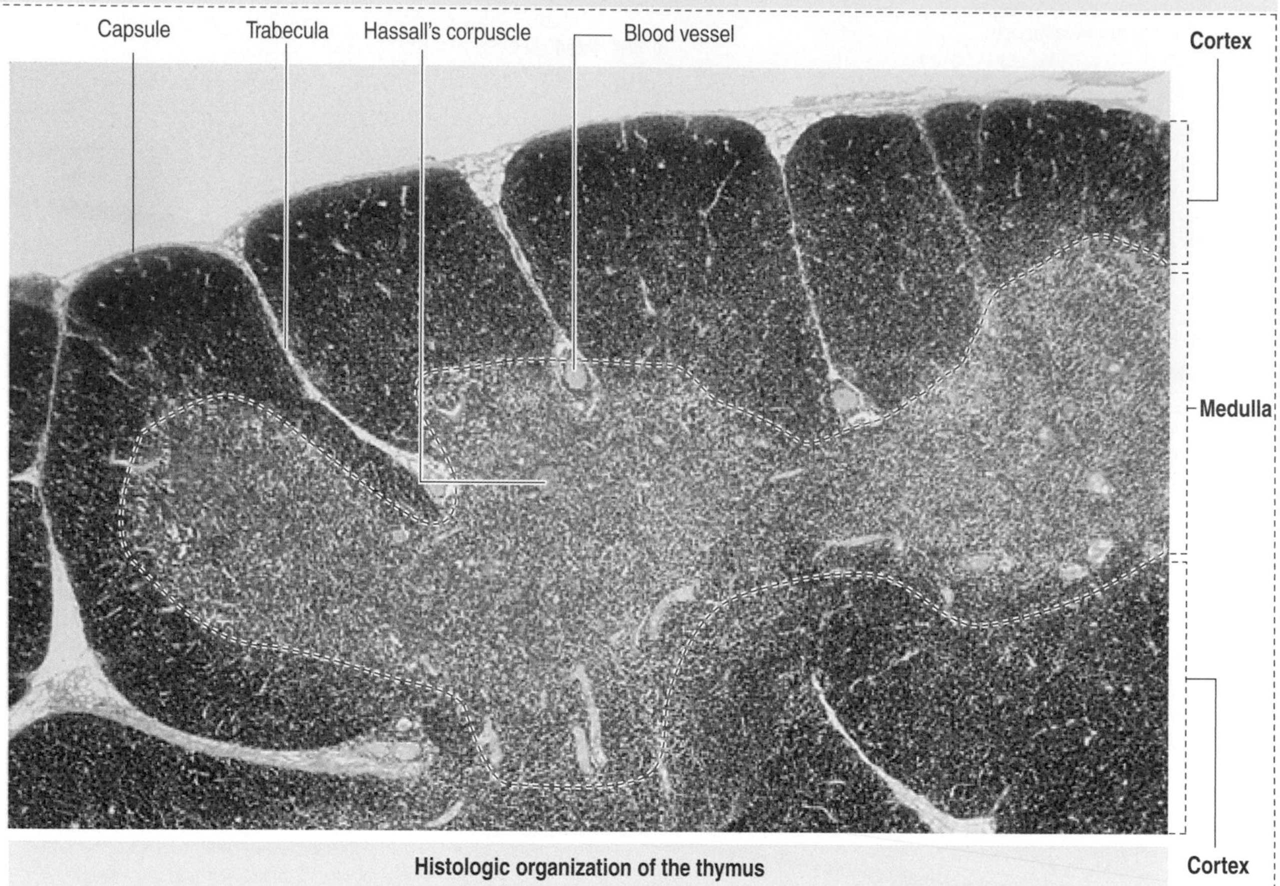
Capsule
Trabecula
Hassall's corpuscle
Blood vessel
Cortex
Medulla
Cortex

Histologic organization of the thymus

The thymus consists of several incomplete lobules. Each lobule contains an independent **outer cortical region**, but the **central medullary region is shared by adjacent lobules**. **Trabeculae**, extensions of the capsule down the **corticomedullary region**, form the boundary of each lobule.

The **cortex** consists of stromal cells and developing T cells (thymocytes), macrophages, and cortical epithelial cells. **MHC class I and II** molecules are present on the surface of the cortical epithelial cells. The characteristic deep-blue nuclear staining of the cortex in histologic preparations reflects the predominant population of T cells as compared to the less basophilic medulla containing a lower number of thymocytes.

Hassall's corpuscles are a characteristic component of the **medulla. Hassall's corpuscles are not seen in the cortex.**

Figure 10-12). The hilum is a concave surface of the lymph node where **efferent lymphatic vessels** and a single **vein** leave and an **artery** enters the lymph node.

The medulla contains two major components:

1. **Medullary sinusoids**, spaces lined by endothelial cells surrounded by reticular cells and macrophages.

2. **Medullary cords**, with B cells, macrophages, and **plasma cells.** Activated B cells migrate from the cortex as plasma cells and enter the medullary sinuses. This is a strategic location because plasma cells can secrete immunoglobulins directly into the medullary sinuses without leaving the lymph node.

Clinical significance: Distribution of B and T cells in the lymph node

Lymph nodes constitute a defense site against lymph-borne microorganisms (bacteria, viruses, parasites) entering the node through afferent lymphatic vessels. This defense mechanism depends on the close interaction of B cells in the follicle nodules with $CD4^+$ T cells in the inner or deep cortex, and it complies with the basic principles of immune responsiveness illustrated in Figure 10-6. The segregation of B and T cells appears dictated by cytokines responsible for the recruitment and histologic distribution of these two cell populations in the

Figure 10-16. **Thymus**

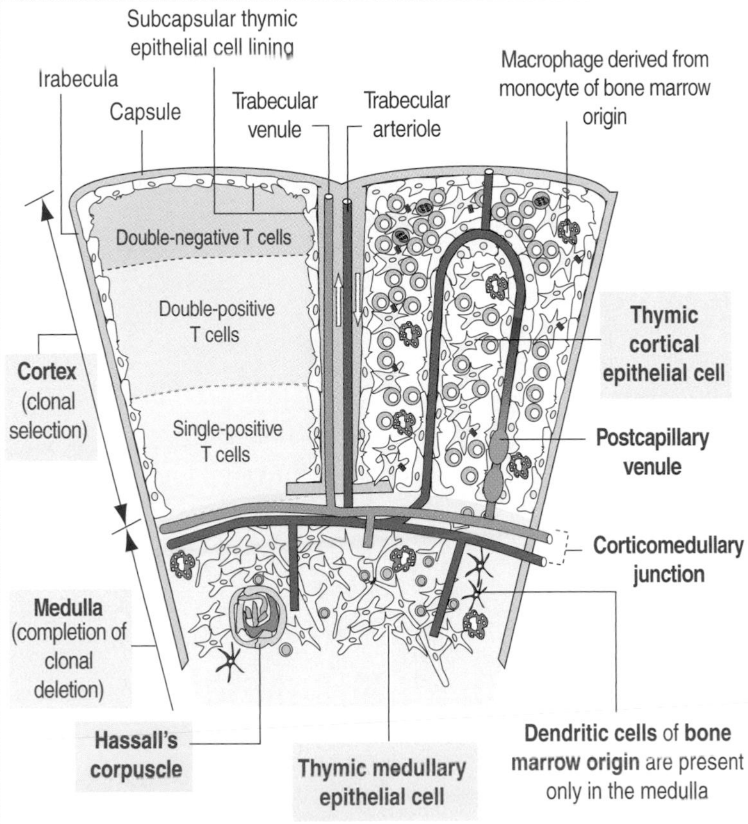

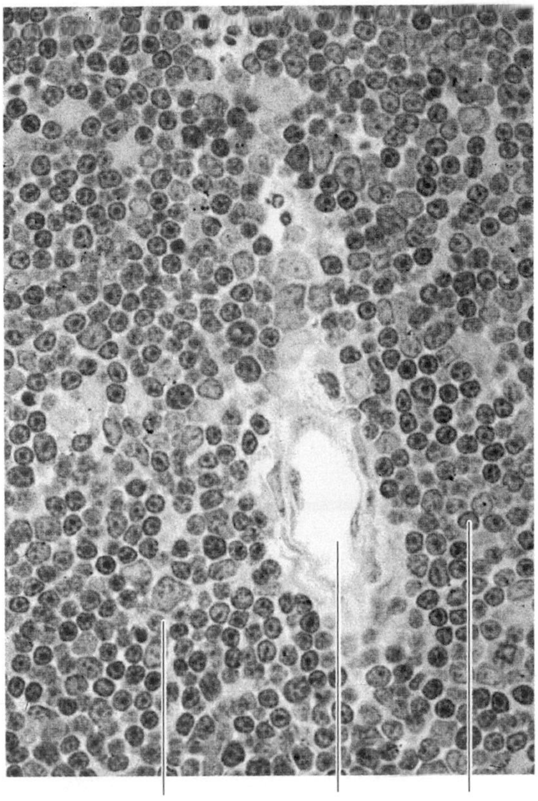

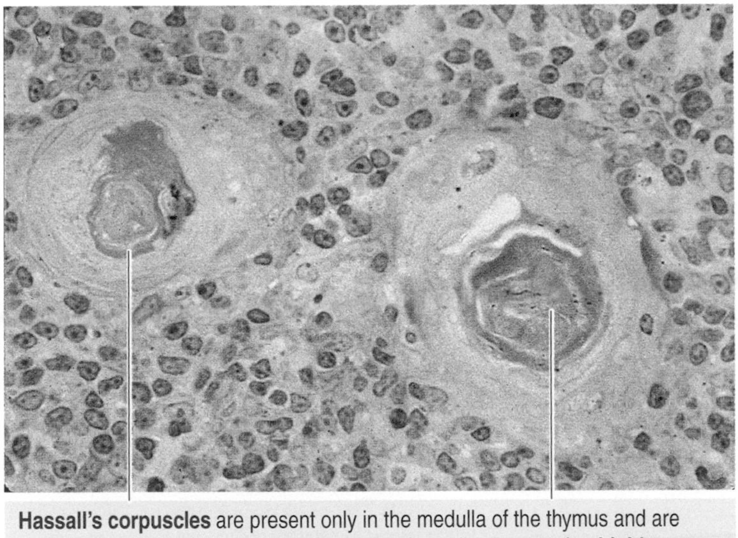

Hassall's corpuscles are present only in the medulla of the thymus and are composed of closely packed whorls of epithelial cells representing **highly keratinized** medullary epithelial cells.

Hassall's corpuscles produce **cytokine thymic stromal lymphopoietin**, which stimulates thymic dendritic cells that in turn complete the maturation of single-positive T cells to optimize negative selection.

Histology of the thymus

The functional thymus consists of two cell populations: **stromal cells** and **developing T cells**. Stromal cells include (1) the **subcapsular thymic epithelial cells** also lining the trabeculae and perivascular spaces; (2) the **thymic cortical epithelial cells**; (3) the **thymic medullary epithelial cells** that give rise to **Hassall's corpuscles**; (4) **macrophages** present in both cortex and medulla, involved in the removal of apoptotic T cells eliminated during clonal selection and deletion; and (5) **dendritic cells** of **bone marrow origin**, confined to the medulla.

Developing T cells include T cells at different stages of maturation. Immature T cells—**double-negative T cells**—enter the cortex of the thymus through blood vessels and proliferate in the subcapsular area. **Double-positive T cells** move to the outer cortex where they are confronted with epithelial cells with cell surface MHC class I and II molecules for clonal selection. **Single-positive T cells** migrate to the inner cortex. The majority of T cells (80% to 85%) are in the cortex. The medulla contains the remaining 15% to 20% of T cells undergoing **clonal deletion** (elimination of autoreactive T cells).

cortex of the lymph node.

In Chapter 12, Cardiovascular System, we discuss that the interstitial fluid, representing plasma filtrate, is transported into blind sacs corresponding to lymphatic capillaries. This interstitial fluid—entering the lymphatic capillaries as **lymph**—flows into collecting lymphatic vessels becoming afferents to regional

Figure 10-17. Thymus

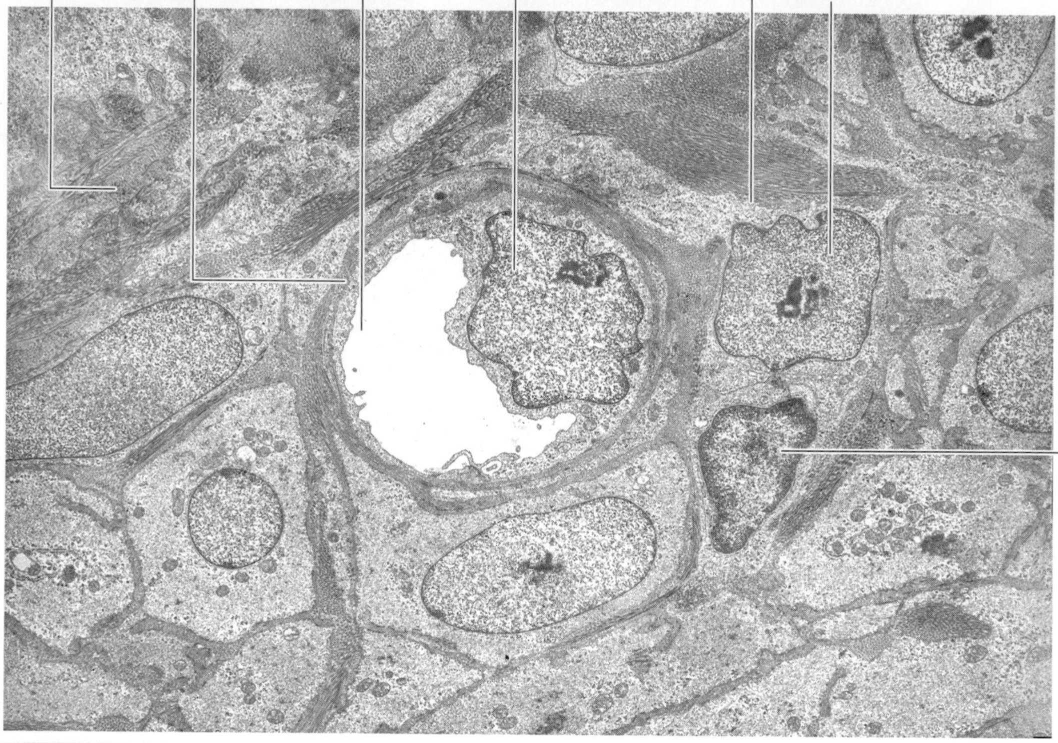

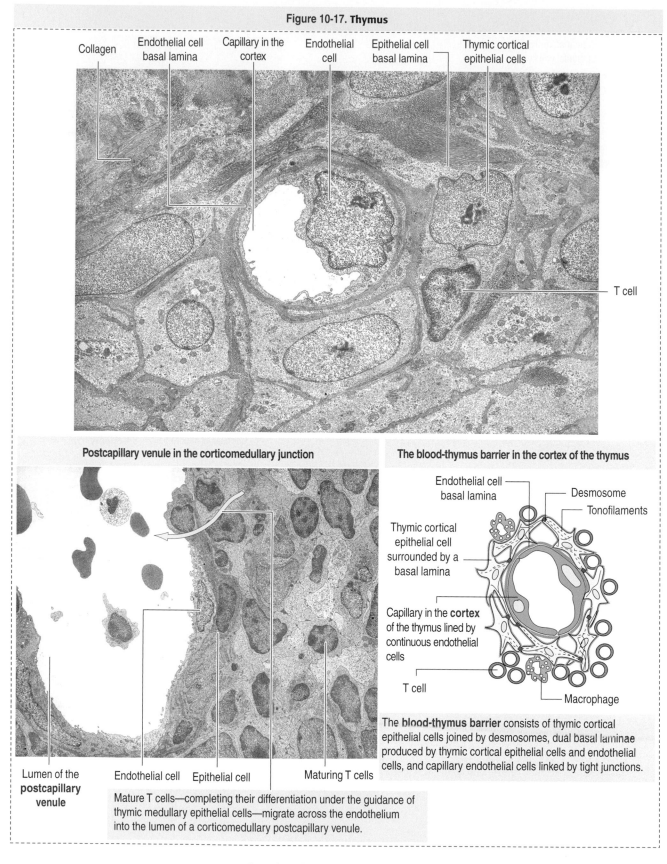

Collagen
Endothelial cell basal lamina
Capillary in the cortex
Endothelial cell
Epithelial cell basal lamina
Thymic cortical epithelial cells
T cell

Postcapillary venule in the corticomedullary junction

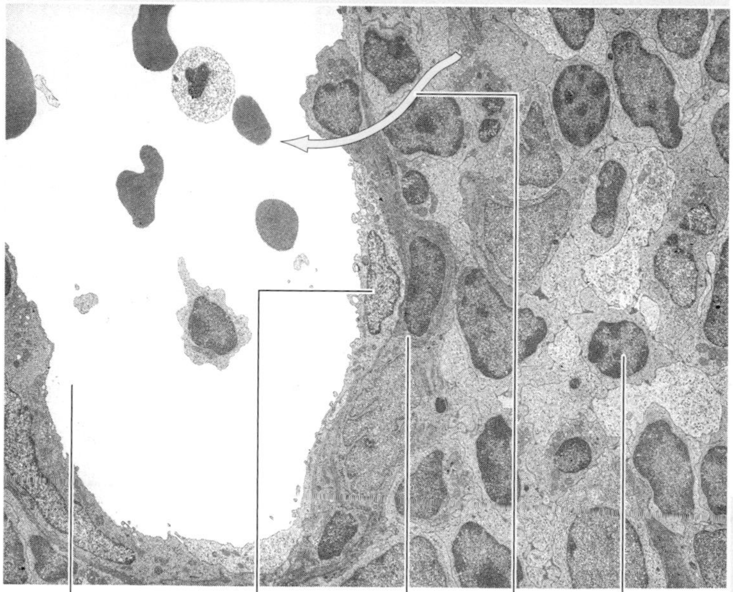

Lumen of the **postcapillary venule**
Endothelial cell
Epithelial cell
Maturing T cells

Mature T cells—completing their differentiation under the guidance of thymic medullary epithelial cells—migrate across the endothelium into the lumen of a corticomedullary postcapillary venule.

The blood-thymus barrier in the cortex of the thymus

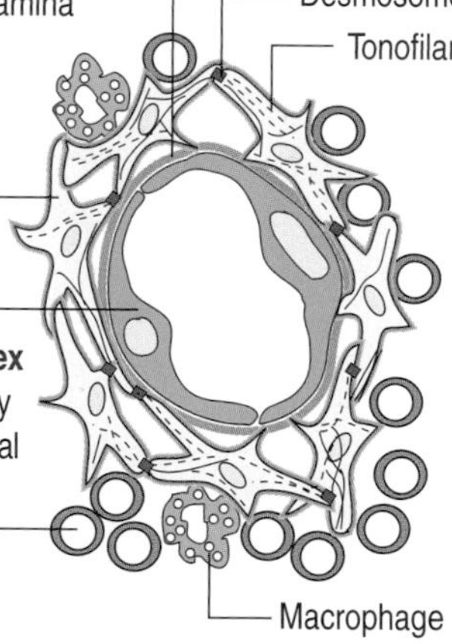

Endothelial cell basal lamina
Desmosome
Tonofilaments
Thymic cortical epithelial cell surrounded by a basal lamina
Capillary in the **cortex** of the thymus lined by continuous endothelial cells
T cell
Macrophage

The **blood-thymus barrier** consists of thymic cortical epithelial cells joined by desmosomes, dual basal laminae produced by thymic cortical epithelial cells and endothelial cells, and capillary endothelial cells linked by tight junctions.

lymph nodes (see Box 10-C). Lymph nodes are linked in series by the lymphatic vessels in such a way that **the efferent lymphatic vessel of a lymph node becomes the afferent lymphatic vessel of a downstream lymph node in the chain.**

Box 10-D | *Aire* gene and autoimmunity

- The human autosomal disorder (autoimmune-polyendocrinopathy–candidiasis–ectodermal dystrophy (APECED; also known as autoimmune polyendocrine syndrome type 1, APS-1) is characterized by the autoimmune destruction of endocrine organs, the inability to eliminate *Candida* yeast infection, and the development of ectodermal dystrophic tissue.
- The production of tissue-specific antibodies and an inflammatory reaction confined to specific structures in several organs (for example, retina, ovary, testis, stomach, and pancreas) are associated with one of the several mutations of the *aire* gene.
- The transcription factor aire enables the expression of several tissue-specific antigens (e.g., thyroglobulin, insulin, retinal S–antigen, zona pellucida glycoprotein in the ovary, proteolipid protein in the central nervous system) by thymic medullary epithelial cells. These self-proteins permit the disposal of autoreactive T cells in the medulla of the thymus.
- In aire-deficient individuals, self-proteins are not expressed and autoreactive T cells are exported to the periphery. The mechanism of self-tolerance is not operational because self-reactive T cells are not eliminated by clonal deletion.

Soluble and particulate antigens drained with the interstitial fluid, as well as antigen-bearing dendritic cells in the skin (Langerhans cells; see Chapter 11, Integumentary System), enter the lymphatic vessels and are transported to lymph nodes. Antigen-bearing dendritic cells enter the $CD4^+$ helper T cell–rich inner cortex. Soluble and particulate antigens are detected in the percolating lymph by resident macrophages and dendritic cells strategically located along the subcapsular and paratrabecular sinuses.

Macrophages display preferential phagocytosis for particulate and opsonized antigens. B cells in the follicle nodule can recognize soluble antigens. The lymph node is programmed for the uptake of lymph-borne antigens that can be processed by B cells, dendritic cells, and macrophages for recognition by helper T cells. A similar antigen uptake process occurs in the white pulp of the spleen, except that antigens are blood-borne.

When the immune reaction is acute in response to locally drained bacteria (for example, infections of the teeth or tonsils), local lymph nodes enlarge and become painful because of the distention of the capsule by cellular proliferation and edema. This condition is known as **acute lymphadenitis**.

Thymus

Development of the thymus

A brief review of the development of the thymus facilitates an understanding of the structure and function of this lymphoid organ. A significant difference from the lymph node and the spleen is that **the stroma of the thymus consists of thymic epithelial cells** organized in a dispersed network to allow for intimate contact with developing **thymocytes**, the T cell precursors arriving from bone marrow. In contrast to the thymus, the stroma of the lymph node and the spleen contains reticular cells and reticular fibers but not epithelial cells.

There are two significant aspects during the development of the thymus with relevance to tolerance for self-antigens and autoimmune diseases:

(1) A single progenitor gives rise to thymic cortical and medullary epithelial cells (Figure 10-14). The transcription factor **Foxn1** (for forkhead box N1) **regulates the differentiation of cortical and medullary thymic cells**, which starts before the arrival of thymocyte precursors from bone marrow. Differentiation includes the expression of cytokeratins and establishment of desmosomal intercellular linkages. In contrast to the stratified squamous epithelium of the epidermis, thymic epithelial cells form an open network that enables a close contact with thymocytes. A mutation of the *Foxn1* gene produces **nude** and **athymic mice**. In an analogous fashion to thymic epithelial cells, Foxn1 regulates the differentiation of epidermal keratinocytes (see Chapter 11, Integumentary System).

(2) The transcription factor **aire** (for autoimmune regulator) enables the expression of a portfolio of tissue-specific self-proteins by thymic **medullary** epithelial cells. The expression of these proteins permits the **elimination of T cells that recognize specific tissue antigens** (autoreactive T cells). The human autosomal disorder called **autoimmune polyendocrinopathy–candidiasis–ectodermal dystrophy (APECED)** is associated with a mutation in the *aire* gene (see Box 10-D).

Thymic cortical epithelial cells are involved in the **clonal selection** of T cells. **Medullary epithelial cells** are involved in the **clonal deletion** of potentially autoreactive T cells.

The **mesenchyme** from the pharyngeal arch gives rise to the capsule, trabeculae, and vessels of the thymus (Figure 10-15). The **thymic epithelial rudiment** attracts **bone marrow–derived thymocyte precursors**, **dendritic cells**, and **macrophages** required for normal thymic function.

During **fetal life**, the thymus contains lymphocytes derived from the liver. T cell progenitors formed in the bone marrow during hematopoiesis enter the thymus as **immature thymocytes** and mature to become immunocompetent T cells (predominantly $CD4^+$ or $CD8^+$), which are then carried by the blood into lymph nodes, spleen, and other lymphoid tissues (Figure 10-16).

The thymus in humans is fully developed before birth. The production of T cells is significant before puberty. After puberty, the thymus begins to involute and the production of T cells in the adult decreases. The progenies of T cells become established, and immunity is maintained without the need to produce new T cells.

Clinical significance: DiGeorge syndrome

DiGeorge syndrome is an **inherited immunodeficiency disease** in which thymic epithelial cells fail to develop, and the thymus and parathyroid glands are rudimentary or absent. Patients have congenital heart defects, hypoparathyroidism, behavioral and psychiatric problems, and increased susceptibility to infections.

When thymic epithelial cells fail to organize the thymus, bone marrow–derived T cell precursors cannot differentiate. Thymic epithelial cells express MHC class I and class II molecules on their surface, and these molecules are required for the clonal selection of T cells. Their absence in DiGeorge syndrome affects the production of functional T cells. The development of B cells is not affected in DiGeorge syndrome.

The **nude (athymic) mouse**—a strain of mice lacking the expression of the **transcription factor Foxn1** necessary for the differentiation of thymic epithelial cells and epidermal cells involved in the normal development of the thymus and **hair follicles**—is the equivalent of DiGeorge syndrome. This syndrome and the nude mouse demonstrate the role of the thymus in cell-mediated immunity and autoimmune disease.

Structure of the thymus

The thymus consists of **two lobes** subdivided into **incomplete lobules**, each separated into an **outer cortex** and a **central medulla** (see Figure 10-15). A connective tissue **capsule** with small arterioles surrounds the lobules. The capsule projects **septa** or **trabeculae**. Blood vessels (**trabecular arterioles** and **venules**) within the trabeculae gain access to the thymic stroma.

The cortex contains **thymic epithelial cells** forming a three-dimensional network supported by collagen fibers. Thymic epithelial cells, linked to each other by **desmosomes**, surround capillaries. A **dual basal lamina** is present in the space between epithelial cells and capillaries. One basal lamina is produced by the cortical thymic epithelial cells. The other basal lamina is of endothelial cell origin. Macrophages may also be present in proximity (Figure 10-17).

Thymic cortical epithelial cells, basal laminae, and endothelial cells form the **functional blood-thymus barrier** (see Figure 10-17). Macrophages adjacent to the capillaries ensure that antigens escaping from blood vessels into the thymus do not react with developing T cells in the cortex, thus preventing the risk of an autoimmune reaction.

Most T cell development takes place in the cortex. In the outer area of the cortex adjacent to the capsule, double-negative thymocytes proliferate and begin the process of gene rearrangement leading to the expression of the pre-TCR along with coreceptors CD4 and CD8 (see Figure 10-16).

Deep in the cortex, maturing T cells are double-positive ($CD4^+$ and $CD8^+$) and become receptive to peptide-MHC complexes. The process of **positive selection** of T cells now starts in the presence of thymic cortical epithelial cells expressing both MHC class I and class II molecules on their surface (see Figure 10-16). MHC class II molecules are required for the development of $CD4^+$ T cells; MHC class I molecules are necessary for the development of $CD8^+$ T cells.

T cells that recognize self-MHC molecules but not self-antigens are allowed to mature by positive selection. T cells unable to recognize MHC molecules are not selected and are eliminated by **programmed cell death**, or **apoptosis** (see Chapter 3, Cell Signaling).

T cells that recognize both self-MHC and self-antigens—produced by thymic

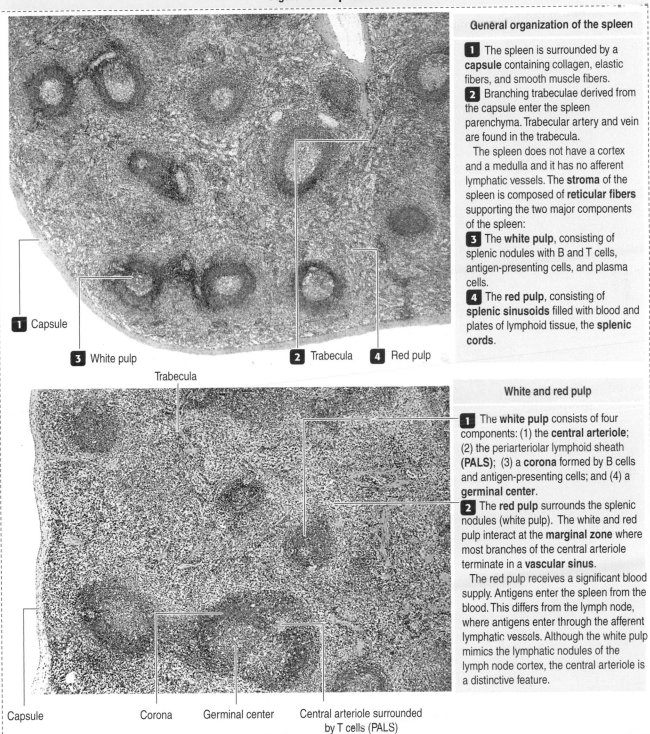

Figure 10-18. Spleen

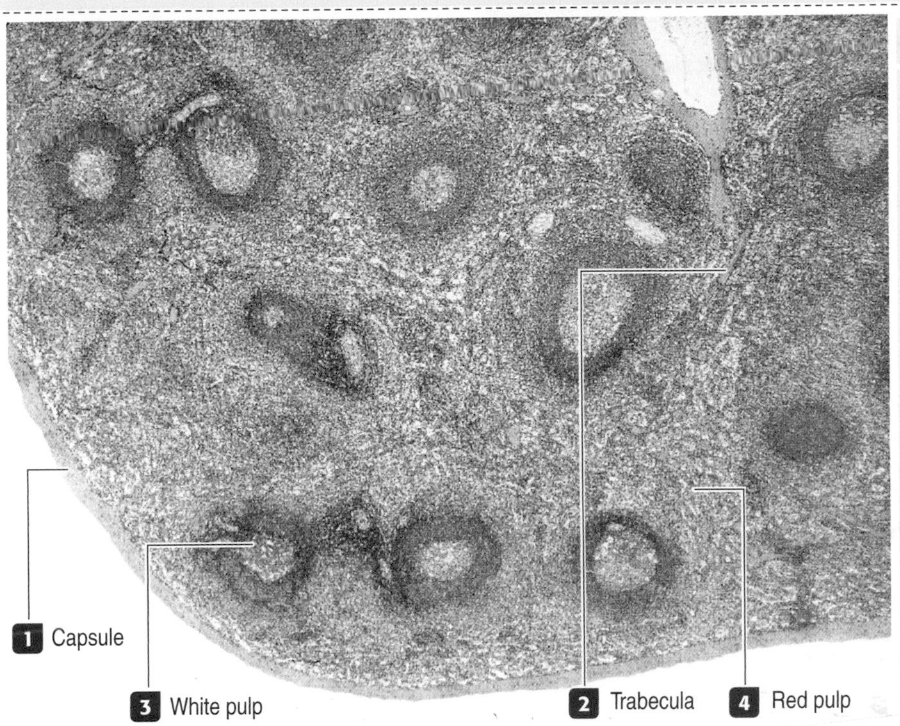
1 Capsule
3 White pulp
2 Trabecula
4 Red pulp

General organization of the spleen

1 The spleen is surrounded by a **capsule** containing collagen, elastic fibers, and smooth muscle fibers.
2 Branching trabeculae derived from the capsule enter the spleen parenchyma. Trabecular artery and vein are found in the trabecula.

The spleen does not have a cortex and a medulla and it has no afferent lymphatic vessels. The **stroma** of the spleen is composed of **reticular fibers** supporting the two major components of the spleen:
3 The **white pulp**, consisting of splenic nodules with B and T cells, antigen-presenting cells, and plasma cells.
4 The **red pulp**, consisting of **splenic sinusoids** filled with blood and plates of lymphoid tissue, the **splenic cords**.

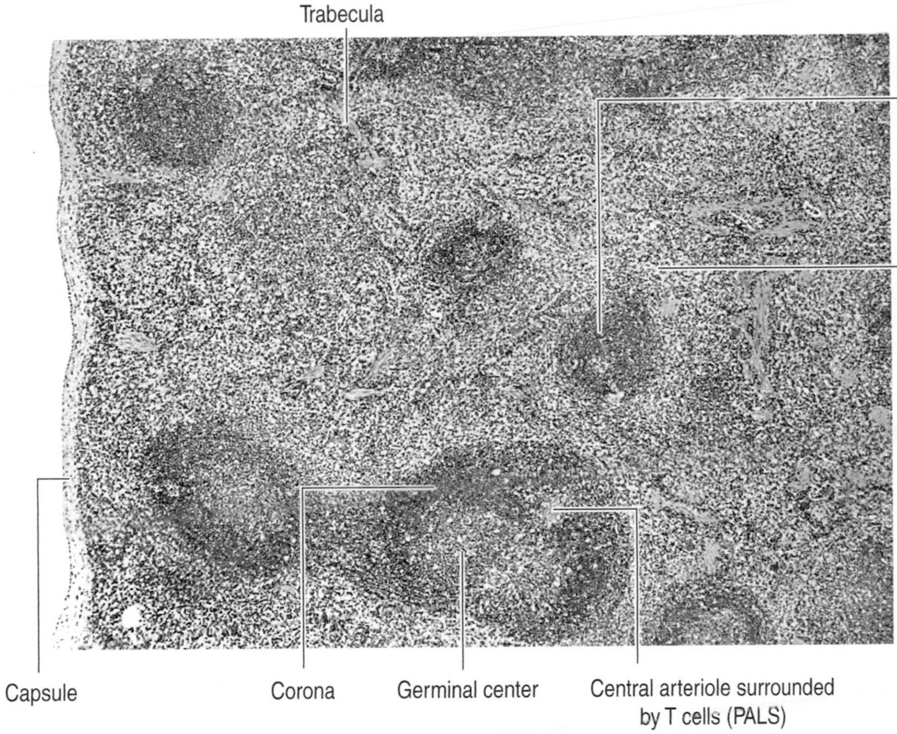
Trabecula
Capsule
Corona
Germinal center
Central arteriole surrounded by T cells (PALS)

White and red pulp

1 The **white pulp** consists of four components: (1) the **central arteriole**; (2) the periarteriolar lymphoid sheath **(PALS)**; (3) a **corona** formed by B cells and antigen-presenting cells; and (4) a **germinal center**.
2 The **red pulp** surrounds the splenic nodules (white pulp). The white and red pulp interact at the **marginal zone** where most branches of the central arteriole terminate in a **vascular sinus**.

The red pulp receives a significant blood supply. Antigens enter the spleen from the blood. This differs from the lymph node, where antigens enter through the afferent lymphatic vessels. Although the white pulp mimics the lymphatic nodules of the lymph node cortex, the central arteriole is a distinctive feature.

medullary epithelial cells under the regulation of the *aire* gene—are eliminated by **negative selection (clonal deletion)**, a task carried out by dendritic cells and macrophages.

About 95% of the developing T cells die within the cortex of the thymus without ever maturing. Double-positive T cells undergo apoptosis within three days in the absence of a surviving signal; positive signals enable the progression to single-positive. Within 1 week, single-positive cells will be eliminated by apoptosis unless they receive a positive signal for survival and export to the periphery. Functional T cells, surviving the selection process, can exit to the peripheral

Figure 10-19. Vascularization of the spleen

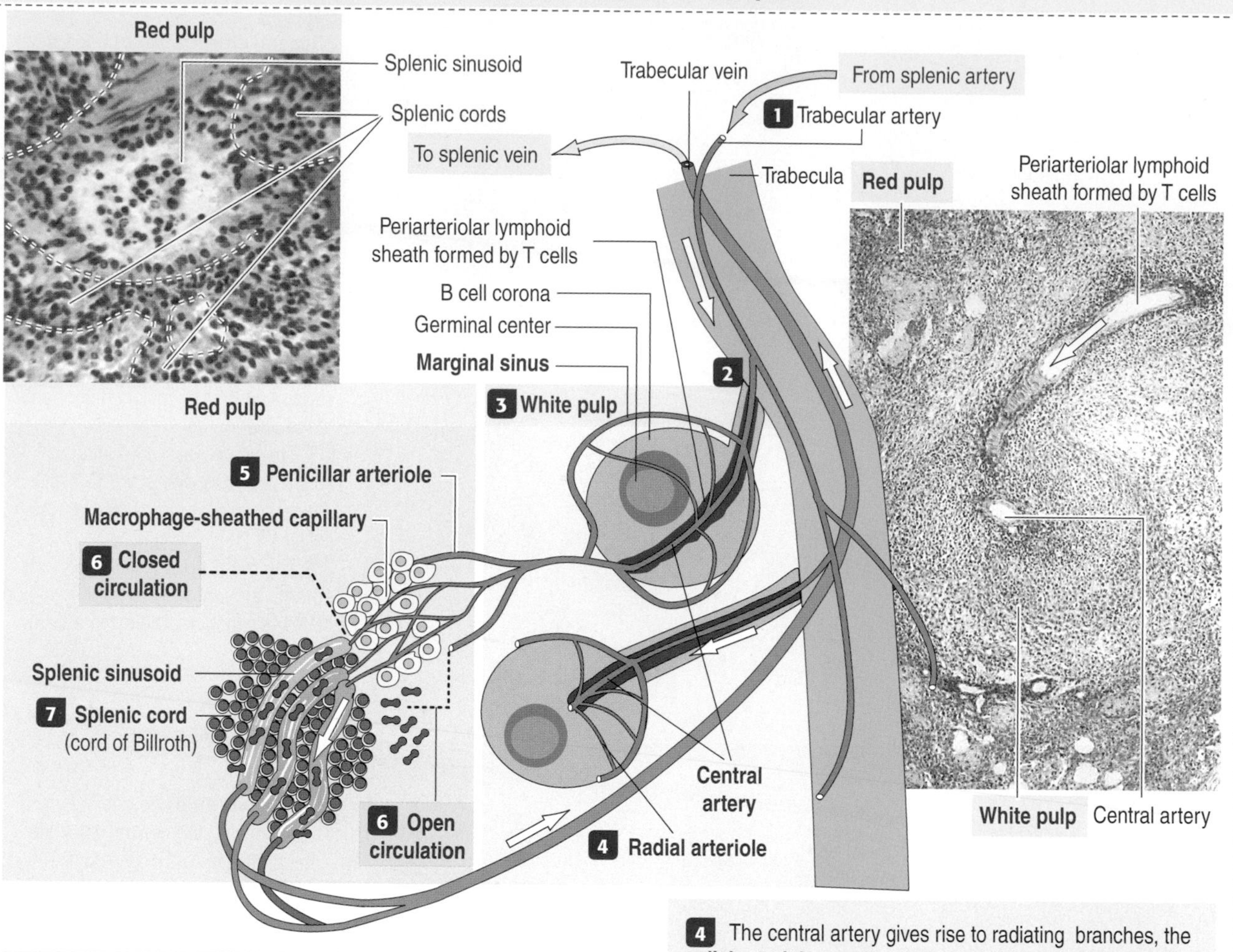

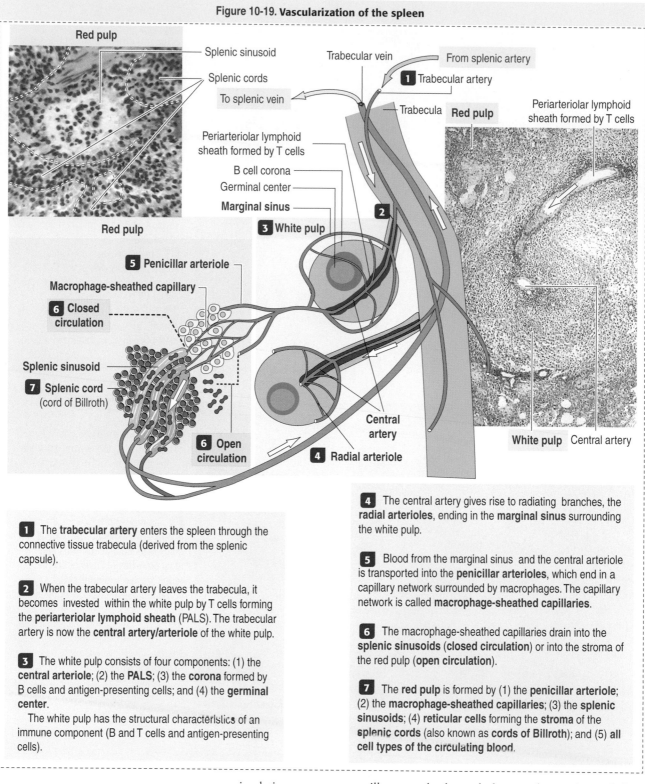

Red pulp
Splenic sinusoid
Splenic cords
To splenic vein
Trabecular vein
From splenic artery
1 Trabecular artery
Trabecula
Red pulp
Periarteriolar lymphoid sheath formed by T cells
Periarteriolar lymphoid sheath formed by T cells
B cell corona
Germinal center
Marginal sinus
2
3 White pulp
Red pulp
5 Penicillar arteriole
Macrophage-sheathed capillary
6 Closed circulation
Splenic sinusoid
7 Splenic cord
(cord of Billroth)
6 Open circulation
4 Radial arteriole
Central artery
White pulp
Central artery

1 The **trabecular artery** enters the spleen through the connective tissue trabecula (derived from the splenic capsule).

2 When the trabecular artery leaves the trabecula, it becomes invested within the white pulp by T cells forming the **periarteriolar lymphoid sheath** (PALS). The trabecular artery is now the **central artery/arteriole** of the white pulp.

3 The white pulp consists of four components: (1) the **central arteriole**; (2) the **PALS**; (3) the **corona** formed by B cells and antigen-presenting cells; and (4) the **germinal center**.

The white pulp has the structural characteristics of an immune component (B and T cells and antigen-presenting cells).

4 The central artery gives rise to radiating branches, the **radial arterioles**, ending in the **marginal sinus** surrounding the white pulp.

5 Blood from the marginal sinus and the central arteriole is transported into the **penicillar arterioles**, which end in a capillary network surrounded by macrophages. The capillary network is called **macrophage-sheathed capillaries**.

6 The macrophage-sheathed capillaries drain into the **splenic sinusoids** (**closed circulation**) or into the stroma of the red pulp (**open circulation**).

7 The **red pulp** is formed by (1) the **penicillar arteriole**; (2) the **macrophage-sheathed capillaries**; (3) the **splenic sinusoids**; (4) **reticular cells** forming the **stroma** of the **splenic cords** (also known as **cords of Billroth**); and (5) **all cell types of the circulating blood**.

circulation across postcapillary venules located close to the corticomedullary junction (see Figure 10-17).

The **medulla** of one lobule is continuous with the medulla of an adjacent lobule. The medulla displays few almost **mature T cells** (single-positive) migrating from the cortex. Maturation of T cells is completed in the medulla, and functional T cells enter postcapillary venules in the corticomedullary junction to exit the thymus toward the peripheral lymphoid organs.

Thymic epithelial cells populate the medulla, many of them forming **Hassall's**

Figure 10-20. **White pulp**

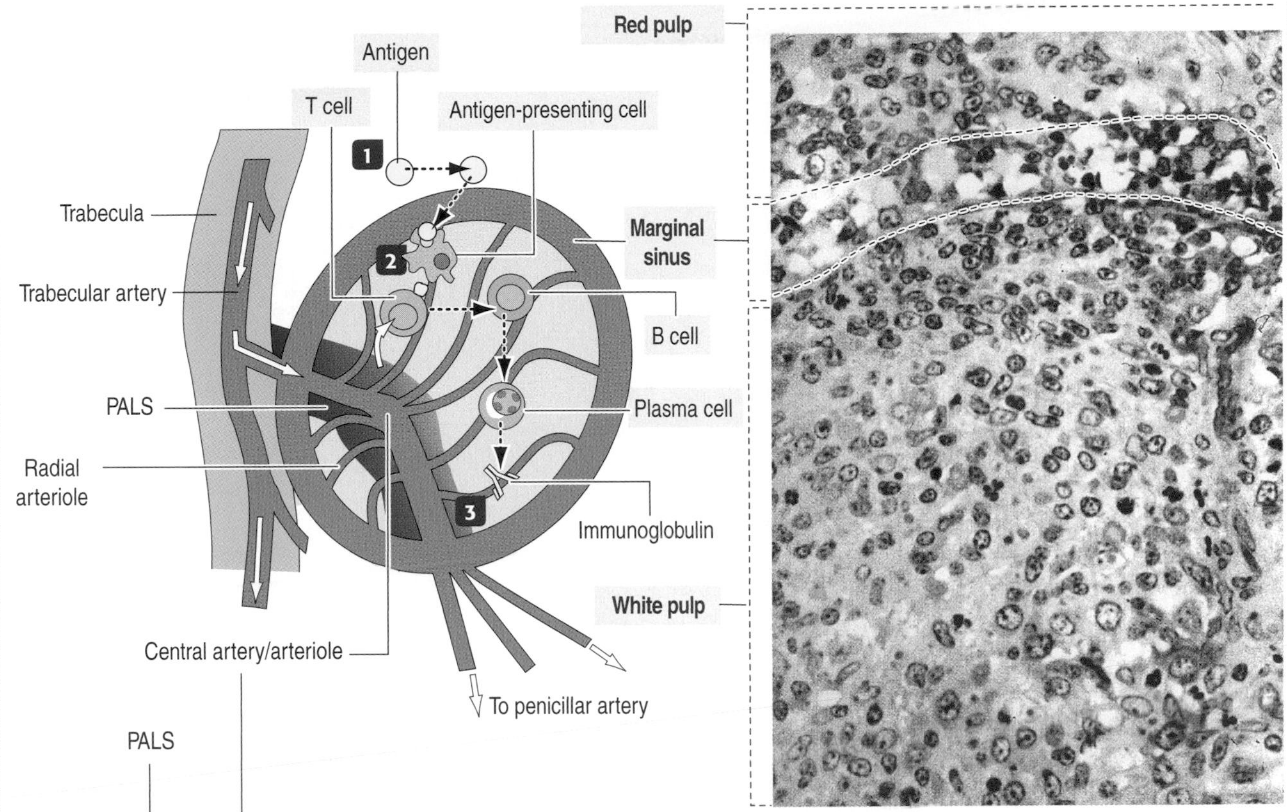

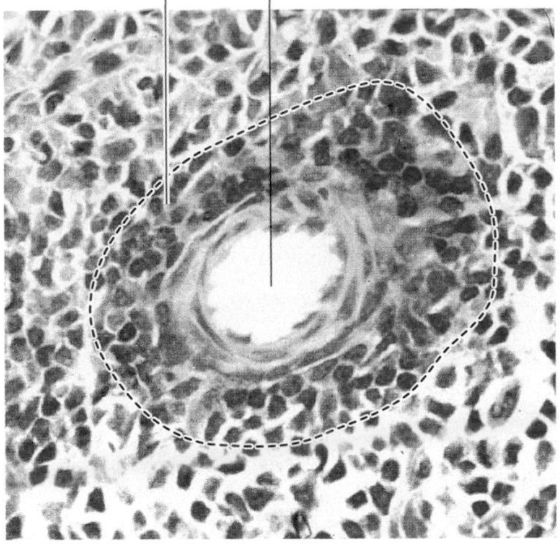

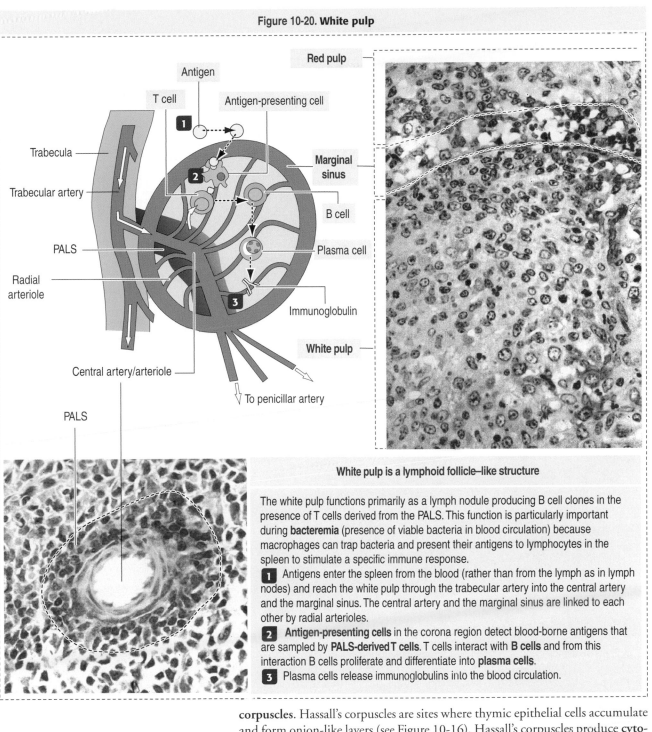

White pulp is a lymphoid follicle–like structure

The white pulp functions primarily as a lymph nodule producing B cell clones in the presence of T cells derived from the PALS. This function is particularly important during **bacteremia** (presence of viable bacteria in blood circulation) because macrophages can trap bacteria and present their antigens to lymphocytes in the spleen to stimulate a specific immune response.

1 Antigens enter the spleen from the blood (rather than from the lymph as in lymph nodes) and reach the white pulp through the trabecular artery into the central artery and the marginal sinus. The central artery and the marginal sinus are linked to each other by radial arterioles.

2 **Antigen-presenting cells** in the corona region detect blood-borne antigens that are sampled by **PALS-derived T cells**. T cells interact with **B cells** and from this interaction B cells proliferate and differentiate into **plasma cells**.

3 Plasma cells release immunoglobulins into the blood circulation.

corpuscles. Hassall's corpuscles are sites where thymic epithelial cells accumulate and form onion-like layers (see Figure 10-16). Hassall's corpuscles produce **cytokine thymic stromal lymphopoietin**, which stimulates thymic dendritic cells to complete the maturation of single-positive T cells to optimize negative selection and ensure tolerance.

Note that **the blood-thymus barrier is not present in the medulla** and that **Hassall's corpuscles can be seen only in the medulla.**

Spleen

The spleen is the largest secondary lymphoid organ of the body. The spleen **lacks a cortex and a medulla.**

Instead, the spleen has two major components with distinct functions (Figure 10-18): the **red pulp** and the **white pulp**.

Figure 10-21. Red pulp

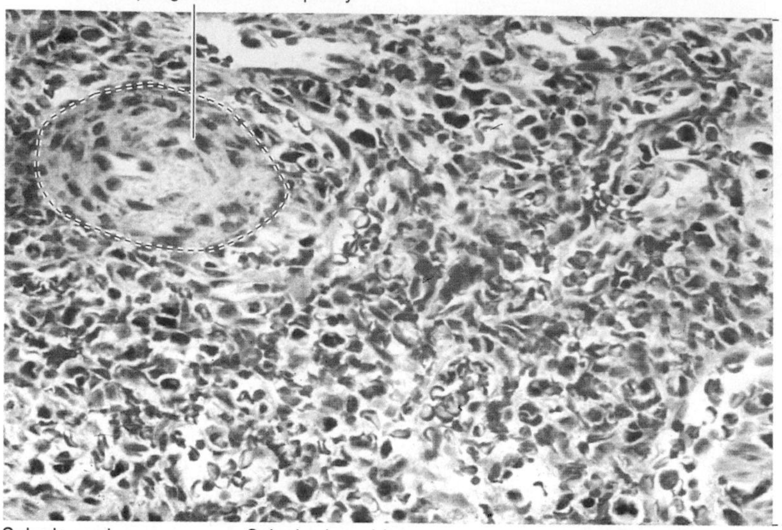

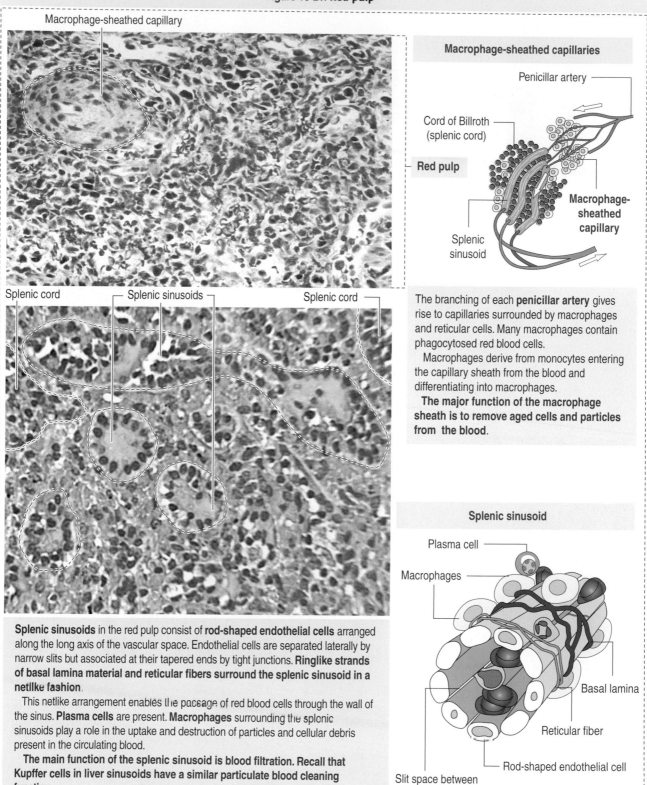

Macrophage-sheathed capillaries

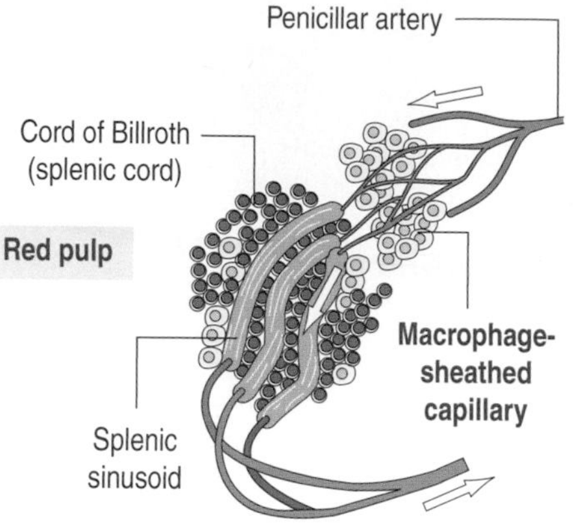

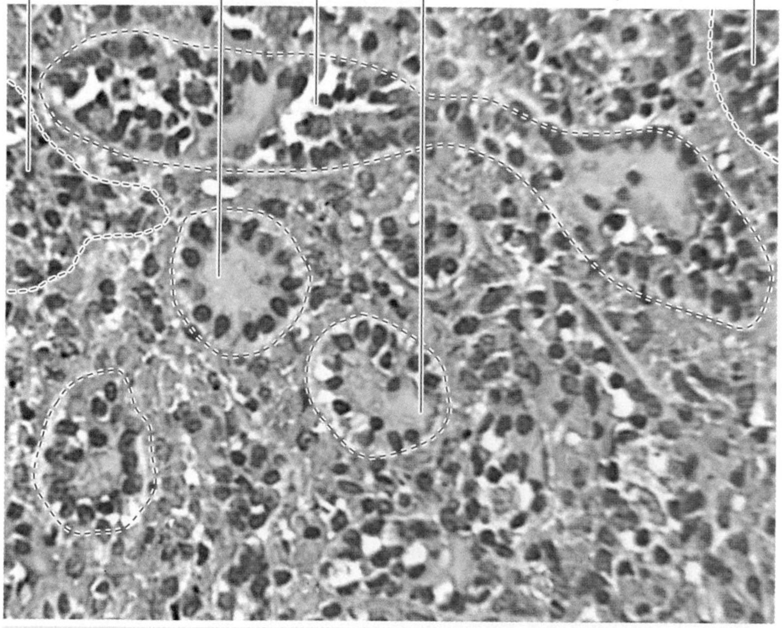

The branching of each **penicillar artery** gives rise to capillaries surrounded by macrophages and reticular cells. Many macrophages contain phagocytosed red blood cells.

Macrophages derive from monocytes entering the capillary sheath from the blood and differentiating into macrophages.

The major function of the macrophage sheath is to remove aged cells and particles from the blood.

Splenic sinusoid

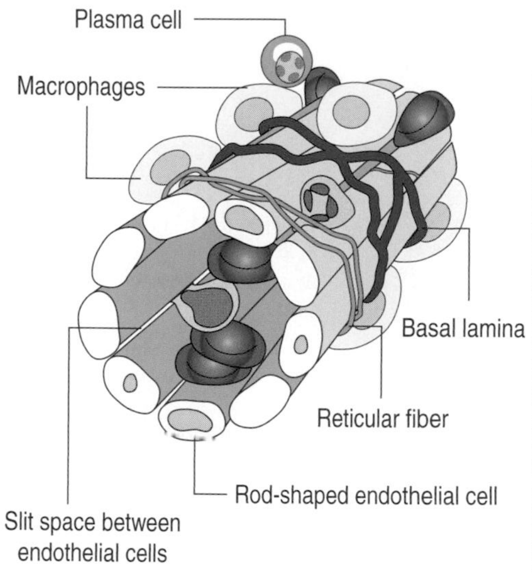

Splenic sinusoids in the red pulp consist of **rod-shaped endothelial cells** arranged along the long axis of the vascular space. Endothelial cells are separated laterally by narrow slits but associated at their tapered ends by tight junctions. **Ringlike strands of basal lamina material and reticular fibers surround the splenic sinusoid in a netlike fashion**.

This netlike arrangement enables the passage of red blood cells through the wall of the sinus. **Plasma cells** are present. **Macrophages** surrounding the splenic sinusoids play a role in the uptake and destruction of particles and cellular debris present in the circulating blood.

The main function of the splenic sinusoid is blood filtration. Recall that Kupffer cells in liver sinusoids have a similar particulate blood cleaning function.

The red pulp is a **filter that removes aged and damaged red blood cells and microorganisms from circulating blood.** It also is a **storage site for red blood cells.** Bacteria can be recognized by macrophages of the red pulp and removed directly or after they are coated with complement proteins (produced in the liver) and immunoglobulins (produced in the white pulp). The clearance of complement–immunoglobulin coated bacteria or viruses by macrophages is very rapid and prevents infections of the kidney, meninges, and lung.

The **white pulp is the immune component of the spleen.** The cell components of the white pulp are similar to those of the lymph node, except that antigens enter the spleen from the blood rather than from the lymph.

Vascularization of the spleen

The spleen is covered by a **capsule** consisting of dense, irregular connective tissue with elastic and smooth muscle fibers (it varies with the species).

Trabeculae derived from the capsule carry blood vessels (**trabecular arteries** and **veins**) and nerves to and from the splenic red pulp (Figure 10-19). A brief review of vascularization of the spleen, which is similar to that of many organs with a significant blood supply such as the kidneys and lung, provides a useful background for understanding the function and structure of this organ.

The **splenic artery** enters the hilum, giving rise to **trabecular arteries,** which are distributed to the splenic pulp along the connective tissue trabeculae. As an artery leaves the trabecula, it becomes invested by a sheath of T cells forming a **periarteriolar lymphoid sheath** (PALS) and penetrates a lymphatic nodule (the **white pulp**). The blood vessel is designated the **central artery** (also called the **follicular arteriole,** because of the nodular or follicular arrangement of the white pulp).

The **central artery** leaves the white pulp to become the **penicillar artery.** Penicillar arteries end as **macrophage-sheathed capillaries.**

Terminal capillaries either drain directly into **splenic sinusoids** (**closed circulation**) or terminate as open-ended vessels within the **red pulp** (**open circulation**). Splenic sinusoids are drained by pulp veins, to trabecular veins, to splenic veins.

White pulp

This component of the spleen is an equivalent of the nodular lymphoid tissue found in lymph nodes except that **it contains a central artery** (also called a central **arteriole**).

The white pulp includes (see Figure 10-19) (1) the **central artery or arteriole** surrounded by a sheath of T cells (PALS) and (2) the **lymphatic nodules,** consisting of B cells. Antigen-presenting cells and macrophages are also present in the white pulp.

There is a **marginal sinus zone** between the red and white pulps that receives **radial arterioles** from the central artery or arteriole (see Figures 10-19 and 10-20). This marginal sinus zone drains into **small sinusoids** located on the outer portion of the marginal zone. At the marginal zone, blood contacts the splenic parenchyma, which contains phagocytic macrophages and antigen-presenting cells, and T and B cells enter the spleen before becoming segregated in their specific splenic location.

Red pulp

The red pulp contains an interconnected network of **splenic sinusoids** lined by elongated endothelial cells. **Splenic cords,** also known as the **cords of Billroth,** separate splenic sinusoids (Figure 10-21; see Figure 10-19).

The **splenic cords** contain **plasma cells, macrophages,** and **blood cells,** all supported by a stroma of **reticular cells** and **fibers.** Cytoplasmic processes of macrophages lie adjacent to the sinusoids and may project into the lumen of the sinusoids through the interendothelial cell slits to sample particulate material.

Splenic sinusoids are discontinuous vascular spaces lined by **rib-shaped endothelial cells** oriented in parallel along the long axis of the sinusoids (see Figure 10-21). Junctional complexes can be found at the tapering ends of the endothelial cells.

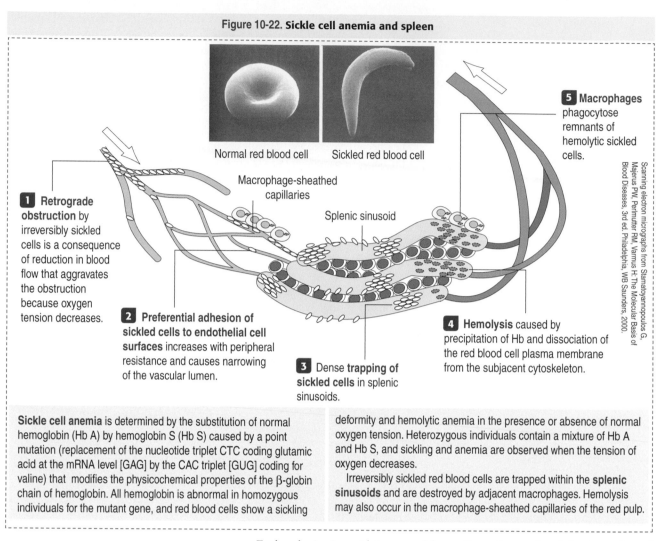

Figure 10-22. Sickle cell anemia and spleen

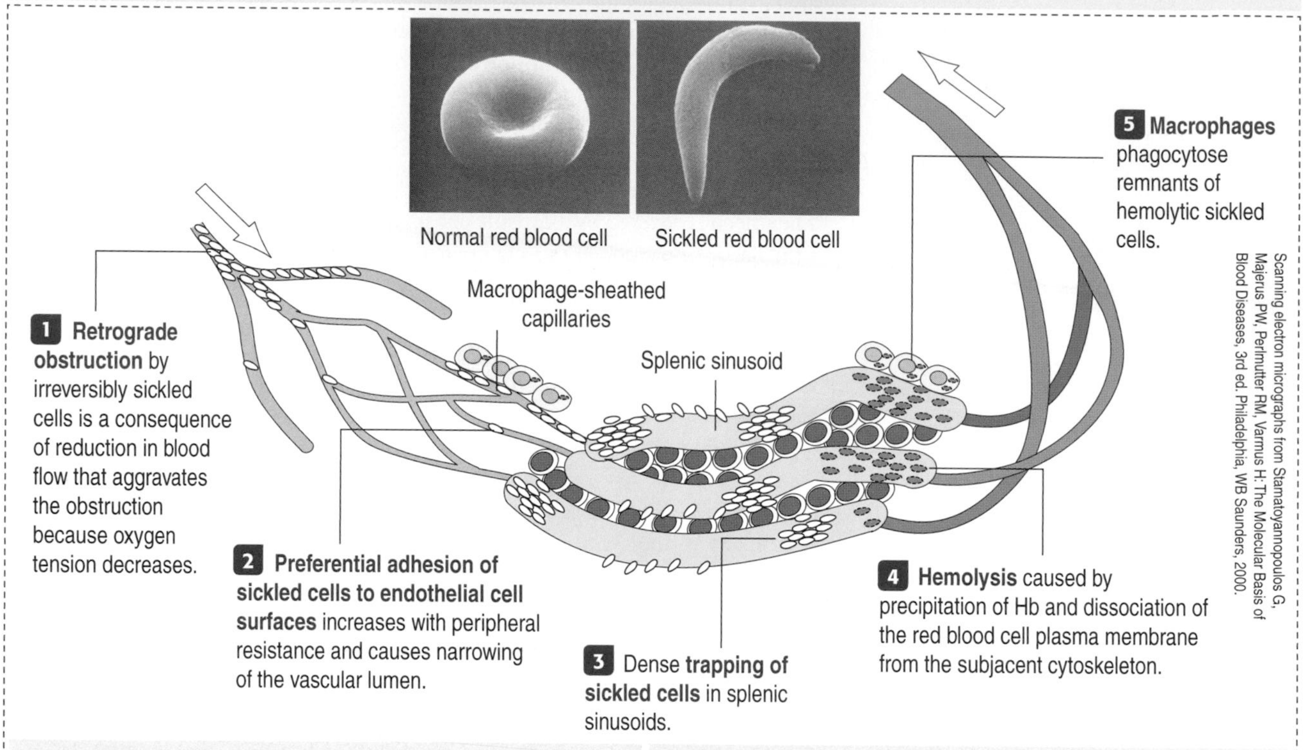
Normal red blood cell
Sickled red blood cell
Macrophage-sheathed capillaries
Splenic sinusoid
1 Retrograde obstruction by irreversibly sickled cells is a consequence of reduction in blood flow that aggravates the obstruction because oxygen tension decreases.
2 Preferential adhesion of sickled cells to endothelial cell surfaces increases with peripheral resistance and causes narrowing of the vascular lumen.
3 Dense trapping of sickled cells in splenic sinusoids.
4 Hemolysis caused by precipitation of Hb and dissociation of the red blood cell plasma membrane from the subjacent cytoskeleton.
5 Macrophages phagocytose remnants of hemolytic sickled cells.
Scanning electron micrographs from Stamatoyannopoulos G, Majerus PW, Perlmutter RM, Varmus H: The Molecular Basis of Blood Diseases, 3rd ed. Philadelphia, WB Saunders, 2000.

Sickle cell anemia is determined by the substitution of normal hemoglobin (Hb A) by hemoglobin S (Hb S) caused by a point mutation (replacement of the nucleotide triplet CTC coding glutamic acid at the mRNA level [GAG] by the CAC triplet [GUG] coding for valine) that modifies the physicochemical properties of the β-globin chain of hemoglobin. All hemoglobin is abnormal in homozygous individuals for the mutant gene, and red blood cells show a sickling deformity and hemolytic anemia in the presence or absence of normal oxygen tension. Heterozygous individuals contain a mixture of Hb A and Hb S, and sickling and anemia are observed when the tension of oxygen decreases.

Irreversibly sickled red blood cells are trapped within the **splenic sinusoids** and are destroyed by adjacent macrophages. Hemolysis may also occur in the macrophage-sheathed capillaries of the red pulp.

Each splenic sinusoid is covered by a discontinuous **basal lamina** oriented around the endothelial cells like ribs or barrel hoops (see Figure 10-21). Adjacent hoops are cross-linked by strands of basal lamina material. In addition, a network of loose **reticular fibers** also encircles the splenic sinusoids. Consequently, blood cells have an unobstructed access to the sinusoids through the narrow slits between the fusiform endothelial cells and the loose basal lamina–reticular fiber network.

Two types of blood circulations have been described in the red pulp (see Figure 10-19): (1) a **closed circulation**, in which arterial vessels connect directly to splenic sinusoids; and (2) an **open circulation**, characterized by blood vessels opening directly into the red pulp spaces, with the blood flowing through these spaces and then entering through the interendothelial cell slits of the splenic sinusoids.

Clinical significance: Sickle cell disease

Sickle cell anemia is discussed briefly in Chapter 6, Blood and Hematopoiesis, within the context of the structure of the red blood cell. Here, we focus on the fate of irreversibly sickled red blood cells when they travel through the narrow passages of the red pulp. We also consider the function of macrophages associated with the splenic sinuses in the disposal of destroyed sickle cells.

When the oxygen tension decreases, sickle cells show preferential adhesion to postcapillary venules followed by trapping of irreversibly sickled cells and retrograde obstruction of the blood vessel (Figure 10-22).

An increased destruction of sickle cells leads to anemia and to an increase in the formation of bilirubin from the released hemoglobin (chronic hyperbilirubinemia). The **occlusion of splenic sinuses** by sickle cells is associated with **splenomegaly**

Figure 10-23. **Homing during inflammation**

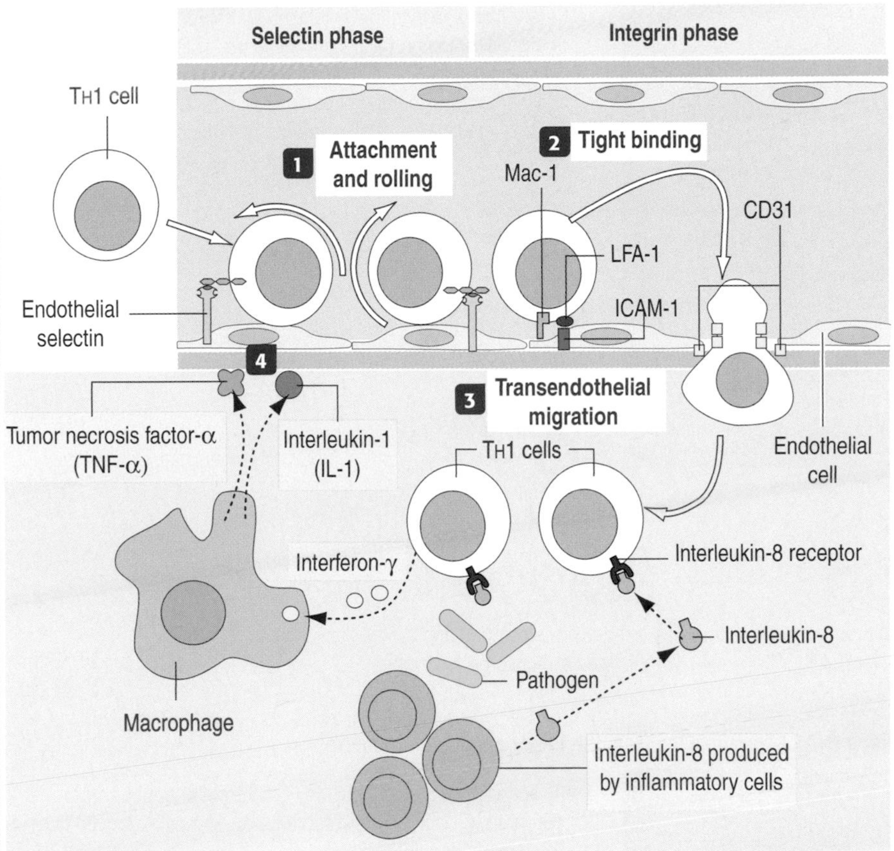

Selectin phase
Integrin phase
TH1 cell
1 Attachment and rolling
2 Tight binding
Mac-1
CD31
LFA-1
ICAM-1
Endothelial selectin
4
3 Transendothelial migration
Tumor necrosis factor-α (TNF-α)
Interleukin-1 (IL-1)
TH1 cells
Endothelial cell
Interleukin-8 receptor
Interferon-γ
Interleukin-8
Pathogen
Macrophage
Interleukin-8 produced by inflammatory cells

1 Attachment and rolling
Leukocytes (TH1 cell in the diagram) establish reversible binding between selectins induced in the endothelial cell surface and carbohydrate ligands on the T cell surface. This binding is not strong and the cell keeps rolling.

2 Tight binding
A strong interaction occurs between the TH1 cell and the endothelial cell. This interaction is mediated by cell adhesion molecules **ICAM-1** (intercellular adhesion molecule) on the endothelium and the T cell integrins **LFA-1** (lymphocyte function–associated antigen) and **Mac-1**.

3 Transendothelial migration
TH1 cells migrate across the endothelium along an **interleukin-8** concentration gradient produced by inflammatory cells. **CD31** contributes to diapedesis.

4 TH1 cells secrete **interferon-γ** to activate macrophages, which in turn secrete **TNF-α** and **IL-1** to stimulate the expression of **selectins** by endothelial cells.

(enlargement of the spleen), disrupted bacterial clearance function of the spleen in cases of bacteremia, and **painful crises** in the affected region. Similar vascular occlusions can also occur in kidney, liver, bones, and retina.

Asplenia (lack of development of the spleen) is a clear demonstration of the function of the spleen in bacteremia. To a certain extent, the Kupffer cells of the liver sinusoids complement the role of the white pulp in the detection and removal of bacteria circulating in blood.

The spleen can be removed surgically (**splenectomy**) in cases of traumatic rupture, as part of the treatment of autoimmune diseases, or because of a malignant tumor of the spleen. Adults who already have antibodies to microorganisms are less prone to bacteremia. Children who have not developed antibodies are more vulnerable.

Clinical significance: Homing during inflammation

In Chapter 1, Epithelium, we discuss the homing process to emphasize the role of cell adhesion molecules in the transendothelial migration of leukocytes. In Chapter 6, Blood and Hematopoiesis, we discuss homing of neutrophils to the connective tissue. Here, we focus on the significance of homing during inflammatory responses to pathogens.

The migration of leukocytes through the body facilitates immune surveillance as well as directs immune responses to antigen-challenged tissues. **Distinct subsets of leukocytes respond to particular types of antigens at different stages during an inflammatory response.**

The migration of leukocytes during inflammation is regulated by a variety of **adhesion molecules** and **chemotactic cytokine receptors** and by the expression of

Figure 10-24. **Adoptive cellular immunotherapy**

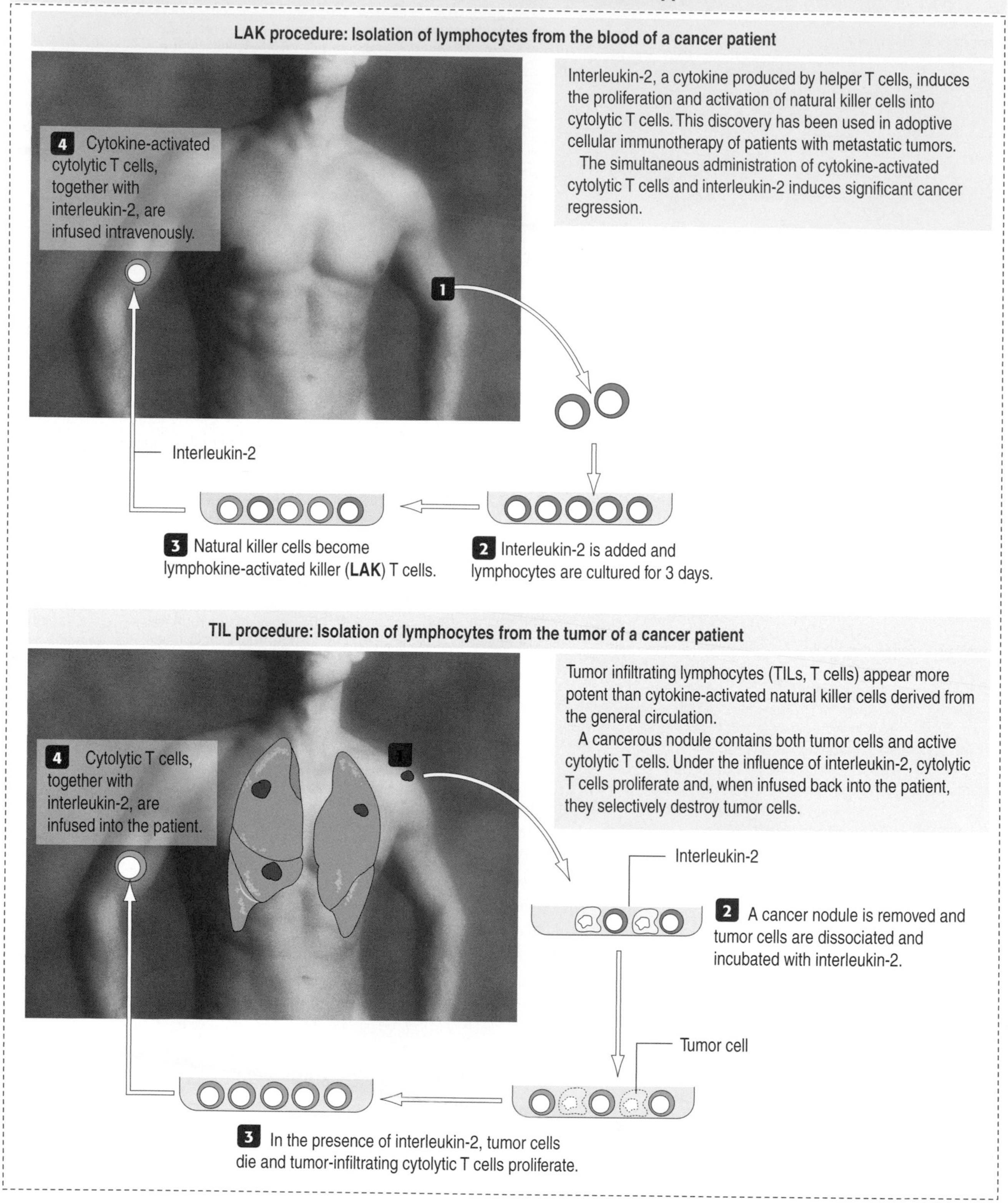

LAK procedure: Isolation of lymphocytes from the blood of a cancer patient
Interleukin-2, a cytokine produced by helper T cells, induces the proliferation and activation of natural killer cells into cytolytic T cells. This discovery has been used in adoptive cellular immunotherapy of patients with metastatic tumors.
The simultaneous administration of cytokine-activated cytolytic T cells and interleukin-2 induces significant cancer regression.
4 Cytokine-activated cytolytic T cells, together with interleukin-2, are infused intravenously.
1
Interleukin-2
3 Natural killer cells become lymphokine-activated killer (LAK) T cells.
2 Interleukin-2 is added and lymphocytes are cultured for 3 days.
TIL procedure: Isolation of lymphocytes from the tumor of a cancer patient
Tumor infiltrating lymphocytes (TILs, T cells) appear more potent than cytokine-activated natural killer cells derived from the general circulation.
A cancerous nodule contains both tumor cells and active cytolytic T cells. Under the influence of interleukin-2, cytolytic T cells proliferate and, when infused back into the patient, they selectively destroy tumor cells.
4 Cytolytic T cells, together with interleukin-2, are infused into the patient.
1
Interleukin-2
2 A cancer nodule is removed and tumor cells are dissociated and incubated with interleukin-2.
Tumor cell
3 In the presence of interleukin-2, tumor cells die and tumor-infiltrating cytolytic T cells proliferate.

leukocyte **adhesion ligands** on the endothelial cell surface (Figure 10–23). **Tumor necrosis factor-α** and **interleukin-1**, produced by antigen-presenting cells in the perivascular space, stimulate the production of cell adhesion ligands by endothelial cells. **Endothelial cells are the regulators of lymphocyte traffic.**

There are two types of endothelium to which leukocytes bind: (1) the **specialized high endothelial venule** of lymphoid tissues and (2) the **flat endothelial cells** of normal and acutely inflamed tissues.

The migration of leukocytes through HEVs is substantial (about one in every four lymphocytes circulating in blood). Different HEVs throughout the body recruit different subsets of lymphocytes into tissues. Migration across flat endothelial cells is minimal, except in cases of inflammation.

Clinical significance: Adoptive cellular immunotherapy

Strategies are being developed to enhance immune response against tumor cells expressing tumor-related antigens. One strategy, called **adoptive cellular immunotherapy**, consists of the transfer of activated immune cells with antitumoral activity into a tumor-bearing host.

Two procedures have been used (Figure 10-24):

1. The **LAK cell procedure** consists of the isolation of lymphokine-activated killer (LAK) cells from the blood of a cancerous patient and their treatment with the cytokine **interleukin-2 (IL-2)** to induce their proliferation in vitro. Activated LAK cells are infused into the patient, together with IL-2. A key issue in this procedure is the isolation of lymphocytes from the same patient, since the infusion of killer T cells from a second patient is not successful. The LAK procedure yields modest benefits when compared with the administration of IL-2 only.

2. The **TIL procedure**, which consists of the isolation of tumor-infiltrating lymphocytes (TILs). In this procedure, a tumor nodule is removed and the cells are dissociated with enzymes. Dissociated cells are cultured with IL-2. This treatment results in the death of cancerous cells and the proliferation of TILs that have already been in contact with tumor cells. TILs are then returned to the patient by transfusion, together with IL-2. About 34% of patients with advanced melanoma receiving TIL treatment had partial or complete tumor regression. A difficulty of the TIL procedure is the isolation of sufficient number of TILs from all tumor specimens for adoptive transfer.

Essential concepts | Immune-Lymphatic System

• Organization of the immune-lymphatic system. The lymphatic system consists of primary and secondary lymphoid organs. The primary lymphoid organs are the bone marrow and the thymus. The secondary lymphoid organs include the lymph nodes, the spleen, the tonsils, and aggregates of lymphoid tissue in several organs, in particular Peyer's patches in the digestive tract (called gut-associated lymphoid tissue [GALT]) and in the lung (called bronchial-associated lymphoid tissue [BALT]).

• The main function of the immune-lymphatic system is to protect the body against pathogens or antigens (bacteria, virus, and parasites). The basis for this defense mechanism, or immune response, is the ability to distinguish between self-antigens and non-self (foreign) antigens.

The two key cell components of the immune system are the lymphocytes and the accessory cells. Lymphocytes include two major groups: (1) B cells, originated and differentiated in the bone marrow and responding to cell-bound or cell-free antigens and (2) T cells, originated in the bone marrow, differentiated in the thymus, and responding to cell-bound antigens.

Accessory cells include the monocyte-derived cells: macrophages and dendritic cells. The follicular dendritic cells, present in lymphatic nodules in lymph nodes, do not derive from bone marrow.

• There are two types of immunity: (1) Innate or natural immunity. This form of immunity, which does not require previous exposure to a pathogen or antigen, involves the epithelial barriers, phagocytic cells (macrophages and neutrophils), natural killer cells, and proteins of the complement system (synthesized by hepatocytes). (2) Adaptive or acquired immunity. This form of immunity, which does require previous exposure to a pathogen or antigen, can be mediated by antibodies produced by plasma cells (humoral immunity), or requires the uptake of a pathogen by an antigen-presenting cell interacting with T cells and B cells (cell-mediated or cellular immunity).

Passive immunity is a temporary form of immunity provided by immunoglobulins produced by another individual in response to an exposure to a pathogen or antigen. Active immunity is a permanent form of immunity developed by an individual after direct exposure to a pathogen or antigen. Adaptive or acquired immunity has the following characteristics: (1) It is specific for an antigen. (2) It is diverse, because responding cells can detect several regions of the same antigen. (3) It produces memory cells after the first encounter with the antigen. Memory cells can react more rapidly when the same antigen reappears. (4) The immune response has a self-limitation; it stops when the antigen is neutralized or eliminated. (5) The immune response has tolerance for self-antigens. A lack of tolerance results in autoimmune diseases.

• B cells originate and mature in the bone marrow. Under the influence of interleukin-7 (produced by stromal cells of the marrow), a pro–B cell gives rise to a pre–B cell. Pre–B cells give rise to immature B cells, which are released into the bloodstream as mature B cells. Maturation includes the expression of cell receptors with the purpose of recognizing and binding self-antigens. B cells that bind strongly to a self-antigen are eliminated by apoptosis. A less strong binding enables the B cell to survive, complete its maturation, and be released into the bloodstream.

• The presentation of antigens by macrophages (called antigen-presenting cells) to T cells is the basis of cell-mediated immunity, and the mechanism of clonal selection of immunocompetent T cells in the thymus. In the mouse, the presentation of antigens is carried out by a cell surface protein complex called major histocompatibility complex (MHC). The MHC-equivalent in humans is called human leukocyte antigen (HLA).

There are two types of MHC molecules: class I MHC (formed by two polypeptide chains, α chain and β_2-microglobulin), and class II MHC (consisting of two polypeptide chains, α chain and β chain). The coreceptor CD8, present on the surface of cytolytic T cells, binds to class I MHC; the coreceptor CD4, present on the surface of helper T cells, binds to class II MHC.

In humans the class I MHC-equivalents consist of three variants, designated HLA-A, HLA-B, and HLA-C. The class II MHC-equivalents also consist of three variants, designated HLA-DR, HLA-DQ, and HLA-DP.

• In addition to coreceptors, members of the immunoglobulin superfamily, T cells have a TCR complex on their surface. Antigen recognition requires the participation of three components: class I or II MHC, TCR, and coreceptor CD4 or CD8. The TCR consists of two chains: α and β chains. Each chain has a variable domain (Vα and Vβ) and a constant domain (Cα and Cβ). The rearrangement at random of gene segments encoding the TCR enables recognition of different regions of a foreign (non-self) antigen.

• The maturation of bone marrow–derived thymocytes in the thymus requires recognition by maturing T cells of class I MHC and class II MHC, present on the surface of thymic epithelial cells, as well as an exposure to self-antigens and non-self (foreign) antigens. Maturation requires the expression of TCR and coreceptors CD4 and CD8 on the surface of the maturing T cells undergoing a selection process. These molecule are the bases of clonal selection and clonal deletion.

During the maturation process, thymocytes arrive at the thymus without coreceptors or TCR on their surface (they are "double-negative" cells). As the maturation process advances, they express TCR and CD4 and CD8 coreceptors ("double-positive" cells). Finally, they become "single-positive" cells ($CD4^+$ or $CD8^+$).

During the maturation process, T cells must be MHC-restricted, tolerant to self-antigens, and bind to non-self antigens to undergo a positive selection. T cells that do not bind to MHC or bind to a self-antigen undergo a negative selection (they are discarded by apoptosis).

The final test takes place in the medullary region of the thymus, where thymic epithelial cells, regulated by the transcription factor aire, express a number of self-antigens that are sampled by the maturing T cells. Mutations of the *aire* gene are associated with the human autosomal disorder **polyendocrinopathy–candidiasis–ectodermal dystrophy (APECED)**, also known as **polyendocrine syndrome type-1**, **(APS-1)**. Autoreactive T cells are exported to the periphery and determine a number of **autoimmune diseases**.

• Helper and cytolytic T cells. There are two subclasses of helper T cells: TH1 cells (involved in reactions caused by intracellular pathogens) and TH2 cells (involved in reactions caused by parasites). After exposure to a fragment of an antigen presented by an antigen-presenting cell, the population of T cells expands by mitosis and recruits B cells. The population of B cells, under the influence of T cells, expands by mitosis. Some of the B cells become memory cells; others differentiate into plasma cells, which secrete immunoglobulins to neutralize an extracellular antigen. Plasma cells are effector cells. Helper T cells are regulatory cells; the do not participate directly in a response. TH1 and TH2 are suppressor cells, a function mediated by their secretory cytokines.

Helper T cells are targets of HIV-type 1 infection and the cause of the **acquired immunodeficiency syndrome (AIDS)**.

An antigen-presenting cell can recruit a cytolytic T cell (CTL), which undergoes mitotic expansion. The cytolytic T cell can bind to an antigen-presenting cell (for example, infected with a virus) and cause its destruction by the release of perforin (to alter water and ionic permeability of the affected cell) and Fas ligand (to induce apoptosis). CTLs are effector cells. Natural killer (NK) cells, which do not belong to the T cell and B cell types, are not activated by antigens—as helper and cytolytic cells are—and lack TCR. NK cells are activated in response to interferons or macrophage-derived cytokines.

• The complement system enables the destruction of pathogens by a mechanism known as opsonization. Proteins of the complement system, most of them produced by hepatocytes, "complement" the effect of antibodies, mannose-binding lectin, and spontaneous activation of C3. A number of complement proteins construct a membrane attack complex (MAC) to induce the lysis of infected cells.

Complement regulators (CRegs) modulate the activity of the complement cascade to protect unintended bystanders. The CReg CD59 is particularly important because it prevents the final assembly of MAC. **Paroxysmal nocturnal hemoglobinuria** is caused by the destruction of red blood cells lacking CD59. Unprotected red blood cells are destroyed by the complement cascade.

• Lymph nodes. The main function of lymph nodes is the filtration of the lymph. A lymph node is surrounded by a connective tissue capsule that sends partitions (trabeculae) inside the lymph node. The stroma of the lymph node consists of a three-dimensional network of reticular fibers (type III collagen). The convex side of the lymph node is the entry side of several afferent lymphatic vessels with valves. Lymph percolates through the subcapsular sinus and the paratrabecular sinus. The concave side of the lymph node is the hilum, the site where an artery enters the lymph node and vein and efferent lymphatic vessel drain the structure.

The lymph node consists of a cortex and a medulla. The cortex is subdivided into an outer cortex, where B cell–containing lymphatic nodules are present, and a deep cortex, where T cells ($CD4^+$) predominate. A lymphatic nodule or follicle consists of a mantle (facing the capsule) and a germinal center, containing proliferating B cells interacting with follicular dendritic cells (FDCs). Macrophages are also present. Macrophages take up particulate matter in the lymph and opsonized antigens and phagocytose apoptotic B cells. FDCs have an antigen-presenting function. B and T cells reach the lymph node through the postcapillary venules present in the inner cortex.

The medulla contains medullary cords, housing B cells, plasma cells, and macrophages, separated by medullary sinuses, endothelial cell–lined spaces containing lymph arriving from the cortical region of the node. Large blood vessels are present in the medulla close to the hilum.

• Thymus. The main function of the thymus is the production of T cells from thymocytes derived from bone marrow.

The thymus derives from the endodermic third pharyngeal pouch (also the site of origin of the inferior parathyroid gland). The thymus is surrounded by a connective tissue capsule projecting trabeculae inside the tissue. Blood vessels are present in the trabeculae and capsule.

The thymus consists of several incomplete lobules. Each lobule has a complete cortex and a medulla shared with adjacent lobules. Two important features are (1) The lack of lymphatic nodules in the cortex. (2) The presence of Hassall's corpuscles in the medulla. Two relevant functional characteristics are the blood-thymus barrier, present in the cortex of the thymus, and postcapillary venules at the corticomedullary junction.

The stroma of the thymus consists of a three-dimensional network of thymic epithelial cells (TECs) interconnected by desmosomes. TECs derive from a common precursor, which gives rise to thymic cortical and medullary epithelial cells when the transcription factor Foxn1 is active. Inactivation of the ***Foxn1*** gene prevents the development of the thymus, resulting in the failure of T cell development leading to a **congenital immunodeficiency**. Cortical TECs express on their surface MHC molecules required for clonal selection. Medullary TECs, activated by the *aire* gene, express self-proteins necessary for clonal deletion of autoreactive T cells. Mutations in the *aire* gene cause a number of autoimmune diseases (including autoimmune polyendocrinopathy–candidiasis–ectodermal dystrophy **[APECED]**, also known as autoimmune polyendocrine type-1 **[APS-1]**) because autoreactive T cells can reach several organs and tissues.

• Spleen. The spleen has a dual function: (1) The white pulp is the immune component of the spleen; components of the white pulp react to blood-borne antigens. (2) The red pulp is a filter that removes aged and damaged red blood cells and microorganisms from circulating blood.

The spleen has distinctive structural features: (1) It lacks a cortex and a medulla. (2) Similar to the lymph node, it has a lymphatic nodule with a germinal center and a mantle populated by B cells and antigen-presenting cells. Contrary to the lymphatic nodule, it has an artery/arteriole surrounded by T cells, the periarteriolar lymphoid sheath (PALS).

The red pulp has two components: (1) The splenic sinuses, formed by elongated endothelial cells separated by narrow slits that allow the passage of cells, are surrounded by an incomplete basal lamina and loose reticular fibers. (2) The splenic cords separate splenic sinuses. They contain macrophages, plasma cells, and blood cells.

There are two types of blood circulation: (1) open circulation, in which red blood cells enter the red pulp spaces, and (2) closed circulation, in which arterial vessels are continuous with the splenic sinusoids.

11. INTEGUMENTARY SYSTEM

The integument is the largest organ of the body. It consists of two components: (1) the **skin** and (2) the **epidermal derivatives**, such as nails, hair, and glands (sweat and sebaceous glands and the mammary gland).

The skin is of particular significance in a clinical physical examination. For example, the color of the skin may indicate the existence of a pathologic condition: a yellow color indicates **jaundice**; a blue-gray color may indicate **cyanosis**, reflecting a pathologic condition of cardiovascular and respiratory function; a pale color is indicative of **anemia**; lack of skin pigmentation suggests **albinism**, a genetic trait characterized by lack of the enzyme tyrosinase, involved in the conversion of the amino acid tyrosine to melanin. Many infectious and immunologic diseases produce characteristic skin changes leading to a correct diagnosis. In addition, the skin has diseases peculiar to itself.

The skin has several **functions**: (1) **protection** (mechanical function); (2) as a **water barrier**; (3) **regulation of body temperature** (conservation and dissipation of heat); (4) **nonspecific defense** (barrier to microorganisms); (5) **excretion of salts**; (6) **synthesis of vitamin D**; (7) as a **sensory organ**, and (8) **sexual signaling**.

Skin types and general organization

The skin consists of three layers firmly attached to one another (Figure 11-1): (1) the outer **epidermis**—derived from ectoderm; (2) the deeper **dermis**—derived from mesoderm; and (3) the **hypodermis** or **subcutaneous layer**—corresponding to the **superficial fascia** of gross anatomy.

Skin is generally classified into two types: (1) **thick skin** and (2) **thin skin**.

Thick skin (more than 5 mm thick) covers the palms of the hands and the soles of the feet and has a thick epidermis and dermis. Thin skin (1 to 2 mm in thickness) lines the rest of the body; the epidermis is thin.

The surface of the skin of the palms and soles and digits of hands and feet has narrow **epidermal ridges** separated by **furrows**. Each epidermal ridge corresponds to an underlying dermal papilla. Ridges and papillae are permanent, have a constant pattern, and are unique to each individual. Impressions of the ridges create **fingerprint** patterns, useful for forensic identification.

The epidermis and dermis display a tight fit interface at the dermal-epidermal junction, where a basal lamina and hemidesmosomes are located. A **primary epidermal ridge** interlocks with a subjacent **primary dermal ridge** (see Figure 11-1). An epidermal **interpapillary peg**, projecting downward from the primary epidermal ridge, interlocks with the primary dermal ridge, which is subdivided into two **secondary dermal ridges**. A number of **dermal papillae** project upward from the surface of each secondary dermal ridge into the epidermal region, interlocking with downward projections of the epidermis. This arrangement is predominant in hairless thick skin. Dermal papillae are numerous and branched. In thin skin, papillae are low and their number is reduced.

Epidermis

The **stratified squamous epithelial layer** of the epidermis consists of four distinct cell types (Figure 11-2):

1. The predominant cell type is the **keratinocyte**, so called because its major product is **keratin**, an intermediate filament protein.

2. **Melanocytes**—neural crest–derived cells responsible for the production of **melanin** (Figure 11-3).

3. **Langerhans cells**—dendritic cells derived from a bone marrow precursor, acting as antigen-trapping cells interacting with T cells.

Figure 11-1. **General organization of the skin**

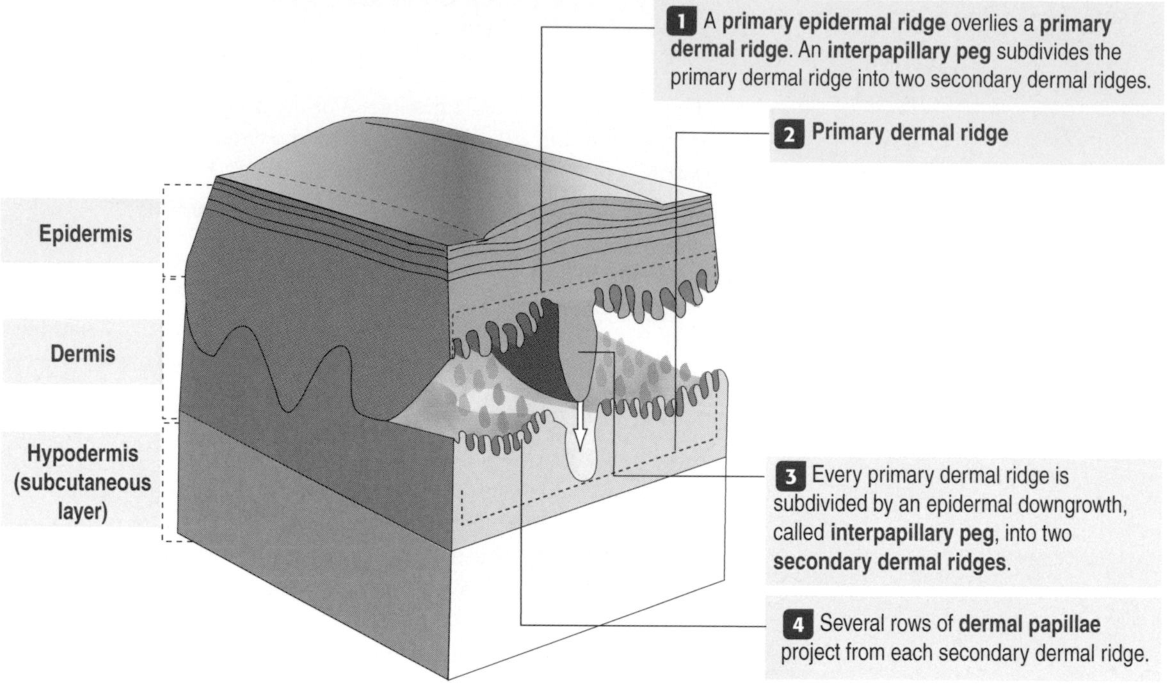

1 A **primary epidermal ridge** overlies a **primary dermal ridge**. An **interpapillary peg** subdivides the primary dermal ridge into two secondary dermal ridges.
2 Primary dermal ridge
Epidermis
Dermis
Hypodermis (subcutaneous layer)
3 Every primary dermal ridge is subdivided by an epidermal downgrowth, called **interpapillary peg**, into two **secondary dermal ridges**.
4 Several rows of **dermal papillae** project from each secondary dermal ridge.

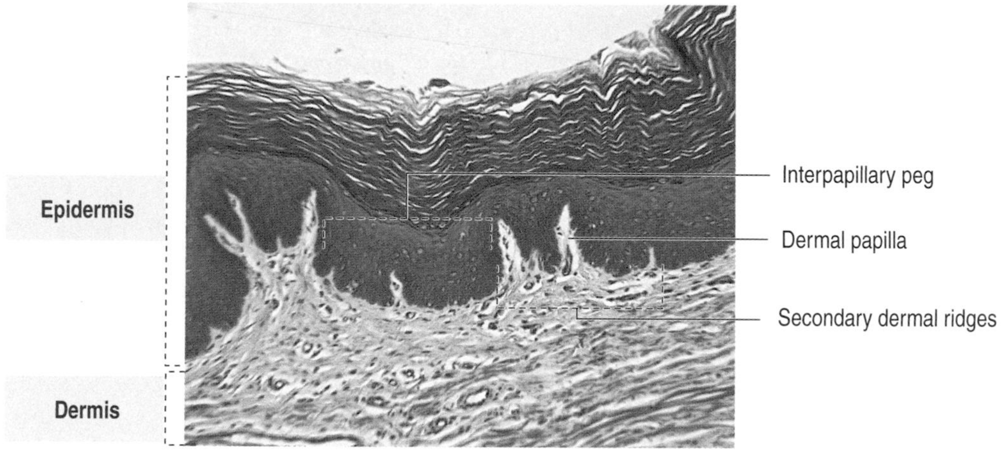

Epidermis
Dermis
Interpapillary peg
Dermal papilla
Secondary dermal ridges

4. **Merkel cells**—neural crest–derived cells involved in tactile sensation.

Keratinocytes are arranged in **five layers** or **strata:** (1) the **stratum basale** (basal cell layer); (2) the **stratum spinosum** (spinous or prickle cell layer); (3) the **stratum granulosum** (granular cell layer); (4) the **stratum lucidum** (clear cell layer); and (5) the **stratum corneum** (cornified cell layer). The first cell layers consist of metabolically active cells; cells of the last two layers undergo **keratinization**, or **cornification**, a process that involves cellular and intercellular molecular changes.

Both the stratum basale and stratum spinosum form the **stratum of Malpighi**. The **stratum basale** (or **stratum germinativum**) consists of a single layer of columnar or high cuboidal keratinocytes resting on a basement membrane. The cytoplasm contains intermediate filaments associated with **desmosomes.** Bundles of intermediate filaments, visible under the light microscope, are called **tonofilaments. Hemidesmosomes** and associated intermediate filaments anchor the basal domain of basal cells to the basement membrane.

The cells of the stratum basale undergo mitosis. While some of the dividing cells add to the population of **stem cells** of the stratum basale, others migrate

Figure 11-2. **Layers of the epidermis of thick skin**

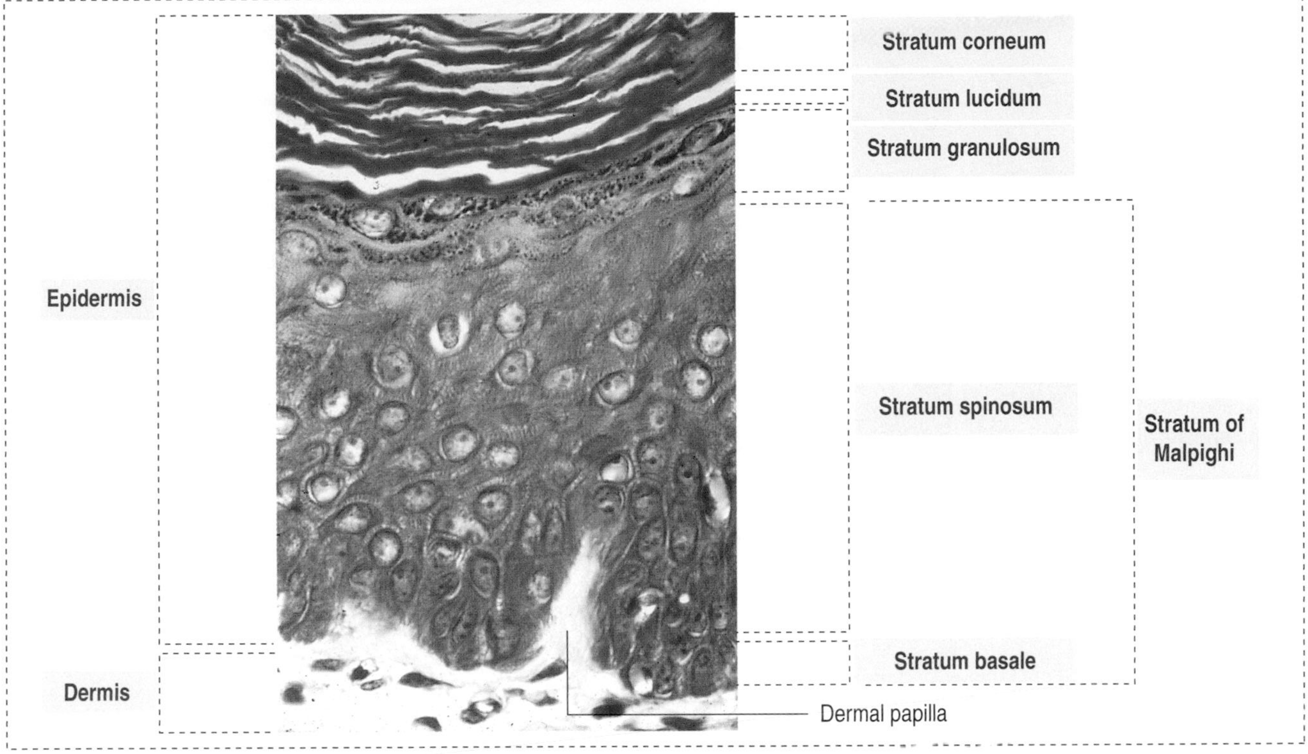

into the stratum spinosum to initiate the differentiation process, ending with the formation of the stratum corneum.

Clinical significance: Wound healing

Skin is an efficient protective barrier. If a portion of epidermis is damaged or destroyed, it must be repaired rapidly by a sequential mechanism called wound healing. This mechanism consists of four stages: (1) the **formation of a fibrin-platelet clot**; (2) **leukocyte recruitment**; (3) **neovascularization and cellular proliferation**; and (4) **tissue remodeling**.

Wound healing starts with the formation of a **blood clot** covering temporarily the open wound. We discuss in Chapter 6, Blood and Hematopoiesis, that the blood clot consists of platelets embedded in a fibrous mesh of cross-linked fibrin molecules formed when thrombin cleaves fibrinogen. We also discuss in Chapter 6 that platelets contain platelet-derived growth factor (PDGF) stored in alpha granules. PDGF and other growth factors are released when platelets degranulate and leukocytes arrive at the wound site. Keratinocytes and endothelial cells express **cytokine CXC** (for cysteine-x-cysteine) and **CXC receptor**, which recruit neutrophils, monocytes, and lymphocytes to the wound site. A deletion of *CXC receptor* gene results in **delayed wound healing.**

Neutrophils arrive within minutes of injury and release proinflammatory cytokines to activate local fibroblasts in the dermis and keratinocytes in the epidermis. Monocytes are recruited next and become **macrophages**, which produce cytokines, growth factors, and angiogenic factors. New blood vessels develop (**angiogenic response**) and organize **granulation tissue**. The pink granular appearance of the granulation tissue is determined by the formation of numerous blood capillaries.

Reepithelialization starts when keratinocytes of the stratum basale layer migrate from the edges of the wound by the formation of F-actin–containing lamellopodia. We discuss in Chapter 1, Epithelium, that hemidesmosomes anchor basal cells to the basal lamina. Leading edge keratinocytes facilitate their displacement by disrupting hemidesmosome attachment to the basal lamina and by dissolving the

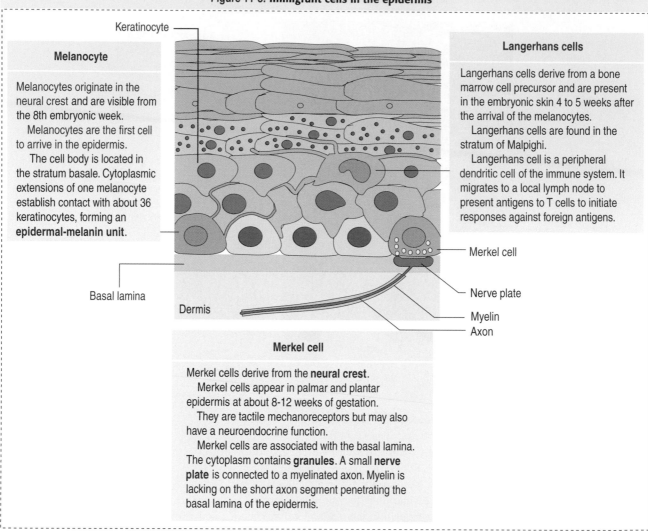

Figure 11-3. Immigrant cells in the epidermis

Melanocyte

Melanocytes originate in the neural crest and are visible from the 8th embryonic week.

Melanocytes are the first cell to arrive in the epidermis.

The cell body is located in the stratum basale. Cytoplasmic extensions of one melanocyte establish contact with about 36 keratinocytes, forming an **epidermal-melanin unit**.

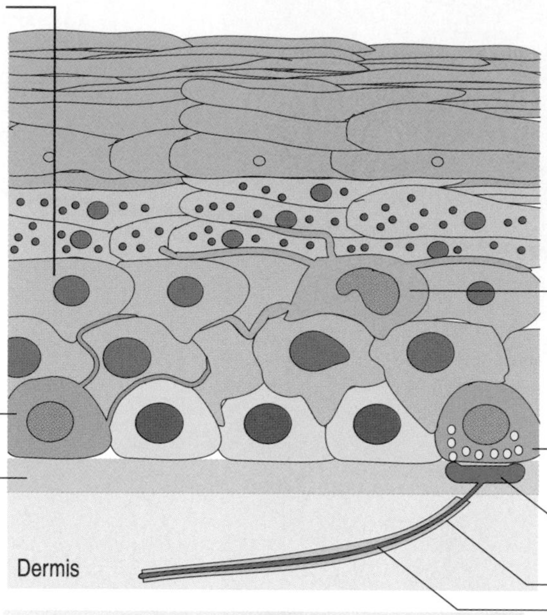

Keratinocyte
Basal lamina
Dermis
Merkel cell
Nerve plate
Myelin
Axon

Langerhans cells

Langerhans cells derive from a bone marrow cell precursor and are present in the embryonic skin 4 to 5 weeks after the arrival of the melanocytes.

Langerhans cells are found in the stratum of Malpighi.

Langerhans cell is a peripheral dendritic cell of the immune system. It migrates to a local lymph node to present antigens to T cells to initiate responses against foreign antigens.

Merkel cell

Merkel cells derive from the **neural crest**.

Merkel cells appear in palmar and plantar epidermis at about 8-12 weeks of gestation.

They are tactile mechanoreceptors but may also have a neuroendocrine function.

Merkel cells are associated with the basal lamina. The cytoplasm contains **granules**. A small **nerve plate** is connected to a myelinated axon. Myelin is lacking on the short axon segment penetrating the basal lamina of the epidermis.

fibrin clot barrier. To accomplish the dissolution of the fibrin clot, keratinocytes upregulate the expression of **plasminogen activator** to convert **plasminogen** within the clot into the fibrinolytic enzyme **plasmin**. Keratinocytes become free from hemidesmosome anchorage with the help of members of the **matrix metalloproteinase family** produced by fibroblasts in the dermis. We discuss the importance of matrix metalloproteinases in Chapter 4, Connective Tissue.

Members of the **epidermal growth factor family** (including epidermal growth factor, transforming growth factor-α, and heparin binding epidermal growth factor) and **keratinocyte growth factor** drive reepithelialization. After the wound surface has been covered by a monolayer of keratinocytes, a new stratified squamous epithelium is established from the margin of the wound toward the center. New hemidesmosomes are formed with the inactivation of matrix metalloproteinases.

Within 3 to 4 days after the wound injury, the underlying connective tissue of the dermis contracts, bringing the wound margins toward one another. Stimulated by local levels of PDGF and transforming growth factor-β, dermal fibroblasts begin to proliferate, infiltrate the blood clot, and deposit type III collagen and extracellular matrix. About 1 week after wounding, a number of wound fibroblasts change into **myofibroblasts** (resembling smooth muscle cells), wound contraction takes place, and healing with a scar occurs.

Retinol (vitamin A) is a precursor of retinoic acid, a hormone-like agent required for the differentiation of epithelia, including epidermis. Retinoids have a

Figure 11-4. Psoriasis

Psoriasis is a chronic epidermal-dermal disease characterized by:
1. Persistent hyperplasia of the epidermis by abnormal cell proliferation and differentiation. Keratinocytes move from the basal layer to the superficial layer in 3 to 5 days, instead of the 28 to 30 days in normal skin. The stratum granulosum may be absent.
2. Abnormal angiogenesis in the dermis capillary plexus. Blood vessels are dilated and convoluted.
3. Infiltration of inflammatory cells in the epidermis and dermis, in particular activated T cells. Neutrophils migrate to the epidermis and form microabscesses.

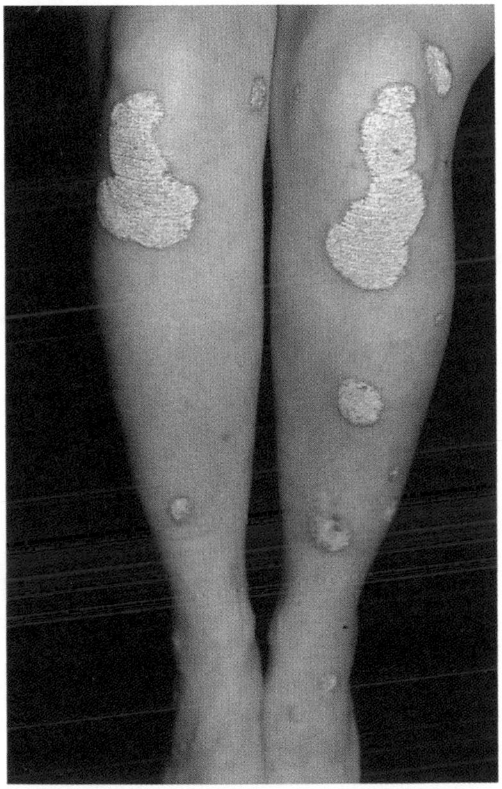

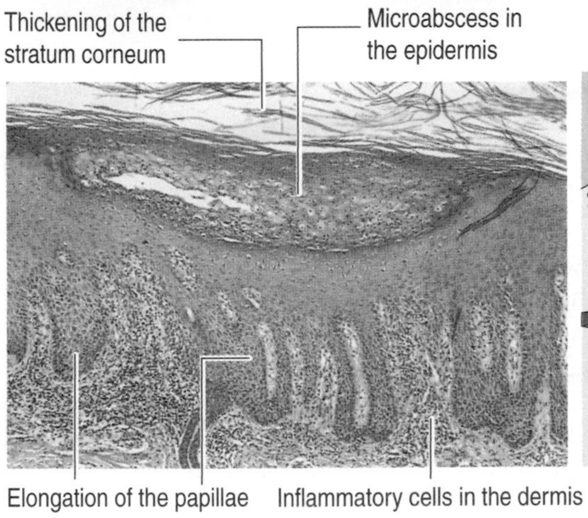

Thickening of the stratum corneum
Microabscess in the epidermis
Elongation of the papillae
Inflammatory cells in the dermis

Pathogenesis of psoriatic plaques

1 Langerhans cells in the epidermis take up antigens and migrate to regional lymph nodes.
2 Langerhans cells interact with T cells (deep cortex of the lymph node).
3 T cells become activated (they express CD2 and CD58, together with either CD80 or CD86 or both). T cells differentiate and express the skin homing receptor cutaneous lymphocyte–associated antigen (CLA).
4 Activated T $CD45^+CLA^+$ cells reenter the blood circulation and home at sites of cutaneous inflammation.
5 In the psoriatic skin, T $CD45^+CLA^+$ cells secrete proinflammatory cytokines, which produce chronically developing psoriatic plaques.

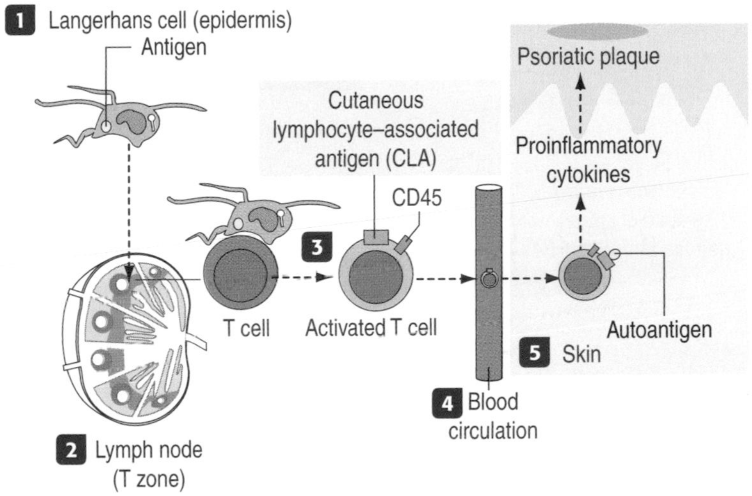

1 Langerhans cell (epidermis)
Antigen
Cutaneous lymphocyte–associated antigen (CLA)
CD45
3
Psoriatic plaque
Proinflammatory cytokines
T cell
Activated T cell
Autoantigen
5 Skin
4 Blood circulation
2 Lymph node (T zone)

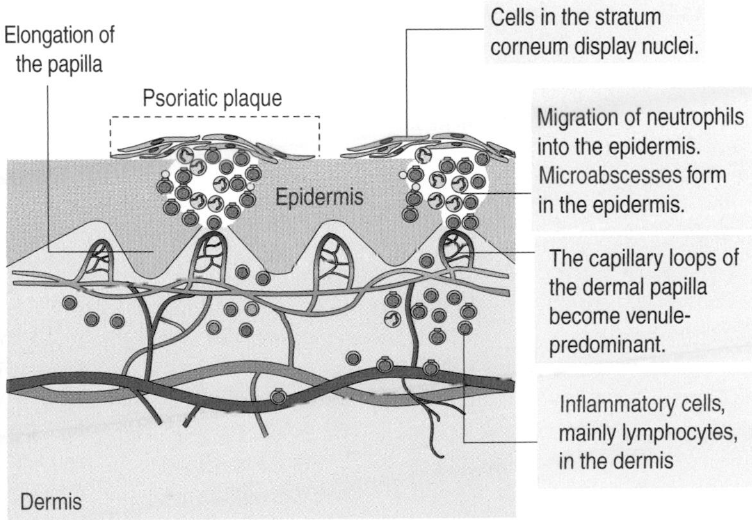

Elongation of the papilla
Cells in the stratum corneum display nuclei.
Psoriatic plaque
Epidermis
Migration of neutrophils into the epidermis. Microabscesses form in the epidermis.
The capillary loops of the dermal papilla become venule-predominant.
Inflammatory cells, mainly lymphocytes, in the dermis
Dermis

Photographs from Callen JP, et al.: Color Atlas of Dermatology. Philadelphia, WB Saunders, 1993.

proliferative effect on the epidermis of normal skin. This effect is mediated at the messenger RNA (mRNA) level by inhibiting cell differentiation and stimulating cell proliferation.

Similar to steroid and thyroid hormones, retinoic acid binds to nuclear recep-

Figure 11-5. **Differentiation of keratinocytes: Expression of keratins**

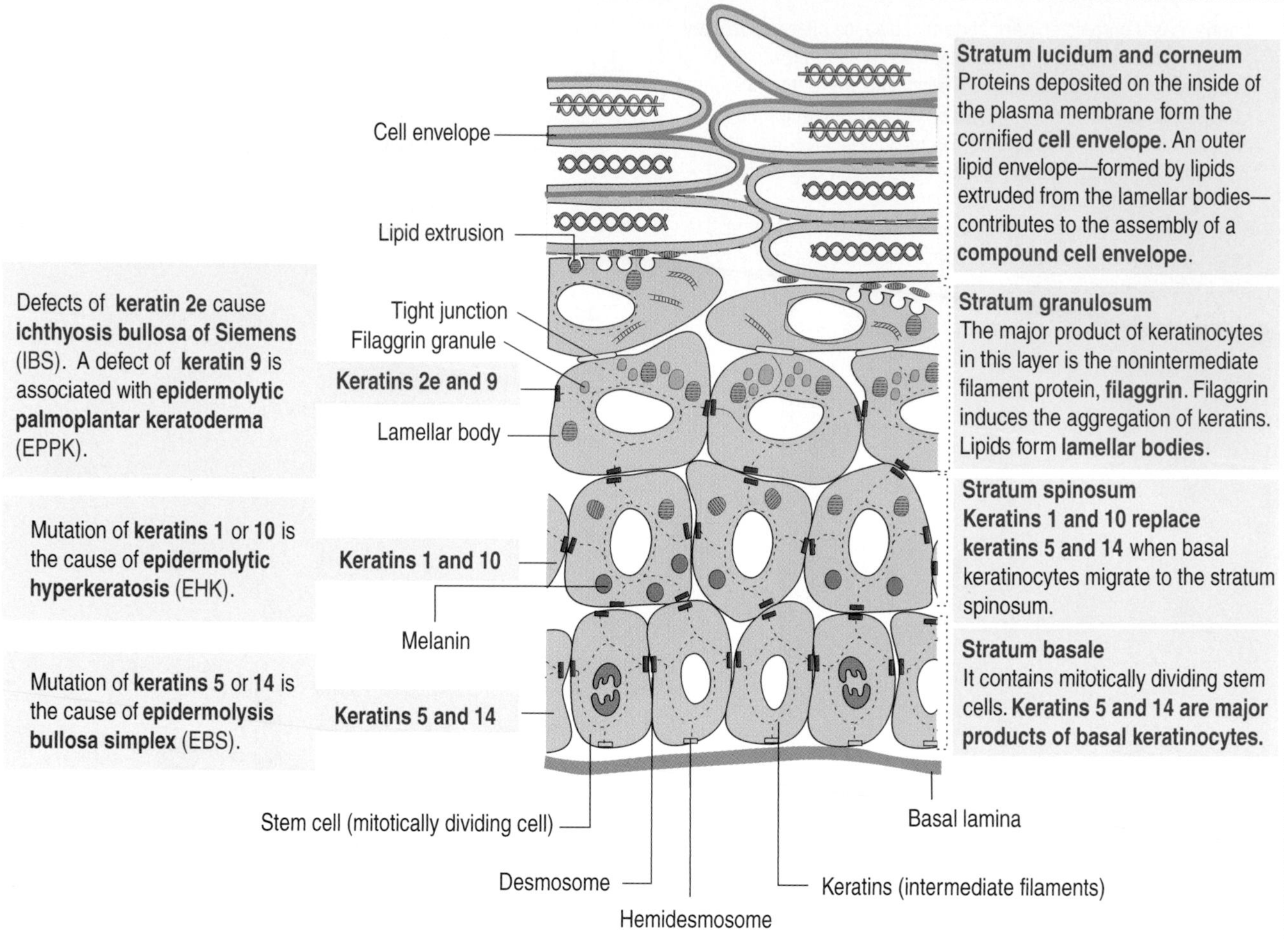

Stratum lucidum and corneum
Proteins deposited on the inside of the plasma membrane form the cornified cell envelope. An outer lipid envelope—formed by lipids extruded from the lamellar bodies—contributes to the assembly of a compound cell envelope.
Cell envelope
Lipid extrusion
Tight junction
Filaggrin granule
Keratins 2e and 9
Lamellar body
Stratum granulosum
The major product of keratinocytes in this layer is the nonintermediate filament protein, filaggrin. Filaggrin induces the aggregation of keratins. Lipids form lamellar bodies.
Defects of keratin 2e cause ichthyosis bullosa of Siemens (IBS). A defect of keratin 9 is associated with epidermolytic palmoplantar keratoderma (EPPK).
Stratum spinosum
Keratins 1 and 10 replace keratins 5 and 14 when basal keratinocytes migrate to the stratum spinosum.
Mutation of keratins 1 or 10 is the cause of epidermolytic hyperkeratosis (EHK).
Keratins 1 and 10
Melanin
Stratum basale
It contains mitotically dividing stem cells. Keratins 5 and 14 are major products of basal keratinocytes.
Mutation of keratins 5 or 14 is the cause of epidermolysis bullosa simplex (EBS).
Keratins 5 and 14
Stem cell (mitotically dividing cell)
Basal lamina
Desmosome
Keratins (intermediate filaments)
Hemidesmosome

tors (**retinoic acid receptor** [**RAR**]). In addition, retinoic acid binds to **cytosolic retinoic acid protein** (**CRAB**), presumably involved in the regulation of the intracellular concentration of retinoic acid.

The retinoic acid–receptor complex has binding affinity for **retinoic acid–responsive elements** (**RAREs**) on DNA and inhibits the expression of genes during keratinocyte differentiation in favor of proliferation. Retinoids are used in the prevention of acne scarring, psoriasis, and other scaling diseases of the skin.

Clinical significance: Psoriasis

Psoriasis is an inflammatory skin disorder. It is characterized by sharply demarcated plaques, called **psoriatic plaques**, covered by white scales commonly seen on the elbows, knees, scalp, umbilicus, and lumbar region. Physical trauma may produce psoriatic plaques at the sites of injury.

The histologic characteristics of the psoriatic plaque include **excessive proliferation of epidermal keratinocytes** (caused by an accelerated migration of keratinocytes from the stratum basale to the stratum corneum), presence of inflammatory cells (T cells and neutrophils) in the dermis and epidermis (**microabscesses**), elongation of epidermic papillae, and prominent **angiogenesis** (Figure 11-4).

Langerhans cells initiate the psoriatic process. The role of Langerhans cells in the activation of T cells in regional lymph nodes is summarized in Figure 11-4.

Cytokines play a significant role in the trafficking and distribution of T cells in the psoriatic skin. Effector T cells are characterized by the expression of the skin homing receptor **cutaneous lymphocyte-associated** (**CLA**) antigen and CD45. $CD45^{+}CLA^{+}$ T cells arrive at sites of cutaneous inflammation, secrete proinflam-

Figure 11-6. Components of the epidermal permeability barrier

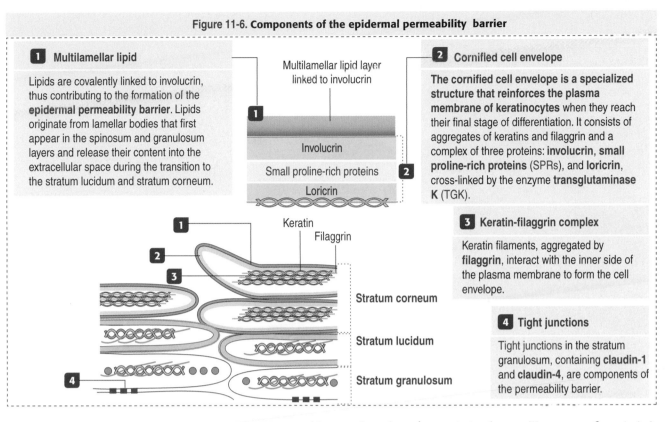

1 Multilamellar lipid

Lipids are covalently linked to involucrin, thus contributing to the formation of the **epidermal permeability barrier**. Lipids originate from lamellar bodies that first appear in the spinosum and granulosum layers and release their content into the extracellular space during the transition to the stratum lucidum and stratum corneum.

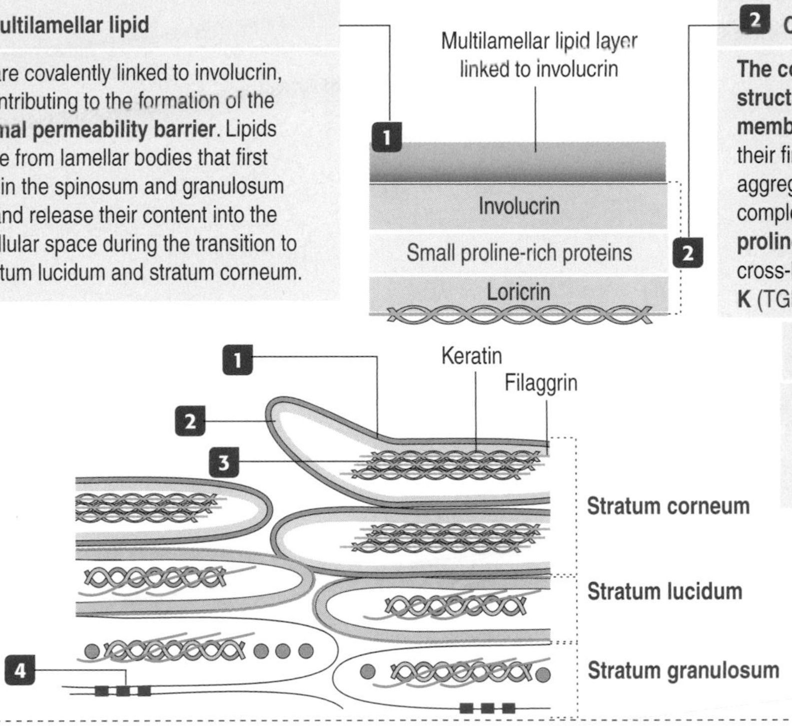

2 Cornified cell envelope

The cornified cell envelope is a specialized structure that reinforces the plasma membrane of keratinocytes when they reach their final stage of differentiation. It consists of aggregates of keratins and filaggrin and a complex of three proteins: **involucrin, small proline-rich proteins** (SPRs), and **loricrin**, cross-linked by the enzyme **transglutaminase K** (TGK).

3 Keratin-filaggrin complex

Keratin filaments, aggregated by **filaggrin**, interact with the inner side of the plasma membrane to form the cell envelope.

4 Tight junctions

Tight junctions in the stratum granulosum, containing **claudin-1** and **claudin-4**, are components of the permeability barrier.

matory cytokines, and produce the psoriatic plaques. Treatment of psoriasis is targeted to the therapeutic inhibition of T cell activation (determined by Langerhans cells in the lymph node), depletion of activated T cells (by monoclonal antibodies directed to cell surface molecules expressed by Langerhans cell–activated T cells), and preventing the recruitment of $CD45^+CLA^+$ T cells (by monoclonal antibodies blocking specific homing).

Differentiation of a keratinocyte

Keratinocytes of the **stratum spinosum** have a flattened polygonal shape with a distinct ovoid nucleus. The cytoplasm displays small granules with a lamellar core, called **membrane-coating granules**, or **lamellar bodies**. Bundles of intermediate filaments—**tonofibrils**—extend into the cytoplasmic spinous-like processes and attach to the **dense plaque** of a desmosome.

The **stratum granulosum** consists of a multilayered assembly of flattened nucleated keratinocytes with characteristic irregularly shaped **keratohyalin granules** without a limiting membrane and associated with the tonofilaments. The **lamellar bodies**, which first appear in keratinocytes of the stratum spinosum, increase in number in the stratum granulosum, and the lamellar product, the **glycolipid acylglucosylceramide**, is released into the intercellular spaces (Figure 11-5). **Tight junctions**, containing **claudin-1** and **claudin-4**, are found in the stratum granulosum (Figure 11-6). In the intercellular space, the lamellar lipid material forms a multilayered structure arranged in wide sheets, coating the surface of keratinocytes of the upper layer, the stratum lucidum. The glycolipid coating provides the water barrier of the epidermis.

The **stratum lucidum** is recognized by some histologists as an intermediate layer above the stratum granulosum and beneath the **stratum corneum**. However, no distinctive cytologic features are significantly apparent.

Both the stratum lucidum and stratum corneum consist of several layers of keratinocytes without nuclei and a cytoplasm containing aggregated intermediate filaments of keratin cross-linked with **filaggrin** (see Figure 11-6) by a process catalyzed by **transglutaminases**. Filaggrin aggregates keratin intermediate fila-

Box 11-A | Cornified cell envelope disorders

- About 50% of patients with lamellar ichthyosis (Greek *ichthys*, fish; *osis*, condition) carry mutations in the *transglutaminase-1* gene. Affected individuals display a collodion membrane (dryness and scaling of the skin seen at birth). This condition is caused by defective cross-linking of cornified cell envelope proteins.
- Vohwinkel syndrome and progressive symmetric erythrokeratodermia are caused by defects in loricrin. Hyperkeratosis (increase in the thickness of the stratum corneum) of the palms and soles is observed.
- X-linked ichthyosis is an autosomal recessive disease associated with a lipid metabolic defect. Thick dark scales in the palms and soles, and corneal opacities, are caused by a defect in the enzyme steroid sulfatase. Accumulation of cholesterol sulfate in the extracellular space of the stratum corneum prevents desquamation and cross-linking of involucrin to the extracellular lipid layer. Cholesterol sulfate inhibits proteases involved in desquamation.

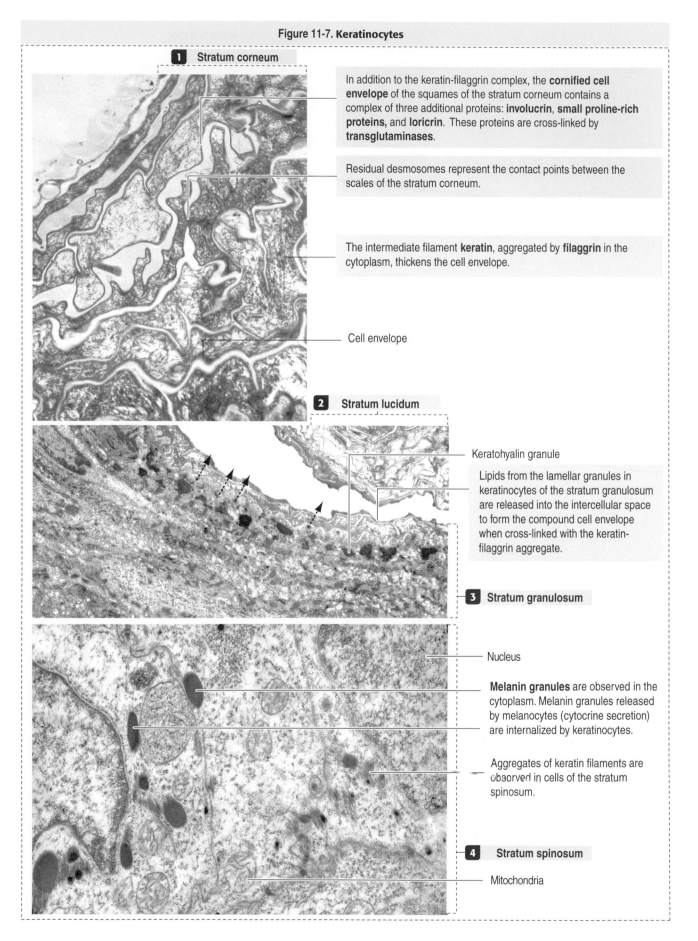

Figure 11-7. Keratinocytes

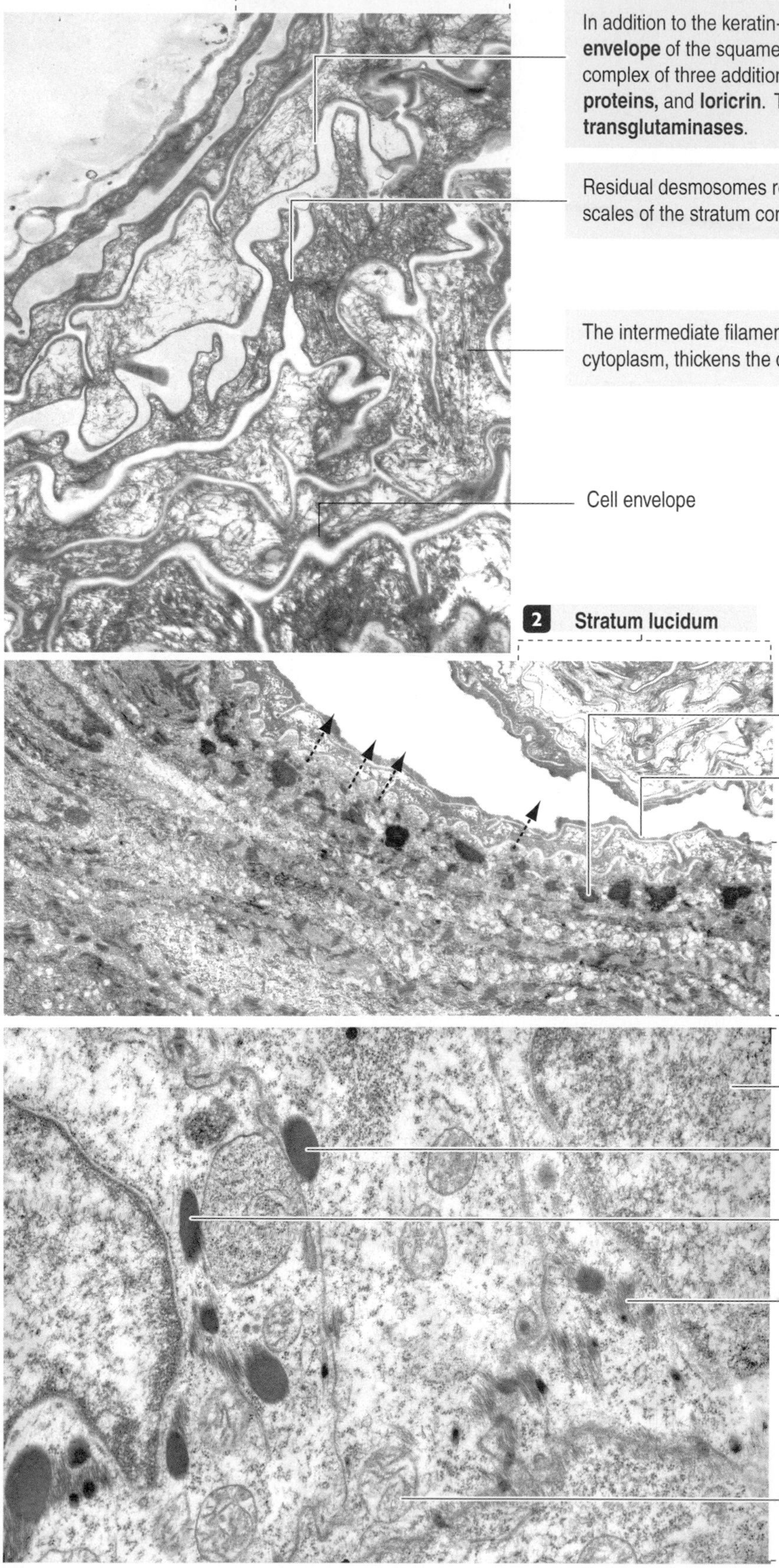

1 Stratum corneum
In addition to the keratin-filaggrin complex, the **cornified cell envelope** of the squames of the stratum corneum contains a complex of three additional proteins: **involucrin**, **small proline-rich proteins,** and **loricrin**. These proteins are cross-linked by **transglutaminases**.
Residual desmosomes represent the contact points between the scales of the stratum corneum.
The intermediate filament **keratin**, aggregated by **filaggrin** in the cytoplasm, thickens the cell envelope.
Cell envelope
2 Stratum lucidum
Keratohyalin granule
Lipids from the lamellar granules in keratinocytes of the stratum granulosum are released into the intercellular space to form the compound cell envelope when cross-linked with the keratin-filaggrin aggregate.
3 Stratum granulosum
Nucleus
Melanin granules are observed in the cytoplasm. Melanin granules released by melanocytes (cytocrine secretion) are internalized by keratinocytes.
Aggregates of keratin filaments are observed in cells of the stratum spinosum.
4 Stratum spinosum
Mitochondria

Figure 11-8. Melanocytes, derived from the neural crest, pigment and protect the skin

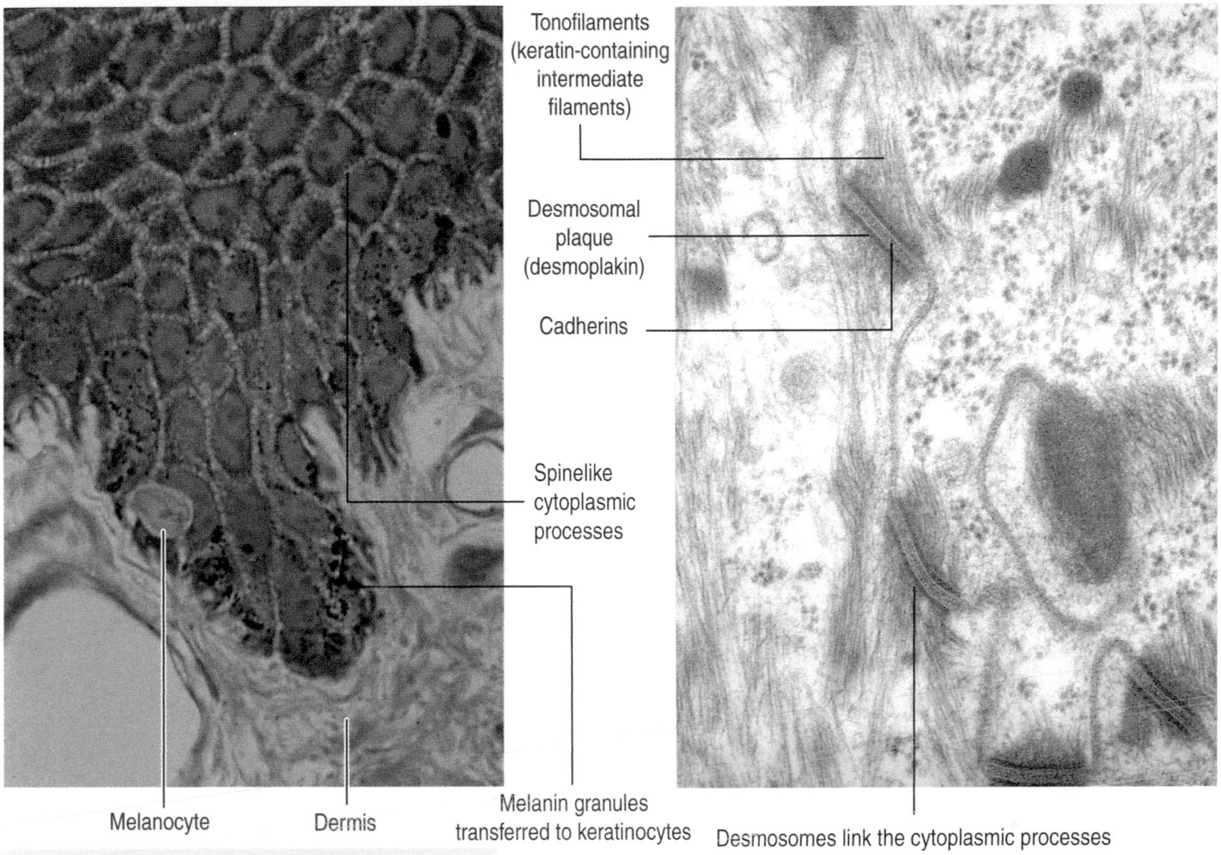

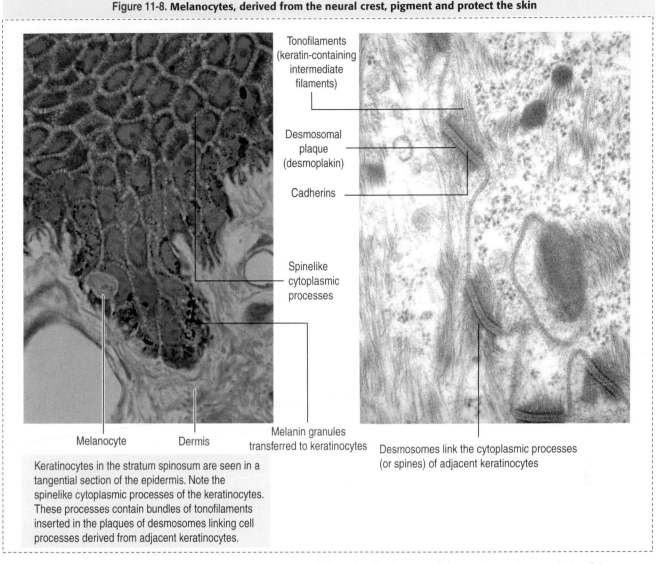

Tonofilaments (keratin-containing intermediate filaments)
Desmosomal plaque (desmoplakin)
Cadherins
Spinelike cytoplasmic processes
Melanocyte
Dermis
Melanin granules transferred to keratinocytes

Desmosomes link the cytoplasmic processes (or spines) of adjacent keratinocytes

Keratinocytes in the stratum spinosum are seen in a tangential section of the epidermis. Note the spinelike cytoplasmic processes of the keratinocytes. These processes contain bundles of tonofilaments inserted in the plaques of desmosomes linking cell processes derived from adjacent keratinocytes.

Box 11-B | **Disorders of keratinization**

- Stratum basale
  Predominant keratins: Keratins 5 and 14
  Disorder: Epidermolysis bullosa simplex
- Stratum spinosum
  Predominant keratins: Keratins 1 and 10
  Disorder: Epidermolytic hyperkeratosis
- Stratum granulosum/stratum corneum
  Predominant keratin: Keratin 9 (palms and soles)
  Disorder: Epidermolytic plantopalmar keratoderma
- Desmosomal defects
  Desmoplakins; cadherins
  Disorder: Striate palmoplantar keratoderma
- Cornified cell envelope (CCE)
  Loricrin and transglutaminase-1 (TGA-1)
  Disorder: Vohwinkel syndrome (loricrin) and congenital ichthyosiform erythroderma (TGA-1)
- Abnormal lipid metabolism affecting the CCE
  Disorder: Sjögren-Larsson syndrome

ments into tight bundles, leading to cell flattening, a characteristic of the stratum corneum.

The keratin-filaggrin complex is deposited on the inside of the plasma membrane forming a structure called the **cornified cell envelope** (Figure 11-7). Additional proteins—**involucrin**, **small proline–rich proteins (SPRs)**, and **loricrin**—are cross-linked by several transglutaminases and reinforce the cornified cell envelope just beneath the plasma membrane. On the outside of the cell, a complex of lipids extruded from lamellar bodies cross-link the cell envelope, forming the **compound cornified cell envelope**.

In summary, keratinocytes of the stratum corneum consist of a keratin-filaggrin matrix surrounded by a reinforcing involucrin–SPRs–loricrin complex that provides elasticity and mechanical resistance. Extracellular insoluble lipids, cross-linked to involucrin, make the cell membrane impermeable to fluids (permeability barrier). See Box 11-A.

The terminally differentiated keratinocytes of the stratum corneum consist of flattened squames with a highly resistant compound cell envelope. Squames are sloughed from the surface of the epidermis and are continually replaced by keratinocytes of the inner strata.

Two additional characteristics of the epidermis are (1) the cell layer–specific expression of keratins observed during differentiation of keratinocytes (see Figure 11-5) and (2) the presence of **tight junctions** and **desmosomes** in the epidermis.

Figure 11-9. **Synthesis and transport of melanin from melanocytes to keratinocytes**

1 Premelanosomes—derived from the Golgi apparatus—contain melanin, a pigment resulting from the **oxidation of tyrosine to DOPA (1,3,4-dihydroxy-phenylalanine), to melanin.**

Melanin has a filamentous structure within the premelanosome **(melanofilaments)**. Melanofilaments are not visible in melanosomes.

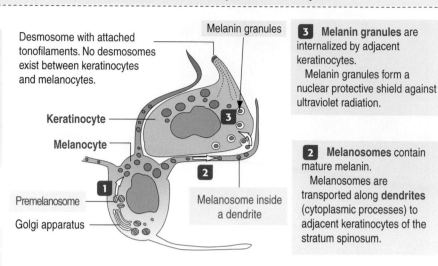

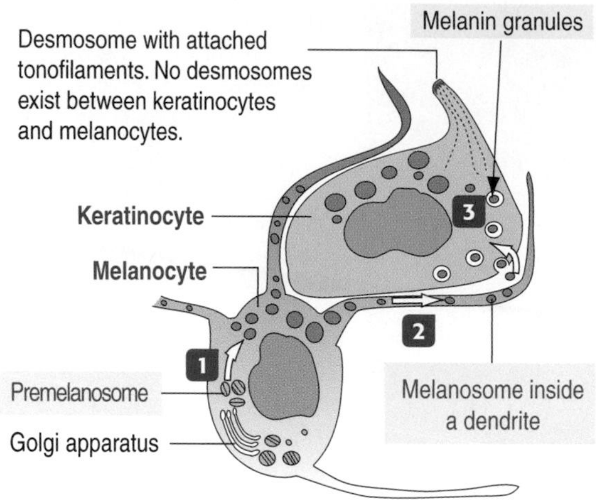

3 Melanin granules are internalized by adjacent keratinocytes.

Melanin granules form a nuclear protective shield against ultraviolet radiation.

2 Melanosomes contain mature melanin.

Melanosomes are transported along **dendrites** (cytoplasmic processes) to adjacent keratinocytes of the stratum spinosum.

Melanocyte differentiation

Melanocytes undergo cell cycle arrest and express proteins required for the synthesis of melanin.

The **microphthalmia-associated transcription factor** (**MITF**) maintains the pool of melanocyte progenitors in adults and **regulates the differentiation of melanocytes.**

The expression of MITF occurs after **α-melanocyte-stimulating hormone** (**α-MSH**) binds to **melanocortin receptor 1 (MC1R)** on melanocytes.

Transport of melanosomes

Melanosomes move inside a dendrite along microtubules through an interaction with **kinesin.**

Once at the periphery, melanosomes detach from microtubules and bind to **F-actin** (located at the subcortical region of dendrites) through an interaction with the molecular motor **myosin Va** recruited to the melanosome by **melanophilin** (an adapter) bound to **Rab27a** (present on the membrane of the melanosome).

Melanosomes are transferred to surrounding keratinocytes.

Griscelli syndrome, associated with partial albinism of hair and skin, results from mutations in the *myosin Va* gene. A subset of Griscelli syndrome patients also have mutations in the *Rab27a* and *melanophilin* genes.

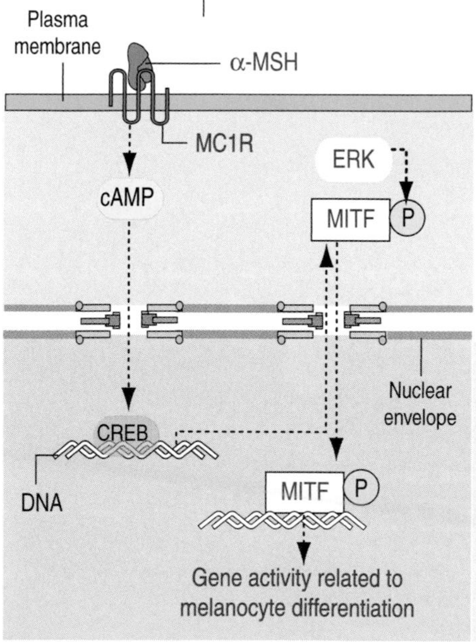

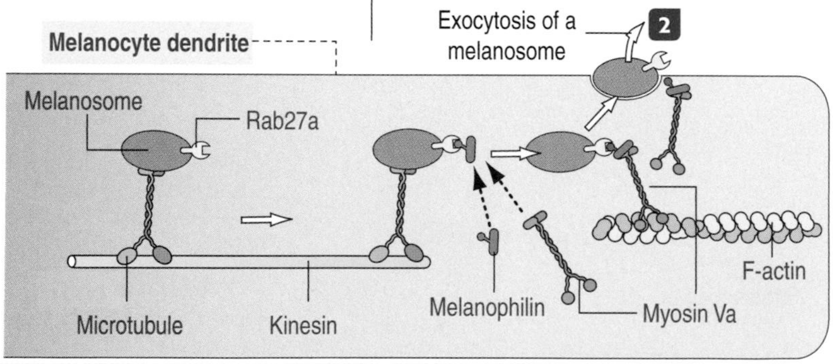

Binding of α-MSH to MC1R results in cyclic adenosine monophosphate (cAMP) production, activation of the cAMP response-element binding (CREB) protein on DNA, and increased expression of MITF.

MITF is released into the cytoplasm, where it is phosphorylated by the extracellular-related kinase (ERK) pathway.

Phosphorylated MITF translocates to the nucleus and stimulates the expression of enzymes (for example, tyrosinase) involved in melanin synthesis, cell cycle arrest, and melanocyte survival.

A lack of functional MITF produces albinism or premature graying. **Excess of MITF production occurs in melanoma.**

The maintenance of a three-dimensional lattice of tightly attached keratinocytes is essential for the protective nature of the permeability barrier.

In Chapter 1, Epithelium, we discuss the structure and components of tight junctions, desmosomes, and intermediate filament keratins, including pathologic conditions such as blistering, epidermolytic, and proliferative diseases (Box 11-B).

Figure 11-10. Langerhans cell, an antigen-presenting dendritic cell of the epidermis

1 The Langerhans cell derives from a **monocyte precursor** of the bone marrow. Monocytes in the epidermis become **Langerhans cells (dendritic cells)** and interact with keratinocytes through **E-cadherins** on their surface.
As antigen-presenting cells, Langerhans cells monitor foreign antigens coming in contact with the epidermis. Dendritic cells are also present in the dermis.

2 Langerhans cells take up an epidermal antigen through **langerin** (a C-type lectin binding to mannose residues) and **CD1a**.

3 Langerhans cells leave the epidermis, enter the lymphatic system, and are transported to a regional lymph node.

4 In the lymph node, Langerhans cells interact with T cells in the deep cortex.
T cells, activated by the epidermal antigen, reenter the blood circulation, extravasate at the site where the epidermal antigen is present, and secrete proinflammatory cytokines.

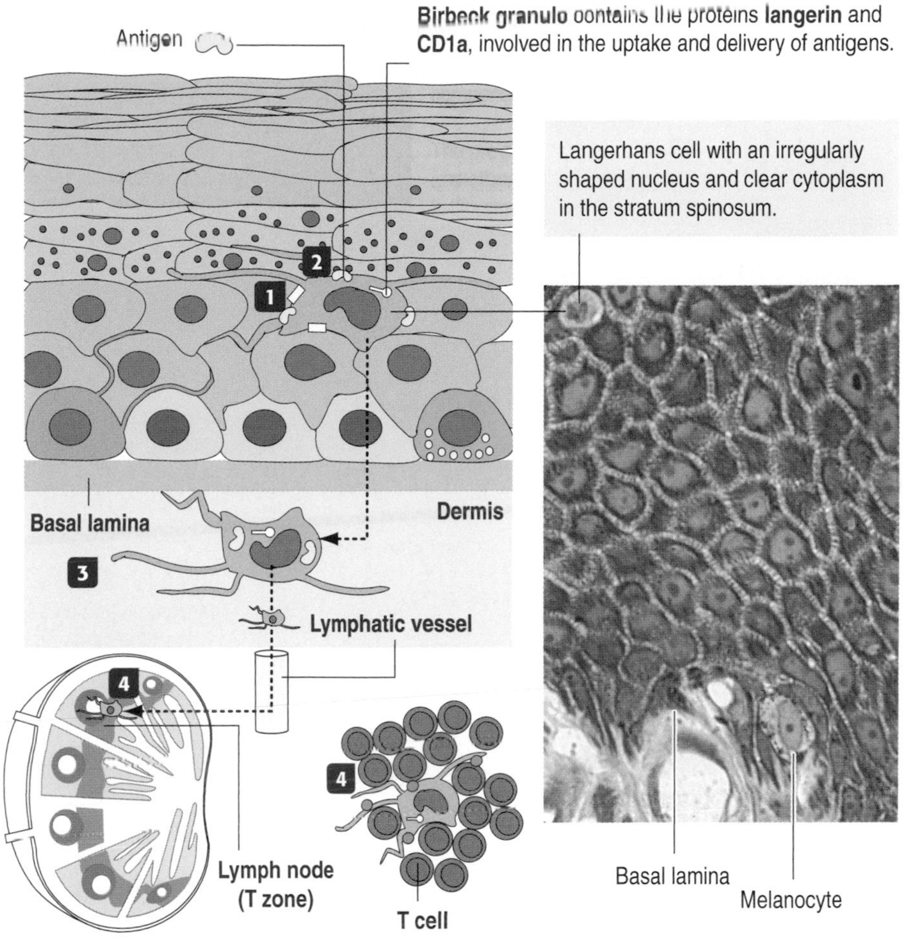

Antigen
Birbeck granule contains the proteins **langerin** and **CD1a**, involved in the uptake and delivery of antigens.
Langerhans cell with an irregularly shaped nucleus and clear cytoplasm in the stratum spinosum.
1
2
Basal lamina
Dermis
3
Lymphatic vessel
4
4
Lymph node (T zone)
T cell
Basal lamina
Melanocyte

Box 11-C | Melanocyte differentiation

- The process of melanocyte differentiation is regulated by MITF. MITF has two major roles: (1) melanocyte cell cycle arrest and (2) to stimulate the expression of genes encoding proteins involved in melanin production.
- Binding of α-MSH to MC1R stimulates cAMP production, which activates the gene expression of MITF after binding to CREB. MITF translocates to the cytoplasm of the melanocyte, is phosphorylated by the ERK pathway, returns to the cell nucleus, and increases the expression of proteins to arrest the melanocyte cell cycle, extend cell survival, and produce melanin.
- MITF overexpression occurs in patients with melanoma. Melanoma accounts for 4% of skin malignant tumors and is responsible for 80% of deaths from skin cancer. Patients with MITF overexpression have a negative clinical prognosis and are usually chemotherapy-resistant. Inhibition of MITF function is a desirable target for treatment of melanoma.

Melanocytes

Melanocytes are branching cells located in the stratum basale of the epidermis (Figure 11-8; see Figure 11-3). Melanocytes derive from **melanoblasts**, a cell precursor migrating from the **neural crest**.

The development of the melanoblast into melanocytes is under the control of the ligand **stem cell factor** interacting with the **c-kit receptor**, a membrane-bound tyrosine kinase. The development of mast cells, primordial germinal cells, and hematopoietic stem cells is also dependent on the interaction of stem cell factor with the c-kit receptor.

Melanocytes enter the developing epidermis and remain as independent cells without desmosome attachment to the differentiating keratinocytes. The turnover of melanocytes is slower than that of keratinocytes.

Melanocytes produce **melanin**, contained in **melanosomes**, which are transferred to neighboring keratinocytes through their branching cell processes, called **melanocyte dendrites**, and released by **cytocrine** secretion (Figure 11-9; Box 11-C).

Melanin is initially stored in a membrane-bound **premelanosome** derived from the Golgi apparatus. Melanin is produced by oxidation of **tyrosine** to **3,4-dihydroxyphenylalanine** (**DOPA**) by the enzyme **tyrosinase**. DOPA is then transformed to melanin, which accumulates in **melanosomes**, the mature melanin granules that are distributed along the melanocyte dendrites.

Cytocrine secretion is preceded by the transport of melanosomes along cytoplasmic **microtubules** by the motor protein **kinesin**. Melanosomes are then transferred to a network of F-actin tracks located beneath the plasma membrane.

Figure 11-11. Hemidesmosomes are the target of autoantibodies causing blistering diseases

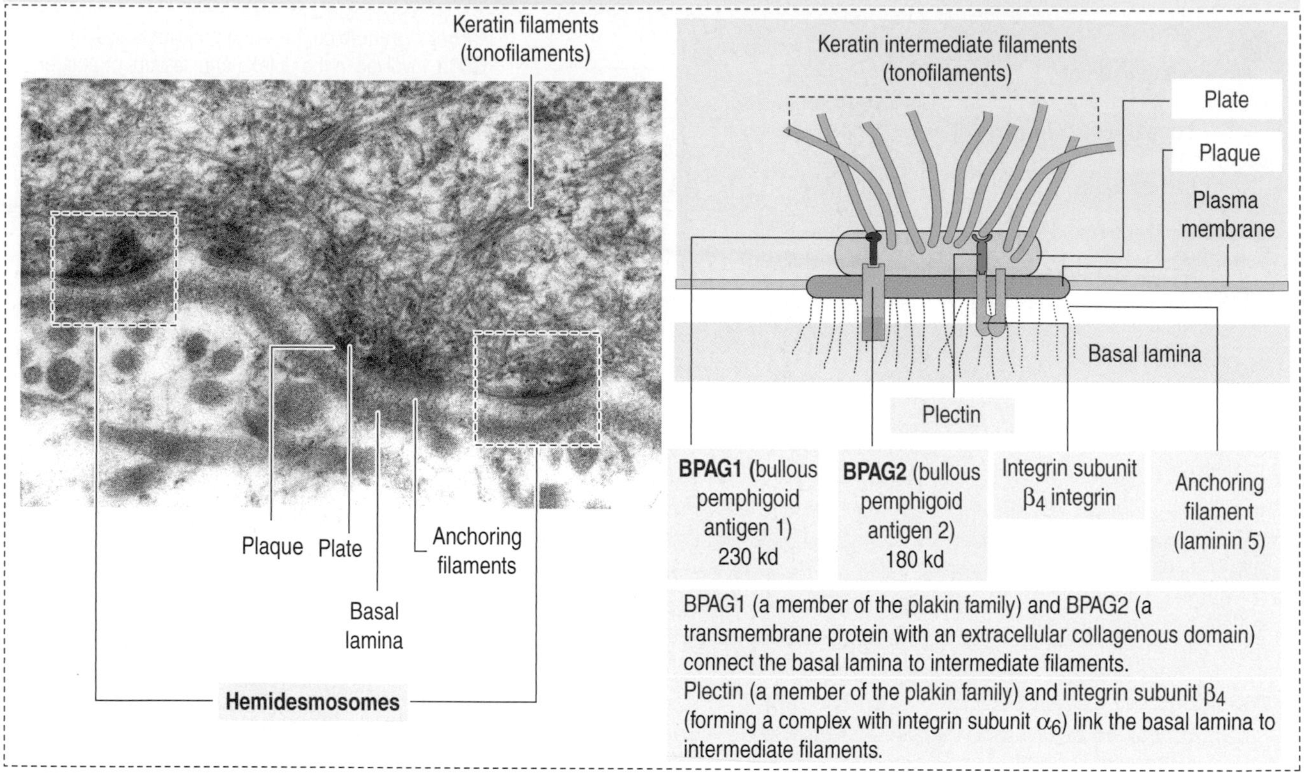
Keratin filaments
(tonofilaments)
Plaque
Plate
Anchoring
filaments
Basal
lamina
Hemidesmosomes
Keratin intermediate filaments
(tonofilaments)
Plate
Plaque
Plasma
membrane
Basal lamina
Plectin
BPAG1 (bullous pemphigoid antigen 1) 230 kd
BPAG2 (bullous pemphigoid antigen 2) 180 kd
Integrin subunit β4 integrin
Anchoring filament (laminin 5)
BPAG1 (a member of the plakin family) and BPAG2 (a transmembrane protein with an extracellular collagenous domain) connect the basal lamina to intermediate filaments.
Plectin (a member of the plakin family) and integrin subunit β4 (forming a complex with integrin subunit α6) link the basal lamina to intermediate filaments.

Melanosome transfer occurs when **melanophilin**, an adapter protein, binds to **Rab27a**, a protein inserted in the melanosome membrane. The F-actin–based molecular motor **myosin Va** binds to the Rab27a-melanophilin complex and transports the melanosome to the plasma membrane. Extruded melanin by exocytosis is captured by adjacent keratinocytes and internalized by endocytosis. The molecular characteristics of the unconventional myosin V are discussed in Chapter 1, Epithelium.

In addition to melanocytes, melanin-producing cells are present in the **choroid plexus**, **retina**, and **ciliary body of the eye**. **Albinism** results from the inability of cells to form melanin. **Griscelli syndrome** is determined by mutations of the *myosin Va* gene. Patients with Griscelli syndrome have silvery hair, partial albinism, occasional neurologic defects, and immunodeficiency (due to a defective vesicular transport and secretion in cytolytic T cells). Similar pigmentation disorders are determined by mutations in the *Rab27a* and *melanophilin* genes.

Langerhans cells (dendritic cells)

Langerhans cells are bone marrow–derived cells present in the epidermis as immunologic sentinels, involved in immune responses, in particular the presentation of antigens to T cells (Figure 11-10).

Langerhans cells, containing an epidermal antigen, enter a lymphatic vessel in the dermis and migrate to a regional lymph node where they interact with T cells in the deep cortex (T cell zone). T cells, activated by the epidermal antigen, reenter the blood circulation, reach the site where the epidermal antigen is present, and release proinflammatory cytokines in an attempt to neutralize the antigen.

Similar to melanocytes, Langerhans cells have cytoplasmic processes (dendritic cells) extending among keratinocytes of the stratum spinosum without establishing desmosomal contact but associating with keratinocytes through **E-cadherin**. Langerhans cells express **CD1a**, a cell surface marker. CD1a mediates the presentation of nonpeptide antigens (for example, α-galactosylceramide) to T cells.

The nucleus of a Langerhans cell is indented, and the cytoplasm contains char-

Figure 11-12. **Blood supply to the skin**

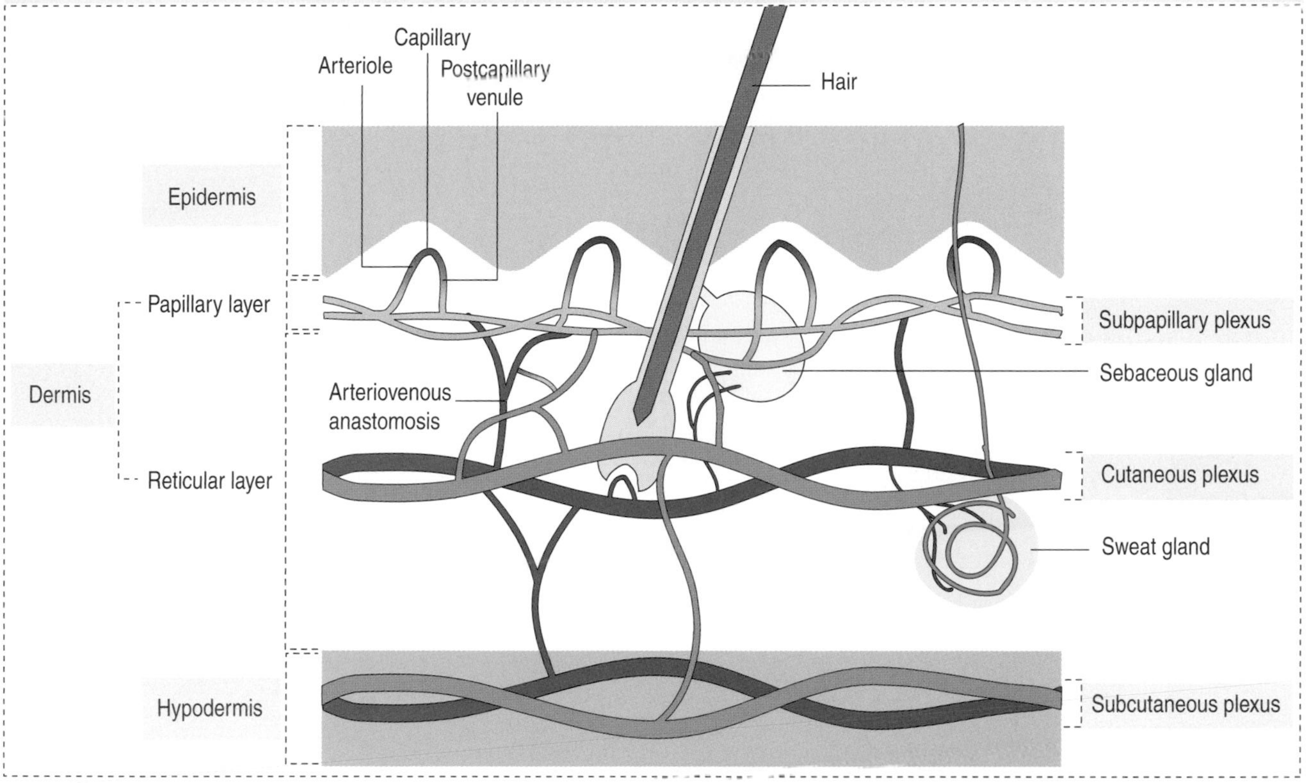

acteristic tennis racket–shaped inclusions (**Birbeck granules**) associated with the protein **langerin**. Langerin is a transmembrane C-type lectin (calcium-dependent) that facilitates the uptake of mannose-containing microbial fragments for their delivery to the endosomal compartment.

Langerhans cells use CD1a and langerin to trigger cellular immune responses to *Mycobacterium leprae*, the causative agent of **leprosy**, also known as **Hansen's disease**, a neurologic disease affecting the extremities. Myelin-producing Schwann cells are the primary target. In the early stages, infected individuals have skin nodules in the face and all over the body, followed by paralysis or loss of sensation in the affected areas, and eventually loss of fingers and toes. Blindness occurs in advanced stages of the disease. Multidrug therapy, consisting of rifampicin, clofazimine, and dapsone, is used to treat all cases of leprosy.

Merkel cells

Merkel cells resemble modified keratinocytes, are found in the stratum basale, and are numerous in the fingertips. Merkel cells are **mechanoreceptor cells** linked to adjacent keratinocytes by desmosomes and in contact with an afferent myelinated nerve fiber projecting from the dermis into the epidermis. The nerve fiber becomes unmyelinated after passing through the basal lamina of the epidermis and expands into a platelike sensory ending, the **nerve plate**, in contact with the Merkel cell (see Figure 11-3).

The nucleus is irregularly shaped and the cytoplasm contains abundant **granules**, presumably neurotransmitters.

Dermis

The dermis is formed by two layers without distinct boundaries: (1) the **papillary layer**, consisting of numerous papillae interdigitating with epidermal pegs forming the dermal-epidermal junction. The junctional interface is stabilized by hemidesmosomes anchoring basal keratinocyte cells to the basal lamina. Loose connective tissue (fibroblasts, collagen fibers, and thin elastic fibers) provides

Figure 11-13. **Sensory receptors of the skin**

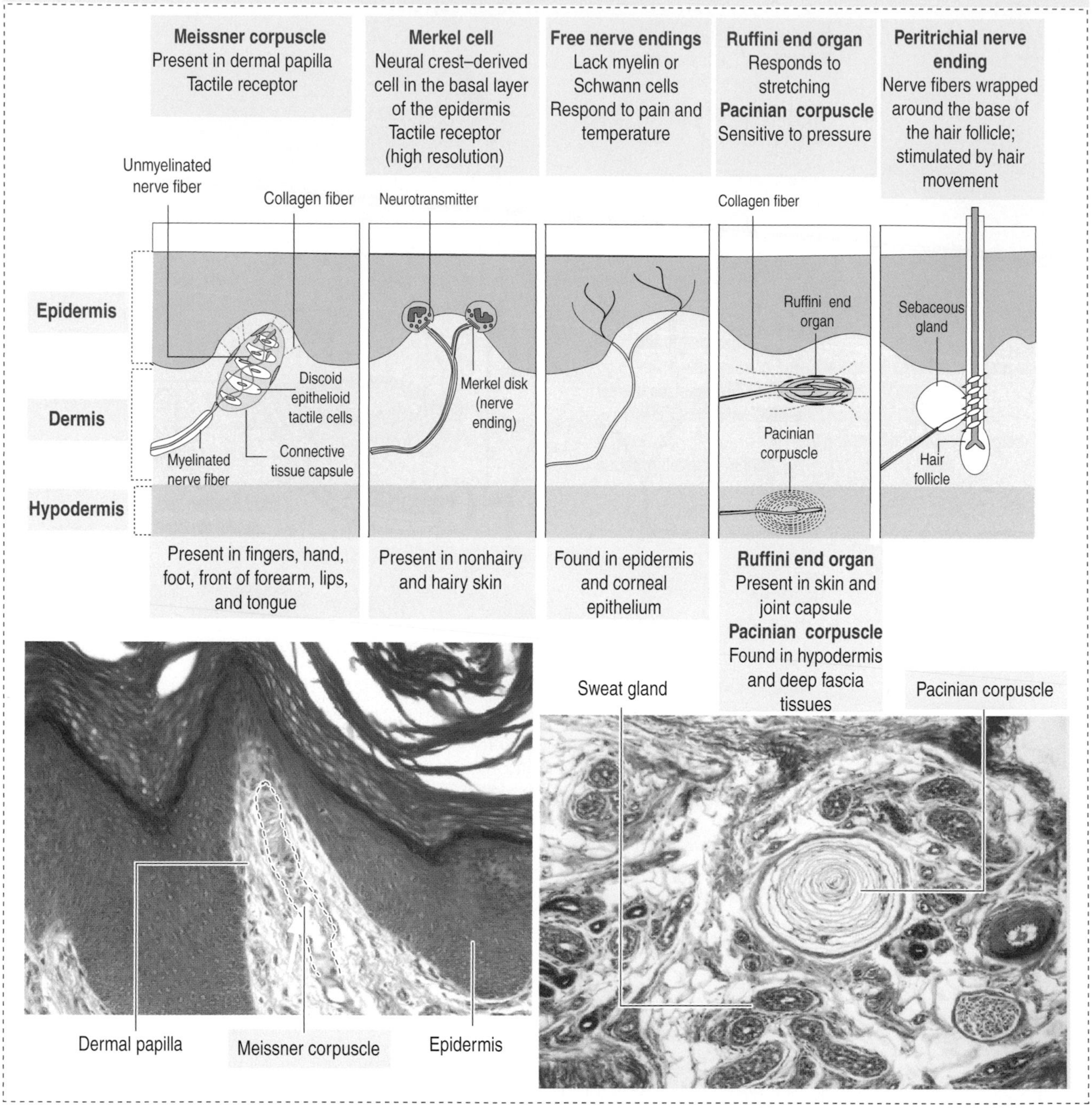

Meissner corpuscle
Present in dermal papilla
Tactile receptor
Merkel cell
Neural crest–derived cell in the basal layer of the epidermis
Tactile receptor (high resolution)
Free nerve endings
Lack myelin or Schwann cells
Respond to pain and temperature
Ruffini end organ
Responds to stretching
Pacinian corpuscle
Sensitive to pressure
Peritrichial nerve ending
Nerve fibers wrapped around the base of the hair follicle; stimulated by hair movement
Unmyelinated nerve fiber
Collagen fiber
Neurotransmitter
Collagen fiber
Epidermis
Dermis
Hypodermis
Discoid epithelioid tactile cells
Myelinated nerve fiber
Connective tissue capsule
Merkel disk (nerve ending)
Ruffini end organ
Pacinian corpuscle
Sebaceous gland
Hair follicle
Present in fingers, hand, foot, front of forearm, lips, and tongue
Present in nonhairy and hairy skin
Found in epidermis and corneal epithelium
Ruffini end organ
Present in skin and joint capsule
Pacinian corpuscle
Found in hypodermis and deep fascia tissues
Sweat gland
Pacinian corpuscle
Dermal papilla
Meissner corpuscle
Epidermis

mechanical anchorage and nutrients to the overlying epidermis. (2) The **reticular layer**, containing thick bundles of collagen fibers and coarse elastic fibers.

Hemidesmosomes on the basal domain of keratinocytes of the stratum basale attach the epidermis to the basement membrane and the papillary layer of the dermis by a **plate/plaque–anchoring filament complex** summarized in Figure 11-11. The molecular and structural components of the hemidesmosome are of considerable importance for understanding the cause of **blistering diseases** of the skin. We discuss in Chapter 1, Epithelium, the clinical significance of hemidesmosomes and intermediate filaments (see Figures 1-36 and 1-37, and Box 11-B).

Hair follicles and **sweat** and **sebaceous glands** are epidermal derivatives present at various levels of the dermis.

Blood and lymphatic supply

The cutaneous vascular supply has a primary function: **thermoregulation**. The

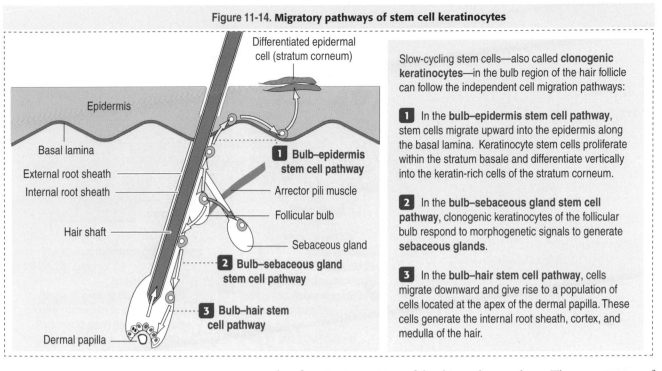

Figure 11-14. **Migratory pathways of stem cell keratinocytes**

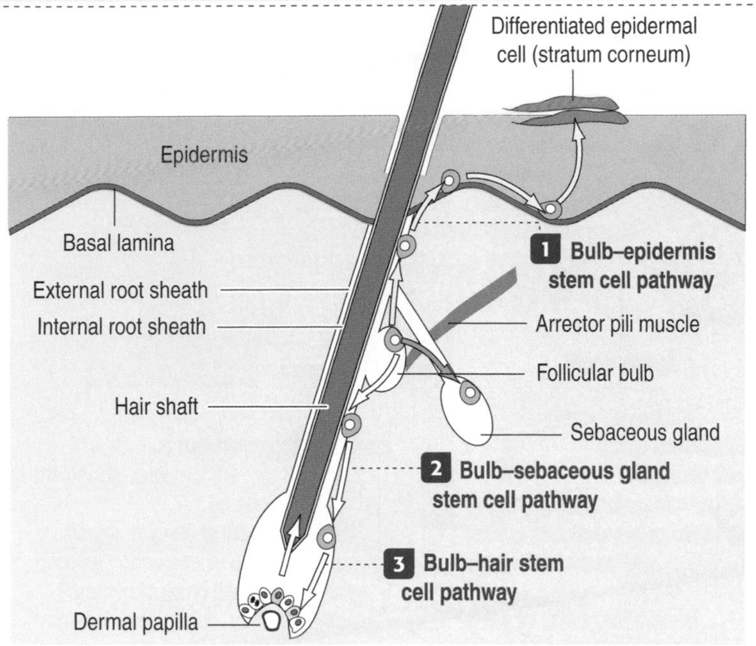

Differentiated epidermal cell (stratum corneum)
Epidermis
Basal lamina
External root sheath
Internal root sheath
Hair shaft
Dermal papilla
1 Bulb–epidermis stem cell pathway
Arrector pili muscle
Follicular bulb
Sebaceous gland
2 Bulb–sebaceous gland stem cell pathway
3 Bulb–hair stem cell pathway

Slow-cycling stem cells—also called **clonogenic keratinocytes**—in the bulb region of the hair follicle can follow the independent cell migration pathways:

1 In the **bulb–epidermis stem cell pathway**, stem cells migrate upward into the epidermis along the basal lamina. Keratinocyte stem cells proliferate within the stratum basale and differentiate vertically into the keratin-rich cells of the stratum corneum.

2 In the **bulb–sebaceous gland stem cell pathway**, clonogenic keratinocytes of the follicular bulb respond to morphogenetic signals to generate **sebaceous glands**.

3 In the **bulb–hair stem cell pathway**, cells migrate downward and give rise to a population of cells located at the apex of the dermal papilla. These cells generate the internal root sheath, cortex, and medulla of the hair.

secondary function is nutrition of the skin and appendages. The arrangement of blood vessels permits rapid modification of blood flow according to the required loss or conservation of heat.

Three interconnected networks are recognized in the skin (Figure 11-12):

1. The **subpapillary plexus**, running along the papillary layer of the dermis.

2. The **cutaneous plexus**, observed at the boundary of the papillary and reticular layers of the dermis.

3. The **hypodermic** or **subcutaneous plexus**, present in the hypodermis or subcutaneous adipose tissue.

The subpapillary plexus gives rise to single loops of capillaries within each dermal papilla. Venous blood from the subpapillary plexus drains into veins of the cutaneous plexus.

Branches of the hypodermic and cutaneous plexuses nourish the adipose tissue of the hypodermis, the sweat glands, and the deeper segment of the hair follicle.

Arteriovenous anastomoses (shunts) between the arterial and venous circulation bypass the capillary network. They are common in the reticular and hypodermic regions of the extremities (hands, feet, ears, lips, nose) and play a role in thermoregulation of the body. The vascular shunts, under autonomic vasomotor control, restrict flow through the superficial plexuses to reduce heat loss, ensuring deep cutaneous blood circulation. In some areas of the body (for example, the face), cutaneous blood circulation is also affected by an emotional state.

A special form of arteriovenous shunt occurring in the periphery is the **glomus apparatus**. The glomus consists of an endothelial-lined channel surrounded by cuboidal glomus cells and a rich nerve supply.

Lymphatic vessels are blind endothelial cell–lined spaces located below the papillary layer of the dermis, collecting interstitial fluid for return to the blood circulation. They also transport Langerhans cells to regional lymph nodes.

Clinical significance: Vascular diseases

Local and generalized vascular diseases affect the cutaneous vascular network. Noninflammatory **purpuras** (extravasation of blood in the dermis from small vessels) can be small (**petechiae**; less than 3 mm in diameter), or large (**ecchymoses**). Coagulation disorders, red blood cell diseases (sickle cell disease), and

Figure 11-15. **Structure of the hair**

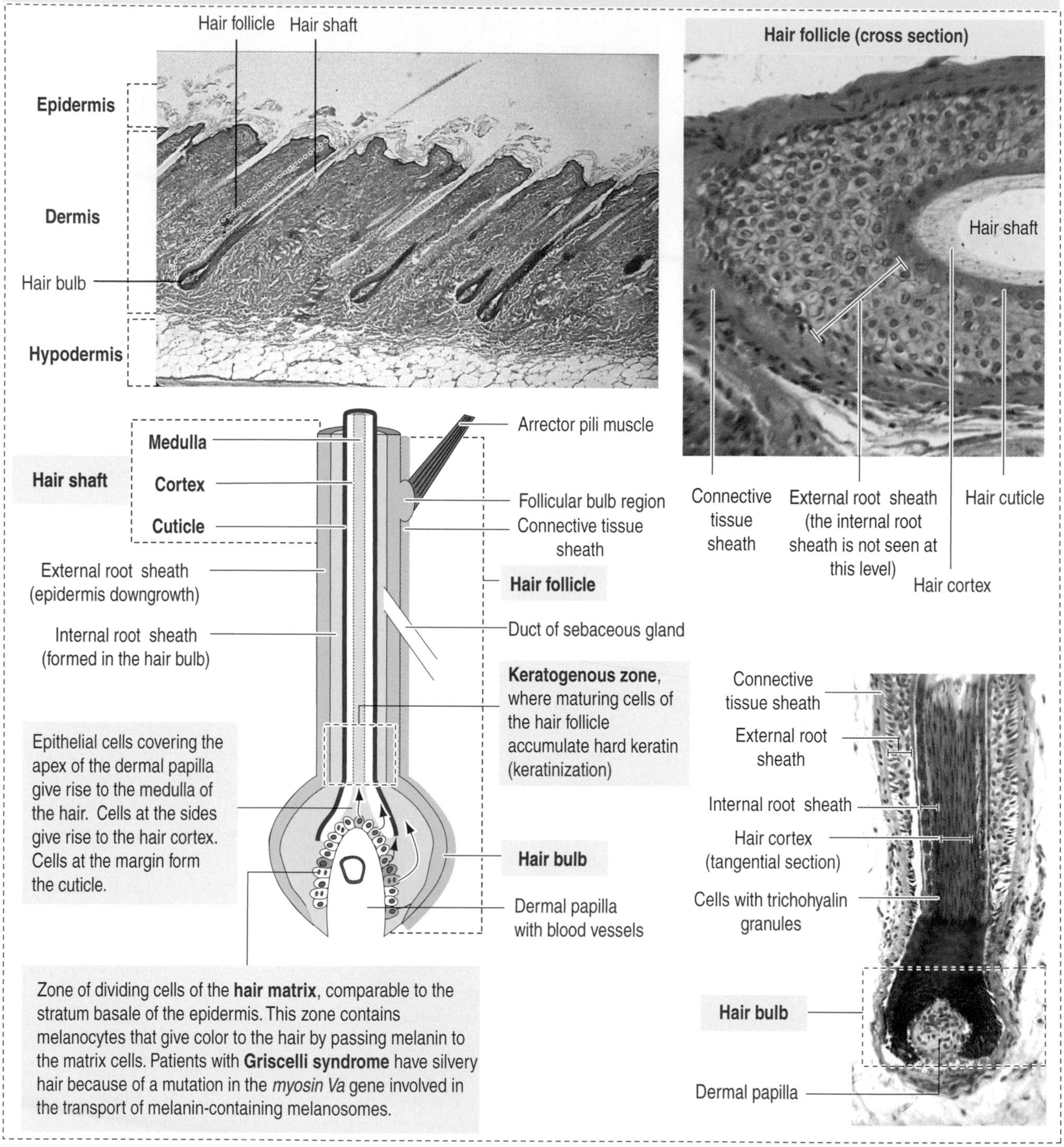

Hair follicle
Hair shaft
Epidermis
Dermis
Hair bulb
Hypodermis
Hair follicle (cross section)
Hair shaft
Connective tissue sheath
External root sheath (the internal root sheath is not seen at this level)
Hair cuticle
Hair cortex
Medulla
Hair shaft
Cortex
Cuticle
Arrector pili muscle
Follicular bulb region
Connective tissue sheath
External root sheath (epidermis downgrowth)
Hair follicle
Internal root sheath (formed in the hair bulb)
Duct of sebaceous gland
Keratogenous zone, where maturing cells of the hair follicle accumulate hard keratin (keratinization)
Epithelial cells covering the apex of the dermal papilla give rise to the medulla of the hair. Cells at the sides give rise to the hair cortex. Cells at the margin form the cuticle.
Hair bulb
Dermal papilla with blood vessels
Zone of dividing cells of the hair matrix, comparable to the stratum basale of the epidermis. This zone contains melanocytes that give color to the hair by passing melanin to the matrix cells. Patients with Griscelli syndrome have silvery hair because of a mutation in the myosin Va gene involved in the transport of melanin-containing melanosomes.
Connective tissue sheath
External root sheath
Internal root sheath
Hair cortex (tangential section)
Cells with trichohyalin granules
Hair bulb
Dermal papilla

trauma are common causes.

Acute **urticaria** is a transient reaction caused by increased vascular permeability associated with edema in the dermis. In Chapter 4, Connective Tissue, we discuss the mechanism of degranulation of mast cells and release of histamine as determinants. **Vasculitis** includes a group of disorders in which there is inflammation of and damage to blood vessel walls. Most cases of cutaneous vasculitis affect small vessels, predominantly venules.

Sensory receptors

Three categories of sensory receptors are present in the skin and other organs (Figure 11-13): (1) **exteroceptors**, (2) **proprioceptors**, and (3) **interoceptors**.

Exteroceptors provide information about the external environment. **Proprioceptors** are located in muscles (muscle spindle), tendons, and joint capsules and provide information about the position and movement of the body. **Interoceptors** provide sensory information from the internal organs of the body.

Another classification of sensory receptors is based on the **type of stimulus** to which a receptor responds: (1) **mechanoreceptors**, (2) **thermoreceptors**, and (3) **nociceptors**.

Mechanoreceptors respond to mechanical deformation of the tissue or the receptor itself (for example, stretch, vibration, pressure, and touch). The mechanoreceptors include both exteroceptors and proprioceptors.

Thermoreceptors respond to warmth or cold.

Nociceptors (or pain receptors) respond to painful stimuli. The skin and the subcutaneous tissue contain receptors that respond to stimuli such as **touch**, **pressure**, **heat**, **cold**, and **pain**.

The simplest mechanoreceptor is the **naked nerve ending**, which lacks a myelin covering. Naked nerve endings are found in the **epidermis** of the skin and the **cornea** of the eye. Naked nerve endings respond to light pressure and touch stimuli.

The second type of mechanoreceptor is the **Merkel disk**. The nerve ending of this receptor discriminates touch and forms a flattened discoid structure attached to the **Merkel cell** found in the stratum basale of the epidermis.

The third type of mechanoreceptor includes two **encapsulated receptors**: (1) the **Meissner corpuscle** and (2) the **pacinian corpuscle**.

The Meissner corpuscle is found in the dermal papillae and accounts for half the tactile receptors of the digits and hand. This receptor is well suited for the detection of shape and texture during active touch.

The pacinian corpuscle is found in the hypodermis, or deep dermis. It responds to transient vibratory stimuli and is the receptor for deep pressure.

The fourth type is the very sensitive **peritrichial nerve ending** wrapped around the base and shaft of the hair follicle. The movement of the hair is sufficient to stimulate the nerve ending of this receptor.

Hypodermis (superficial fascia)

The hypodermis, or subcutaneous layer of the skin, is a deeper continuation of the dermis. It consists of loose connective tissue and adipose cells forming a layer of variable thickness depending on its location in the body.

The hypodermis facilitates mobility of the skin, and the adipose tissue contributes to thermal insulation and storage of metabolic energy and acts as a shock absorber. The hypodermis contains muscles in the head and neck (for example, platysma). No adipose tissue is found in the subcutaneous portion of the eyelids, clitoris, or penis.

Skin appendages: Hair

During development, the epidermis and dermis interact to develop sweat glands and appendages, such as hairs. A hair follicle primordium (called the **hair germ**) forms as a cell aggregate in the basal layer of the epidermis, induced by signaling molecules derived from fibroblasts of the dermal mesoderm.

As basal epidermal cell clusters extend into the dermis, dermal fibroblasts form a small nodule (called a **dermal papilla**) under the hair germ. The dermal papilla pushes into the core of the hair germ, whose cells divide and differentiate to form the keratinized hair shaft. Melanocytes present in the hair germ produce and transfer melanin into the shaft.

A bulbous swelling (called the **follicular bulb**) on the side of the hair germ contains stem cells—**clonogenic keratinocytes**—that can migrate and regenerate the hair shaft, the epidermis, and sebaceous glands (Figure 11-14) in response to morphogenetic signals.

The first hair in the human embryo is thin, unpigmented, and spaced, and is

Figure 11-16. Sebaceous gland: Holocrine secretion

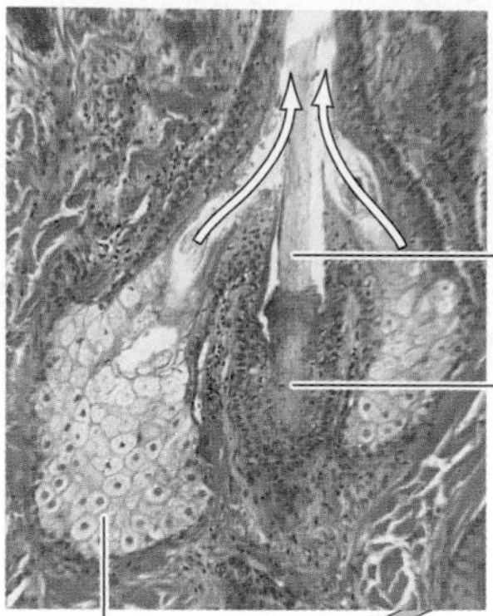
Hair shaft
Tangential section of the hair bulb
Sebaceous gland

Sebaceous glands are appendages of the hair follicle. Their short ducts—lined by a stratified squamous epithelium continuous with the external root sheath of the hair—open into the hair canal. Hair-independent sebaceous glands can be found on the lips, areolae of the nipples, the labia minora, and the inner surface of the prepuce.

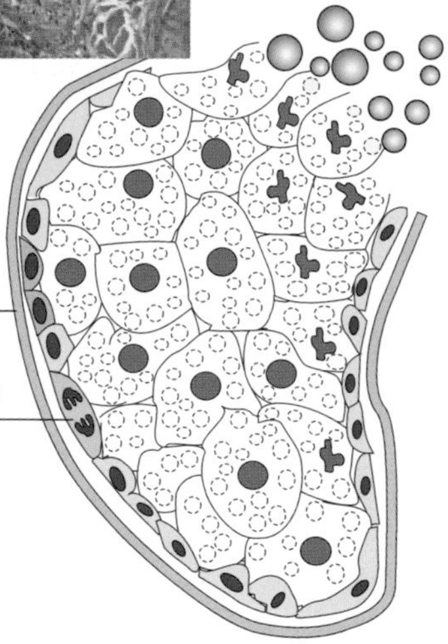
Basal lamina

1 **Basal cells** regenerate sebum-producing cells lost during the **holocrine** secretory process.

2 Sebum-secreting cells on top of the basal cells begin to store the oily secretion within cytoplasmic droplets.

3 In proximity to the acinar duct, the nuclei of the sebum-secreting cells shrink and degenerate, and coalescing droplets of sebum are released into the short duct. The acini lack a proper lumen.

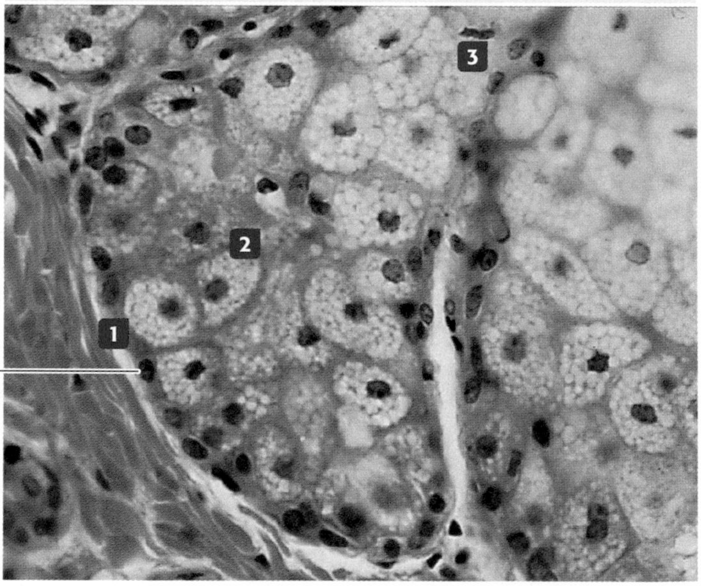
3
2
1

Basal cells divide by mitosis and accumulate lipids as they move into the central part of the acinus.

Sebum is the oily secretion of sebaceous cells. Sebum is released by a **holocrine mechanism**, resulting in the destruction of entire cells that become part of the secretion.

called **lanugo**. Lanugo is shed before birth and replaced by short colorless hair called **vellus**. Terminal hair replaces vellus, which remains in the so-called hairless parts of the skin (such as the forehead of the adult and armpits of infants).

Hair follicles are tubular invaginations of the epidermis responsible for the growth of hair. Hair follicles are constantly renewing, alternating phases of growth (**anagen**) with regression (**catagen**) and rest (**telogen**).

Each **hair follicle** consists of two parts (Figure 11-15): (1) the **hair shaft** and (2) the **hair bulb**.

The hair shaft is a filamentous keratinized structure present almost all over the body surface, except on the thick skin of the palms and soles, the sides of fingers and toes, the nipples, and the glans penis and the clitoris, among others. A cross section of the hair shaft of thick hair reveals three concentric zones containing keratinized cells: (1) the **cuticle**, (2) the **cortex**, and (3) the **medulla** (the last is absent in thin hair). The hair shaft consists of **hard keratin**.

The **hair bulb** is the expanded end portion of the invaginated hair follicle. A vascularized connective tissue core (**dermal papilla**) projects into the hair bulb.

The hair shaft is surrounded by (1) the **external root sheath**, a downgrowth of the epidermis; and (2) the **internal root sheath**, generated by the hair bulb (the **hair matrix**), and is made up of three layers of **soft keratin** (which from the

Figure 11-17. Eccrine sweat glands: Merocrine secretion

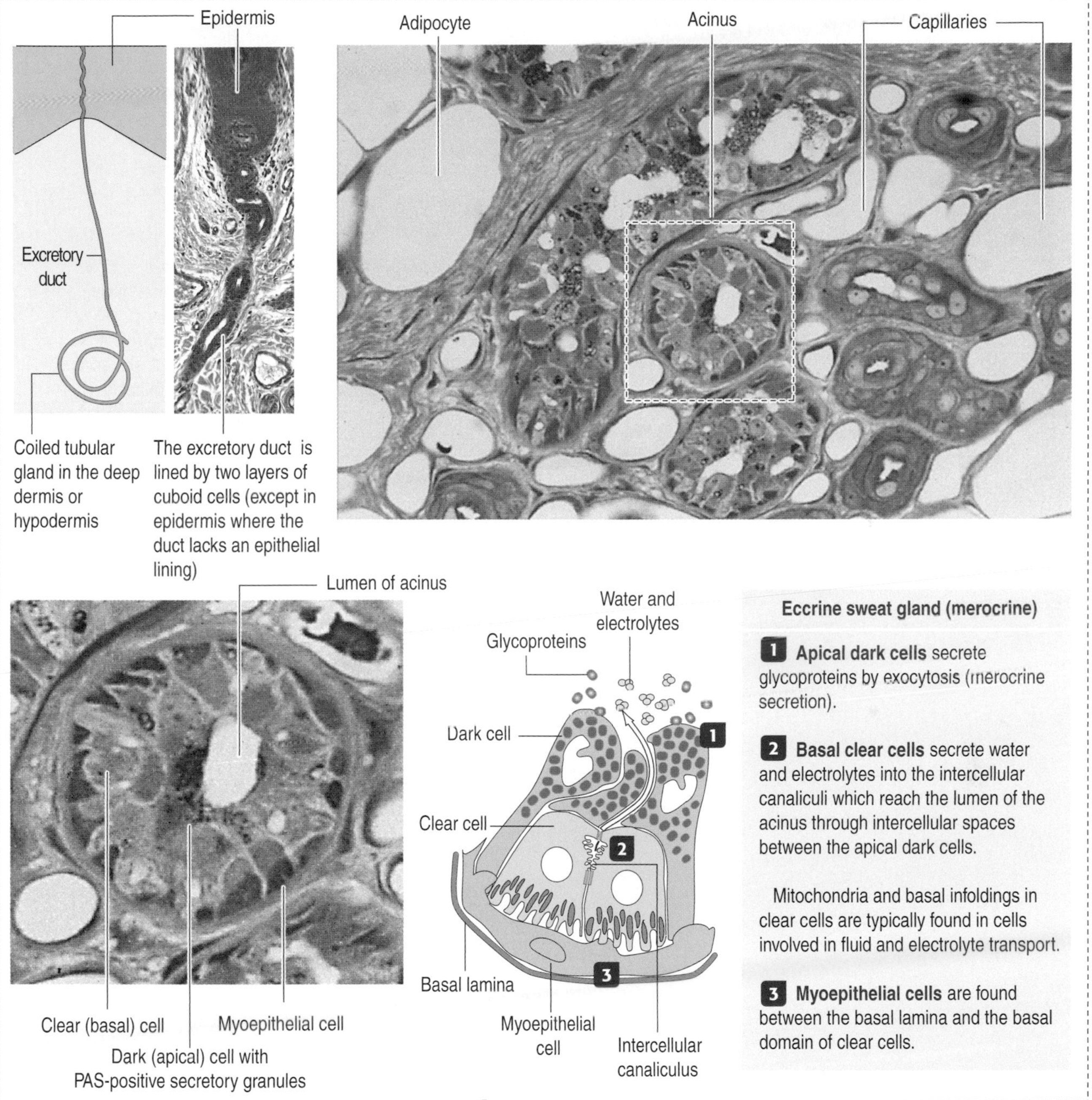
Epidermis
Excretory duct
Coiled tubular gland in the deep dermis or hypodermis
The excretory duct is lined by two layers of cuboid cells (except in epidermis where the duct lacks an epithelial lining)
Adipocyte
Acinus
Capillaries
Lumen of acinus
Clear (basal) cell
Myoepithelial cell
Dark (apical) cell with PAS-positive secretory granules
Water and electrolytes
Glycoproteins
Dark cell
Clear cell
Basal lamina
Myoepithelial cell
Intercellular canaliculus
1
2
3
Eccrine sweat gland (merocrine)
1 Apical dark cells secrete glycoproteins by exocytosis (merocrine secretion).
2 Basal clear cells secrete water and electrolytes into the intercellular canaliculi which reach the lumen of the acinus through intercellular spaces between the apical dark cells.
Mitochondria and basal infoldings in clear cells are typically found in cells involved in fluid and electrolyte transport.
3 Myoepithelial cells are found between the basal lamina and the basal domain of clear cells.

outside to the inside are Henle's layer, Huxley's layer, and the cuticle of the inner root sheath, adjacent to the cuticle of the hair shaft).

The keratinization of the hair and internal root sheath occurs in a region called the **keratogenous zone**, the transition zone between maturing epidermal cells and hard keratin. The external root sheath is not derived from the hair bulb.

The hair follicle is surrounded by a connective tissue layer and associated with the **arrector pili muscle**, a bundle of smooth muscle fibers aligned at an oblique angle to the hair follicle and attached to the **follicular bulb**. The **autonomic nervous system** controls the arrector pili muscle, which contracts during fear, strong emotions, and cold temperature.

The hair follicle is associated with **sebaceous glands** with their excretory duct connected to the lumen of the hair follicle. When the arrector pili muscle contracts, the hair stands up and forces sebum out of the sebaceous gland into the

Figure 11-18. Apocrine sweat glands: Merocrine secretion

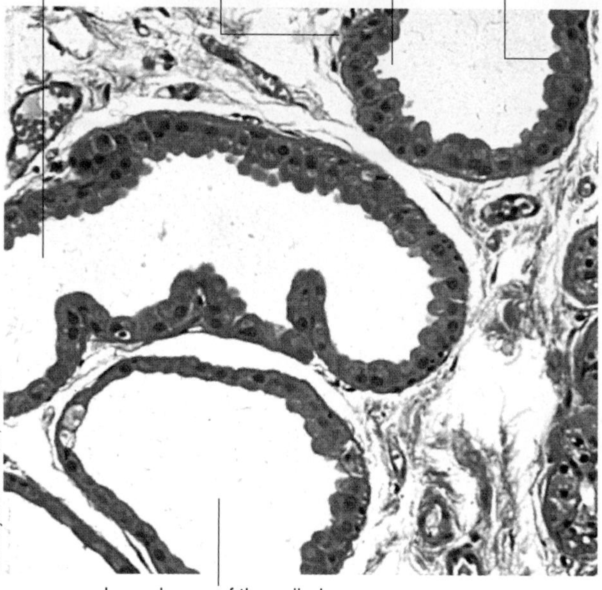
Lumen
Location of myoepithelial cells
Lumen
Cuboidal epithelial cell lining
Large lumen of the coiled secretory portion
Courtesy of E.W. Gresik, New York.

Apocrine sweat gland

Apocrine sweat glands are found in the **axilla**, **circumanal region**, and **mons pubis**.

The **coiled region of apocrine glands is larger** (~ 3 mm in diameter) than that of the eccrine sweat glands (~0.4 mm in diameter).

Apocrine sweat glands are located in the dermis, and the **excretory duct opens into the canal of the hair follicle.**

The secretory cells are cuboid and **associated with myoepithelial cells at their basal surface**—as in the eccrine sweat glands. The **secretory activity starts at puberty**. Their secretion acquires a conspicuous odor after being modified by local bacteria.

Although called apocrine—because of the incorrect interpretation that the apical domain of the secretory cells is shed during secretion—these sweat glands **release their secretion by a merocrine process**.

lumen of the hair follicle.

The color of the hair depends on the amount and distribution of melanin in the hair shaft. Few melanosomes are seen in blond hair. Few melanocytes and melanin are seen in gray hair. Red hair has a chemically distinct melanin, and melanosomes are round rather than ellipsoid.

A structure that is not recognized in routine histologic sections of hairs is the **peritrichial nerve endings** wrapped around the base of the hair follicle. The nerve is stimulated by hair movement (see Figure 11-13).

We discussed earlier in this chapter the participation of myosin Va in the transport of melanin-containing melanosomes to keratinocytes (called **matrix cells** in the hair bulb) and the lack of hair pigmentation in patients with **Griscelli syndrome** caused by mutations of *myosin Va*, *Rab27a*, and *melanophilin* genes.

Keratinocyte stem cells and the hair follicle

The epidermis is contiguous with the external root sheath of the hair follicle, a structure responsible for developing the hair shaft. When the epidermis is lost in severely burned patients, **keratinocyte stem cells** migrate upward from the **follicular bulb** to reestablish the **epidermis** by populating the highly proliferative and self-renewing cells of the stratum basale (see Figure 11-14). These stem cells can also give rise to **hair follicles** and **sebaceous glands**.

There are two signaling pathways that stimulate stem cells to enter the epidermal differentiation pathway: (1) the **Wnt** (wingless-related) **signaling pathway** and (2) the **Notch signaling pathway**. The Wnt signaling pathway is important for the morphogenesis of the hair follicle. The Notch signaling pathway stimulates epidermal differentiation in the postnatal epidermis.

During embryogenesis, the **bone morphogenetic protein** (**BMP**) pathway promotes ectodermal differentiation to an epidermal cell fate.

Glands

The glands of the skin are (1) the **sebaceous glands** (Figure 11-16), (2) the **sweat glands** (eccrine and apocrine sweat glands) (Figures 11-17 and 11-18), and (3) the

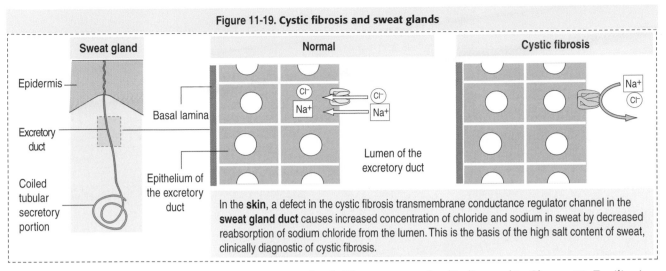

Figure 11-19. **Cystic fibrosis and sweat glands**

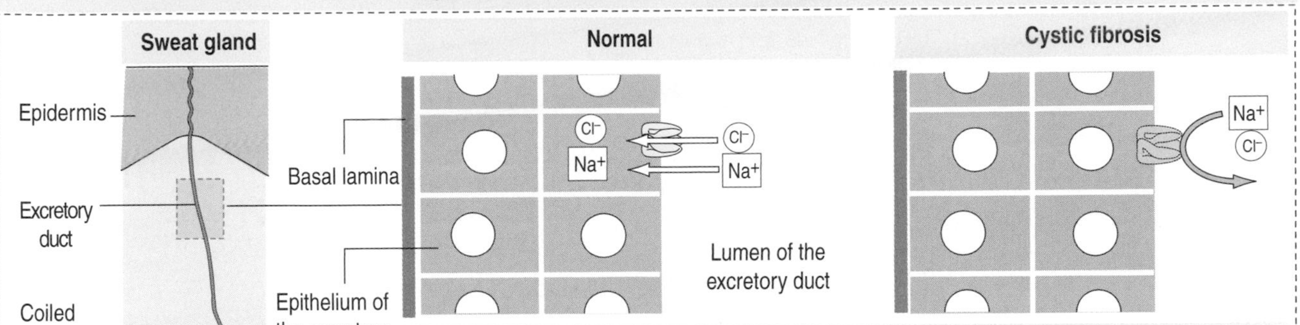
Sweat gland
Epidermis
Excretory duct
Coiled tubular secretory portion
Basal lamina
Epithelium of the excretory duct
Normal
Cl⁻
Na⁺
Cl⁻
Na⁺
Lumen of the excretory duct
Cystic fibrosis
Na⁺
Cl⁻

In the **skin**, a defect in the cystic fibrosis transmembrane conductance regulator channel in the **sweat gland duct** causes increased concentration of chloride and sodium in sweat by decreased reabsorption of sodium chloride from the lumen. This is the basis of the high salt content of sweat, clinically diagnostic of cystic fibrosis.

mammary glands. The mammary gland is discussed in Chapter 23, Fertilization, Placentation, and Lactation.

The **sebaceous gland** is a **holocrine simple saccular gland** extending over the entire skin except for the palms and soles. The **secretory portion** of the sebaceous gland lies in the **dermis**, and the **excretory duct opens into the neck of the hair follicle.** Sebaceous glands can be independent of the hairs and open directly on the surface of the skin of the lips, the corner of the mouth, the glans penis, the labia minora, and the mammary nipple.

The secretory portion of the sebaceous gland consists of groups of alveoli connected to the excretory duct by a short ductule. Each alveolus is lined by cells resembling multilocular adipocytes with numerous small lipid droplets. The excretory duct is lined by stratified squamous epithelium continuous with the external root sheath of the hair and the epidermis (the malpighian layer). The oily secretion of the gland (**sebum**) is released on the surface of the hair and the epidermis.

Sweat glands

There are two types of sweat glands: (1) **eccrine (merocrine) sweat glands** (see Figure 11-17) and (2) **apocrine sweat glands** (see Figure 11-18).

The **eccrine sweat gland** is a **simple coiled tubular gland** with a role in the **control of body temperature**. Eccrine sweat glands are innervated by **cholinergic nerves.** The **secretory portion** of the eccrine sweat gland (see Figure 11-17) is a convoluted tube composed of three cell types: (1) **clear cells**, (2) **dark cells**, and (3) **myoepithelial cells.**

The **clear cells** are separated from each other by **intercellular canaliculi**, show an infolded basal domain with abundant mitochondria, rest on a basal lamina, and secrete most of the water and electrolytes (mainly Na^+ and Cl^-) of sweat.

The **dark cells** rest on top of the clear cells. Dark cells secrete glycoproteins.

Myoepithelial cells are found between the basal lamina and the clear cells.

The **excretory portion** of the eccrine sweat gland is lined by a **bilayer of cuboid cells** that partially reabsorb NaCl and water under the influence of **aldosterone.** The reabsorption of NaCl by the excretory duct is deficient in patients with cystic fibrosis (see next section). The duct follows a **helical path** when it approaches the epidermis and opens on its surface at a **sweat pore.** Within the epidermis, the excretory duct loses its epithelial wall and is surrounded by keratinocytes.

Apocrine sweat glands (see Figure 11-18) are coiled and occur in the axilla, mons pubis, and circumanal area. Apocrine sweat glands contain secretory acini larger than those in the eccrine sweat glands. The secretory portion is located in the dermis and hypodermis. The **excretory duct opens into the hair follicle** (instead of into the epidermis as in the eccrine sweat glands). Apocrine sweat glands are

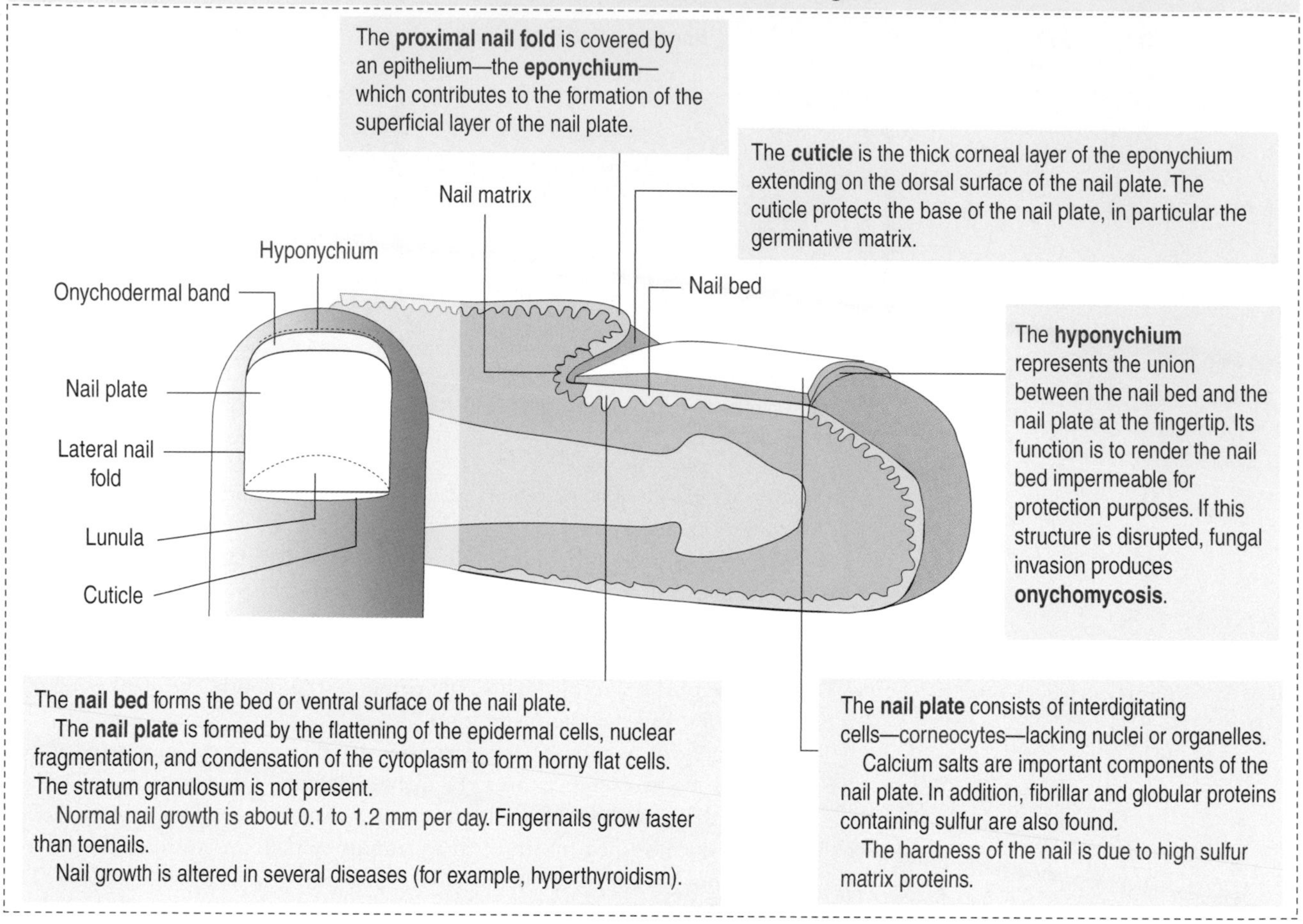
The **proximal nail fold** is covered by an epithelium—the **eponychium**—which contributes to the formation of the superficial layer of the nail plate.
The **cuticle** is the thick corneal layer of the eponychium extending on the dorsal surface of the nail plate. The cuticle protects the base of the nail plate, in particular the germinative matrix.
Nail matrix
Hyponychium
Onychodermal band
Nail bed
Nail plate
Lateral nail fold
Lunula
Cuticle
The **hyponychium** represents the union between the nail bed and the nail plate at the fingertip. Its function is to render the nail bed impermeable for protection purposes. If this structure is disrupted, fungal invasion produces **onychomycosis**.
The **nail bed** forms the bed or ventral surface of the nail plate.
The **nail plate** is formed by the flattening of the epidermal cells, nuclear fragmentation, and condensation of the cytoplasm to form horny flat cells. The stratum granulosum is not present.
Normal nail growth is about 0.1 to 1.2 mm per day. Fingernails grow faster than toenails.
Nail growth is altered in several diseases (for example, hyperthyroidism).
The **nail plate** consists of interdigitating cells—corneocytes—lacking nuclei or organelles.
Calcium salts are important components of the nail plate. In addition, fibrillar and globular proteins containing sulfur are also found.
The hardness of the nail is due to high sulfur matrix proteins.
Figure 11-20. **Structure and formation of the fingernail**

functional after puberty and are supplied by **adrenergic nerves**.

Two special examples of apocrine sweat glands are the **ceruminous glands** in the external auditory meatus and the **glands of Moll** of the margin of the eyelids.

The ceruminous glands produce **cerumen**, a pigmented lipid; the excretory duct opens, together with the ducts of sebaceous glands, into the hair follicles of the external auditory meatus.

The excretory duct of the glands of Moll opens into the free surface of the epidermis of the eyelid, or the eyelashes.

Clinical significance: Sweat glands and cystic fibrosis

Cystic fibrosis is a genetic disorder of epithelial transport of Cl^- by the channel protein **CFTR** (**cystic fibrosis transmembrane conductance regulator**), encoded by the *cystic fibrosis* gene located on chromosome 7.

Exocrine glands and the epithelial lining of the respiratory, gastrointestinal, and reproductive tracts are affected by a mutation of CFTR. Recurrent pulmonary infections, pancreatic insufficiency, steatorrhea, hepatic cirrhosis, intestinal obstruction, and male infertility are clinical features of cystic fibrosis.

The **excretory ducts of sweat glands** are lined by epithelial cells containing CFTR involved in the transport of Cl^- (Figure 11-19). The CFTR channel opens when an agonist, such as acetylcholine, induces an increase in cyclic adenosine monophosphate (cAMP), followed by activation of protein kinase A, production of adenosine triphosphate (ATP) (see Chapter 3, Cell Signaling), and binding of ATP to two ATP-binding domains of CFTR.

A defect in CFTR in sweat gland ducts leads to a **decrease in the reabsorption of sodium chloride from the lumen**, resulting in **increased concentrations of chloride in sweat.**

In the respiratory epithelium (see Chapter 13, Respiratory System), a defect in CFTR results in a **reduction or loss of chloride secretion into the airways**, active reabsorption of sodium and water, and a consequent decrease in the water content of the protective mucus blanket. Dehydrated mucus causes defective mucociliary action and predisposes to recurrent pulmonary infections.

Fingernails

The nails are hard keratin plates on the dorsal surface of the terminal phalanges of the fingers and toes (Figure 11-20). The **nail plate** covers the **nail bed**, the surface of the skin that consists of the stratum basale and stratum spinosum only.

The body of the plate is surrounded by lateral **nail folds** having a structure similar to that of the adjacent epidermis of the skin. When the lateral nail folds break down, an inflammatory process develops. This process is called **onychocryptosis** and is frequently observed in the nail of the first toe (ingrown nail).

The proximal edge of the plate is the **root** or **matrix** of the nail (where the whitish crescent-shaped **lunula** is located), in close proximity to the **nail matrix**, a region of the epidermis responsible for the formation of the nail substance. The distal portion of the plate is the free edge of the nail.

The nail plate consists of compact scales corresponding to cornified epithelial cells. The proximal edge of the nail plate is covered by the **eponychium**, a projecting fold of the stratum corneum of the skin, the **cuticle**. A loss of the cuticle facilitates inflammatory and infective processes of the nail matrix, leading to **nail plate dystrophies.**

Under the distal and free edge of the nail plate, the stratum corneum of the epidermis forms a thick structure, the **hyponychium**. The hyponychium protects the matrix bed of the nail from bacterial and fungal invasion.

Essential concepts | Integumentary System

• Skin consists of three layers: (1) epidermis, (2) dermis, and (3) hypodermis or subcutaneous layer. There are two types of skin: (1) thick skin (for example, palms and soles) and (2) thin skin.

The epidermis and dermis are tightly interlocked. Primary epidermal ridges interact with primary dermal ridges. An epithelial-derived interpapillary peg divides the primary dermal ridge into secondary dermal ridges. Each secondary dermal ridge has numerous dermal papillae interlocking with the epidermal region. The dermal-epidermal interface is stabilized by hemidesmosomes.

• The epidermis is a stratified squamous epithelium consisting of four different cell types: (1) keratinocytes (ectoderm-derived), (2) melanocytes (neural crest–derived), (3) Langerhans cells (bone marrow–derived dendritic cells), and (4) Merkel cells (neural crest–derived).

Keratinocytes are distributed in five strata or layers: (1) stratum basale (basal layer, which contains stem cells), (2) stratum spinosum (spinous or prickle cell layer), (3) stratum granulosum (granular cell layer), (4) stratum lucidum (clear cell layer), and (5) stratum corneum (cornified cell layer). Keratinocytes are associated with each other by desmosomes and tight junctions.

• **Wound healing**. Skin is repaired rapidly to maintain an efficient protective barrier. Wound healing consists of four stages: (1) Formation of a fibrin-platelet clot at the site of injury. (2) Recruitment of leukocytes to protect the site from infection. Keratinocytes and endothelial cells express **cytokine CXC** (cysteine-x-cysteine) and its receptor to recruit leukocytes. Monocytes recruited to the injury site become macrophages. (3) Neovascularization and cellular proliferation. **Granulation tissue**, rich in blood capillaries, is seen. (4) Tissue remodeling. Keratinocytes express plasminogen activator to convert plasminogen within the fibrin clot into plasmin. Plasmin and matrix metalloproteinases (produced by fibroblasts in the dermis) free basal keratinocytes from their basal lamina anchorage site and reepithelialization starts. Epidermal growth factor and keratinocyte growth factor stimulate reepithelialization. Fibroblasts in the dermis, stimulated by platelet-derived growth factor (PDGF) and transforming growth factor-β, start to proliferate. A number of fibroblasts change into myofibroblasts, and contraction of the dermis occurs (healing with a scar).

• **Psoriasis** is an inflammatory skin disorder producing a characteristic **psoriatic plaque**, commonly seen on the elbows, knees, scalp, umbilicus, and lumbar region. Persistent hyperplasia of the epidermis caused by abnormal cell proliferation and differentiation is observed. Keratinocytes move from the basal layer to the superficial layer in 3 to 5 days (instead of 28 to 30 days in normal skin).

Langerhans cells in the epidermis take up antigens and migrate to regional lymph nodes, where they interact in the deep cortex with T cells. T cells are activated (express homing receptor cutaneous lymphocyte-associated antigen [CLA] and CD45), reenter the bloodstream, home at sites of cutaneous inflammation, and produce the characteristic psoriatic plaques.

• The differentiation of keratinocytes is characterized by (1) the expression of specific keratin pairs in each layer (keratins 5 and 14 in the stratum basale; keratins 1 and 10 in the stratum spinosum, and keratins 2e and 9 in the stratum granulosum); (2) the presence of lamellar bodies (containing the glycolipid acetylglucosylceramide extruded into the extracellular space to form a multilamellar lipid layer) and keratohyalin granules in the stratum granulosum; (3) the presence in the stratum corneum of the cornified cell envelope (an involucrin–small proline-rich–loricrin protein complex associated with keratin-filaggrin aggregates inside the cell, associated with the extracellular multilamellar lipid layer anchored to involucrin); and (4) the presence of desmosomes and tight junctions (containing claudin-1 and claudin-4).

• Melanocytes are branching cells located in the stratum basale. They migrate from the neural crest under control of c-kit receptor (a tyrosine kinase) and its ligand, stem cell factor. Melanocytes produce melanin contained in melanosomes. Melanin is produced by oxidation of tyrosine to DOPA (1,3,4-dihydroxyphenylalanine) by tyrosinase. DOPA is transformed into melanin.

Melanosomes are transported along melanocyte dendritic processes. Kinesin transports melanosomes along microtubules to F-actin aggregates located under the plasma membrane. The microtubule–F-actin switch involves the attachment of the adapter melanophilin to Rab27a, a receptor on the melanosome membrane. Myosin Va recruits the melanosome–Rab27a–melanophilin complex, which is transported along F-actin tracks and released into the intercellular space by an exocrine mechanism (cytocrine secretion). Keratinocytes of the stratum spinosum take up the melanin-containing melanosomes by endocytosis.

A genetic defect in myosin Va, melanophilin, and Rab27a disrupts the transport of melanin. **Griscelli syndrome** and its variants determine partial albinism, occasional neurologic defects, and immunodeficiency. Microphthalmia-associated transcription factor (MITF) regulates the differentiation of melanocytes (cell cycle arrest, melanin production, and cell survival).

• Langerhans cells are dendritic cells of the epidermis derived from the bone marrow. Similar to melanocytes, Langerhans cells have dendritic processes in contact with keratinocytes through E-cadherin. Langerhans cells have on their surface langerin, a transmembrane C-type lectin, and CD1a. Langerin participates in the uptake of antigens; CD1a mediates the presentation of nonpeptide antigens to T cells. A characteristic landmark of Langerhans cells is the Birbeck granule.

• Merkel cells are found in the stratum basale. They are mechanoreceptors linked to adjacent keratinocytes by desmosomes.

• The dermis consists of two layers: (1) the papillary layer (loose connective tissue with collagen bundles and thin elastic fibers) and (2) the reticular layer (dense connective tissue with collagen bundles and thick elastic fibers).

Three interconnected blood vessel plexuses are seen in the dermis: (1) the subpapillary plexus (along the papillary layer), (2) the cutaneous plexus (at the papillary-reticular layer interface), and (3) the hypodermic or subcutaneous plexus (in the hypodermis). The primary function of the vascular network is thermoregulation; the secondary function is nutrition of the skin and appendages.

• Sensory receptors can be classified as exteroceptors (provide information about the external environment), proprioceptors (provide information about the position and movements of the body), and interoceptors (provide information from the internal organs of the body).

Based on the type of stimulus, sensory receptors can be classified as (1) mechanoreceptors (respond to mechanical stimulation from outside or inside the body; this group includes nerve free endings, the Merkel cell, the encapsulated Meissner corpuscle and pacinian corpuscle), and the peritrichial nerve endings of the hair; (2) thermoreceptors (respond to temperature changes); and (3) nociceptors (respond to pain).

• Skin appendages: hair. The first type of hair of the human embryo is called lanugo and is thin and unpigmented. Lanugo is replaced by vellus before birth. Terminal hair replaces vellus, which remains in the hairless regions of the skin (for example, forehead).

Hair follicles are tubular invaginations of the epidermis. Each hair follicle consists of two components: (1) the hair shaft (which includes the medulla, cortex, and cuticule, the latter associated with the internal root sheath) and (2) the hair bulb, the expanded portion of the hair follicle. The hair follicle is surrounded by connective tissue (associated with the external root sheath, a downgrowth of the epidermis). The dermal papilla extends into the hair bulb.

Hair is generated from the base of the hair bulb. The hair bulb has two layers: the matrix zone (where all mitotic activity occurs), and the keratogenous zone (where hair cells undergo keratinization).

Two structures are associated with the hair follicle: the arrector pili muscle (attached to the follicular bulb), and sebaceous glands, with their excretory ducts connected to the lumen of the hair follicle.

• Development of the skin. There are two signaling pathways that stimulate stem cells to enter the epidermal differentiation pathway: (1) the Wnt (wingless-related) signaling pathway and (2) The Notch signaling pathway. The Wnt signaling pathway is important for the morphogenesis of the hair follicle. The Notch signaling pathway stimulates epidermal differentiation in the postnatal epidermis.

• Glands of the skin include (1) sebaceous glands, (2) sweat glands (eccrine and apocrine), and (3) mammary gland.

Sebaceous glands are holocrine simple saccular glands. The secretory portion is located in the dermis; the excretory duct opens into the neck of the hair follicle. Cells of the secretory portion (alveoli) contain small lipid droplets (sebum).

Eccrine (merocrine) sweat glands are simple coiled tubular glands. Their primary function is control of body temperature. The secretory portion consists of three cell types: (1) basal clear cells (separated from each other by intercellular canaliculi; they secrete water and electrolytes); (2) apical dark cells (secrete glycoproteins); and (3) myoepithelial cells. The excretory portion is lined by a stratified cuboidal epithelium (except in the epidermis, where keratinocytes constitute the wall of the excretory duct).

Cystic fibrosis is a genetic disorder of epithelial transport of chloride ions by the channel protein cystic fibrosis transmembrane conductance regulator (CFTR). The lining epithelium of the excretory duct of eccrine sweat glands contains CFTR. A defect in CFTR causes a decrease in the reabsorption of sodium chloride from the lumen, resulting in increased concentrations of Cl^- in sweat.

Apocrine sweat glands are coiled and occur in the axilla, mons pubis, and circumanal area. The secretory acini are larger than in eccrine sweat glands. The excretory duct opens into the hair follicle (instead of into the epidermis as in the eccrine sweat glands). Ceruminous glands in the external auditory meatus and glands of Moll of the margin of the eyelids, are examples of apocrine sweat glands.

• Fingernails. The nails are hard keratin plates covering the nail bed, the surface of the skin consisting of the stratum basale and stratum spinosum only. Nail plates are formed by scales of cornified epithelial cells. The stratum corneum of the epidermis forms the hyponychium, a thick structure, under the distal and free edge of the nail plate. The proximal edge of the plate is covered by the eponychium, a projection of the stratum corneum of the skin.

12. CARDIOVASCULAR SYSTEM

General characteristics of the cardiovascular system

The cardiovascular system is a continuous, completely closed system of endothelial tubes. The general purpose of the cardiovascular system is the perfusion of capillary beds permeating all organs with fresh blood over a narrow range of hydrostatic pressures. Local functional demands determine the structural nature of the wall surrounding the endothelial tubes.

The circulation is divided into the **systemic** or **peripheral circulation** and the **pulmonary circulation**.

Arteries transport blood under high pressure and their muscular walls are thick (Figure 12-1). The veins are conduits for transport of the blood from tissues back to the heart. The pressure in the venous system is very low and the walls of the veins are thin.

There are variations in blood pressure in various parts of the cardiovascular system (see Figure 12-1). Because the heart pumps blood continuously in a pulsatile fashion into the aorta, the pressure in the aorta is high (about 100 mm Hg) and the arterial pressure fluctuates between a **systolic level** of 120 mm Hg and a **diastolic level** of 80 mm Hg.

As the blood flows through the systemic circulation, its pressure reaches the lowest value (0 mm Hg) when it returns to the right atrium of the heart through the terminal vena cava. In the capillaries, the pressure is about 35 mm Hg at the arteriolar end and lower (10 mm Hg) at the venous end. Although the pressure in the pulmonary arteries is pulsatile, as in the aorta, the systolic pressure is less (about 25 mm Hg), and the diastolic pressure is 8 mm Hg. The pressure in the pulmonary capillaries is only 7 mm Hg, as compared with an average pressure of 17 mm Hg in the capillary bed of the systemic circulation.

Heart

The heart is a folded endothelial tube whose wall is thickened to act as a regulated

Figure 12-1. Blood pressure and vascular anatomy

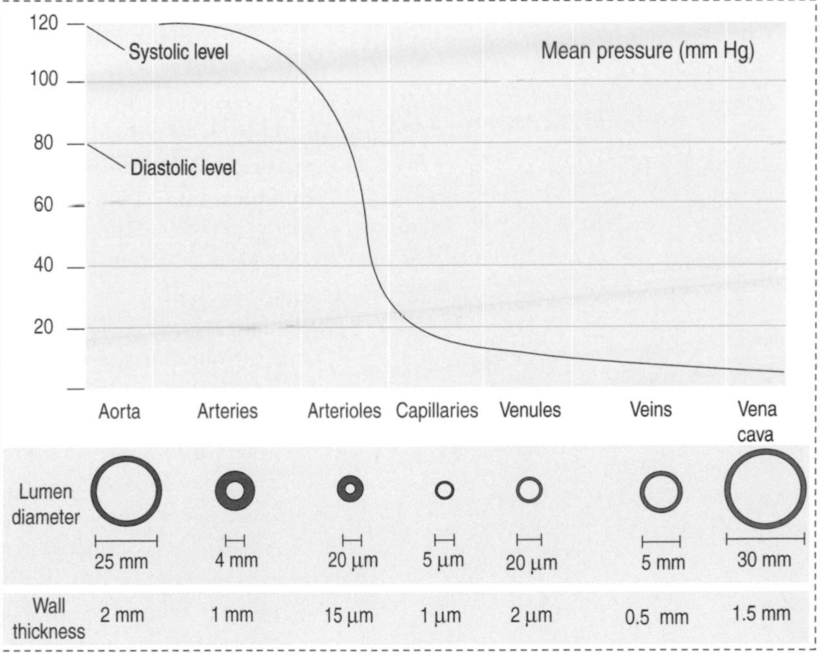

Figure 12-2. **Heart: Purkinje fibers**

Purkinje fibers are bundles of impulse-conducting cardiac fibers extending from the atrioventricular node. They can be found beneath the endocardium lining the interventricular septum.

Purkinje fibers can be distinguished from regular cardiocytes by their **location**, their **larger size**, and **lighter cytoplasmic staining** (glycogen content).

The **subendocardial connective tissue layer** consists of collagen and elastic fibers synthesized by fibroblasts.

This layer contains small blood vessels, nerves, and bundles of the conduction system (**Purkinje fibers**). The subendocardial layer is not present in papillary muscles and chordae tendineae inserted at the free edges of the mitral and tricuspid valves.

Endocardium (endothelial cell lining)

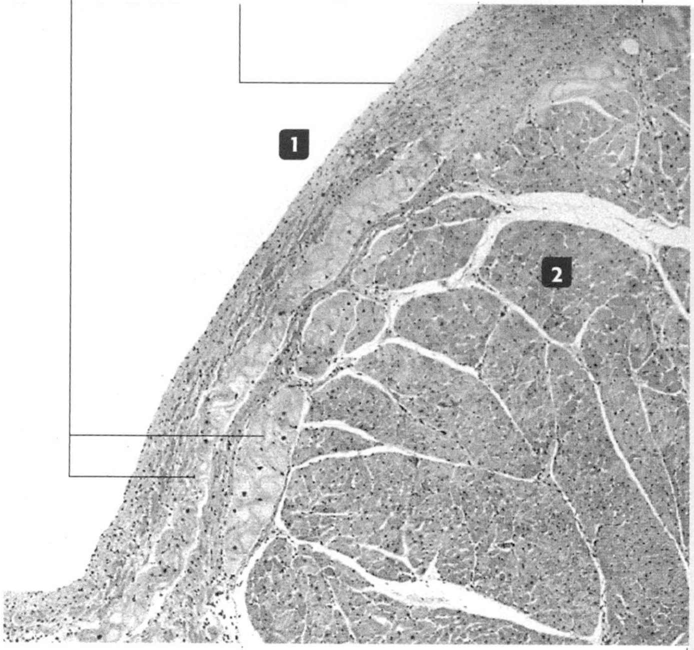

Myocardium (cardiac muscle)

Heart

The wall of the heart consists of three layers:

1 **Endocardium**, homologous to the tunica intima of blood vessels.

2 **Myocardium**, continuous with the tunica media of blood vessels.

3 **Epicardium**, similar to the tunica adventitia of blood vessels (not shown in the illustration).

The myocardium consists of three cell types:

1. **Contractile cardiocytes**, which contract to pump blood through the circulation.
2. **Myoendocrine cardiocytes**, producing atrial natriuretic factor.
3. **Nodal cardiocytes**, specialized to control the rhythmic contraction of the heart. These cells are located in (1) the **sinoatrial node**, at the superior vena cava–right atrium junction; and (2) the **atrioventricular node**, present under the endocardium of the interatrial and interventricular septa.

pump. The heart is the major determinant of systemic blood pressure.

The cardiac wall consists of three layers:

1. **Endocardium**, consisting of an **endothelial lining** and **subendothelial connective tissue**.

2. **Myocardium**, a functional syncytium of striated cardiac muscle fibers forming three major types of cardiac muscle: **atrial muscle**, **ventricular muscle**, and **specialized excitatory** and **conductive muscle fibers**.

3. **Epicardium**, a low-friction surface lined by a **mesothelium** in contact with the serosal pericardial space.

The heart is composed of two syncytia of muscle fibers: (1) the **atrial syncytium**, forming the walls of the two atria; and (2) the **ventricular syncytium**, forming the wall of the two ventricles. Atria and ventricles are separated by **fibrous connective tissue** surrounding the valvular openings between the atria and the ventricles.

Conductive system of the heart

The heart has two specialized conductive systems:

1. The **sinus node**, or **sinoatrial** (S-A) node, which generates impulses to cause rhythmic contractions of the cardiac muscle.

2. A specialized **conductive system**, consisting of the **internodal pathway**, which conducts the impulse from the S-A node to the atrioventricular (A-V) node); the **A-V node**, in which the atrial impulse is delayed before reaching the ventricles; the **atrioventricular bundle**, which conducts the impulse from the atria to the

Figure 12-3. **Atrial natriuretic factor**

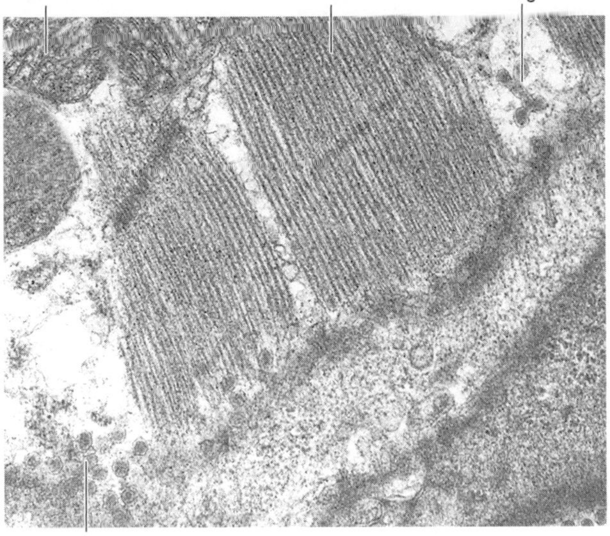
Mitochondria
Sarcomere
Atrial cell granules
Atrial cell granules

Atrial cardiocytes contain membrane-bound storage granules and a more highly developed Golgi apparatus and rough endoplasmic reticulum than their ventricular counterparts. The density of these granules in atrial cells can be altered by varying the intake of salt and water.

Atrial cell granules contain a potent polypeptide hormone, named **atrial natriuretic factor** (**ANF**), that stimulates diuresis (Greek *diourein*, to urinate) and natriuresis (Latin *natrium*, sodium + Greek *diourein*).

ANF also relaxes the cardiovascular muscle by antagonizing the actions of **vasopressin** (a polypeptide released from the neurohypophysis) and **angiotensin II** (a peptide derived from the **renin**-induced breakdown of **angiotensinogen**, a protein produced in liver and released into the systemic blood).

ANF prevents sodium and water reabsorption from causing **hypervolemia** (abnormal increase in the volume of circulating fluid in the body) and **hypertension** that can result in cardiac failure.

Increasing pressure across the atrial wall seems to be the principal mediator of ANF release as a prohormone. Once outside the atrial cell, the ANF prohormone undergoes a rapid enzymatic cleavage to produce the principal form of circulating ANF.

ventricles; and the **left and right bundles of Purkinje fibers**, which conduct the impulse to all parts of the ventricles (Figure 12-2).

When stretched, cardiac muscle cells of the atrium (atrial cardiocytes) secrete a peptide called **atrial natriuretic factor** (ANF) (Figure 12-3) that stimulates both diuresis and excretion of sodium in urine (natriuresis) by increasing the glomerular filtration rate. By this mechanism, the blood volume is reduced and the stretching of the atrial cardiocytes is relieved.

Histologically (see Figure 7-18 in Chapter 7, Muscle Tissue), individual cardiac muscle cells have a central nucleus and are linked to each other by **intercalated disks**. The presence of **gap junctions** in the longitudinal segment of the intercalated disks between connected cardiac muscle cells allows free diffusion of ions and the rapid spread of the action potential from cell to cell. The electrical resistance is low because gap junctions bypass the **transverse** components of the intercalated disk (**fasciae adherentes** and **desmosomes**).

Differences between cardiac muscle fibers and Purkinje fibers

The **Purkinje fibers** lie **beneath the endocardium** lining the two sides of the interventricular septum (see Figure 12-2). They can be distinguished from cardiac muscle fibers because they contain a **reduced number of myofibrils located at the periphery of the fiber** and the **diameter of the fiber is larger.** In addition, they give a positive reaction for **acetylcholinesterase**, and they contain abundant **glycogen**. Purkinje fibers lose these specific characteristics when they merge with cardiac muscle fibers. Like cardiac muscle fibers, Purkinje fibers are striated and are linked to each other by atypical intercalated disks.

Arteries

Arteries conduct blood from the heart to the capillaries. They store some of the pumped blood during each cardiac systole to ensure continued flow through the capillaries during cardiac diastole.

Arteries are organized in three major **tunics** or layers (Figure 12-4):

1. The **tunica intima** is the innermost coat. It consists of an **endothelial lining** continuous with the endocardium, the inner lining of the heart; an intermediate layer of loose connective tissue, the **subendothelium**; and an external layer of elastic fibers, the **internal elastic lamina**.

2. The **tunica media** is the middle coat. It consists mainly of smooth muscle

Figure 12-4. Structure of a muscular artery

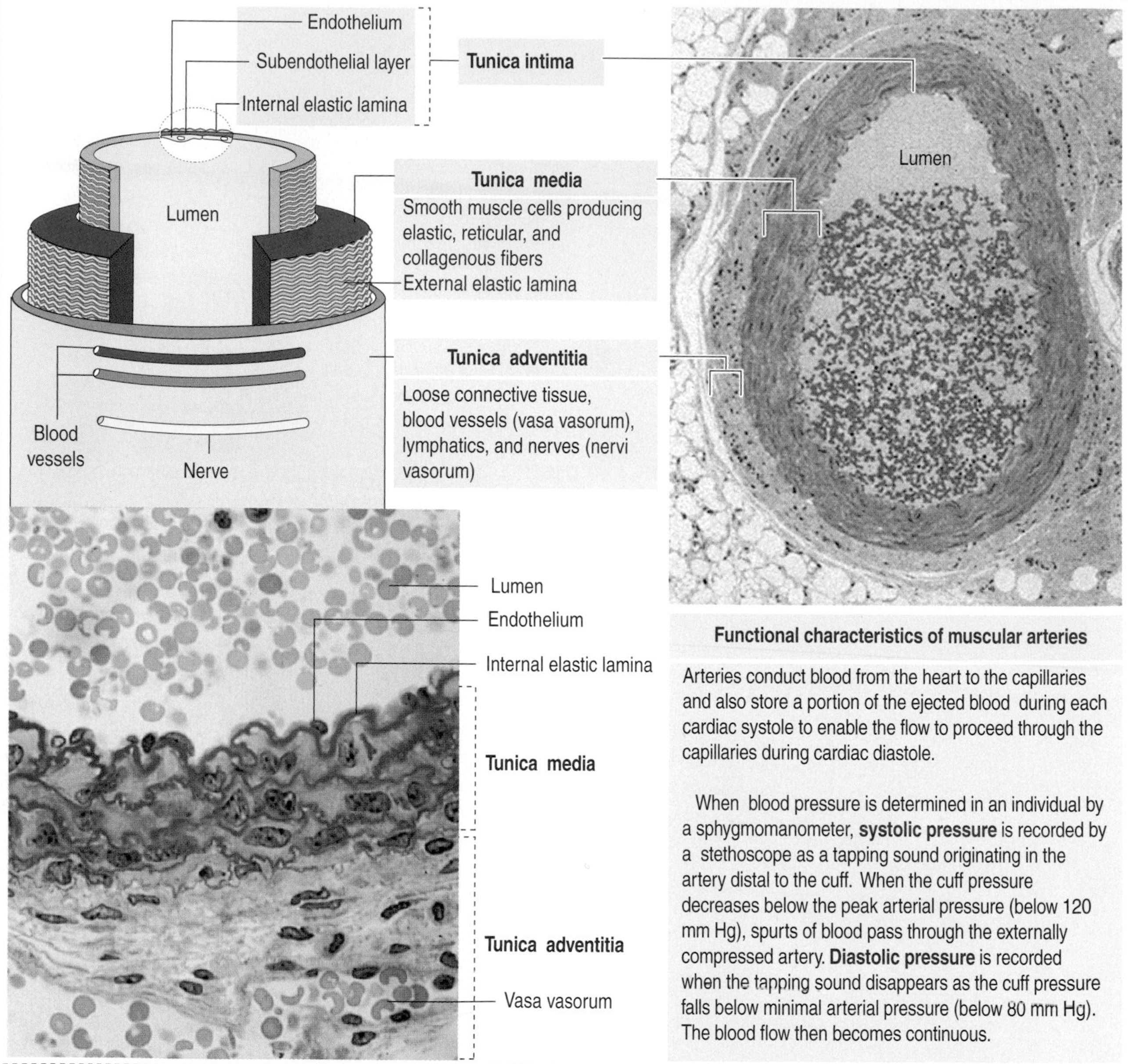

Endothelium
Subendothelial layer
Internal elastic lamina
Tunica intima
Lumen
Tunica media
Smooth muscle cells producing elastic, reticular, and collagenous fibers
External elastic lamina
Tunica adventitia
Loose connective tissue, blood vessels (vasa vasorum), lymphatics, and nerves (nervi vasorum)
Blood vessels
Nerve
Lumen
Lumen
Endothelium
Internal elastic lamina
Tunica media
Tunica adventitia
Vasa vasorum

Functional characteristics of muscular arteries

Arteries conduct blood from the heart to the capillaries and also store a portion of the ejected blood during each cardiac systole to enable the flow to proceed through the capillaries during cardiac diastole.

When blood pressure is determined in an individual by a sphygmomanometer, **systolic pressure** is recorded by a stethoscope as a tapping sound originating in the artery distal to the cuff. When the cuff pressure decreases below the peak arterial pressure (below 120 mm Hg), spurts of blood pass through the externally compressed artery. **Diastolic pressure** is recorded when the tapping sound disappears as the cuff pressure falls below minimal arterial pressure (below 80 mm Hg). The blood flow then becomes continuous.

cells surrounded by a variable number of collagen fibers, extracellular matrix, and elastic sheaths with irregular gaps (fenestrated elastic membranes).

Collagen fibers provide a supporting framework for smooth muscle cells and limit the distensibility of the wall of the vessel. Veins have a higher content of collagen than arteries.

3. The **tunica externa**, or **adventitia**, is the outer coat and consists mainly of connective tissue. An external elastic lamina can be seen separating the tunica media from the adventitia. The adventitia of large vessels (arteries and veins) contains small vessels (**vasa vasorum**) that penetrate the outer portion of the tunica media to supply oxygen and nutrients.

From the heart to the capillaries, arteries can be classified into three major groups: (1) **large elastic arteries**, (2) **medium-sized muscular arteries** (see Figure 12-4), and (3) **small arteries** and **arterioles**.

Large elastic arteries are conducting vessels

The **aorta** and its largest branches (the **brachiocephalic**, **common carotid**, **sub-**

Figure 12-5. **Structure of an elastic artery (aorta)**

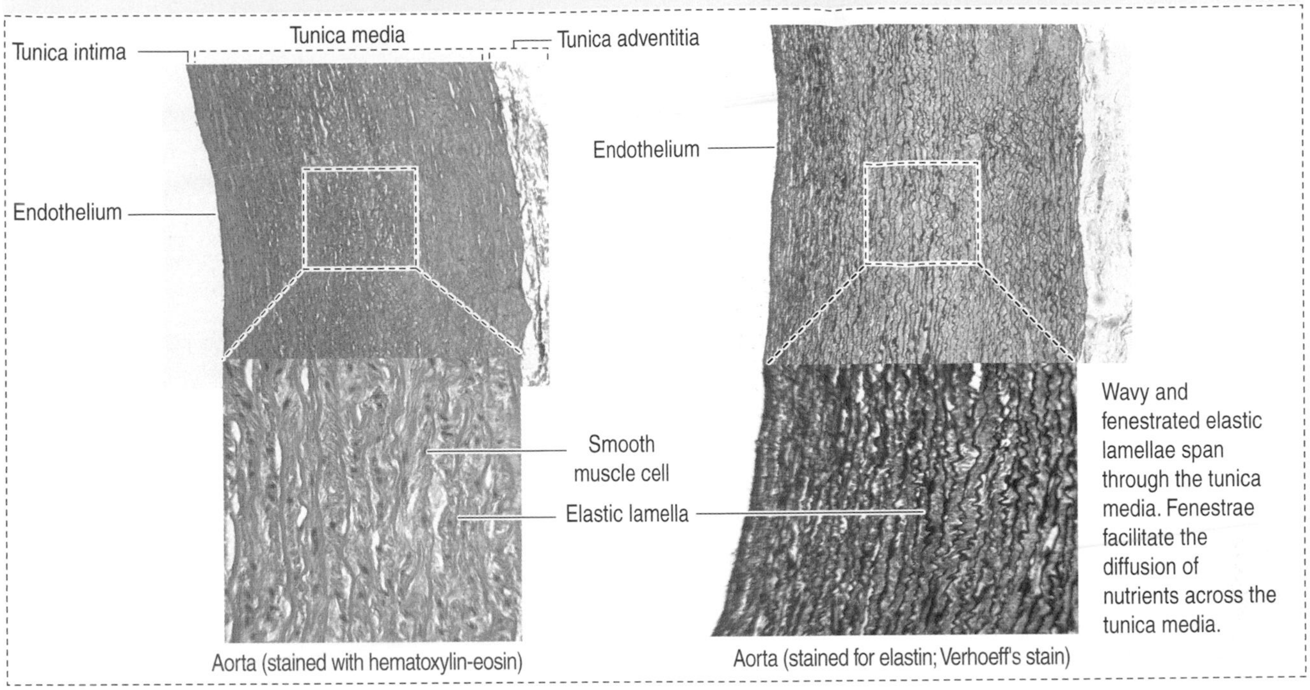
Tunica intima
Tunica media
Tunica adventitia
Endothelium
Endothelium
Smooth muscle cell
Elastic lamella
Wavy and fenestrated elastic lamellae span through the tunica media. Fenestrae facilitate the diffusion of nutrients across the tunica media.
Aorta (stained with hematoxylin-eosin)
Aorta (stained for elastin; Verhoeff's stain)

clavian, and **common iliac** arteries) are **elastic arteries** (Figure 12-5). They are **conducting arteries** because they conduct blood from the heart to the medium-sized **distributing arteries**.

Large elastic arteries have two major characteristics: (1) They receive blood from the heart under high pressure. (2) They keep blood circulating continuously while the heart is pumping intermittently. Because they distend during systole and recoil during diastole, elastic arteries can sustain a continuous blood flow despite the intermittent pumping action of the heart.

The **tunica intima** of the elastic arteries consists of the endothelium and the subendothelial connective tissue.

Large amounts of **fenestrated elastic sheaths** are found in the **tunica media**, with bundles of smooth muscle cells permeating the narrow spaces between the elastic lamellae. Collagen fibers are present in all tunics, but especially in the adventitia. We have seen in Chapter 4, Connective Tissue, that smooth muscle cells can synthesize **both elastic and collagen fibers**. Blood vessels (**vasa vasorum**), nerves (**nervi vasorum**), and **lymphatics** can be recognized in the tunica adventitia of large elastic arteries.

Clinical significance: Aortic aneurysms

The two major types of aortic aneurysm are the **syphilitic aneurysm** (relatively rare because syphilis is no longer common) and the **abdominal aneurysm**. The latter is caused by a weakening of the aortic wall produced by atherosclerosis (see Figure 12-14). Aortic aneurysms generate murmurs caused by blood turbulence in the dilated aortic segment. A severe complication is rupture of the aneurysm followed by immediate death.

Marfan syndrome (see Chapter 4, Connective Tissue) is an autosomal dominant defect associated with aortic dissecting aneurysm and skeletal and ocular abnormalities due to mutations in the *fibrillin 1* gene. Fibrillins are major components of the elastic fibers found in the aorta, periosteum, and suspensory ligament of the lens.

Medium-sized muscular arteries are distributing vessels

There is a gradual transition from large arteries, to medium-sized arteries, to small

Figure 12-6. Arterioles: Resistance vessels

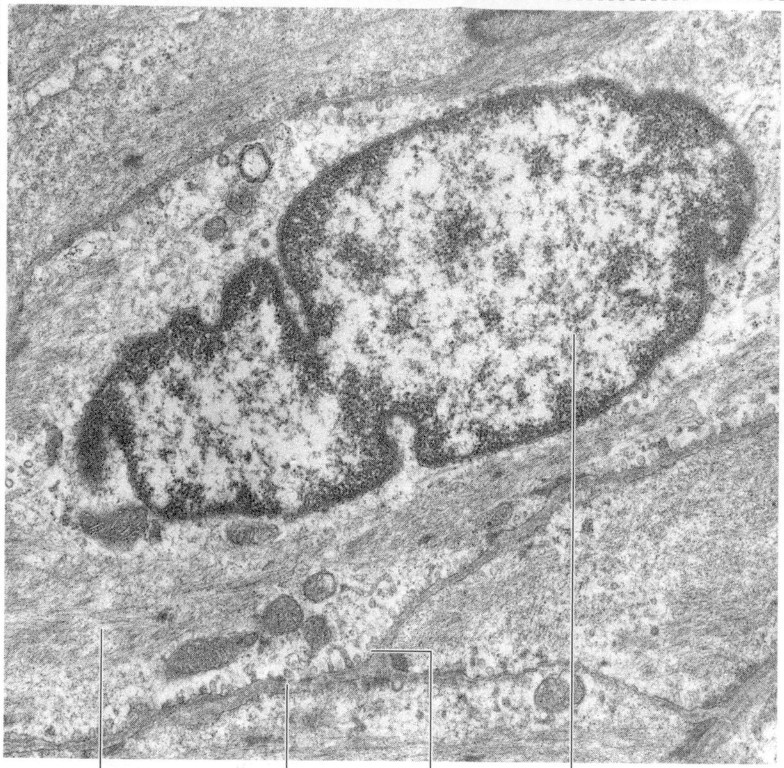
Actin-myosin bundle
Basal lamina
Pinocytosis
Nucleus

Vascular smooth muscle cells of arterioles

Vascular smooth muscle cells have a significant role in the control of total peripheral resistance, arterial and venous tone, and blood distribution throughout the body.

The cytoplasm of vascular smooth muscle cells contains actin and myosin filaments whose contraction is controlled by calcium. The increase in calcium concentration occurs through voltage-gated calcium channels (known as **electromechanical coupling**) and through receptor-mediated calcium channels (known as **pharmacomechanical coupling**). Both channels are present in the plasma membrane. Calcium can also be released from cytoplasmic storage sites (endoplasmic reticulum). Smooth muscle cells lack troponin.

The constant blood flow depends on a **myogenic mechanism**: arteriolar smooth muscle cells contract in response to increased transmural pressure and relax when the pressure decreases.

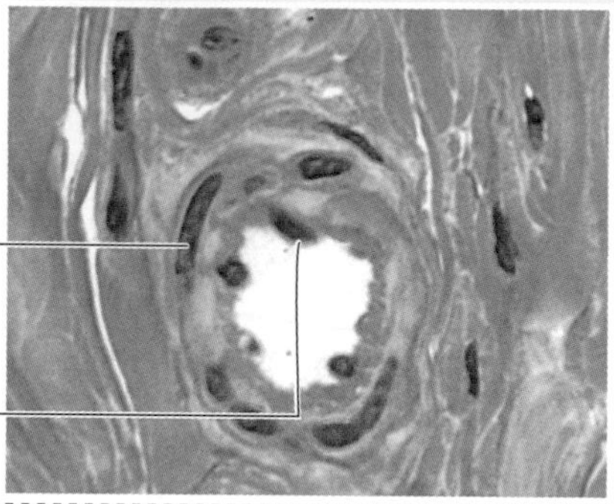
Vascular smooth muscle cell
Endothelial cell

arteries and arterioles. Medium-sized arteries are **distributing vessels**, allowing a selective distribution of blood to different organs in response to functional needs. Examples of medium-sized arteries include the radial, tibial, popliteal, axillary, splenic, mesenteric, and intercostal arteries. The diameter of medium-sized muscular arteries is about 3 mm or greater.

The **tunica intima** consists of three layers: (1) the **endothelium**, (2) the **subendothelium**, and (3) the **internal elastic lamina** (see Figure 12-4).

The internal elastic lamina is a fenestrated band of elastic fibers that often shows folds in sections of fixed tissue owing to contraction of the smooth muscle cell layer (tunica media).

The **tunica media** shows a significant reduction in elastic components and an increase in smooth muscle fibers. In the larger vessels of this group, a fenestrated **external elastic lamina** can be seen at the junction of the tunica media and the adventitia.

Arterioles are resistance vessels

Arterioles are the final branches of the arterial system. Arterioles regulate the distribution of blood to different capillary beds by **vasoconstriction** and **vasodilation** in localized regions. Partial contraction (known as **tone**) of the vascular smooth muscle exists in arterioles. Arterioles are structurally adapted for vasoconstriction and vasodilation because their walls contain circularly arranged smooth muscle fibers. Arterioles are regarded as **resistance vessels** and are the major determinants of systemic blood pressure (Figure 12-6).

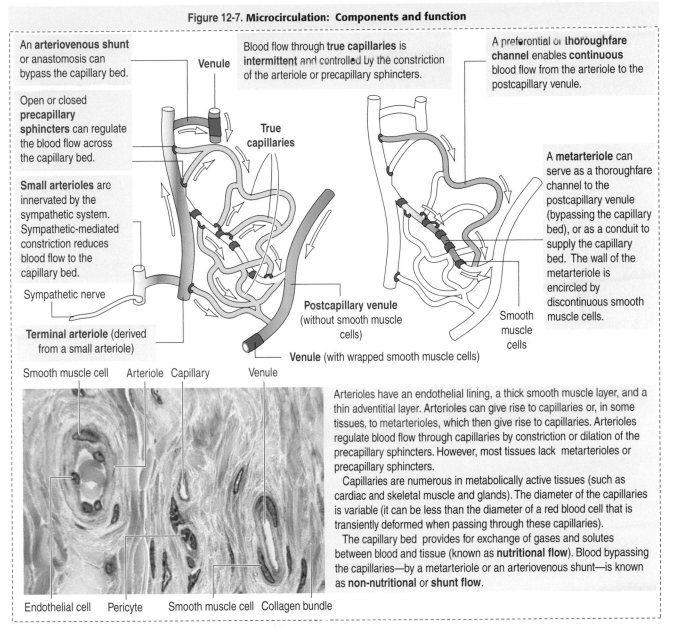

Figure 12-7. Microcirculation: Components and function

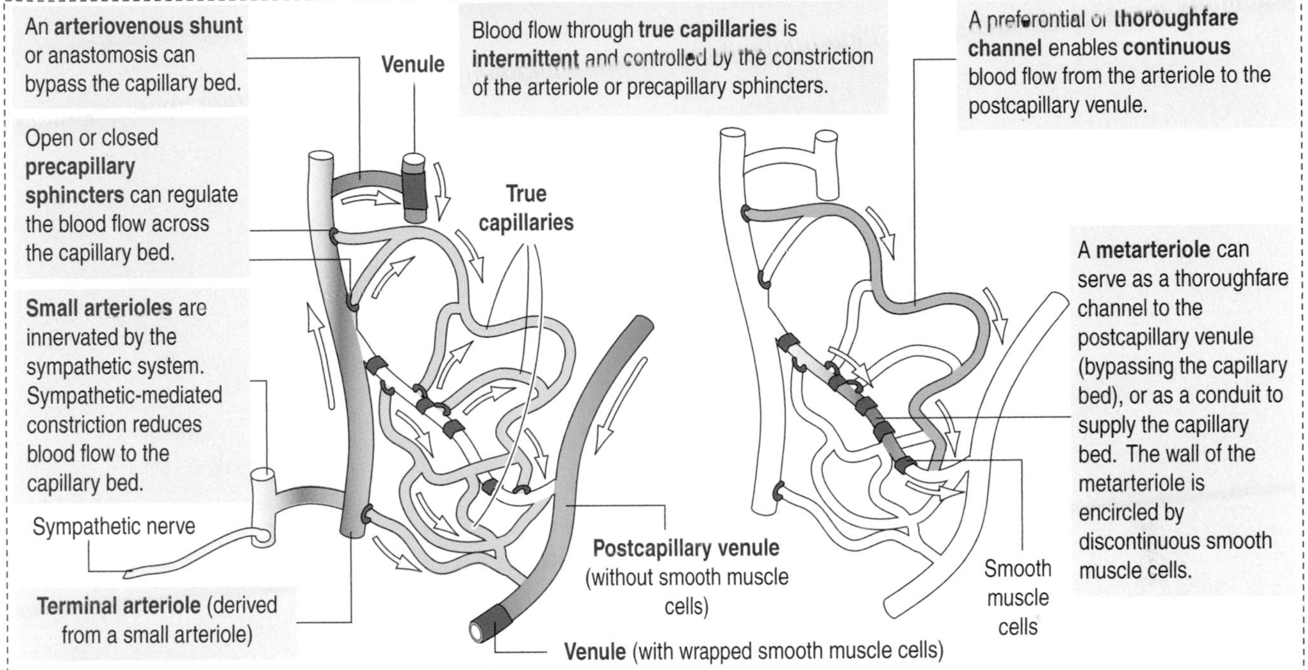
An **arteriovenous shunt** or anastomosis can bypass the capillary bed.
Venule
Blood flow through **true capillaries** is **intermittent** and controlled by the constriction of the arteriole or precapillary sphincters.
A preferential or **thoroughfare channel** enables **continuous** blood flow from the arteriole to the postcapillary venule.
Open or closed **precapillary sphincters** can regulate the blood flow across the capillary bed.
True capillaries
Small arterioles are innervated by the sympathetic system. Sympathetic-mediated constriction reduces blood flow to the capillary bed.
A **metarteriole** can serve as a thoroughfare channel to the postcapillary venule (bypassing the capillary bed), or as a conduit to supply the capillary bed. The wall of the metarteriole is encircled by discontinuous smooth muscle cells.
Sympathetic nerve
Postcapillary venule (without smooth muscle cells)
Smooth muscle cells
Terminal arteriole (derived from a small arteriole)
Venule (with wrapped smooth muscle cells)

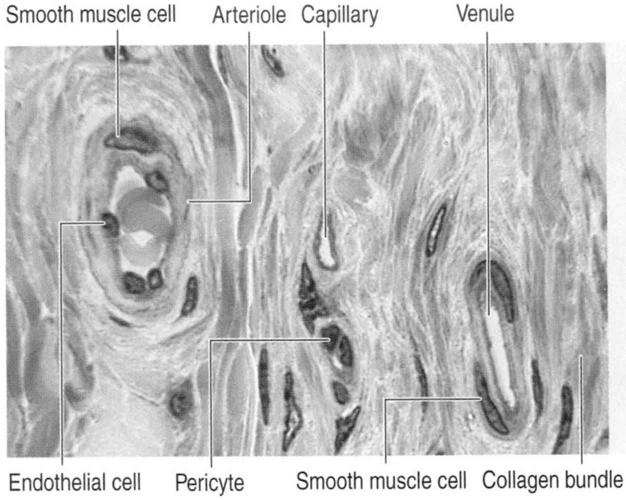
Smooth muscle cell
Arteriole
Capillary
Venule
Endothelial cell
Pericyte
Smooth muscle cell
Collagen bundle

Arterioles have an endothelial lining, a thick smooth muscle layer, and a thin adventitial layer. Arterioles can give rise to capillaries or, in some tissues, to metarterioles, which then give rise to capillaries. Arterioles regulate blood flow through capillaries by constriction or dilation of the precapillary sphincters. However, most tissues lack metarterioles or precapillary sphincters.

Capillaries are numerous in metabolically active tissues (such as cardiac and skeletal muscle and glands). The diameter of the capillaries is variable (it can be less than the diameter of a red blood cell that is transiently deformed when passing through these capillaries).

The capillary bed provides for exchange of gases and solutes between blood and tissue (known as **nutritional flow**). Blood bypassing the capillaries—by a metarteriole or an arteriovenous shunt—is known as **non-nutritional** or **shunt flow**.

The diameter of arterioles and small arteries ranges from 20 to 130 μm. Since the lumen is small, these blood vessels can be closed down to generate high resistance to blood flow. The **tunica intima** has an endothelium, subendothelium, and internal elastic lamina. The **tunica media** consists of two to five concentric layers of smooth muscle cells. The **tunica adventitia**, or **tunica externa**, contains slight collagenous tissue, binding the vessel to its surroundings.

The segment beyond the arteriole proper is the **metarteriole**, the terminal branch of the arterial system. It consists of one layer of muscle cells, often **discontinuous**, and represents an important local regulator of blood flow.

Capillaries are exchange vessels

Capillaries are extremely thin tubes formed by a single layer of highly permeable **endothelial cells** surrounded by a basal lamina. The diameter range of a capillary is about 5 to 10 μm, large enough to accommodate one red blood cell, and thin enough (0.5 μm) for gas diffusion.

The **microvascular bed**, the site of the **microcirculation** (Figure 12-7), is composed of the **terminal arteriole** (and **metarteriole**), the **capillary bed**, and the

Figure 12-8. Structure of capillaries

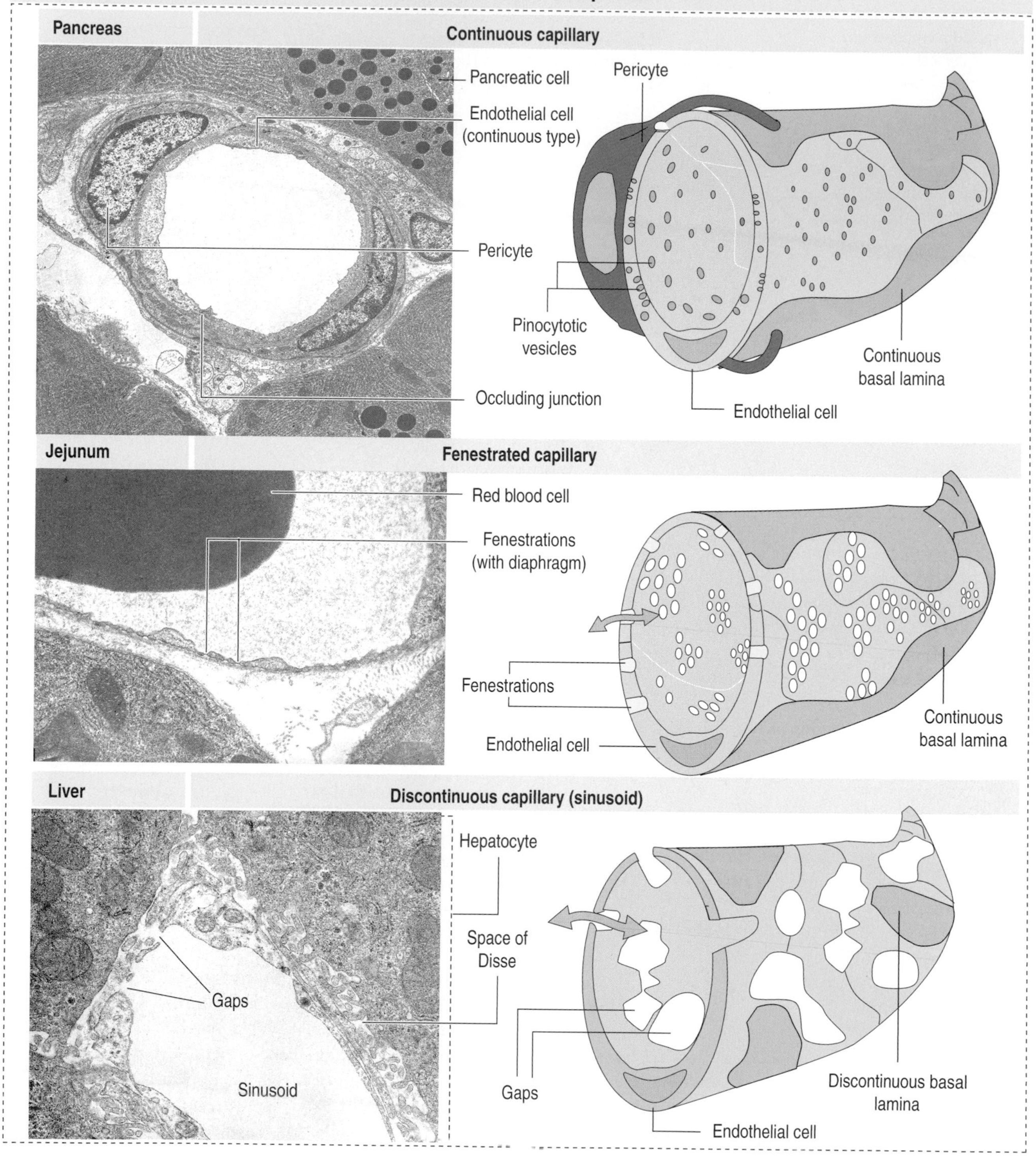

Pancreas
Continuous capillary
Pancreatic cell
Endothelial cell (continuous type)
Pericyte
Pericyte
Pinocytotic vesicles
Occluding junction
Endothelial cell
Continuous basal lamina
Jejunum
Fenestrated capillary
Red blood cell
Fenestrations (with diaphragm)
Fenestrations
Endothelial cell
Continuous basal lamina
Liver
Discontinuous capillary (sinusoid)
Hepatocyte
Space of Disse
Gaps
Sinusoid
Gaps
Discontinuous basal lamina
Endothelial cell

postcapillary venules. The capillary bed consists of slightly large capillaries (called **preferential** or **thoroughfare channels**), where blood flow is **continuous**, and small capillaries, called the **true capillaries**, where blood flow is **intermittent**.

The amount of blood entering the microvascular bed is regulated by the contraction of smooth muscle fibers of the **precapillary sphincters** located where true capillaries arise from the arteriole or metarteriole. The capillary circulation can be bypassed by channels (**through channels**) connecting terminal arterioles to postcapillary venules.

When functional demands decrease, most precapillary sphincters are closed,

Figure 12-9. Types of capillaries

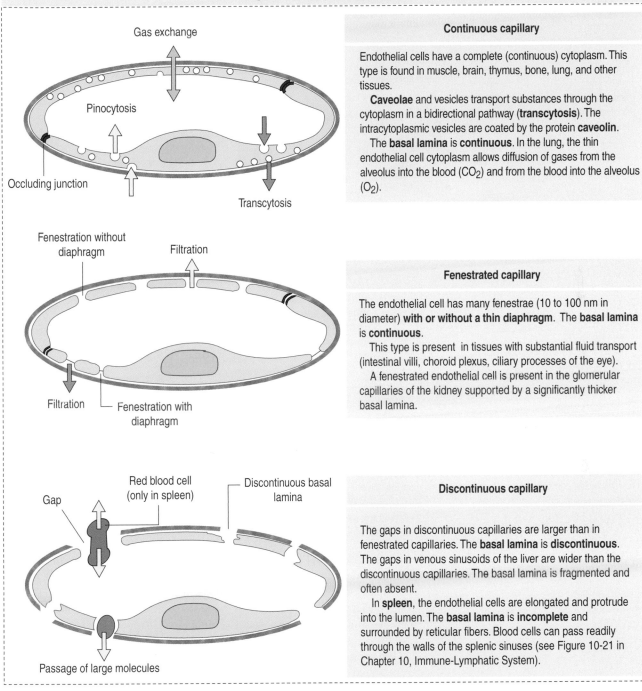

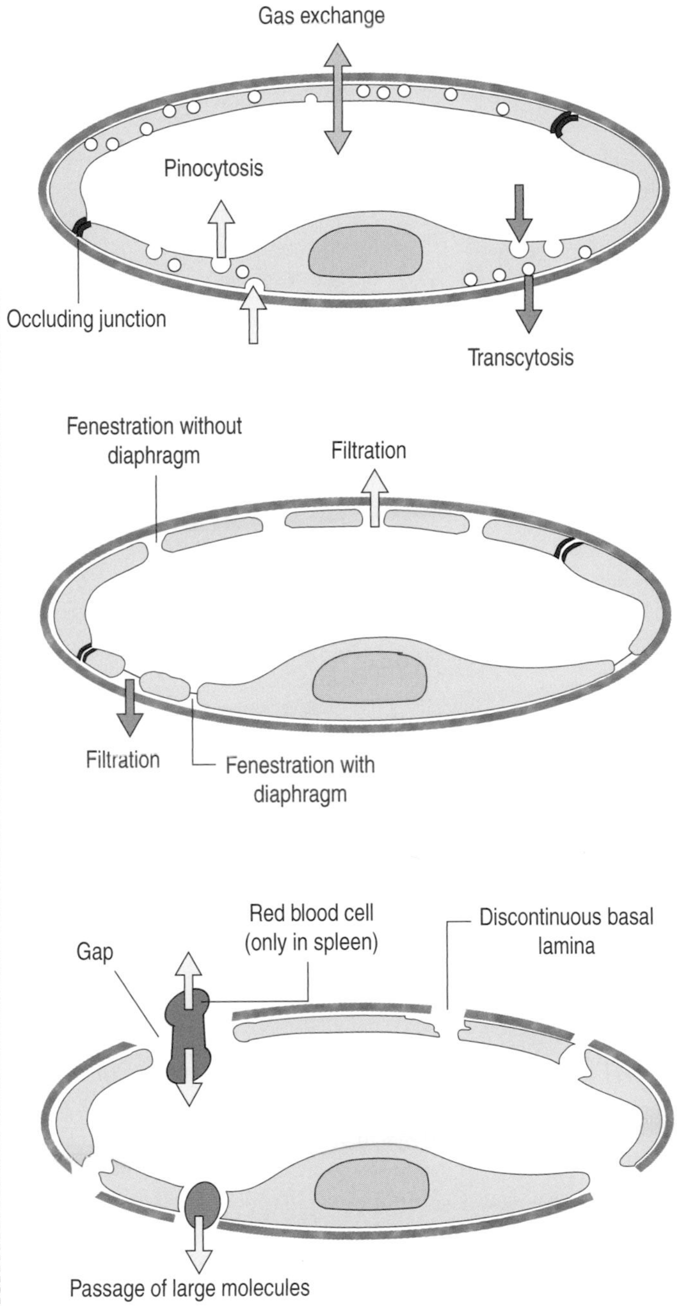

Gas exchange
Pinocytosis
Occluding junction
Transcytosis
Fenestration without diaphragm
Filtration
Filtration
Fenestration with diaphragm
Red blood cell (only in spleen)
Discontinuous basal lamina
Gap
Passage of large molecules

Continuous capillary

Endothelial cells have a complete (continuous) cytoplasm. This type is found in muscle, brain, thymus, bone, lung, and other tissues.

Caveolae and vesicles transport substances through the cytoplasm in a bidirectional pathway (**transcytosis**). The intracytoplasmic vesicles are coated by the protein **caveolin**.

The **basal lamina** is **continuous**. In the lung, the thin endothelial cell cytoplasm allows diffusion of gases from the alveolus into the blood (CO_2) and from the blood into the alveolus (O_2).

Fenestrated capillary

The endothelial cell has many fenestrae (10 to 100 nm in diameter) **with or without a thin diaphragm**. The **basal lamina** is **continuous**.

This type is present in tissues with substantial fluid transport (intestinal villi, choroid plexus, ciliary processes of the eye).

A fenestrated endothelial cell is present in the glomerular capillaries of the kidney supported by a significantly thicker basal lamina.

Discontinuous capillary

The gaps in discontinuous capillaries are larger than in fenestrated capillaries. The **basal lamina** is **discontinuous**. The gaps in venous sinusoids of the liver are wider than the discontinuous capillaries. The basal lamina is fragmented and often absent.

In **spleen**, the endothelial cells are elongated and protrude into the lumen. The **basal lamina** is **incomplete** and surrounded by reticular fibers. Blood cells can pass readily through the walls of the splenic sinuses (see Figure 10-21 in Chapter 10, Immune-Lymphatic System).

forcing the flow of blood into thoroughfare channels. **Arteriovenous shunts**, or **anastomoses**, are direct connections between arterioles and postcapillary venules and bypass the microvascular bed.

The three-dimensional design of the microvasculature varies from organ to organ. The local conditions of the tissues (concentration of nutrients and metabolites and other substances) can control local blood flow in small portions of a tissue area.

Three types of capillaries: Continuous, fenestrated, and discontinuous

Three morphologic types of capillaries are recognized (Figures 12-8 and 12-9): **continuous**, **fenestrated**, and **discontinuous** (**sinusoids**).

Continuous capillaries are lined by a complete simple squamous endothelium

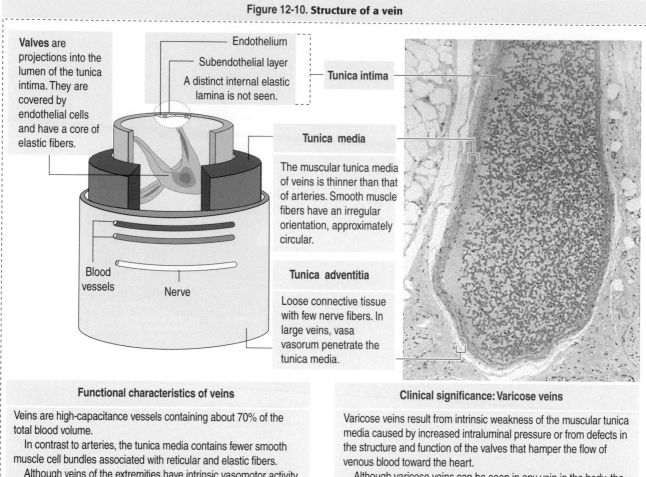

Figure 12-10. Structure of a vein

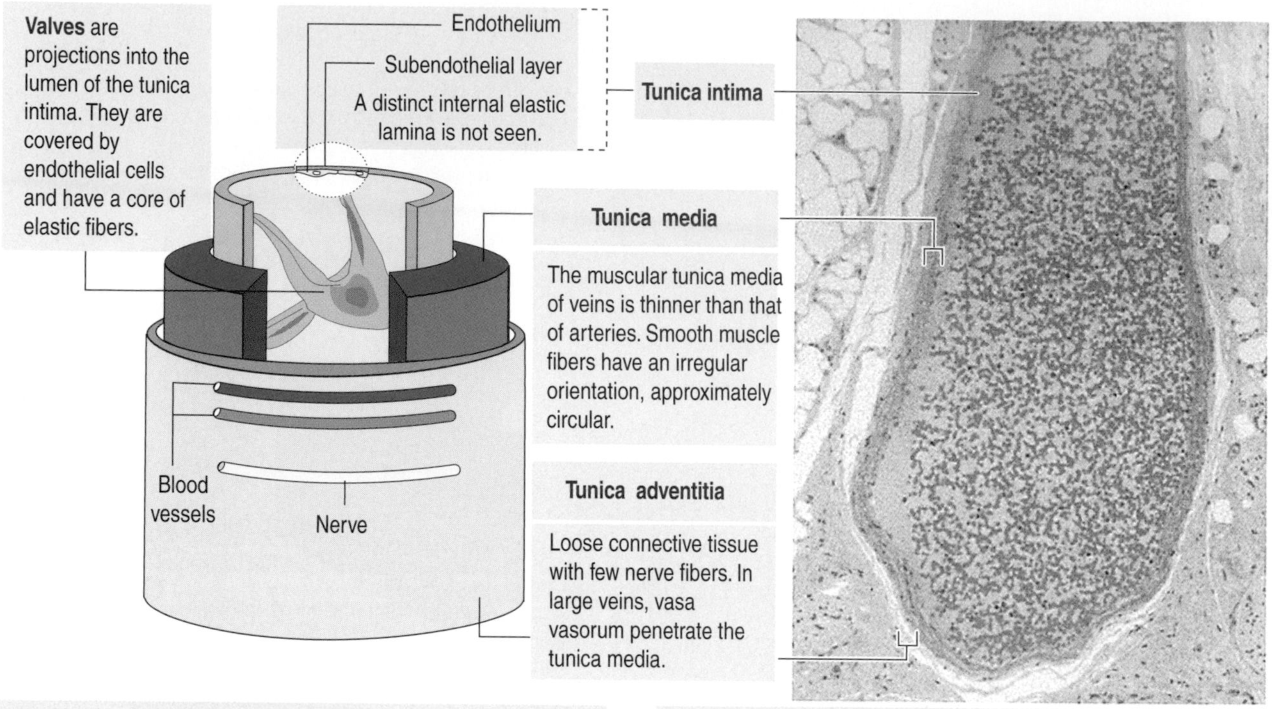
Valves are projections into the lumen of the tunica intima. They are covered by endothelial cells and have a core of elastic fibers.
Endothelium
Subendothelial layer
A distinct internal elastic lamina is not seen.
Tunica intima
Tunica media
The muscular tunica media of veins is thinner than that of arteries. Smooth muscle fibers have an irregular orientation, approximately circular.
Tunica adventitia
Loose connective tissue with few nerve fibers. In large veins, vasa vasorum penetrate the tunica media.
Blood vessels
Nerve

Functional characteristics of veins

Veins are high-capacitance vessels containing about 70% of the total blood volume.

In contrast to arteries, the tunica media contains fewer smooth muscle cell bundles associated with reticular and elastic fibers.

Although veins of the extremities have intrinsic vasomotor activity, the transport of blood back to the heart depends on external forces provided by the contraction of surrounding skeletal muscles and on valves that ensure one-way blood flow.

Clinical significance: Varicose veins

Varicose veins result from intrinsic weakness of the muscular tunica media caused by increased intraluminal pressure or from defects in the structure and function of the valves that hamper the flow of venous blood toward the heart.

Although varicose veins can be seen in any vein in the body, the most common are the saphenous veins of the legs, veins in the anorectal region (**hemorrhoids**), the veins of the lower esophagus (**esophageal varices**), and veins in the spermatic cord (**varicocele**).

and a basal lamina. **Pericytes** can occur between the endothelium and the basal lamina. Pericytes are undifferentiated cells that resemble modified smooth muscle cells and are distributed at random intervals in close contact with the basal lamina. Endothelial cells are linked by tight junctions and transport fluids and solutes by **caveolae** and **pinocytotic vesicles**. Continuous capillaries occur in brain, muscle, skin, thymus, and lung.

Fenestrated capillaries have **pores**, or **fenestrae**, with or without **diaphragms**. Fenestrated capillaries with a diaphragm are found in intestines, endocrine glands, and around kidney tubules. Fenestrated capillaries without a diaphragm are characteristic of the renal glomerulus. In this particular case, the basal lamina constitutes an important permeability barrier, as we will analyze in Chapter 14, Urinary System.

Discontinuous capillaries are characterized by an incomplete endothelial lining and basal lamina, with **gaps** or **holes** between and within endothelial cells. Discontinuous capillaries and sinusoids are found where an intimate relation is needed between blood and parenchyma (for example, in the liver and spleen).

Veins are capacitance or reservoir vessels

The venous system starts at the end of the capillary bed with a **postcapillary venule** that structurally resembles continuous capillaries but with a wider lumen. Postcapillary venules, the preferred site of migration of blood cells into tissues by

Figure 12-11. "Blind sac" origin of lymphatic capillaries

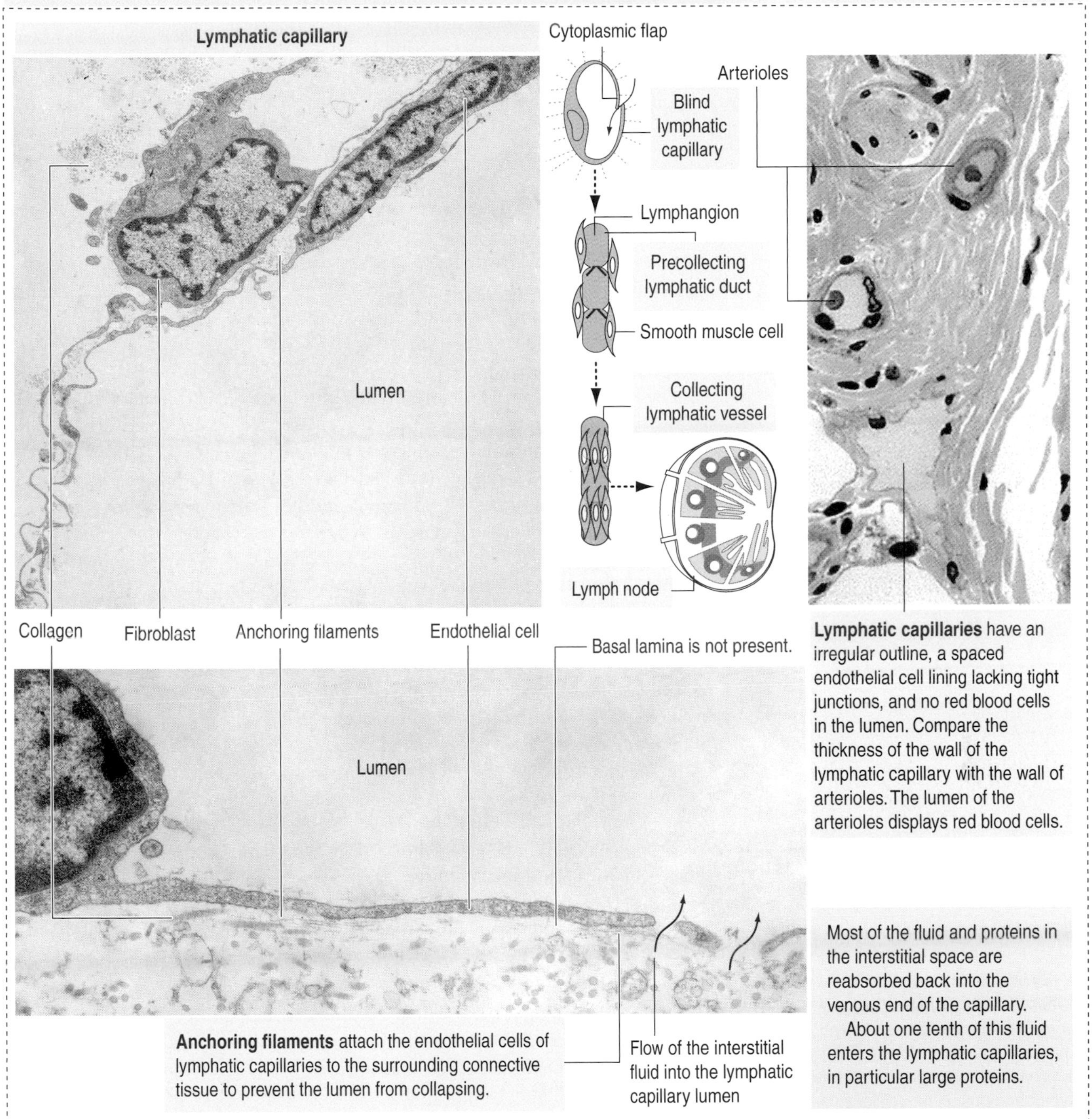

Lymphatic capillary
Cytoplasmic flap
Arterioles
Blind lymphatic capillary
Lymphangion
Precollecting lymphatic duct
Smooth muscle cell
Collecting lymphatic vessel
Lymph node
Lumen
Collagen
Fibroblast
Anchoring filaments
Endothelial cell
Basal lamina is not present.
Lymphatic capillaries have an irregular outline, a spaced endothelial cell lining lacking tight junctions, and no red blood cells in the lumen. Compare the thickness of the wall of the lymphatic capillary with the wall of arterioles. The lumen of the arterioles displays red blood cells.
Lumen
Most of the fluid and proteins in the interstitial space are reabsorbed back into the venous end of the capillary.
About one tenth of this fluid enters the lymphatic capillaries, in particular large proteins.
Anchoring filaments attach the endothelial cells of lymphatic capillaries to the surrounding connective tissue to prevent the lumen from collapsing.
Flow of the interstitial fluid into the lymphatic capillary lumen

a mechanism called **diapedesis** (Greek *dia*, through; *pedan*, to leap), are tubes of endothelial cells supported by a basal lamina and an adventitia of collagen fibers and fibroblasts.

In lymphatic tissues, the endothelial cells are taller. **High endothelial venules are associated with the mechanism of homing of lymphocytes in lymphoid organs** (see Chapter 10, Immune-Lymphatic System).

Postcapillary venules converge to form **muscular venules**, which converge into **collecting venules**, leading to a series of **veins** of progressively larger diameter.

Veins have a relatively thin wall in comparison to arteries of the same size (Figure 12–10). The high capacitance of veins is attributable to the distensibility of their wall (**compliance vessels**) and, therefore, the content of blood is large relative to the volume of the veins. A small increase in the intraluminal pressure results in a large increase in the volume of contained blood.

Similar to arteries, veins consist of tunics. However, the distinction of a tunica media from a tunica adventitia is often not clear. The lumen is lined by an endothelium and a subjacent basal lamina. **A distinct internal elastic lamina is not seen.**

The **muscular tunica media** is thinner than in arteries, and smooth muscle cells have an irregular orientation, approximately circular. A longitudinal orientation is observed in the iliac vein, brachiocephalic vein, superior and inferior venae cavae, portal vein, and renal vein.

The **tunica adventitia** consists of collagen fibers and fibroblasts with few nerve fibers. In large veins, the vasa vasorum penetrate the wall.

A typical characteristic of veins is the presence of **valves** to prevent reflux of blood. A valve is a projection into the lumen of the tunica intima, covered by endothelial cells and strengthened by elastic and collagen fibers.

Lymphatic vessels

The functions of the lymphatic vascular system are to (1) conduct immune cells and lymph to lymph nodes, 2) remove excess fluid accumulated in interstitial spaces, and (3) transport chylomicrons, lipid-containing particles, through lacteal lymphatic vessels inside the intestinal villi (see Chapter 16, Lower Digestive Segment). The flow of lymph is under low pressure and unidirectional.

Lymphatic capillaries form networks in tissue spaces and begin as dilated tubes with closed ends (blind tubes) in proximity to blood capillaries. Lymphatic capillaries collect tissue fluid, the **lymph**. The wall of a **lymphatic capillary** consists of a single layer of endothelial cells **lacking a complete basal lamina** (Figure 12-11). Bundles of **anchoring filaments** associated to the endothelium prevent the lymphatic capillaries from collapsing during changes in interstitial pressure and enable the uptake of soluble tissue components. **Lymphatic capillaries can be found in most tissues. Exceptions are cartilage, bone, epithelia, the central nervous system, bone marrow, and placenta.**

The accumulation of fluid in the interstitial space is a normal event of circulation and blind-ended lymphatic capillaries take up the excess fluid. An increase in the intraluminal volume in the lymphatic capillary opens the overlapping cytoplasmic flaps drawing fluid in. When the lymphatic capillary fills, the overlapping flaps, acting as a primary valve opening, close, preventing fluid backflow into the interstitium.

Lymphatic capillaries converge into **precollecting lymphatic vessels** draining lymph into **collecting lymphatic vessels. The collecting vessels are surrounded by smooth muscle cells, which provide intrinsic pumping activity.** Movement in the surrounding tissue provides a passive extrinsic pump.

The collecting vessels consist of bulblike segments separated by luminal valves. The sequential contraction of each segment, called **lymphangions**, propels the unidirectional flow of lymph (see Box 12-A). A collecting lymphatic vessel gives rise to **terminal lymphatic vessels** in the proximity of a lymph node. These terminal lymphatic vessels branch and become lymphatic afferent vessels, which penetrate the lymph node capsule and release lymph and its contents into the subcapsular sinus. Lymph nodes are distributed along the pathway of the lymph vessels to filter the lymph before reaching the thoracic and right lymphatic ducts. A total of 2 to 3 L of lymph is produced each day.

Lymph is returned to the bloodstream via two main trunks: (1) the large **thoracic duct** and (2) the smaller **right lymphatic duct**.

Larger lymphatic vessels have three layers, similar to those of the small veins, but the lumen is larger.

The **tunica intima** consists of an endothelium and a thin subendothelial layer of connective tissue.

The **tunica media** contains a few smooth muscle cells in a concentric arrange-

Box 12-A | **How lymph flows**

- **By intrinsic contraction**

When collecting lymphatics or larger lymphatic vessels become expanded by lymph, the smooth muscle of the wall contracts. Each segment of the lymphatic vessel between successive valves, called **lymphangions**, behaves like an automatic pump: When the segment is filled with lymph, the wall contracts, the valve opens, and lymph flows into the next segment. This process continues along the entire length of the lymph vessel until the fluid is finally emptied.

- **By extrinsic contraction**

In addition to the intrinsic contraction mechanism, external factors such as contraction of the surrounding muscles during exercise, arterial pulsations, and compression of tissues by forces outside the body compress the lymph vessel and cause pumping. When lymph drainage is impaired, excess fluid accumulates in the tissue spaces (**edema**).

Figure 12-12. **Glomerulus and portal systems**

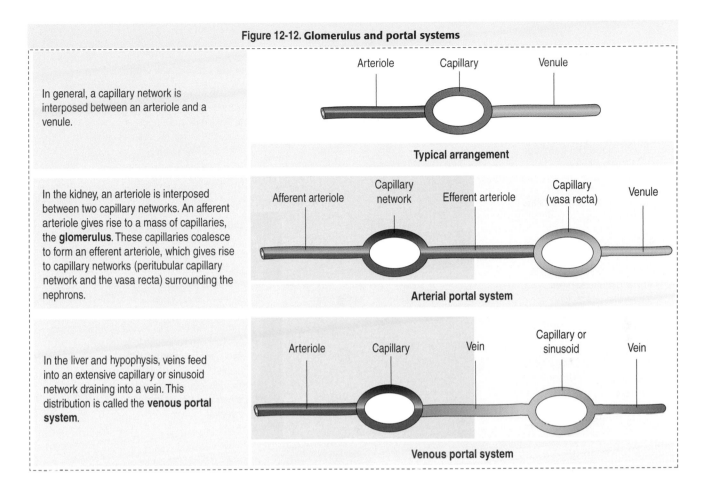

In general, a capillary network is interposed between an arteriole and a venule.

In the kidney, an arteriole is interposed between two capillary networks. An afferent arteriole gives rise to a mass of capillaries, the **glomerulus**. These capillaries coalesce to form an efferent arteriole, which gives rise to capillary networks (peritubular capillary network and the vasa recta) surrounding the nephrons.

In the liver and hypophysis, veins feed into an extensive capillary or sinusoid network draining into a vein. This distribution is called the **venous portal system**.

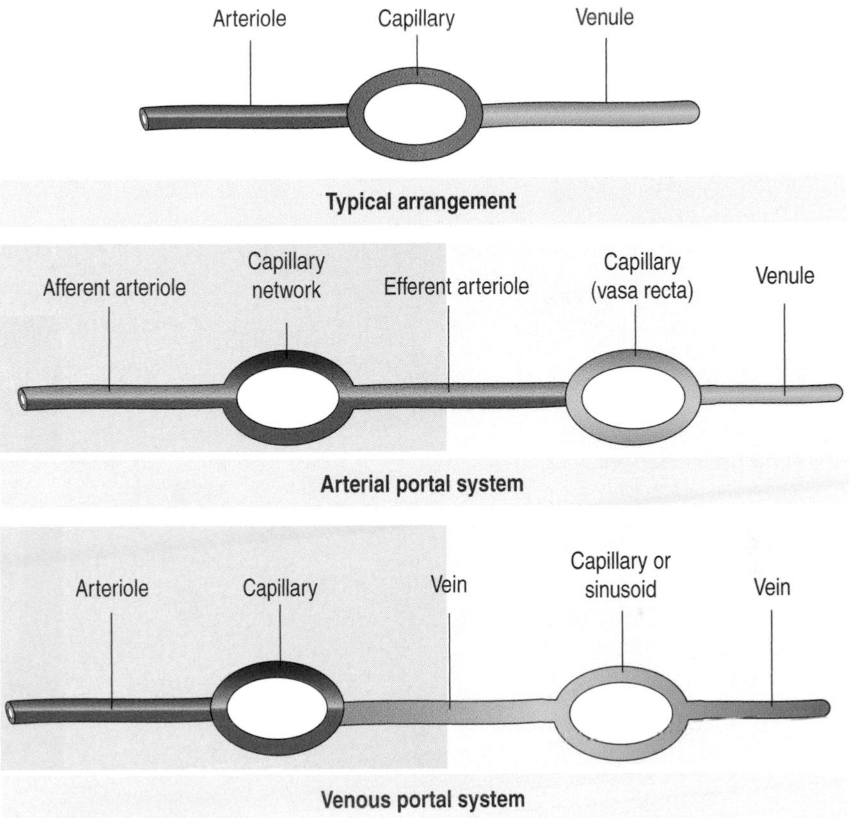

Arteriole
Capillary
Venule
Typical arrangement
Afferent arteriole
Capillary network
Efferent arteriole
Capillary (vasa recta)
Venule
Arterial portal system
Arteriole
Capillary
Vein
Capillary or sinusoid
Vein
Venous portal system

ment separated by collagenous fibers.

The **tunica adventitia** is connective tissue with fibroelastic fibers.

Like veins, lymphatic vessels have **valves**, but their number is larger. The structure of the **thoracic duct** is similar to that of a medium-sized vein, but the muscular tunica media is more prominent.

Box 12-B | **Lymphatic vascular disorders**

- **Lymphedema** is caused by a defect in the transport of lymph because of abnormal vessel development or damaged lymphatic vessels. Accumulation of fluid and proteins in the interstitial spaces leads to lymphedema. Protein-rich fluid in the interstitial space initiates an inflammatory reaction causing fibrosis, impaired immune responses, and adipose degeneration of the connective tissue.
- **Filariasis (elephantiasis)** is a parasitic infection of lymphatic vessels by *Wuchereria bancrofti* or *Brugia malayi* worms, transmitted by mosquito bites. This condition causes damage to the lymphatic vessels with chronic lymphedema of legs and genitals. Filariasis occurs in tropical countries.
- **Chylous ascites** and **chylothorax** are caused by the accumulation of high fat containing fluid, or chyle, in the abdomen or thorax as a result of trauma, obstruction, or abnormal development of lymphatic vessels.

Clinical significance: Edema

Edema occurs when the volume of interstitial fluid increases and exceeds the drainage capacity of the lymphatics, or lymphatic vessels become blocked. Subcutaneous tissue has the capacity to accumulate interstitial fluid and gives rise to clinical edema (see Box 12-B).

In patients with extensive capillary injury (burns), both intravascular fluid and plasma proteins escape into the interstitial space. Proteins accumulating in the interstitial compartment increase the oncotic pressure, leading to additional fluid loss due to the greater osmotic force outside the capillary bed.

Special capillary arrangements: Glomerulus and portal systems

In general, blood from an arteriole flows into a capillary network and is drained by a venule. There are two specialized capillary systems that depart from this standard arrangement (Figure 12-12): (1) the **glomerulus** and (2) the **portal system**.

In the kidney, an **afferent arteriole** drains into a capillary network called the **glomerulus**. The glomerular capillaries coalesce to form an **efferent arteriole**, which branches into another capillary network called the **vasa recta**. The vasa recta surround the limbs of the loop of Henle and play a significant role in the formation of urine. The glomerulus system is essential for blood filtration in the renal corpuscle (see Chapter 14, Urinary System).

Figure 12-13. Endothelium

Endothelial cells produce prostacyclin

1 Prostacyclin is formed by endothelial cells from arachidonic acid by a process catalyzed by prostacyclin synthase. Prostacyclin prevents the adhesion of platelets to the endothelium, and **avoids blood clot formation**. Prostacyclin is also a **vasodilator**.

Endothelial cells control vascular cell growth

Angiogenesis occurs during normal wound healing and vascularization of tumors. Endothelial cells secrete factors that stimulate angiogenesis.

Some of these factors induce endothelial cell proliferation and migration; others activate endothelial cell differentiation or induce a secondary cell type to produce angiogenic factors.

Endothelial cells modulate smooth muscle activity

2 Endothelial cells secrete smooth muscle cell relaxing factors (such as **nitric oxide**), and smooth muscle cell contraction factors (such as **endothelin 1**).

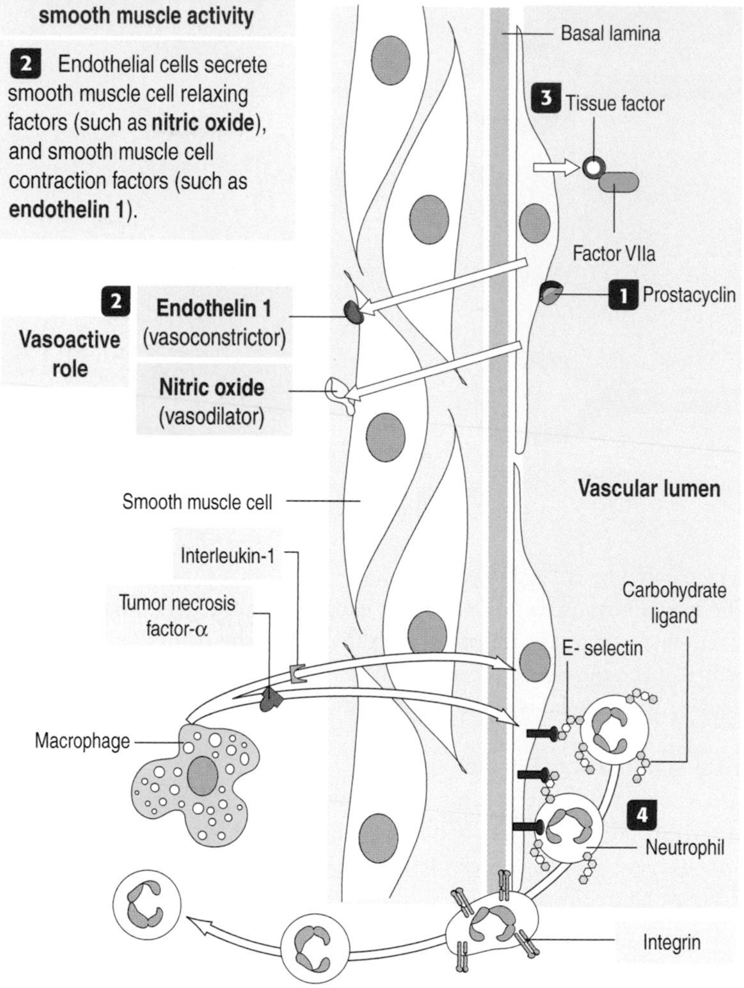

2
Vasoactive role
Endothelin 1
(vasoconstrictor)
Nitric oxide
(vasodilator)
Smooth muscle cell
Interleukin-1
Tumor necrosis factor-α
Macrophage
Basal lamina
3 Tissue factor
Factor VIIa
1 Prostacyclin
Vascular lumen
Carbohydrate ligand
E- selectin
4
Neutrophil
Integrin

Endothelial cells trigger blood coagulation

3 Endothelial cells release **tissue factor** that binds to factor VIIa to convert factor X into factor Xa and initiate the common pathway of blood clotting (see Blood Coagulation in Chapter 6, Blood and Hematopoiesis).

Thrombin (bound to its receptor on platelet surfaces) acts on fibrinogen to form fibrin monomers. **Fibrin monomers** self-aggregate to form a soft fibrin clot cross-linked by factor XIII.

Both platelets and fibrin form a hemostatic plug when there is an injury to the wall of a blood vessel.

Endothelial cells regulate the traffic of inflammatory cells

4 Endothelial cells facilitate transendothelial migration of cells involved in an inflammatory reaction (for example, **neutrophils**) in the surrounding extravascular connective tissue.

Activated macrophages secrete tumor necrosis factor-α and interleukin-1, which induce the expression of **E-selectin** by endothelial cells.

In the **portal system**, intestinal capillaries are drained by the portal vein to the liver. In the **liver**, the portal vein branches into venous sinusoids between cords of hepatocytes. Blood flows from the sinusoids into a collecting vein and then back to the heart via the inferior vena cava.

A similar portal system is observed in the hypophysis. Venules connect the primary sinusoidal plexus of the hypothalamus (median eminence) with the secondary plexus in the anterior lobe of the hypophysis, forming the **hypophysial-portal system.** This system transports releasing factors from the hypothalamus to stimulate the secretion of hormones into the bloodstream by cells of the anterior hypophysis.

Endothelial cell–mediated regulation of blood flow

The general assumption that the endothelium is just an inert simple squamous

Figure 12-14. **Formation of an atheroma**

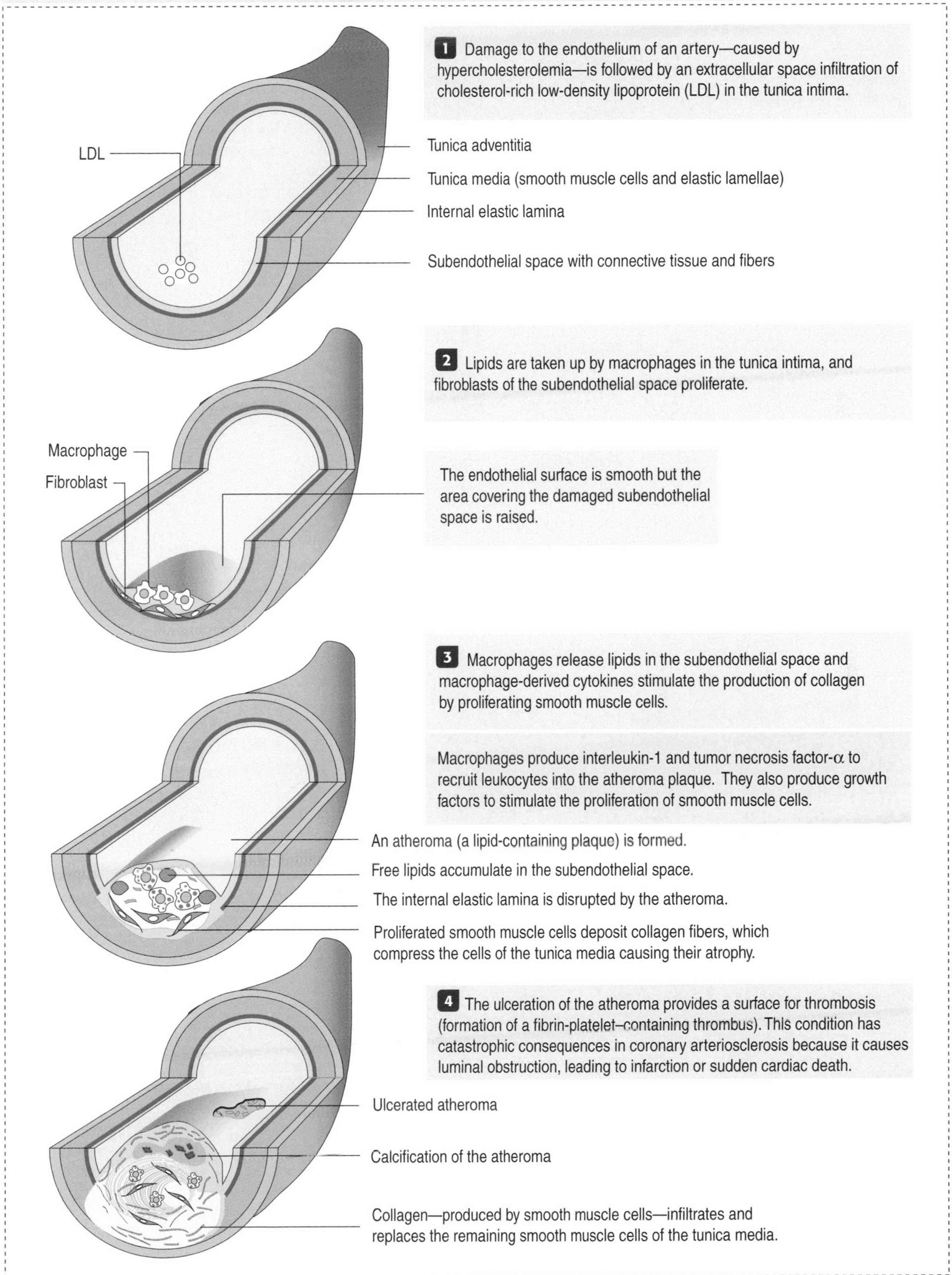
1 Damage to the endothelium of an artery—caused by hypercholesterolemia—is followed by an extracellular space infiltration of cholesterol-rich low-density lipoprotein (LDL) in the tunica intima.
LDL
Tunica adventitia
Tunica media (smooth muscle cells and elastic lamellae)
Internal elastic lamina
Subendothelial space with connective tissue and fibers
2 Lipids are taken up by macrophages in the tunica intima, and fibroblasts of the subendothelial space proliferate.
Macrophage
Fibroblast
The endothelial surface is smooth but the area covering the damaged subendothelial space is raised.
3 Macrophages release lipids in the subendothelial space and macrophage-derived cytokines stimulate the production of collagen by proliferating smooth muscle cells.
Macrophages produce interleukin-1 and tumor necrosis factor-α to recruit leukocytes into the atheroma plaque. They also produce growth factors to stimulate the proliferation of smooth muscle cells.
An atheroma (a lipid-containing plaque) is formed.
Free lipids accumulate in the subendothelial space.
The internal elastic lamina is disrupted by the atheroma.
Proliferated smooth muscle cells deposit collagen fibers, which compress the cells of the tunica media causing their atrophy.
4 The ulceration of the atheroma provides a surface for thrombosis (formation of a fibrin-platelet–containing thrombus). This condition has catastrophic consequences in coronary arteriosclerosis because it causes luminal obstruction, leading to infarction or sudden cardiac death.
Ulcerated atheroma
Calcification of the atheroma
Collagen—produced by smooth muscle cells—infiltrates and replaces the remaining smooth muscle cells of the tunica media.

Figure 12-15. Angiogenesis

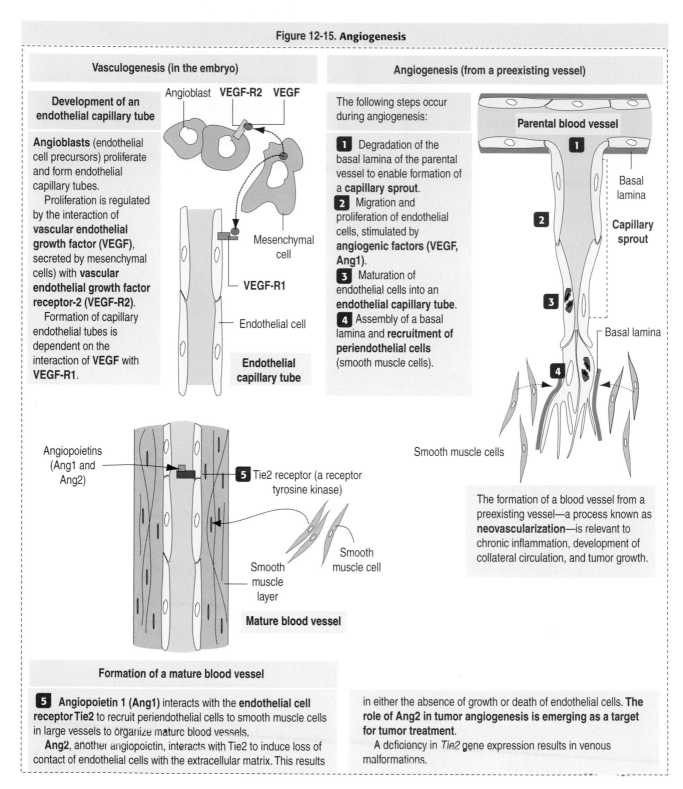

Vasculogenesis (in the embryo)

Development of an endothelial capillary tube

Angioblasts (endothelial cell precursors) proliferate and form endothelial capillary tubes.

Proliferation is regulated by the interaction of **vascular endothelial growth factor (VEGF)**, secreted by mesenchymal cells) with **vascular endothelial growth factor receptor-2 (VEGF-R2)**.

Formation of capillary endothelial tubes is dependent on the interaction of **VEGF** with **VEGF-R1**.

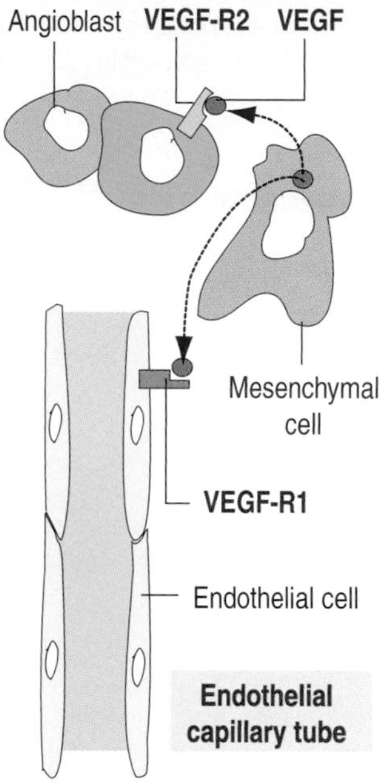

Angioblast
VEGF-R2
VEGF
Mesenchymal cell
VEGF-R1
Endothelial cell
Endothelial capillary tube

Angiogenesis (from a preexisting vessel)

The following steps occur during angiogenesis:

1 Degradation of the basal lamina of the parental vessel to enable formation of a **capillary sprout**.

2 Migration and proliferation of endothelial cells, stimulated by **angiogenic factors (VEGF, Ang1)**.

3 Maturation of endothelial cells into an **endothelial capillary tube**.

4 Assembly of a basal lamina and **recruitment of periendothelial cells** (smooth muscle cells).

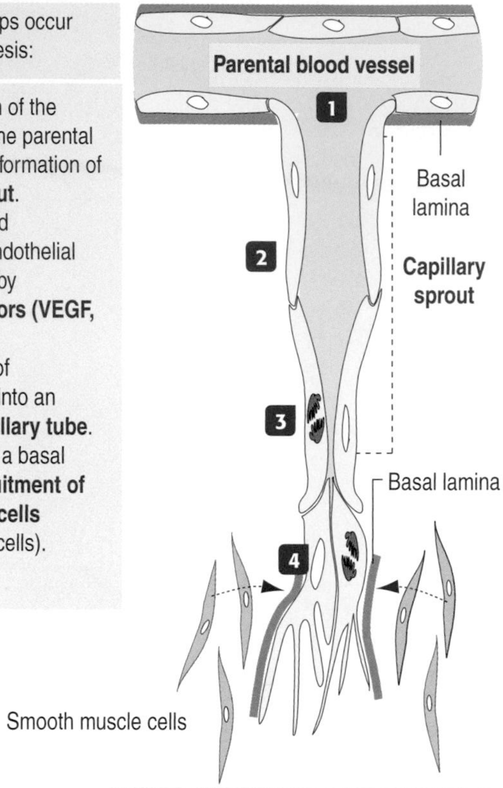

Parental blood vessel
1
Basal lamina
2
Capillary sprout
3
Basal lamina
4
Smooth muscle cells

The formation of a blood vessel from a preexisting vessel—a process known as **neovascularization**—is relevant to chronic inflammation, development of collateral circulation, and tumor growth.

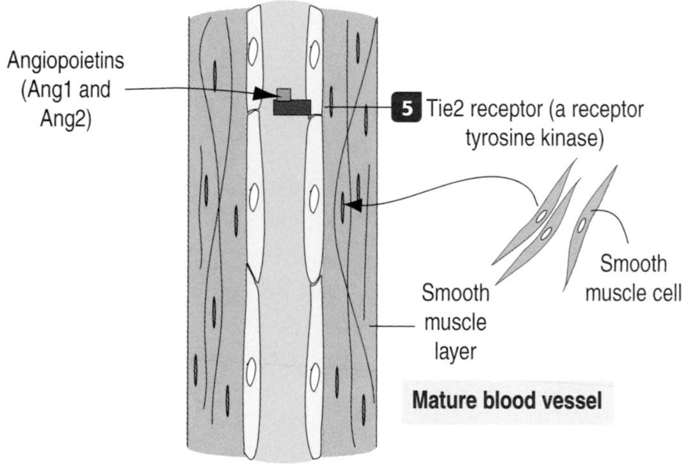

Angiopoietins (Ang1 and Ang2)
5 Tie2 receptor (a receptor tyrosine kinase)
Smooth muscle cell
Smooth muscle layer
Mature blood vessel

Formation of a mature blood vessel

5 **Angiopoietin 1 (Ang1)** interacts with the **endothelial cell receptor Tie2** to recruit periendothelial cells to smooth muscle cells in large vessels to organize mature blood vessels.

Ang2, another angiopoietin, interacts with Tie2 to induce loss of contact of endothelial cells with the extracellular matrix. This results in either the absence of growth or death of endothelial cells. **The role of Ang2 in tumor angiogenesis is emerging as a target for tumor treatment**.

A deficiency in *Tie2* gene expression results in venous malformations.

epithelium lining blood vessels is no longer correct. In addition to enabling the passage of molecules and gases and retaining blood cells and large molecules, endothelial cells produce **vasoactive substances** that can induce contraction and relaxation of the smooth muscle vascular wall (Figure 12-13).

Nitric oxide, synthesized by endothelial cells from L-arginine upon stimulation by acetylcholine or other agents, activates guanylate cyclase and consequently cyclic guanosine monophosphate (cGMP) production, which induces **relaxation** of the smooth muscle cells of the vascular wall. **Endothelin 1** is a very potent **vasoconstrictor** peptide produced by endothelial cells.

Figure 12-16. Tumor angiogenesis

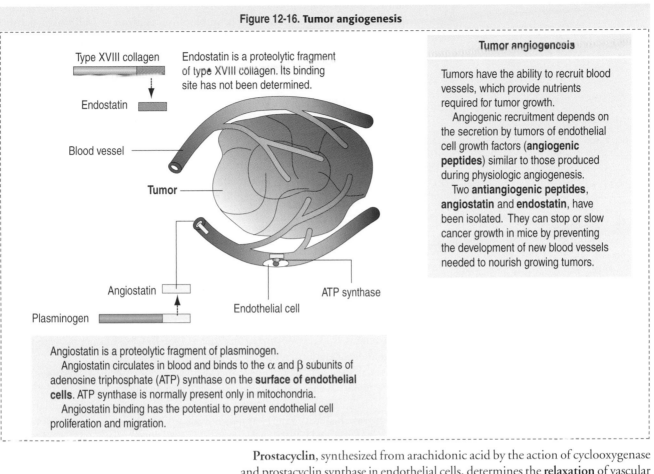

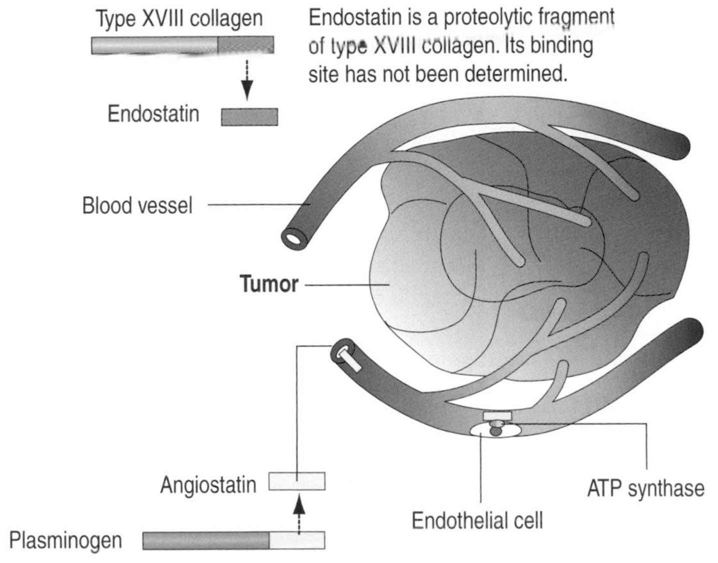
Type XVIII collagen
Endostatin is a proteolytic fragment of type XVIII collagen. Its binding site has not been determined.
Endostatin
Blood vessel
Tumor
Angiostatin
Plasminogen
Endothelial cell
ATP synthase

Tumor angiogenesis

Tumors have the ability to recruit blood vessels, which provide nutrients required for tumor growth.

Angiogenic recruitment depends on the secretion by tumors of endothelial cell growth factors (**angiogenic peptides**) similar to those produced during physiologic angiogenesis.

Two **antiangiogenic peptides**, **angiostatin** and **endostatin**, have been isolated. They can stop or slow cancer growth in mice by preventing the development of new blood vessels needed to nourish growing tumors.

Angiostatin is a proteolytic fragment of plasminogen.

Angiostatin circulates in blood and binds to the α and β subunits of adenosine triphosphate (ATP) synthase on the **surface of endothelial cells.** ATP synthase is normally present only in mitochondria.

Angiostatin binding has the potential to prevent endothelial cell proliferation and migration.

Prostacyclin, synthesized from arachidonic acid by the action of cyclooxygenase and prostacyclin synthase in endothelial cells, determines the **relaxation** of vascular smooth muscle cells by the action of cyclic adenosine monophosphate (cAMP). Synthetic prostacyclin is used to produce vasodilation in severe **Raynaud's phenomenon** (pain and discoloration of fingers and toes produced by vasospasm), **ischemia**, and in the treatment of **pulmonary hypertension**. Prostacyclin also **prevents platelet adhesion and clumping leading to blood clotting.**

The endothelium has a **passive role** in the transcapillary exchange of solvents and solutes by **diffusion**, **filtration**, and **pinocytosis**. The permeability of capillary endothelial cells is tissue-specific. Liver sinusoids are more permeable to albumin than are the capillaries of the renal glomerulus. In addition there is a topographic permeability. The endothelial cells at the venous end are more permeable than those at the arterial end. Postcapillary venules have the greatest permeability to leukocytes.

Clinical significance: Arterial diseases

Arteriosclerosis designates the thickening and loss of elasticity of the arterial walls. **Arteriolosclerosis** is the thickening of the walls of **small arteries** and **arterioles**, mainly of the kidneys and brain, and is usually associated with hypertension or diabetes.

The thickening and hardening of the walls of arteries caused by an **atheroma** (Greek *athere*, gruel; *oma*, tumor)—a plaque of lipids, cells, and connective tissue in the **tunica intima**— is known as **atherosclerosis** (Figure 12-14). Atherosclerosis is frequently seen in arteries sustaining high blood pressure. Atherosclerosis does not affect veins.

Atherosclerosis correlates with the serum levels of cholesterol or **low-density lipoprotein** (LDL). A genetic defect in lipoprotein metabolism (**familial hypercholesterolemia**) is associated with atherosclerosis and myocardial infarction before patients reach 20 years of age. We discuss in Chapter 2, Epithelial Glands, that familial hypercholesterolemia is caused by defects in the LDL receptor, resulting in increasing LDL circulating levels in blood. In contrast to LDL, **high-density lipoprotein (HDL)** transports cholesterol to the liver for excretion in the bile (see in the gallbladder section of Chapter 17, Digestive Glands).

Atheromas protrude into the lumen, weakening the underlying tunica media, and undergo a series of complications that predispose to **thrombosis**. The major blood vessels involved are the **abdominal aorta** and the **coronary** and **cerebral arteries. Coronary arteriosclerosis** causes **ischemic heart disease** and, when the arterial lesions are complicated by thrombosis, **myocardial infarction** occurs. Atherothrombosis of the cerebral vessels is the major cause of **brain infarct**, so-called **stroke**, one of the most common causes of neurologic disease. Arteriosclerosis of the abdominal aorta leads to **abdominal aortic aneurysm**, a dilation that sometimes ruptures to produce massive fatal hemorrhage.

Vasculogenesis and angiogenesis

After birth, angiogenesis contributes to organ growth. In the adult, most blood vessels remain stable and angiogenesis occurs in the endometrium and ovary during the menstrual cycle, and in the placenta during pregnancy. Endothelial cells retain a proliferating potential in response to physiologic stimulation (blood vessels) and inflammation (lymphatic vessels), and during wound healing and repair (see Chapter 11, Integumentary System). Under pathologic conditions, angiogenesis is excessive during malignant (see Box 12-C), ocular (age-related macular degeneration), and inflammatory conditions.

Arterial angiogenesis during embryogenesis is controlled by members of the Notch family. Venous angiogenesis is regulated by the orphan receptor COUP-TFII. The homeobox gene *Prox-1* specifies lymphangiogenesis. **Vascular endothelial growth factor** (**VEGF**) and its homolog **VEGF-C** are regulators of vascular and lymphatic endothelial cell sprouting, respectively. **Platelet-derived growth factor** (**PDGF**) and **angiopoietin 1** recruit cells to construct the walls around endothelial channels.

An understanding of vasculogenesis and angiogenesis is relevant to develop therapeutic strategies to produce revascularization of ischemic tissues or inhibit angiogenesis in cancer, ocular, joint, or skin disorders.

The vascular system is formed by two processes (Figure 12-15):

1. **Vasculogenesis**, a process initiated by the coalescence of free and migratory **vascular endothelial progenitors**, or **angioblasts**, during **embryogenesis** to form a **primitive vascular network in the yolk sac and trunk axial vessels.** Vasculogenesis is essential for embryonic survival. Embryonic arterial and venous endothelial cells are molecularly distinct: **ephrin-B2** and its receptor are expressed in arterial vessels; **ephrin-B4** is expressed in venous vessels.

2. **Angiogenesis**, a process initiated in a **preexisting vessel** and observed in the embryo and adult. Angiogenesis in the adult occurs during the uterine menstrual cycle, placental growth, wound healing, and inflammatory responses. As we will discuss below, tumor angiogenesis is a specific form of angiogenesis with important clinical implications.

Endothelial cells are involved in vasculogenesis and angiogenesis. Endothelial cells migrate, proliferate, and assemble into tubes to contain the blood. Periendothelial cells (smooth muscle cells, pericytes, and fibroblasts) are recruited to surround the newly formed endothelial tubes.

The following molecules are central to vascular morphogenesis: (1) **Tie2**, a receptor tyrosine kinase that modulates a signaling cascade required for the induction or inhibition of endothelial cell proliferation; (2) **VEGFs**, with binding affinity to two different receptors, **VEGF-R1** and **VEGF-R2**, present on endothelial cells; and (3) **angiopoietins 1** and **2** (**Ang1** and **Ang2**), with binding affinity to **Tie2**.

Ang1 mediates vascular maturation. In the absence of VEGF, Ang2 blocks Ang1 effects, resulting in either endothelial cell remodeling or apoptosis. Ang2 is selectively expressed in the ovary, uterus, and placenta, three tissues in which

Box 12-C | Kaposi sarcoma

- **Kaposi sarcoma** is a tumor characterized by vascular nodules in the skin, mucosa, and internal organs, frequently found in AIDS patients.
- The vascular nodules consist of spindle-shaped tumor cells and highly developed vascular spaces. The spindle cells express blood and lymphatic endothelial cell markers, suggesting the endothelial origin of these cells. Transcriptional products of Kaposi sarcoma tumor cells are closely related to normal lymphatic endothelial cells.
- Kaposi sarcoma is associated with infections by the human herpesvirus-8.

angiogenesis is relevant to female reproductive physiology.

Clinical significance: Tumor angiogenesis

In Chapter 4, Connective Tissue, we discuss the molecular biology of tumor invasion. We briefly mention that tumors secrete **angiogenic factors** that increase the vascularization and nutrition of an invading tumor. These angiogenic factors are similar to those produced during normal wound healing. In addition, we indicated that newly formed blood vessels facilitate the dissemination of tumor cells to distant tissues (**metastasis**).

Certain tumors can release **antiangiogenic peptides** that prevent their distant metastases from recruiting blood vessels. Two antiangiogenic peptides have been isolated (Figure 12-16): (1) **angiostatin**, a breakdown product of **plasminogen**; and (2) **endostatin**, a breakdown peptide of **type XVIII collagen**. When administered to mice, these peptides can slow down or stop the growth of established tumors.

Angiostatin binds to the enzyme a**denosine triphosphate** (ATP) **synthase** present on the surface of endothelial cells. This enzyme is not found on the surface of other cells. ATP synthase synthesizes ATP. When angiostatin binds to ATP synthase, its enzymatic activity is blocked and the growth of blood vessels is prevented.

Essential concepts | **Cardiovascular System**

• Heart. The wall of the heart consists of three layers: (1) Endocardium, formed by an endothelial lining and subendothelial connective tissues. (2) Myocardium, formed by three types of cardiac muscle: atrial muscle, ventricular muscle, and conducting muscle fibers of Purkinje. (3) Epicardium, lined by a mesothelium facing the serosal pericardial space. Cardiocytes of the atrium secrete atrial natriuretic factor, a protein that stimulates diuresis and natriuresis.

The conductive systems of the heart are the sinus node (or sinoatrial [S-A] node); the internodal pathway, linking the sinus node to the atrioventricular (A-V) node; the atrioventricular bundle, linking the atria to the ventricles; and the left and right bundles of Purkinje fibers.

Cardiocytes are striated cells with a central nucleus and are linked to each other by intercalated disks. The transverse components of the intercalated disk are fasciae adherentes and desmosomes; gap junctions are present in the longitudinal component. The cytoplasm contains myofibrils. Purkinje cells lie beneath the endocardium along the two sides of the interventricular septum. Compared to cardiocytes, the number of myofibrils in Purkinje fibers is reduced, the diameter of the fibers is larger, and the cytoplasm contains abundant glycogen.

• Circulation is divided into the systemic or peripheral circulation, and the pulmonary circulation.

Arteries conduct blood from the heart to the capillaries. The wall of arteries consists of three layers: (1) Tunica intima (endothelium, subendothelial connective tissue, and the internal elastic lamina). (2) Tunica media (smooth muscle cells surrounded by collagen fibers, and elastic sheaths). (3) Tunica externa or adventitia (connective tissue, vessels, and nerves).

There are three major groups of arteries: (1) large elastic arteries; (2) medium-sized arteries; and (3) small arteries and arterioles.

Large elastic arteries are conducting vessels. The aorta is an example. Fenestrated elastic sheaths and elastic-producing smooth muscle cells are present in the tunica media. **Aortic aneurysms** are produced by atherosclerosis or defective synthesis and assembly of elastic fibers (**Marfan syndrome, dissecting aneurysm**).

Medium-sized arteries are distributing vessels. The tunica media shows a reduction in elastic fibers and an increase in smooth muscle fibers. An external elastic lamina is seen at the tunica media–adventitia junction.

Arterioles are resistance vessels. Arterioles regulate blood distribution to the microcirculation by vasoconstriction and vasodilation. Arterioles are the major determinants of systemic blood pressure. The tunica media consists of two to five layers of smooth muscle.

Capillaries are exchange vessels. The microvascular bed, the site of microcirculation, consists of the terminal arteriole, metarteriole, the capillary bed, and the postcapillary venules. The capillary bed consists of slightly larger capillaries (called preferential or thoroughfare channels) characterized by continuous blood flow, and small capillaries (called true capillaries), where blood flow is intermittent. Precapillary sphincters (smooth muscle cells) are located at the origin site of true capillaries from the arteriole or metarteriole. Capillary circulation can be bypassed by through channels connecting terminal arterioles to postcapillary venules. Arteriovenous shunts, or anastomoses, connect arterioles to postcapillary venules, bypassing the microvascular bed.

There are three types of capillaries: continuous, fenestrated, and discontinuous (sinusoids). Continuous capillaries are lined by a complete simple squamous endothelium and basal lamina. Pericytes, smooth muscle cell–like, can be present between the endothelium and the basal lamina. Endothelial cells have two characteristics: they are linked by tight junctions, and the transport of solutes and fluids occurs by caveolae and pinocytotic vesicles.

Fenestrated capillaries have pores, or fenestrae, with or without diaphragms.

Discontinuous capillaries have an incomplete endothelial cell lining and basal lamina. Gaps are seen between and within endothelial cells.

Veins are capacitance or reservoir vessels. The venous system starts with a postcapillary venule (the site of migration of blood cells into tissues by diapedesis), consisting of an endothelial tube surrounded by a basal lamina, and a loose connective tissue adventitia. In lymphatic tissues, endothelial cells of postcapillary venules are taller (high endothelial venules). Postcapillary venules converge to form muscular venules, which give rise to collecting venules, leading to veins of increasing diameter.

Veins have the following characteristics: (1) Distinction of a tunica media from a tunica adventitia is often not discernible. (2) A distinct internal elastic lamina is not visualized. (3) Veins have valves, projections into the lumen of the tunica intima, to prevent blood reflux.

Lymphatic vessels conduct immune cells and lymph to lymph nodes, remove excess fluid accumulated in interstitial spaces, and transport chylomicrons collected by lacteal lymphatic vessels. Lymph flow is under low pressure and unidirectional.

Lymphatic capillaries begin as dilated, blind endothelial cell–lined tubes lacking a basal lamina and maintained open by bundles of anchoring filaments. Lymphatic vessels are not found in cartilage, bone, epithelia, central nervous system, and placenta.

Lymphatic capillaries converge into precollecting lymphatic vessels draining lymph into collecting lymphatic vessels surrounded by smooth muscle cells, providing intrinsic pumping activity. Lymphangions are bulblike segments separated by luminal valves. Terminal lymphatic vessels are seen in the proximity of a lymph node. Lymph returns to the bloodstream through the large thoracic duct, and the smaller right lymphatic duct.

Lymphedema is caused by a defect in the transport of lymph determined by abnormal development or a damaged lymphatic vessel. **Filariasis** (elephantiasis) is caused by a parasitic infection of lymphatic vessels. Chronic lymphedema of the legs and genitals is characteristic. **Chylous ascites** and **chylothorax** is the accumulation of lymph with high fat content (chyle) in the abdomen and thorax, caused by trauma, obstruction, or abnormal development of lymphatic vessels.

• Special capillary arrangements. (1) Arterial portal system: afferent arteriole followed by a capillary network draining into an efferent arteriole (instead of a venule). (2) Venous portal system: capillary drained by a vein, which gives rise to venous capillaries or sinusoids and continues with a vein.

• Endothelial cell functions. (1) Production of prostacyclin (from arachidonic acid) to avoid adhesion of platelets to the endothelium and intravascular blood clot formation, and to determine the relaxation of the smooth muscle cell wall. (2) Production of angiogenic factors during normal wound healing and vascularization of tumors. (3) Initiation of blood coagulation by releasing tissue factor to activate factor VIIa to convert factor X into factor Xa. (4) Regulation of smooth muscle activity (nitric oxide produces vasodilation; endothelin 1 triggers vasoconstriction). (5) Regulation of inflammatory cell trafficking. Macrophages in the connective tissue produce tumor necrosis factor-α (TNF-α) and interleukin-1 to accelerate homing of inflammatory cells to block the action of pathogens.

• **Arterial diseases**. **Arteriosclerosis** is the thickening and loss of elasticity of the arterial walls. **Arteriolosclerosis** is the thickening of the wall of small arteries and arterioles.

Atherosclerosis is the thickening of the arterial walls caused by atheromas, plaques of lipids, cells, and connective tissue in the tunica intima. **Familial hypercholesterolemia** is a genetic defect in the lipoprotein metabolism caused by a defect in the receptor that internalizes low-density lipoprotein. Atheromas weaken the tunica media and predispose to thrombosis. The abdominal aorta, and the coronary and cerebral arteries are the major blood vessels involved. Abdominal aortic aneurysm, myocardial infarction, and brain infarct (stroke) are complications.

• **Vasculogenesis and angiogenesis**. Vasculogenesis is the process initiated by vascular endothelial progenitors (called angioblasts) during embryogenesis.

Angiogenesis is a process of vessel formation initiated from a preexisting vessel, and it is observed in the embryo and adult.

Endothelial cells are involved in vasculogenesis and angiogenesis.

During vasculogenesis, angioblasts proliferate and assemble into tubes containing blood. Periendothelial cells (smooth muscle cells, pericytes, and fibroblasts) are recruited to complete the formation of the vessel. Endothelial proliferation is regulated by vascular endothelial growth factor (VEGF), secreted by mesenchymal cells, bound to its receptor VEGF-R1. Angiopoietin interacts with the endothelial cell receptor Tie2 to recruit periendothelial cells (smooth muscle cells).

During angiogenesis, a capillary sprout is formed from a preexisting vessel. Endothelial cells, stimulated by VEGF and angiopoietin, form an endothelial tube. The recruitment of periendothelial cells follows.

• **Tumor angiogenesis**. Certain tumors produce angiogenic factors that increase the vascularization and nutrition of an invading tumor. Antiangiogenic peptides angiostatin and endostatin slow down or stop the growth of established tumors by blocking tumor angiogenesis.

13. RESPIRATORY SYSTEM

General outline of the respiratory system

The respiratory system consists of three main portions with distinct functions:

1. An **air-conducting portion.**
2. A **respiratory portion** for gas exchange between blood and air.
3. A **mechanism for ventilation**, driven by the inspiratory and expiratory movements of the thoracic cage.

The **air-conducting portion** consists, sequentially, of the **nasal cavities** and **associated sinuses**, the **nasopharynx**, the **oropharynx**, the **larynx**, the **trachea**, the **bronchi**, and the **bronchioles.** The oropharynx also participates in food transport. The **conducting portion** provides a passage for inhaled and exhaled air in and out of the respiratory portion.

The **respiratory portion** is composed, in sequence, of the **respiratory bronchioles, alveolar ducts, alveolar sacs**, and **alveoli.** The main function is the exchange of gases between air and blood.

Terminal bronchioles and the lung territory they supply constitute a **pulmonary lobule**, composed of several **pulmonary acini.**

A **pulmonary acinus** is formed when **terminal bronchioles** branch to become **respiratory bronchioles.** A respiratory acinus is a triangular-shaped structure with the apex occupied by respiratory bronchioles and the base by its divisions: the alveolar ducts, alveolar sacs, and alveoli.

Respiration involves the participation of a **ventilation mechanism.** The inflow (inspiration) and outflow (expiration) of air occur with the aid of four elements:

1. The **thoracic** or **rib cage.**
2. Associated **intercostal muscles.**
3. The **diaphragm muscle.**
4. The **elastic connective tissue of the lung.**

Nasal cavities and paranasal sinuses

The nasal cavities and paranasal sinuses provide an extensive surface area for (1) warming and moistening air and (2) filtering dust particles present in the inspired air. In addition, the roof of each nasal cavity and part of the superior concha

Figure 13-1. **Nasal cavities**

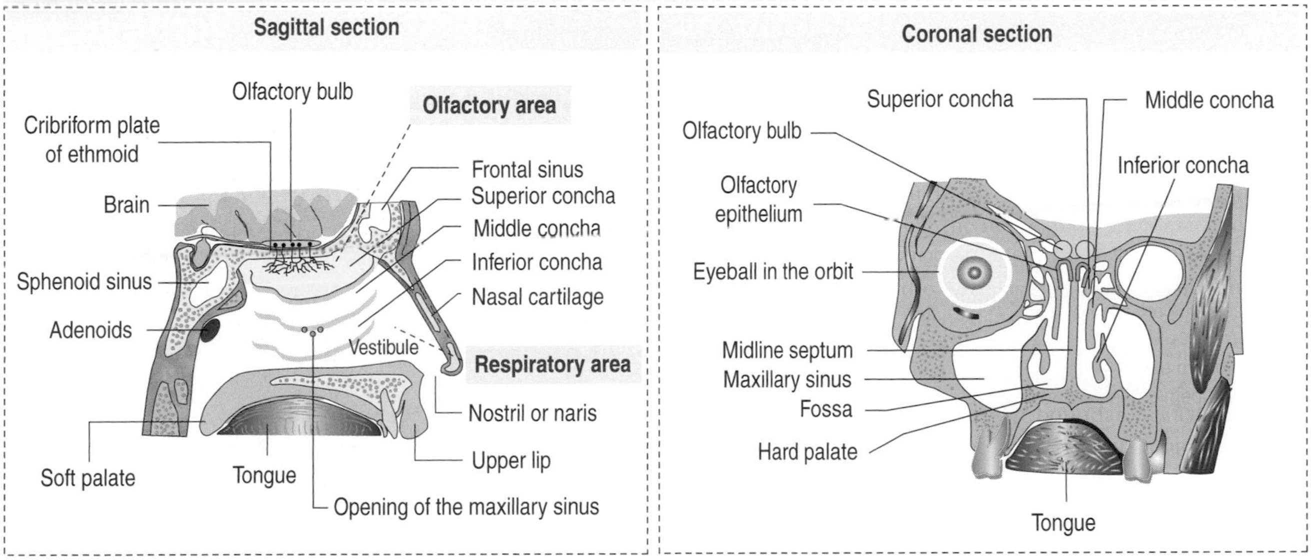

Figure 13-2. **Olfactory mucosa**

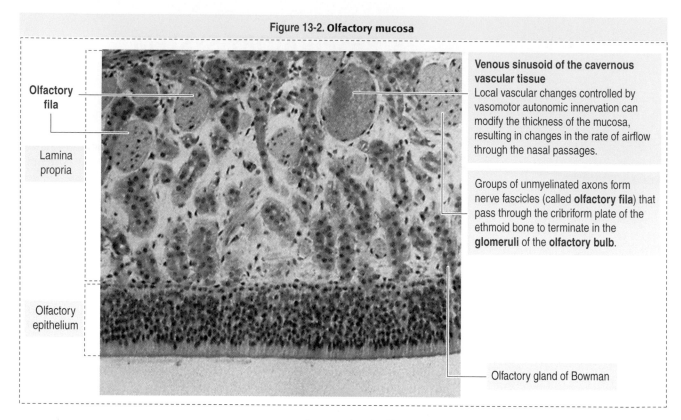

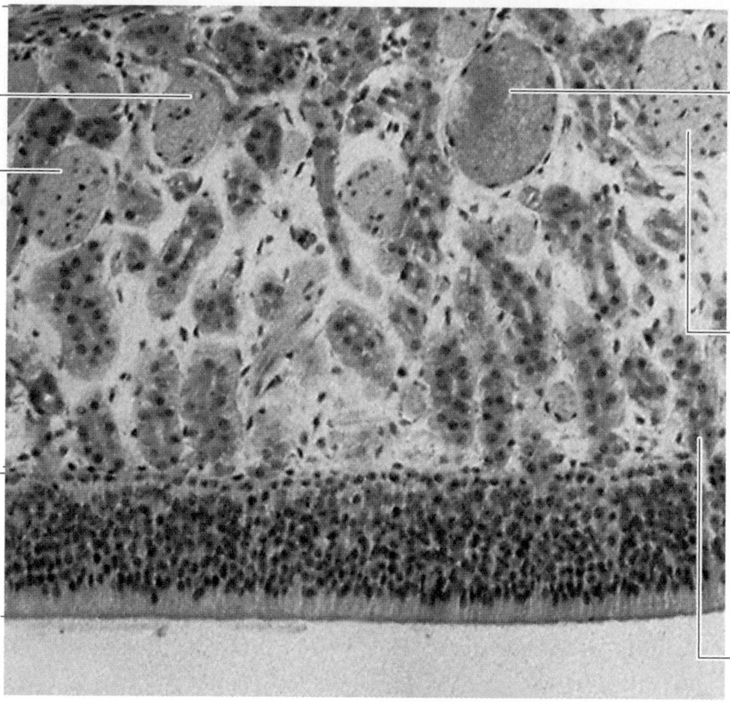
Olfactory fila
Lamina propria
Olfactory epithelium
Venous sinusoid of the cavernous vascular tissue
Local vascular changes controlled by vasomotor autonomic innervation can modify the thickness of the mucosa, resulting in changes in the rate of airflow through the nasal passages.
Groups of unmyelinated axons form nerve fascicles (called olfactory fila) that pass through the cribriform plate of the ethmoid bone to terminate in the glomeruli of the olfactory bulb.
Olfactory gland of Bowman

contain the specialized **olfactory mucosa**.

Each nasal cavity, separated from the other by the **septum**, consists of the **vestibule**, the **respiratory portion**, and the **olfactory area** (Figure 13-1).

Air enters through the **nostril**, or **naris**, whose external surface is lined by **keratinized squamous epithelium**. At the **vestibule**, the epithelium becomes **nonkeratinized**.

The **respiratory portion** is lined by a **pseudostratified ciliated epithelium with goblet cells** supported by the lamina propria, which consists of connective tissue with **seromucous glands**. The lamina propria has a **rich superficial venous plexus**, known as **cavernous** or **erectile tissue**. The lamina propria is continuous with the periosteum or perichondrium of bone or cartilage, respectively, forming the wall of the nasal cavities.

Projecting into each nasal cavity from the lateral wall are three curved plates of bone covered by a mucosa: the **superior**, **middle**, and **inferior turbinate bones**, or **conchae** (Latin *concha*, shell).

Secretions from goblet cells and seromucous glands maintain the mucosal surface moist and humidify the inspired air. Incoming air is warmed by blood in the venous plexus, which flows in a direction opposite to that of the inspired air (**countercurrent flow**). The highly vascular nature of the nasal mucosa, in particular of the anterior septum, accounts for common bleeding (**epistaxis**) after trauma or acute inflammation (**rhinitis**).

Conchae cause airflow turbulence, thus facilitating contact between the air and the mucus blanket covering the respiratory region of each nasal cavity. The mucus blanket traps particulates in the air that are transported posteriorly by ciliary action to the nasopharynx, where they are swallowed with the saliva.

Paranasal sinuses are air-containing cavities within the bones of the skull. They are the **maxillary**, **frontal**, **ethmoidal**, and **sphenoid sinuses**. The sinuses are lined by a thin **pseudostratified columnar ciliated epithelium**, with fewer goblet cells and glands in the lamina propria. No erectile tissue is present in the paranasal sinuses. Sinuses communicate with the nasal cavity by openings lined by an epithelium similar to that of the main nasal cavity. The ethmoidal sinuses open beneath the superior conchae and the maxillary sinus opens under the middle concha.

Nasopharynx

The posterior portion of the nasal cavities is the nasopharynx, which at the level of the soft palate becomes the oropharynx.

The **auditory tubes** (**eustachian tubes**), extending from the middle ear, open into the lateral walls of the oropharynx.

The **nasopharynx** is lined by a **pseudostratified columnar epithelium** like the nasal cavities, and changes into **nonkeratinizing squamous epithelium** at the oropharynx. Abundant **mucosa-associated lymphoid tissue** is present beneath the nasopharyngeal epithelium, forming **Waldeyer's ring**. The **nasopharyngeal tonsils** (**adenoids**) are present at the posterior and upper regions of the nasopharynx.

Olfactory epithelium

The olfactory epithelium contains three major types of cells (Figures 13-2 and 13-3): (1) **basal cells**, (2) **olfactory cells** (bipolar neurons), and (3) **supporting or sustentacular cells**.

The **basal cells** are mitotically active stem cells, producing daughter cells that differentiate first into **immature olfactory cells** and then into **mature olfactory cells**. Olfactory cells proliferate during adult life. The life span of an olfactory cell is about 30 to 60 days.

The **olfactory cell** is highly polarized (see Figure 13-3). The **apical region**, facing the surface of the mucosa, forms a **knoblike ending** (called **olfactory vesicle** or **olfactory knob**) with 10 to 20 modified cilia. The **basal region** gives rise to an **axon**. Several axons, projecting from the olfactory cells, form small unmyelinated bundles (called **olfactory fila**; from Latin *filum*, thread) surounded by glial-like cells. Nerve bundles cross the **cribriform plate of the ethmoid bone** and contact in the **glomerulus** dendrites of **mitral cells**, neurons of the **olfactory bulb**, to establish appropriate synaptic connections (see Box 13-A).

Olfactory serous glands (called **glands of Bowman**), which are present under the epithelium, secrete a serous fluid in which odoriferous substances are dissolved. The secretory fluid contains the odorant-binding protein (**OBP**) with high binding affinity for a large number of **odorant molecules**. OBP carries odorants to receptors present on the surface of the modified cilia and removes them after they have been sensed. In addition, the secretory product of the glands of Bowman contains protective substances such as **lysozyme** and immunoglobulin A (**IgA**) secreted by plasma cells.

Box 13-A | Olfactory epithelium

- The olfactory epithelium consists of olfactory cells (bipolar neurons), basal cells (a stem cell that differentiates into olfactory cells), and sustentacular or supporting cells. These cells can be identified on the basis of the position and shape of their nuclei (see Figure 13-3).
- An olfactory cell has two portions: an apical dendrite with a knob bearing about 10 to 20 olfactory nonmotile modified cilia and a basal axon, forming bundles that will pass through the cribriform plate of the ethmoid bone.
- Cilia contain the odorant receptor (OR). There are about 1000 genes expressing ORs but each olfactory receptor cell expresses only one OR gene.
- Secretions of the serous glands of Bowman contain odorant-binding protein.
- Axons from olfactory cells with the same OR terminate in one to three glomeruli present in the olfactory bulb. Dendritic endings of predominantly mitral cells extend into the glomeruli. Axons of mitral cells form the olfactory tract, the initiation of cranial nerve I.
- Olfactory receptor cells have a lifespan of 30 to 60 days and can regenerate from basal cells.
- Temporary or permanent damage to the olfactory epithelium causes anosmia (Greek *an*, not; *osme*, sense of smell).

Larynx

The two main functions of the larynx are (1) to produce sound and (2) to close the trachea during swallowing to prevent food and saliva from entering the airway.

The **wall of the larynx** is made up of the **thyroid** and **cricoid hyaline cartilage** and the **elastic cartilage core of the epiglottis** extending over the lumen (Figure 13-4).

Extrinsic laryngeal muscles attach the larynx to the **hyoid bone** to raise the larynx during swallowing.

Intrinsic laryngeal muscles (**abductor**, **adductors**, and **tensors**), innervated by the recurrent laryngeal nerve, link the thyroid and cricoid cartilages. When intrinsic muscles contract, the tension on the vocal cords changes to modulate phonation. The middle and lower laryngeal arteries (derived from the superior and inferior thyroid artery) supply the larynx. Lymphatic plexuses drain to the upper cervical lymph nodes and to the nodes along the trachea.

The larynx can be subdivided into three regions:

1. The **supraglottis**, which includes the epiglottis, false vocal cords (or folds), and laryngeal ventricles.

Figure 13-3. Olfactory epithelium

1 **Olfactory nerve filaments** are bundled in groups of 10 to 100 and penetrate the cribriform plate of the ethmoid bone reaching the **olfactory bulb**. In the olfactory bulb, the axon terminals connect with synaptic terminals of **mitral cells** forming synaptic structures called **glomeruli**.

2 The olfactory signal is sent by **mitral cells—**through the **olfactory nerve tract**—to the **corticomedial amygdala portion of the brain.**

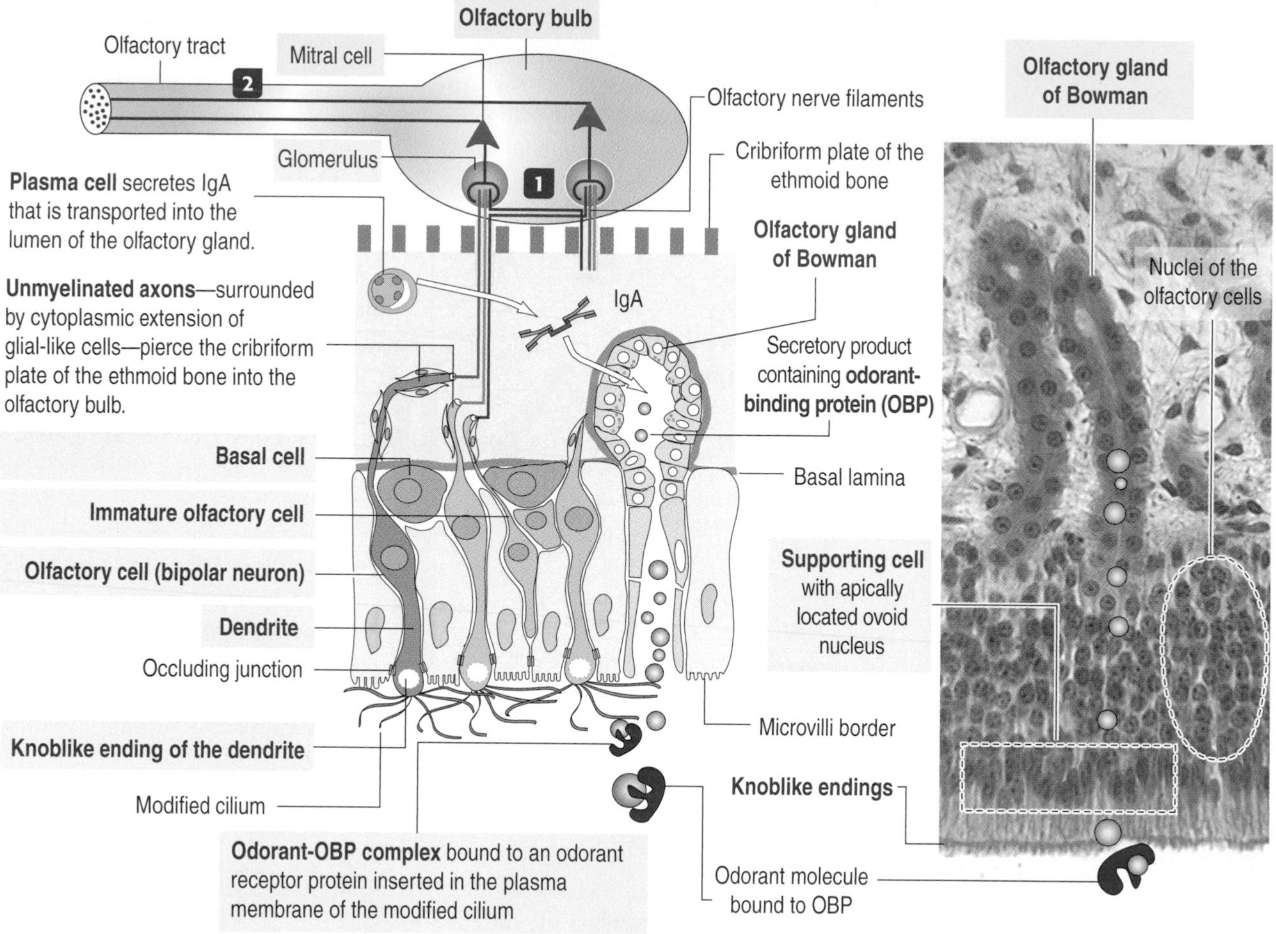

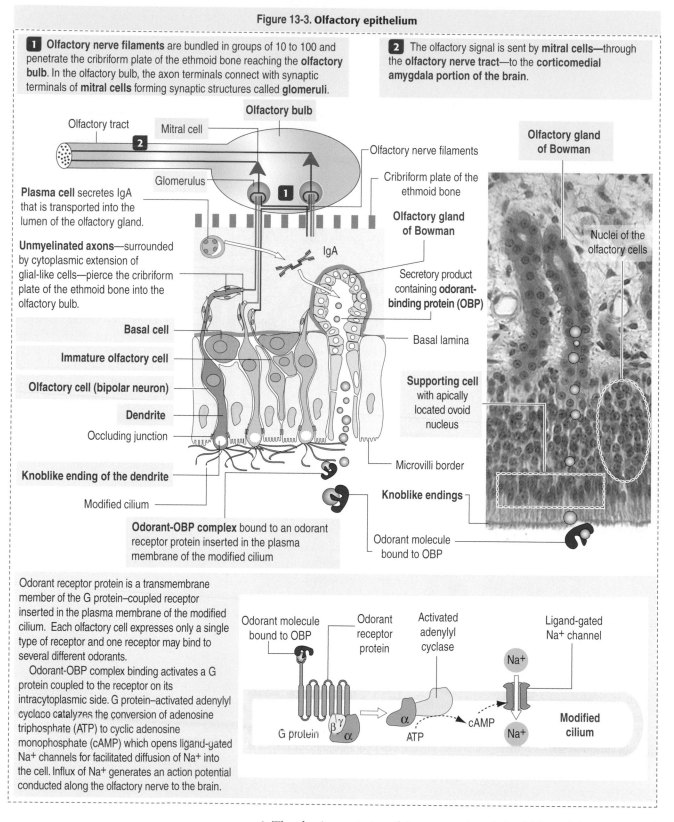

Olfactory bulb
Olfactory tract
Mitral cell
2
Olfactory nerve filaments
Olfactory gland of Bowman
Glomerulus
1
Cribriform plate of the ethmoid bone
Plasma cell secretes IgA that is transported into the lumen of the olfactory gland.
Olfactory gland of Bowman
Nuclei of the olfactory cells
Unmyelinated axons—surrounded by cytoplasmic extension of glial-like cells—pierce the cribriform plate of the ethmoid bone into the olfactory bulb.
IgA
Secretory product containing odorant-binding protein (OBP)
Basal cell
Basal lamina
Immature olfactory cell
Olfactory cell (bipolar neuron)
Supporting cell with apically located ovoid nucleus
Dendrite
Occluding junction
Microvilli border
Knoblike ending of the dendrite
Knoblike endings
Modified cilium
Odorant-OBP complex bound to an odorant receptor protein inserted in the plasma membrane of the modified cilium
Odorant molecule bound to OBP

Odorant receptor protein is a transmembrane member of the G protein–coupled receptor inserted in the plasma membrane of the modified cilium. Each olfactory cell expresses only a single type of receptor and one receptor may bind to several different odorants.

Odorant-OBP complex binding activates a G protein coupled to the receptor on its intracytoplasmic side. G protein–activated adenylyl cyclase catalyzes the conversion of adenosine triphosphate (ATP) to cyclic adenosine monophosphate (cAMP) which opens ligand-gated Na^+ channels for facilitated diffusion of Na^+ into the cell. Influx of Na^+ generates an action potential conducted along the olfactory nerve to the brain.

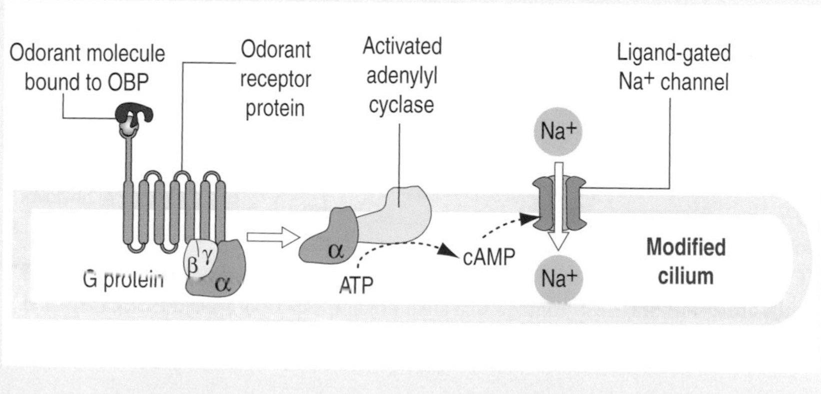

Odorant molecule bound to OBP
Odorant receptor protein
Activated adenylyl cyclase
Ligand-gated Na+ channel
Na+
G protein
β γ
α
α
ATP
cAMP
Na+
Modified cilium

2. The **glottis**, consisting of the true vocal cords (or folds) and the anterior and posterior commissures.

3. The **subglottis**, the region below the true vocal cords, extending down to the lower border of the cricoid cartilage.

During forced inspiration, vocal cords are **abducted**, and the space between the vocal cords widens.

Box 13-B | True vocal cords or folds

• The true vocal cords or folds consist of two regions—the cover and the core—with different structural properties.
• The cover consists of stratified squamous epithelium and the superficial layer of the lamina propria (the space of Reinke). The core is composed of the intermediate and deep layers of the lamina propria (representing the vocal ligament) and the vocalis or thyroarytenoid muscle.

The cover is flexible, whereas the core is stiff and has contractile properties allowing adjustment of stiffness.
• During phonation, the cover of the vocal cords displays horizontal movements and vertical undulation (known as mucosal wave). Changes in the stiffness in the core of the cords modify the mucosal wave. As the stiffness of the cord increases, the velocity of the mucosal wave increases and the pitch rises.

During phonation, the vocal cords are **adducted** and the space between the vocal cords changes into a linear slit. The vibration of the free edges of the cords (a cover consisting of both the stratified squamous epithelial covering and the superficial layer of the lamina propria, known as **Reinke's space**) during passage of air between them produces sound. The contraction of the intrinsic muscles of the larynx, forming the body of the cords, increases tension on the vocal cords, changing the pitch of the produced sound (see Box 13-B).

The mucosa of the larynx is continuous with that of the pharynx and the trachea. A **stratified squamous epithelium** covers the **lingual surface** and a small extension of the pharyngeal surface of the epiglottis and the **true vocal cords**. Elsewhere, the epithelium is **pseudostratified ciliated, with goblet cells**.

Laryngeal seromucous glands are found throughout the lamina propria, except at the level of the true vocal cords. The lamina propria of the **true vocal cords** consists of three layers (see Figure 13-4): (1) a superficial layer containing extracellular matrix and few elastic fibers. This layer is known as **Reinke's space**; (2) an intermediate layer with an increased content of elastic fibers; and (3) a deep layer with abundant elastic and collagen fibers.

Reinke's space and the epithelial covering are responsible for vocal cord vibration. **Reinke's edema** results when viral infection, trauma (laryngeal endoscopy), or severe coughing spells cause fluid to accumulate in the superficial layer of the lamina propria. Both the intermediate and deep layer of the lamina propria constitute the **vocal ligament**.

The lamina propria is usually rich in **mast cells**. Mast cells participate in hypersensitivity reactions leading to edema and laryngeal obstruction, a potential medical emergency. **Croup** designates a laryngotracheobronchitis in children, in which an inflammatory process narrows the airway and produces **inspiratory stridor**.

Trachea

The trachea, the major segment of the **conducting region** of the respiratory system, is the continuation of the larynx.

The trachea branches to form the right and left primary bronchi entering the hilum of each lung. The **hilum** is the region where the primary bronchus, **pulmonary artery**, **pulmonary vein**, **nerves**, and **lymphatics** enter and leave the lung. Secondary divisions of the bronchi and accompanying connective tissue septa divide each lung into lobes.

The right lung has three lobes, whereas the left lung has two lobes.

Subsequent bronchial divisions further subdivide each lobe into bronchopulmonary segments. **The bronchopulmonary segment is the gross anatomic unit of the lung that can be removed surgically**. Successive bronchial branching gives rise to several generations of **bronchopulmonary subsegments**.

The trachea and main bronchi are lined by **pseudostratified columnar ciliated epithelium** resting on a distinct basal lamina. Several types of cells can be identified (Figure 13-5):

1. **Columnar ciliated cells** are the predominant cell population, extending from the lumen to the basal lamina.
2. **Goblet cells** are abundant nonciliated cells, also in contact with the lumen and the basal lamina.
3. **Basal cells** rest on the basal lamina but do not extend to the lumen.
4. **Cells of Kulchitsky** are neuroendocrine cells also resting on the basal lamina and are predominantly found at the bifurcation of lobar bronchi. They give rise to bronchial carcinoid tumors within the bronchial mucosa. These cells secrete peptide hormones such as serotonin, calcitonin, antidiuretic hormone (ADH) and adrenocorticotropic hormone (ACTH).

The lamina propria contains elastic fibers. The **submucosa** displays **mucous** and **serous glands**.

Figure 13-4. Structure of the larynx

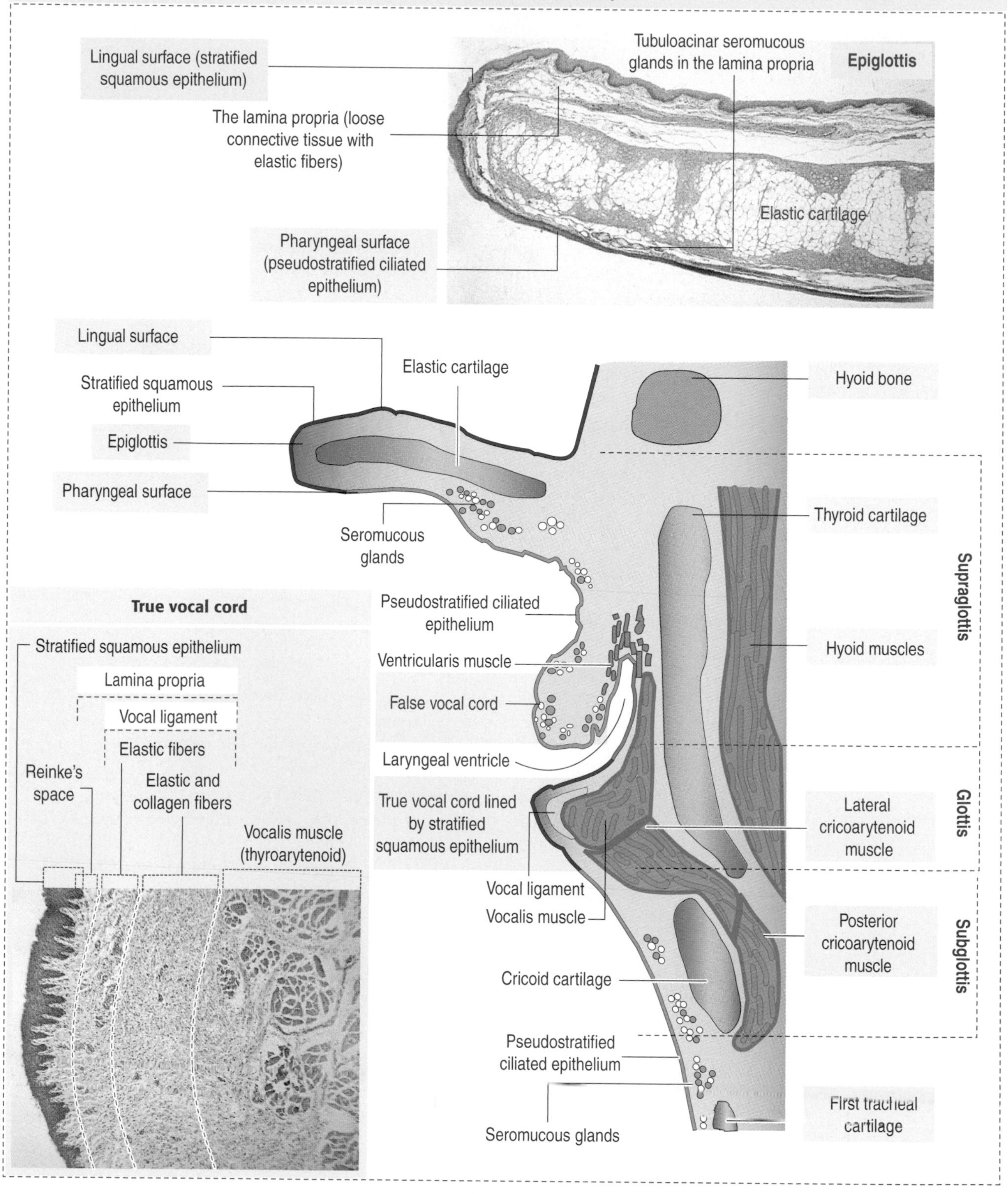

Epiglottis
Lingual surface (stratified squamous epithelium)
Tubuloacinar seromucous glands in the lamina propria
The lamina propria (loose connective tissue with elastic fibers)
Elastic cartilage
Pharyngeal surface (pseudostratified ciliated epithelium)
Lingual surface
Elastic cartilage
Hyoid bone
Stratified squamous epithelium
Epiglottis
Pharyngeal surface
Seromucous glands
Thyroid cartilage
Supraglottis
Pseudostratified ciliated epithelium
Hyoid muscles
Ventricularis muscle
False vocal cord
Laryngeal ventricle
True vocal cord lined by stratified squamous epithelium
Lateral cricoarytenoid muscle
Glottis
Vocal ligament
Vocalis muscle
Posterior cricoarytenoid muscle
Subglottis
Cricoid cartilage
Pseudostratified ciliated epithelium
Seromucous glands
First tracheal cartilage
True vocal cord
Stratified squamous epithelium
Lamina propria
Vocal ligament
Elastic fibers
Reinke's space
Elastic and collagen fibers
Vocalis muscle (thyroarytenoid)

The framework of the trachea and extrapulmonary bronchi consists of a stack of **C-shaped hyaline cartilages**, each surrounded by a **fibroelastic layer** blending with the perichondrium. In the **trachea** and **primary bronchi**, the open ends of the cartilage rings point posteriorly to the esophagus. The lowest tracheal cartilage is the **carinal cartilage**. Transverse fibers of the **trachealis muscle** attach to the inner ends of the cartilage. In branching bronchi, cartilage **rings** (see Figure 13-5) are replaced by irregularly shaped cartilage **plates** (Figure 13-6), surrounded by

Figure 13-5. Structure of the trachea

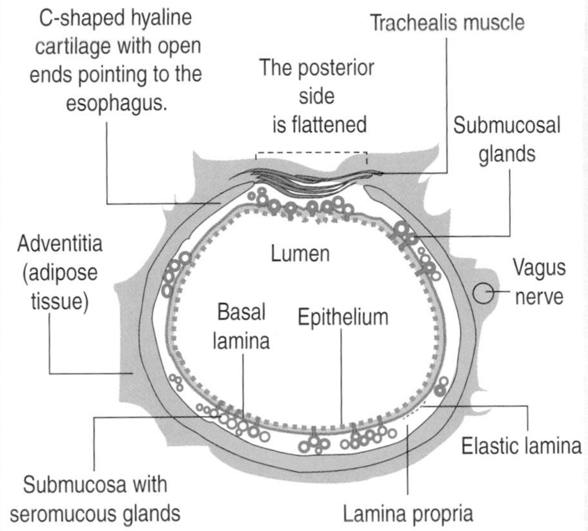

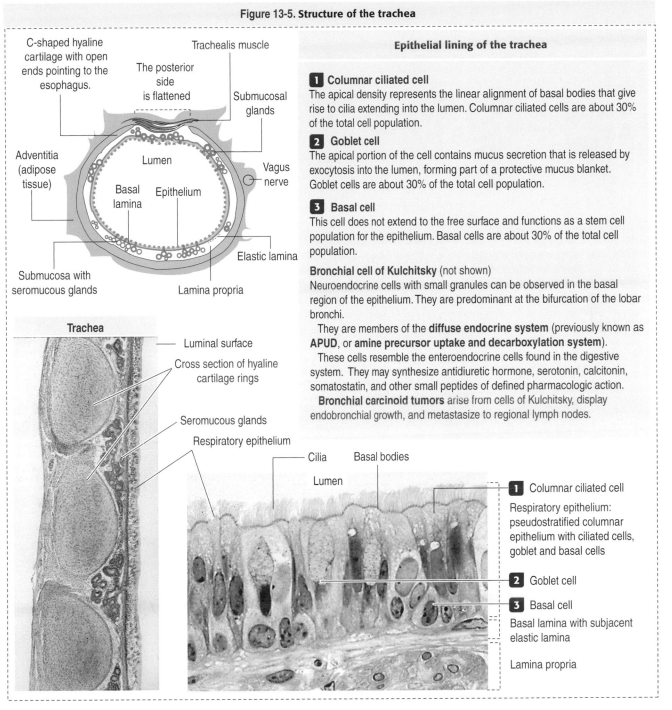

C-shaped hyaline cartilage with open ends pointing to the esophagus.
Trachealis muscle
The posterior side is flattened
Submucosal glands
Adventitia (adipose tissue)
Lumen
Vagus nerve
Basal lamina
Epithelium
Elastic lamina
Submucosa with seromucous glands
Lamina propria

Epithelial lining of the trachea

1 Columnar ciliated cell
The apical density represents the linear alignment of basal bodies that give rise to cilia extending into the lumen. Columnar ciliated cells are about 30% of the total cell population.

2 Goblet cell
The apical portion of the cell contains mucus secretion that is released by exocytosis into the lumen, forming part of a protective mucus blanket. Goblet cells are about 30% of the total cell population.

3 Basal cell
This cell does not extend to the free surface and functions as a stem cell population for the epithelium. Basal cells are about 30% of the total cell population.

Bronchial cell of Kulchitsky (not shown)
Neuroendocrine cells with small granules can be observed in the basal region of the epithelium. They are predominant at the bifurcation of the lobar bronchi.

They are members of the **diffuse endocrine system** (previously known as **APUD**, or **amine precursor uptake and decarboxylation system**).

These cells resemble the enteroendocrine cells found in the digestive system. They may synthesize antidiuretic hormone, serotonin, calcitonin, somatostatin, and other small peptides of defined pharmacologic action.

Bronchial carcinoid tumors arise from cells of Kulchitsky, display endobronchial growth, and metastasize to regional lymph nodes.

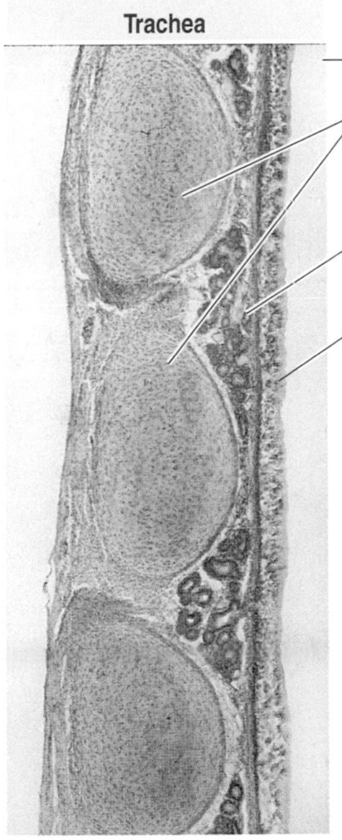

Trachea
Luminal surface
Cross section of hyaline cartilage rings
Seromucous glands
Respiratory epithelium

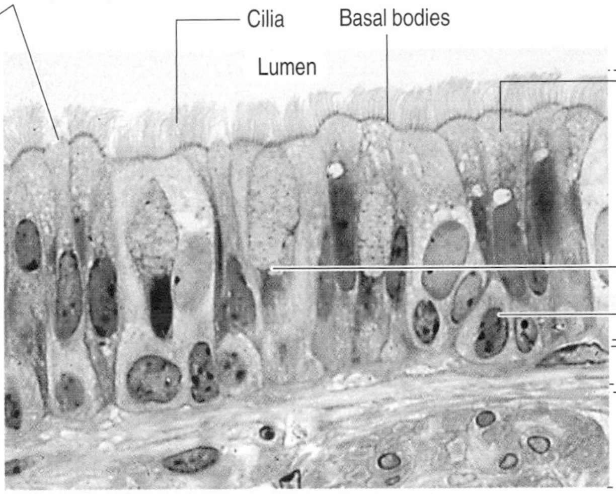

Cilia
Basal bodies
Lumen
1 Columnar ciliated cell
Respiratory epithelium: pseudostratified columnar epithelium with ciliated cells, goblet and basal cells
2 Goblet cell
3 Basal cell
Basal lamina with subjacent elastic lamina
Lamina propria

smooth muscle bundles in a spiral arrangement.

Intrapulmonary segmentation of the bronchial tree

Within the pulmonary parenchyma, a segmental bronchus gives rise to large and small subsegmental bronchi. A small subsegmental bronchus is continuous with a bronchiole. This transition involves **the loss of cartilage plates in the bronchiole and a progressive increase in the number of elastic fibers.**

The intrapulmonary segmentation results in the organization of a **pulmonary lobule** and a **pulmonary acinus** (Figure 13-7; see also Figure 13-6).

Pulmonary lobule and pulmonary acinus

A terminal bronchiole and the associated region of pulmonary tissues that it sup-

Figure 13-6. Segmentation of the intrapulmonary bronchial tree

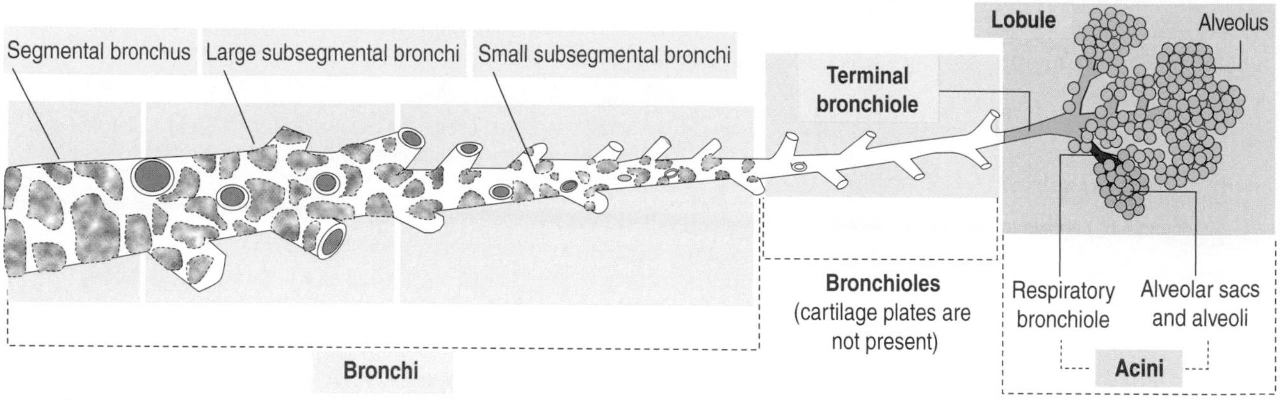

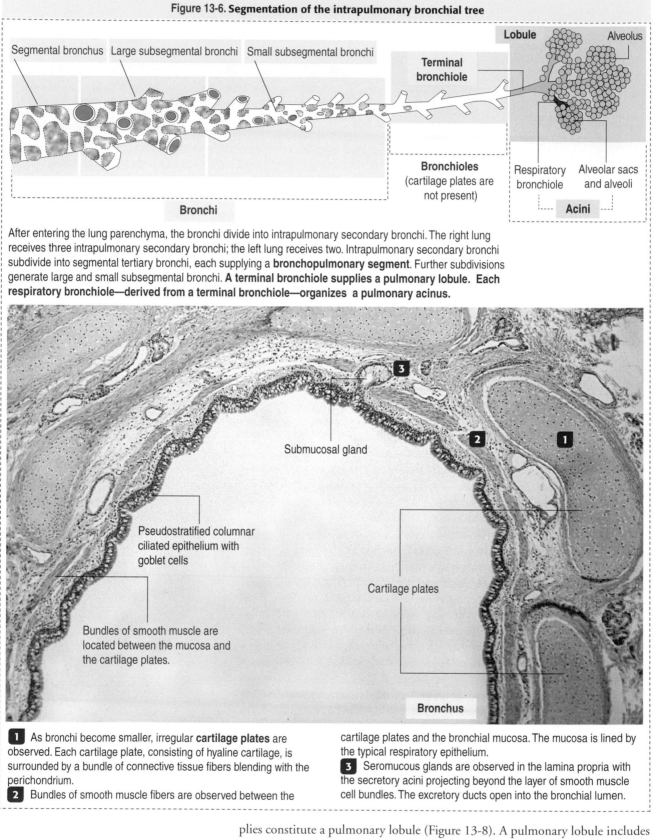

Segmental bronchus
Large subsegmental bronchi
Small subsegmental bronchi
Terminal bronchiole
Lobule
Alveolus
Bronchi
Bronchioles (cartilage plates are not present)
Respiratory bronchiole
Alveolar sacs and alveoli
Acini

After entering the lung parenchyma, the bronchi divide into intrapulmonary secondary bronchi. The right lung receives three intrapulmonary secondary bronchi; the left lung receives two. Intrapulmonary secondary bronchi subdivide into segmental tertiary bronchi, each supplying a **bronchopulmonary segment**. Further subdivisions generate large and small subsegmental bronchi. **A terminal bronchiole supplies a pulmonary lobule. Each respiratory bronchiole—derived from a terminal bronchiole—organizes a pulmonary acinus.**

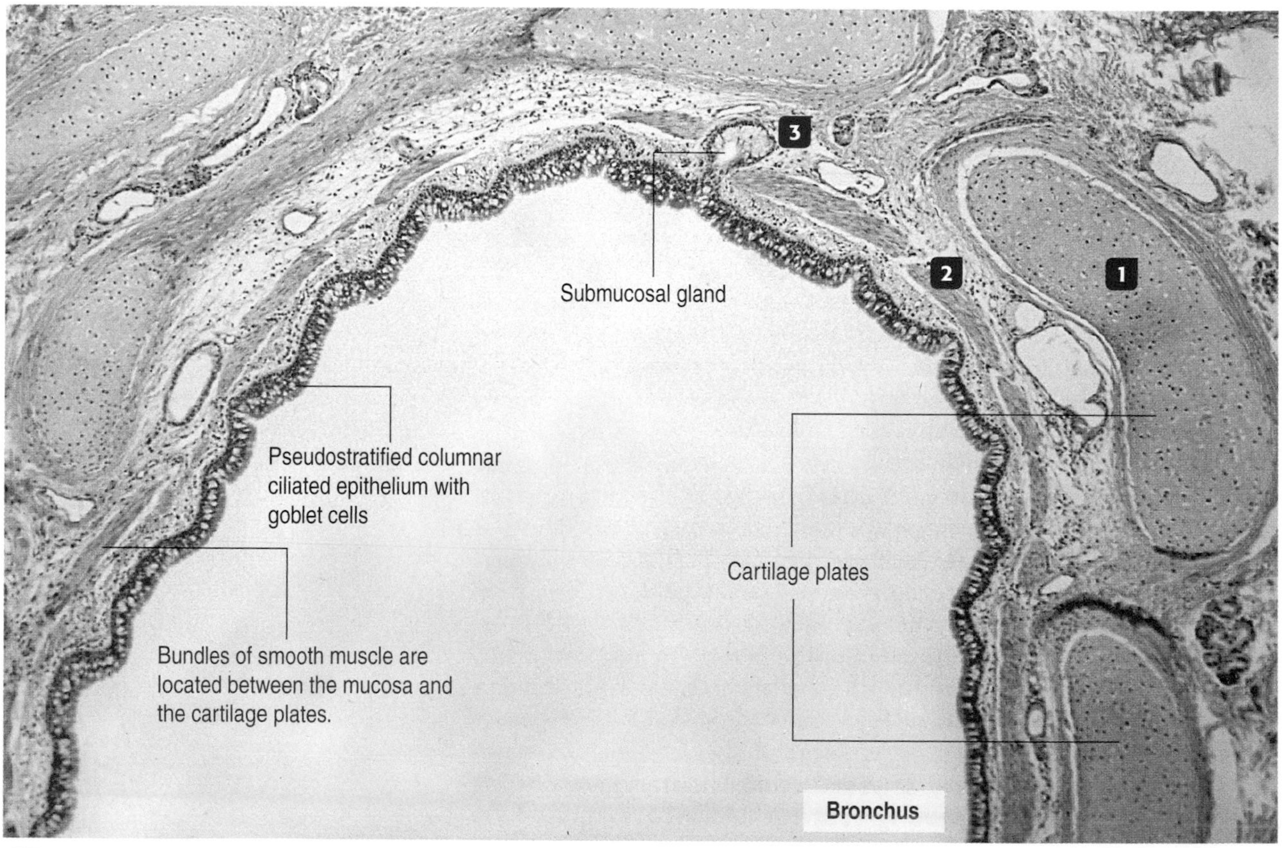

3
Submucosal gland
2
1
Pseudostratified columnar ciliated epithelium with goblet cells
Cartilage plates
Bundles of smooth muscle are located between the mucosa and the cartilage plates.
Bronchus

1 As bronchi become smaller, irregular **cartilage plates** are observed. Each cartilage plate, consisting of hyaline cartilage, is surrounded by a bundle of connective tissue fibers blending with the perichondrium.

2 Bundles of smooth muscle fibers are observed between the cartilage plates and the bronchial mucosa. The mucosa is lined by the typical respiratory epithelium.

3 Seromucous glands are observed in the lamina propria with the secretory acini projecting beyond the layer of smooth muscle cell bundles. The excretory ducts open into the bronchial lumen.

plies constitute a pulmonary lobule (Figure 13-8). A pulmonary lobule includes the respiratory bronchioles, alveolar ducts, alveolar sacs, and alveoli.

Physiologists designate the pulmonary acinus as the portion of the lung supplied by a respiratory bronchiole. Therefore, respiratory acini are subcomponents of a respiratory lobule. In contrast to the acinus, the pulmonary lobule includes

Figure 13-7. Histology of the intrapulmonary bronchial tree

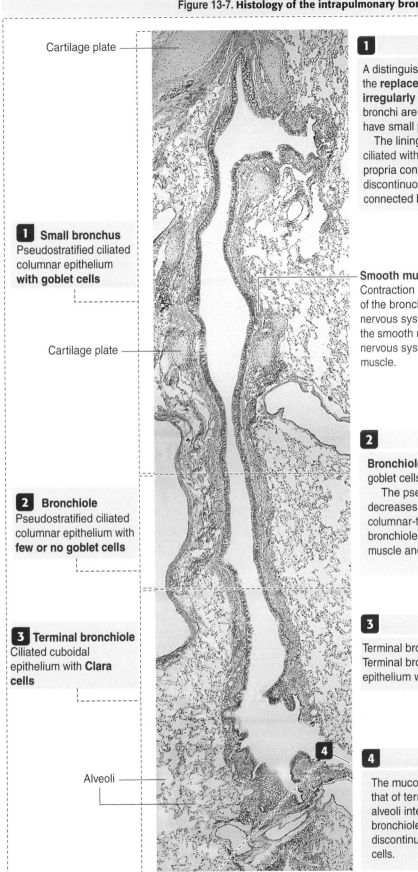

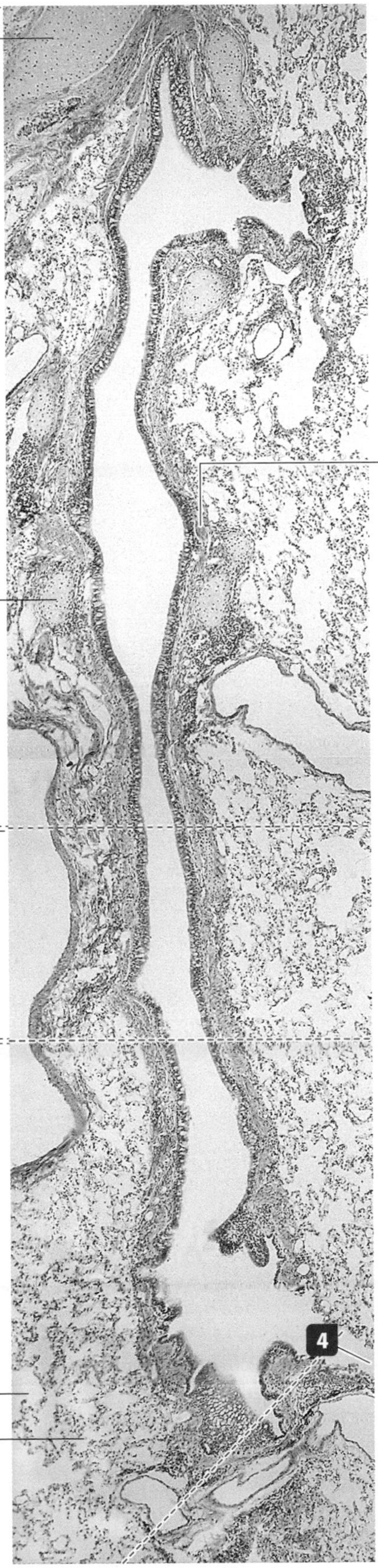

1 Small bronchi

A distinguishing feature between trachea and bronchi is the **replacement of hyaline cartilage rings by irregularly shaped cartilaginous plates** in bronchi. Large bronchi are encircled by the plates, but smaller bronchi have small plates.

The lining epithelium is pseudostratified columnar ciliated with mucus-secreting goblet cells. The lamina propria contains a layer of circularly arranged but discontinuous smooth muscle, and seromucous glands connected by excretory ducts to the epithelial surface.

Smooth muscle bundles

Contraction of the smooth muscle decreases the lumen of the bronchus. Stimulation of the parasympathetic nervous system (vagus nerve) produces contraction of the smooth muscle. Stimulation of the sympathetic nervous system inhibits contraction of the smooth muscle.

2 Bronchioles

Bronchioles lack cartilage and glands, but a few goblet cells may be found in the initial portions.

The pseudostratified ciliated columnar epithelium decreases in height to finally become simple columnar-to-cuboidal ciliated at the terminal bronchioles. The lamina propria is composed of smooth muscle and elastic and collagenous fibers.

3 Terminal bronchioles

Terminal bronchioles give rise to respiratory bronchioles. Terminal bronchioles are lined by a ciliated cuboidal epithelium with Clara cells.

4 Respiratory bronchioles

The mucosa of the respiratory bronchioles is similar to that of terminal bronchioles, except for the presence of alveoli interrupting the continuity of the wall of the bronchiole. The low cuboidal epithelium is replaced discontinuously by squamous type I alveolar epithelial cells.

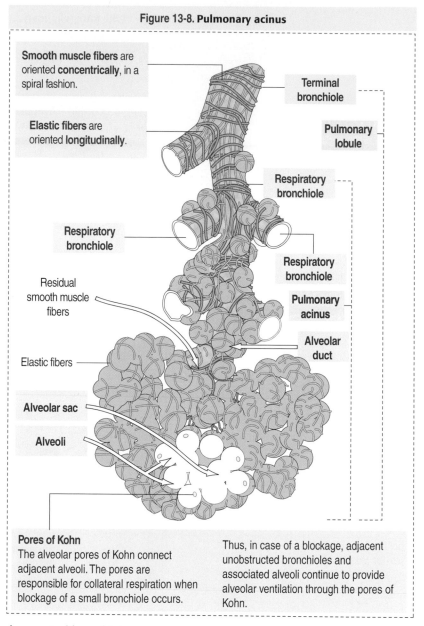

Figure 13-8. **Pulmonary acinus**

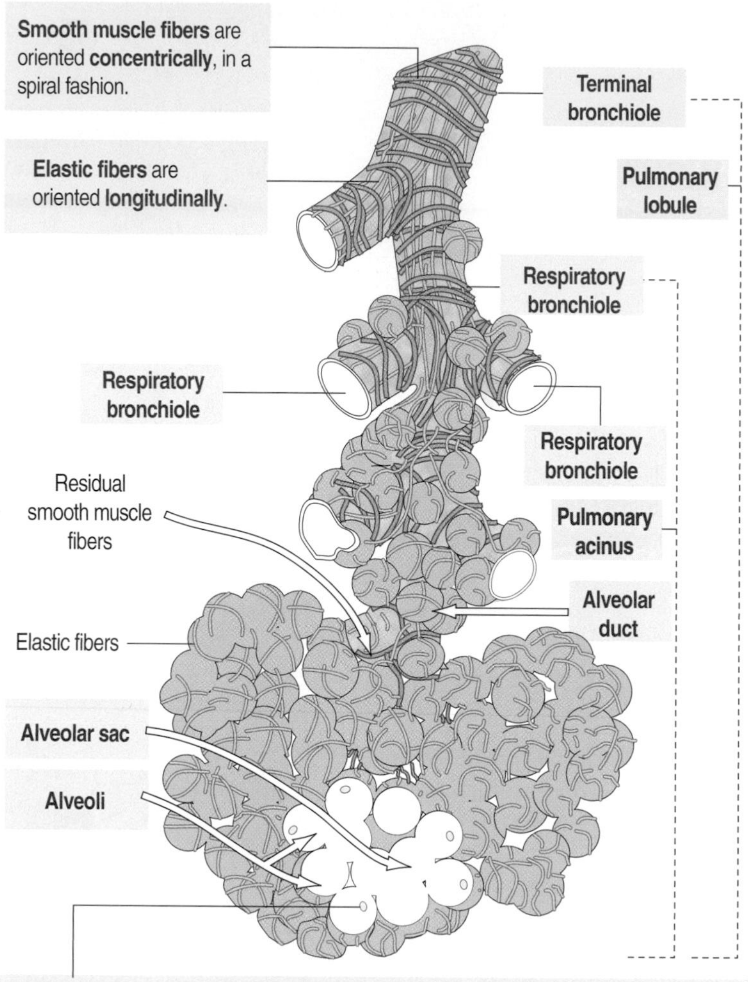
Smooth muscle fibers are oriented **concentrically**, in a spiral fashion.
Elastic fibers are oriented **longitudinally**.
Terminal bronchiole
Pulmonary lobule
Respiratory bronchiole
Respiratory bronchiole
Respiratory bronchiole
Residual smooth muscle fibers
Pulmonary acinus
Alveolar duct
Elastic fibers
Alveolar sac
Alveoli

Pores of Kohn
The alveolar pores of Kohn connect adjacent alveoli. The pores are responsible for collateral respiration when blockage of a small bronchiole occurs.

Thus, in case of a blockage, adjacent unobstructed bronchioles and associated alveoli continue to provide alveolar ventilation through the pores of Kohn.

the terminal bronchiole.

The pulmonary lobule–acinus concept is important for understanding the types of **emphysema**—permanent enlargement of the air spaces distal to the terminal bronchioles, associated with the destruction of their walls.

Distal to the respiratory bronchiole is the **alveolar duct**. The alveolar duct is characterized by an interrupted wall with typical **smooth muscle knobs** bulging into the lumen (Figure 13-9).

At the distal end, the smooth muscle knobs disappear and the lining epithelium is primarily **type I alveolar epithelial cells**. Alveolar ducts branch to form two or more **alveolar sacs**. Alveolar sacs are formed by the **alveoli**, the terminal part of the airway.

Clinical significance: Emphysema

Chronic obstructive pulmonary disease (**COPD**) is characterized by progressive and often irreversible airflow limitations. COPD includes **emphysema** and **asthma**.

COPD occurs in the **peripheral airways**—the bronchioles—and **lung parenchyma. Elastic fibers** are important components of bronchioles and alveolar

Figure 13-9. **Transition from terminal bronchiole to respiratory bronchiole**

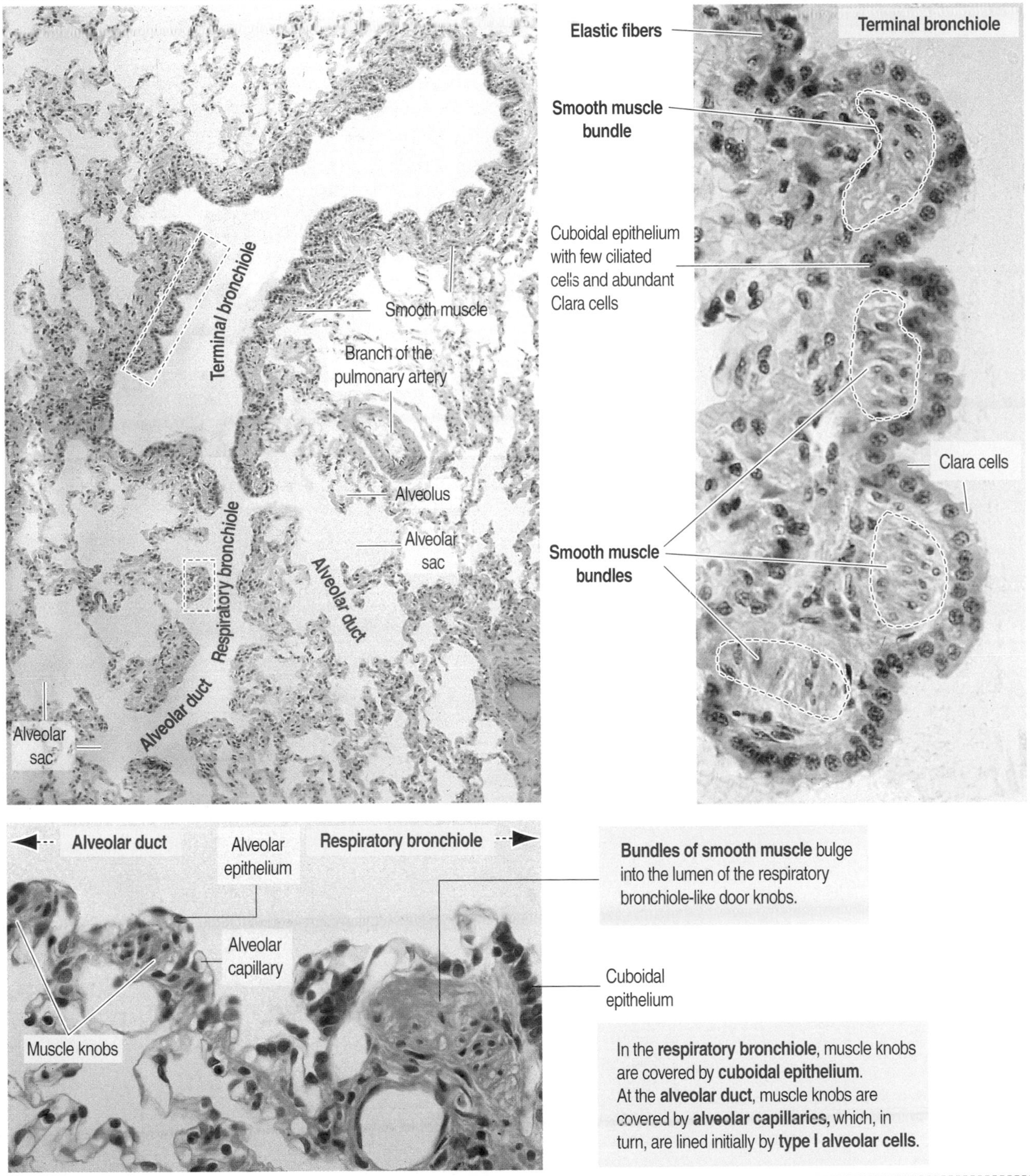
Terminal bronchiole
Smooth muscle
Branch of the pulmonary artery
Alveolus
Alveolar sac
Respiratory bronchiole
Alveolar duct
Alveolar duct
Alveolar sac
Elastic fibers
Terminal bronchiole
Smooth muscle bundle
Cuboidal epithelium with few ciliated cells and abundant Clara cells
Clara cells
Smooth muscle bundles
Alveolar duct
Alveolar epithelium
Respiratory bronchiole
Alveolar capillary
Muscle knobs
Cuboidal epithelium

Bundles of smooth muscle bulge into the lumen of the respiratory bronchiole-like door knobs.

In the **respiratory bronchiole**, muscle knobs are covered by **cuboidal epithelium**.
At the **alveolar duct**, muscle knobs are covered by **alveolar capillaries,** which, in turn, are lined initially by **type I alveolar cells**.

walls. A loss of elasticity and breakdown of elastic fibers gives rise to **emphysema**, characterized by chronic airflow obstruction. As a result, adjacent alveoli become confluent, creating large **air spaces**, or **blebs** (Figure 13-10).

Terminal and respiratory bronchioles are also affected by the loss of elastic tissue. As a result of the loss of elastic fibers, the small airways tend to collapse during expiration, leading to chronic airflow obstruction and secondary infections.

Let us review the concepts of the pulmonary lobule and the acinus to understand the types of emphysema. Figures 13-6 and 13-8 show that a **pulmonary lobule**

Figure 13-10. Elastic fibers and emphysema

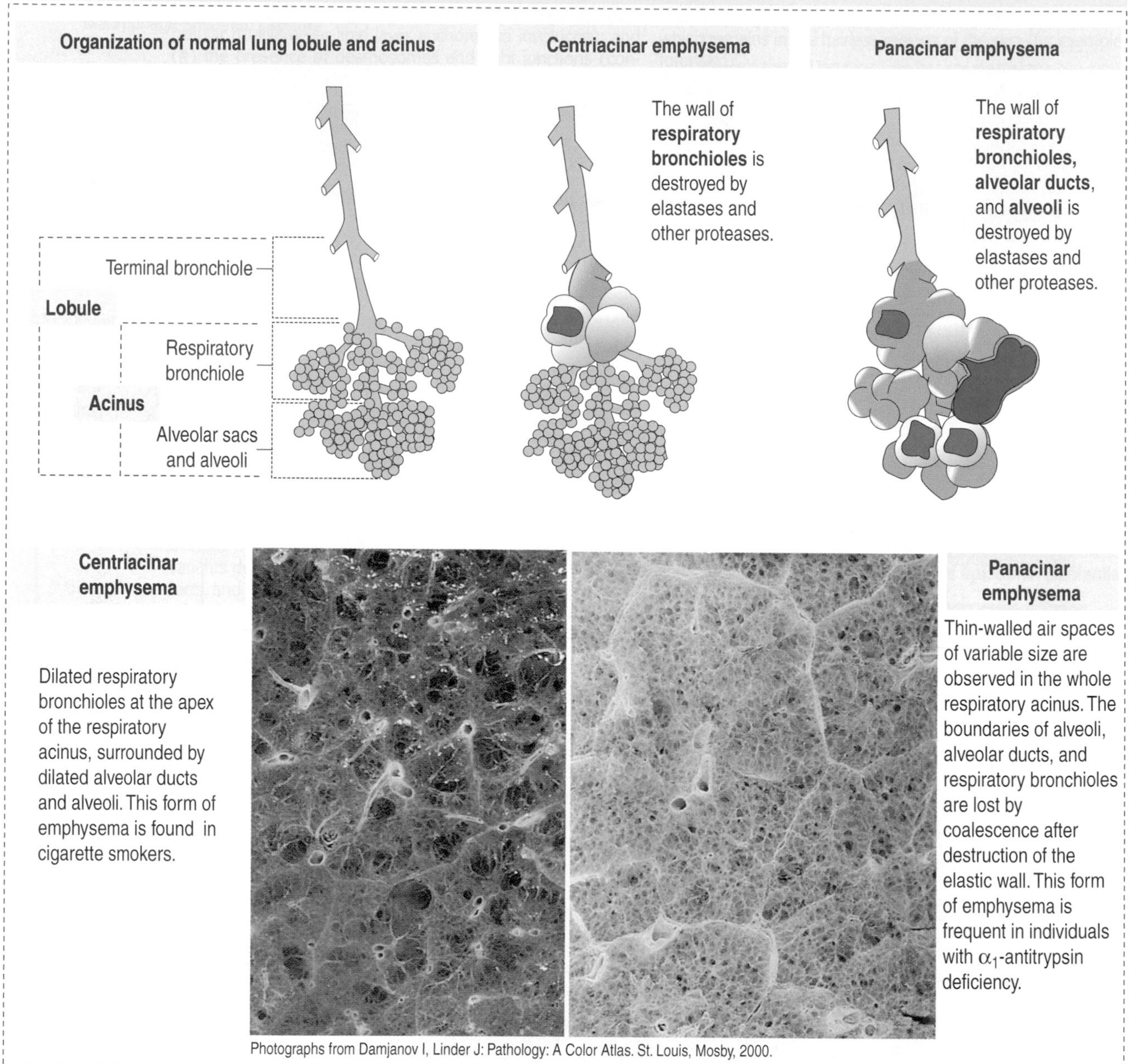
Organization of normal lung lobule and acinus
Terminal bronchiole
Lobule
Respiratory bronchiole
Acinus
Alveolar sacs and alveoli
Centriacinar emphysema
The wall of **respiratory bronchioles** is destroyed by elastases and other proteases.
Panacinar emphysema
The wall of **respiratory bronchioles, alveolar ducts**, and **alveoli** is destroyed by elastases and other proteases.
Centriacinar emphysema
Dilated respiratory bronchioles at the apex of the respiratory acinus, surrounded by dilated alveolar ducts and alveoli. This form of emphysema is found in cigarette smokers.
Panacinar emphysema
Thin-walled air spaces of variable size are observed in the whole respiratory acinus. The boundaries of alveoli, alveolar ducts, and respiratory bronchioles are lost by coalescence after destruction of the elastic wall. This form of emphysema is frequent in individuals with α_1-antitrypsin deficiency.

Photographs from Damjanov I, Linder J: Pathology: A Color Atlas. St. Louis, Mosby, 2000.

includes the terminal bronchiole and the first to third generations of derived respiratory bronchioles. Each respiratory bronchiole gives rise to alveolar ducts and alveoli, an arrangement known as the **acinus**—so called because aggregates of alveoli cluster like acini in connection with the ductlike respiratory bronchiole. Because a pulmonary lobule generates several respiratory bronchioles, each resolved into an acinus, a pulmonary lobule is made up of several acini.

Centriacinar (or centrilobular) emphysema originates when the **respiratory bronchioles** are affected. The more distal alveolar duct and alveoli are intact. Thus, emphysematous and normal air spaces coexist within the same lobule and acini.

In panacinar (or panlobular) emphysema, blebs are observed from the respiratory bronchiole down to the alveolar sacs. This type of emphysema is more common in patients with a **deficiency in the** ***α_1-antitrypsin*** **gene** encoding a serum protein.

Protein α_1-antitrypsin is a major inhibitor of proteases, in particular **elastase**, secreted by neutrophils during inflammation (Figure 13-11). Under the influence of a stimulus, such as cigarette smoke, **macrophages** in the alveolar wall and

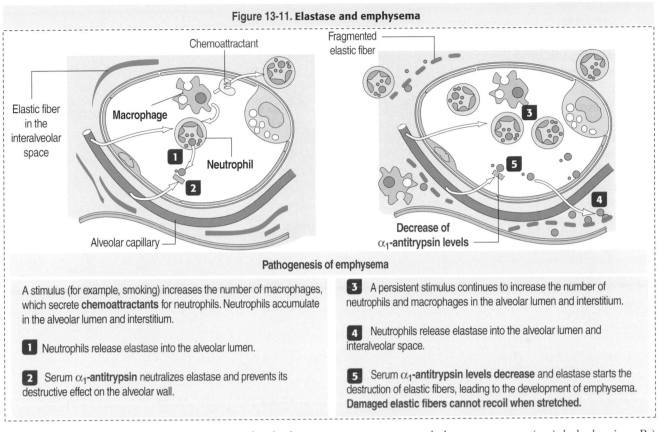

Figure 13-11. Elastase and emphysema

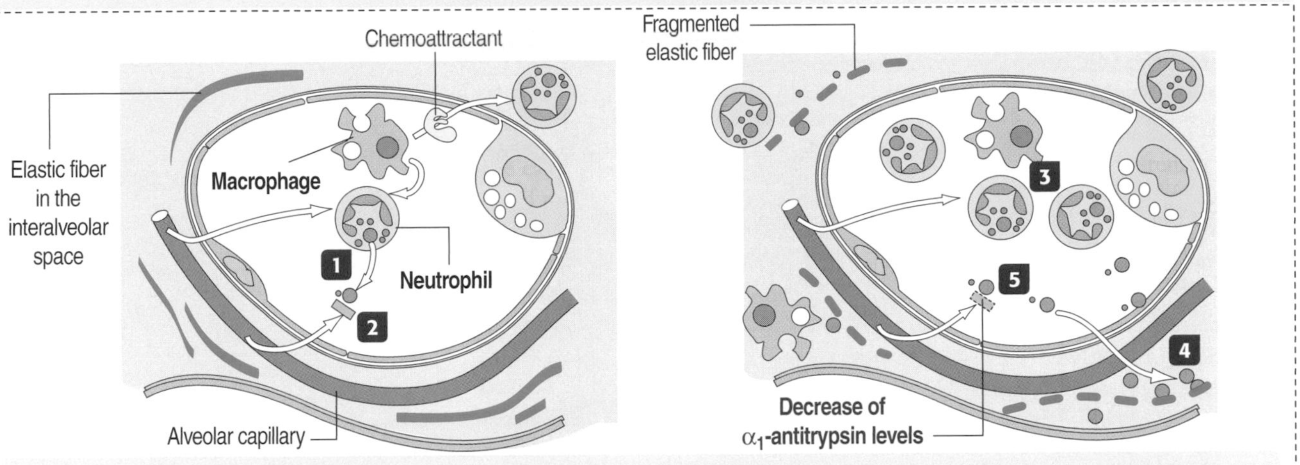

Chemoattractant
Fragmented elastic fiber
Elastic fiber in the interalveolar space
Macrophage
Neutrophil
1
2
3
4
5
Alveolar capillary
Decrease of α_1-antitrypsin levels

Pathogenesis of emphysema

A stimulus (for example, smoking) increases the number of macrophages, which secrete **chemoattractants** for neutrophils. Neutrophils accumulate in the alveolar lumen and interstitium.

1 Neutrophils release elastase into the alveolar lumen.

2 Serum **α_1-antitrypsin** neutralizes elastase and prevents its destructive effect on the alveolar wall.

3 A persistent stimulus continues to increase the number of neutrophils and macrophages in the alveolar lumen and interstitium.

4 Neutrophils release elastase into the alveolar lumen and interalveolar space.

5 Serum **α_1-antitrypsin levels decrease** and elastase starts the destruction of elastic fibers, leading to the development of emphysema. **Damaged elastic fibers cannot recoil when stretched.**

alveolar lumen secrete proteases and chemoattractants (mainly leukotriene B_4) to recruit **neutrophils**.

Chemoattracted neutrophils appear in the alveolar lumen and wall and release **elastase**, normally neutralized by **α_1-antitrypsin**. Chronic smokers have low serum levels of α_1-antitrypsin, and elastase continues the unopposed destruction of elastic fibers present in the alveolar wall. This process develops in 10% to 15% of smokers and leads to emphysema.

Asthma is a chronic inflammatory process characterized by the **reversible narrowing of the airways** (**bronchoconstriction**) in response to various stimuli. The classic **symptoms of asthma** are **wheezing**, **cough**, and **shortness of breath** (**dyspnea**).

Emphysema differs from asthma in that the abnormalities limiting airflow are predominantly **irreversible** and a **destructive process** targets the lung parenchyma.

Clinical significance: Asthma

Asthma is characterized by **airway hyperresponsiveness**, defined by three salient features (Figure 13-12): (1) Airway wall inflammation involving **neutrophils**, **T cells** ($CD8^+$), and **macrophages.** Asthma is characterized by the recruitment of **T cells** ($CD4^+$) and **eosinophils** (see Figure 13-12); (2) luminal obstruction of airways by mucus, caused by hypersecretion of bronchial mucous glands, along with infiltration by inflammatory cells; and (3) vasodilation of the bronchial microvasculature with increased vascular permeability and edema.

Asthma can be triggered by repeated antigen exposure (**allergic asthma**) or by an abnormal autonomic neural regulation of airway function (**nonallergic asthma**).

The pathophysiologic aspects of asthma appear to result from the aberrant proliferation of $CD4^+$ helper T_H2 cells producing three cytokines: **interleukin (IL)-4**, IL-5, and IL-13. IL-4 stimulates immature T cells to develop into the T_H2 cell type, which produces IL-13 to precipitate an asthma attack.

Figure 13-12. **Pathogenesis of asthma**

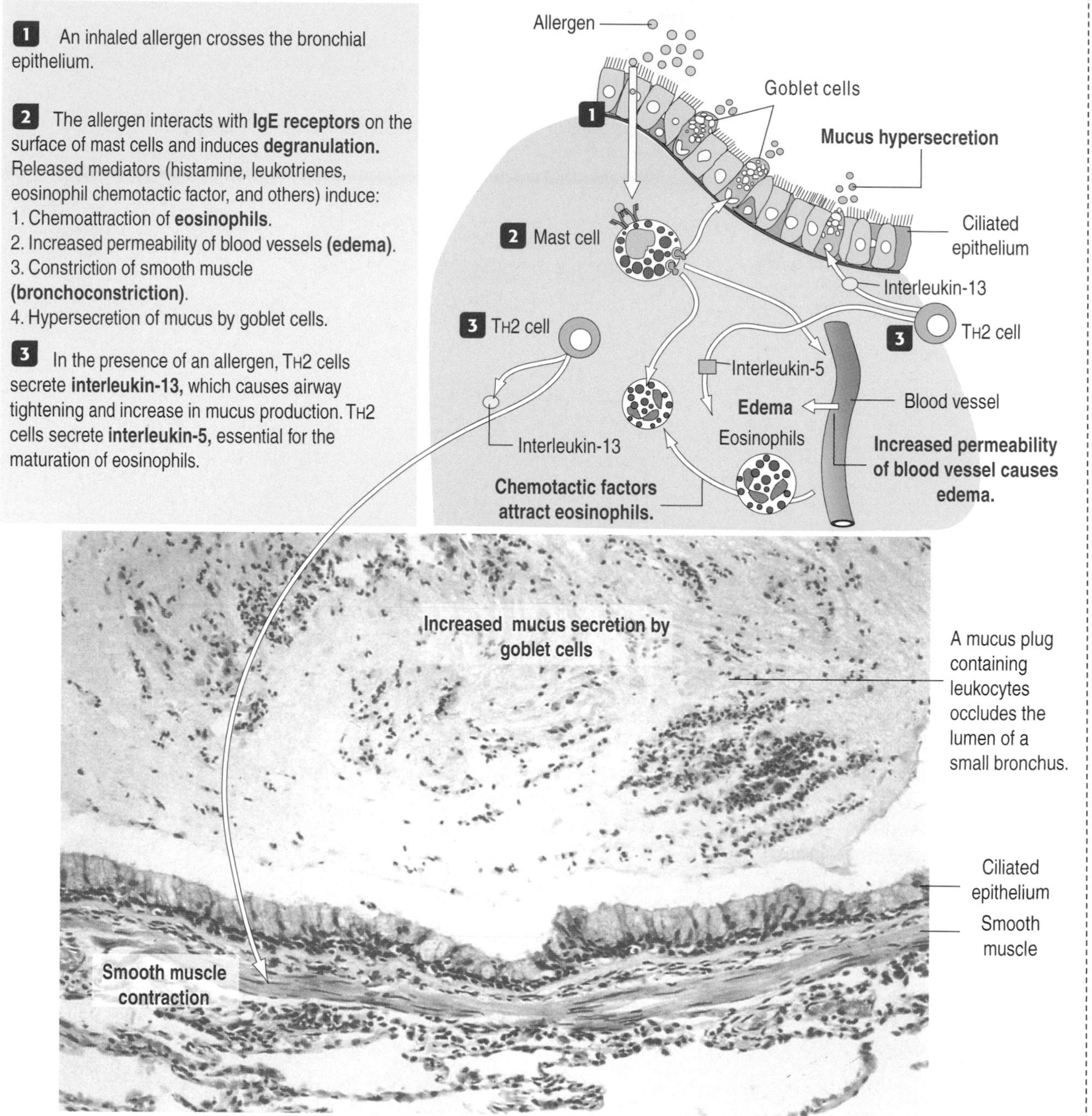
1 An inhaled allergen crosses the bronchial epithelium.
2 The allergen interacts with **IgE receptors** on the surface of mast cells and induces **degranulation.** Released mediators (histamine, leukotrienes, eosinophil chemotactic factor, and others) induce:
1. Chemoattraction of **eosinophils**.
2. Increased permeability of blood vessels **(edema)**.
3. Constriction of smooth muscle **(bronchoconstriction)**.
4. Hypersecretion of mucus by goblet cells.
3 In the presence of an allergen, TH2 cells secrete **interleukin-13,** which causes airway tightening and increase in mucus production. TH2 cells secrete **interleukin-5,** essential for the maturation of eosinophils.
Allergen
Goblet cells
Mucus hypersecretion
Ciliated epithelium
2 Mast cell
Interleukin-13
3 TH2 cell
3 TH2 cell
Interleukin-5
Edema
Blood vessel
Eosinophils
Interleukin-13
Increased permeability of blood vessel causes edema.
Chemotactic factors attract eosinophils.
Increased mucus secretion by goblet cells
A mucus plug containing leukocytes occludes the lumen of a small bronchus.
Ciliated epithelium
Smooth muscle
Smooth muscle contraction

Photograph from Curran RC: Colour Atlas of Histopathology, 3rd ed. New York, Oxford University Press, 1985.

Nonciliated Clara cells in terminal bronchioles secrete surfactant

Clara cells represent **80% of the epithelial cell population** of the **terminal bronchiole** (Figure 13-13). Clara cells secrete a component of the surfactant material covering the alveoli. More recently, **Clara cells have been associated with Cl^- release mediated by a chloride channel regulated by a cyclic guanosine monophosphate (cGMP)–guanylyl cyclase C mechanism.**

Clinical significance: Cystic fibrosis

Cystic fibrosis is a recessive genetic disease affecting children and young adults. The genetic defect responsible for cystic fibrosis is on the long arm of chromosome 7. **A characteristic of the disease is the production of abnormally thick mucus by epithelial cells lining the respiratory and gastrointestinal tracts** (Figure 13-

Figure 13-13. Structure and function of Clara cells

Clara cells

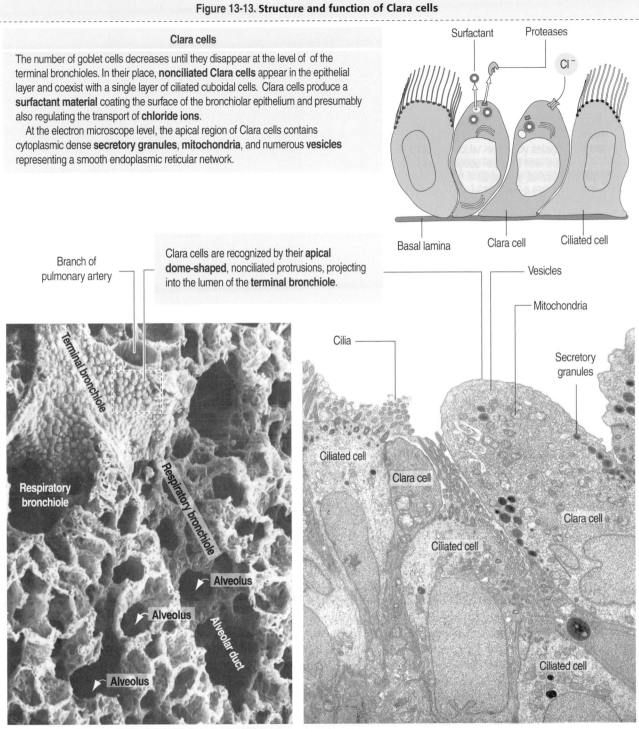

The number of goblet cells decreases until they disappear at the level of of the terminal bronchioles. In their place, **nonciliated Clara cells** appear in the epithelial layer and coexist with a single layer of ciliated cuboidal cells. Clara cells produce a **surfactant material** coating the surface of the bronchiolar epithelium and presumably also regulating the transport of **chloride ions**.

At the electron microscope level, the apical region of Clara cells contains cytoplasmic dense **secretory granules**, **mitochondria**, and numerous **vesicles** representing a smooth endoplasmic reticular network.

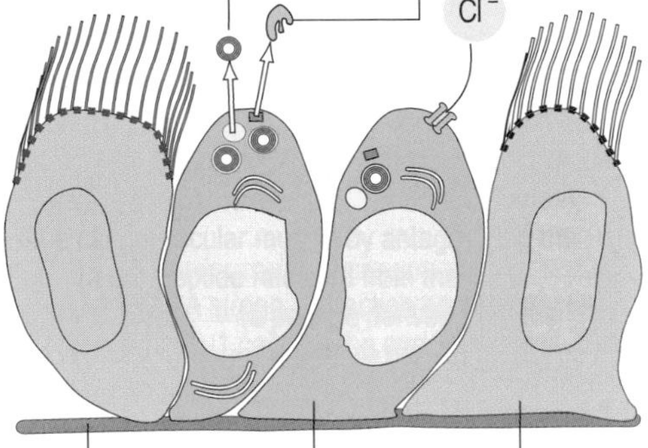

Surfactant
Proteases
Cl⁻
Basal lamina
Clara cell
Ciliated cell

Clara cells are recognized by their **apical dome-shaped**, nonciliated protrusions, projecting into the lumen of the **terminal bronchiole**.

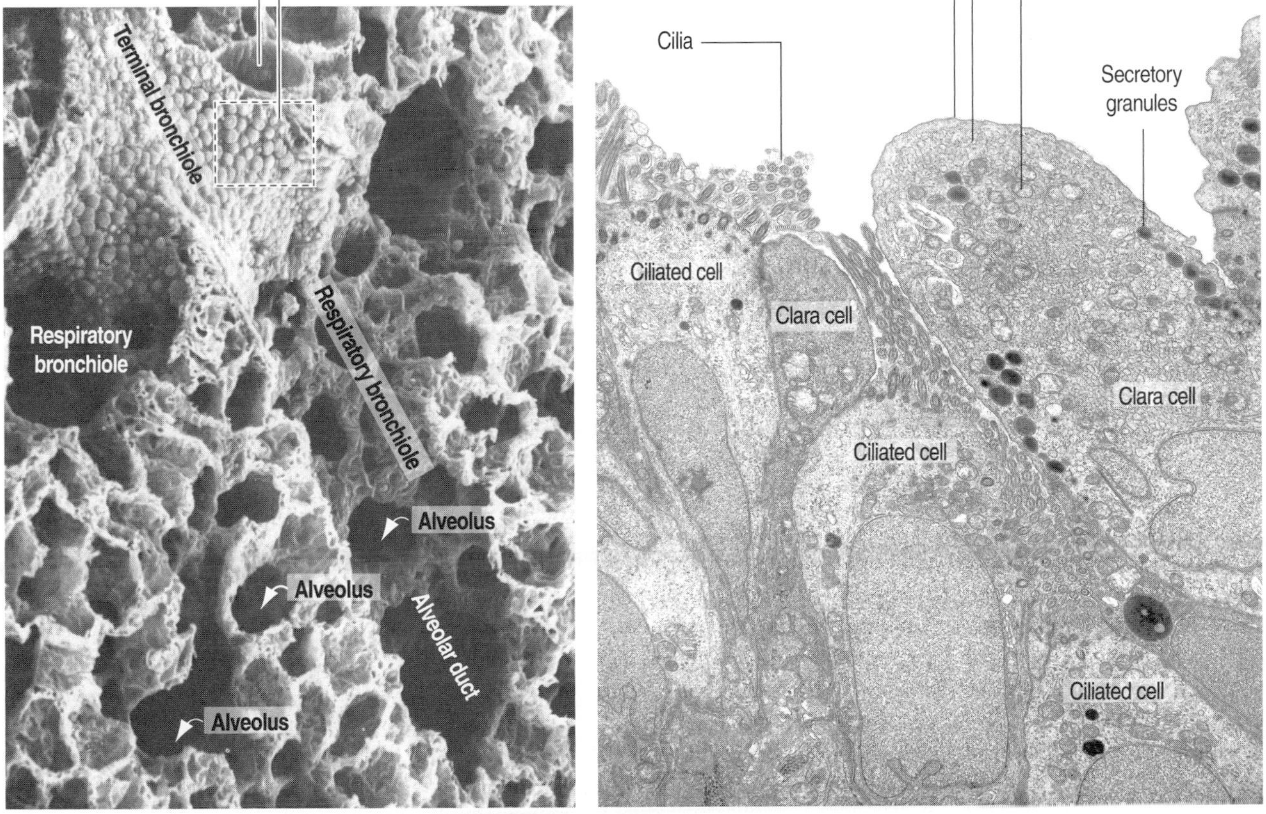

Branch of pulmonary artery
Terminal bronchiole
Respiratory bronchiole
Respiratory bronchiole
Alveolus
Alveolus
Alveolar duct
Alveolus
Vesicles
Mitochondria
Cilia
Secretory granules
Ciliated cell
Clara cell
Clara cell
Ciliated cell
Ciliated cell

Scanning electron micrograph from Kessel RG, Kardon RH: Tissues and Organs. New York, WH Freeman, 1979.

14). Respiratory disease results from the obstruction of the pulmonary airways by thick mucus plugs, followed by bacterial infections. Cough, chronic purulent secretions, and dyspnea are typical symptoms of this COPD.

In most patients, the blockage of pancreatic ducts by mucus causes pancreatic dysfunction. Pancreatic ductules release a bicarbonate-rich fluid under regulation of secretin. Secretin is produced by enteroendocrine cells in response to acidic gastric contents entering the duodenum (see Chapter 17, Digestive Glands).

In the skin, the excessive presence of salt secretion by sweat glands is diagnostic of cystic fibrosis (see Chapter 11, Integumentary System).

Figure 13-14. Cystic fibrosis

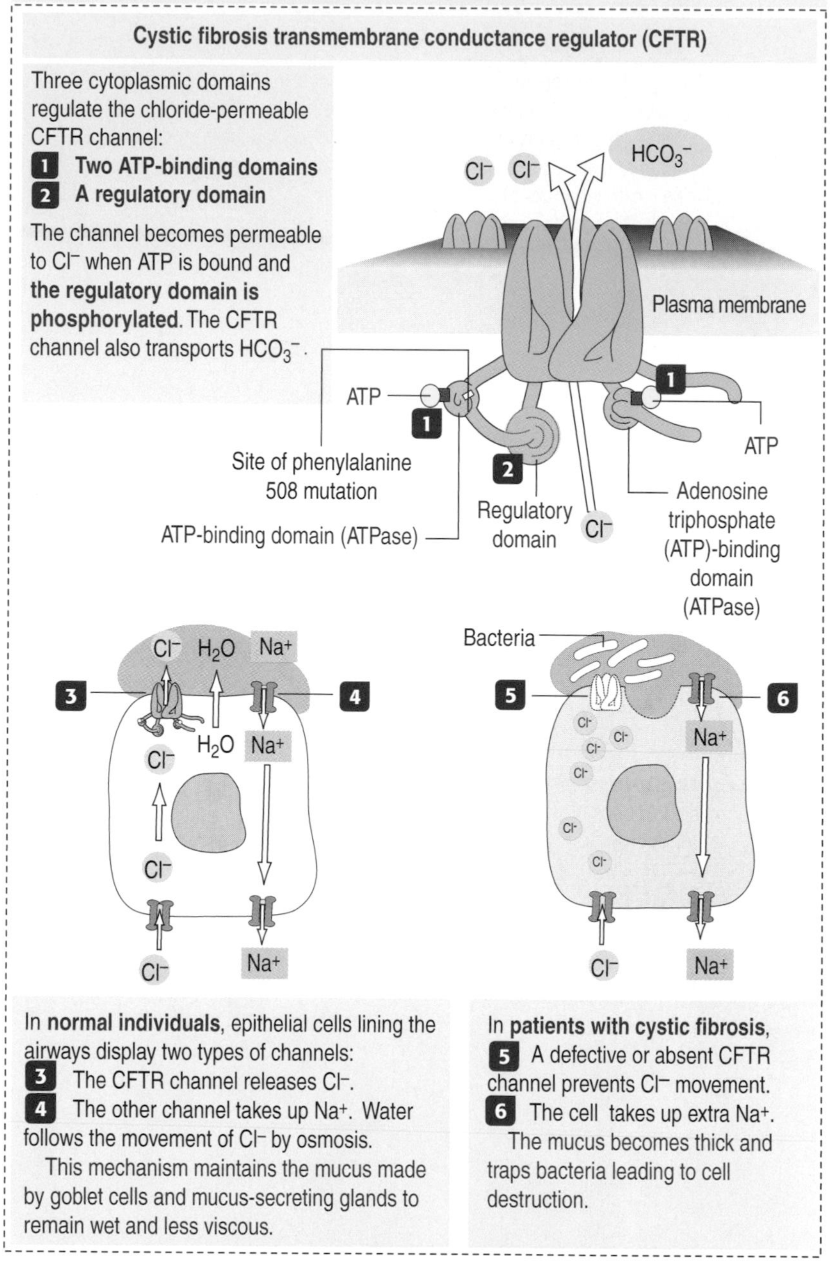
Cystic fibrosis transmembrane conductance regulator (CFTR)
Three cytoplasmic domains regulate the chloride-permeable CFTR channel:
1 Two ATP-binding domains
2 A regulatory domain
The channel becomes permeable to Cl⁻ when ATP is bound and the regulatory domain is phosphorylated. The CFTR channel also transports HCO3⁻.
Cl⁻ Cl⁻
HCO3⁻
Plasma membrane
ATP
1
Site of phenylalanine 508 mutation
ATP-binding domain (ATPase)
2
Regulatory domain
Cl⁻
1
ATP
Adenosine triphosphate (ATP)-binding domain (ATPase)
Cl⁻ H2O Na+
3
4
H2O Na+
Cl⁻
Cl⁻
Cl⁻
Na+
Bacteria
5
6
Cl⁻
Na+
Cl⁻
Na+
In normal individuals, epithelial cells lining the airways display two types of channels:
3 The CFTR channel releases Cl⁻.
4 The other channel takes up Na+. Water follows the movement of Cl⁻ by osmosis.
This mechanism maintains the mucus made by goblet cells and mucus-secreting glands to remain wet and less viscous.
In patients with cystic fibrosis,
5 A defective or absent CFTR channel prevents Cl⁻ movement.
6 The cell takes up extra Na+.
The mucus becomes thick and traps bacteria leading to cell destruction.

Treatment of the disease consists of physical therapy to facilitate bronchial drainage, antibiotic treatment of infections, and pancreatic enzyme replacement.

A defective transport of Cl^- by the submucosal glands of the respiratory mucosa, excretory ducts of sweat glands, and other epithelia is the cause of cystic fibrosis (see Figure 13-14).

The sequence of the **cystic fibrosis gene** on chromosome 7 shows that it encodes a protein called **cystic fibrosis transmembrane conductance regulator (CFTR)**, belonging to the **ABC transporter family**—so called because it contains adenosine triphosphate (ATP)-binding domains, or **A**TP-**b**inding **c**assettes, and requires ATP hydrolysis to transport ions, sugars, and amino acids. In 70% of patients with cystic fibrosis, the amino acid 508—of a total of 1480 amino acids in CFTR protein—is missing.

As a member of the ABC transporter family, CFTR is rather unusual because it appears to require both ATP hydrolysis and cyclic adenosine monophosphate (cAMP)–dependent phosphorylation to function as a Cl^- channel.

Figure 13-15. Subdivisions of the respiratory bronchiole: Alveolar duct, alveolar sac, and alveoli

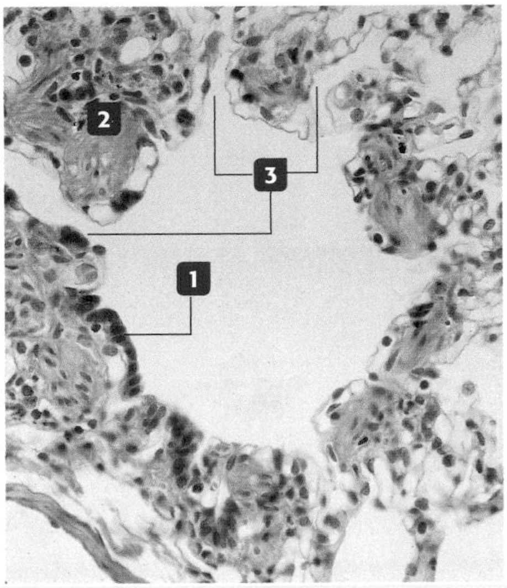

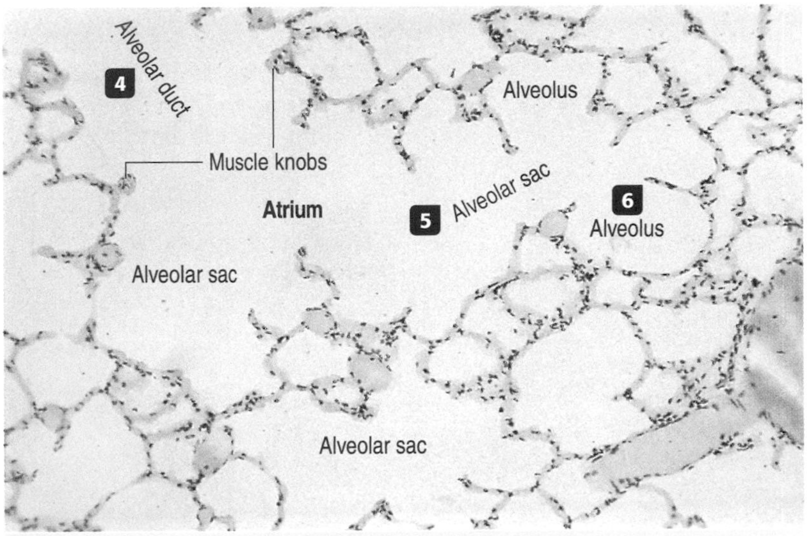

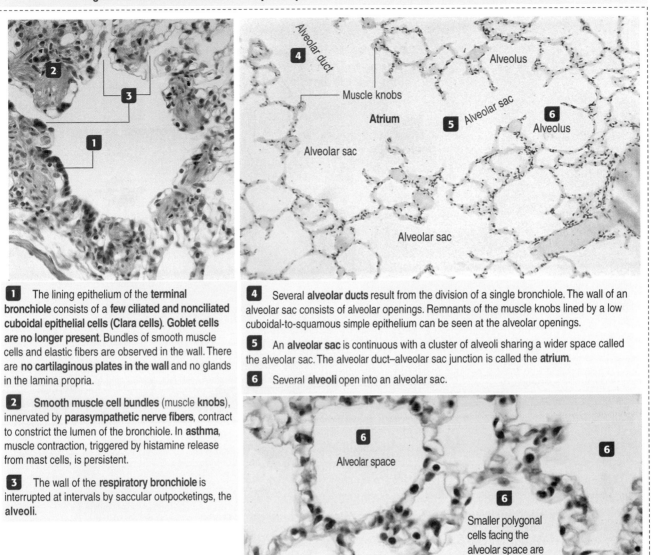

1 The lining epithelium of the **terminal bronchiole** consists of a **few ciliated and nonciliated cuboidal epithelial cells (Clara cells)**. **Goblet cells are no longer present**. Bundles of smooth muscle cells and elastic fibers are observed in the wall. There are **no cartilaginous plates in the wall** and no glands in the lamina propria.

2 **Smooth muscle cell bundles** (muscle **knobs**), innervated by **parasympathetic nerve fibers**, contract to constrict the lumen of the bronchiole. In **asthma**, muscle contraction, triggered by histamine release from mast cells, is persistent.

3 The wall of the **respiratory bronchiole** is interrupted at intervals by saccular outpocketings, the **alveoli**.

4 Several **alveolar ducts** result from the division of a single bronchiole. The wall of an alveolar sac consists of alveolar openings. Remnants of the muscle knobs lined by a low cuboidal-to-squamous simple epithelium can be seen at the alveolar openings.

5 An **alveolar sac** is continuous with a cluster of alveoli sharing a wider space called the alveolar sac. The alveolar duct–alveolar sac junction is called the **atrium**.

6 Several **alveoli** open into an alveolar sac.

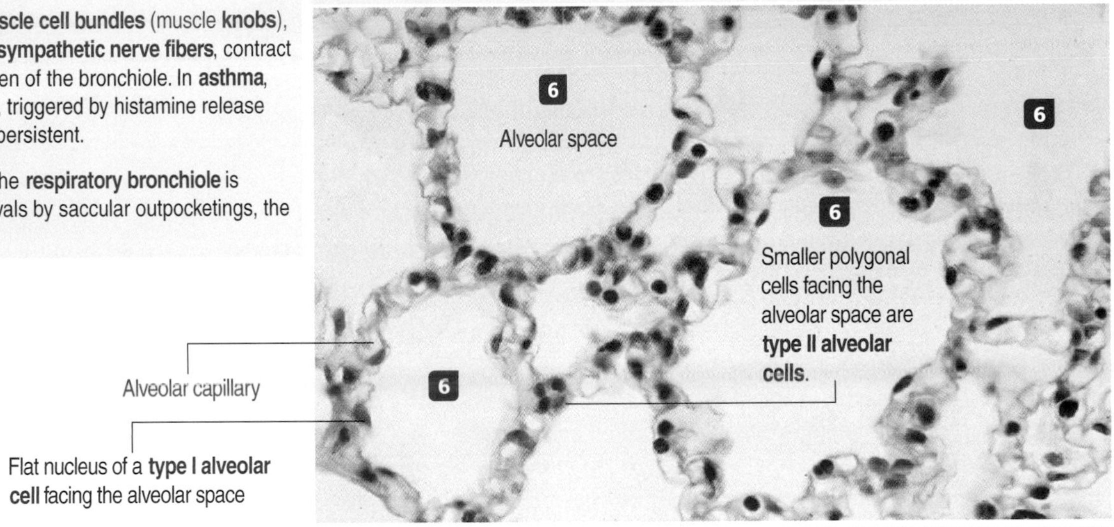

Inherited mutations of CFTR in patients with cystic fibrosis result in defective chloride transport and increased sodium absorption. The CFTR channel also transports **bicarbonate ions.** Inherited mutations of CFTR have now been shown to disrupt bicarbonate transport. We have mentioned above that the exocrine pancreas secretes digestive enzymes in a bicarbonate-rich fluid. The recently recognized role of **Clara cells in chloride transport** is of clinical significance.

The respiratory portion of the lung

Terminal bronchioles give rise to three generations of **respiratory bronchioles** (0.5 to 0.2 mm in diameter).

Respiratory bronchioles represent the transition from the conducting to the respiratory portion of the lung (Figure 13-15). They are lined initially by **simple cuboidal epithelial cells**, some of which are ciliated. The epithelium becomes **low cuboidal** and **nonciliated** in subsequent branches. The respiratory bronchiole

Figure 13-16. **Structure of the alveolus**

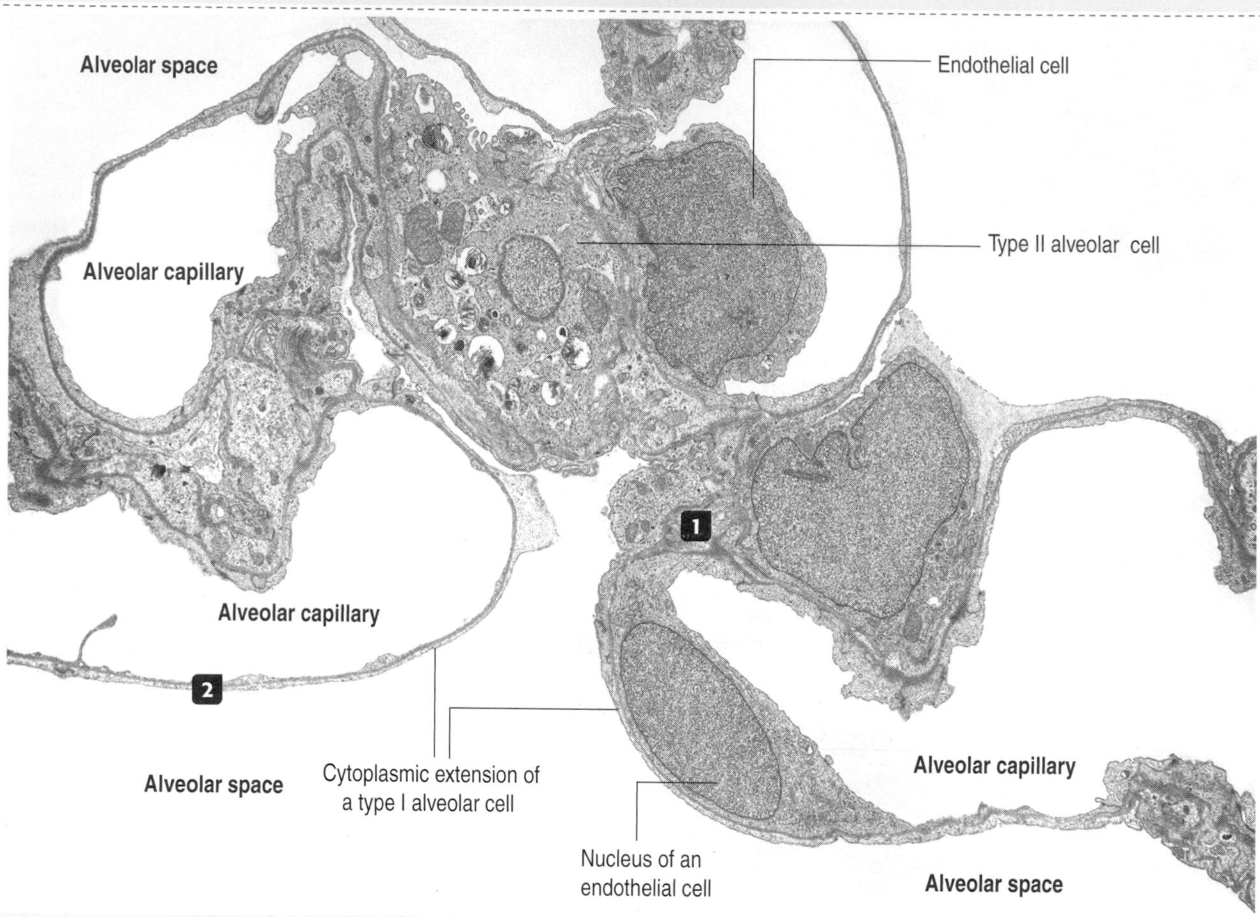

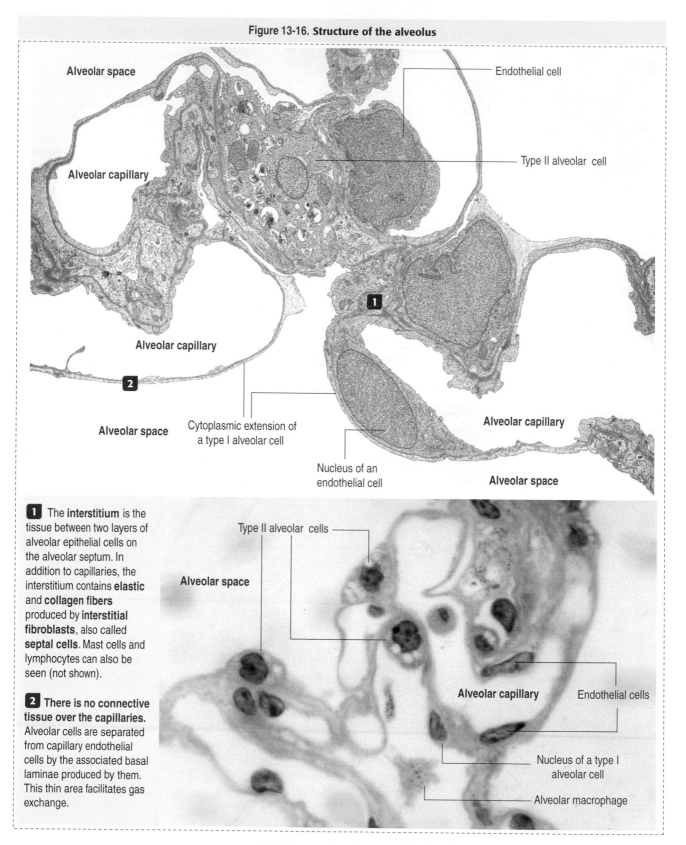

Alveolar space
Endothelial cell
Type II alveolar cell
Alveolar capillary
1
Alveolar capillary
2
Alveolar space
Cytoplasmic extension of a type I alveolar cell
Alveolar capillary
Nucleus of an endothelial cell
Alveolar space

1 The **interstitium** is the tissue between two layers of alveolar epithelial cells on the alveolar septum. In addition to capillaries, the interstitium contains **elastic** and **collagen fibers** produced by **interstitial fibroblasts**, also called **septal cells**. Mast cells and lymphocytes can also be seen (not shown).

2 There is no connective tissue over the capillaries. Alveolar cells are separated from capillary endothelial cells by the associated basal laminae produced by them. This thin area facilitates gas exchange.

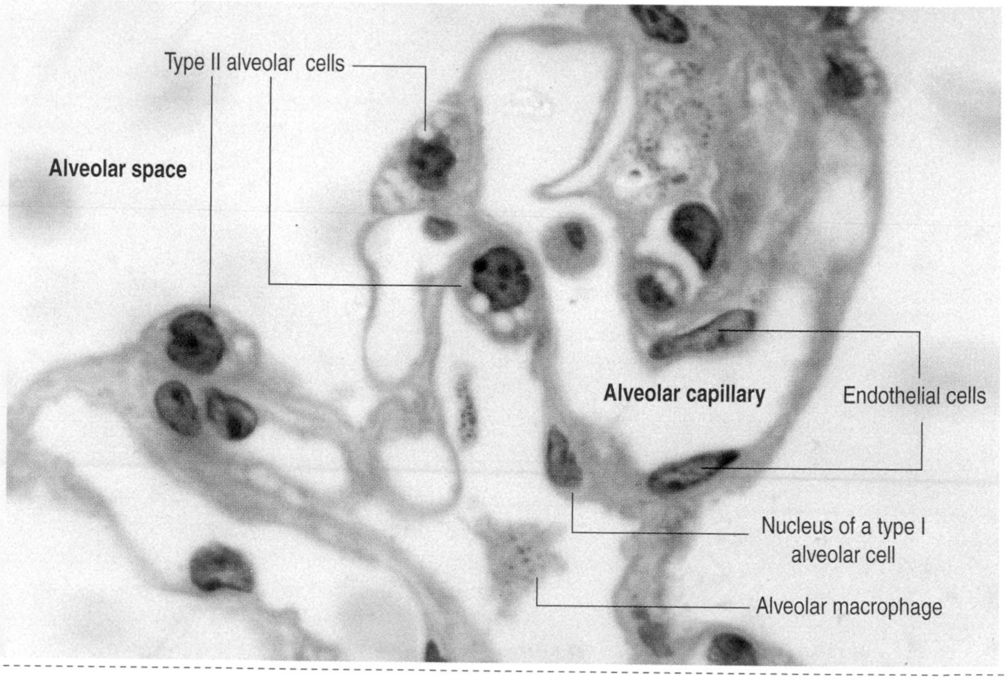

Type II alveolar cells
Alveolar space
Alveolar capillary
Endothelial cells
Nucleus of a type I alveolar cell
Alveolar macrophage

subdivides to give rise to an **alveolar duct** (see Figure 13-15). The alveolar duct is continuous with the **alveolar sac. Several alveoli open into an alveolar sac.**

The alveolus is the functional unit of the pulmonary acinus

About 300 million air sacs, or **alveoli,** in each lung provide a total surface area

Figure 13-17. Air-blood barrier

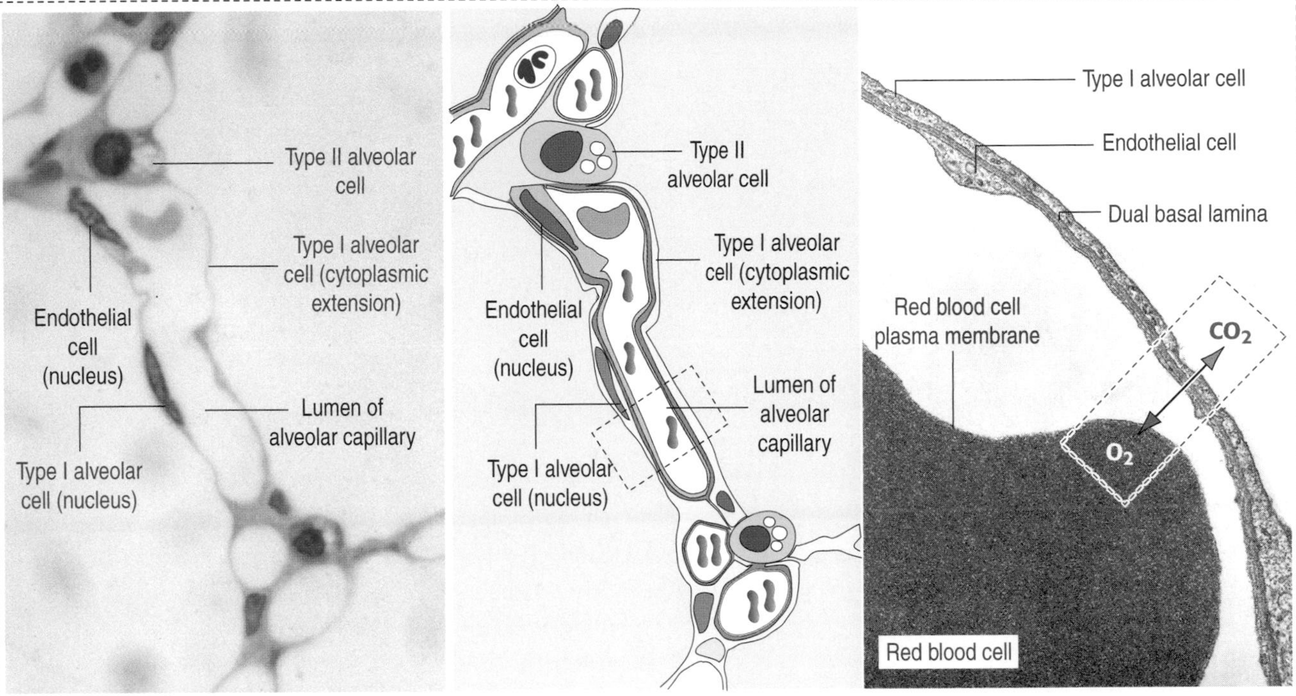

The lung is a gas-exchanging organ for the provision of O_2 to the blood and removal of CO_2 from the blood. Alveolar capillaries are closely apposed to the alveolar lumen.

Gas exchange by **passive diffusion** occurs across the **air-blood barrier** consisting of (1) cytoplasmic extensions of **type I alveolar cells**; (2) a **dual basal lamina**, synthesized by type I alveolar cells and endothelial cells; (3) cytoplasmic extensions of continuous **endothelial cells**; and (4) the plasma membrane of **red blood cells**.

Type II alveolar cells contribute indirectly to the gas-exchange process by secreting **surfactant**, a lipid-protein complex that reduces the surface tension of the alveolus and prevents alveolar collapsing.

Clinical significance: Alveolar gas exchange and acid-base balance

Changes in **partial pressure of CO_2** (designated Pco_2) caused by inadequate ventilation leads to **acid-base balance** disturbances and, consequently, to an alteration in **blood pH**.

An increase in Pco_2 decreases blood pH; a decrease of Pco_2 increases pH. An increase in ventilation decreases Pco_2. Pco_2 increases as ventilation decreases.

Both blood pH and Pco_2 are critical regulators of the ventilation rate sensed by **chemoreceptors**, located in the brain (medulla) and carotid and aortic bodies.

of 75 m^2 for oxygen and carbon dioxide exchange. Each alveolus has a thin wall with capillaries lined by **simple squamous epithelial cells** (Figure 13-16) forming part of the **air-blood barrier** (Figure 13-17).

The **alveolar epithelium** consists of two cell types (see Figures 13-16 and 13-17): (1) **type I alveolar cells**, representing about **40%** of the epithelial cell population but lining **90%** of the alveolar surface; and (2) **type II alveolar cells**, approximately **60%** of the cells, covering only **10%** of the alveolar surface area.

Each alveolus opens into an alveolar sac. However, a few of them open directly into the respiratory bronchiole (see Figure 13-15). **This particular feature distinguishes the respiratory bronchiole from the terminal bronchiole, whose wall is not associated with alveoli.**

The low cuboidal epithelium of the respiratory bronchiole is continuous with the squamous type I alveolar cells of the alveolus (see Figure 13-9).

Additional cells of the alveolar septa are the **alveolar macrophages** (Figure 13-18) (also called **dust cells**; they are derived from bone-marrow monocytes and frequently seen in the alveolar lumen), **fibroblasts** (producing elastic fibers), and **mast cells**. Alveolar capillaries are lined by continuous endothelial cells juxtaposed to type I alveolar cells through a dual basal lamina produced by these two cells. Alveolar endothelial cells contain **angiotensin-converting enzyme** for

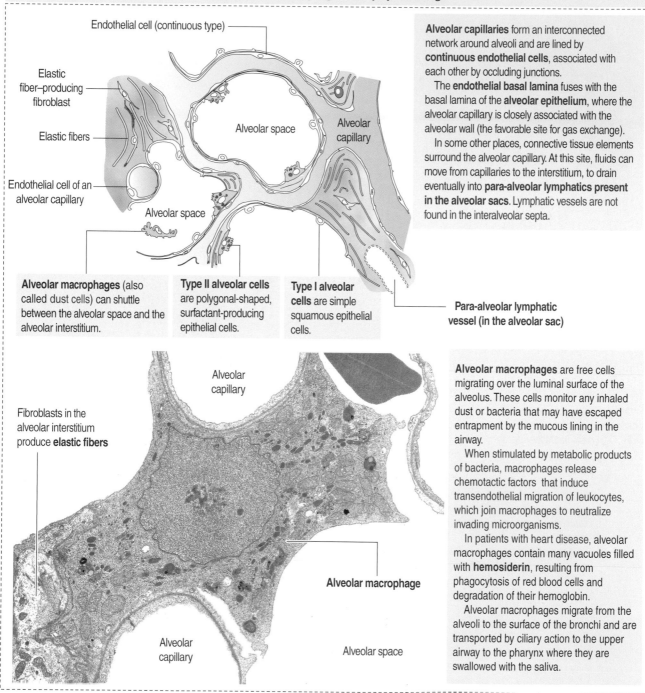

Figure 13-18. Macrophages and lymph drainage

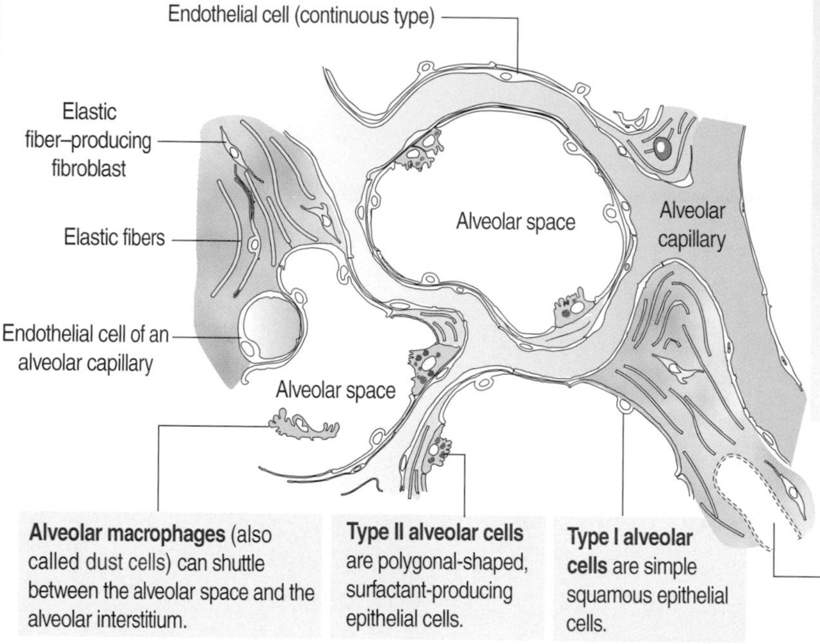

Endothelial cell (continuous type)
Elastic fiber–producing fibroblast
Elastic fibers
Endothelial cell of an alveolar capillary
Alveolar space
Alveolar capillary
Alveolar space
Alveolar macrophages (also called dust cells) can shuttle between the alveolar space and the alveolar interstitium.
Type II alveolar cells are polygonal-shaped, surfactant-producing epithelial cells.
Type I alveolar cells are simple squamous epithelial cells.
Para-alveolar lymphatic vessel (in the alveolar sac)

Alveolar capillaries form an interconnected network around alveoli and are lined by **continuous endothelial cells**, associated with each other by occluding junctions.

The **endothelial basal lamina** fuses with the basal lamina of the **alveolar epithelium**, where the alveolar capillary is closely associated with the alveolar wall (the favorable site for gas exchange).

In some other places, connective tissue elements surround the alveolar capillary. At this site, fluids can move from capillaries to the interstitium, to drain eventually into **para-alveolar lymphatics present in the alveolar sacs.** Lymphatic vessels are not found in the interalveolar septa.

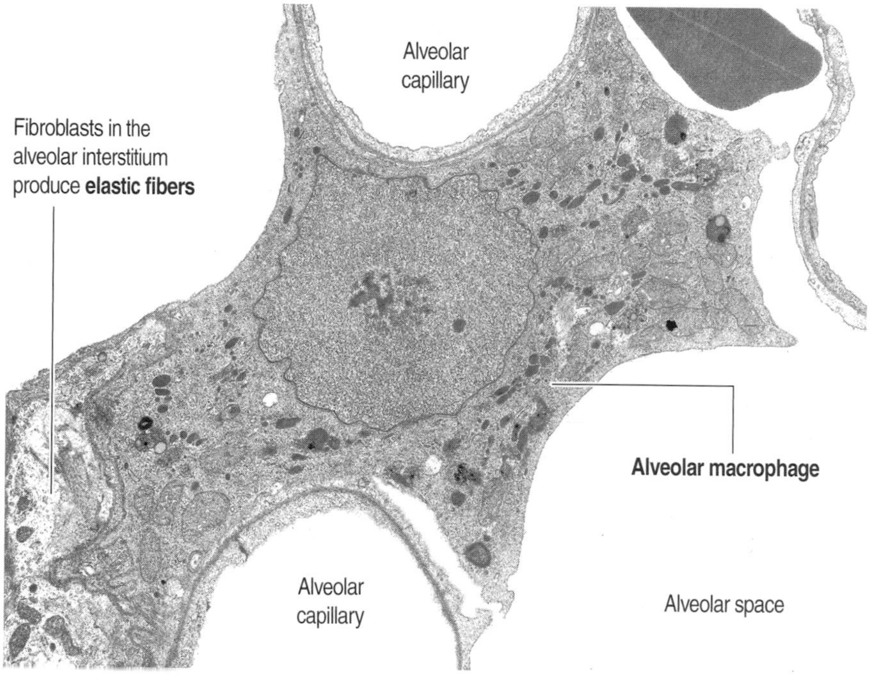

Alveolar capillary
Fibroblasts in the alveolar interstitium produce **elastic fibers**
Alveolar macrophage
Alveolar capillary
Alveolar space

Alveolar macrophages are free cells migrating over the luminal surface of the alveolus. These cells monitor any inhaled dust or bacteria that may have escaped entrapment by the mucous lining in the airway.

When stimulated by metabolic products of bacteria, macrophages release chemotactic factors that induce transendothelial migration of leukocytes, which join macrophages to neutralize invading microorganisms.

In patients with heart disease, alveolar macrophages contain many vacuoles filled with **hemosiderin**, resulting from phagocytosis of red blood cells and degradation of their hemoglobin.

Alveolar macrophages migrate from the alveoli to the surface of the bronchi and are transported by ciliary action to the upper airway to the pharynx where they are swallowed with the saliva.

the conversion of angiotensin I to angiotensin II (see Figure 14-18 in Chapter 14, Urinary System).

Type II alveolar cells secrete pulmonary surfactant

Type II alveolar cells are predominantly located at the **angles formed by adjacent alveolar septa.** Contrasting with the more squamous type I alveolar cells, type II alveolar cells are polygonal-shaped and extend beyond the level of the surrounding epithelium.

The free surface of type II alveolar cells is covered by short microvilli. The cytoplasm displays dense membrane-bound **lamellar bodies**, representing secretory granules containing **pulmonary surfactant** (Figure 13-19).

Figure 13-19. **Type II alveolar cell**

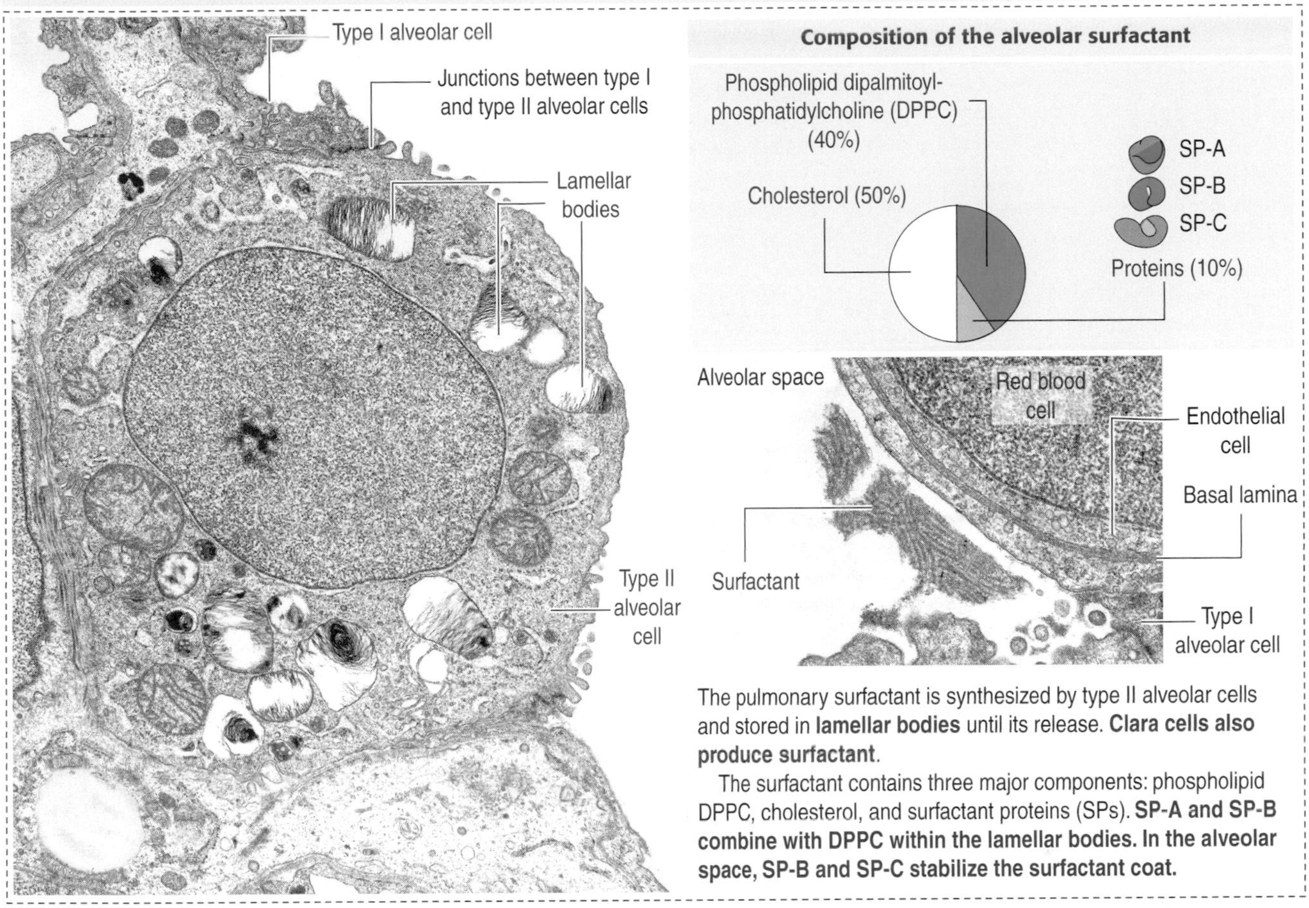

Type I alveolar cell
Junctions between type I and type II alveolar cells
Lamellar bodies
Type II alveolar cell
Composition of the alveolar surfactant
Phospholipid dipalmitoyl-phosphatidylcholine (DPPC) (40%)
Cholesterol (50%)
SP-A
SP-B
SP-C
Proteins (10%)
Alveolar space
Red blood cell
Endothelial cell
Basal lamina
Surfactant
Type I alveolar cell

The pulmonary surfactant is synthesized by type II alveolar cells and stored in **lamellar bodies** until its release. **Clara cells also produce surfactant.**

The surfactant contains three major components: phospholipid DPPC, cholesterol, and surfactant proteins (SPs). **SP-A and SP-B combine with DPPC within the lamellar bodies. In the alveolar space, SP-B and SP-C stabilize the surfactant coat.**

Surfactant is released by exocytosis and spreads over a thin layer of fluid that normally coats the alveolar surface. By this mechanism, the **pulmonary surfactant lowers the surface tension at the air-fluid interface and thus reduces the tendency of the alveolus to collapse at the end of expiration.** Clara cells, located in terminal bronchioles, also secrete pulmonary surfactant.

The pulmonary surfactant contains (1) **phospholipids**, (2) **cholesterol**, and (3) **proteins** (see Figure 13-19).

Specific surfactant proteins (SPs) consist of one **hydrophilic glycoprotein** (SP-A) and two **hydrophobic proteins** (**SP-B** and **SP-C**).

Within the lamellar bodies, SP-A and SP-B transform the **phospholipid dipalmitoylphosphatidylcholine** (**DPPC**) into a mature surfactant molecule.

In the alveolar space, SP-B and SP-C **stabilize** the phospholipid layer and enhance the surfactant action of the phospholipid DPPC–protein complex (Figure 13–20).

Surfactant turnover is facilitated by the phagocytic function of alveolar macrophages (see Figures 13-18 and 13-20).

An additional function of type II alveolar cells is the **maintenance and repair of the alveolar epithelium when injury occurs.** When type I alveolar cells are damaged, type II alveolar cells increase in number and differentiate into type I alveolar-like cells (see Figure 13-20).

Clinical significance: Acute respiratory distress syndrome

The significance of the cell components of the alveolus becomes clear when we analyze the relevant aspects of the acute respiratory distress syndrome (ARDS).

ARDS results from a disruption of the normal barrier that prevents leakage of fluid of the alveolar capillaries into the interstitium and alveolar spaces.

Figure 13-20. Assembly and degradation of alveolar surfactant

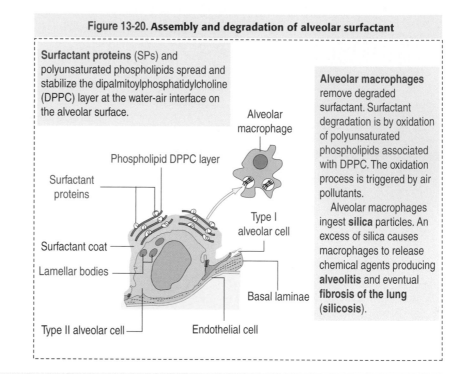

Surfactant proteins (SPs) and polyunsaturated phospholipids spread and stabilize the dipalmitoylphosphatidylcholine (DPPC) layer at the water-air interface on the alveolar surface.

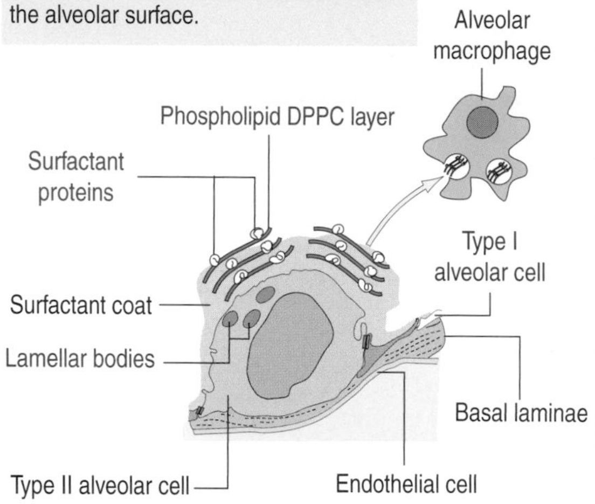

Alveolar macrophages remove degraded surfactant. Surfactant degradation is by oxidation of polyunsaturated phospholipids associated with DPPC. The oxidation process is triggered by air pollutants.

Alveolar macrophages ingest **silica** particles. An excess of silica causes macrophages to release chemical agents producing **alveolitis** and eventual **fibrosis of the lung** (**silicosis**).

Figure 13-21. Acute respiratory distress syndrome (ARDS) and pulmonary edema

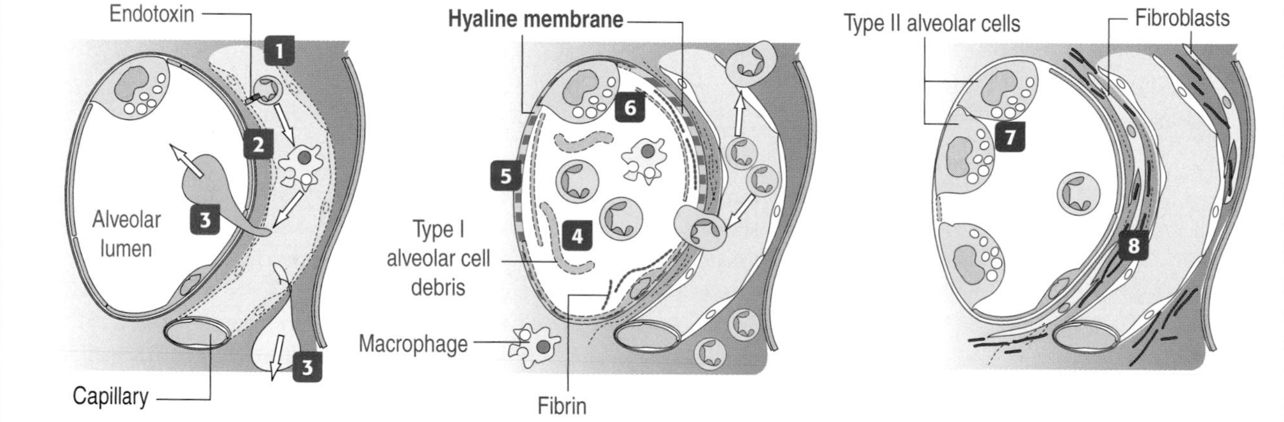

1 Endotoxin induces the release of proinflammatory substances that induce the attachment of neutrophils to endothelial cells.

2 Neutrophils release proteolytic enzymes and, together with endotoxin, damage the endothelial cells. Macrophages are activated by inflammatory cytokines and contribute to the endothelial cell damage.

3 The alveolar-capillary barrier becomes permeable and cells and fluid enter the interstitium and alveolar space.

4 Following the endothelial cell injury, type I alveolar cells die, denuding the alveolar side of the barrier. Neutrophils and macrophages are seen in the alveolar lumen and interstitium.

5 Fibrin and cell debris accumulated in the alveolar lumen form a **hyaline membrane**.

6 Fibrin inhibits the synthesis of surfactant by type II alveolar cells.

7 A repair process can restore normal function or cause progressive fibrosis. Type II alveolar cells proliferate, reestablish the production of surfactant, and differentiate into type I alveolar cells.

8 If the initial damage is severe, interstitial fibroblasts proliferate, progressive interstitial and intra-alveolar fibrosis develops, and gas exchange is seriously affected.

Cardiogenic pulmonary edema

A dysfunction of the left ventricle is the main cause of this type of pulmonary edema.

Pulmonary capillaries are dilated and an increase in hydrostatic pressure leads to interstitial and alveolar edema.

Abundant leukocytes and red blood cells and protein-rich fluid are visualized in the lumen of dilated alveoli.

Figure 13-22. Neonatal respiratory distress syndrome

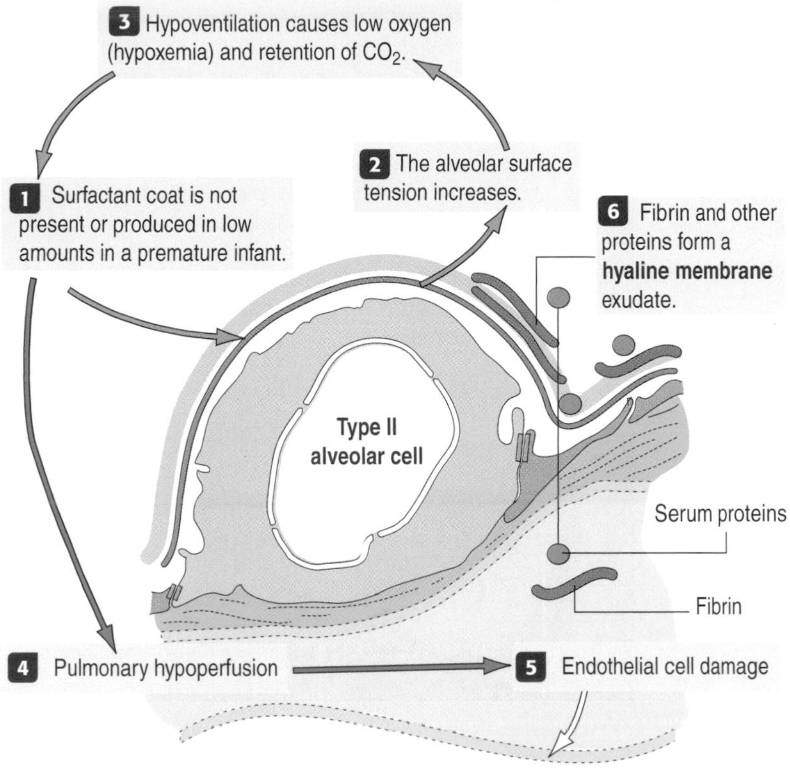

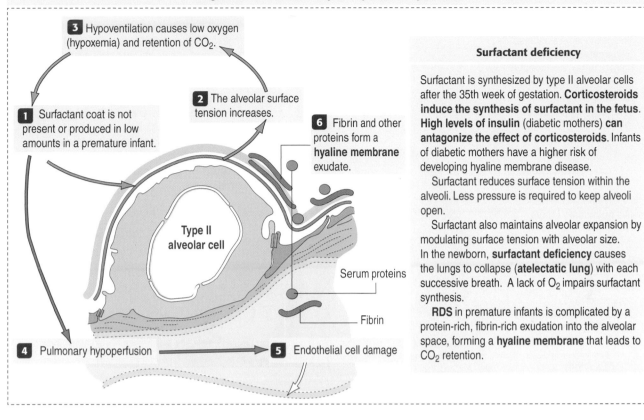

3 Hypoventilation causes low oxygen (hypoxemia) and retention of CO_2.
2 The alveolar surface tension increases.
1 Surfactant coat is not present or produced in low amounts in a premature infant.
6 Fibrin and other proteins form a hyaline membrane exudate.
Type II alveolar cell
Serum proteins
Fibrin
4 Pulmonary hypoperfusion
5 Endothelial cell damage

Surfactant deficiency

Surfactant is synthesized by type II alveolar cells after the 35th week of gestation. **Corticosteroids induce the synthesis of surfactant in the fetus. High levels of insulin** (diabetic mothers) **can antagonize the effect of corticosteroids.** Infants of diabetic mothers have a higher risk of developing hyaline membrane disease.

Surfactant reduces surface tension within the alveoli. Less pressure is required to keep alveoli open.

Surfactant also maintains alveolar expansion by modulating surface tension with alveolar size. In the newborn, **surfactant deficiency** causes the lungs to collapse (**atelectatic lung**) with each successive breath. A lack of O_2 impairs surfactant synthesis.

RDS in premature infants is complicated by a protein-rich, fibrin-rich exudation into the alveolar space, forming a **hyaline membrane** that leads to CO_2 retention.

Two mechanisms can alter the alveolar barrier. In the first mechanism, an **increase in hydrostatic pressure in the alveolar capillaries**—caused, for example, by failure of the left ventricle or stenosis of the mitral valve—results in increased fluid and proteins in the alveolar spaces. The resulting edema is called **cardiogenic** or **hydrostatic pulmonary edema**.

In the second mechanism, the hydrostatic pressure is normal, but the endothelial lining of the alveolar capillaries or the epithelial lining of the alveoli is damaged. Inhalation of agents such as smoke, water (near drowning), or bacterial endotoxins (resulting from sepsis); or trauma can cause a defect in **permeability**. A cardiac component may or may not be involved. Although the resulting edema is called **noncardiogenic**, it can coexist with a cardiogenic condition.

A common pathologic pattern of diffuse alveolar damage (Figure 13-21) can be observed in cardiogenic and noncardiogenic ARDS. The **first phase** of ARDS is an **acute exudative process** defined by interstitial and alveolar edema, neutrophil infiltration, hemorrhage, and deposits of fibrin. Cellular debris, resulting from dead type I alveolar cells, and fibrin deposited in the alveolar space form **hyaline membranes** (Figure 13-22).

The **second phase** is a **proliferative process** in which alveolar cells proliferate and differentiate to restore the epithelial alveolar lining, returning gas exchange to normal in most cases. In other cases, the interstitium displays inflammatory cells and fibroblasts. Fibroblasts proliferate and invade the alveolar spaces through gaps of the basal lamina. The hyaline membranes either are removed by phagocytosis by macrophages or are invaded by fibroblasts.

The **third phase** is **chronic fibrosis** and occlusion of blood vessels. Because ARDS is part of a systemic inflammatory response, the outcome of the lung process depends on improvement of the systemic condition. The prognosis for return to normal lung function is good.

The diagnosis of ARDS is based on clinical (dyspnea, cyanosis, and tachypnea) and radiologic examination. Treatment is focused on neutralizing the disorder

Figure 13-23. Blood supply and lymph drainage of the pulmonary lobule

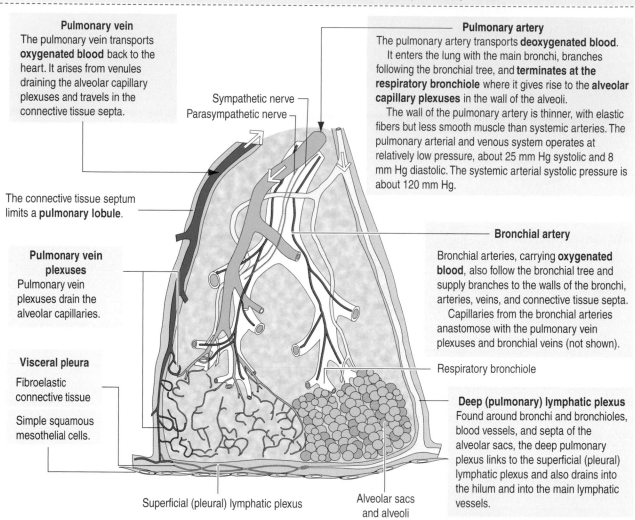

Pulmonary vein
The pulmonary vein transports **oxygenated blood** back to the heart. It arises from venules draining the alveolar capillary plexuses and travels in the connective tissue septa.

Pulmonary artery
The pulmonary artery transports **deoxygenated blood**.
It enters the lung with the main bronchi, branches following the bronchial tree, and **terminates at the respiratory bronchiole** where it gives rise to the **alveolar capillary plexuses** in the wall of the alveoli.
The wall of the pulmonary artery is thinner, with elastic fibers but less smooth muscle than systemic arteries. The pulmonary arterial and venous system operates at relatively low pressure, about 25 mm Hg systolic and 8 mm Hg diastolic. The systemic arterial systolic pressure is about 120 mm Hg.

The connective tissue septum limits a **pulmonary lobule**.

Pulmonary vein plexuses
Pulmonary vein plexuses drain the alveolar capillaries.

Bronchial artery
Bronchial arteries, carrying **oxygenated blood**, also follow the bronchial tree and supply branches to the walls of the bronchi, arteries, veins, and connective tissue septa.
Capillaries from the bronchial arteries anastomose with the pulmonary vein plexuses and bronchial veins (not shown).

Visceral pleura
Fibroelastic connective tissue
Simple squamous mesothelial cells.

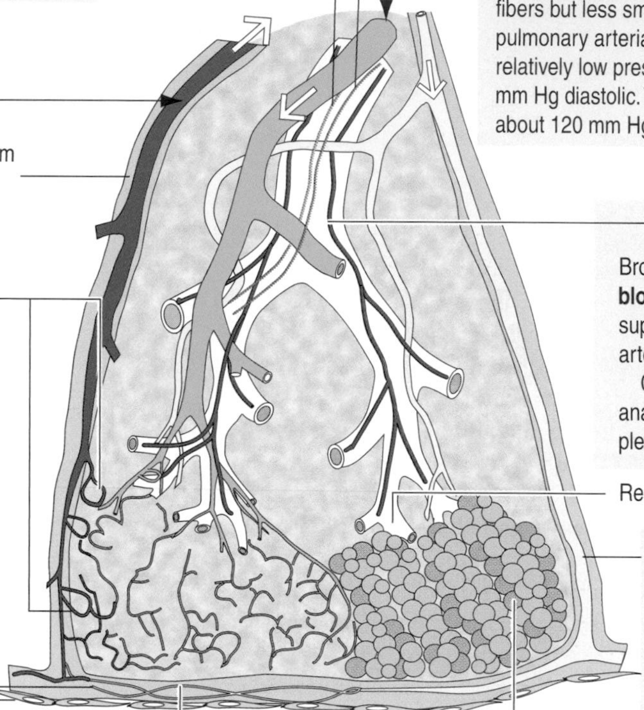

Deep (pulmonary) lymphatic plexus
Found around bronchi and bronchioles, blood vessels, and septa of the alveolar sacs, the deep pulmonary plexus links to the superficial (pleural) lymphatic plexus and also drains into the hilum and into the main lymphatic vessels.

Disorders of the pleura

Pleuritic chest pain: A symptom resulting from inflammation of the pleural surfaces. The pain originates in the parietal pleura, innervated by the intercostal nerves.
Pleural effusion: Abnormal accumulation of liquid in the pleural space. Large pleural effusion restricts pulmonary function because air spaces and pulmonary circulation are compressed.
Hydrothorax: Accumulation of water may be an early sign of congestive heart failure. It is also observed in cirrhosis, malignant disease, and pulmonary embolism.
Hemothorax: Direct hemorrhage into the pleural space resulting from trauma to the thorax (rib fracture or penetrating object).
Chylothorax: Accumulation of chyle, a lipid-rich liquid transported from intestinal lacteals to systemic veins in the thorax through the thoracic duct. Obstruction or disruption of the thoracic duct by mediastinal tumors are the most common cause of chylothorax.
Pneumothorax: Accumulation of air in the pleural space indicates disruption of the visceral or parietal pleura after tracheobronchial rupture or focal pulmonary destructive processes (AIDS).

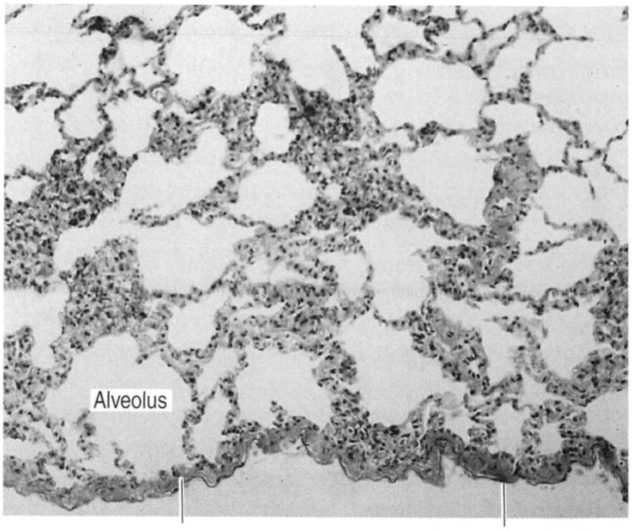

Fibroelastic connective tissue with blood and lymphatic vessels and nerves

Mesothelial cell lining

Visceral pleura

causing ARDS and providing support of gas exchange until the condition improves.

Pleura

The pleura consists of two layers: (1) a **visceral layer** and (2) a **parietal layer.**

The **visceral layer** is closely attached to the lung. It is lined by a **simple squamous epithelium**, called **mesothelium**, and consists of cells with **apical microvilli** resting on a basal lamina applied to a connective tissue rich in **elastic fibers** (Figure 13-23). This connective tissue is continuous with the interlobular and interlobar septa of the lung. The parietal layer is also lined by the mesothelium.

The **visceral layer** seals the lung surface, preventing leakage of air into the thoracic cavity. The **parietal layer** is thicker and lines the inner surface of the thoracic cavity. A very thin liquid film in between the visceral and parietal layers permits the smooth gliding of one layer against the other.

Blood vessels to the visceral pleura derive from pulmonary and bronchial blood vessels (see Figure 13-23). The vascular supply to the parietal pleura derives from the systemic blood vessels. Branches of the phrenic and intercostal nerves are found in the parietal pleura; the visceral pleura receives branches of the vagus and sympathetic nerves supplying the bronchi.

Clinical significance: Disorders of the pleura

Under **normal conditions**, the visceral pleura glides smoothly on the parietal pleura during respiration. However, during an **inflammatory process**, characteristic friction sounds can be detected during the physical examination.

If fluid accumulates in the pleural cavity (**hydrothorax**), the lung collapses gradually and the mediastinum is displaced toward the opposite site. The presence of air in the pleural cavity (**pneumothorax**), caused by a penetrating wound, rupture of the lung, or injections for therapeutic reasons (to immobilize the lung in the treatment of tuberculosis), also collapses the lung.

Collapse of the lung is caused by the recoil properties of its elastic fibers. In the normal lung, such a recoil is prevented by negative intrapleural pressure and the close association of the parietal and visceral layers of the pleura.

Mesothelioma is a tumor that originates in the mesothelial cell lining of the pleura, the peritoneum, and the pericardium. Mesothelioma is associated with previous long exposure (15 to 40 years) to asbestos. Pleural mesothelioma spreads within the thoracic cavity (pericardium or diaphragm) and metastasis can involve any organ, including brain. Symptoms include pleural effusion, chest pain, or dyspnea. Organ imaging studies of the thorax can detect thickening of the pleura (asbestos plaques) and fluid containing tumoral cells.

• The respiratory system consists of three portions: (1) an air-conducting portion; (2) a respiratory portion for gas exchange between blood and air; and (3) a mechanism of ventilation, controlled by the inspiratory and expiratory movements of the thoracic cage.

• The air-conducting portion consists of the nasal cavities and associated sinuses, the nasopharynx, the oropharynx, the larynx, the trachea, the bronchi, and the bronchioles. The respiratory portion includes the respiratory bronchioles, alveolar ducts, alveolar sacs, and alveoli. The ventilation mechanism involves the thoracic or rib cage, intercostal muscles, the diaphragm muscle, and the elastic connective tissue of the lung.

• The functions of the nasal cavity and paranasal sinuses is warming and moistening air and filtering dust particles present in the inspired air. The respiratory portion is lined by pseudostratified ciliated epithelium with goblet cells supported by a lamina propria consisting of connective tissue, seromucous glands, and a rich superficial venous plexus (called cavernous or erectile tissue). Incoming air is warmed by blood in the venous plexus and moistened by secretions of the seromucous glands and goblet cells. The superior, middle, and inferior turbinate bones, or conchae, determine airflow disturbance to facilitate warming and moistening of air. Paranasal sinuses (maxillary, frontal, ethmoidal, and sphenoidal sinuses) are lined by a thin pseudostratified columnar ciliated epithelium with few goblet cells.

• The nasopharynx is lined by a pseudostratified columnar epithelium that changes to nonkeratinizing squamous epithelium at the oropharynx. Aggregates of mucosa-associated lymphoid tissue, forming part of Waldeyer's ring, are present at the nasopharynx.

• The olfactory area is present on the roof of the nasal cavity. The mucosa of the olfactory area consists of pseudostratified ciliated columnar epithelium with goblet cells flanking the olfactory epithelium. The olfactory epithelium consists of three cell types: olfactory cells (bipolar neurons), basal cells (stem cells that differentiate into olfactory cells), and sustentacular or supporting cells. The underlying lamina propria contains the superficial venous plexus, the glands of Bowman, and nerve bundles (called fila olfactoria).

The olfactory cell has two regions: an apical region (the dendrite) characterized by an apical knob bearing nonmotile olfactory cilia. Olfactory cilia contain odorant receptors that bind to odorant-binding proteins (produced by the gland of Bowman) carrying an inhaled odorant particle. On the opposite site of the ciliary dendritic region, olfactory cells form small fascicles of unmyelinated axons surrounded by ensheathing glial cells. Axons penetrate the cribriform plate of the ethmoid bone and synapse with neurons in the olfactory bulb. The axons of the olfactory cells converge to one or more glomeruli and interact predominantly with dendrites of mitral cells. The olfactory bulb also contains interneurons called granule cells and tufted cells. Axons from mitral cells and tufted cells form the olfactory tract (olfactory nerve or cranial nerve I), which carries olfactory information to the olfactory cortex.

The odorant–odorant binding protein complex attaches to receptors on cilia. Binding of the odorant receptor activates G protein coupled to the receptor. G protein activates adenylyl cyclase, which catalyzes the production of cAMP from ATP. Ligand-gated Na^+ channels are opened by cAMP to facilitate the diffusion of Na^+ into the cell. The influx of Na^+ across the plasma membrane generates an action potential conducted to the brain along the olfactory nerve.

Anosmia refers to deprivation of the sense of smell by disease or injury. Olfactory cells have a lifespan of about 1 to 2 months and are replaced throughout life by undifferentiated basal cells. Sensory endings of the trigeminal nerve, found in the olfactory epithelium, are responsible for the harmful sensation caused by irritants such as ammonia.

• The larynx consists of cartilages (epiglottis, thyroid cartilage, cricoid cartilage, and arytenoid cartilage), intrinsic muscles (abductor, adductors, and tensors involved in phonation), and extrinsic muscles (involved in swallowing). A nonkeratinizing stratified squamous epithelium covers the lingual surface of the epiglottis and the true vocal cords (also called folds). The rest is lined by a pseudostratified ciliated epithelium with goblet cells and seromucous glands in the lamina propria.

The lamina propria of the true vocal cords has special characteristics of clinical significance. The superficial layer (under the stratified squamous epithelium) consists of extracellular matrix and very few elastic fibers and fibroblasts. This layer, called Reinke's space, can accumulate fluid (Reinke's edema). The subjacent layers contain elastic and collagen fibers corresponding to the vocal ligament. Deep in the lamina propria is the vocalis (thyroarytenoid) muscle. There are no seromucous glands in the lamina propria of the true vocal cord.

• The trachea is lined by pseudostratified columnar ciliated epithelium with goblet cells. Basal cells and cells of Kulchitsky (neuroendocrine cells) rest on the basal lamina but do not extend to the lumen. The lamina propria contains elastic fibers. Seromucous glands are observed in the submucosa. A stack of C-shaped hyaline cartilage forms the framework of the trachea. The trachealis muscle (smooth muscle) connects the free ends of the C-shaped hyaline cartilage.

Bronchial carcinoid tumors arise from cells of Kulchitsky. These cells secrete peptide hormones (serotonin, somatostatin, calcitonin, antidiuretic hormone [ADH], adrenocorticotropic hormone [ACTH], and others). Bronchial carcinoid tumors (including small-cell lung carcinoma) can invade locally and metastasize to regional lymph nodes.

• As bronchi divide into intrapulmonary bronchi, the tracheal C-shaped rings break down into cartilage plates (distributed around the lumen) and smooth muscle bundles shift between the mucosa and the cartilage plates.

Aggregates of lymphoid tissue are observed in the wall of intrapulmonary bronchi (known collectively as BALT, bronchial-associated lymphoid tissue).

Further subdivisions give rise to terminal bronchioles, each supplying a pulmonary lobule. Each respiratory bronchiole, subdivisions of a terminal bronchiole, gives rise to a pulmonary or lung acinus. Essentially, a pulmonary lobule consists of several pulmonary acini. Relevant features of the wall of the terminal and respiratory bronchioles are the spiral-like arrangement of smooth muscle fibers and the longitudinal distribution of elastic fibers.

Branches of the pulmonary artery, transporting deoxygenated blood, run parallel to the bronchial tree. Branches of the bronchial artery provide nutrients to the walls of the bronchial tree. Recall that the pulmonary vein, carrying oxygenated blood, travels in the connective tissue septa limiting pulmonary lobules.

Asthma, characterized by both reversible bronchoconstriction of the smooth muscle bundles encircling the bronchiolar lumen and mucus hypersecretion by goblet cells triggered by allergens or autonomic neural factors, leads to a reduction in the lumen of the airways. Wheezing, cough, and shortness of breath (dyspnea) are classic symptoms.

• Terminal bronchioles lack cartilage and submucosal glands

and the pseudostratified columnar ciliated epithelium decreases in height to finally become low columnar-to-cuboidal with few ciliated cells. Surfactant-secreting Clara cells predominate in the terminal bronchiole. Remember that the terminal bronchiole is the initiation site of a pulmonary lobule.

Cystic fibrosis results in the production of abnormally thick mucus by glands lining the respiratory and gastrointestinal tracts. Inherited mutations of cystic fibrosis transmembrane conductance regulator (CFTR) result in defective Cl^- transport and increased Na^+ absorption. Bacterial infections are associated with the thick mucus plugs. Cough, purulent secretions, and dyspnea are typical symptoms.

• The wall of a respiratory bronchiole is discontinuous, interrupted by the saccular outpocketing of alveoli. Note that the wall of terminal bronchioles is not associated with alveoli. Bundles of smooth muscle fibers form knobs bulging into the lumen and the lining epithelium is cuboidal-to-simple squamous. Elastic fibers are important components of the bronchioles and alveolar walls.

Emphysema is caused by a permanent enlargement of the air spaces distal to the terminal bronchioles due to the progressive and irreversible destruction of elastic tissue of the alveolar walls. Elastic tissue in the interalveolar wall can be destroyed by elastase released by neutrophils present in the alveolar lumen. Serum α_1-antitrypsin neutralizes elastase. A persistent stimulus increases the number of neutrophils in the alveolar lumen, the source of elastase. Serum levels of α_1-antitrypsin decrease and elastase starts the destruction of elastic fibers. Damaged elastic fibers cannot recoil when stretched and, as a result, adjacent alveoli become confluent, producing large air spaces, or blebs, the structural landmark of emphysema. The loss of elastic tissue also affects terminal and respiratory bronchioles.

Chronic obstructive pulmonary disease (COPD) includes emphysema and asthma.

• The respiratory bronchiole represents the interface between the conducting and respiratory portions of the respiratory tract. The respiratory bronchiole is regarded as the beginning of the respiratory portion. Remember that the respiratory bronchiole is the initiation site of a pulmonary or lung acinus.

Each respiratory bronchiole gives rise to alveolar ducts, alveolar sacs, and alveoli. The alveolar epithelium consists of two cell types lining the surface of the capillaries (terminal branches of the pulmonary artery), and the alveolar wall. Type I alveolar cells represent about 40% of the alveolar epithelial cell population and cover 90% of the alveolar surface. Type II alveolar cells, about 60% of the cells, cover only 10% of the alveolar surface and are preferentially located at the angles formed by adjacent alveolar septa. Type II alveolar cells produce surfactant.

Pulmonary surfactant contains cholesterol (50%), phospholipids (40%), and SP (surfactant protein) SP-A, SP-B, and SP-C (10%). Clara cells also produce surfactant. Surfactant maintains alveolar expansion by modulating surface tension.

Additional components of the alveolus include endothelial cells (lining the alveolar capillaries), macrophages (alveolar phagocytes or dust cells), fibroblasts in the interalveolar septum (producing elastic fibers), and mast cells.

Neonatal respiratory distress syndrome (RDS) in premature infants is caused by surfactant deficiency leading to the collapse of the alveolar walls. The development of a fibrin-rich exudation, covering with a hyaline membrane the alveolar surface, complicates the RDS condition. Corticosteroids induce the synthesis of surfactant in the fetus. High levels of insulin in diabetic mothers antagonize the effect of corticosteroids.

• The air-blood barrier consists of (1) the thin cytoplasmic extensions of type I alveolar cells, (2) a dual basal lamina produced by type I alveolar cells and subjacent endothelial cells lining the alveolar capillaries, (3) cytoplasmic extensions of endothelial cells, and (4) the plasma membrane of red blood cells. Recall that the biconcave shape of red blood cells favors the rapid O_2-CO_2 exchange in the alveolar capillaries. Also note that surfactant contributes indirectly to an effective gas exchange by preventing alveolar collapse.

Acute respiratory distress syndrome (ARDS) results from an increase in the hydrostatic pressure in the alveolar capillaries (cardiogenic) or damage to the alveolar epithelial lining caused by bacterial endotoxins or trauma (noncardiogenic). These mechanisms result in an increase in fluid and proteins in the alveolar spaces (pulmonary edema).

• The pleura consists of two layers: (1) a visceral layer closely attached to the lung and lined by a simple squamous epithelium (mesothelium) and (2) a parietal layer also lined by mesothelial cells and supported by connective tissue rich in fat. The visceral pleura glides on the parietal pleura during respiration.

Disorders of the pleura include inflammatory processes, and accumulation of fluid (hydrothorax), blood (hemothorax), or air (pneumothorax).

Mesothelioma is a localized or diffuse malignant tumor of the pleura associated with asbestos exposure for long periods of time. Symptoms include pleural effusion, chest pain, or dyspnea. Mesothelioma can also affect the peritoneum and pericardium.

14. URINARY SYSTEM

The urinary system has three critical functions: (1) to clear the blood of nitrogenous and other waste metabolic products by **filtration** and **excretion**; (2) to balance the concentration of body fluids and electrolytes, also by **filtration** and **excretion**; and (3) to recover by **reabsorption** small molecules (amino acids, glucose, and peptides), ions (Na^+, Cl^-, Ca^{2+}, PO^{3-}), and water, in order to maintain blood **homeostasis** (Greek *homoios,* similar; *stasis,* standing).

The kidney regulates **blood pressure** by producing the enzyme **renin**. Renin initiates the conversion of **angiotensinogen** (a plasma protein produced in liver) to the active component **angiotensin II**.

The kidney is also an **endocrine organ**. It produces **erythropoietin**, a stimulant of red blood cell production in bone marrow (for the role of erythropoietin, see Chapter 6, Blood and Hematopoiesis). It also activates **1,25-hydroxycholecalciferol**, a vitamin D derivative involved in the control of calcium metabolism (see vitamin D metabolism in Chapter 19, Endocrine System).

Kidney

The urinary system consists of paired kidneys and ureters and a single urinary bladder and urethra. Each kidney has a **cortex** (subdivided into **outer cortex** and **juxtamedullary cortex**) and a **medulla** (subdivided into **outer medulla** and **inner medulla**).

The medulla is formed by conical masses, the **medullary pyramids**, with their bases located at the corticomedullary junction. A medullary pyramid, together with the associated covering cortical region, constitutes a **renal lobe**. The base of the renal lobe is the renal capsule. The lateral boundaries of each renal lobe are the **renal columns** (of Bertin), residual structures representing the fusion of primitive lobes within the metanephric blastema. The apex of each renal lobe terminates in a conic-shaped **papilla** surfaced by the **area cribrosa** (the opening site of the papillary ducts). The papilla is surrounded by a **minor calyx.** Each minor calyx collects the urine from a papilla dripping from the area cribrosa. Minor calyces converge to form the **major calyces** which, in turn, form the **pelvis.**

Organization of the renal vascular system

The main function of the kidney is to **filter the blood** supplied by the renal arteries branching from the descending aorta.

The kidneys receive about 20% of the cardiac output per minute and filter about 1.25 L of blood per minute. Essentially, all the blood of the body passes through the kidneys every 5 minutes.

About 90% of the cardiac output goes to the renal cortex; 10% of the blood goes to the medulla. Approximately 125 mL of filtrate is produced per minute, but 124 mL of this amount is reabsorbed.

About 180 L of fluid ultrafiltrate is produced in 24 hours and transported through the uriniferous tubules. Of this amount, 178.5 L is recovered by the tubular cells and returned to the blood circulation, whereas only 1.5 L is excreted as **urine**.

We start our discussion by focusing on the vascularization of the kidney (Figure 14-1).

Oxygenated blood is supplied by the **renal artery**. The renal artery gives rise to several **interlobar arteries**, running across the medulla through the renal columns along the sides of the pyramids.

At the corticomedullary junction, interlobar arteries give off several branches at right angles, changing their vertical path to a horizontal direction to form

Figure 14-1. **Vascularization of the kidney**

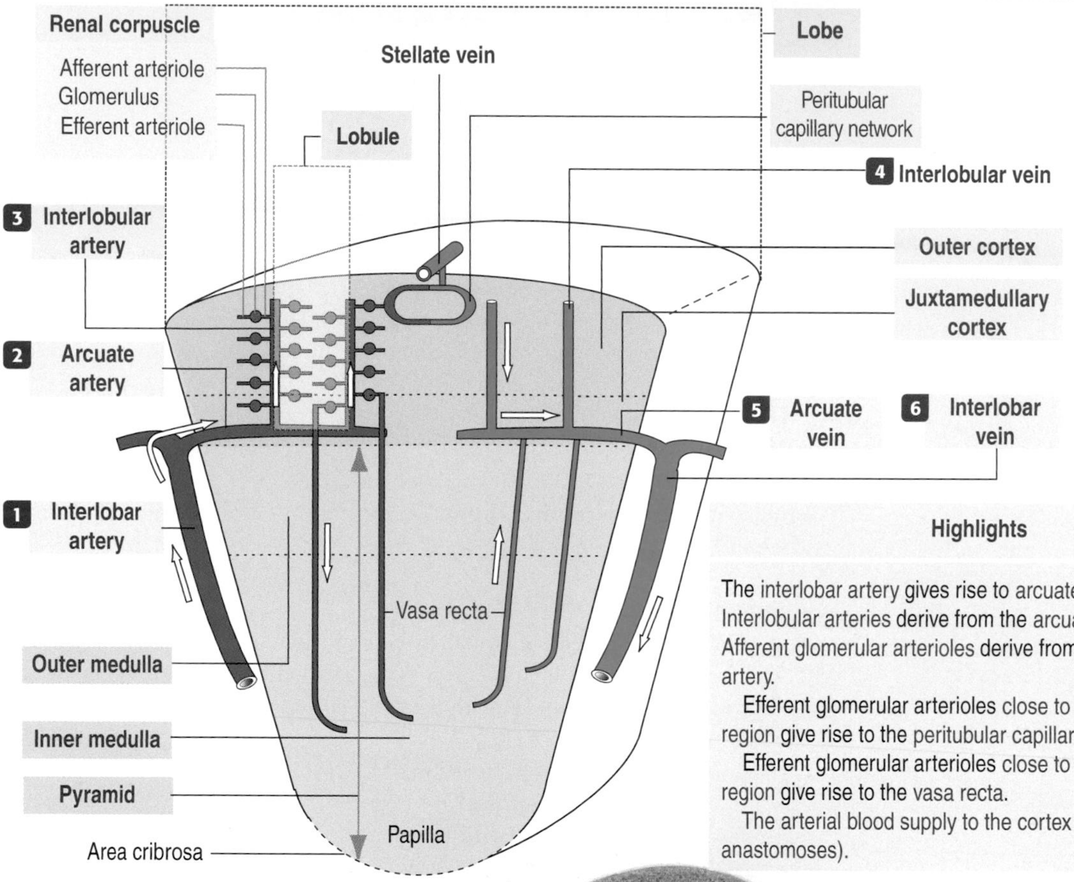

Renal corpuscle
Afferent arteriole
Glomerulus
Efferent arteriole
Stellate vein
Lobe
Lobule
Peritubular capillary network
4 Interlobular vein
3 Interlobular artery
Outer cortex
Juxtamedullary cortex
2 Arcuate artery
5 Arcuate vein
6 Interlobar vein
1 Interlobar artery
Vasa recta
Outer medulla
Inner medulla
Pyramid
Papilla
Area cribrosa

Highlights

The interlobar artery gives rise to arcuate arteries. Interlobular arteries derive from the arcuate artery. Afferent glomerular arterioles derive from an interlobular artery.

Efferent glomerular arterioles close to the subcapsular region give rise to the peritubular capillary network.

Efferent glomerular arterioles close to the juxtamedullary region give rise to the vasa recta.

The arterial blood supply to the cortex is terminal (no anastomoses).

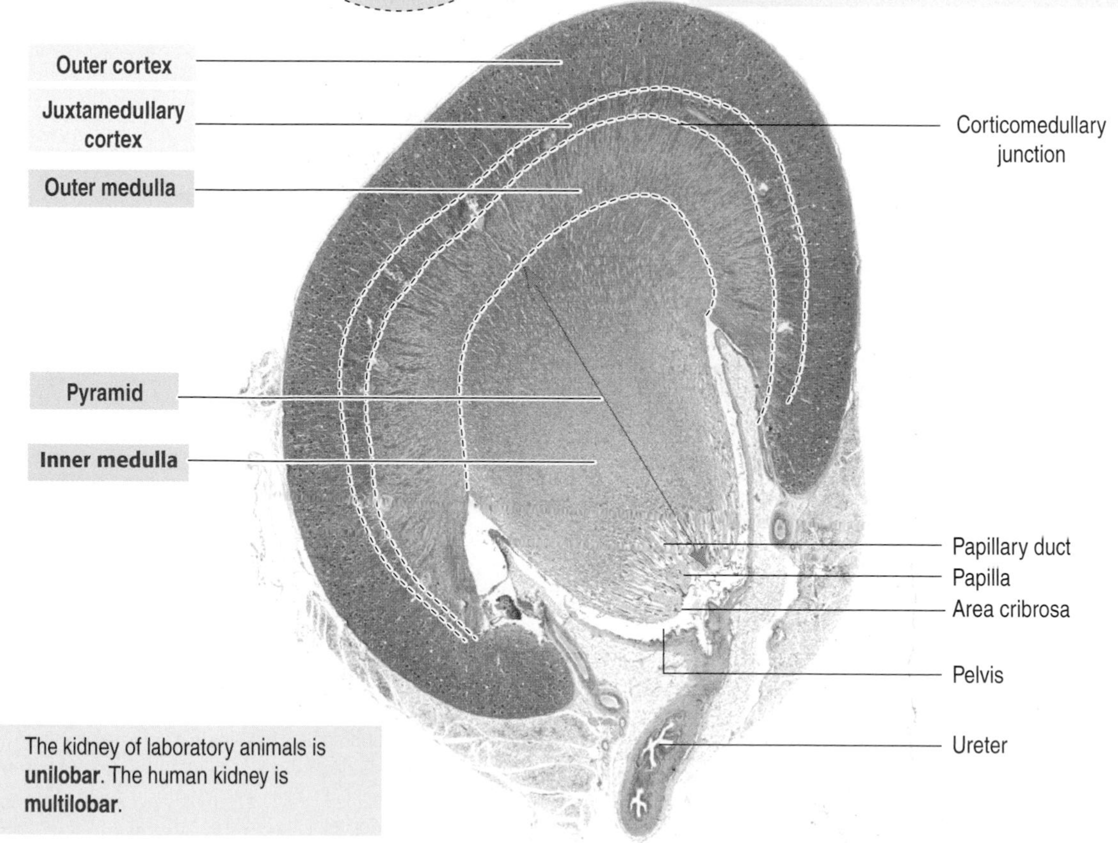

Outer cortex
Juxtamedullary cortex
Outer medulla
Corticomedullary junction
Pyramid
Inner medulla
Papillary duct
Papilla
Area cribrosa
Pelvis
Ureter

The kidney of laboratory animals is **unilobar**. The human kidney is **multilobar**.

Figure 14-2. Arterial and venous portal systems

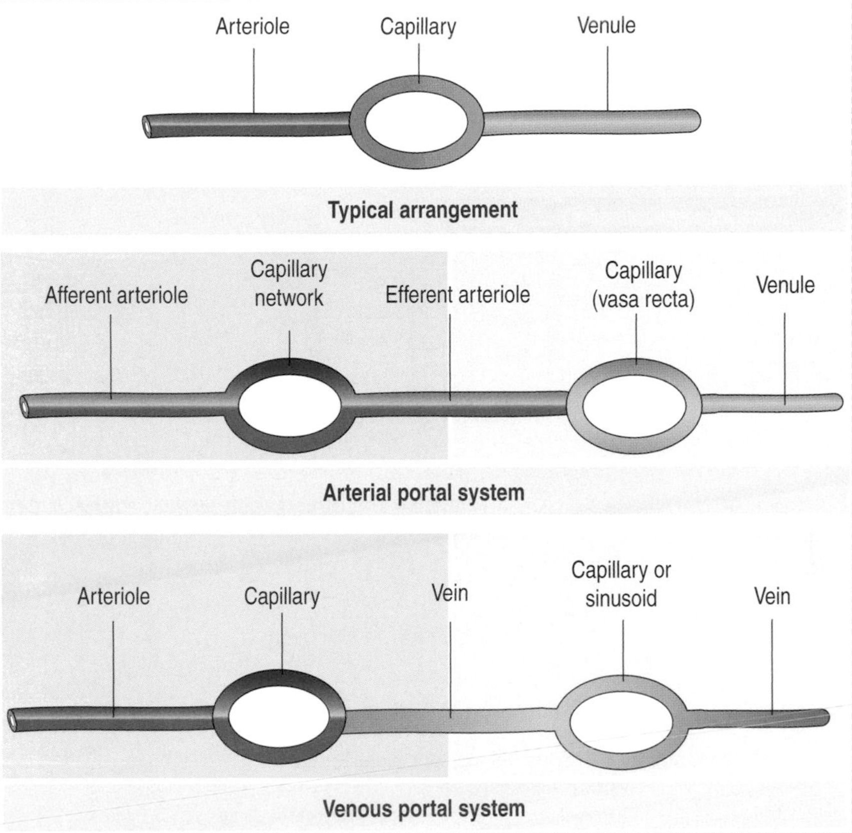

In general, a capillary network is interposed between an arteriole and a venule.

In the kidney, an arteriole is interposed between two capillary networks. An afferent arteriole gives rise to a mass of capillaries, the **glomerulus**. These capillaries coalesce to form an efferent arteriole, which gives rise to capillary networks (peritubular capillary network and the vasa recta) surrounding the nephrons.

In the liver and hypophysis, veins feed into an extensive capillary or sinusoid network draining into a vein. This distribution is called the **venous portal system**.

the **arcuate arteries**, running along the corticomedullary boundary. The renal arterial architecture is **terminal**. There are no anastomoses between interlobular arteries. This is an important concept in renal pathology for understanding **focal necrosis** as a consequence of an arterial obstruction. For example, **renal infarct** can be caused by atherosclerotic plaques in the renal artery or embolization of atherosclerotic plaques derived from the aorta.

Vertical branches emerging from the arcuate arteries, the **interlobular arteries**, penetrate the cortex. As interlobular arteries ascend toward the outer cortex, they branch several times to form the **afferent glomerular arterioles** (see Figure 14-1).

The afferent glomerular arteriole, in turn, forms the **glomerular capillary network**, enveloped by the two-layered **capsule of Bowman**, and continues as the **efferent glomerular arteriole**. This particular arrangement, a capillary network flanked by two arterioles (instead of an arteriole and a venule) is called the **glomerulus** or **arterial portal system**.

The glomerular **arterial portal system** (Figure 14-2) is structurally and functionally distinct from the **venous portal system** of the liver. Both the glomerulus and the surrounding capsule of Bowman form the **renal corpuscle** (also called the malpighian corpuscle).

The smooth muscle cell wall of the **afferent glomerular arteriole** contains epithelial-like cells, called **juxtaglomerular cells**, with secretory granules containing **renin**. A few juxtaglomerular cells may be found in the wall of the efferent glomerular arteriole.

Vasa recta

Depending upon the location of the renal corpuscle, the efferent glomerular arteriole forms two different capillary networks:

1. A **peritubular capillary network**, surrounding the **cortical** segments of

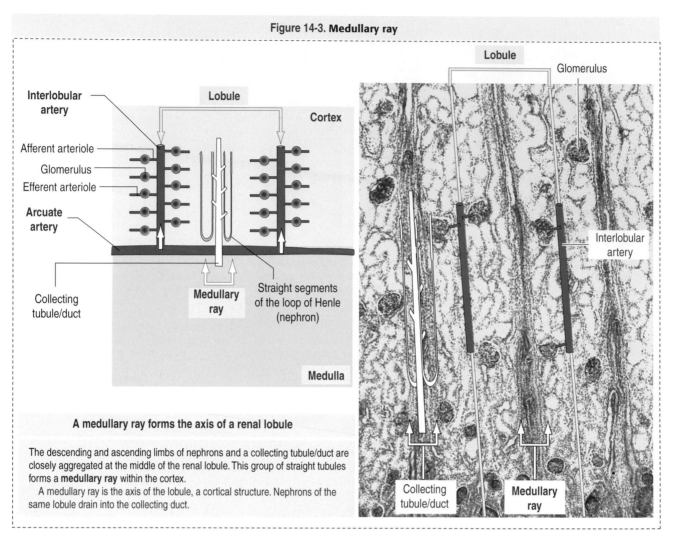

Figure 14-3. **Medullary ray**

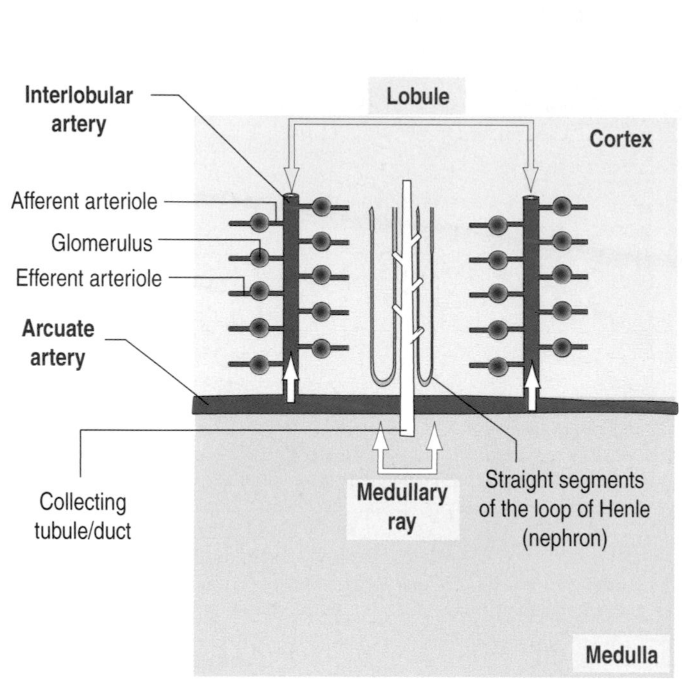

Interlobular artery
Lobule
Cortex
Afferent arteriole
Glomerulus
Efferent arteriole
Arcuate artery
Collecting tubule/duct
Medullary ray
Straight segments of the loop of Henle (nephron)
Medulla

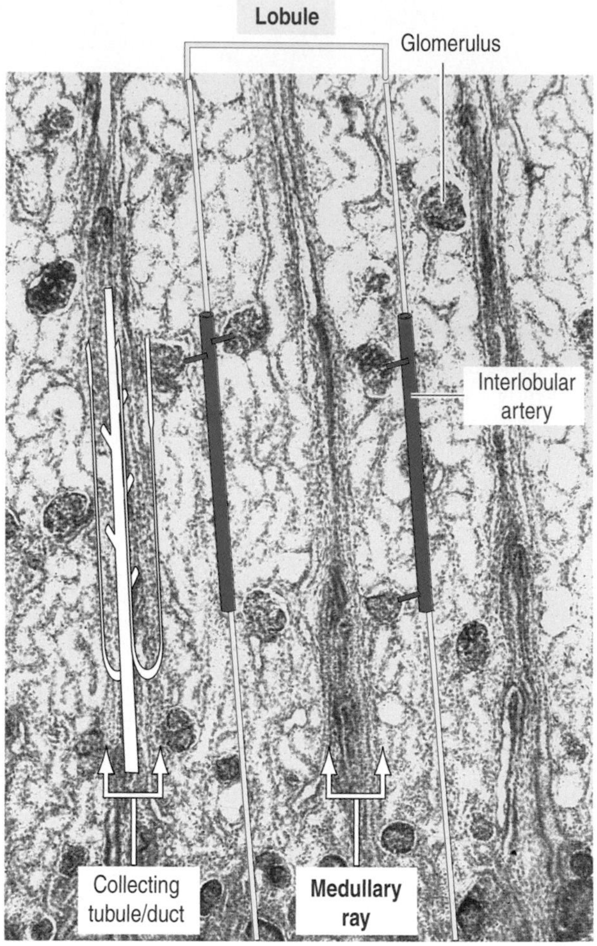

Lobule
Glomerulus
Interlobular artery
Collecting tubule/duct
Medullary ray

A medullary ray forms the axis of a renal lobule

The descending and ascending limbs of nephrons and a collecting tubule/duct are closely aggregated at the middle of the renal lobule. This group of straight tubules forms a **medullary ray** within the cortex.

A medullary ray is the axis of the lobule, a cortical structure. Nephrons of the same lobule drain into the collecting duct.

the superficial uriniferous tubules. The peritubular capillary network, lined by fenestrated endothelial cells, drains into the **interlobular vein** converging to the **arcuate vein**. Arcuate veins drain into the **interlobar veins**, which are continuous with the **renal vein.**

2. The **vasa recta (straight vessels)**, formed by multiple branching of the efferent arterioles located close to the corticomedullary junction. The **descending** components of the vasa recta (**arterial capillaries lined by continuous endothelial cells**) extend into the **medulla**, parallel to the medullary segments of the uriniferous tubules, make a hairpin turn, and return to the corticomedullary junction as **ascending venous capillaries lined by fenestrated endothelial cells.**

Note that the vascular supply to the renal medulla is largely derived from the efferent glomerular arterioles. The descending vasa recta bundles penetrate to varying depths of the renal medulla, alongside the **descending** and **ascending limbs** of the **loop of Henle** and the **collecting ducts**. Side branches connect the returning ascending vasa recta to the **interlobular** and **arcuate veins**. Remember the close relationship of the vasa recta with each other and adjacent tubules and ducts. This is the structural basis of the countercurrent exchange and multiplier mechanism of urine formation as we will discuss later.

Difference between lobe and lobule

A **renal medullary pyramid** is a **medullary** structure limited by interlobar arteries at the sides. The corticomedullary junction is the base and the papilla is the apex of the pyramid.

A **renal lobule** is a **cortical** structure that can be defined in two different ways

Figure 14-4. Uriniferous tubule

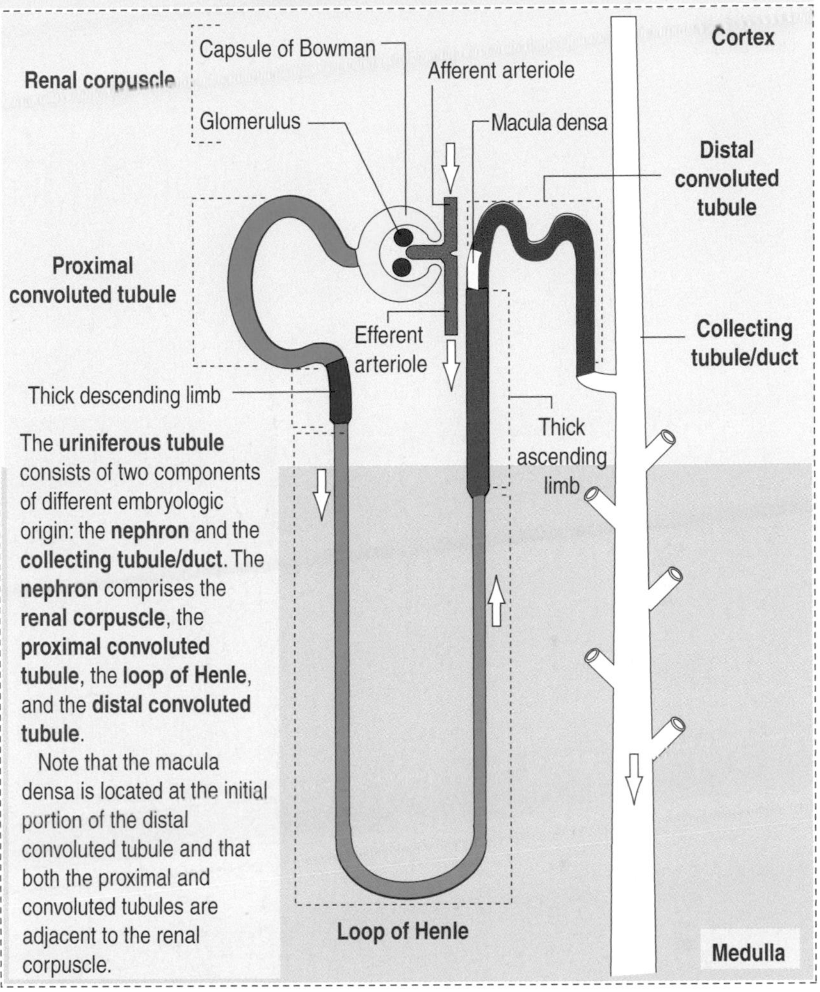
Renal corpuscle
Capsule of Bowman
Glomerulus
Afferent arteriole
Macula densa
Cortex
Distal convoluted tubule
Proximal convoluted tubule
Efferent arteriole
Collecting tubule/duct
Thick descending limb
Thick ascending limb
Loop of Henle
Medulla

The **uriniferous tubule** consists of two components of different embryologic origin: the **nephron** and the **collecting tubule/duct**. The **nephron** comprises the **renal corpuscle**, the **proximal convoluted tubule**, the **loop of Henle**, and the **distal convoluted tubule**.

Note that the macula densa is located at the initial portion of the distal convoluted tubule and that both the proximal and convoluted tubules are adjacent to the renal corpuscle.

(see Figure 14-1): (1) The renal lobule is a portion of the cortex **flanked by two adjacent ascending interlobular arteries**. Each interlobular artery gives rise to a series of glomeruli, each consisting of an afferent glomerular arteriole, a capillary network, and the efferent glomerular arteriole. (2) The renal lobule consists of a single **collecting duct** (of Bellini) and the surrounding nephrons that drain into it. The straight portions of the nephrons, together with the single collecting duct, is called a **medullary ray** (of Ferrein). A **medullary ray** is the **axis of the lobule** (Figure 14-3).

Note that the **cortex has many lobules** and that **each lobule has a single medullary ray**.

The uriniferous tubule consists of a nephron and a collecting duct

Each kidney has about 1.3 million uriniferous tubules surrounded by a stroma containing loose connective tissue, blood vessels, lymphatics, and nerves. Each uriniferous tubule consists of two embryologically distinct segments (Figure 14-4): (1) the **nephron** and (2) the **collecting duct**.

The **nephron** consists of two components: (1) the **renal corpuscle** (300 μm in diameter) and (2) a long **renal tubule** (5 to 7 mm long).

The **renal tubule** consists of several regions: (1) the **proximal convoluted tubule**, (2) the **loop of Henle**, and (3) the **distal convoluted tubule**, which empties into the **collecting tubule**.

Collecting tubules have three distinct topographic distributions: a **cortical collecting tubule** (found in the renal cortex as the centerpiece of the medullary ray), an **outer medullary collecting tubule** (present in the outer medulla), and

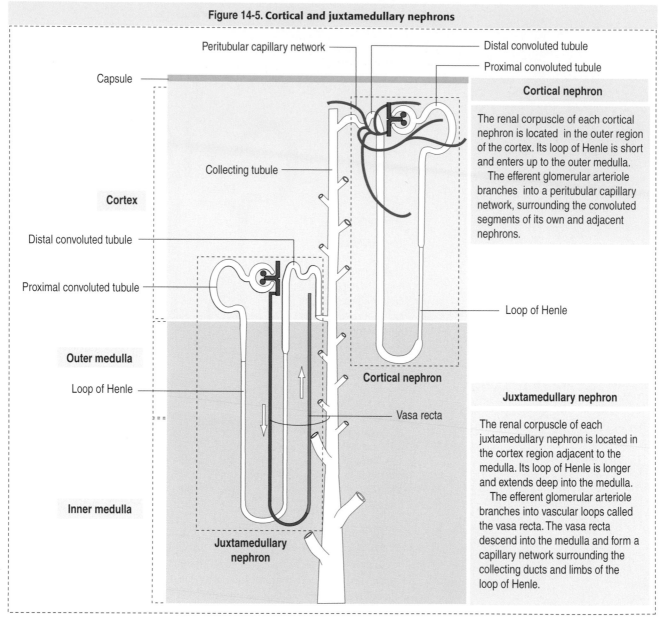

Figure 14-5. Cortical and juxtamedullary nephrons

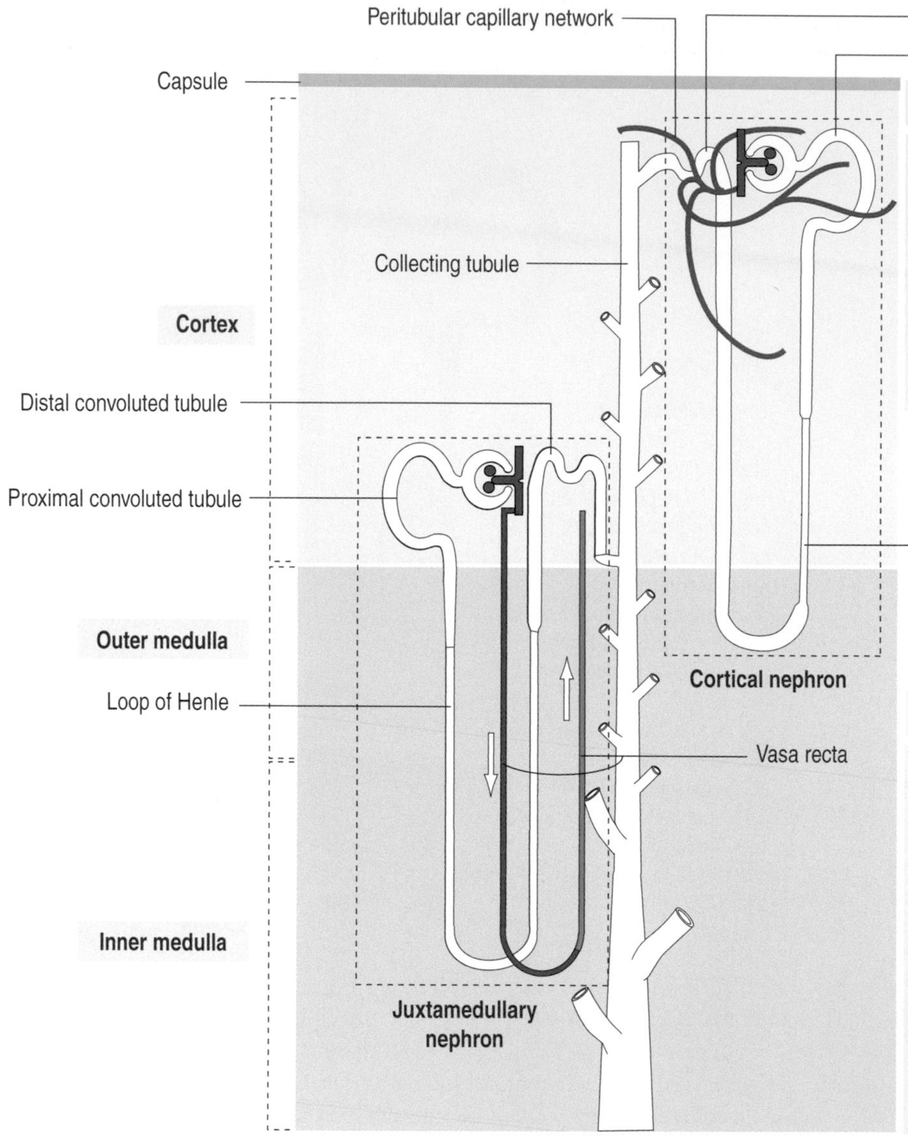

Cortical nephron

The renal corpuscle of each cortical nephron is located in the outer region of the cortex. Its loop of Henle is short and enters up to the outer medulla.

The efferent glomerular arteriole branches into a peritubular capillary network, surrounding the convoluted segments of its own and adjacent nephrons.

Juxtamedullary nephron

The renal corpuscle of each juxtamedullary nephron is located in the cortex region adjacent to the medulla. Its loop of Henle is longer and extends deep into the medulla.

The efferent glomerular arteriole branches into vascular loops called the vasa recta. The vasa recta descend into the medulla and form a capillary network surrounding the collecting ducts and limbs of the loop of Henle.

an **inner medullary** segment (located in the inner medulla).

Depending on the distribution of renal corpuscles, nephrons can be either **cortical** or **juxtamedullary**. Renal tubules derived from **cortical nephrons** have a **short** loop of Henle that penetrates just up to the outer medulla. Renal tubules from **juxtamedullary nephrons** have a **long** loop of Henle projecting into the inner medulla (Figure 14-5).

Nephron: The renal corpuscle is the filtering unit

The **renal corpuscle,** or **malpighian corpuscle** (Figure 14-6), consists of the **capsule of Bowman** investing a capillary tuft, the **glomerulus.**

The **capsule of Bowman** has two layers: (1) the **visceral layer**, attached to the capillary glomerulus, and (2) the **parietal layer**, associated with the connective tissue stroma.

The visceral layer is lined by epithelial cells called **podocytes**, reinforced by a basal lamina. The parietal layer is covered by a basal lamina supported by **simple squamous epithelium** and is continuous with the **simple cuboidal epithelium** of the proximal convoluted tubule.

A **urinary space (Bowman's space or capsular space)**, containing the **plasma**

Figure 14-6. Renal corpuscle

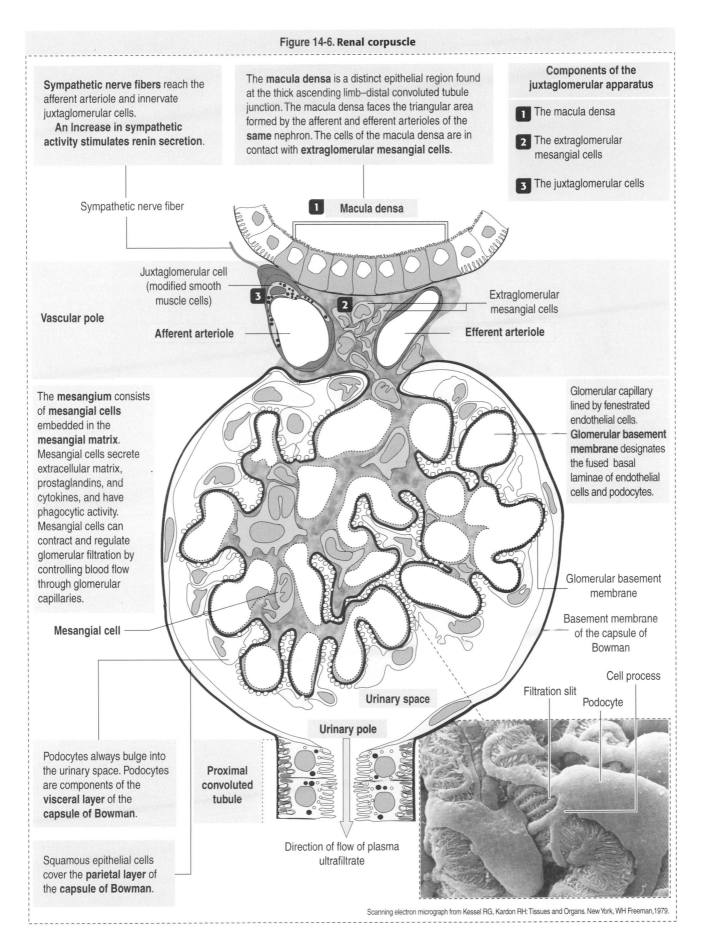

Sympathetic nerve fibers reach the afferent arteriole and innervate juxtaglomerular cells.
An Increase in sympathetic activity stimulates renin secretion.

The **macula densa** is a distinct epithelial region found at the thick ascending limb–distal convoluted tubule junction. The macula densa faces the triangular area formed by the afferent and efferent arterioles of the **same** nephron. The cells of the macula densa are in contact with **extraglomerular mesangial cells**.

Components of the juxtaglomerular apparatus

1. The macula densa
2. The extraglomerular mesangial cells
3. The juxtaglomerular cells

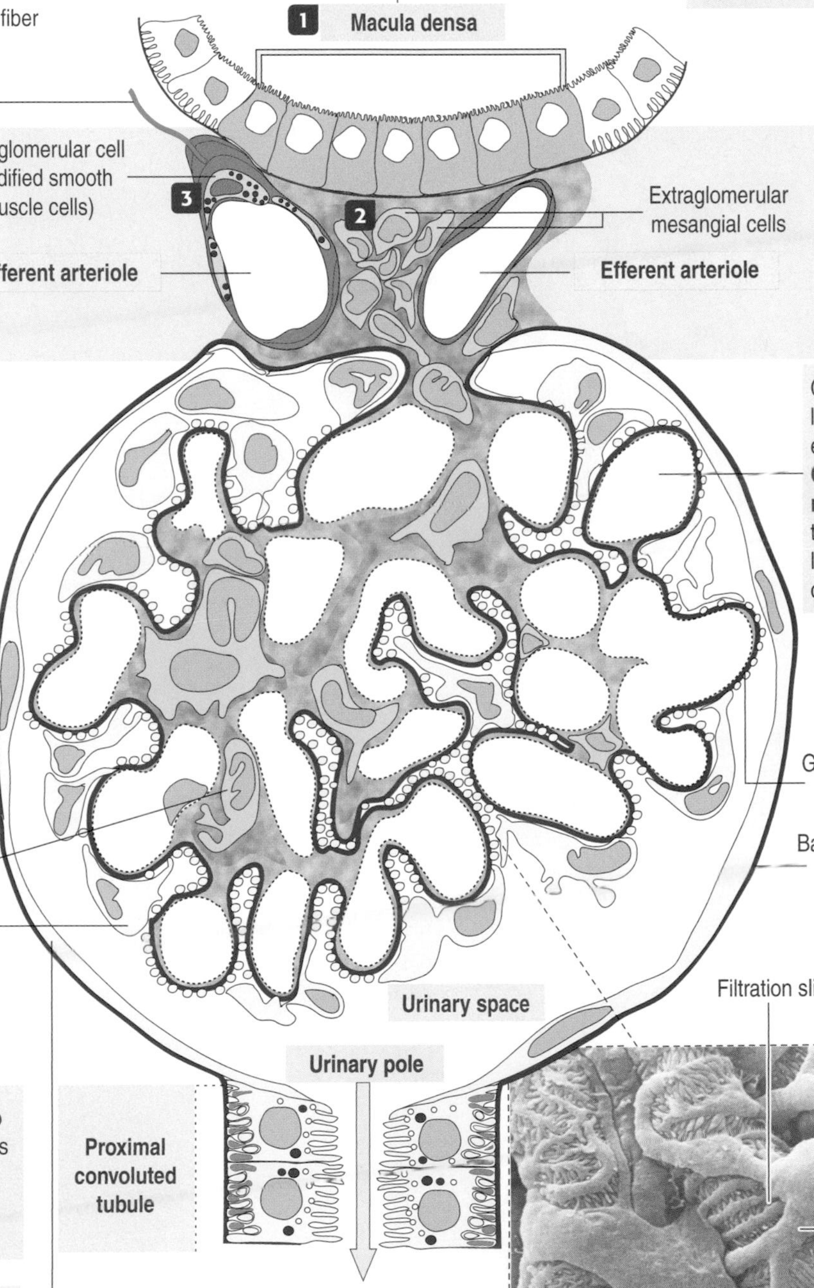

Sympathetic nerve fiber
1 Macula densa
Juxtaglomerular cell (modified smooth muscle cells)
3
2
Extraglomerular mesangial cells
Vascular pole
Afferent arteriole
Efferent arteriole
Mesangial cell
Glomerular basement membrane
Basement membrane of the capsule of Bowman
Urinary space
Urinary pole
Proximal convoluted tubule
Direction of flow of plasma ultrafiltrate

The **mesangium** consists of **mesangial cells** embedded in the **mesangial matrix**. Mesangial cells secrete extracellular matrix, prostaglandins, and cytokines, and have phagocytic activity. Mesangial cells can contract and regulate glomerular filtration by controlling blood flow through glomerular capillaries.

Glomerular capillary lined by fenestrated endothelial cells. **Glomerular basement membrane** designates the fused basal laminae of endothelial cells and podocytes.

Podocytes always bulge into the urinary space. Podocytes are components of the **visceral layer** of the **capsule of Bowman**.

Squamous epithelial cells cover the **parietal layer** of the **capsule of Bowman**.

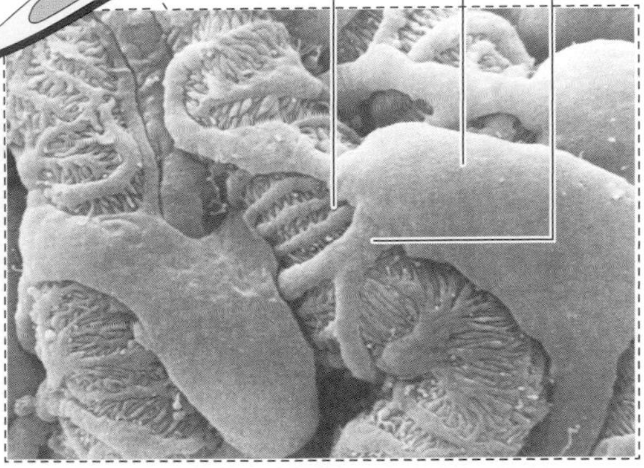

Cell process
Filtration slit
Podocyte

Scanning electron micrograph from Kessel RG, Kardon RH: Tissues and Organs. New York, WH Freeman, 1979.

Figure 14-7. Components of the renal corpuscle visualized by light and electron microscopy

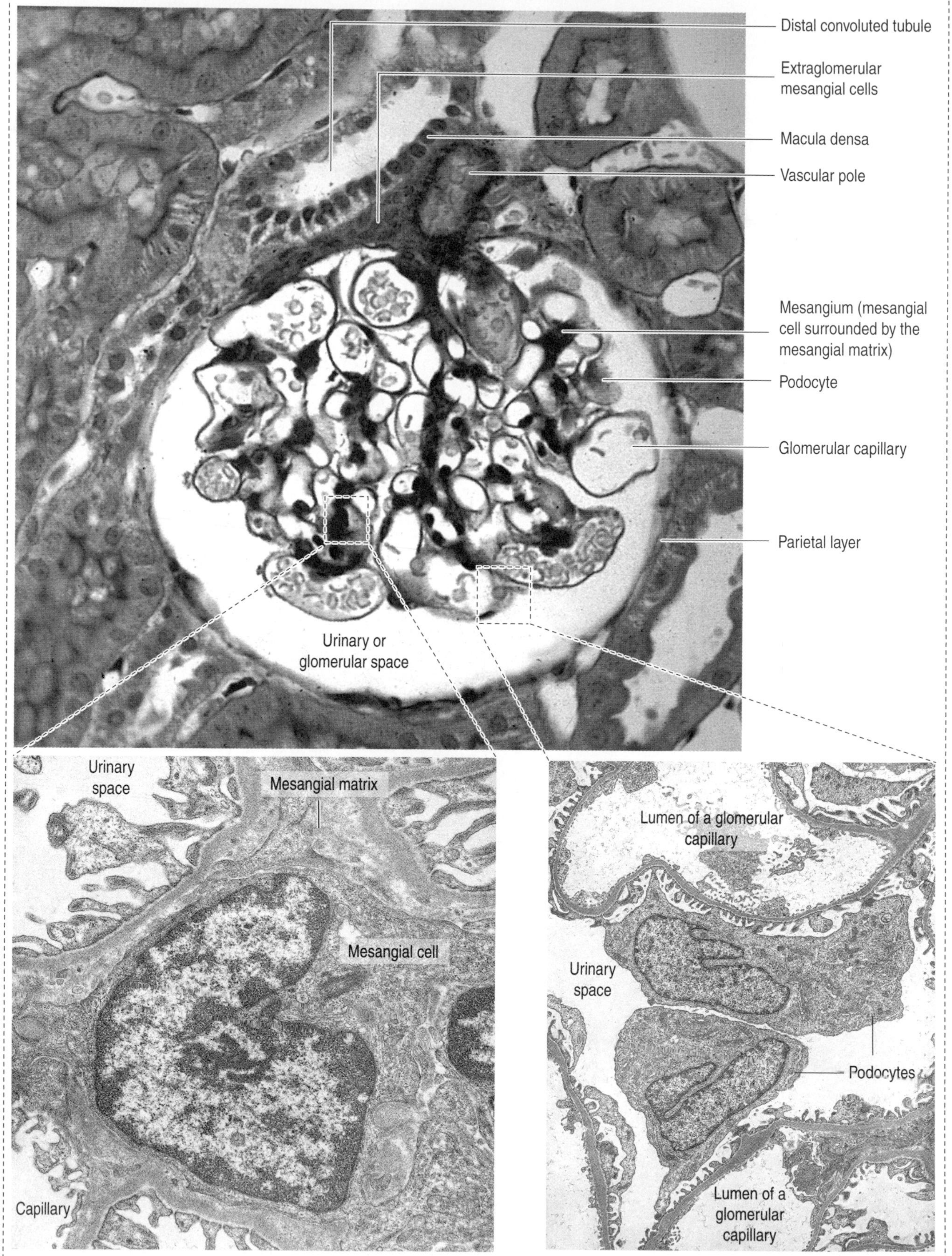

Distal convoluted tubule
Extraglomerular mesangial cells
Macula densa
Vascular pole
Mesangium (mesangial cell surrounded by the mesangial matrix)
Podocyte
Glomerular capillary
Parietal layer
Urinary or glomerular space
Urinary space
Mesangial matrix
Mesangial cell
Capillary
Lumen of a glomerular capillary
Urinary space
Podocytes
Lumen of a glomerular capillary

ultrafiltrate (primary urine), exists between the visceral and parietal layers of the capsule. The plasma ultrafiltrate contains trace amounts of protein. The urinary space is continuous with the lumen of the proximal convoluted tubule at the **urinary pole**, the gate through which the plasma ultrafiltrate flows into the proximal convoluted tubule. The opposite pole, the site of entry and exit of the afferent and efferent glomerular arterioles, is called the **vascular pole**.

The **glomerulus** consists of three components (Figure 14-7):

1. The glomerular **capillaries**, lined by **fenestrated endothelial cells.**

2. The **mesangium**, formed by **mesangial cells** embedded in the **mesangial matrix.**

3. The **podocytes**, constituents of the **visceral layer** of the capsule of Bowman. Recall that the **parietal layer** of the capsule of Bowman is a simple squamous epithelium.

Podocytes

The podocytes have long and branching cell processes that completely encircle the surface of the glomerular capillary. Both podocytes and fenestrated endothelial cells and their corresponding basal laminae constitute the **glomerular filtration barrier.**

The endings of the cell processes, the pedicels, from the same podocyte or adjacent podocytes, interdigitate to cover the basal lamina and are separated by gaps, the **filtration slits.** Filtration slits are bridged by a membranous material, the **filtration slit diaphragm** (Figure 14-8). Pedicels are attached to the basal lamina by $\alpha_3\beta_1$ **integrin.**

The podocyte filtration slit diaphragm consists of the protein **nephrin** interacting with nephrin molecules in a homophilic manner, and with the nephrin-related transmembrane proteins **Neph1** and **Neph2. Nephrin** is anchored to actin filaments (within the pedicel) by the proteins **podocin** and CD2-associated proteins (**CD2AP**). The interaction of nephrin in the middle of the slit creates a filtering structure retarding the passage of molecules crossing the endothelial fenestrations and the basal laminae.

In addition to the components of the glomerular filtration barrier, other limiting factors controlling the passage of molecules in the plasma ultrafiltrate are size and electric charge. Molecules with a size less than 3.5 nm and positively charged or neutral are filtered more readily. Albumin (3.6 nm and anionic) filters poorly.

Clinical significance: Alport's syndrome

The **fenestrated endothelial cells** of the glomerular capillaries are covered by a basal lamina to which the foot processes of the podocytes attach (see Figure 14-8). Podocytes produce **glomerular endothelial growth factor** to stimulate the development of the endothelium and maintenance of its fenestrations.

The endothelium is permeable to water, urea, glucose, and small proteins. The surface of the endothelial cells is coated with negatively charged glycoproteins that block the passage of large anionic proteins.

The endothelial cell **basal lamina**, closely associated with the basal lamina produced by podocytes, contains **type IV collagen**, **fibronectin**, **laminin**, and **heparan sulfate** as major proteins.

Each type IV collagen monomer consists of three α chains forming a triple helix. There are six chains (α1 to α6) encoded by six genes (*COL4A1* through *COL4A6*). Two domains of each monomer are important: (1) the noncollagenous (**NC1**) **domain** at the C-terminal and (2) the **7S domain** at the N-terminal. The NC1 and 7S domains, separated by a long collagenous domain, are cross-linking domains required for formation of the type IV collagen network. A correctly assembled network is critical for maintaining the integrity of the glomerular basal lamina and its permeability function.

Figure 14-8. **Glomerular filtration barrier**

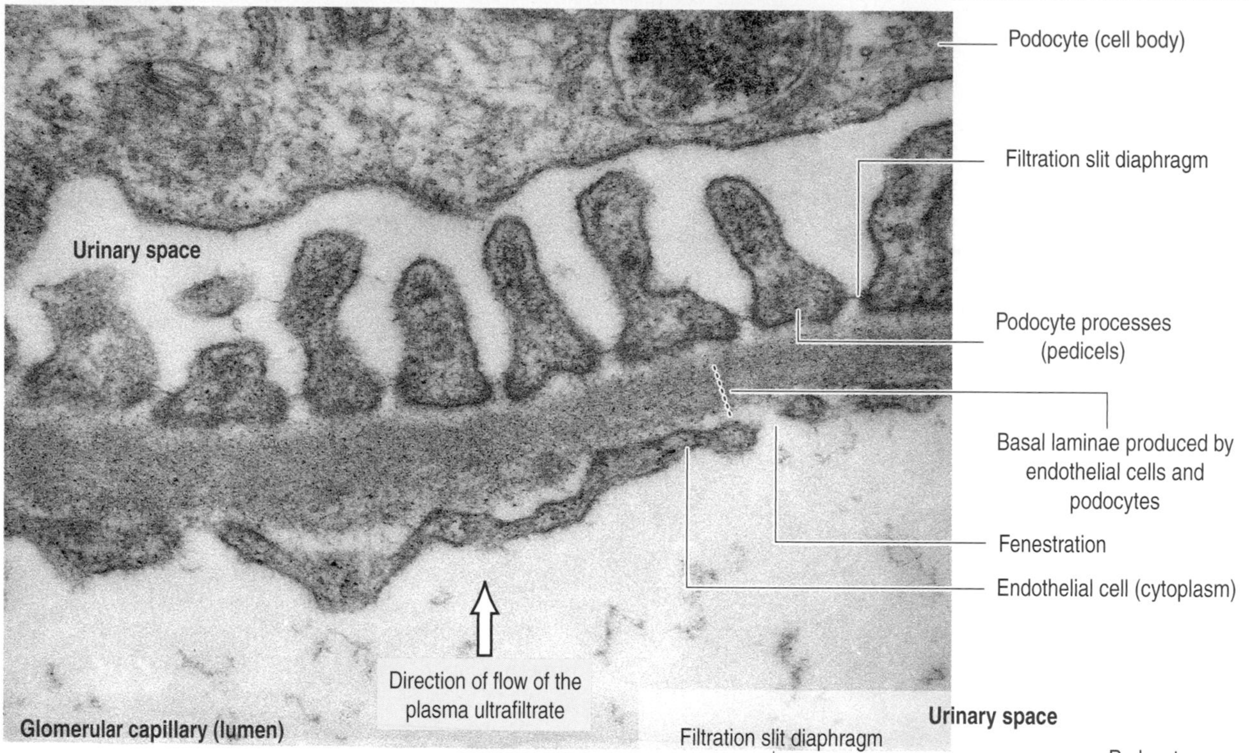

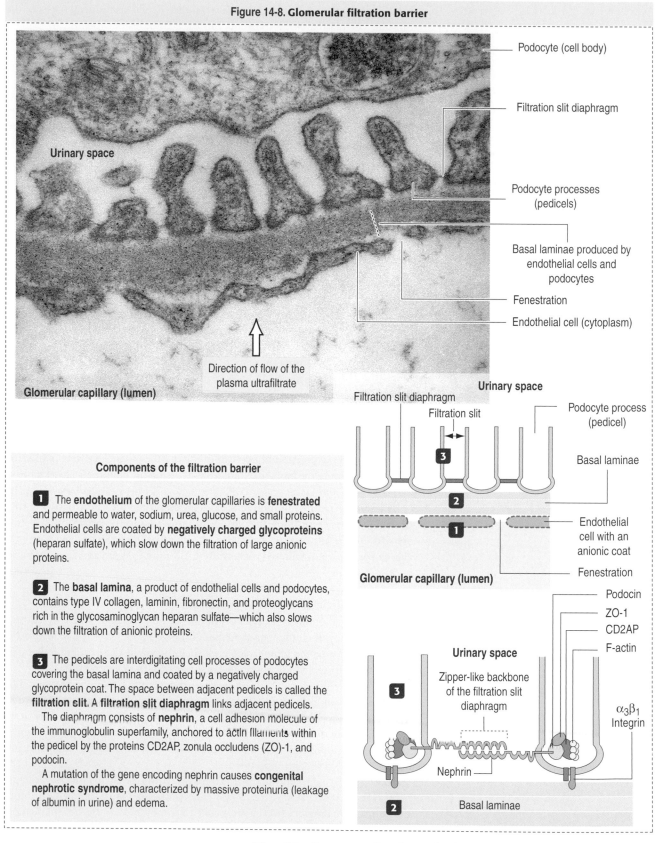

Podocyte (cell body)
Filtration slit diaphragm
Urinary space
Podocyte processes (pedicels)
Basal laminae produced by endothelial cells and podocytes
Fenestration
Endothelial cell (cytoplasm)
Direction of flow of the plasma ultrafiltrate
Glomerular capillary (lumen)

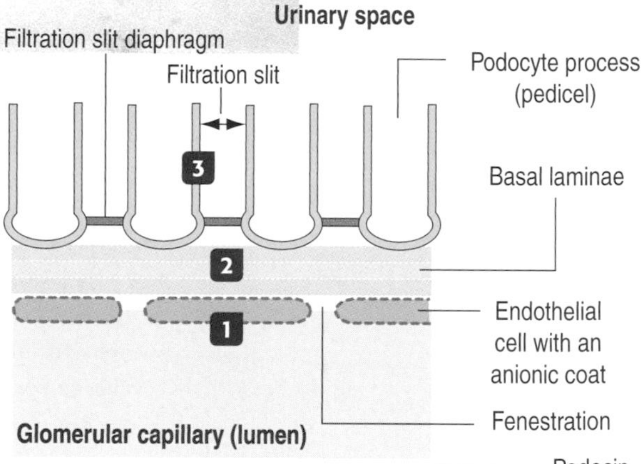

Urinary space
Filtration slit diaphragm
Filtration slit
Podocyte process (pedicel)
3
Basal laminae
2
Endothelial cell with an anionic coat
1
Glomerular capillary (lumen)
Fenestration

Components of the filtration barrier

1 The **endothelium** of the glomerular capillaries is **fenestrated** and permeable to water, sodium, urea, glucose, and small proteins. Endothelial cells are coated by **negatively charged glycoproteins** (heparan sulfate), which slow down the filtration of large anionic proteins.

2 The **basal lamina**, a product of endothelial cells and podocytes, contains type IV collagen, laminin, fibronectin, and proteoglycans rich in the glycosaminoglycan heparan sulfate—which also slows down the filtration of anionic proteins.

3 The pedicels are interdigitating cell processes of podocytes covering the basal lamina and coated by a negatively charged glycoprotein coat. The space between adjacent pedicels is called the **filtration slit**. A **filtration slit diaphragm** links adjacent pedicels.

The diaphragm consists of **nephrin**, a cell adhesion molecule of the immunoglobulin superfamily, anchored to actin filaments within the pedicel by the proteins CD2AP, zonula occludens (ZO)-1, and podocin.

A mutation of the gene encoding nephrin causes **congenital nephrotic syndrome**, characterized by massive proteinuria (leakage of albumin in urine) and edema.

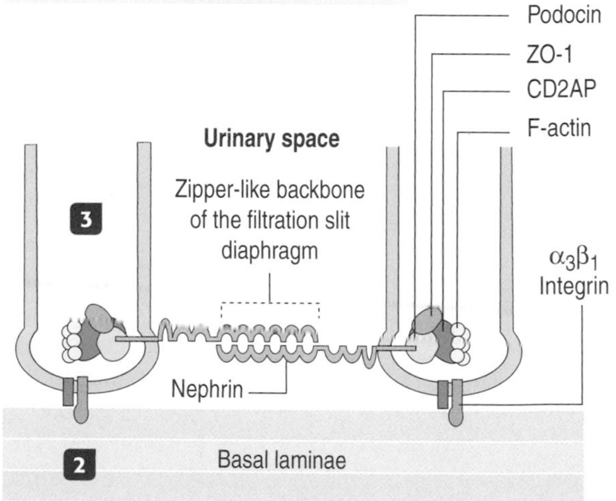

Podocin
ZO-1
CD2AP
F-actin
Urinary space
3
Zipper-like backbone of the filtration slit diaphragm
$\alpha_3\beta_1$ Integrin
Nephrin
2
Basal laminae

Type IV collagens are directly involved in the pathogenesis of three diseases. (1) **Goodpasture syndrome**, an autoimmune disorder consisting in progressive glomerulonephritis and pulmonary hemorrhage, caused by anti-α3(IV) antibodies binding to the glomerular and alveolar basal laminae. (2) **Alport's syndrome**, a

Figure 14-9. **Functions and organization of the mesangium**

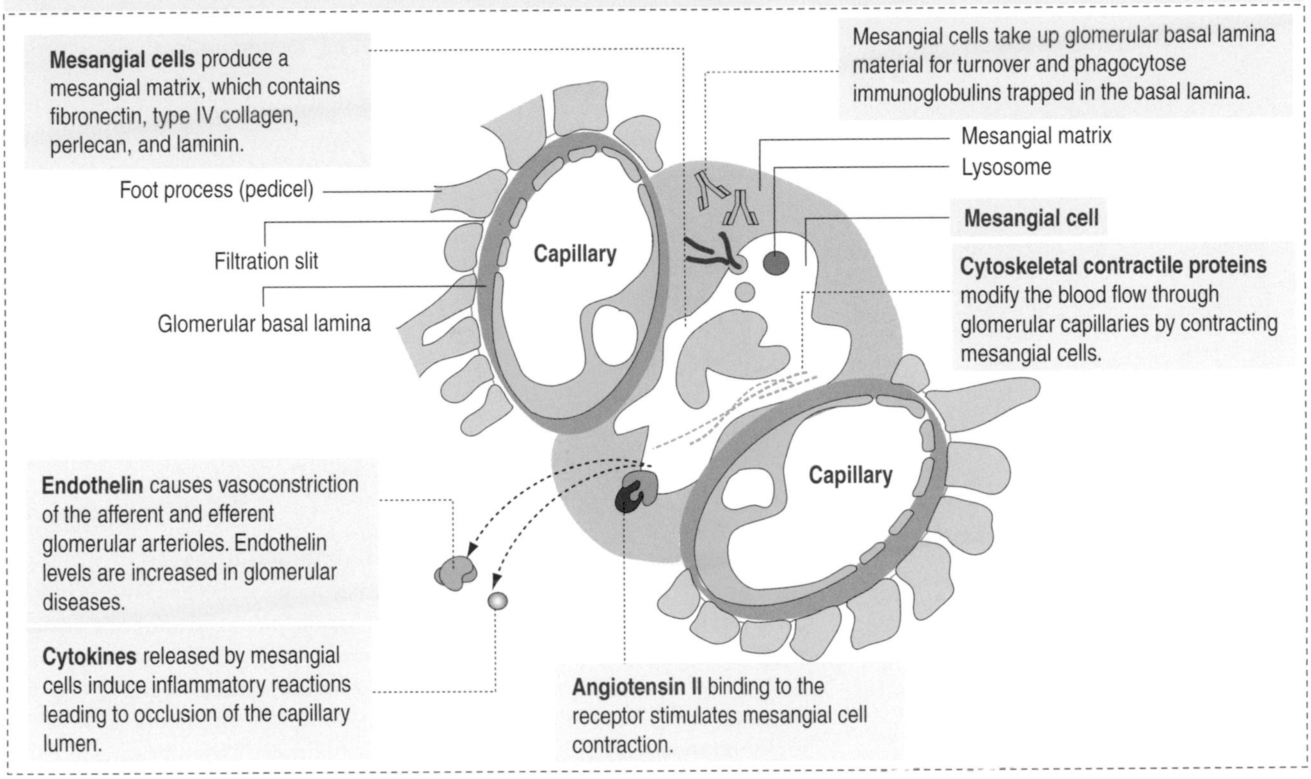

Mesangial cells produce a mesangial matrix, which contains fibronectin, type IV collagen, perlecan, and laminin.
Foot process (pedicel)
Filtration slit
Glomerular basal lamina
Capillary
Mesangial cells take up glomerular basal lamina material for turnover and phagocytose immunoglobulins trapped in the basal lamina.
Mesangial matrix
Lysosome
Mesangial cell
Cytoskeletal contractile proteins modify the blood flow through glomerular capillaries by contracting mesangial cells.
Capillary
Endothelin causes vasoconstriction of the afferent and efferent glomerular arterioles. Endothelin levels are increased in glomerular diseases.
Cytokines released by mesangial cells induce inflammatory reactions leading to occlusion of the capillary lumen.
Angiotensin II binding to the receptor stimulates mesangial cell contraction.

progressive inherited nephropathy, characterized by irregular thinning, thickening, and splitting of the glomerular basal lamina. Alport's syndrome is transmitted by an **X-linked recessive** trait, is predominant in **males**, and involves mutations of the *COL4A5* gene. Patients with Alport's syndrome—often associated with hearing loss (defective function of the stria vascularis of the cochlea) and ocular symptoms (defect of the lens capsule)—have **hematuria** (blood in the urine) and **progressive glomerulonephritis** leading to renal failure. The abnormal glomerular filtration membrane enables the passage of red blood cells and proteins. (3) **Benign familial hematuria**, caused by a dominant inherited mutation of the *COL4A4* gene, which does not lead to renal failure.

Clinical significance: Congenital nephrotic syndrome

Congenital nephrotic syndrome is caused by a mutation in the ***nephrin*** gene leading to the absence or malfunction of the podocyte slit filtration diaphragm. About 70 different mutations have been described. Affected children have massive proteinuria even in utero and the nephrotic syndrome develops soon after birth. Infants display abdominal distention, hypoalbuminemia, hyperlipidemia, and edema. Congenital nephrotic syndrome, particularly common in Finland, is lethal.

Mesangium

The mesangium is an **intraglomerular** structure interposed between the glomerular capillaries, consisting of two components: (1) the **mesangial cells** and (2) the **mesangial matrix**.

In addition, mesangial cells aggregate outside the glomerulus (**extraglomerular mesangial cells**; see Figures 14-7 and 14-15) in a space limited by the macula densa and the afferent and efferent glomerular arterioles. Intraglomerular mesangial cells may be continuous with **extraglomerular mesangial cells**.

Mesangial cells are specialized **pericytes** with characteristics of smooth muscle cells and macrophages.

Mesangial cells are (1) **contractile**, (2) **phagocytic**, and (3) capable of **proliferation**. They synthesize **both matrix and collagen**, and secrete **biologically active substances** (prostaglandins and endothelins). Endothelins induce the constriction of afferent and efferent glomerular arterioles.

Mesangial cells participate indirectly in the glomerular filtration process by:

1. **Providing mechanical support for the glomerular capillaries.**
2. **Controlling the turnover of the glomerular basal lamina material** by their phagocytic activity.
3. **Regulating blood flow** by their contractile activity.
4. **Secreting prostaglandins and endothelins.**
5. **Responding to angiotensin II.**

The glomerular filtration membrane does not completely surround the capillaries (Figure 14-9). Immunoglobulins and complement molecules, unable to cross the filtration barrier, can enter the mesangial matrix. The accumulation of immunoglobulin complexes in the matrix induces the production of cytokines by mesangial cells that trigger an immune response leading to the eventual occlusion of the glomerulus.

Clinical significance of the glomerulus: Glomerular diseases

The damage to the glomerulus can be initiated by immune mechanisms. **Antibodies against glomerular components** (cells and basal lamina) and **antibody-antigen complexes circulating in blood** can cause glomerular injury or **glomerulonephritis** (Figure 14-10). Antibody-antigen complexes are not immunologically targeted to glomerular components. They are trapped in the glomerulus because of the filtration properties of the glomerular filtration barrier. A complicating factor is that trapped antibody-antigen complexes provide binding sites to complement proteins, which also contribute to the glomerular damage (see Chapter 10, Immune-Lymphatic System, for a review of the complement cascade).

As we have seen, autoantibodies can target domains of type IV collagen, a component of the glomerular filtration barrier. The binding of antibodies to specific domains of type IV collagen generates a **diffuse linear pattern** detected by immunofluorescence microscopy (see Figure 14-10). In addition, the deposit of circulating antibody-antigen complexes produces a **granular pattern**. Systemic lupus erythematosus and bacterial (streptococci) and viral (hepatitis B virus) infections generate antibody-antigen complexes circulating in blood.

Immune complexes can deposit between the endothelial cells of the glomerular capillaries and the basal lamina (**subendothelial deposits**), in the mesangium, and less frequently between the basal lamina and the foot processes of podocytes (**subepithelial deposits**).

Immune complexes produced after bacterial infection can cause the proliferation of glomerular cells (endothelial and mesangial cells) and attract neutrophils and monocytes. This condition, known as **acute proliferative glomerulonephritis**, is observed in children and is generally reversible with treatment. This disease is more severe in adults: it can evolve into **rapidly progressive (crescentic) glomerulonephritis** (Figure 14-11).

A typical feature of crescentic glomerulonephritis is the presence of glomerular cell debris, causing severe glomerular injury. The proliferation of parietal cells of the capsule of Bowman and migrating neutrophils and lymphocytes into the space of Bowman occur. Both the cellular crescents and deposits of fibrin compress the glomerular capillaries.

Juxtaglomerular apparatus

The juxtaglomerular apparatus is a small endocrine structure consisting of:

1. The **macula densa** (see Figure 14-7), a distinct region of the initial portion of the distal convoluted tubule.
2. The **extraglomerular mesangial cells** (see Figure 14-7).

Figure 14-10. Pathology of the mesangium

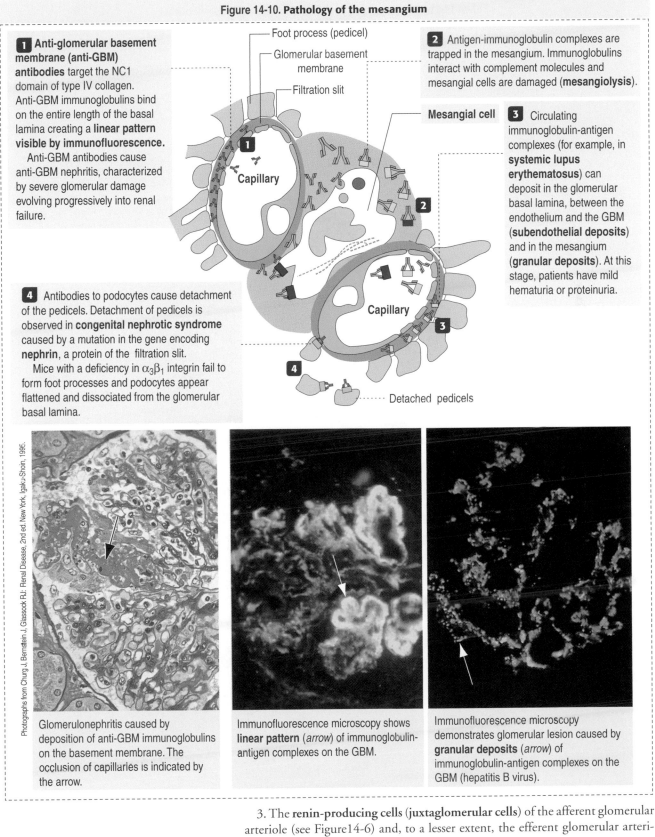

1 **Anti-glomerular basement membrane (anti-GBM) antibodies** target the NC1 domain of type IV collagen. Anti-GBM immunoglobulins bind on the entire length of the basal lamina creating a **linear pattern visible by immunofluorescence.**

Anti-GBM antibodies cause anti-GBM nephritis, characterized by severe glomerular damage evolving progressively into renal failure.

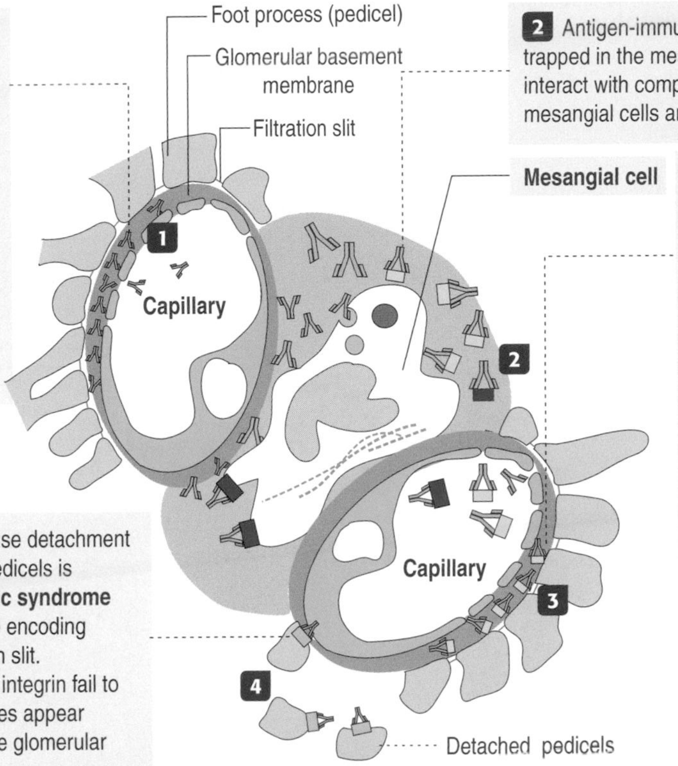

2 Antigen-immunoglobulin complexes are trapped in the mesangium. Immunoglobulins interact with complement molecules and mesangial cells are damaged (**mesangiolysis**).

3 Circulating immunoglobulin-antigen complexes (for example, in **systemic lupus erythematosus**) can deposit in the glomerular basal lamina, between the endothelium and the GBM (**subendothelial deposits**) and in the mesangium (**granular deposits**). At this stage, patients have mild hematuria or proteinuria.

4 Antibodies to podocytes cause detachment of the pedicels. Detachment of pedicels is observed in **congenital nephrotic syndrome** caused by a mutation in the gene encoding **nephrin**, a protein of the filtration slit.

Mice with a deficiency in $\alpha_3\beta_1$ integrin fail to form foot processes and podocytes appear flattened and dissociated from the glomerular basal lamina.

Photographs from Churg J, Bernstein J, Glassock RJ: Renal Disease, 2nd ed. New York, Igaku-Shoin, 1995.

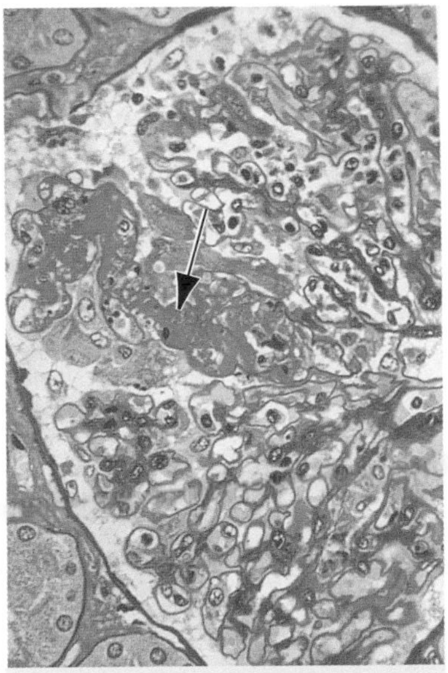

Glomerulonephritis caused by deposition of anti-GBM immunoglobulins on the basement membrane. The occlusion of capillaries is indicated by the arrow.

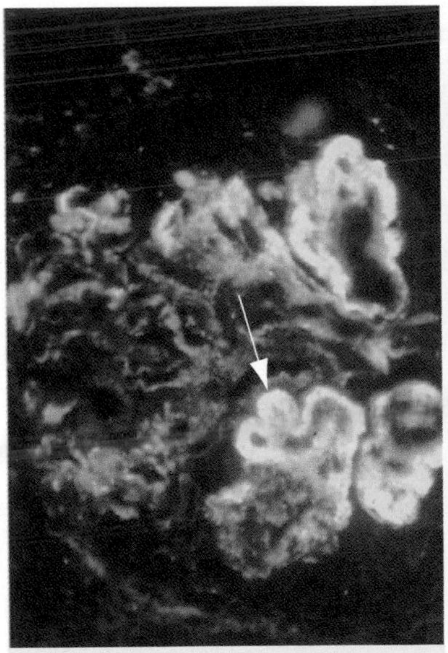

Immunofluorescence microscopy shows **linear pattern** (*arrow*) of immunoglobulin-antigen complexes on the GBM.

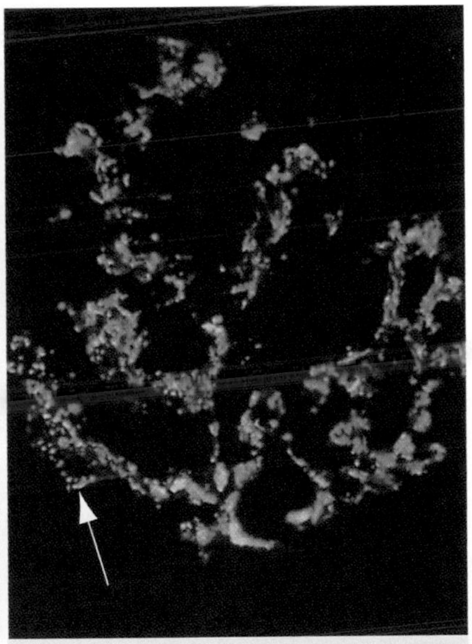

Immunofluorescence microscopy demonstrates glomerular lesion caused by **granular deposits** (*arrow*) of immunoglobulin-antigen complexes on the GBM (hepatitis B virus).

3. The **renin-producing cells** (**juxtaglomerular cells**) of the afferent glomerular arteriole (see Figure14-6) and, to a lesser extent, the efferent glomerular arteriole.

The macula densa is sensitive to changes in NaCl concentration and affects renin release by juxtaglomerular cells. Renin is secreted when the NaCl concentration or blood pressure falls. Extraglomerular mesangial cells (also called **lacis cells**) are

Figure 14-11. **Pathology of the renal corpuscle: Glomerulonephritis**

Acute proliferative diffuse glomerulonephritis

The deposition of immune complexes in the glomerular basement membrane (GBM) (resulting from a bacterial, viral, or protozoal infection) triggers the proliferation of endothelial and mesangial cells. In the presence of complement proteins, neutrophils accumulate in the lumen of the capillaries, which become occluded.

A **nephritic syndrome**, characterized by hematuria, oliguria, hypertension, and edema, is diagnosed. Children are predominantly affected.

The nephritic syndrome is reversible: Immune complexes are removed from the GBM, endothelial cells are shed, and the population of proliferative mesangial cells returns to normal. The renal function is reestablished.

Rapidly progressive (crescentic) glomerulonephritis

The proliferation of the epithelial cells of the capsule of Bowman and infiltration of macrophages produce a crescent-like mass in most glomeruli. The crescent enlarges and compresses the glomerular capillaries, which are displaced and stop functioning. This condition progresses rapidly to renal failure.

The accumulation of fibrin and other serum proteins and the necrosis of the glomerular capillaries stimulate the proliferative process.

Rapidly progressive glomerulonephritis is an immune-mediated process and is detected in a number of conditions, such as **Goodpasture syndrome** (caused by antibodies binding to the 7S domain of type IV collagen of the GBM), **systemic lupus erythematosus**, or of unknown cause (**idiopathic**).

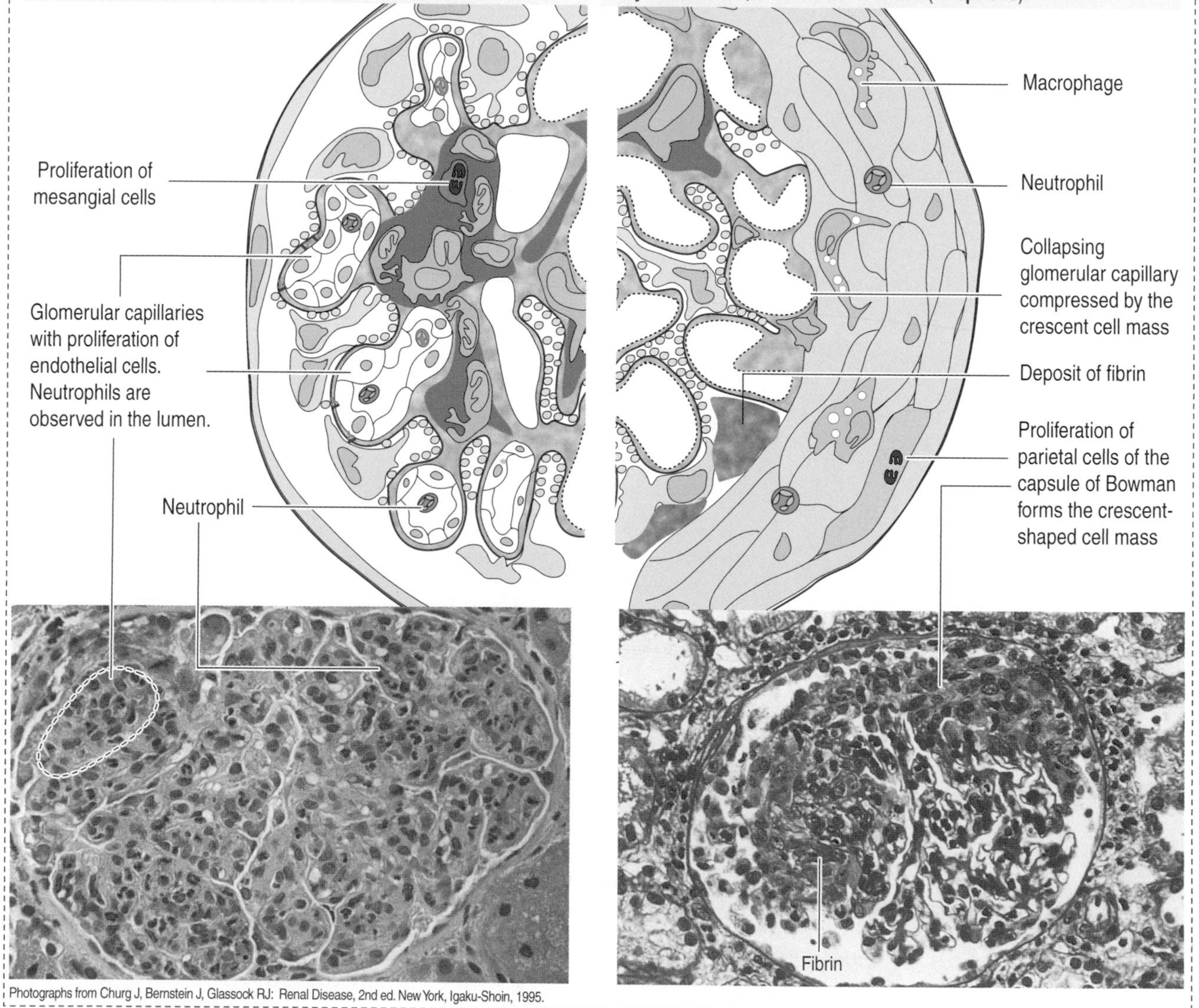
Proliferation of mesangial cells
Glomerular capillaries with proliferation of endothelial cells. Neutrophils are observed in the lumen.
Neutrophil
Macrophage
Neutrophil
Collapsing glomerular capillary compressed by the crescent cell mass
Deposit of fibrin
Proliferation of parietal cells of the capsule of Bowman forms the crescent-shaped cell mass
Fibrin

Photographs from Churg J, Bernstein J, Glassock RJ: Renal Disease, 2nd ed. New York, Igaku-Shoin, 1995.

connected to each other and to juxtaglomerular cells by gap junctions.

The juxtaglomerular apparatus is one of the components of the **tubuloglomerular feedback mechanism** involved in the autoregulation of **renal blood flow** and **glomerular filtration**.

The other component is the **sympathetic nerve fibers** (adrenergic) innervating the juxtaglomerular cells. Renin secretion is enhanced by **norepinephrin**e and

Figure 14-12. Proximal convoluted tubule (PCT)

Proximal convoluted tubule

The PCT reabsorbs about 70% of filtered water. The osmotic gradient established by reabsorbed glucose and NaCl is the driving force for water reabsorption across tight junctions and the proximal tubular cells.

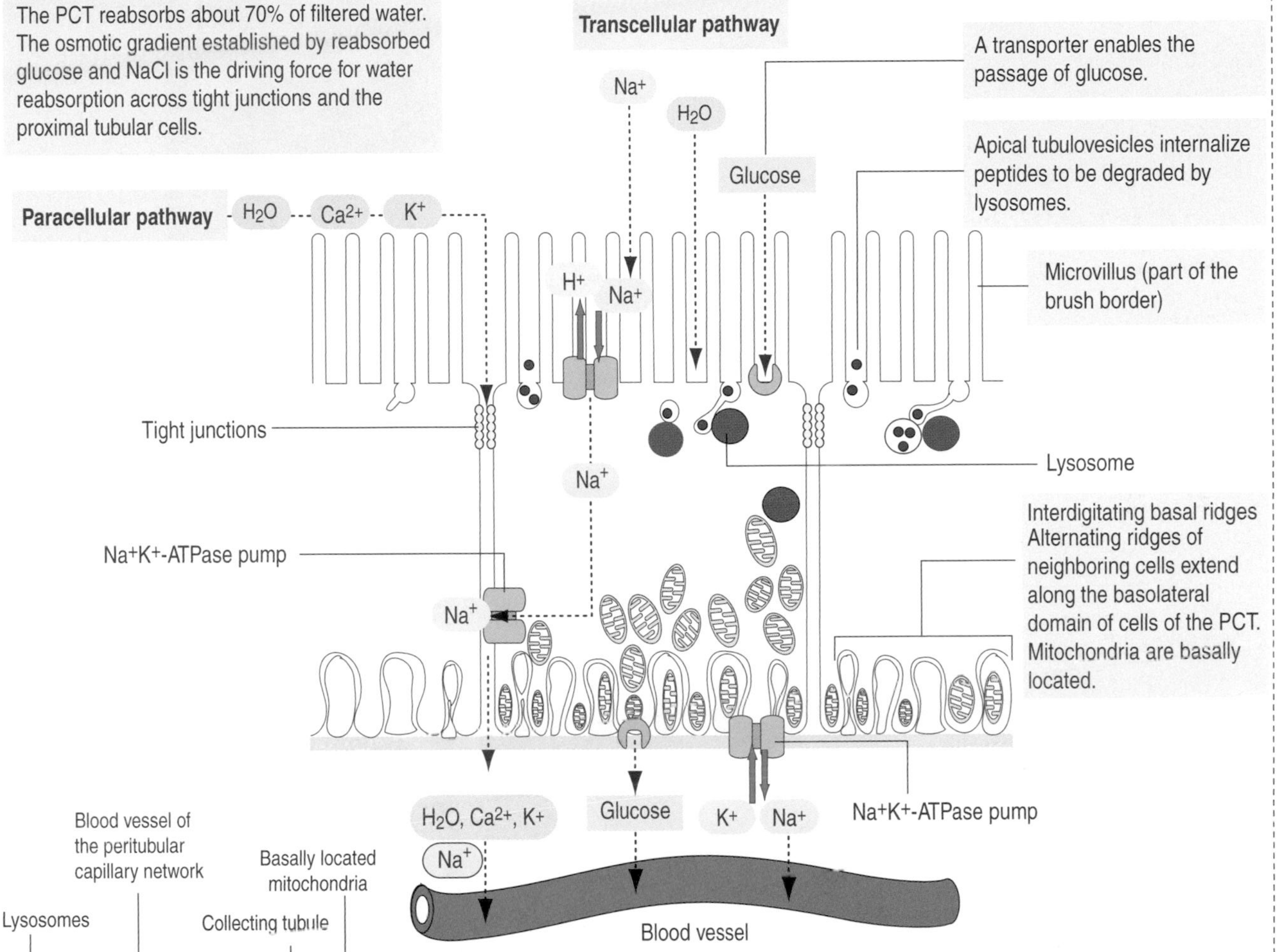

Transcellular pathway
Na+
H2O
Glucose
A transporter enables the passage of glucose.
Apical tubulovesicles internalize peptides to be degraded by lysosomes.
Paracellular pathway
H2O
Ca2+
K+
H+
Na+
Microvillus (part of the brush border)
Tight junctions
Lysosome
Na+
Interdigitating basal ridges Alternating ridges of neighboring cells extend along the basolateral domain of cells of the PCT. Mitochondria are basally located.
Na+K+-ATPase pump
Na+
H2O, Ca2+, K+
Na+
Glucose
K+
Na+
Na+K+-ATPase pump
Blood vessel

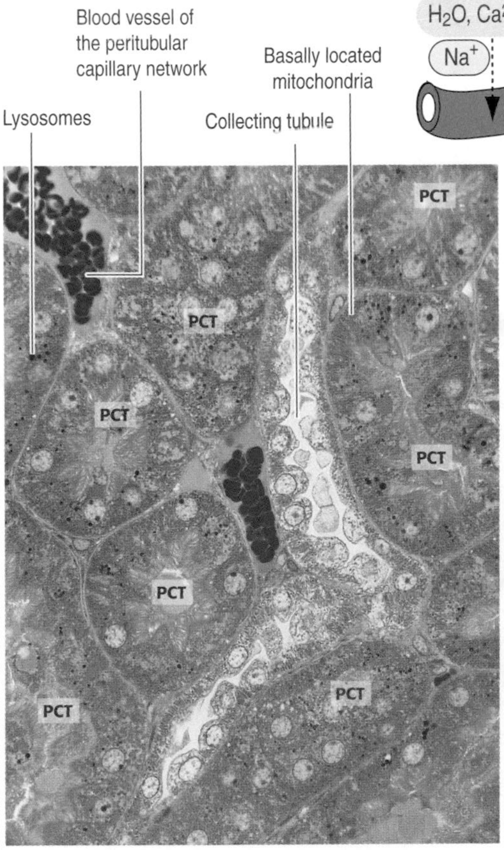

Blood vessel of the peritubular capillary network
Basally located mitochondria
Lysosomes
Collecting tubule
PCT
PCT
PCT
PCT
PCT
PCT
PCT
PCT

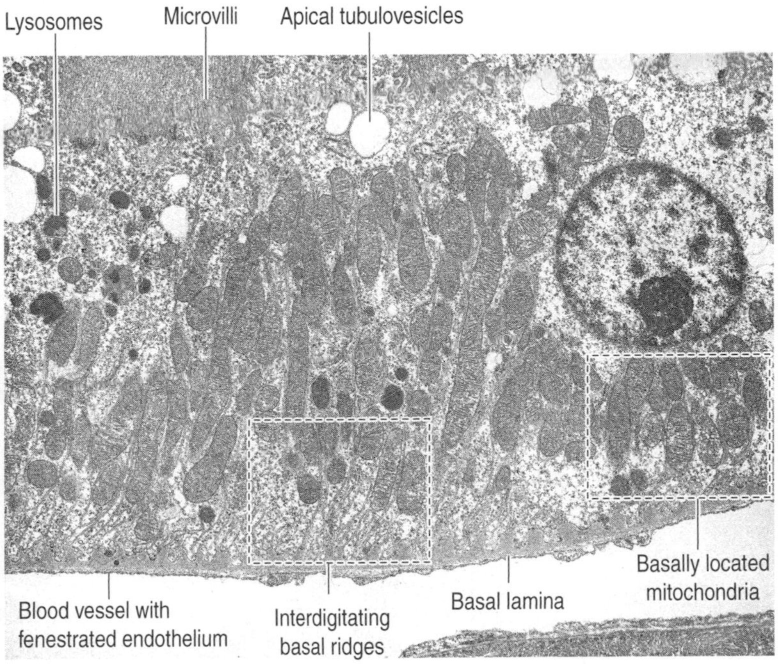

Lysosomes
Microvilli
Apical tubulovesicles
Blood vessel with fenestrated endothelium
Interdigitating basal ridges
Basal lamina
Basally located mitochondria

Figure 14-13. **Loop of Henle**

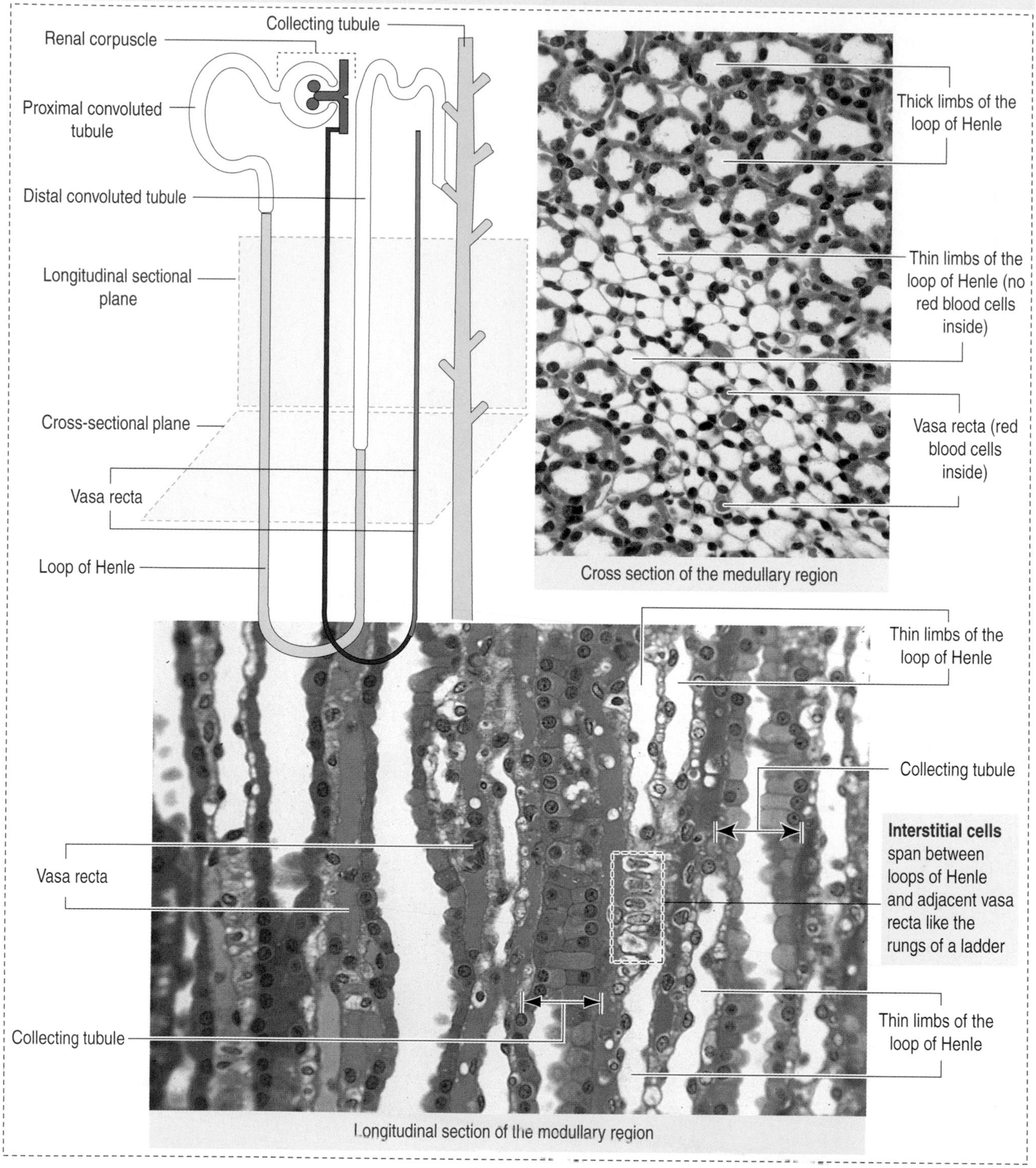

Renal corpuscle
Collecting tubule
Proximal convoluted tubule
Distal convoluted tubule
Longitudinal sectional plane
Cross-sectional plane
Vasa recta
Loop of Henle
Thick limbs of the loop of Henle
Thin limbs of the loop of Henle (no red blood cells inside)
Vasa recta (red blood cells inside)
Cross section of the medullary region
Thin limbs of the loop of Henle
Collecting tubule
Interstitial cells span between loops of Henle and adjacent vasa recta like the rungs of a ladder
Vasa recta
Thin limbs of the loop of Henle
Collecting tubule
Longitudinal section of the medullary region

dopamine secreted by adrenergic nerve fibers. Norepinephrine binds to α_1-adrenergic receptors in the afferent glomerular arteriole to cause vasoconstriction. There is no parasympathetic innervation.

We come back to the tubuloglomerular feedback mechanism when we discuss the renin-angiotensin-aldosterone regulatory mechanism (see Figure 14-18).

Proximal convoluted tubule: The reabsorption component

The plasma ultrafiltrate in the urinary space is transported by **active** and **passive** mechanisms to the proximal convoluted tubule (PCT), where about 70% of

Figure 14-14. Distal convoluted tubule (DCT)

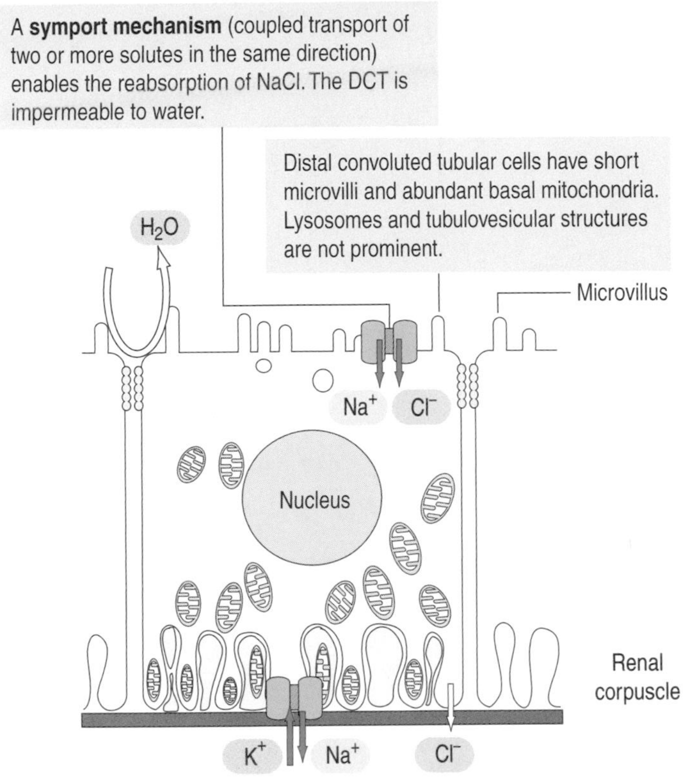
A **symport mechanism** (coupled transport of two or more solutes in the same direction) enables the reabsorption of NaCl. The DCT is impermeable to water.
Distal convoluted tubular cells have short microvilli and abundant basal mitochondria. Lysosomes and tubulovesicular structures are not prominent.
H_2O
Microvillus
Na^+
Cl^-
Nucleus
K^+
Na^+
Cl^-

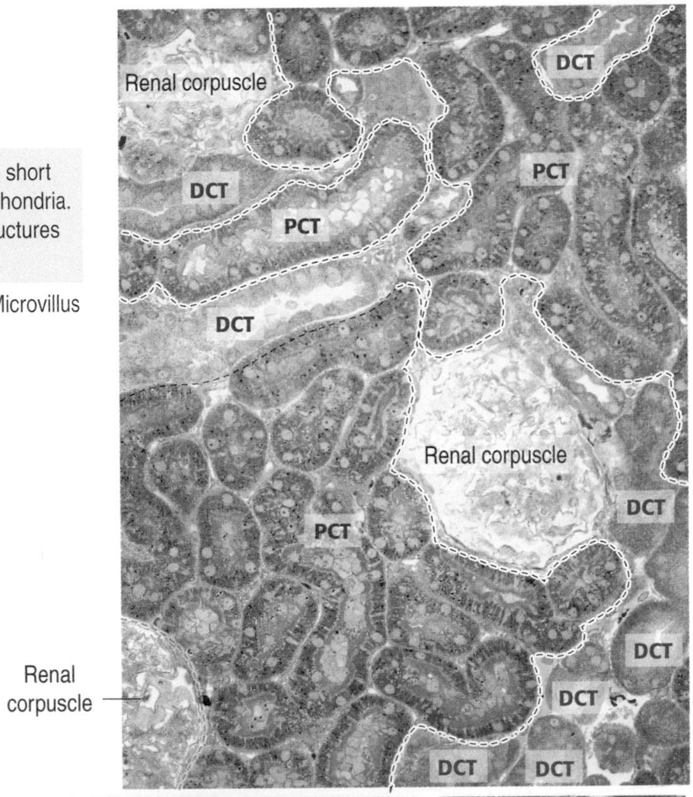
Renal corpuscle
DCT
PCT
DCT
PCT
PCT
DCT
Renal corpuscle
DCT
PCT
DCT
Renal corpuscle
DCT
DCT
DCT

Identification parameters of PCTs and DCTs

The identification of proximal convoluted tubules (PCTs) and DCTs is facilitated by the following parameters:

1. Both are adjacent to renal corpuscles.

2. PCTs contain cells with abundant **lysosomes** (stained dark in both light microscope illustrations).

3. The **apical domain** of PCTs has a prominent **brush border (microvilli)** and **vesicles**. In contrast, the apical domain of DCTs has sparce microvilli and vesicles.

4. Cells lining the PCTs and DCTs contain abundant basally located **mitochondria**.

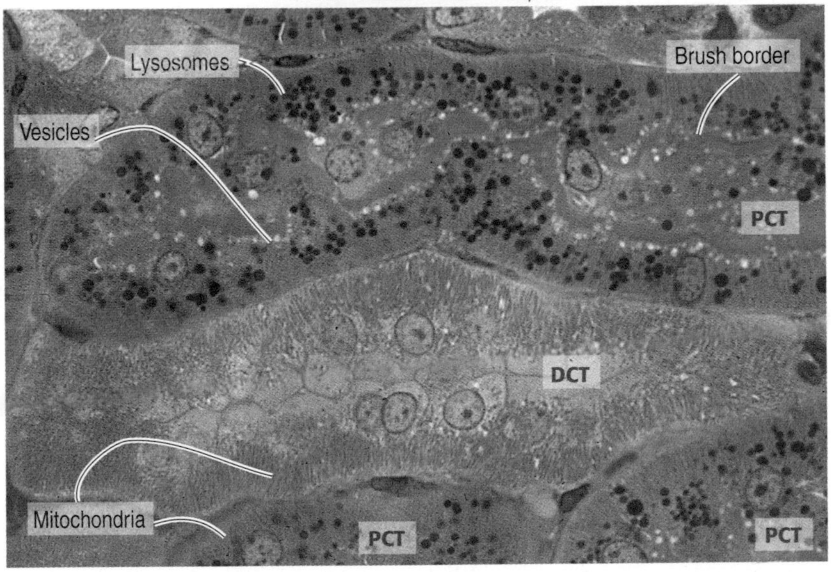
Lysosomes
Brush border
Vesicles
PCT
DCT
Mitochondria
PCT
PCT

filtered water, glucose, Na^+, Cl^-, and K^+, and other solutes are reabsorbed.

Cuboidal epithelial cells, held together by apical **tight junctions**, line the PCT and have structural characteristics suitable for reabsorption. They display the following features (Figure 14-12):

1. An apical domain with a well-developed **brush border** consisting of **microvilli.**

2. A basolateral domain with extensive plasma membrane **infoldings** and **interdigitations**.

3. Long mitochondria located between the plasma membrane folds provide adenosine triphosphate (ATP) for active transport of ions mediated by an **Mg^{2+}-dependent Na^+ K^+-activated pump.**

Figure 14-15. Juxtaglomerular cells and extramesangial cells

Juxtaglomerular cell

1. It is predominant in the **afferent arteriole** of the glomerulus.
2. It is a modified smooth muscle cell producing the enzyme **renin**.
3. Together with extraglomerular mesangial cells and the macula densa of the distal convoluted tubule, it is part of the **juxtaglomerular apparatus**.
4. Is innervated by **sympathetic nerve fibers**. Renin secretion is enhanced by **norepinephrine** and **dopamine** secreted by adrenergic nerve fibers.

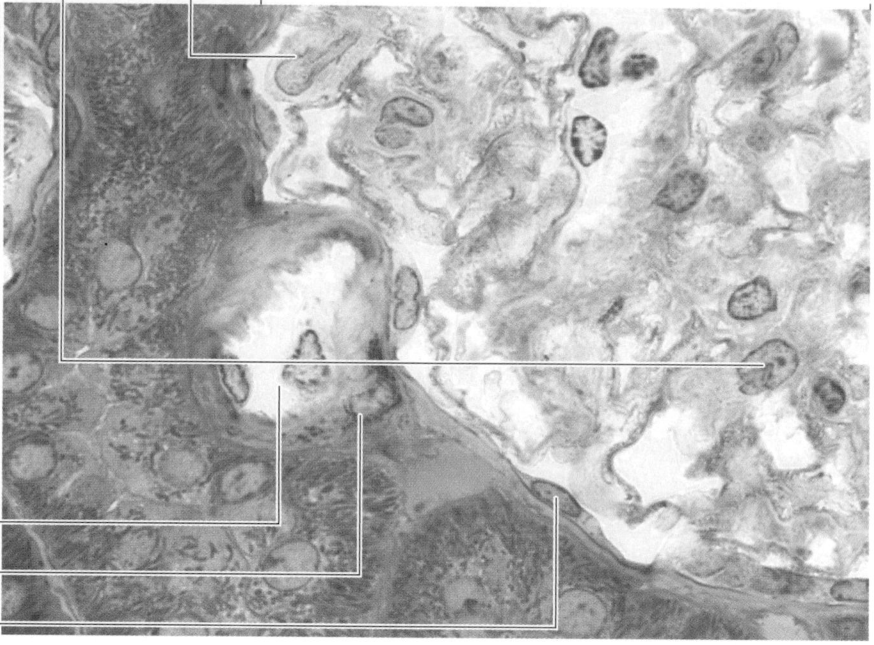

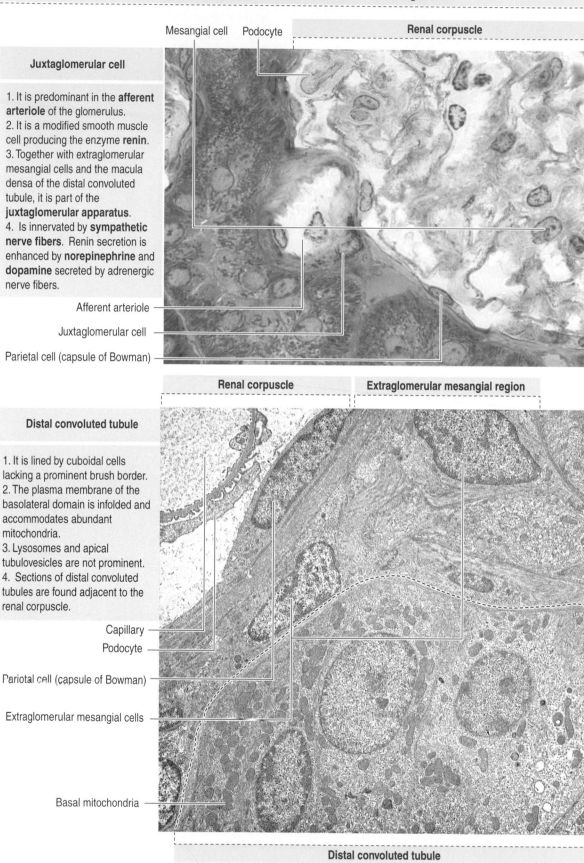

Mesangial cell
Podocyte
Renal corpuscle
Afferent arteriole
Juxtaglomerular cell
Parietal cell (capsule of Bowman)

Distal convoluted tubule

1. It is lined by cuboidal cells lacking a prominent brush border.
2. The plasma membrane of the basolateral domain is infolded and accommodates abundant mitochondria.
3. Lysosomes and apical tubulovesicles are not prominent.
4. Sections of distal convoluted tubules are found adjacent to the renal corpuscle.

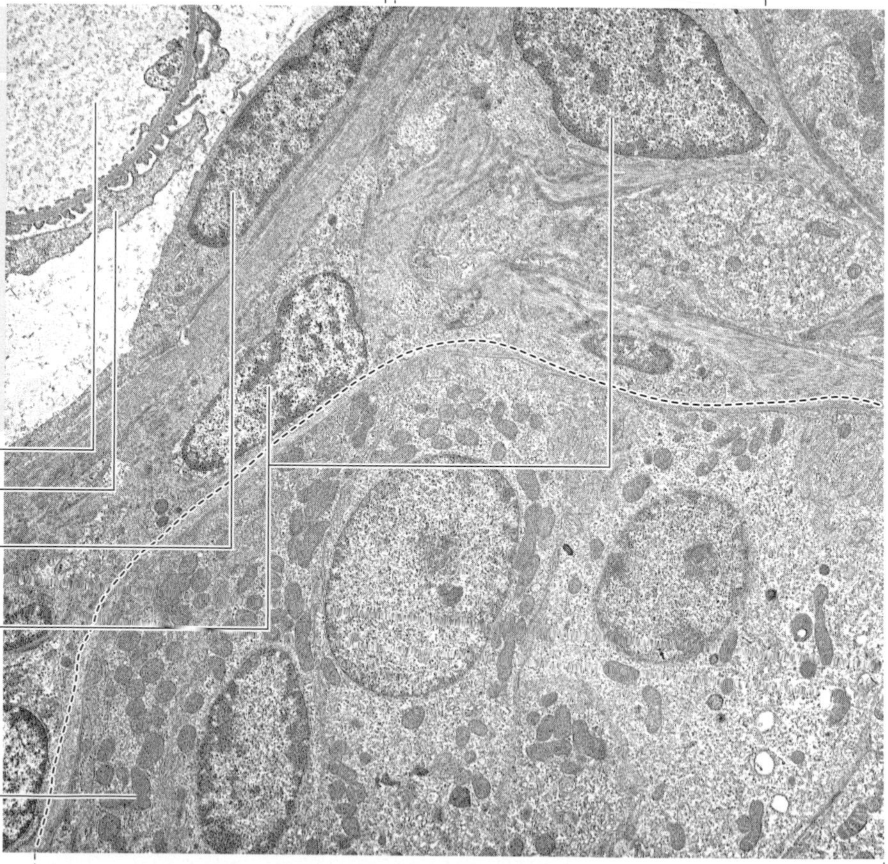

Renal corpuscle
Extraglomerular mesangial region
Capillary
Podocyte
Parietal cell (capsule of Bowman)
Extraglomerular mesangial cells
Basal mitochondria
Distal convoluted tubule

4. Apical **tubulovesicles** and **lysosomes** provide a mechanism for endocytosis and breakdown of small proteins into amino acids. The movement of **urea** and **glucose** across the plasma membrane is mediated by a **transport protein**. Reabsorbed material enters the peritubular capillary network.

The driving force for water reabsorption is a **transcellular** osmotic gradient established by the reabsorption of solutes, such as NaCl and glucose. Because the PCT is highly permeable to water, water passes by osmosis across tight junctions (**paracellular pathway**) into the lateral intercellular space. An increase in the hydrostatic pressure in the intercellular compartment forces fluids and solutes to move into the capillary network.

The **Fanconi syndrome** is a renal hereditary (primary) or acquired (secondary) disease in which PCTs fail to reabsorb amino acids and glucose. Consequently, these substances are excreted in urine. The cause is a defective cellular energy metabolism resulting from a decrease in ATP levels attributed to the impaired activity of the Mg^{2+}-dependent Na^+ K^+-activated ATPase pump. **Cystinosis,** caused by the accumulation of cystine in renal tubule cells, is the most common cause of Fanconi syndrome in children.

Loop of Henle

The loop of Henle reabsorbs about 15% of the filtered water and 25% of the filtered NaCl, K^+, Ca^{2+}, and HCO_3^-.

The loop of Henle consists of a **descending limb** and an **ascending limb**. Each limb is formed by a **thick segment** and a **thin segment** (Figure 14-13).

The thick descending segment is a continuation of the PCT. The thick ascending segment is continuous with the distal convoluted tubule (DCT).

The length of the thin segments varies in cortical and juxtamedullary nephrons. Because **the ascending limb is impermeable to water**, filtered water reabsorption occurs exclusively in the descending limb, driven by an osmotic gradient between the tubular fluid and the interstitial fluid.

As in the PCT, an **Na^+, K^+-ATPase pump** in the ascend-ing limb is a key element in the reabsorption of solutes. Inhibition of this pump by **diuretics** such as **furosemide** (Lasix) inhibits the reabsorption of NaCl and increases urinary excretion of both NaCl and water by reducing the osmolality of the interstitial fluid in the medulla.

The thick segments of the limbs are lined by a low cuboidal epithelium in transition with the epithelial lining of the proximal tubules. The thin segments are lined by a squamous simple epithelium.

Distal convoluted tubule

The DCT and the collecting duct reabsorb approximately 7% of the filtered NaCl. The **distal portion** of the DCT and the **collecting ducts** are permeable to water in the presence of **antidiuretic hormone** (ADH, or vasopressin).

NaCl enters the cell across the apical domain and leaves the cell by an **Na^+, K^+-ATPase pump** (Figure 14-14). The reabsorption of NaCl is reduced by **thiazide diuretics** that inhibit the apical domain transporting mechanism (see Figure 14-20).

The active dilution of the tubular fluid initiated in the ascending segments of the loop of Henle continues in the DCT. Because the ascending segment of the loop of Henle is the major site where water and solutes are separated, the excretion of both dilute and concentrated urine requires the normal function of the loop of Henle.

The cuboidal epithelial cell lining of the DCT has the following characteristics (Figure 14-15; see also Figure14-14):

1. **Cuboidal cells are shorter** than those in the PCT and **lack a prominent brush border**.

2. As in the PCT, the plasma membrane of the basolateral domain is infolded

Figure 14-16. Collecting tubule/duct

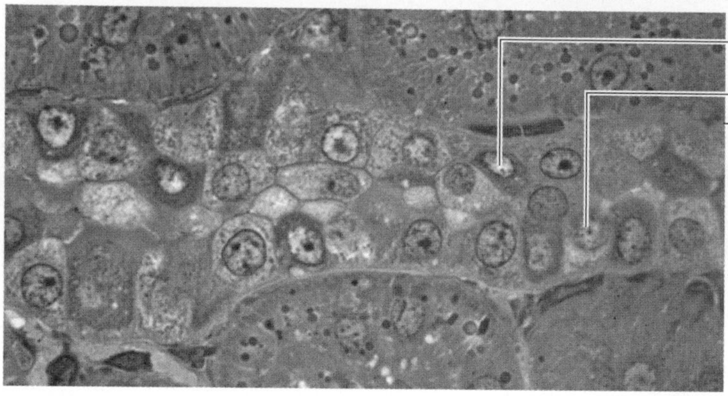

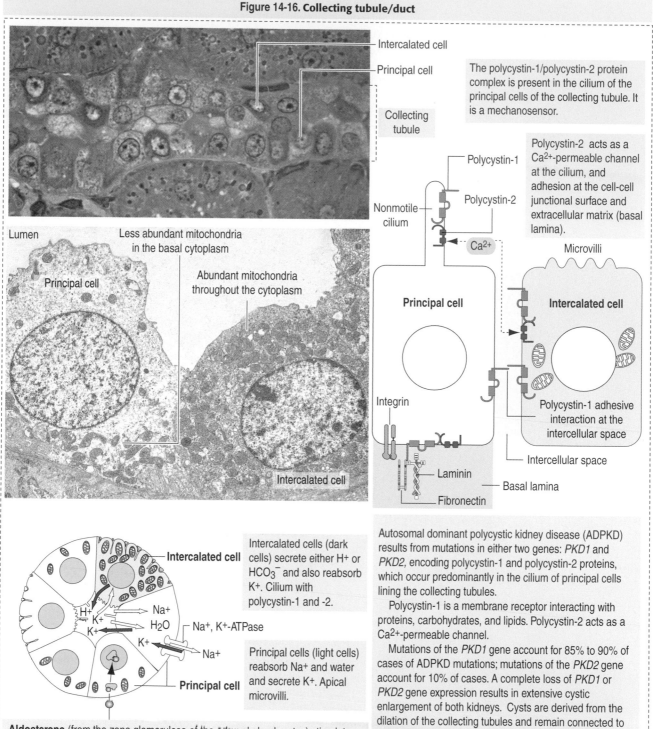

Intercalated cell
Principal cell
Collecting tubule

The polycystin-1/polycystin-2 protein complex is present in the cilium of the principal cells of the collecting tubule. It is a mechanosensor.

Polycystin-2 acts as a Ca^{2+}-permeable channel at the cilium, and adhesion at the cell-cell junctional surface and extracellular matrix (basal lamina).

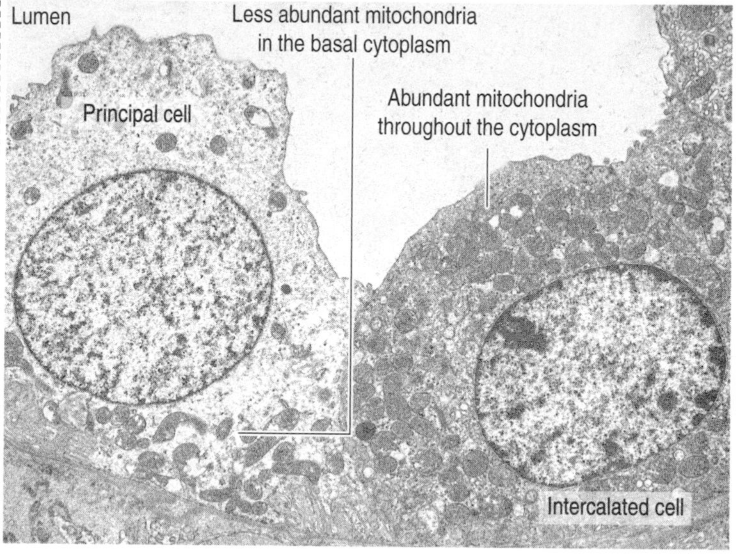

Lumen
Less abundant mitochondria in the basal cytoplasm
Principal cell
Abundant mitochondria throughout the cytoplasm
Intercalated cell

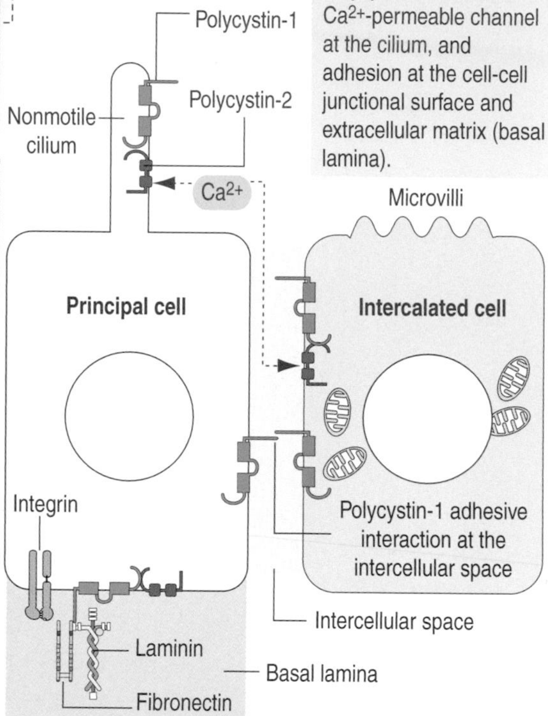

Polycystin-1
Polycystin-2
Nonmotile cilium
Ca2+
Microvilli
Principal cell
Intercalated cell
Integrin
Polycystin-1 adhesive interaction at the intercellular space
Intercellular space
Laminin
Basal lamina
Fibronectin

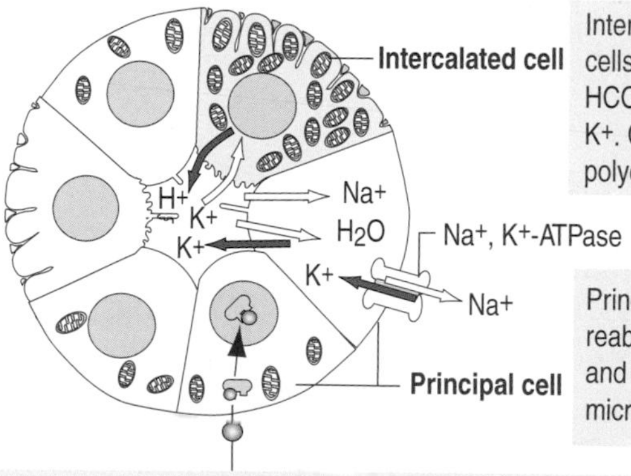

Intercalated cell
H+
K+
K+
Na+
H2O
Na+, K+-ATPase
K+
Na+
Principal cell

Intercalated cells (dark cells) secrete either H^+ or HCO_3^- and also reabsorb K^+. Cilium with polycystin-1 and -2.

Principal cells (light cells) reabsorb Na^+ and water and secrete K^+. Apical microvilli.

Aldosterone (from the zona glomerulosa of the adrenal gland cortex) stimulates the reabsorption of Na^+ at the collecting tubule. Retention of Na^+ results in water retention, helping to correct hypovolemia (decrease in total body water) and hyponatremia (decrease in total body Na^+).

Autosomal dominant polycystic kidney disease (ADPKD) results from mutations in either two genes: *PKD1* and *PKD2,* encoding polycystin-1 and polycystin-2 proteins, which occur predominantly in the cilium of principal cells lining the collecting tubules.

Polycystin-1 is a membrane receptor interacting with proteins, carbohydrates, and lipids. Polycystin-2 acts as a Ca^{2+}-permeable channel.

Mutations of the *PKD1* gene account for 85% to 90% of cases of ADPKD mutations; mutations of the *PKD2* gene account for 10% of cases. A complete loss of *PKD1* or *PKD2* gene expression results in extensive cystic enlargement of both kidneys. Cysts are derived from the dilation of the collecting tubules and remain connected to the nephron of origin. Nephron segments also show cystic dilations.

Hypertension and renal failure are clinical manifestations

and lodges mitochondria.

3. In the **macula densa**, the cells display a **reversed polarity**: the nucleus occupies an apical position and the basal domain, containing a Golgi apparatus, faces the juxtaglomerular cells and extraglomerular mesangial cells. The macula densa, located at the junction of the ascending thick segment with the DCT, senses changes in Na^+ concentration in the tubular fluid.

Collecting tubule (duct)

The collecting tubule (also called duct) is lined by a cuboidal epithelium composed of two cell types: **principal cells** and **intercalated cells** (Figure 14-16). Principal cells have an apical nonmotile cilium and a basolateral domain with moderate infoldings and mitochondria. They reabsorb Na^+ and water and secrete K^+ in an Na^+,K^+-ATPase pump-dependent manner. Intercalated cells have apical microvilli and abundant mitochondria and secrete either H^+ or HCO_3^-. Therefore, they are important regulators of acid-base balance. They also reabsorb K^+.

The nonmotile cilium of principal cells is a **mechanosensor** of fluid flow and contents. The ciliary plasma membrane contains membrane-associated proteins **polycystin-1** and **polycystin-2.** Polycystin-1 is regarded as a cell-cell and cell-extracellular matrix adhesive protein. Polycystin-2 acts as a Ca^{2+}-permeable channel.

A mutation of either the gene *PKD1,* encoding polycystin-1, or *PKD2,* encoding polycystin-2, results in **autosomal dominant polycystic kidney disease (ADPKD)**. A complete loss of *PKD1* or *PKD2* gene expression results in the formation of massive renal cysts derived from dilated collecting ducts. Patients present with blood hypertension and progressive renal failure after their third decade of life. Renal dialysis and renal transplantation can extend the lifetime of patients with ADPKD.

Interstitial cells

We noted in Figure 14-13 the presence of vertical stacks of interstitial cells extending from the loops of Henle to adjacent vasa recta like the rungs of a ladder. There are two populations of interstitial cells: renal cortical and medullary fibroblasts. Their function is the maintenance of renal architecture and production of **erythropoietin**. Synthetic erythropoietin is used in the treatment of anemia resulting from chronic renal failure or cancer chemotherapy.

The cytoplasm of renal medullary fibroblast-like interstitial cells contains actin filaments. It has been suggested that interstitial cells secrete prostaglandins and may regulate papillary blood flow by contracting in response to hormonal stimulation. Lipid droplets can also be seen in their cytoplasm.

Activated interstitial fibroblasts and inflammatory cells (macrophages and lymphocytes) participate in **interstitial nephritis** (tubulointerstitial disease) caused by nephrotoxic drugs (such as heavy metals or hypersensitivity to penicillin) or by an immunologic mechanism (for example, lupus erythematosus).

Excretory passages of urine

The urine released at the openings of the papillary ducts flows from the calyces and pelvis into the ureters and enters the urinary bladder. Peristaltic waves, spreading from the calyces along the ureter, force the urine toward the bladder.

The walls of the ureter and urinary bladder (Figure 14-17) contain folds (rugae). As the bladder fills with urine, the rugae flatten and the volume of the bladder increases with minimal increase in intravesical pressure. The renal calyces, pelvis, ureter, and urinary bladder are lined by a **transitional epithelium**, the **urothelium**, composed of basal and superficial cells. The epithelium and the subjacent lamina propria are surrounded by **combined helical and longitudinal layers of smooth muscle fibers**.

In the bladder, a mixture of randomly arranged smooth muscle cells form the syncytial **detrusor muscle**. At the neck of the urinary bladder, the muscle fibers form a three-layer (inner longitudinal, middle circular, and outer longitudinal) internal functional sphincter.

Micturition, the process of emptying the urinary bladder, involves the micturition reflex, an automatic spinal cord reflex, and the stimulation of the detrusor muscle by parasympathetic fibers to contract.

Nephrolithiasis is a condition in which kidney stones, composed of calcium

Figure 14-17. Urinary bladder

The **mucosa** of the urinary bladder is folded and lined with transitional epithelium (urothelium). Fibroelastic connective tissue extends into the folds (*arrows*).

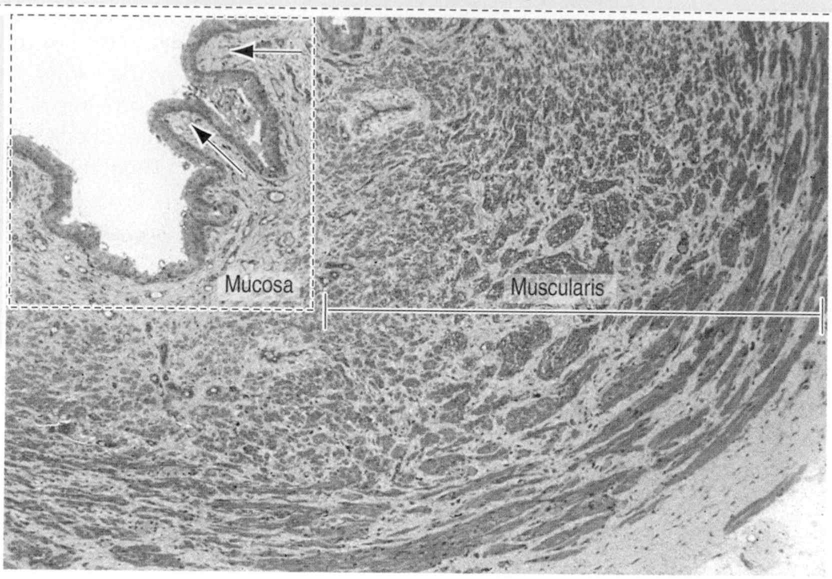
Mucosa
Muscularis

The **muscularis** contains numerous bundles of smooth muscle cells arranged irregularly as outer and inner longitudinal layers and a middle circular layer.

Urothelium of an empty urinary bladder

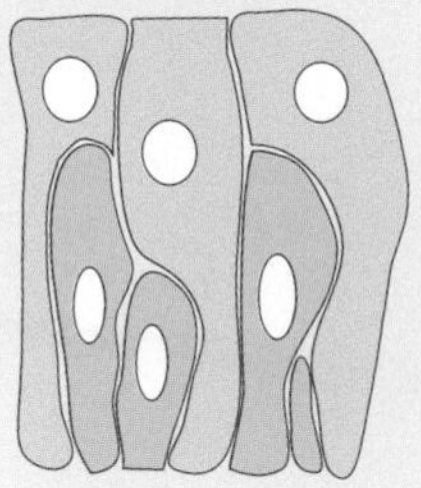

Urothelium of a urinary bladder filled with urine

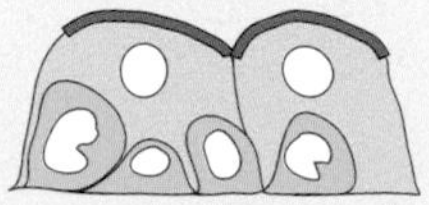

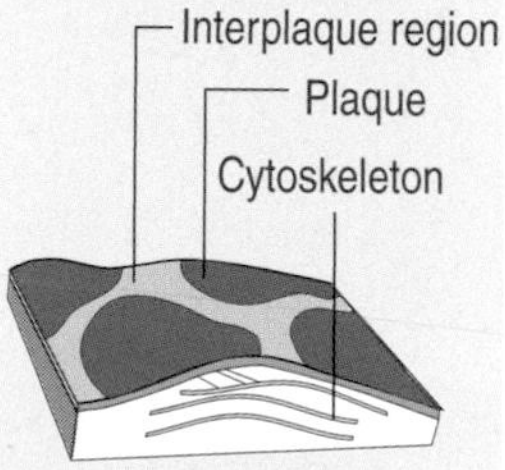
Interplaque region
Plaque
Cytoskeleton

Plaques are formed by the aggregation of hexagonal intramembranous proteins to which cytoskeletal proteins are anchored on the cytoplasmic side.

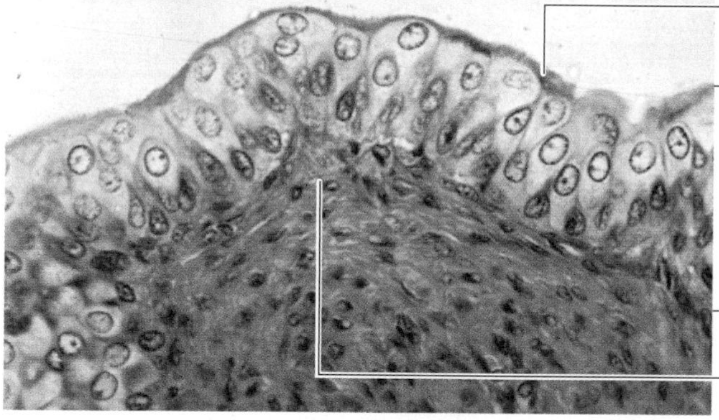
Plaques
Fibroelastic connective tissue

Urothelium

The columnar-like epithelium can stretch and resemble a stratified squamous epithelium when urine is present in the urinary bladder.

Apical plaques generate a thickened domain able to adjust to large changes in surface area.

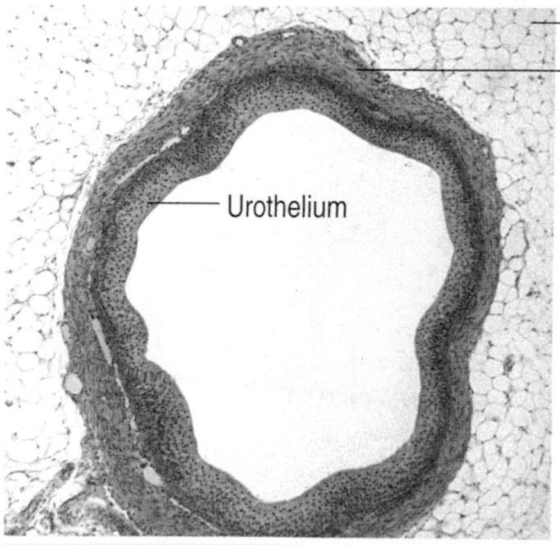
Adventitia
Muscularis
Urothelium

Ureter

The mucosa of the ureter is lined by a transitional epithelium (urothelium). The mucosa is surrounded by a fibroelastic lamina propria and a muscularis with two to three layers of smooth muscle. The ureter is surrounded by an adventitia containing adipose tissue.

salts, uric acid, or magnesium-ammonium acetate, form by crystallization when urine is concentrated. When the ureter is blocked by a stone, the contraction of the smooth muscle generates severe pain in the flank.

The **male urethra** is 20 cm long and consists of three segments. Upon leaving the urinary bladder, the **prostatic urethra**—lined by transitional epithelium—crosses the prostate gland, continues as a short **membranous urethra** segment, and ends as the **penile urethra**, which is enclosed by the corpus spongiosum of the penis (see Figure 21-12 in Chapter 21, Sperm Transport and Maturation). Both the membranous and penile urethra are lined by pseudostratified or stratified columnar epithelium.

The **female urethra** is 4 cm long and its longitudinally microfolded mucosa is covered by a stratified squamous epithelium that becomes moderately keratinized stratified squamous epithelium near the urethral meatus. The lamina propria contains elastic fibers and a venous plexus. An **inner smooth muscle layer** and an **external striated muscle layer** (continuous with the internal sphincter) are present in the wall. Additional structural details of the male and female urethra can be found in Chapter 21, Sperm Transport and Maturation, and Chapter 22, Follicle Development and Menstrual Cycle, respectively.

Regulation of water and NaCl absorption

Several hormones and factors regulate the absorption of water and NaCl (see Box 14-A for a review of terminology related to osmoregulation):

1. **Angiotensin II** stimulates NaCl and water reabsorption in the PCT. A decrease in the extracellular fluid volume activates the renin-angiotensin-aldosterone system and increases the concentration of plasma angiotensin II.

2. **Aldosterone**, synthesized by the glomerulosa cells of the adrenal cortex, stimulates the reabsorption of NaCl at the ascending limb of the loop of Henle, the DCT, and the collecting tubule. An increase in the plasma concentration of angiotensin II and K^+ stimulates aldosterone secretion.

3. **Atrial natriuretic factor** (a 28-amino-acid peptide secreted by atrial cardiocytes; see Figure 12-3 in Chapter 12, Cardiovascular System) and **urodilatin** (a 32-amino-acid peptide analog of atrial natriuretic factor) are encoded by the same gene and have similar amino acid sequences. Atrial natriuretic factor has two main functions: (1) it increases the urinary excretion of NaCl and water and (2) it inhibits the release of ADH from the neurohypophysis.

Urodilatin is secreted by epithelial cells of the DCT and collecting tubule and inhibits NaCl and water reabsorption by the medullary portion of the collecting tubule. Urodilatin is a more potent natriuretic and diuretic hormone than atrial natriuretic factor.

4. **Antidiuretic hormone,** or **vasopressin**, is the most important hormone in the regulation of water balance. ADH is a small peptide (nine amino acids in length) synthesized by neuroendocrine cells located within the **supraoptic** and **paraventricular nuclei** of the **hypothalamus**.

When the extracellular fluid volume decreases (hypovolemia), ADH increases the permeability of the collecting tubule to water, thereby increasing water reabsorption. When ADH is not present, the collecting tubule is impermeable to water. ADH has little effect on the urinary excretion of NaCl.

Diabetes insipidus is a disorder associated with a low production of ADH (central diabetes insipidus) or a failure of the kidney to respond to circulating ADH (nephrogenic diabetes insipidus). In the absence of ADH, water cannot be reabsorbed normally to correct hyperosmolality, and **hypernatremia** (high levels of Na^+ in plasma), **polyuria** (excessive volume of urine and frequency of urination), and **polydipsia** (thirst and increasing drinking) occur.

In **diabetes mellitus,** the concentration of glucose in plasma is abnormally elevated. Glucose overwhelms the reabsorptive capacity of the PCT, and intratubular glucose levels increase. Acting as an effective osmole, intratubular glucose hampers water reabsorption even in the presence of ADH. **Osmotic diuresis** is responsible for **glucosuria** (presence of glucose in urine), polyuria, and polydipsia in the diabetic patient. No glucosuria is observed in patients with diabetes insipidus.

Box 14-A | Review of terminology

- Osmolality is the concentration of solutes in body fluids. Alterations in osmolality depend on the gain or loss of water or on the loss or gain of osmoles (for example, glucose, urea, and salts). Plasma osmolality is kept normalized by the excretion of excess water, recovery of lost water, or by normalization of solute levels in the body.
- Molarity and molality refer to the concentration of a solute in a solution. The units of molarity are mol solute/L solution. The units of molality are mol solute/kg solvent. Osmolality and osmolarity represent the number of moles of solute particles in a solution (for example, Na^+ and Cl^- separately) instead of moles of compound in solution (for example, NaCl).
- Osmosis is the passive diffusion of water (the solvent) across a membrane from an area of low solute concentration to an area of high solute concentration. Osmotic equilibrium is reached when the amount of solute is equal on both sides of a membrane and the influx of water stops. Osmosis depends on the number of free dissolved particles without distinction between different molecular species (for example, Na^+ and Cl^-).
- Osmotic pressure is an indicator of how much water a compartment will draw into it through osmosis. Osmolarity and osmolality of the compartments on either side of a membrane determine the osmotic pressure of a compartment.
- Plasma membrane pumps and channels ensure that solutes are not distributed evenly on either side of a membrane as water does. If solutes distributed evenly, a concentration gradient would not exist to drive osmosis.
- Effective osmoles. A solute such as urea is not an effective osmole because it does not create osmotic pressure. Solutes such as Na^+, K^+, and Cl^- are effective osmoles. Pumps and channels keep Na^+ outside of cells and K^+ inside of cells as effective osmoles.
- Aquaporins. The permeability of cells to water is facilitated by plasma membrane water channels called aquaporins. Different tissues have variable amounts of aquaporins and the cells may be more or less permeable to water than others. Antidiuretic hormone determines the insertion of aquaporins in the collecting duct, increasing its permeability to water.

Renin-angiotensin-aldosterone system

This system is a significant component of the **tubuloglomerular feedback system,** essential for the maintenance of systemic arterial blood pressure when there is a reduction in the vascular volume. A reduction in vascular volume results in a decrease in the rate of glomerular filtration and the amount of filtered NaCl. A reduction in filtered NaCl is sensed by the macula densa, which triggers renin secretion and the production of angiotensin II, a potent vasoconstrictor.

The **tubuloglomerular feedback system** consists of:

1. A **glomerular component**: The **juxtaglomerular cells** predominate in the muscle cell wall of the afferent glomerular arteriole but are also present in smaller number in the efferent glomerular arteriole. Juxtaglomerular cells synthesize, store, and release **renin**. Activation of sympathetic nerve fibers results in the increased secretion of renin.

2. A **tubular component**: The **macula densa** mediates renin secretion after sensing the NaCl content in the incoming urine from the thick ascending seg-

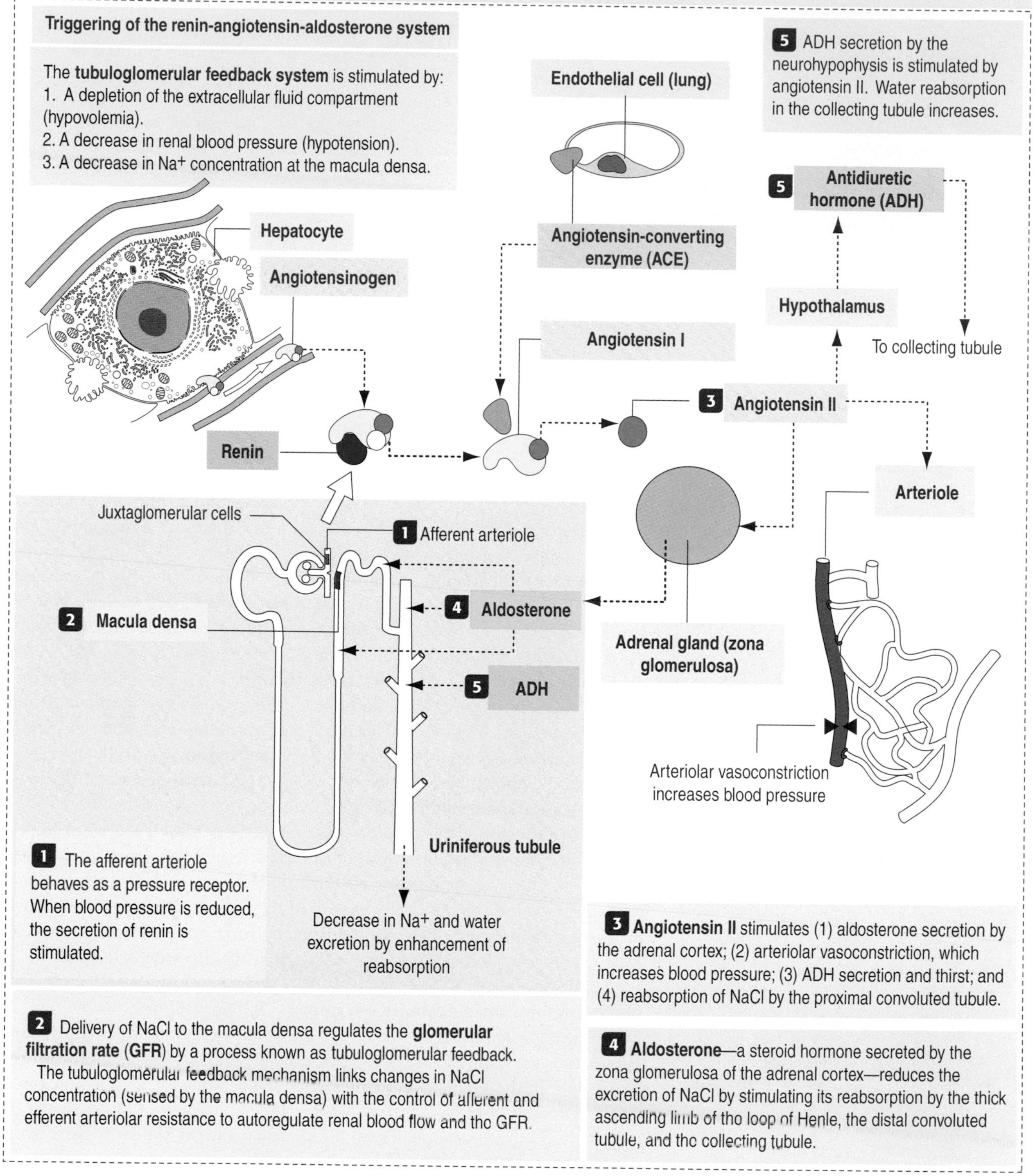

Triggering of the renin-angiotensin-aldosterone system
The tubuloglomerular feedback system is stimulated by:
1. A depletion of the extracellular fluid compartment (hypovolemia).
2. A decrease in renal blood pressure (hypotension).
3. A decrease in Na+ concentration at the macula densa.
Endothelial cell (lung)
5 ADH secretion by the neurohypophysis is stimulated by angiotensin II. Water reabsorption in the collecting tubule increases.
5 Antidiuretic hormone (ADH)
Hepatocyte
Angiotensinogen
Angiotensin-converting enzyme (ACE)
Hypothalamus
Angiotensin I
To collecting tubule
3 Angiotensin II
Renin
Arteriole
Juxtaglomerular cells
1 Afferent arteriole
4 Aldosterone
2 Macula densa
Adrenal gland (zona glomerulosa)
5 ADH
Arteriolar vasoconstriction increases blood pressure
Uriniferous tubule
1 The afferent arteriole behaves as a pressure receptor. When blood pressure is reduced, the secretion of renin is stimulated.
Decrease in Na+ and water excretion by enhancement of reabsorption
3 Angiotensin II stimulates (1) aldosterone secretion by the adrenal cortex; (2) arteriolar vasoconstriction, which increases blood pressure; (3) ADH secretion and thirst; and (4) reabsorption of NaCl by the proximal convoluted tubule.
2 Delivery of NaCl to the macula densa regulates the glomerular filtration rate (GFR) by a process known as tubuloglomerular feedback.
The tubuloglomerular feedback mechanism links changes in NaCl concentration (sensed by the macula densa) with the control of afferent and efferent arteriolar resistance to autoregulate renal blood flow and the GFR.
4 Aldosterone—a steroid hormone secreted by the zona glomerulosa of the adrenal cortex—reduces the excretion of NaCl by stimulating its reabsorption by the thick ascending limb of the loop of Henle, the distal convoluted tubule, and the collecting tubule.

Figure 14-18. Renin-angiotensin-aldosterone system

ment of the limb of Henle. When the delivery of NaCl to the macula densa decreases, renin secretion is enhanced. Conversely, when NaCl increases, renin secretion decreases.

The **renin-angiotensin-aldosterone system** consists of the following components (Figure 14-18):

1. **Angiotensinogen**, a circulating protein in plasma produced by the liver.

2. The **juxtaglomerular cells**, the source of the proteolytic enzyme **renin**, which converts **angiotensinogen** to **angiotensin I**, a decapeptide with no known

Figure 14–19. Countercurrent multiplier and exchanger

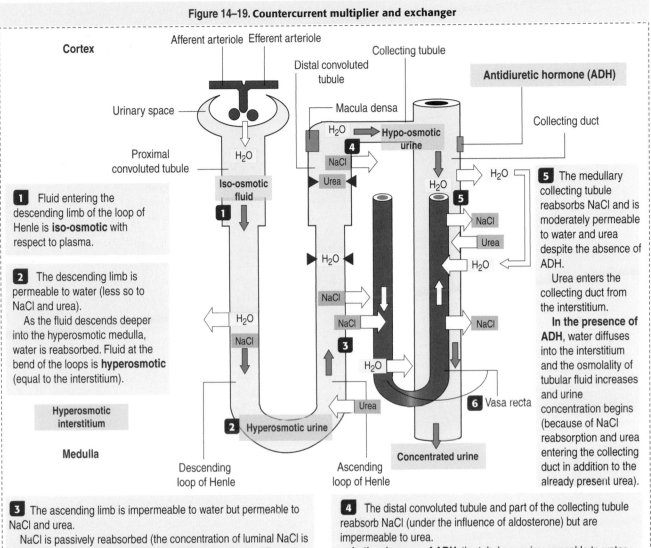

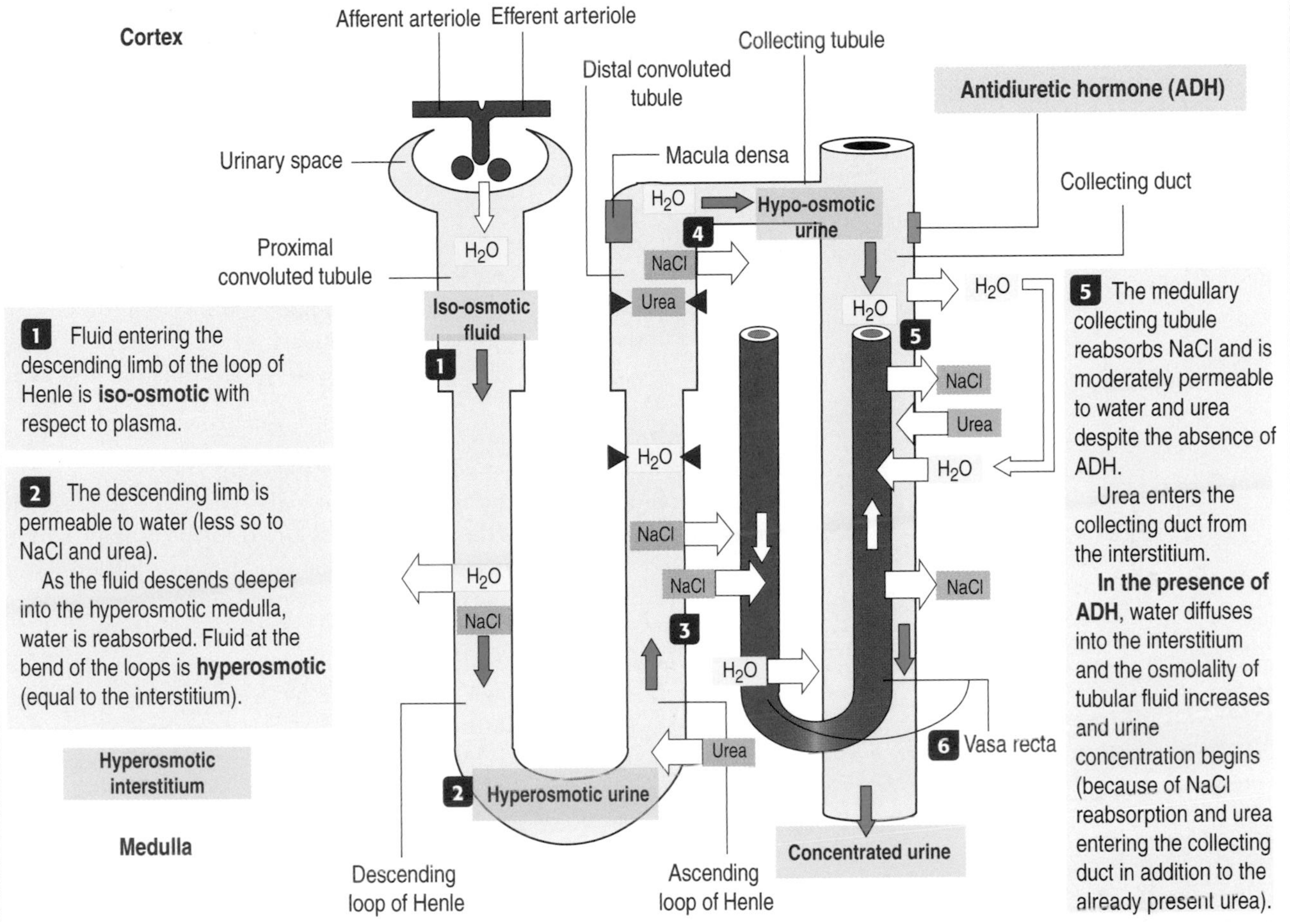
Cortex
Afferent arteriole
Efferent arteriole
Collecting tubule
Distal convoluted tubule
Antidiuretic hormone (ADH)
Urinary space
Macula densa
Collecting duct
H_2O
Hypo-osmotic urine
4
Proximal convoluted tubule
NaCl
Urea
Iso-osmotic fluid
1
5
Urea
H_2O
NaCl
3
2
Hyperosmotic interstitium
Hyperosmotic urine
6 Vasa recta
Medulla
Concentrated urine
Descending loop of Henle
Ascending loop of Henle

1 Fluid entering the descending limb of the loop of Henle is **iso-osmotic** with respect to plasma.

2 The descending limb is permeable to water (less so to NaCl and urea).

As the fluid descends deeper into the hyperosmotic medulla, water is reabsorbed. Fluid at the bend of the loops is **hyperosmotic** (equal to the interstitium).

5 The medullary collecting tubule reabsorbs NaCl and is moderately permeable to water and urea despite the absence of ADH.

Urea enters the collecting duct from the interstitium.

In the presence of ADH, water diffuses into the interstitium and the osmolality of tubular fluid increases and urine concentration begins (because of NaCl reabsorption and urea entering the collecting duct in addition to the already present urea).

3 The ascending limb is impermeable to water but permeable to NaCl and urea.

NaCl is passively reabsorbed (the concentration of luminal NaCl is greater than the interstitial NaCl concentration) and urea diffuses into the tubular fluid (urea concentration in the lumen is less than that in the interstitium).

Dilution of the tubular fluid occurs and urine becomes gradually **hypo-osmotic** with respect to plasma.

Note that NaCl and urea (and other solutes) in the interstitial fluid provide the driving force for reabsorption.

Urea is produced in the liver as a product of protein metabolism and enters the nephron by glomerular filtration.

4 The distal convoluted tubule and part of the collecting tubule reabsorb NaCl (under the influence of aldosterone) but are impermeable to urea.

In the absence of ADH, the tubules are impermeable to water (NaCl is reabsorbed without water) and the osmolality is reduced. The fluid entering the collecting ducts is **hypo-osmotic with respect to plasma**.

6 The **vasa recta** are a capillary network that removes—in a flow-dependent manner—excess of water and solutes continuously added to the interstitium by the nephron segments.

physiologic function.

3. The **angiotensin-converting enzyme** (ACE), a product of pulmonary and renal **endothelial cells**, which converts **angiotensin I** to the octapeptide **angiotensin II**.

Angiotensin has several important functions:

1. It stimulates the secretion of aldosterone by the adrenal cortex.
2. It causes vasoconstriction, which, in turn, increases blood pressure.
3. It enhances the reabsorption of NaCl by the PCTs of the nephron.
4. It stimulates ADH release.

Aldosterone acts primarily on **principal cells of the collecting tubule** and secondarily on the thick ascending limb of Henle to increase the entry of NaCl across the apical membrane. As with all steroid hormones, aldosterone enters the cell and binds to a cytosolic receptor. The aldosterone-receptor complex enters the nucleus and stimulates gene activity required for the reabsorption of NaCl.

Countercurrent multiplier and exchanger

The kidneys regulate water balance and are the major site for the release of water from the body. Water is also lost by evaporation from the skin and the respiratory tract and from the gastrointestinal tract (fecal water and diarrhea).

Water excretion by the kidneys occurs independently of other substances, such as Na^+, Cl^-, K^+, H^+, and urea. The kidney excretes either **concentrated** (hyper-osmotic) or **diluted** (hypo-osmotic) urine.

ADH regulates the volume and osmolality of the urine without modifying the excretion of other solutes. The primary action of ADH is to increase the permeability of the collecting tubule to water. An additional action is to increase the permeability of the collecting ducts at the medullary region to urea.

Figure 14-19 summarizes the **essential steps of urine formation and excretion**:

1. The fluid from the proximal convoluted tubules entering the loop of Henle is **iso-osmotic** with respect to plasma.

2. The **descending limb of the loop of Henle** is **highly permeable to water and, to a lesser extent, to NaCl**. As the fluid descends into the hyperosmotic interstitium, water and NaCl equilibrate and the tubular fluid becomes **hyperosmotic**.

3. When the fluid reaches the **bend of the loop**, its composition is **hyperosmotic**.

4. The **ascending limb of the loop of Henle** is **impermeable to water**. The concentration of NaCl in the lumen, greater than in the interstitium, is reabsorbed and enters the descending (arterial) portion of the vasa recta. Therefore, the fluid leaving this tubular segment is **hypo-osmotic**. This segment of the nephron is called the **diluting segment**.

5. The distal convoluted tubule and cortical portions of the collecting tubule reabsorb NaCl. In the **absence** of ADH, water permeability is low. In the **presence** of ADH, water diffuses out of the collecting tubule into the interstitium and enters the ascending (venous) segment of the vasa recta. The process of urine concentration starts.

6. The **medullary regions** of the collecting tubule reabsorb urea. A small amount of water is reabsorbed and the urine is concentrated.

The mechanism by which the loop of Henle generates the hypertonic interstitial gradient is known as **countercurrent multiplication**. This designation is based on the **flow of fluid in opposite directions** (**countercurrent flow**) within the two parallel limbs of the loop of Henle.

Note that:

1. The fluid flows **into the medulla** in the descending limb and **out of the medulla** in the ascending limb.

2. The countercurrent flow within the descending and ascending limbs of the loop of Henle "multiplies" the osmotic gradient between the tubular fluid in the descending and ascending limbs.

3. A **hyperosmotic interstitium** is generated by the reabsorption of NaCl in the **ascending limb** of the loop of Henle. This is an important step for the uriniferous tubule to excrete urine hyperosmotic with respect to plasma.

4. The concentration of NaCl increases progressively with increasing depth into the medulla. The highest concentration of NaCl is at the level of the papilla. This **medullary gradient** results from the accumulation of NaCl reabsorbed by the process of countercurrent multiplication.

5. The **vasa recta** transport nutrients and oxygen to the uriniferous tubules. They also remove excess water and solutes, continuously added by the countercurrent multiplication process. An increase in blood flow through the vasa recta dissipates the medullary gradient.

Figure 14-20. Diuretics: Mechanism of action

Diuretics are drugs that increase the output of urine **(diuresis)** by acting on specific membrane transport proteins. The common effect of diuretics is the inhibition of Na^+ reabsorption by the nephron leading to an increase in the excretion of Na^+ **(natriuresis).**

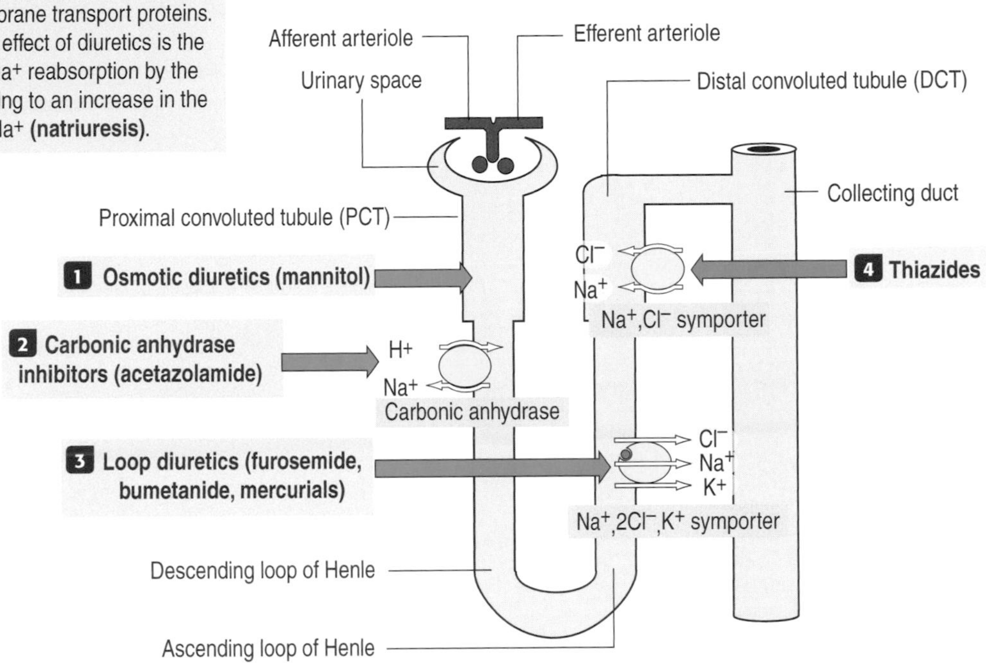

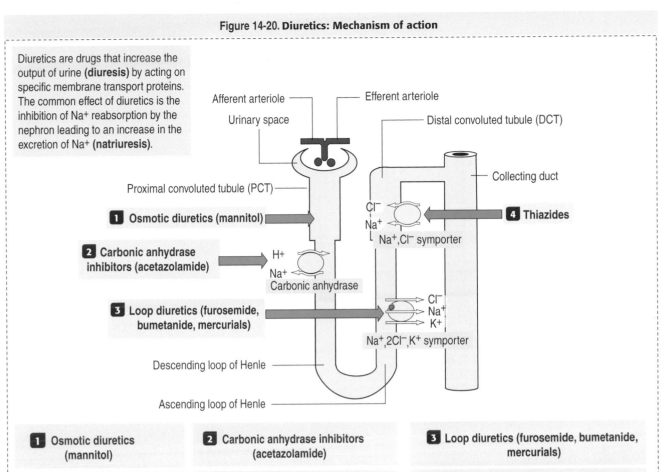

1 Osmotic diuretics (mannitol)

Osmotic diuresis affects the transport of water across the epithelial cells lining the **PCT and thin descending limb of the loop of Henle.** Osmotic diuretics enter the nephron by glomerular filtration and generate an osmotic pressure gradient.

Osmotic diuretics do not inhibit a specific membrane transport protein. When urea and glucose are present in abnormally high concentrations (diabetes mellitus or renal diseases), they can behave as osmotic diuretics.

2 Carbonic anhydrase inhibitors (acetazolamide)

Carbonic acid inhibitors reduce Na^+ reabsorption by their effects on carbonic anhydrase, present mainly in the PCT. The Na^+,H^+ antiporter in the apical membrane of PCT cells depends on H^+ for Na^+ exchange.

H^+ is secreted in the tubular fluid where it combines with filtered HCO_3^- to form H_2CO_3. H_2CO_3 is hydrolyzed to CO_2 and H_2O by carbonic anhydrase located on the apical membrane of the PCT to facilitate CO_2 and H_2O reabsorption. Carbonic anhydrase inhibitors reduce the reabsorption of HCO_3^-. Because the amount of secreted H^+ depends on Na^+, inhibition of carbonic anhydrase causes a decrease in Na^+, H_2O, and HCO_3^- reabsorption, leading to natriuresis.

3 Loop diuretics (furosemide, bumetanide, mercurials)

Loop diuretics are the most potent diuretics available to inhibit Na^+ reabsorption by the **thick ascending limb of Henle's loop** by blocking the Na^+,$2Cl^-$,K^+ symporter located in the apical membrane of the epithelial cells. Loop diuretics also perturb the process of countercurrent multiplication (the ability to dilute or concentrate urine).

4 Thiazides (chlorothiazide)

Thiazide diuretics inhibit Na^+ reabsorption in the **initial portion of the DCT** by blocking the Na^+,Cl^- symporter present in the apical cell membrane. Because water cannot cross this portion of the nephron and this is the site of urine dilution, thiazides reduce the ability to dilute the urine by inhibition of NaCl reabsorption.

Clinical significance: Mechanism of action of diuretics

The main function of diuretics is to increase the excretion of Na^+ by inhibiting Na^+ reabsorption by the nephron. The effect of diuretics depends on the volume of the extracellular fluid (ECF) compartment and the effective circulating volume (ECV). If the ECV decreases, the glomerular filtration rate (GFR) decreases, the load of filtered Na^+ is reduced, and the reabsorption of Na^+ by the PCT increases.

With these events in mind, you realize that the action of diuretics acting on the DCT can be compromised by the presence of lower concentrations of Na^+ when the ECV is reduced.

Figure 14-20 provides a summary of the mechanism of action of osmotic diuretics, carbonic anhydrase inhibitors, loop diuretics, and thiazide diuretics.

Osmotic diuretics inhibit the reabsorption of water and solutes in the PCT and descending thin limb of the loop of Henle.

Carbonic anhydrase inhibitors inhibit Na^+, HCO_3^-, and water reabsorption in the PCT.

Loop diuretics inhibit the reabsorption of NaCl in the thick ascending limb of the loop of Henle. About 25% of the filtered load of Na^+ can be excreted by the action of loop diuretics.

Thiazide diuretics inhibit the reabsorption of NaCl in the DCT.

Essential concepts | Urinary System

• Functions of the urinary system: (1) Filtration of the blood and excretion of waste metabolic products (from proteins, urea; from nucleic acids, uric acid; from muscle, creatinine; from hemoglobin metabolism, urobilin, which gives urine its color). (2) Regulation of water and electrolyte balance. (3) Regulation of arterial blood pressure (by maintaining blood volume and producing renin, a key initiator of the angiotensin-aldosterone cascade). (4) Regulation of erythropoiesis (through erythropoietin, produced by renal interstitial cells) and production of active vitamin D. Chronic renal diseases are associated with anemia because of a decrease in the production of erythropoietin.

• Each kidney consists of a cortex and a medulla. The cortex is subdivided into outer cortex and juxtamedullary cortex. The medulla is subdivided into outer medulla and inner medulla. A **renal lobe** is a triangular-shaped structure consisting of a medullary pyramid—formed by the outer and inner medullary regions—covered by the corresponding cortex. The base of the triangle is lined by the capsule; the papilla is at the apex of the triangle; the lateral boundaries are the renal columns of Bertin. A minor calyx collects urine from each papilla covered by the area cribrosa, the opening site of the papillary ducts.

• The organization of the renal vascular system is key for understanding renal structure and function. After entering the kidney, the renal artery divides into interlobar arteries (running through the renal columns along the sides of the pyramids). At the corticomedullary junction, interlobar arteries change from a vertical to a horizontal direction to form the arcuate arteries. Vertical branches of the arcuate arteries enter the renal cortex and become interlobular arteries.

A **renal lobule** is defined as the portion of the cortex between two adjacent interlobular arteries. The axis of the lobule is occupied by a medullary ray (of Ferrein) consisting of a single collecting duct (of Bellini) collecting the fluid of the correponding intralobular nephrons. As you can see, renal lobules are cortical entities, whereas renal lobes are combined cortical-medullary structures. In fact, renal lobules are subcomponents of the renal lobes.

Interlobular arteries branch several times to form afferent arterioles. Each afferent arteriole forms the glomerular capillary network and continues as an efferent arteriole. This arteriolar-capillary-arteriolar arrangement (instead of arteriole-capillary-venule sequence) is called the glomerular or arterial portal system.

Blood vessels derived from the branching of the glomerular efferent arterioles form two different vascular networks: (1) a peritubular capillary network, surrounding the cortical segments of the uriniferous tubules, and (2) the vasa recta (straight vessels) with a descending arteriolar-capillary component and an ascending capillary-venous component, alongside the descending and ascending limbs of the loops of Henle, respectively. This vascular-tubular arrangement is essential for understanding the countercurrent multiplier and exchange mechanism of urine formation.

• The **uriniferous tubule** consists of two components of different embryologic origin: (1) the nephron and (2) the collecting tubule/duct.

The nephron consists of two components (1) the renal corpuscle and (2) the renal tubule. The renal corpuscle (of Malpighi) is formed by the capsule of Bowman investing the glomerular capillaries (the glomerulus). The renal tubule consists of the proximal convoluted tubule (PCT), the loop of Henle, and the distal convoluted tubule (DCT), which drains into the collecting tubule.

The collecting tubule can be found in the cortex (cortical collecting tubules), the outer medulla (outer medullary collecting tubule), and inner medulla (inner medullary collecting tubule). Depending on the distribution of renal corpuscles, nephrons can be either cortical nephrons or juxtamedullary nephrons.

The capsule of Bowman has two layers: a parietal layer (simple squamous epithelium supported by a basement membrane) and a visceral layer attached to the wall of the glomerular capillaries. The visceral layer consists of branched epithelial cells, the podocytes. The space between the parietal and visceral layers of the capsule of Bowman is the urinary space or Bowman's space. The urinary space is continuous with the lumen of the PCT, the initial segment of the renal tubule. At this region, the urinary pole, the simple squamous epithelium of the parietal layer of the capsule of Bowman, becomes simple cuboidal with apical microvilli (brush border). This is the lining of the PCT.

The glomerulus consists of three components: (1) the glomerular capillaries, lined by fenestrated endothelial cells; (2) the mesangium, consisting of mesangial cells producing the mesangial matrix; and (3) the podocytes. Note that renal corpuscle and glomerulus designate different structures. A renal corpuscle includes the capsule of Bowman and the glomerulus. The designation glomerulus does not include the capsule of Bowman.

Mesangial cells are embedded in an extracellular matrix present between glomerular capillaries. Aggregates of mesangial cells can be seen outside the glomerulus (extraglomerular mesangial cells). Mesangial cells are pericyte-like cells with contractile and phagocytic properties. Mesangial cells participate indirectly in glomerular filtration by providing mechanical support to glomerular capillaries, turning over glomerular basal lamina components, and secreting vasoactive substances (prostaglandins and endothelins).

• An understanding of the structure of the **glomerular filtration barrier** is essential for grasping the clinical characteristics of proteinuria syndromes. The barrier has three layers: (1) the fenestrated endothelial cells of the glomerular capillaries; (2) the dual glomerular basal lamina (produced by endothelial cells and podocytes); and (3) the podocytes, including a filtration slit diaphragm between the interdigitating foot processes of podocytes.

The **podocyte filtration slit diaphragm** has a relevant role in glomerular filtration. Defects in some of its protein components lead to **hereditary proteinuria syndromes.** The filtration slit diaphragm is supported by intracellular F-actin present in pedicels, small podocyte cytoplasmic processes anchored to the dual basal lamina. The C-terminal intracellular segment of the protein nephrin is attached to F-actin by podocin, ZO-1, and CD2AP proteins. The N-terminal extracellular segment of nephrin interacts with another nephrin molecule (homophilic interaction) extending from an adjacent pedicel to form the backbone of the slit diaphragm.

The nephrin gene is mutated in **congenital nephrotic syndrome** of the Finnish type. Affected children display massive proteinuria and edema.

The dual glomerular basal lamina contains type IV collagen, a molecule directly involved in the pathogenesis of **Goodpasture syndrome** (an autoimmune disorder consisting in progressive glomerulonephritis and pulmonary hemorrhage caused by autoantibodies targeting the glomerular and alveolar basal lamina) and **Alport's syndrome** (an inherited X-linked recessive nephropathy, predominant in males, and associated with hematuria, progressive glomerulonephritis, deafness, and ocular symptoms).

Glomerulonephritis defines an inflammatory process of the renal corpuscle. Antibody-antigen complexes circulating in blood trapped in the glomerular filtration barrier contribute to glomerular damage. Antibody-antigen complexes are produced by autoimmune diseases (systemic lupus erythematosus) or bacterial and viral infections (streptococci and hepatitis B virus). **Acute proliferative glomerulonephritis** observed in children is reversible. It is caused by proliferation of endothelial and mesangial cells in the presence of neutrophils. **Rapid progressive (crescentic) glomerulonephritis** consists in proliferation of parietal cells of the capsule of Bowman and infiltration of macrophages forming a crescent-like mass within the glomerulus. This form of glomerulonephritis is observed in Goodpasture syndrome.

• The juxtaglomerular apparatus consists of (1) the macula densa (an Na^+ sensor present in the initial portion of the DCT); (2) the extraglomerular mesangial cells (a supporting cushion of the macula densa located at the vascular pole of the renal corpuscle); and (3) the renin-producing juxtaglomerular cells (modified smooth muscle cells of the wall of the afferent arteriole).

The juxtaglomerular apparatus is one of the components of the tubuloglomerular feedback mechanism participating in the autoregulation of renal blood flow and glomerular filtration.

• The PCT, a continuation of the urinary space (or Bowman's capsular space), is the major reabsorption component of the nephron. The PCT is lined by a simple cuboidal epithelium with well-developed apical microvilli (brush border) and tubulovesicles and lysosomes involved in the endocytosis and breakdown of peptides into amino acids. A basolateral domain displays plasma membrane infoldings and interdigitations that lodge numerous mitochondria providing adenosine triphosphate (ATP) for active ion transport mediated by an Na^+, K^+–activated ATPase pump.

A paracellular transport pathway (across tight junctions) mobilizes, by osmosis, water into the lateral intercellular space. A transcellular transport pathway is involved in the reabsorption of solutes such as NaCl, peptides, and glucose.

Fanconi syndrome is a renal hereditary (primary) or acquired (secondary) disease in which amino acids and glucose are not reabsorbed and are found in urine. The cause appears to be a defect in the cellular energy metabolism decreasing the levels of ATP by the impaired activity of the Na^+, K^+ –activated ATPase pump. The accumulation of cystine in renal tubules (cystinosis leading to renal failure) is the most common cause of Fanconi syndrome in children.

• The loop of Henle consists of a descending limb and an ascending limb. Each limb is formed by a thick segment (lined by simple cuboidal epithelium) and a thin segment (lined by simple squamous epithelium). The descending thick segment is a continuation of the proximal convoluted tubule. The ascending thick segment is continuous with the distal convoluted tubule. The U-shaped thin segment forms most of the loop in juxtamedullary nephrons deep in the medulla. Recall that the loop of Henle of cortical nephrons penetrates up to the outer medulla.

• The DCT is lined by a simple cuboidal epithelium with a less developed apical brush border when compared to the lining epithelium of the PCT.

Tubulovesicles and lysosomes are less prominent. The basolateral domain is infolded and mitochondria are abundant at this location. A distinctive structure is the macula densa, a cluster of cells located at the junction of the ascending thick segment with the DCT. The macula densa faces the extraglomerular mesangial cells and is part of the juxtaglomerular apparatus.

It is important to remember for histologic identification purposes that both PCT and DCT are adjacent to the renal corpuscle. There are specific structural features to remember: although epithelial cells lining the PCT and DCT contain abundant basal mitochondria, epithelial cells of the DCT do not show the characteristic apical tubulovesicles and lysosomes observed in cells of the PCT. In addition, the brush border is more prominent in the PCT than in the DCT.

• The collecting tubules (also called ducts) originate in the cortical medullary rays. We have already seen that a medullary ray is the axis of a renal lobule, a cortical subdivision bordered laterally by adjacent interlobular arteries, branches of the arcuate artery. Cortical medullary rays join others to form wider papillary ducts in the papilla. Papillary ducts open on the surface of the papilla forming a perforated area cribrosa.

The lining epithelium is simple cuboidal and consists of two cell types: (1) principal cells, light cells with an apical nonmotile cilium and (2) intercalated cells, dark cells with apical microvilli and abundant mitochondria. A useful identification feature to recall is that the cell outline of the principal and intercalated cells is very distinct.

Principal cells respond to aldosterone, a mineralocorticoid produced by cells of the zona glomerulosa of the adrenal cortex.

The apical nonmotile cilium of principal cells is a mechanosensor receiving signals from the fluid contents in the tubular lumen. Ciliary bending by fluid flow or mechanical stimulation induce Ca^{2+} release from intracellular storage sites. The ciliary plasma membrane contains the polycystin-1/polycystin-2 protein complex. Polycystin-2 acts as a Ca^{2+}-permeable channel.

Autosomal dominant polycystic kidney disease (ADPKD) results from mutations in either two genes: *PKD1,* encoding polycystin-1, or *PKD2,* encoding polycystin-2. Extensive cystic enlargement of both kidneys results from a complete loss of *PKD1* or *PKD2* gene expression. Blood hypertension preceding progressive renal failure is observed in patients with ADPKD. Renal dialysis and renal transplantation are the indicated treatments.

• Interstitial cells, mainly fibroblasts, can be found in the renal cortex and medulla. Their main function is to maintain the renal architecture and produce erythropoietin, a major regulatory protein of erythropoiesis.

Activated interstitial fibroblasts and inflammatory cells (macrophages and lymphocytes) are involved in interstitial nephritis (also called tubulointerstitial disease) caused by nephrotoxic drugs or by an immunologic mechanism.

• The excretory passages of urine include the renal calyces and pelvis, ureters, and urinary bladder, lined by a transitional epithelium (urothelium) supported by a lamina propria and surrounded by spiral and longitudinally arranged layers of smooth muscle. The male urethra consists of three segments: prostatic urethra (lined by transitional epithelium), membranous urethra, and penile urethra (both lined by pseudostratified-to-stratified columnar epithelium. The penile urethra is surrounded by the corpus spongiosum. The female urethra is lined sequentially by transitional epithelium to stratified squamous epithelium to low keratinized stratified squamous epithelium. The wall of the female urethra consists of an inner smooth muscle layer surrounded by an external striated muscle layer.

• The renin-angiotensin-aldosterone system is essential for the maintenance of systemic blood pressure when there is a reduction in the blood volume or pressure. The system is triggered by a tubuloglomerular feedback mechanism originating in the juxtaglomerular apparatus. The tubular component is the Na^+-sensing macula densa; the glomerular component is the renin-producing juxtaglomerular cells. The immediate objectives of the tubuloglomerular feedback mechanism are the regulation of the glomerular filtration rate (by controlling afferent and efferent arteriolar resistance; recall the glomerular arterial portal arrangement already discussed) and the release of renin from juxtaglomerular cells to produce angiotensin II.

The major steps leading to the production of angiotensin II and its activities are:

1. Renin converts angiotensinogen (produced in hepatocytes) to angiotensin I. Angotensin-converting enzyme (produced by pulmonary and renal endothelial cells) converts angiotensin I to angiotensin II.

2. Angiotensin II targets the hypothalamus to produce antidiuretic hormone (ADH, released by the neurohypophysis). Antidiuretic hormone stimulates water reabsorption in the collecting tubule. In **diabetes insipidus,** water cannot be normally reabsorbed in the collecting tubule because of a low production of antidiuretic hormone. In **diabetes mellitus,** the high concentration of intratubular glucose impairs water reabsorption and osmotic diuresis occurs. Both diabetes insipidus and mellitus are associated with hypernatremia, polydipsia, and polyuria. Glucose in urine (glucosuria) is not observed in patients with diabetes insipidus.

3. Angiotensin II targets the zona glomerulosa of the adrenal cortex to release aldosterone. Aldosterone reduces the excretion of NaCl at the level of the thick ascending segment of the loop of Henle, the DCT, and the collecting tubule.

4. Angiotensin II targets arterioles to produce vasoconstriction, which increases blood pressure.

• The loop of Henle creates an osmotic gradient causing water to flow out the collecting tubule into the surrounding interstitial tissue. A countercurrent multiplication in the loop of Henle maintains high solute concentration in the renal medulla. Countercurrent multiplication occurs because (1) the thin descending segment of the loop of Henle is permeable to water but has low permeability to salt; (2) the thin ascending segment is permeable to salt but not to water; and (3) the thick ascending segment reabsorbs salt by active transport and is impermeable to water. As you can see, countercurrent multiplication results in increasing salt concentration in the medullary interstitium with the descent of the loop of Henle segment. When ADH increases water permeability of the collecting duct, water can flow down its osmotic gradient into the salty medullary interstitium.

Water and some salt must find its way back from the salty interstitium to the bloodstream to reduce plasma osmolality. The parallel arrangement of the peritubular vasa recta with the U-shaped loop of Henle participates in the absorption of solute and water by countercurrent exchange: the arterial descending segment of the vasa recta absorbs some salt and the venous ascending segment of the vasa recta reabsorbs water. In this way, the loop of Henle–dependent countercurrent multiplication does not accumulate salt and water indefinitely in the interstitium with the help of the vasa recta–dependent countercurrent exchange.

• Diuretics are drugs that increase the output of urine (diuresis) by acting on specific membrane transport proteins. Inhibition of Na^+ resorption by the nephron leads to an increase in the excretion of Na^+ (natriuresis) and water.

15. UPPER DIGESTIVE SEGMENT

General outline of the digestive or alimentary tube

Swallowing, **digestion**, and **absorption** take place through the digestive or alimentary tube, a 7- to 10-m hollow muscular conduit. The digestive process converts food material into a **soluble form** easy to absorb by the **small intestine**. The **elimination of insoluble residues** and other materials is the function of the **large intestine**.

Histologically, the digestive tube consists of four major layers: (1) an inner **mucosal** layer encircling the lumen, (2) a **submucosal** layer, (3) a **muscularis externa** layer, and (4) a **serosal/adventitial** layer.

The inner mucosal layer shows significant variations along the digestive tube. It is subdivided into three components: (1) an **epithelial layer**, (2) a connective tissue **lamina propria**, and (3) a smooth muscle **muscularis mucosae**.

Upper digestive segment: Mouth, esophagus, and stomach

We have divided the discussion of the digestive system into two components or chapters: Chapter 15 is focused on the **upper digestive segment** and includes the mouth, esophagus, and stomach. Chapter 16 describes the **lower digestive segment** (small and large intestine). This division is based on the distinctive functions of the upper digestive segment (swallowing and digestion) and lower digestive segment (absorption).

Mouth

The mouth is the entrance to the digestive tube. **Ingestion**, **partial digestion**, and **lubrication** of the food, or **bolus**, are the main functions of the mouth and its associated **salivary glands**. We study the salivary glands in Chapter 17, Digestive Glands.

The **mouth**, or **oral cavity**, includes the lips, cheeks, teeth, gums, tongue, and palate. Except for the teeth, the mouth is lined by a **stratified squamous epithelium**, with a submucosa present only in certain regions.

The **lips** consist of three regions: (1) the **cutaneous region**, (2) the **red region**, and (3) the **oral mucosa region**.

The cutaneous region is covered by thin skin (**keratinized stratified squamous epithelium with hair follicles and sebaceous and sweat glands**). The red region is lined by a stratified squamous epithelium supported by tall papillae containing blood vessels responsible for the red color of this region. The oral mucosa region is continuous with the mucosa of the cheeks and gums.

The stratified squamous epithelium covering the inner surface of the lips and cheeks is supported by a dense lamina propria and a submucosa, closely bound by connective tissue fibers to the underlying skeletal muscles.

The **gums**, or **gingivae**, are similar to the red region of the lips, except on the free margin, where significant keratinization is seen. The lamina propria of the gums binds tightly to the periosteum of the alveolar processes of the maxillae and mandible and to the periodontal membrane. The gums lack submucosa or glands.

The **hard palate** is lined by a keratinizing stratified squamous epithelium similar to that of the free margins of the gums. A submucosa is present in the midline but absent in the area adjacent to the gums. Collagenous fibers in the submucosa bind the mucosa to the periosteum of the hard palate.

Figure 15-1. **Tongue**

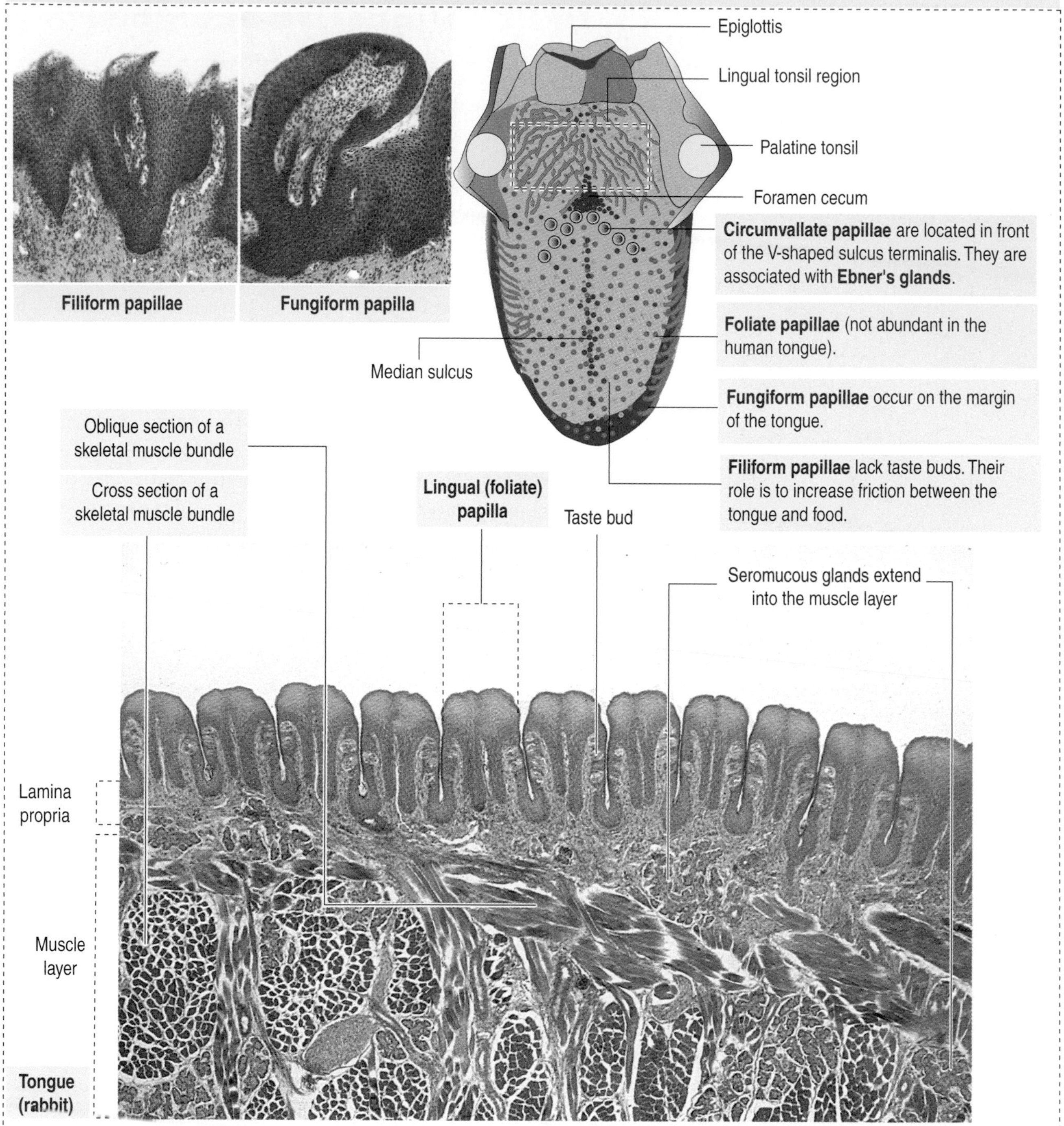

Epiglottis
Lingual tonsil region
Palatine tonsil
Foramen cecum
Circumvallate papillae are located in front of the V-shaped sulcus terminalis. They are associated with **Ebner's glands**.
Foliate papillae (not abundant in the human tongue).
Fungiform papillae occur on the margin of the tongue.
Filiform papillae lack taste buds. Their role is to increase friction between the tongue and food.
Median sulcus
Filiform papillae
Fungiform papilla
Oblique section of a skeletal muscle bundle
Cross section of a skeletal muscle bundle
Lingual (foliate) papilla
Taste bud
Seromucous glands extend into the muscle layer
Lamina propria
Muscle layer
Tongue (rabbit)

The **soft palate** and **uvula** are lined by a nonkeratinized stratified squamous epithelium extending into the oropharynx where it becomes continuous with the pseudostratified ciliated columnar epithelium of the upper respiratory tract. The submucosa is loose and contains abundant mucous and serous glands. Skeletal muscle fibers are present in the soft palate and uvula.

Tongue

The anterior two thirds of the tongue consists of a core mass of **skeletal muscle** oriented in three directions: **longitudinal**, **transverse**, and **oblique**. The posterior one third displays aggregations of lymphatic tissue, the **lingual tonsils**.

The dorsal surface of the tongue is covered by a **nonkeratinized stratified squa-**

mous epithelium supported by a lamina propria associated with the muscle core of the tongue. **Serous** and **mucous glands** extend across the lamina propria and the muscle. Their ducts open into the **crypts** and **furrows** of the **lingual tonsils** and **circumvallate papillae**, respectively.

The dorsal surface of the tongue contains numerous mucosal projections called **lingual papillae** (Figure 15-1). Each **lingual papilla** is formed by a highly vascular connective tissue core and a covering layer of stratified squamous epithelium. According to their shape, lingual papillae can be divided into four types: (1) **filiform papillae** (narrow conical), the most abundant; (2) **fungiform papillae** (mushroom-shaped); (3) **circumvallate papillae**; and (4) **foliate papillae** (leaf-shaped), rudimentary in humans but well developed in rabbits and monkeys.

Taste buds are found in all lingual papillae except the filiform papillae. Taste buds are barrel-shaped epithelial structures containing chemosensory cells called **gustatory receptor cells.** Gustatory receptor cells are in synaptic contact with the terminals of the gustatory nerves.

Circumvallate (wall-like) **papillae** are located in the posterior part of the tongue, aligned **in front of the sulcus terminalis.** The circumvallate papilla occupies a recess in the mucosa and, therefore, it is surrounded by a **circular furrow** or **trench.**

Serous glands, or **Ebner's glands**, in the connective tissue, in contact with the underlying muscle, are associated with the circumvallate papilla. **The ducts of Ebner's glands open into the floor of the circular furrow.**

The sides of the circumvallate papilla and the facing wall of furrow contain several taste buds. Each **taste bud**, depending on the species, consists of 50 to 150 cells, with its narrow apical ends extending into a **taste pore**. A taste bud has three cell components (Figure 15-2): (1) **taste receptor cells**, (2) **supporting cells** (or immature taste cells), and (3) **precursor cells** (or basal cells).

Taste receptor cells have a lifespan of 10 to 14 days. **Precursor cells give rise to supporting cells** (or **immature taste cells) which, in turn, become mature taste receptor cells.** The basal portion of a taste receptor cell makes contact with an **afferent nerve terminal** derived from neurons in the sensory ganglia of the **facial**, **glossopharyngeal**, and **vagus** nerves.

Sweet, **sour**, **bitter**, and **salty** are the four classic taste sensations. A fifth taste is **umami** (the taste of monosodium glutamate). A specific taste sensation is generated by specific taste receptor cells. The **facial nerve** carries the five taste sensations; the **glossopharyngeal nerve** carries sweet and bitter sensations.

Taste is initiated when soluble chemicals, called **tastants**, diffuse through the taste pore and interact with the **G-protein** α, β, and γ **subunits** (called **gustducin**) **linked to the taste receptors** (designated **TR1** and **TR2**), present in the **apical microvilli** of the **taste receptor cells.** As we discussed in Chapter 3, Cell Signaling, guanosine triphosphate (GTP) binding to the α subunit of the G-protein complex activates target molecules (ion channels in the taste receptor cells). Ionic changes within taste cells cause either depolarization (see Figure 15-2) or hyperpolarization of the receptor cells. An increase in intracellular Ca^{2+} triggers the release of neurotransmitters at the afferent synapse with the afferent nerve terminal. Some taste receptor cells respond to only one of the basic taste substances. Others are sensitive to more than one taste substance.

Tooth

In the adult human, dentition consists of 32 permanent teeth. The 16 upper teeth are embedded in **alveolar processes** of the maxilla. The lower 16 teeth are embedded in similar alveolar processes of the mandible. The permanent dentition is preceded by a set of 20 **deciduous teeth**, also called **milk** or **baby teeth.** Deciduous teeth appear at about 6 months of age and the entire set is present by age 6 to 8 years. The deciduous teeth are replaced between ages 10 and 12 by the 32 permanent teeth. This replacement process ends at about age 18.

Figure 15-2. Taste bud

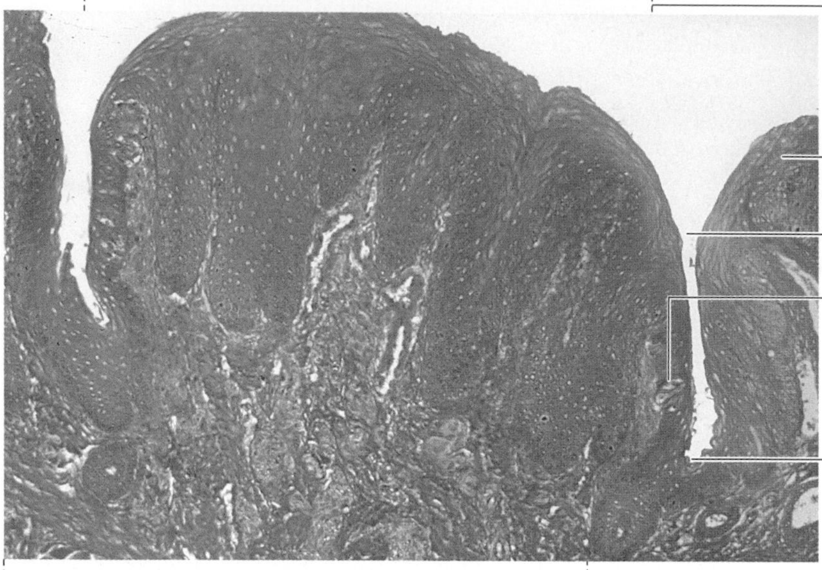

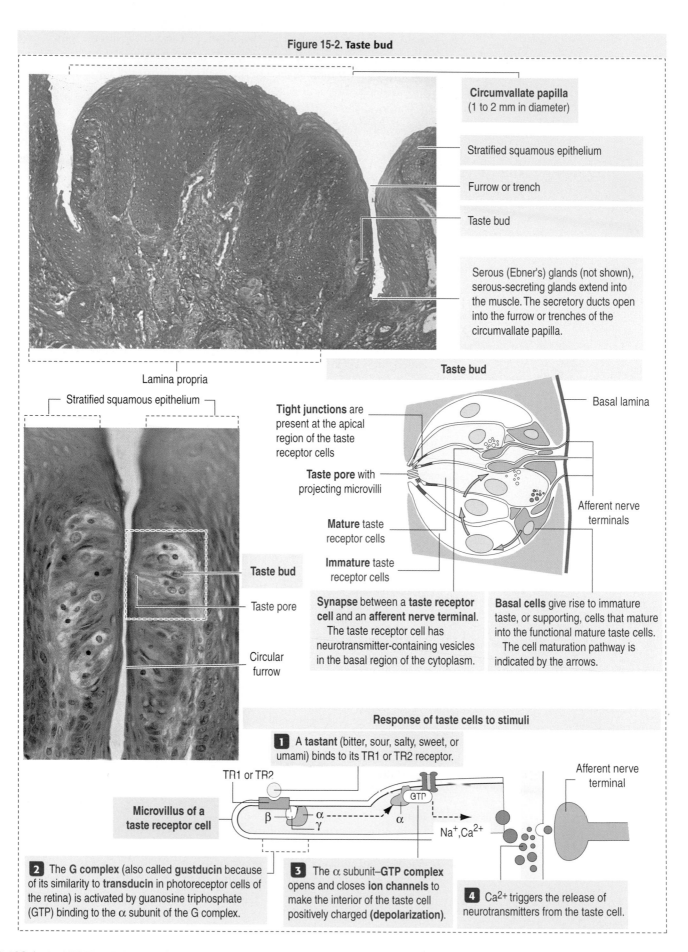

Serous (Ebner's) glands (not shown), serous-secreting glands extend into the muscle. The secretory ducts open into the furrow or trenches of the circumvallate papilla.

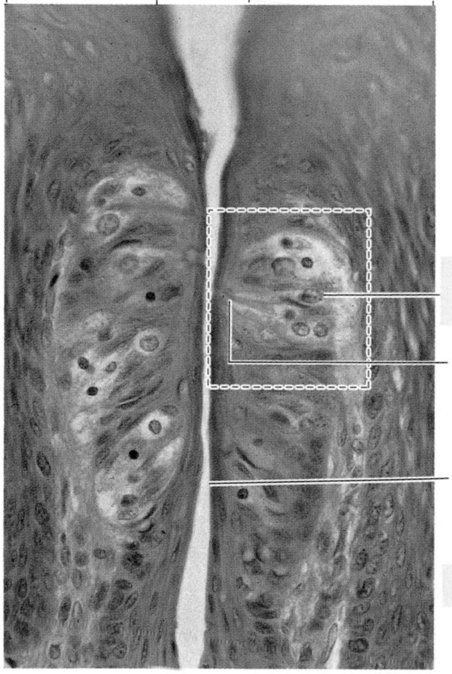

Taste bud

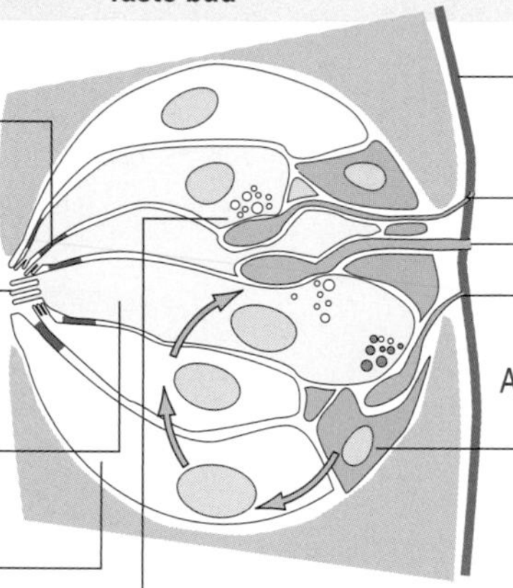

Tight junctions are present at the apical region of the taste receptor cells

Synapse between a **taste receptor cell** and an **afferent nerve terminal**.
The taste receptor cell has neurotransmitter-containing vesicles in the basal region of the cytoplasm.

Basal cells give rise to immature taste, or supporting, cells that mature into the functional mature taste cells.
The cell maturation pathway is indicated by the arrows.

Response of taste cells to stimuli

1 A **tastant** (bitter, sour, salty, sweet, or umami) binds to its TR1 or TR2 receptor.

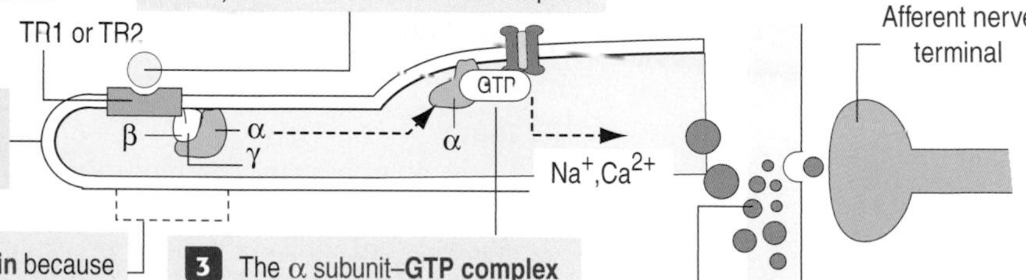

2 The **G complex** (also called **gustducin** because of its similarity to **transducin** in photoreceptor cells of the retina) is activated by guanosine triphosphate (GTP) binding to the α subunit of the G complex.

3 The α subunit–**GTP complex** opens and closes **ion channels** to make the interior of the taste cell positively charged **(depolarization)**.

4 Ca^{2+} triggers the release of neurotransmitters from the taste cell.

Figure 15-3. Longitudinal section of the tooth

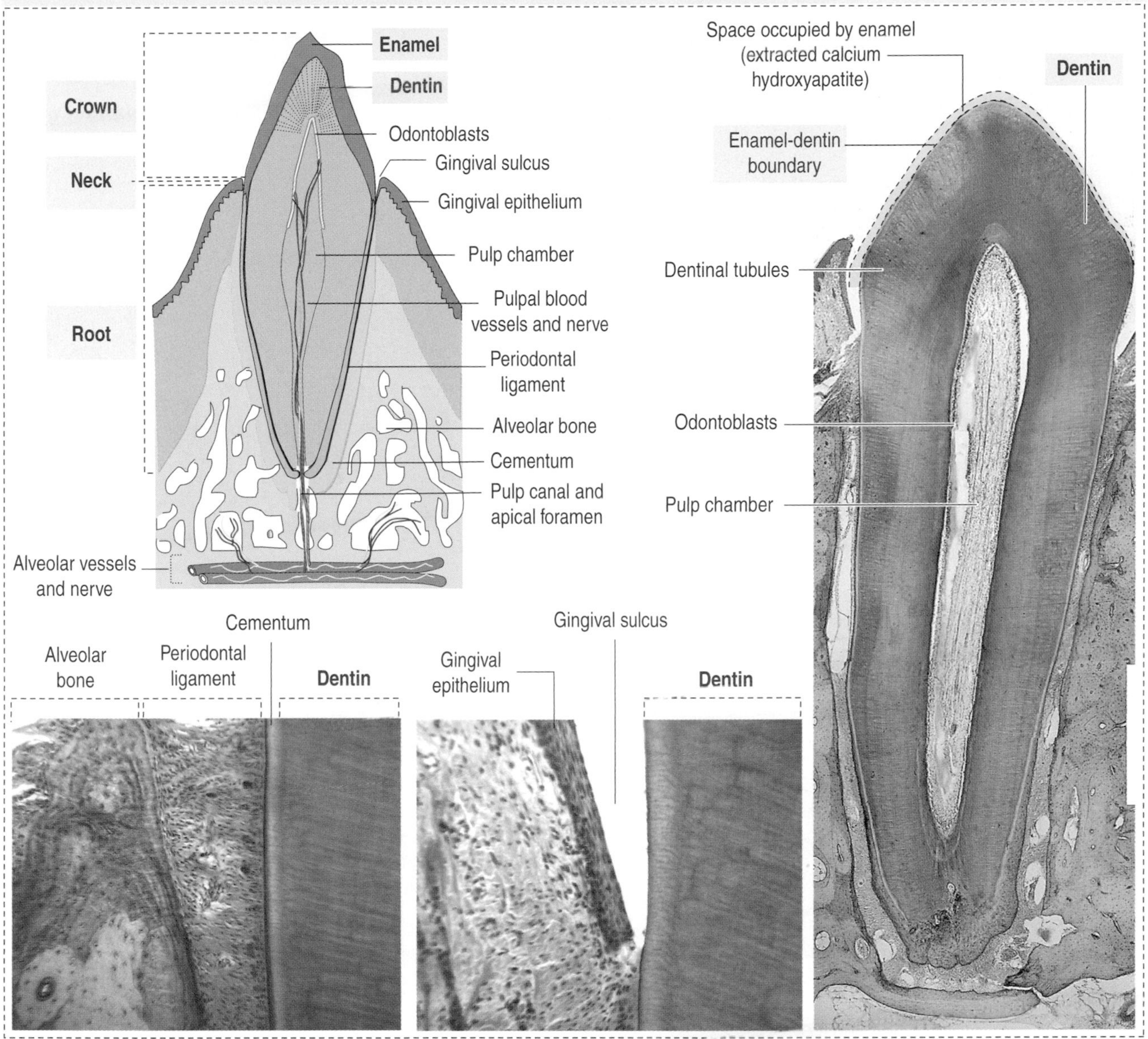

Each of the several types of teeth has a distinctive shape and function: **incisors** are specialized for cutting; **canines,** for puncturing and holding; and **molars,** for crushing.

Each tooth consists of a **crown** and either single or multiple **roots** (Figure 15-3). The crown is covered by highly calcified layers of **enamel** and **dentin.** The outer surface of the root is covered by another calcified tissue called **cementum.** The dentin forms the bulk of the tooth and contains a central chamber filled with soft tissue, the **pulp.** The pulp chamber opens at the **apical foramen** into the bony alveolar process by the **root canal.** Blood vessels, nerves, and lymphatics enter and leave the pulp chamber through the apical foramen. Myelinated nerve fibers run along with the blood vessels.

Tooth development: Differentiation of ameloblasts and odontoblasts

The ectoderm, cranial neural crest, and mesenchyme contribute to the development of the tooth (Figure 15-4). **Ameloblasts** derive from the **ectoderm. Odontoblasts** derive from the **cranial neural crest. Cementocytes** derive from the **mesenchyme.**

Secreted signaling molecules—**activin βA, fibroblast growth factor,** and **bone**

Figure 15-4. Stages of tooth development

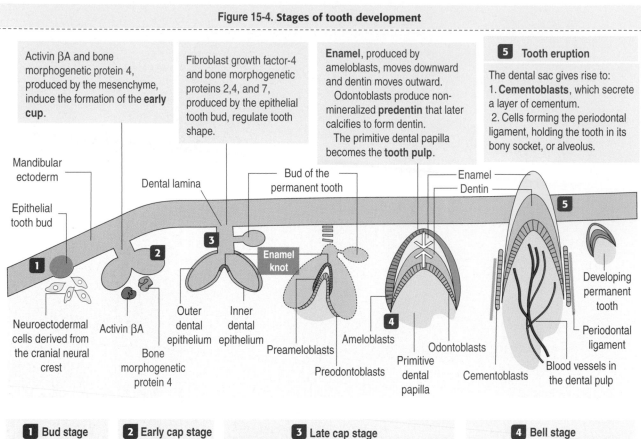

Activin βA and bone morphogenetic protein 4, produced by the mesenchyme, induce the formation of the **early cup**.

Fibroblast growth factor-4 and bone morphogenetic proteins 2,4, and 7, produced by the epithelial tooth bud, regulate tooth shape.

Enamel, produced by ameloblasts, moves downward and dentin moves outward.

Odontoblasts produce non-mineralized **predentin** that later calcifies to form dentin.

The primitive dental papilla becomes the **tooth pulp**.

5 Tooth eruption

The dental sac gives rise to:

1. **Cementoblasts**, which secrete a layer of cementum.
2. Cells forming the periodontal ligament, holding the tooth in its bony socket, or alveolus.

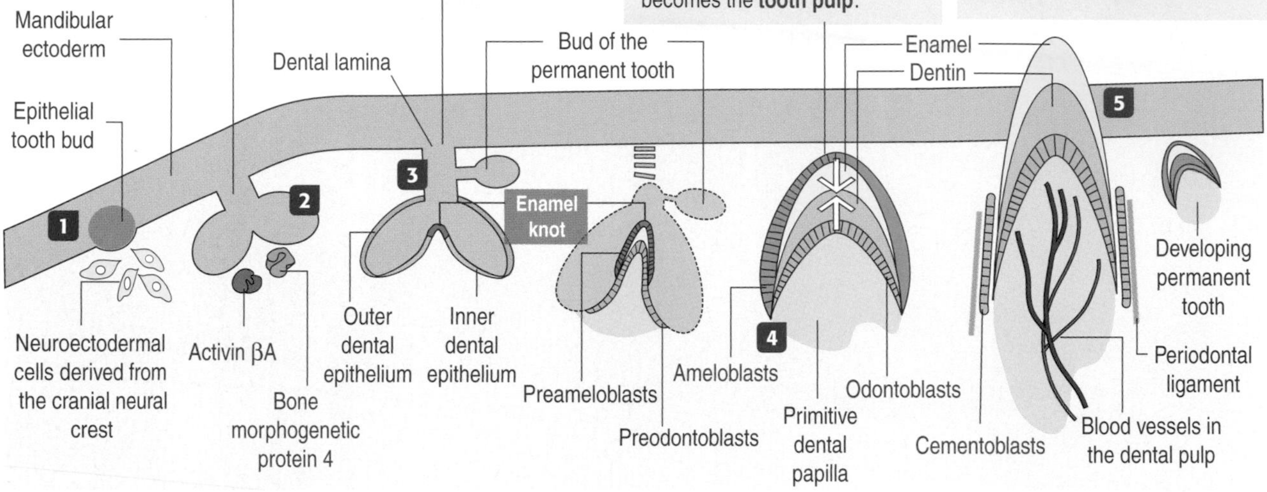

Mandibular ectoderm
Epithelial tooth bud
Dental lamina
Bud of the permanent tooth
Enamel
Dentin
1
2
3
4
5
Enamel knot
Neuroectodermal cells derived from the cranial neural crest
Activin βA
Bone morphogenetic protein 4
Outer dental epithelium
Inner dental epithelium
Preameloblasts
Preodontoblasts
Ameloblasts
Primitive dental papilla
Odontoblasts
Cementoblasts
Blood vessels in the dental pulp
Periodontal ligament
Developing permanent tooth

1 Bud stage

Neuroectodermal cells induce the overlying ectodermic epithelial cells to proliferate and form the epithelial tooth bud. There are 20 buds, one for each of the deciduous teeth.

2 Early cap stage

Cells of the epithelial tooth bud proliferate and invaginate into the underlying mesoderm.

3 Late cap stage

The **dental lamina** connects the downward-growing cells with the ectodermal epithelium.

The cells at the growing end of the dental bud form a caplike structure. The epithelial tooth bud is lined by an **outer** and **inner dental epithelium**.

The bud of the permanent tooth develops from the dental lamina and remains dormant. The **enamel knot** signals tooth development.

4 Bell stage

At the **enamel knot** site, the outermost cells of the dental papilla differentiate into dentin-producing **odontoblasts**. A single layer of enamel-secreting **ameloblasts** develops in the inner dental epithelium portion of the enamel knot.

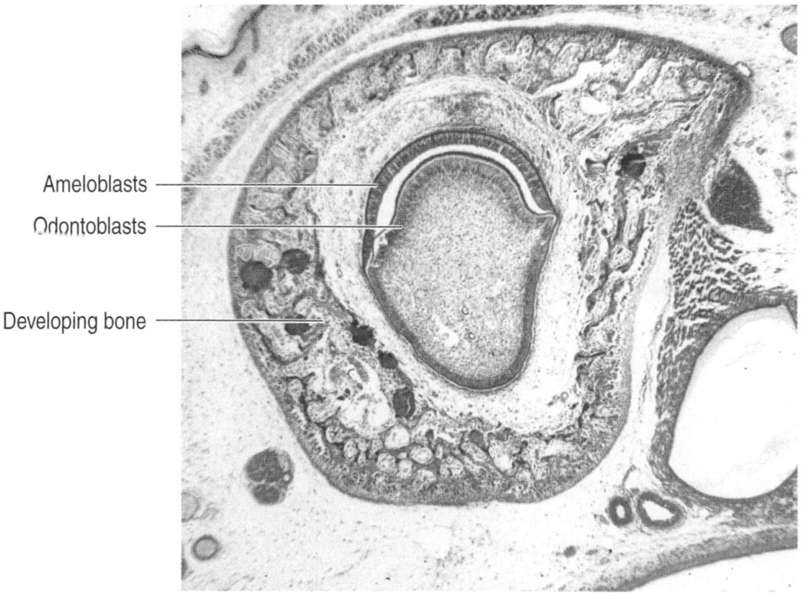

Ameloblasts
Odontoblasts
Developing bone

Figure 15-5. **Odontoblast**

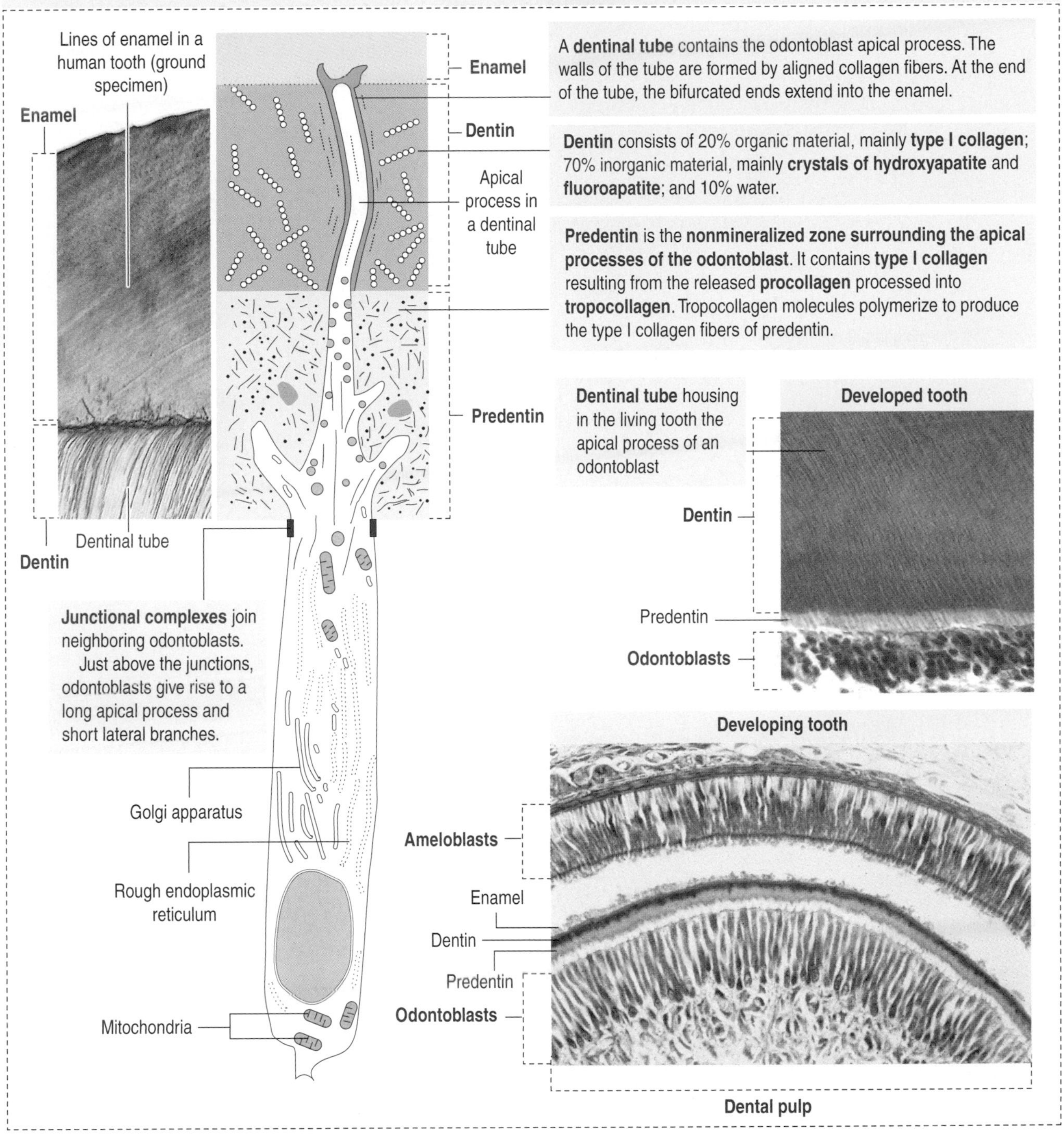
Lines of enamel in a human tooth (ground specimen)
Enamel
Dentinal tube
Dentin
Enamel
Dentin
Apical process in a dentinal tube
Predentin
A **dentinal tube** contains the odontoblast apical process. The walls of the tube are formed by aligned collagen fibers. At the end of the tube, the bifurcated ends extend into the enamel.
Dentin consists of 20% organic material, mainly **type I collagen**; 70% inorganic material, mainly **crystals of hydroxyapatite** and **fluoroapatite**; and 10% water.
Predentin is the **nonmineralized zone surrounding the apical processes of the odontoblast**. It contains **type I collagen** resulting from the released **procollagen** processed into **tropocollagen**. Tropocollagen molecules polymerize to produce the type I collagen fibers of predentin.
Junctional complexes join neighboring odontoblasts.
Just above the junctions, odontoblasts give rise to a long apical process and short lateral branches.
Golgi apparatus
Rough endoplasmic reticulum
Mitochondria
Dentinal tube housing in the living tooth the apical process of an odontoblast
Developed tooth
Dentin
Predentin
Odontoblasts
Developing tooth
Ameloblasts
Enamel
Dentin
Predentin
Odontoblasts
Dental pulp

morphogenetic proteins—mediate the interaction between the dental epithelium and the mesenchyme during tooth morphogenesis. Figure 15-4 illustrates the relevant steps of tooth development.

Odontoblasts

A layer of odontoblasts is present at the periphery of the pulp. Odontoblasts are active secretory cells that synthesize and secrete collagen and noncollagenous material, the organic components of the **dentin**.

The **odontoblast** is a columnar epithelial-like cell located at the **inner side** of the dentin, in the pulp cavity (Figure 15-5). The apical cell domain is embedded in **predentin**, a nonmineralized layer of dentin-like material. The apical domain

Figure 15-6. Ameloblast

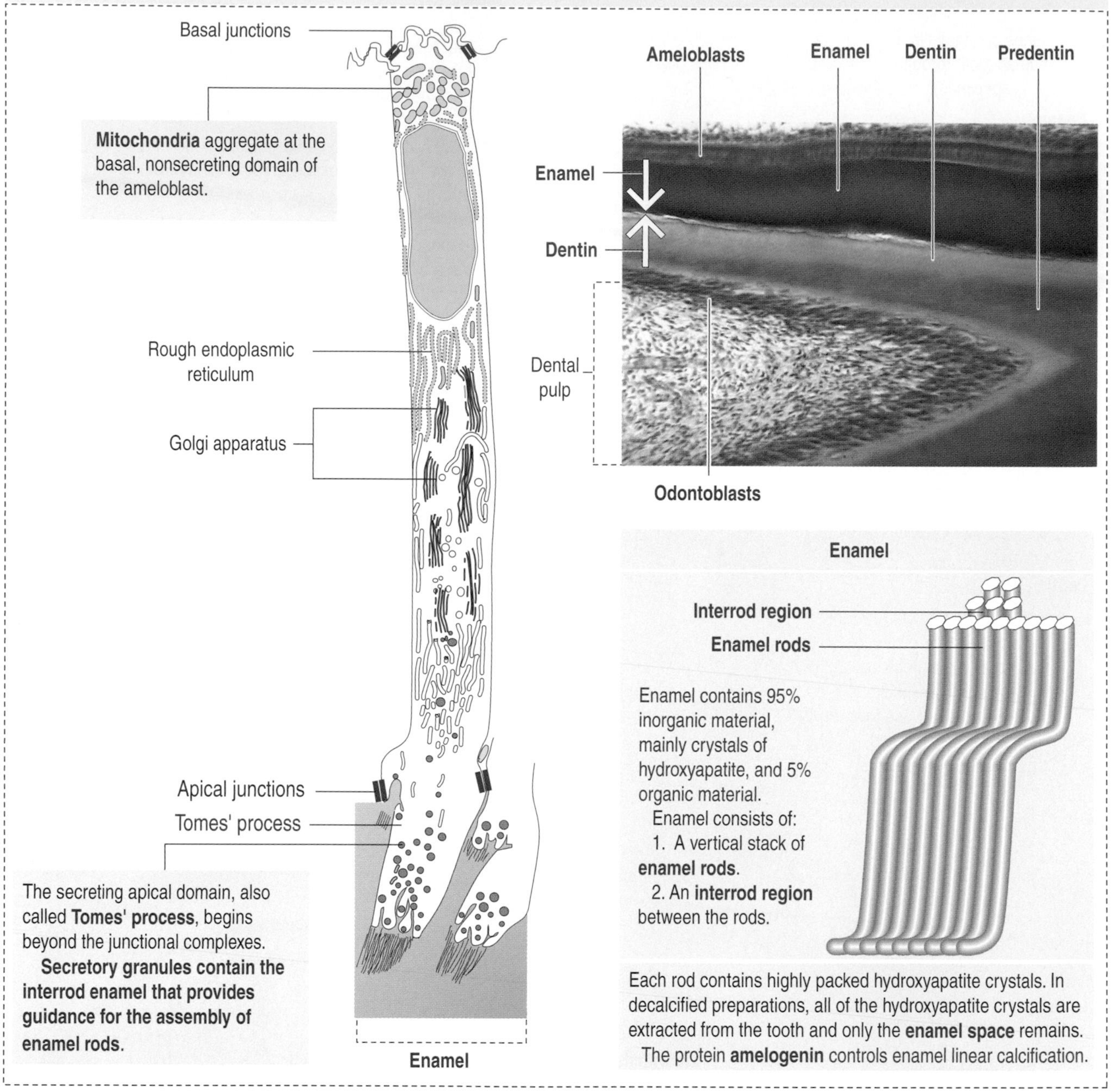

Basal junctions
Mitochondria aggregate at the basal, nonsecreting domain of the ameloblast.
Rough endoplasmic reticulum
Golgi apparatus
Apical junctions
Tomes' process
The secreting apical domain, also called Tomes' process, begins beyond the junctional complexes.
Secretory granules contain the interrod enamel that provides guidance for the assembly of enamel rods.
Enamel
Ameloblasts
Enamel
Dentin
Predentin
Enamel
Dentin
Dental pulp
Odontoblasts
Enamel
Interrod region
Enamel rods
Enamel contains 95% inorganic material, mainly crystals of hydroxyapatite, and 5% organic material.
Enamel consists of:
1. A vertical stack of enamel rods.
2. An interrod region between the rods.
Each rod contains highly packed hydroxyapatite crystals. In decalcified preparations, all of the hydroxyapatite crystals are extracted from the tooth and only the enamel space remains.
The protein amelogenin controls enamel linear calcification.

projects a main **apical cell process** that becomes enclosed within a canalicular system just above the **junctional complexes** linking adjacent odontoblasts.

A well-developed **rough endoplasmic reticulum** and **Golgi apparatus** as well as **secretory granules** are found in the apical region of the odontoblast. The secretory granules contain **procollagen**. When procollagen is released from the odontoblast, it is enzymatically processed to **tropocollagen**, which aggregates into **type I collagen** fibrils.

Predentin is the layer of dentin adjacent to the odontoblast cell body and processes. Predentin is **nonmineralized** and consists mainly of collagen fibrils that will become covered (mineralized) by hydroxyapatite crystals in the dentin region. A demarcation **mineralization front** separates predentin from dentin. **Dentin** consists of 20% organic material, mainly type I collagen; 70% inorganic material, mainly crystals of hydroxyapatite and fluoroapatite; and 10% water.

Coronal dentin dysplasia (also known as **dentin dysplasia, type II**) is a rare inherited autosomal defect characterized by abnormal development of dentin, extremely short roots (rootless teeth), and obliterated pulp chambers.

The **pulp** consists of blood vessels, nerves, and lymphatics surrounded by fibroblasts and mesenchyme-like extracellular elements. Blood vessels (arterioles) branch into a capillary network **among the cell bodies of the odontoblasts**. An inflammation in the pulp causes swelling and pain. Because there is no space for swelling in the pulp cavity, the blood supply is suppressed by compression, leading rapidly to the death of the pulpal cells.

Cementum

The **cementum** is a bonelike mineralized tissue covering the outer surface of the root. Like bone, the cementum consists of calcified collagenous fibrils and trapped osteocyte-like cells called **cementocytes**.

The cementum meets the enamel at the **cementoenamel junction** and separates the crown from the root at the **neck region** of the tooth. The outermost layer of the cementum is uncalcified and is produced by **cementoblasts** in contact with the **periodontal ligament**, a collagen- and fibroblast-rich and vascularized suspensory ligament holding the tooth in the sockets of the alveolar bone (see Figure 15-3). The strength of the periodontal ligament fibers gives teeth mobility and strong bone attachment, both useful in orthodontic treatment.

Ameloblasts

Ameloblasts are enamel-producing cells present only during tooth development. The ameloblast (Figure 15-6) is a polarized columnar cell with mitochondria and a nucleus present in the basal region of the cell. The supranuclear region contains numerous cisternae of rough endoplasmic reticulum and Golgi apparatus.

Beyond apical junctional complexes joining contiguous ameloblasts, the apical domain displays a broad process, **Tomes' process**, in proximity to the calcified enamel matrix. The apical domain has abundant secretory granules containing glycoprotein precursors of the enamel matrix.

The **enamel** is the hardest substance found in the body. About 95% of the enamel is composed of crystals of hydroxyapatite; less than 5% is protein. The newly secreted enamel contains a high content of protein (about 30%), whose concentration decreases to 1% during enamel mineralization. The extracellular matrix of the developing enamel contains two classes of proteins: **amelogenin** and **enamelin**.

Amelogenin is the major constituent, unique to the developing enamel. It controls the calcification of the enamel. Enamelin is a minor component; it has ameloprotease activity, which breaks down amelogenin during enamel assembly. **Amelogenesis imperfecta** is an X chromosome–linked inherited disease affecting the synthesis of amelogenin required for the formation of the tooth enamel; affected enamel does not attain its normal thickness, hardness, and color. **Autosomal-dominant amelogenesis imperfecta** is caused by a mutation of the *enamelin* gene.

Electron microscopic examination shows that the enamel consists of thin undulated **enamel rods** separated by an **interrod region** with a structure similar to that of the enamel rods but with its crystals oriented in a different direction. Each rod is coated with a thin layer of organic matrix, called the **rod sheath**.

General organization of the digestive or alimentary tube

Although we study each segment of the digestive or alimentary tube separately, it is important to discuss first the general organization of the tube to understand that each segment does not function as an independent unit.

We start with the common histologic features of the digestive tube by indicating that, except for the oral cavity, the digestive tube has a uniform histologic organization. This organization is characterized by distinct and significant structural variations reflecting changes in functional activity.

Figure 15-7. **Overall histologic organization of the digestive tube**

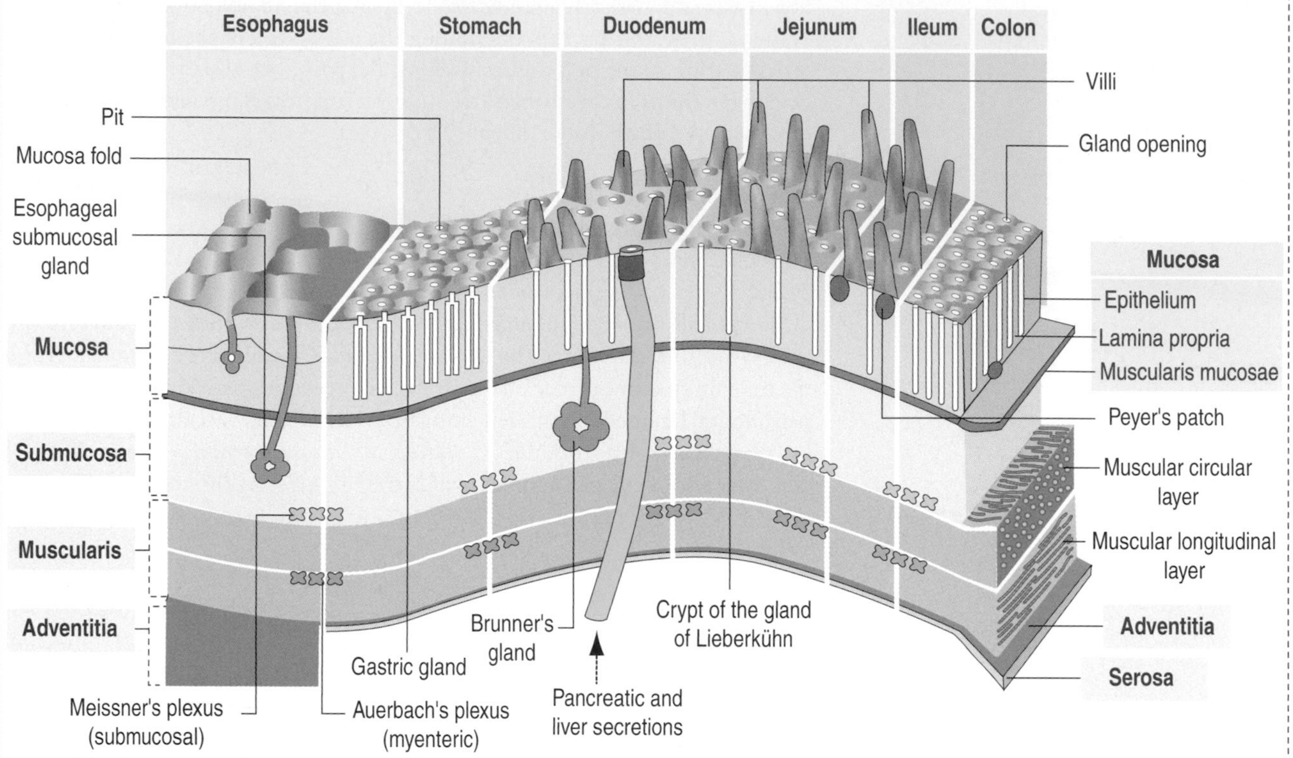

After the oral cavity, the digestive tube is differentiated into four major organs: **esophagus**, **stomach**, **small intestine**, and **large intestine**. Each of these organs is made up of four concentric layers (Figure 15-7): (1) the **mucosa**, (2) the **submucosa**, (3) the **muscularis**, and (4) the **adventitia**, or **serosa**.

The mucosa has three components: a **lining epithelium**, an underlying **lamina propria** consisting of a vascularized loose connective tissue, and a thin layer of smooth muscle, the **muscularis mucosae**.

Lymphatic nodules and scattered immunocompetent cells (lymphocytes, plasma cells, and macrophages) are present in the lamina propria. The lamina propria of the small and large intestines is a relevant site of immune responses (see Chapter 16, Lower Digestive Segment).

The lining epithelium invaginates to form **glands**, extending into the **lamina propria** (**mucosal glands**) or **submucosa** (**submucosal glands**), or **ducts**, transporting secretions from the liver and pancreas through the wall of the digestive tube (duodenum) into its lumen.

In the stomach and small intestine, both the mucosa and submucosa extend into the lumen as folds, called rugae and plicae, respectively. In other instances, the mucosa alone extends into the lumen as fingers, or villi. **Mucosal glands increase the secretory capacity**, whereas **villi increase the absorptive capacity of the digestive tube**.

The **mucosa** shows significant variations from segment to segment of the digestive tract. The submucosa consists of a dense irregular connective tissue with large blood vessels, lymphatics, and nerves branching into the mucosa and muscularis. Glands are present in the submucosa of the esophagus and duodenum.

The **muscularis** contains two layers of smooth muscle: the smooth muscle fibers of the inner layer are arranged around the tube lumen (circular layer); fibers of the outer layer are disposed along the tube (longitudinal layer). **Contraction of the smooth fibers of the circular layer reduces the lumen; contraction of the fibers of the longitudinal layer shortens the tube.** Skeletal muscle fibers are present in

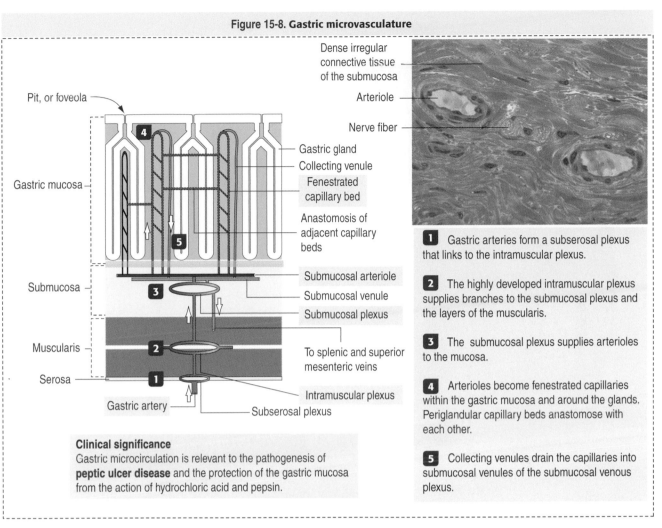

Figure 15-8. Gastric microvasculature

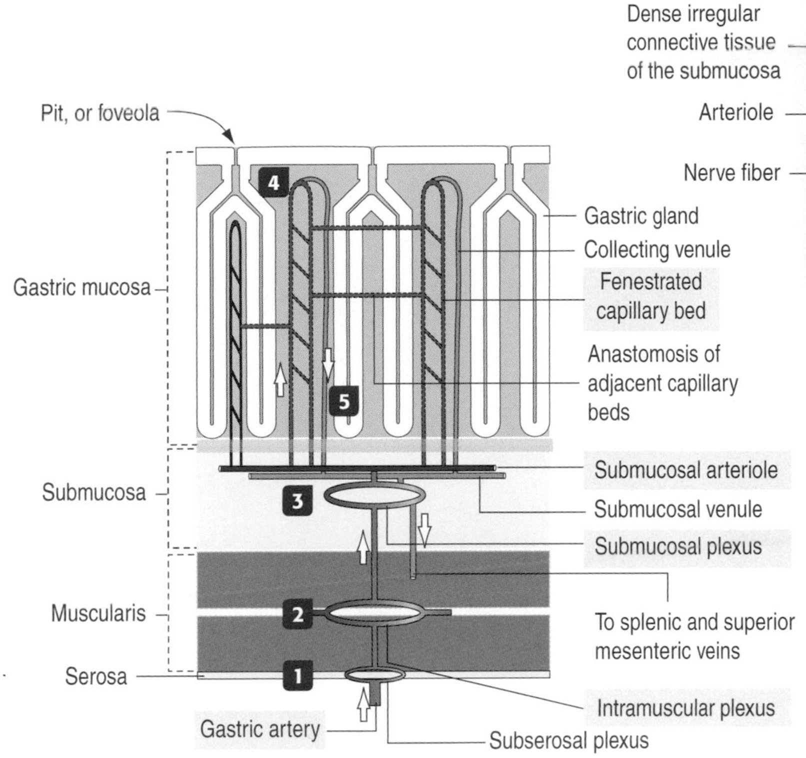

Pit, or foveola
Gastric mucosa
Submucosa
Muscularis
Serosa
Gastric artery
4
5
3
2
1
Gastric gland
Collecting venule
Fenestrated capillary bed
Anastomosis of adjacent capillary beds
Submucosal arteriole
Submucosal venule
Submucosal plexus
To splenic and superior mesenteric veins
Intramuscular plexus
Subserosal plexus

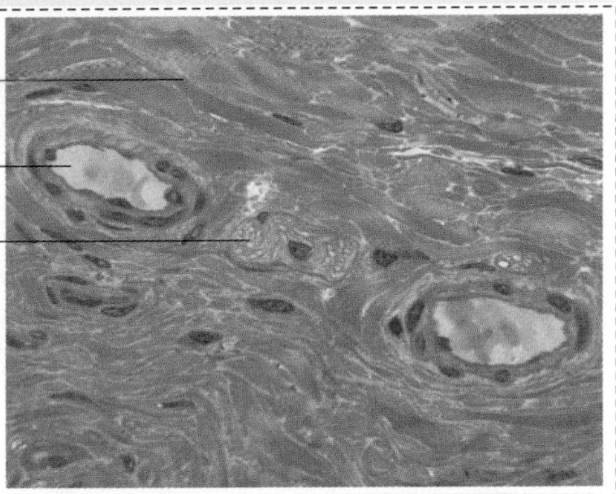

Dense irregular connective tissue of the submucosa
Arteriole
Nerve fiber

1 Gastric arteries form a subserosal plexus that links to the intramuscular plexus.

2 The highly developed intramuscular plexus supplies branches to the submucosal plexus and the layers of the muscularis.

3 The submucosal plexus supplies arterioles to the mucosa.

4 Arterioles become fenestrated capillaries within the gastric mucosa and around the glands. Periglandular capillary beds anastomose with each other.

5 Collecting venules drain the capillaries into submucosal venules of the submucosal venous plexus.

Clinical significance
Gastric microcirculation is relevant to the pathogenesis of **peptic ulcer disease** and the protection of the gastric mucosa from the action of hydrochloric acid and pepsin.

the upper esophagus and the anal sphincter.

The **adventitia** of the digestive tract consists of several layers of connective tissue continuous with adjacent connective tissues. When the digestive tube is suspended by the mesentery or peritoneal fold, the adventitia is covered by a **mesothelium (simple squamous epithelium)** supported by a thin connective tissue layer, together forming a **serosa,** or serous membrane.

Microvasculature of the digestive tube

We start our discussion with the **microvasculature of the stomach.** The **microcirculation of the small intestine** and differences from the gastric microcirculation are discussed in Chapter 16, Lower Digestive Segment (see Figure 16-3).

Blood and lymphatic vessels and nerves reach the walls of the digestive tube through the supporting mesentery or the surrounding tissues. After entering the walls of the stomach, arteries organize three arterial networks: the **subserosal, intramuscular,** and **submucosal plexuses** (Figure 15-8). Some branches from the plexuses run longitudinally in the muscularis and submucosa; other branches extend perpendicularly into the mucosa and muscularis.

In the mucosa, **arterioles** derived from the submucosal plexus supply a bed of **fenestrated capillaries** around the gastric glands and anastomose laterally with each other. The fenestrated nature of the capillaries facilitates bicarbonate delivery to protect the surface epithelial cells against hydrochloric acid damage (see Figure 15-17).

Collecting venules descend from the mucosa into the submucosa as veins, leave the digestive tube through the mesentery, and drain into the splenic and superior

Figure 15-9. Innervation of the digestive tube

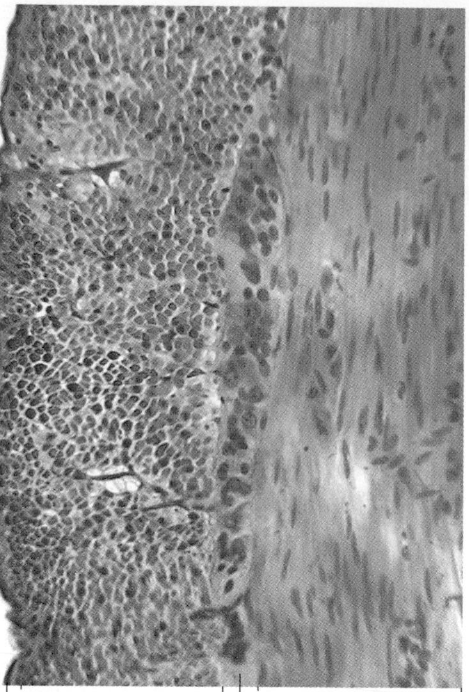
Outer muscle layer (longitudinal)
Inner muscle layer (circular)
Serosa
Myenteric plexus of Auerbach

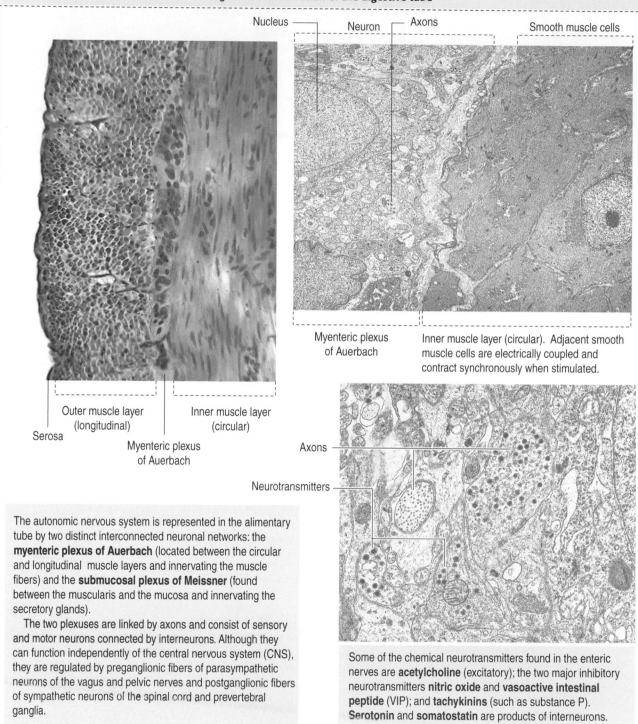

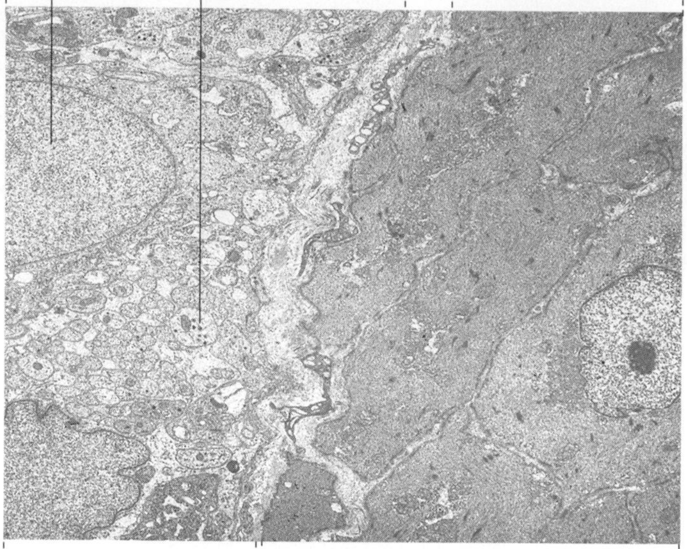
Nucleus
Neuron
Axons
Smooth muscle cells
Myenteric plexus of Auerbach
Inner muscle layer (circular). Adjacent smooth muscle cells are electrically coupled and contract synchronously when stimulated.

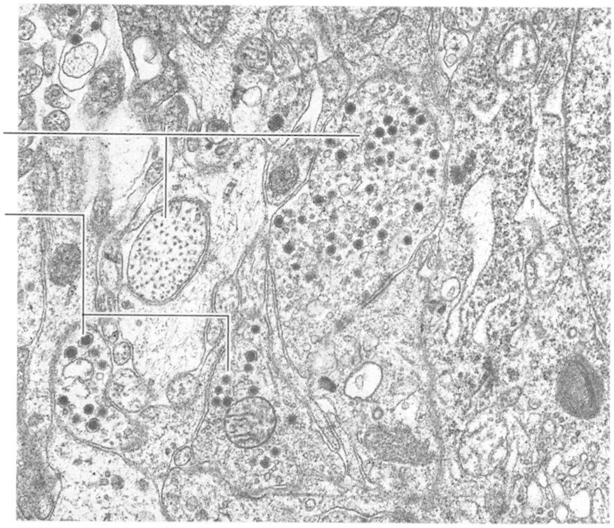
Axons
Neurotransmitters

The autonomic nervous system is represented in the alimentary tube by two distinct interconnected neuronal networks: the **myenteric plexus of Auerbach** (located between the circular and longitudinal muscle layers and innervating the muscle fibers) and the **submucosal plexus of Meissner** (found between the muscularis and the mucosa and innervating the secretory glands).

The two plexuses are linked by axons and consist of sensory and motor neurons connected by interneurons. Although they can function independently of the central nervous system (CNS), they are regulated by preganglionic fibers of parasympathetic neurons of the vagus and pelvic nerves and postganglionic fibers of sympathetic neurons of the spinal cord and prevertebral ganglia.

Some of the chemical neurotransmitters found in the enteric nerves are **acetylcholine** (excitatory); the two major inhibitory neurotransmitters **nitric oxide** and **vasoactive intestinal peptide** (VIP); and **tachykinins** (such as substance P). **Serotonin** and **somatostatin** are products of interneurons.

mesenteric veins. Mesenteric veins drain into the portal vein, leading to the liver (see Chapter 17, Digestive Glands).

Clinical significance: Gastric microcirculation and gastric ulcers

As we discuss later in this chapter, gastric microcirculation plays a significant role in the protection of the integrity of the gastric mucosa. A breakdown in this protective mechanism, including mucus and bicarbonate secretion, allows the destructive action of hydrochloric acid and pepsin and bacterial infection, leading to **peptic ulcer disease** (**PUD**). PUD includes a group of disorders characterized by a partial or total loss of the mucosal surface of the stomach or duodenum or both.

The rich blood supply to the gastric mucosa is of considerable significance in understanding bleeding associated with **stress ulcers.** Stress ulcers are superficial gastric mucosal erosions observed after severe trauma or severe illness and after long-term use of aspirin and corticosteroids. In most cases, stress ulcers are clinically asymptomatic and are detected only when they cause severe bleeding.

Nerve supply of the digestive tube

The digestive tube is innervated by the autonomic nervous system (ANS). The ANS consists of an **extrinsic component** (the parasympathetic and sympathetic innervation) and an **intrinsic**, or **enteric**, **component**.

Sympathetic nerve fibers derive from the thoracic and lumbar spinal cord. **Parasympathetic** nerve fibers derive from the vagal dorsal motor nucleus of the medulla oblongata. **Visceral sensory** fibers originate in the spinal dorsal root ganglia.

The **intrinsic** or **enteric innervation** is represented by two distinct interconnected neuronal circuits formed by sensory and motor neurons linked by interneurons: (1) the **submucosal plexus of Meissner**, present in the **submucosa**; and (2) the **myenteric plexus of Auerbach** (Figure 15-9), located **between the inner circular and outer longitudinal layers of the muscularis**.

Neurons and interneurons of the plexuses give off axons that branch to form the networks. The plexuses are connected to the extrinsic sympathetic and parasympathetic ANS: the plexuses of Auerbach and Meissner receive **preganglionic axons** of the **parasympathetic neurons** and **postganglionic axons** of **sympathetic neurons**.

The intrinsic or enteric nervous system enables the digestive tube to respond to both local stimuli and input from extrinsic nerves of the ANS. The integrated extrinsic and intrinsic (enteric) networks regulate and control (1) **peristaltic contractions of the muscularis and movements of the muscularis mucosae** and (2) **secretory activities of the mucosal and submucosal glands.** Stimulation of **preganglionic parasympathetic nerve fibers** (**cholinergic terminals**) of the muscularis causes **increased motility** as well as glandular secretory activity. Stimulation of **postganglionic sympathetic nerve fibers** (**adrenergic terminals**) on the smooth muscle cells causes **decreased motility**.

Esophagus

The esophagus is a muscular tube linking the pharynx to the stomach. It runs through the thorax, crosses the diaphragm, and enters the stomach. Contractions of the muscularis propel the food down the esophagus—in about 2 seconds. At this velocity, changes of pressure and volume within the thorax are minimal. No disruption of respiration and cardiopulmonary circulation takes place.

The esophageal **mucosa** consists of a **stratified squamous epithelium** overlying a lamina propria with numerous connective tissue papillae (Figure 15-10). The **muscularis mucosae** is not present in the upper portion of the esophagus, but it becomes organized near the stomach. Both the mucosa and the submucosa in the undistended esophagus form **longitudinal folds** that give the lumen an irregular outline. As the bolus of food moves down the esophagus, the folds disappear transiently and then are restored by the recoil of the elastic fibers of the submucosa.

The **submucosa** contains a network of collagen and elastic fibers and many small blood vessels. At the lower end of the esophagus, **submucosal venous plexuses** drain into both the systemic venous system and the portal venous system. An increase in pressure in the portal venous system, caused by chronic liver disease, results in dilation of the submucosal venous sinuses and the formation of **esophageal varices**. Rupture of the varices or ulceration of the overlying mucosa

Figure 15-10. Esophagus

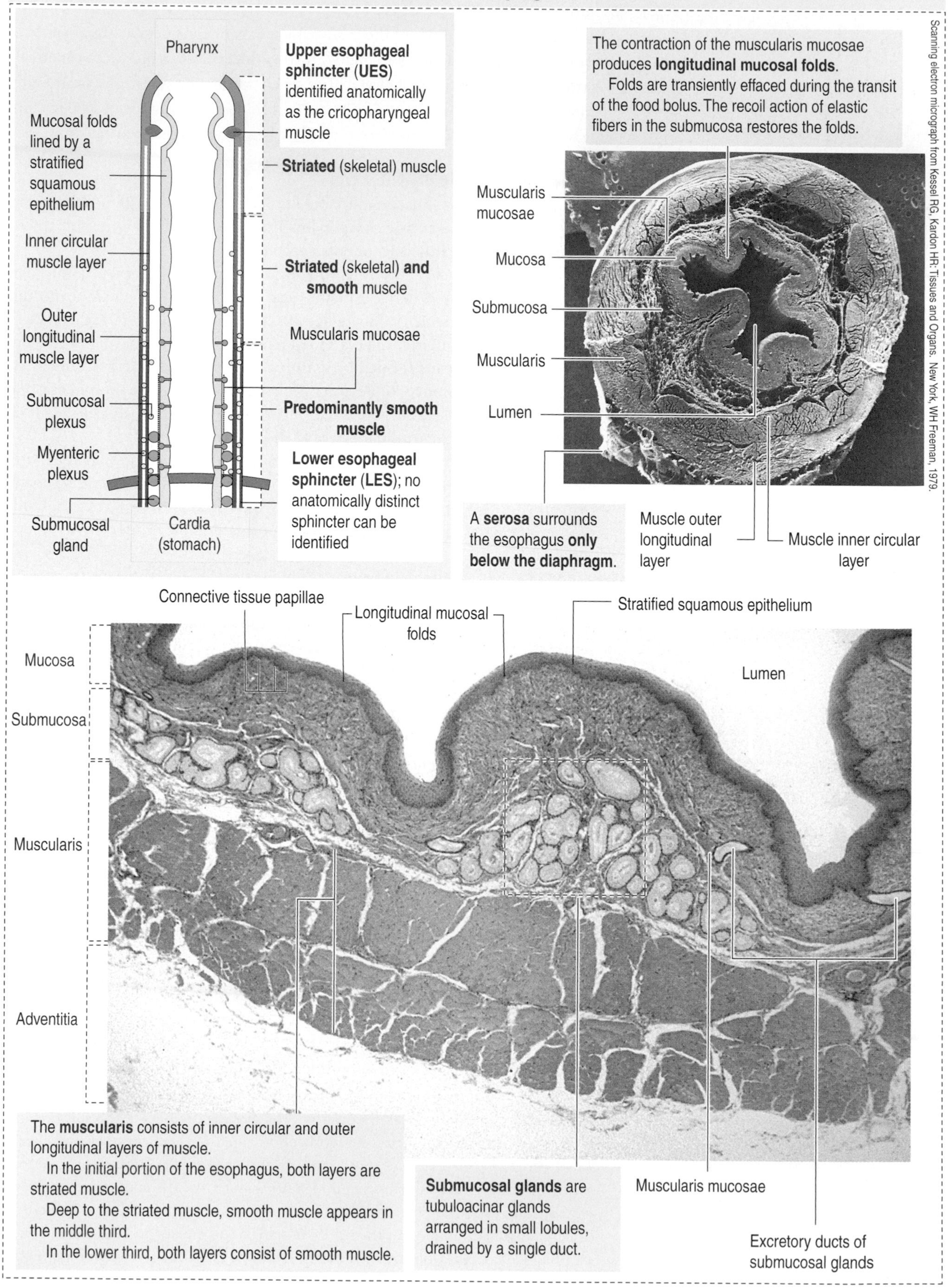
Pharynx
Upper esophageal sphincter (UES) identified anatomically as the cricopharyngeal muscle
Mucosal folds lined by a stratified squamous epithelium
Striated (skeletal) muscle
Inner circular muscle layer
Striated (skeletal) **and smooth** muscle
Outer longitudinal muscle layer
Muscularis mucosae
Submucosal plexus
Predominantly smooth muscle
Myenteric plexus
Lower esophageal sphincter (LES); no anatomically distinct sphincter can be identified
Submucosal gland
Cardia (stomach)
The contraction of the muscularis mucosae produces **longitudinal mucosal folds.**
Folds are transiently effaced during the transit of the food bolus. The recoil action of elastic fibers in the submucosa restores the folds.
Scanning electron micrograph from Kessel RG, Kardon HR: Tissues and Organs. New York, WH Freeman, 1979.
Muscularis mucosae
Mucosa
Submucosa
Muscularis
Lumen
A **serosa** surrounds the esophagus **only below the diaphragm.**
Muscle outer longitudinal layer
Muscle inner circular layer
Connective tissue papillae
Longitudinal mucosal folds
Stratified squamous epithelium
Mucosa
Submucosa
Muscularis
Adventitia
Lumen
The **muscularis** consists of inner circular and outer longitudinal layers of muscle.
In the initial portion of the esophagus, both layers are striated muscle.
Deep to the striated muscle, smooth muscle appears in the middle third.
In the lower third, both layers consist of smooth muscle.
Submucosal glands are tubuloacinar glands arranged in small lobules, drained by a single duct.
Muscularis mucosae
Excretory ducts of submucosal glands

Figure 15-11. Stomach: Ruga

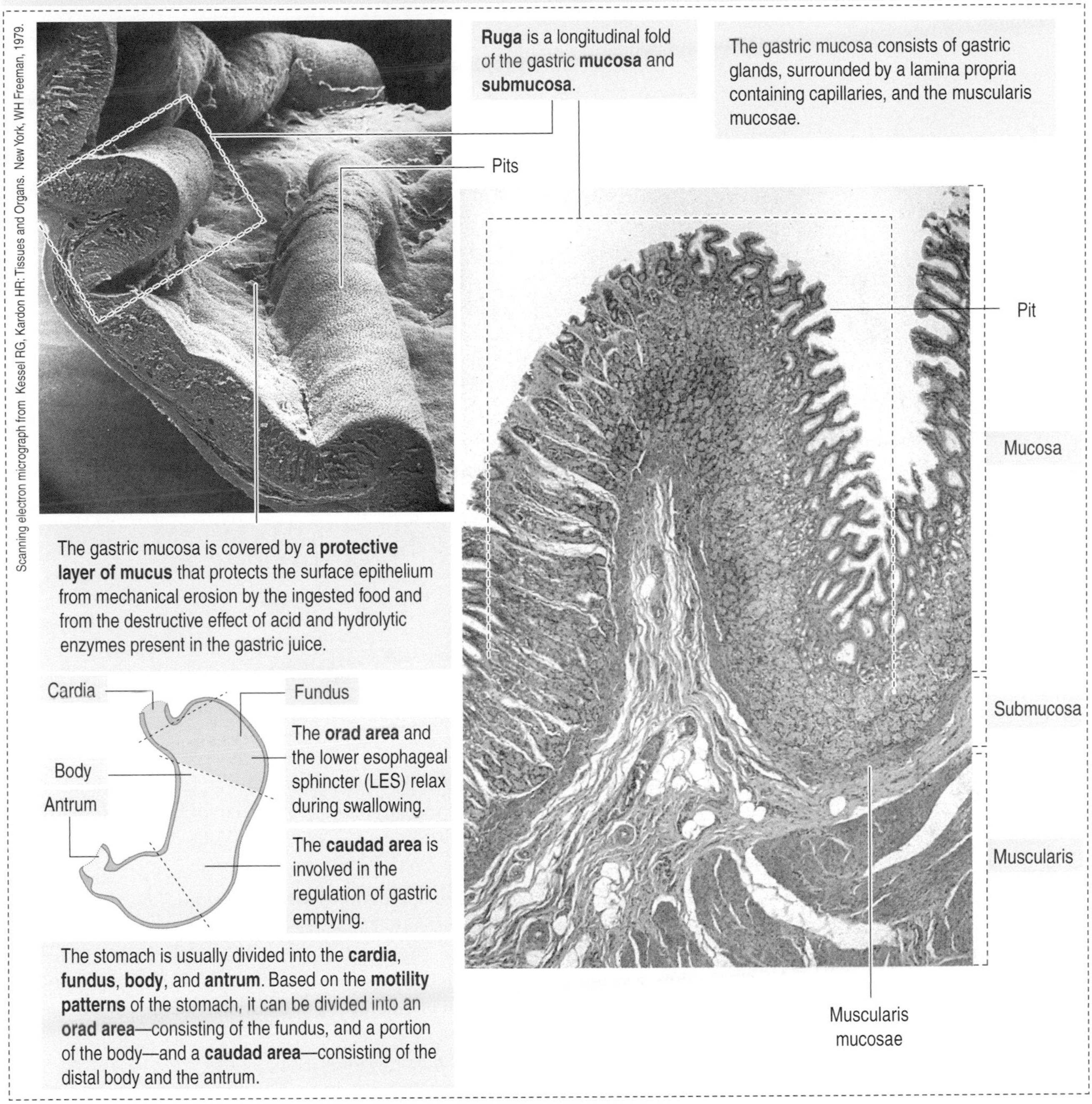

Scanning electron micrograph from Kessel RG, Kardon HR: Tissues and Organs. New York, WH Freeman, 1979.
Ruga is a longitudinal fold of the gastric mucosa and submucosa.
The gastric mucosa consists of gastric glands, surrounded by a lamina propria containing capillaries, and the muscularis mucosae.
Pits
Pit
Mucosa
Submucosa
Muscularis
Muscularis mucosae
The gastric mucosa is covered by a protective layer of mucus that protects the surface epithelium from mechanical erosion by the ingested food and from the destructive effect of acid and hydrolytic enzymes present in the gastric juice.
Cardia
Fundus
Body
Antrum
The orad area and the lower esophageal sphincter (LES) relax during swallowing.
The caudad area is involved in the regulation of gastric emptying.
The stomach is usually divided into the cardia, fundus, body, and antrum. Based on the motility patterns of the stomach, it can be divided into an orad area—consisting of the fundus, and a portion of the body—and a caudad area—consisting of the distal body and the antrum.

can produce hemorrhage into the esophagus and stomach, often causing vomiting (**hematemesis**).

Mucosal and **submucosal glands** are found in the esophagus. Their function is to produce continuously a thin layer of mucus that lubricates the surface of the epithelium.

The **mucosal tubular glands**, restricted to the lamina propria, resemble the cardiac glands of the stomach and are called **cardiac esophageal glands**.

The **submucosal tubuloacinar glands**, found in the submucosa just beneath the muscularis mucosae, are organized into small lobules drained by a single duct (see Figure 15-10). The acini are lined by two secretory cell types: a **mucous** and a **serous** cell type, the latter with secretory granules containing lysozyme.

The composition of the inner circumferential (or circular) and outer longitudinal layers of the **muscularis** shows **segment-dependent variations**. In the **upper**

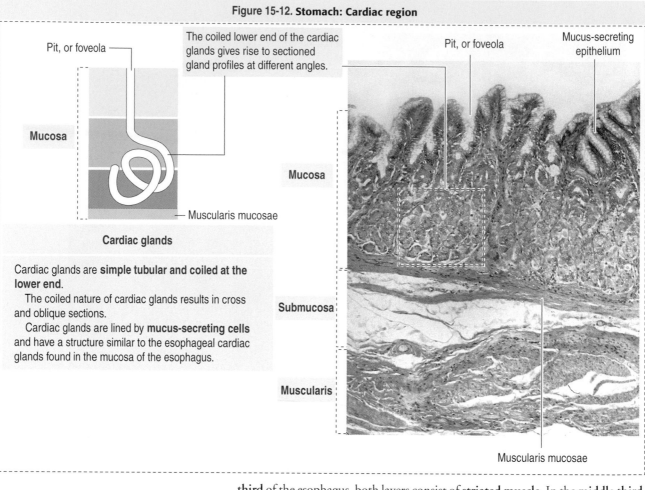

Figure 15-12. **Stomach: Cardiac region**

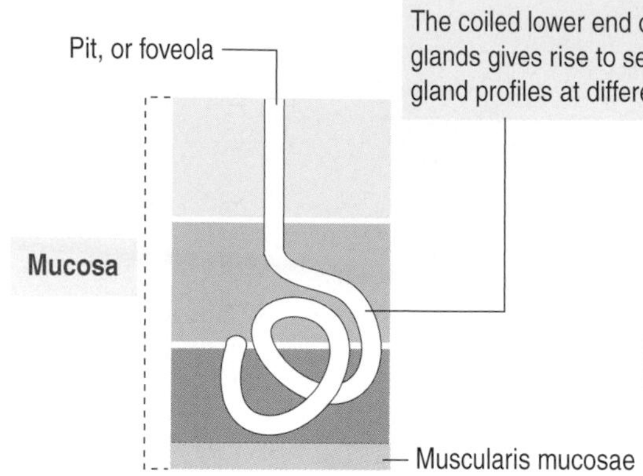

Pit, or foveola
The coiled lower end of the cardiac glands gives rise to sectioned gland profiles at different angles.
Mucosa
Muscularis mucosae

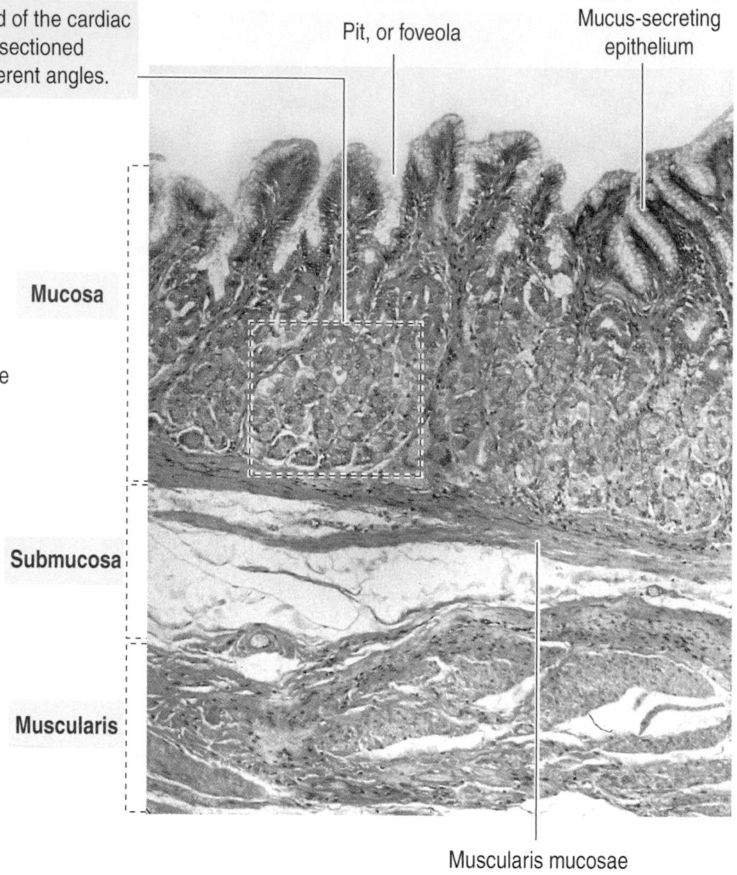

Pit, or foveola
Mucus-secreting epithelium
Mucosa
Submucosa
Muscularis
Muscularis mucosae

Cardiac glands

Cardiac glands are **simple tubular and coiled at the lower end.**

The coiled nature of cardiac glands results in cross and oblique sections.

Cardiac glands are lined by **mucus-secreting cells** and have a structure similar to the esophageal cardiac glands found in the mucosa of the esophagus.

third of the esophagus, both layers consist of **striated muscle**. In the **middle third**, **smooth muscle fibers can be seen deep to the striated muscle**. In the **lower third**, both layers of the muscularis contain **smooth muscle cells**.

Clinical significance: The mechanism of swallowing and dysphagia

The esophagus has **two sphincters**: (1) the anatomically defined **upper esophageal sphincter (UES)**, or **cricopharyngeal sphincter**, and (2) the functionally defined **lower esophageal sphincter** (LES), or **gastroesophageal sphincter**. The **UES participates in the initiation of swallowing**. The **LES prevents reflux of gastric contents into the esophagus**.

Because the esophageal stratified squamous lining epithelium may be replaced at the lower end by a poorly resistant columnar epithelium, a reflux of acidic gastric secretions causes chronic inflammation (**reflux esophagitis**) or ulceration and difficulty in swallowing (**dysphagia**). This persistent condition leads to fibrosis and eventual stricture of the lower esophagus.

When the esophageal hiatus in the diaphragm does not close entirely during development, a **hiatus hernia** enables a portion of the stomach to move into the thoracic cavity. In **sliding hiatus hernia**, the stomach protrudes through the diaphragmatic hiatus, normally occupied by the lower esophagus. Reflux esophagitis and peptic ulceration in the intrathoracic portion of the stomach and lower esophagus leads to difficulty in swallowing and the feeling of a lump in the throat. This condition, commonly seen in family practice patients, affects young and middle-aged women in particular.

The movements involved in swallowing are coordinated by nerves from the cervical and thoracic sympathetic trunks, forming plexuses in the submucosa and in between the inner and outer layers of the muscularis. Diseases affecting

Figure 15-13. **Stomach: Gastric gland**

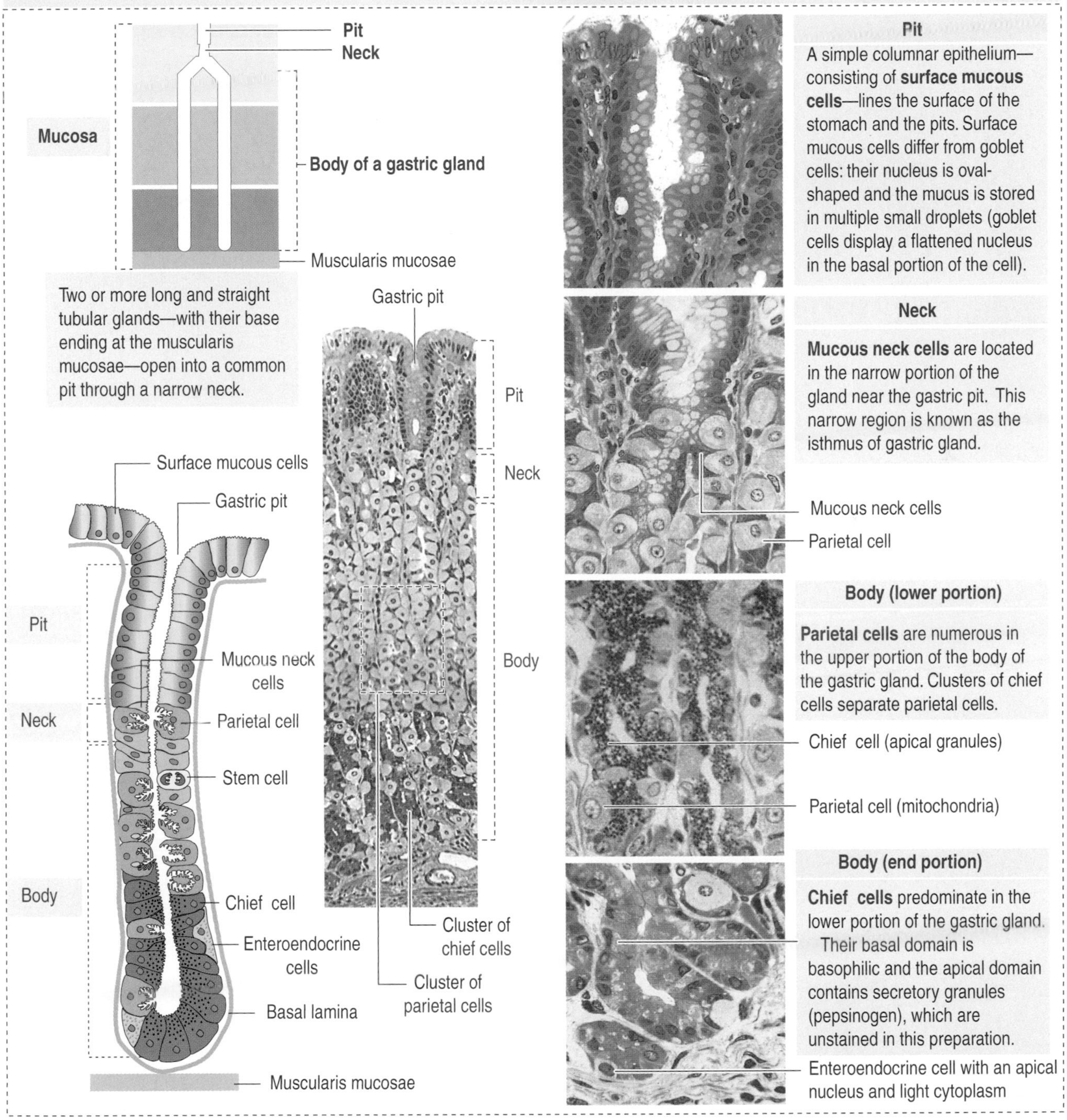

Pit
Neck
Mucosa
Body of a gastric gland
Muscularis mucosae
Two or more long and straight tubular glands—with their base ending at the muscularis mucosae—open into a common pit through a narrow neck.
Gastric pit
Pit
Neck
Body
Surface mucous cells
Gastric pit
Pit
Neck
Body
Mucous neck cells
Parietal cell
Stem cell
Chief cell
Enteroendocrine cells
Basal lamina
Muscularis mucosae
Cluster of chief cells
Cluster of parietal cells
Pit
A simple columnar epithelium—consisting of surface mucous cells—lines the surface of the stomach and the pits. Surface mucous cells differ from goblet cells: their nucleus is oval-shaped and the mucus is stored in multiple small droplets (goblet cells display a flattened nucleus in the basal portion of the cell).
Neck
Mucous neck cells are located in the narrow portion of the gland near the gastric pit. This narrow region is known as the isthmus of gastric gland.
Mucous neck cells
Parietal cell
Body (lower portion)
Parietal cells are numerous in the upper portion of the body of the gastric gland. Clusters of chief cells separate parietal cells.
Chief cell (apical granules)
Parietal cell (mitochondria)
Body (end portion)
Chief cells predominate in the lower portion of the gastric gland. Their basal domain is basophilic and the apical domain contains secretory granules (pepsinogen), which are unstained in this preparation.
Enteroendocrine cell with an apical nucleus and light cytoplasm

this neuromuscular system may result in muscle spasm, difficulty in swallowing, and substernal pain.

Stomach

The stomach extends from the esophagus to the duodenum. At the **gastroesophageal junction**, the epithelium changes from stratified squamous to a simple columnar type. The muscularis mucosae of the esophagus is continuous with that of the stomach. However, the submucosa does not have a clear demarcation line, and glands from the cardiac portion of the stomach may extend under the stratified squamous epithelium and contact the esophageal cardiac glands.

The **function of the stomach is to homogenize and chemically process the swallowed semisolid food**. Both the contractions of the muscular wall of the

Figure 15-14. Gastric gland: Surface and neck cells

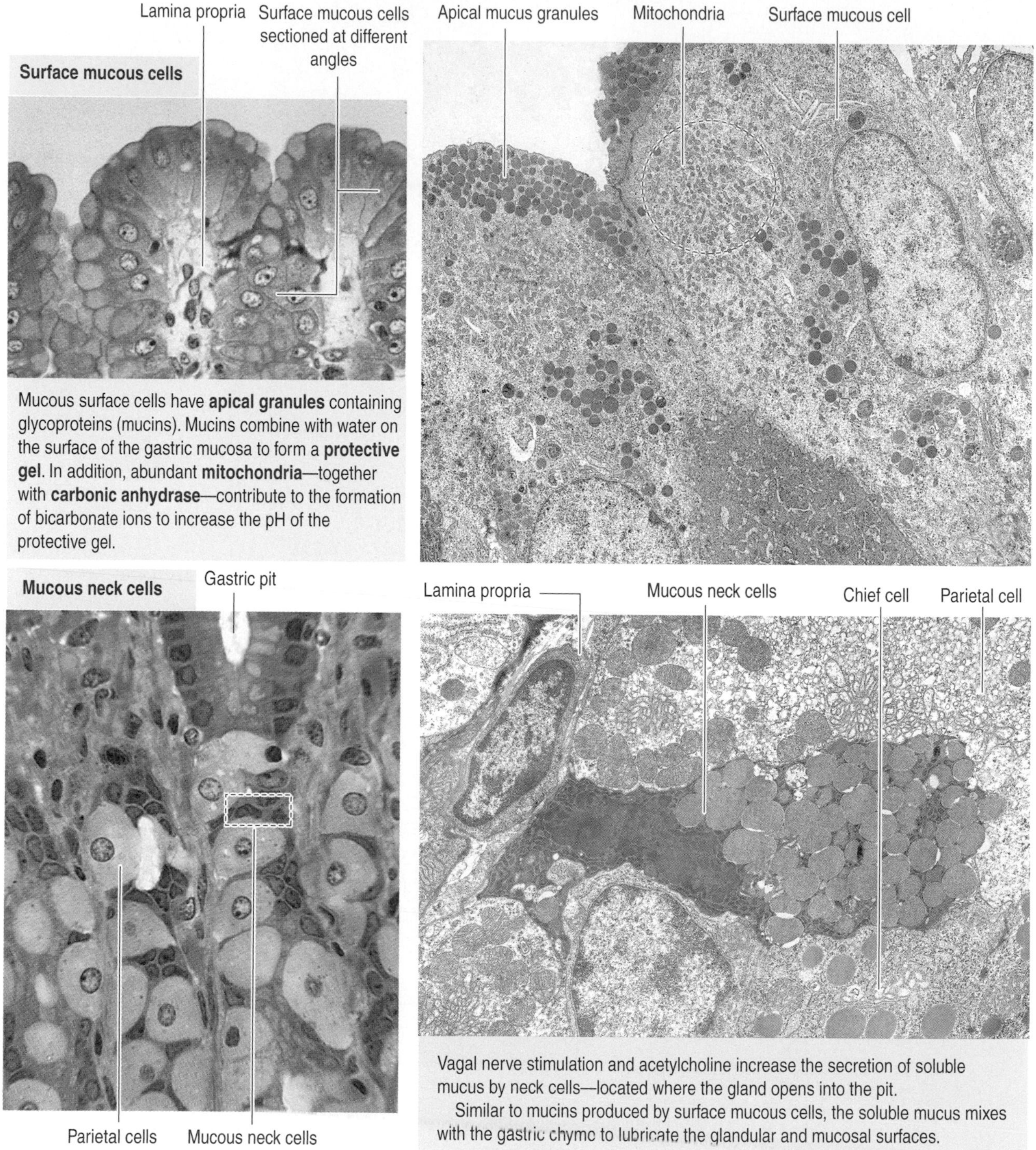

Surface mucous cells
Lamina propria
Surface mucous cells sectioned at different angles
Apical mucus granules
Mitochondria
Surface mucous cell
Mucous neck cells
Gastric pit
Lamina propria
Mucous neck cells
Chief cell
Parietal cell
Parietal cells
Mucous neck cells

Mucous surface cells have **apical granules** containing glycoproteins (mucins). Mucins combine with water on the surface of the gastric mucosa to form a **protective gel**. In addition, abundant **mitochondria**—together with **carbonic anhydrase**—contribute to the formation of bicarbonate ions to increase the pH of the protective gel.

Vagal nerve stimulation and acetylcholine increase the secretion of soluble mucus by neck cells—located where the gland opens into the pit.

Similar to mucins produced by surface mucous cells, the soluble mucus mixes with the gastric chyme to lubricate the glandular and mucosal surfaces.

stomach and the acid and enzymes secreted by the gastric mucosa contribute to this function. Once the food is transformed into a thick fluid, it is released gradually into the duodenum.

Four regions are recognized in the stomach: (1) the **cardia**, a 2- to 3-cm-wide zone surrounding the esophageal opening; (2) the **fundus**, projecting to the left of the opening of the esophagus; (3) the **body**, an extensive central region; and (4) the **pyloric antrum** (Greek *pyloros*, gatekeeper), ending at the gastroduodenal orifice. Based on the **motility** characteristics of the stomach, the **orad area**, consisting of the fundus and the upper part of the body, relaxes during swallowing.

Figure 15-15. Gastric gland: Chief and parietal cells

Chief cell

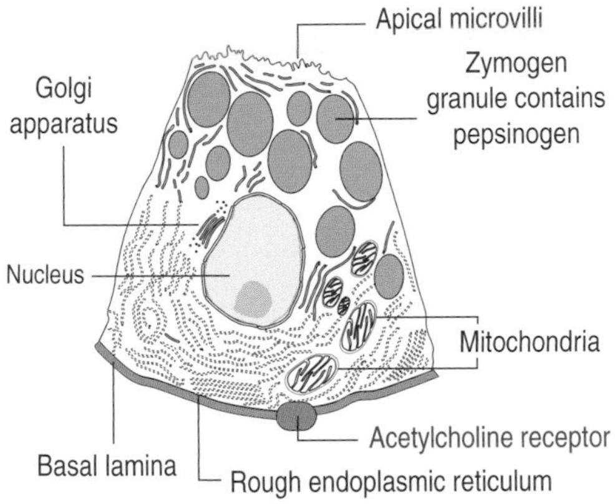

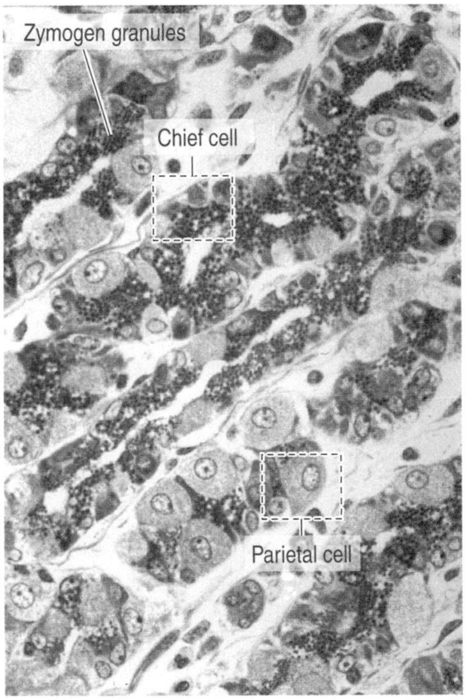

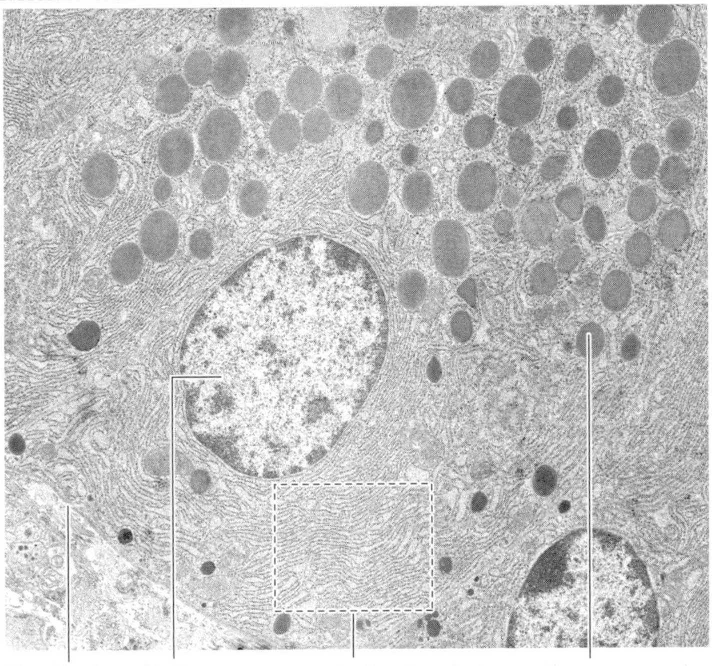

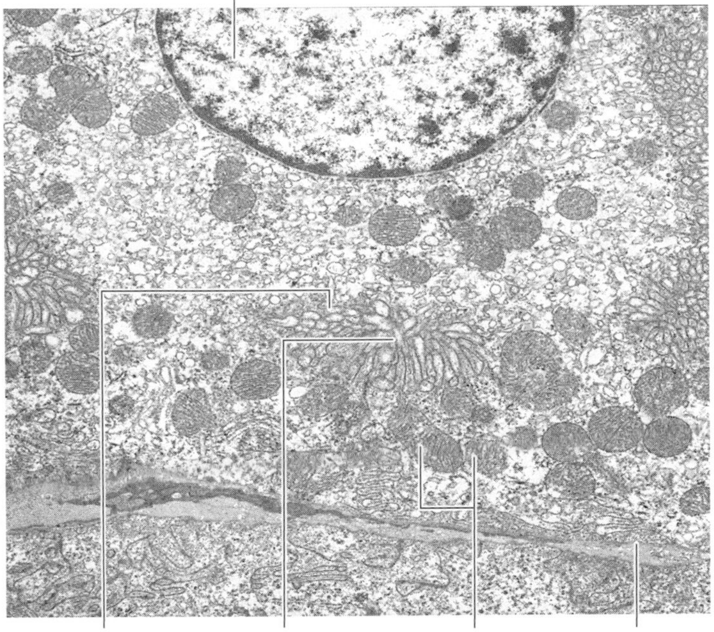

Parietal cell

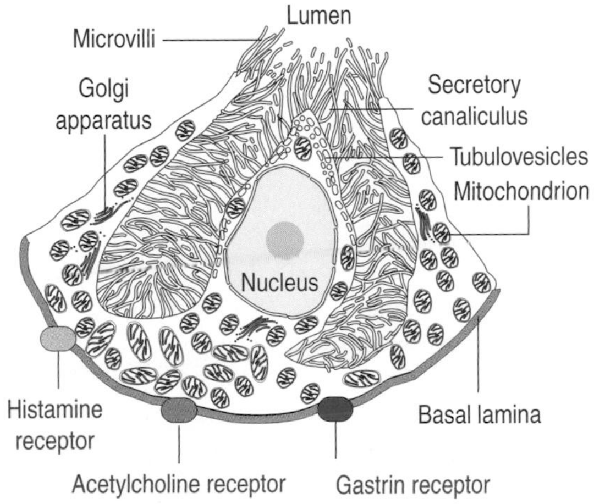

The gastric glands of the fundus-body region contain two major cell types:

1. **Chief** or **peptic cells**, which produce and secrete **pepsinogen** (42.5 kd), a precursor of the proteolytic enzyme **pepsin** (35 kd) produced in the gastric juice when the pH is below 5.0. Pepsin can catalyze the formation of additional pepsin from pepsinogen. **Acetylcholine** stimulates the secretion of pepsinogen.

2. **Parietal** or **oxyntic cells**, which secrete **hydrochloric acid** and **intrinsic factor** in humans (in some species, chief cells secrete intrinsic factor). The cytoplasm of parietal cells displays numerous **tubulovesicles** and an **intracellular canaliculus** continuous with the lumen of the gastric gland.

After stimulation, the tubulovesicles fuse with the plasma membrane of the intracellular canaliculus. **Carbonic anhydrase** and **H^+,K^+-ATPase** are localized in the microvilli projecting into the lumen of the intracellular canaliculus.

The **caudad area**, consisting of the lower portion of the body and the antrum, participates in the regulation of gastric emptying.

The empty stomach shows gastric mucosal folds, or **rugae**, covered by **gastric pits** or **foveolae** (Figure 15-11). A **gastric mucosal barrier**, produced by **surface mucous cells**, protects the mucosal surface. The surface mucous cells contain apical periodic acid–Schiff (PAS)-positive granules and are linked to each other by apical tight junctions.

Cardia region

Glands of the cardia region are **tubular**, with a **coiled end** and an **opening continuous with the gastric pits** (Figure 15-12). A mucus-secreting epithelium lines the cardiac glands.

Functions of the gastric gland

Gastric glands of the fundus-body region are the major contributors to the gastric juice. About 15 million gastric glands open into 3.5 million gastric pits. From two to seven gastric glands open into a single gastric pit, or foveola.

A gastric gland consists of three regions (Figure 15-13): (1) The **pit**, or **foveola**, lined by surface mucous cells; (2) the **neck**, containing mucous neck cells, mitotically active stem cells, and parietal cells; and (3) the **body**, representing the major length of the gland. The upper and lower portions of the body contain different proportions of cells lining the gastric gland.

The surface mucous cells line the surface of the gastric mucosa and the gastric pits (Figure 15-14; see also Figure 15-13).

The gastric glands proper house five major cell types: (1) **mucous neck cells** (see Figure 15-13), (2) **chief cells** (also called **peptic cells**), (3) **parietal cells** (also called **oxyntic cells**), (4) **stem cells**, and (5) **gastroenteroendocrine cells** (called **enterochromaffin cells** because of their staining affinity for chromic acid salts).

The upper portion of the main body of the gastric gland contains abundant parietal cells. Chief cells and gastroenteroendocrine cells predominate in the lower portion (see Figure 15-13).

The gastric mucosa of the fundus-body has two classes of mucus-producing cells (see Figure 15-14): (1) the **surface mucous cells** lining the pit and (2) the **mucous neck cells** located at the opening of the gastric gland into the pit. Both cells produce mucins, glycoproteins with high molecular mass. A mucus layer, containing 95% water and 5% mucins, forms an insoluble gel that attaches to the surface of the gastric mucosa, forming a 100-μm-thick protective gastric mucosal barrier. This protective mucus blanket traps **bicarbonate ions** and neutralizes the microenvironment adjacent to the apical region of the surface mucous cells to an alkaline pH.

Na^+, K^+, and Cl^- are additional constituents of the protective mucosal barrier. Patients with chronic vomiting or undergoing continuous aspiration of gastric juice require intravenous replacement of NaCl, dextrose, and K^+ to prevent hypokalemic metabolic acidosis.

Chief cells (Figure 15-15) predominate in the lower third of the gastric gland. **Chief cells are not present in cardiac glands and are seldom found in the pyloric antrum.** Chief cells have a structural similarity to the zymogenic cells of the exocrine pancreas: the basal region of the cytoplasm contains an extensive rough endoplasmic reticulum. Pepsinogen-containing secretory granules (**zymogen granules**) are observed in the apical region of the cell. **Pepsinogen**, a proenzyme stored in the zymogen granules, is released into the lumen of the gland and converted in the acid environment of the stomach to **pepsin**, a proteolytic enzyme capable of digesting most proteins. Exocytosis of pepsinogen is rapid and stimulated by

Figure 15-16. **Hydrochloric acid secretion by parietal cells**

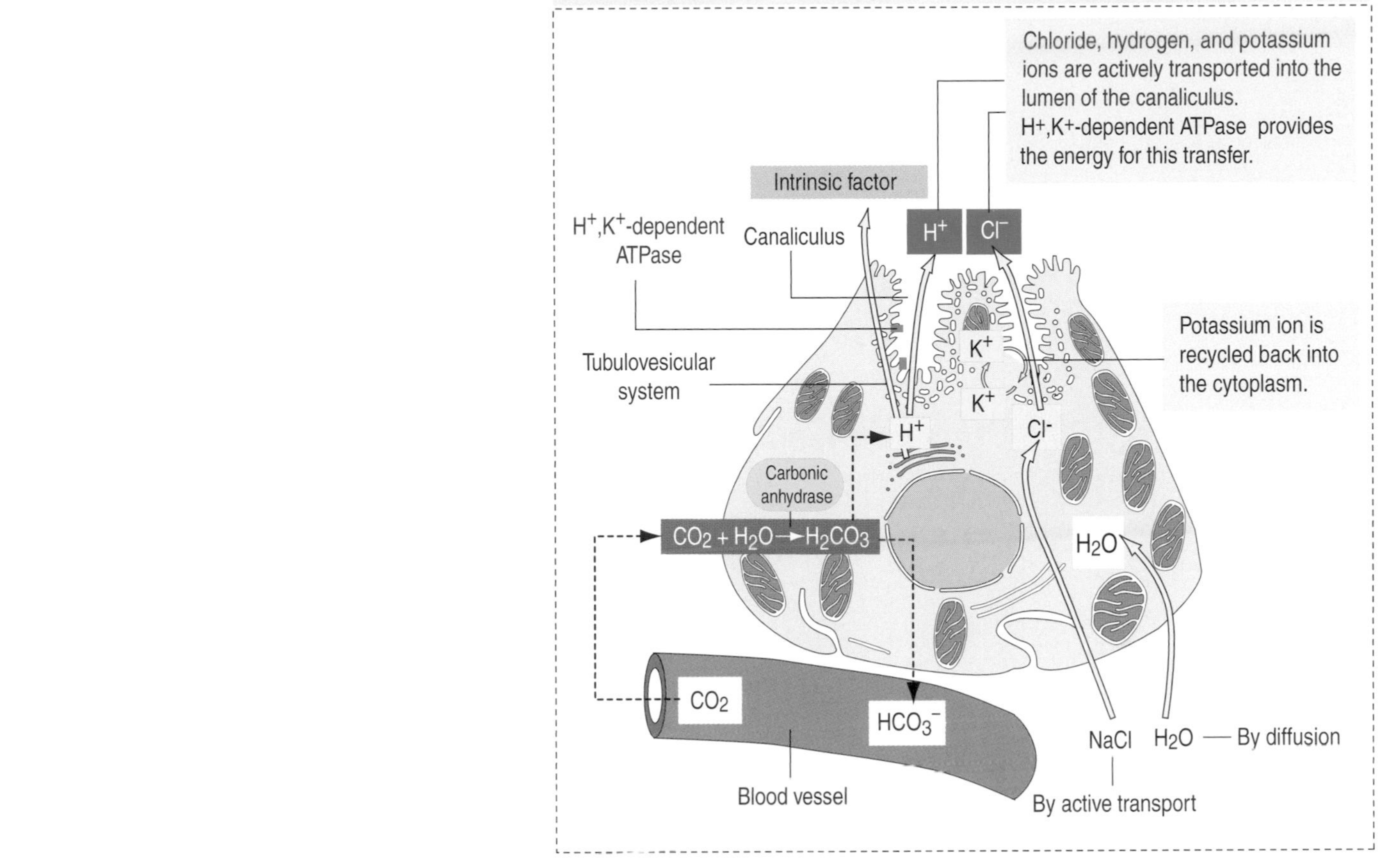

Chloride, hydrogen, and potassium ions are actively transported into the lumen of the canaliculus.
H+,K+-dependent ATPase provides the energy for this transfer.
Intrinsic factor
H+,K+-dependent ATPase
Canaliculus
H+
Cl−
Potassium ion is recycled back into the cytoplasm.
K+
K+
Tubulovesicular system
H+
Cl-
Carbonic anhydrase
CO2 + H2O → H2CO3
H2O
CO2
HCO3−
NaCl
H2O — By diffusion
Blood vessel
By active transport

feeding (after fasting).

Parietal cells predominate near the neck and in the upper segment of the gastric gland and are linked to chief cells by junctional complexes. Parietal cells produce the **hydrochloric acid** of the gastric juice and **intrinsic factor**, a glycoprotein that binds to vitamin B_{12}. Vitamin B_{12} binds in the stomach to the transporting binding protein intrinsic factor. In the small intestine, the vitamin B_{12}–intrinsic factor complex binds to intrinsic factor receptor on the surface of enterocytes in the ileum and is transported to the liver through the portal circulation.

Autoimmune gastritis is caused by autoantibodies to H^+,K^+-dependent ATPase, a parietal cell antigen, and intrinsic factor. Destruction of parietal cells causes a reduction in hydrochloric acid in the gastric juice (**achlorhydria**) and a lack of synthesis of intrinsic factor. The resulting vitamin B_{12} deficiency disrupts the formation of red blood cells in the bone marrow, leading to a condition known as **pernicious anemia**, identified by examination of peripheral blood as **megaloblastic anemia** characterized by **macrocytic red blood cells** and **hypersegmented large neutrophils** (see Chapter 6, Blood and Hematopoiesis).

Parietal cells have three distinctive features (see Figure 15-15): (1) **abundant mitochondria**, which occupy about 40% of the cell volume and provide the adenosine triphosphate (ATP) required to pump **H^+ ions** into the lumen of the intracellular canaliculus; (2) an **intracellular canaliculus**, formed by an invagination of the apical cell surface and continuous with the lumen of the gastric gland, which is lined by numerous **microvilli**; and (3) an **H^+,K^+**-dependent **ATPase-rich tubulovesicular system**, which is distributed along the secretory canaliculus during the resting state of the parietal cell.

After stimulation, the tubulovesicular system fuses with the membrane of the secretory canaliculus, and numerous microvilli project into the canalicular space. Membrane fusion increases the amount of H^+,K^+-ATPase and expands the intracellular canaliculus. H^+,K^+-ATPase represents about 80% of the protein

Figure 15-17. **Protective gastric mucus blanket**

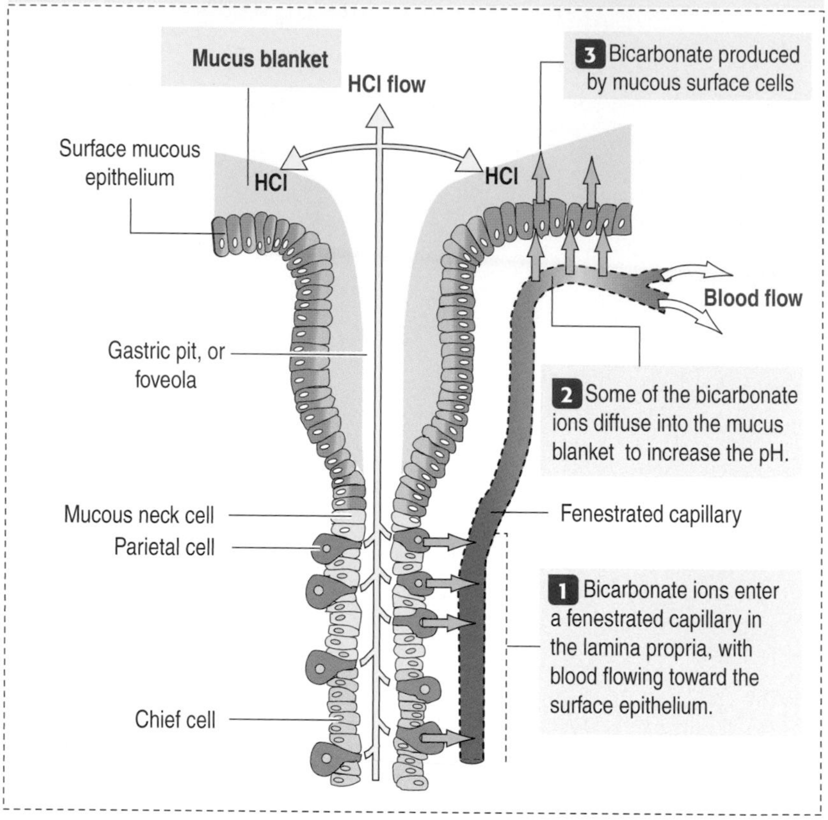

Mucus blanket
HCl flow
3 Bicarbonate produced by mucous surface cells
Surface mucous epithelium
HCl
HCl
Blood flow
Gastric pit, or foveola
2 Some of the bicarbonate ions diffuse into the mucus blanket to increase the pH.
Mucous neck cell
Fenestrated capillary
Parietal cell
1 Bicarbonate ions enter a fenestrated capillary in the lamina propria, with blood flowing toward the surface epithelium.
Chief cell

content of the plasma membrane of the microvilli.

Secretion of hydrochloric acid by parietal cells

Parietal cells produce an acidic secretion (pH 0.9 to 2.0) rich in hydrochloric acid, with a concentration of H^+ ions one million times greater than that of blood (Figure 15-16). The release of H^+ ions and Cl^- by the parietal cell involves the membrane fusion of the tubulovesicular system with the intracellular canaliculus.

The parasympathetic mediator **acetylcholine** and the peptide **gastrin**, produced by enteroendocrine cells of the pyloric antrum, stimulate parietal cells to secrete HCl (see Figure 15-19). Acetylcholine also stimulates the release of gastrin. **Histamine** potentiates the effects of acetylcholine and gastrin on parietal cell secretion after binding to the **histamine H_2 receptor**. Histamine is produced by **enterochromaffin-like (ECL) cells** within the lamina propria surrounding the gastric glands. **Cimetidine** is an H_2 receptor antagonist that inhibits histamine-dependent acid secretion.

H^+,K^+-dependent ATPase facilitates the exchange of H^+ and K^+. Cl^- and Na^+ (derived from the dissociation of NaCl) are actively transported into the lumen of the intracellular canaliculus, leading to the production of HCl. K^+ and Na^+ are recycled back into the cell by separate pumps once H^+ has taken their place. **Omeprazole**, with binding affinity to H^+,K^+-dependent ATPase, inactivates acid secretion and is an effective agent in the treatment of peptic ulcer.

Water enters the cell by osmosis—because of the secretion of ions into the canaliculus—and dissociates into H^+ and hydroxyl ions (HO^-). **Carbon dioxide**, entering the cell from the blood or formed during metabolism of the cell, combines with HO^- to form **carbonic acid** under the influence of **carbonic anhydrase**. Carbonic acid dissociates into **bicarbonate ions** (HCO_3^-) and **hydrogen ions**. HCO_3^- diffuses out of the cell into the blood and accounts for the increase in blood plasma pH during digestion.

Figure 15-18. *Helicobacter pylori* and chronic gastric inflammation and ulcers

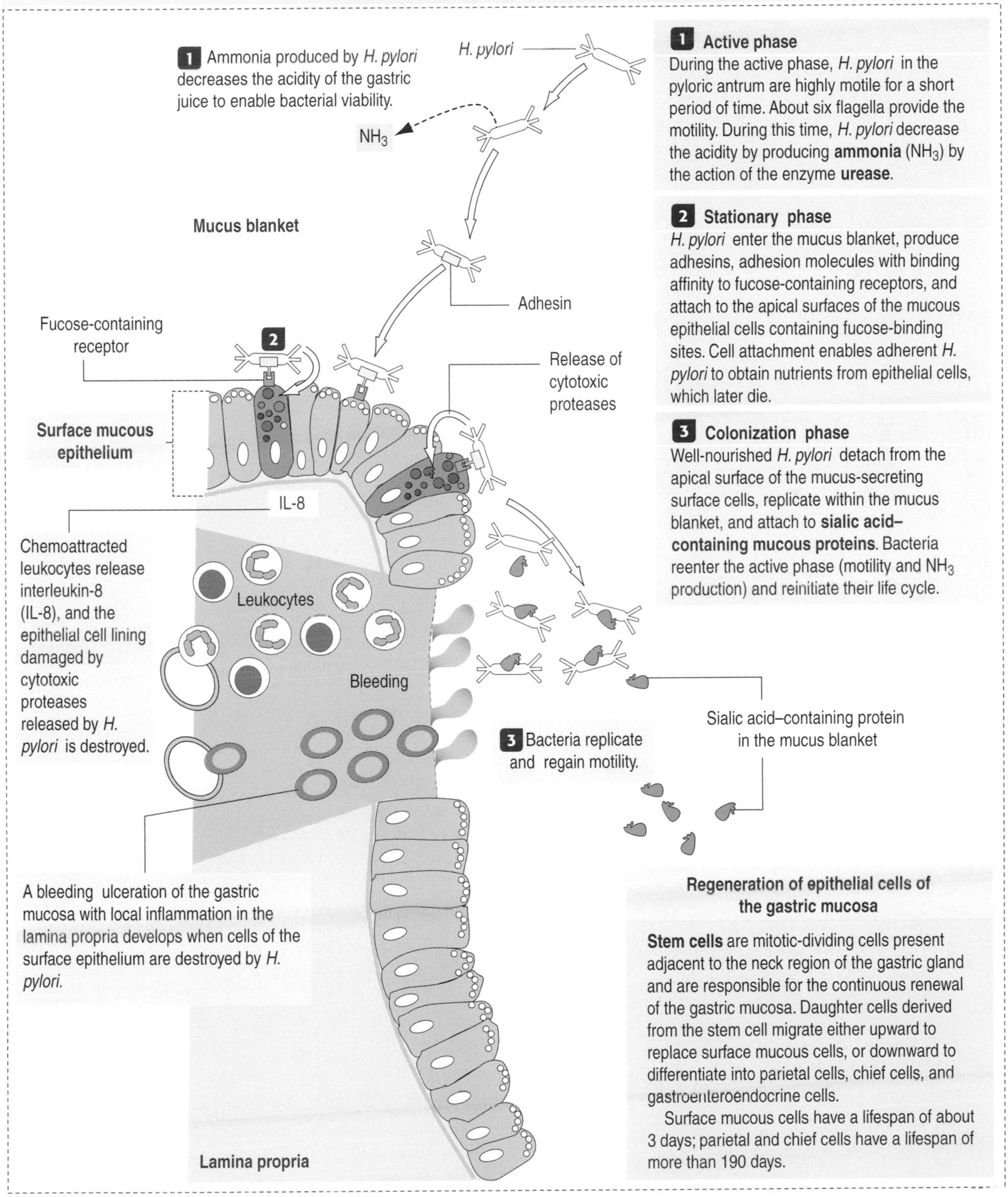

1 Ammonia produced by H. pylori decreases the acidity of the gastric juice to enable bacterial viability.
H. pylori
NH3
Mucus blanket
Adhesin
Fucose-containing receptor
2
Release of cytotoxic proteases
Surface mucous epithelium
IL-8
Chemoattracted leukocytes release interleukin-8 (IL-8), and the epithelial cell lining damaged by cytotoxic proteases released by H. pylori is destroyed.
Leukocytes
Bleeding
3 Bacteria replicate and regain motility.
Sialic acid–containing protein in the mucus blanket
A bleeding ulceration of the gastric mucosa with local inflammation in the lamina propria develops when cells of the surface epithelium are destroyed by H. pylori.
Lamina propria
1 Active phase
During the active phase, H. pylori in the pyloric antrum are highly motile for a short period of time. About six flagella provide the motility. During this time, H. pylori decrease the acidity by producing ammonia (NH3) by the action of the enzyme urease.
2 Stationary phase
H. pylori enter the mucus blanket, produce adhesins, adhesion molecules with binding affinity to fucose-containing receptors, and attach to the apical surfaces of the mucous epithelial cells containing fucose-binding sites. Cell attachment enables adherent H. pylori to obtain nutrients from epithelial cells, which later die.
3 Colonization phase
Well-nourished H. pylori detach from the apical surface of the mucus-secreting surface cells, replicate within the mucus blanket, and attach to sialic acid–containing mucous proteins. Bacteria reenter the active phase (motility and NH3 production) and reinitiate their life cycle.
Regeneration of epithelial cells of the gastric mucosa
Stem cells are mitotic-dividing cells present adjacent to the neck region of the gastric gland and are responsible for the continuous renewal of the gastric mucosa. Daughter cells derived from the stem cell migrate either upward to replace surface mucous cells, or downward to differentiate into parietal cells, chief cells, and gastroenteroendocrine cells.
Surface mucous cells have a lifespan of about 3 days; parietal and chief cells have a lifespan of more than 190 days.

Clinical significance: *Helicobacter pylori* infection

It is convenient to regard the gastric juice as a combination of two separate secretions: (1) an **alkaline mucosal gel protective component**, produced by surface mucous cells and mucous neck cells; and (2) HCl and pepsin, two **parietal–chief cell–derived potentially aggressive components**. The protective component is **constitutive**; it is always present. The aggressive component is **facultative** because

Figure 15-19. **G cell (pyloric antrum)**

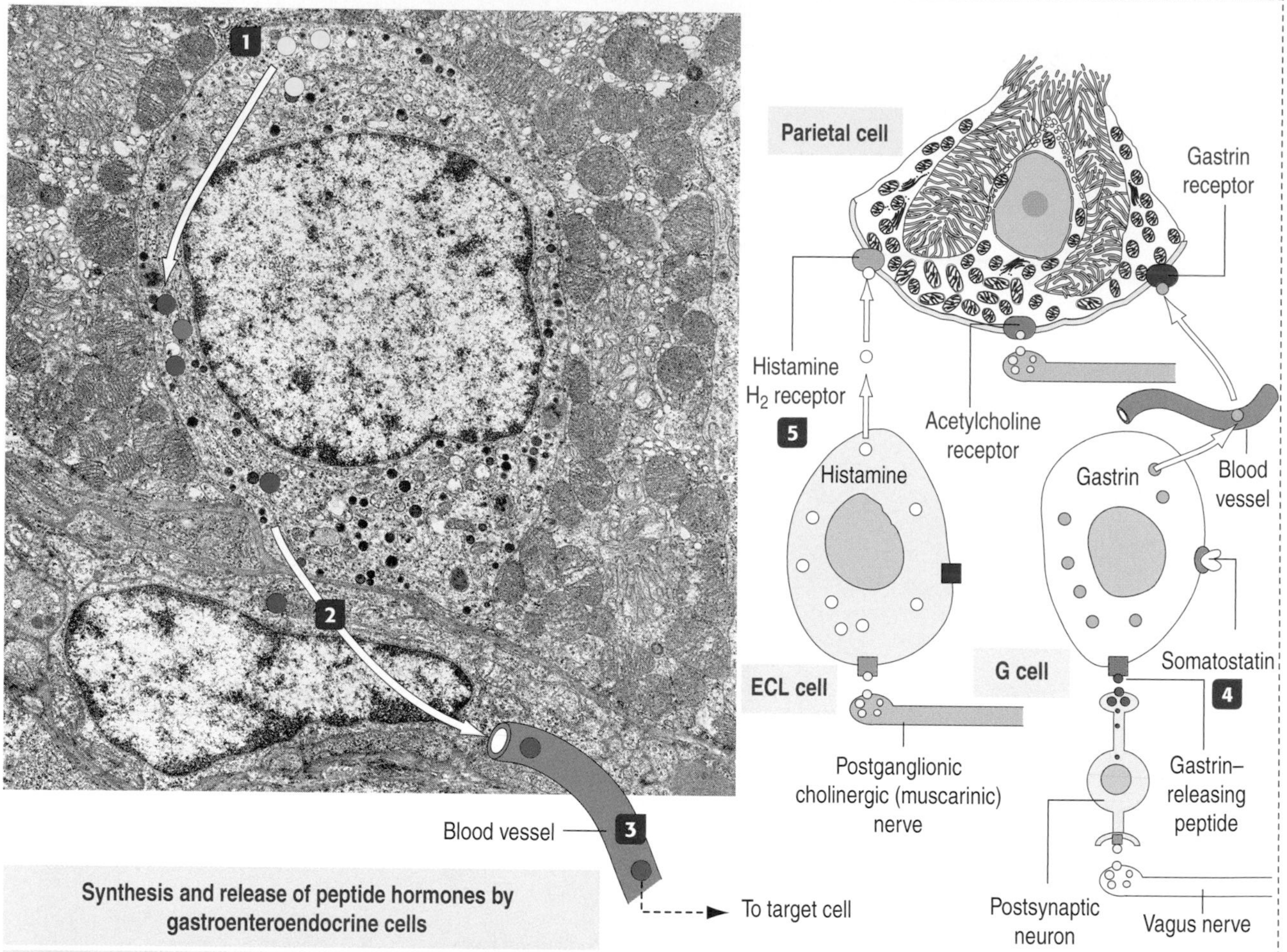

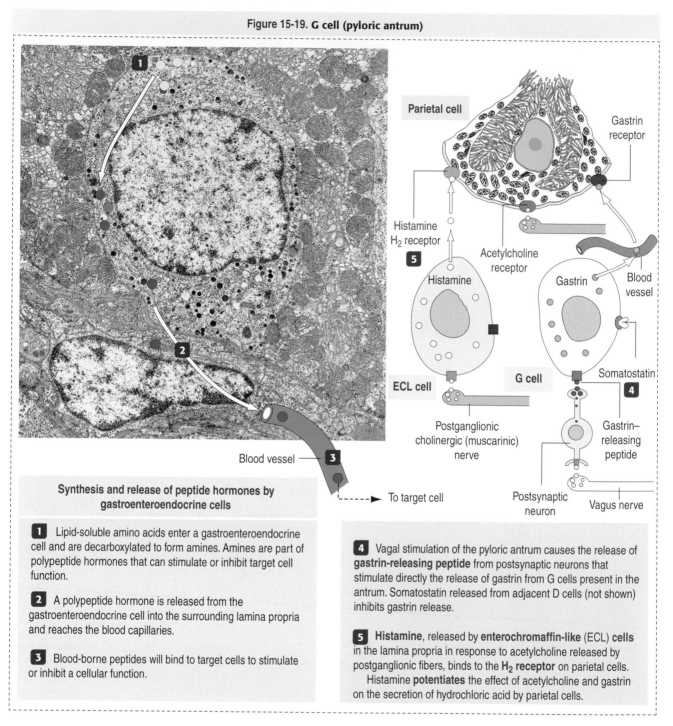

Synthesis and release of peptide hormones by gastroenteroendocrine cells

1 Lipid-soluble amino acids enter a gastroenteroendocrine cell and are decarboxylated to form amines. Amines are part of polypeptide hormones that can stimulate or inhibit target cell function.

2 A polypeptide hormone is released from the gastroenteroendocrine cell into the surrounding lamina propria and reaches the blood capillaries.

3 Blood-borne peptides will bind to target cells to stimulate or inhibit a cellular function.

4 Vagal stimulation of the pyloric antrum causes the release of **gastrin-releasing peptide** from postsynaptic neurons that stimulate directly the release of gastrin from G cells present in the antrum. Somatostatin released from adjacent D cells (not shown) inhibits gastrin release.

5 **Histamine**, released by **enterochromaffin-like** (ECL) **cells** in the lamina propria in response to acetylcholine released by postganglionic fibers, binds to the **H_2 receptor** on parietal cells.
Histamine **potentiates** the effect of acetylcholine and gastrin on the secretion of hydrochloric acid by parietal cells.

hydrochloric acid and pepsin levels increase above basal levels after food intake.

The viscous, highly glycosylated gastric mucus blanket—produced by surface mucous cells and mucous neck cells—maintains a neutral pH at the epithelial cell surfaces of the stomach. In addition, the mitochondrial-rich surface mucous cells (see Figure 15-14) produce HCO_3^- ions diffusing into the surface mucus gel. Recall the clinical significance during chronic vomiting of Na^+, K^+, and Cl^- present in the protective mucosal barrier and gastric juice (see section on functions of the gastric gland).

HCO_3^- ions, produced by parietal cells, enter the fenestrated capillaries of the lamina propria. Some of the HCO_3^- ions diffuse into the mucus blanket and neutralize the low pH created by the HCl content of the gastric lumen at the vicinity of the surface mucous cells (Figure 15-17).

However, the mucus blanket lining the gastric epithelium, in particular in the **pyloric antrum**, is the site where the flagellated bacterium *Helicobacter pylori* resides in spite of the hostile environment.

H. pylori survives and replicates in the gastric lumen. Its presence has been associated with **acid peptic ulcers** and **adenocarcinoma of the stomach.**

Three phases define the pathogenesis of *H. pylori* (Figure 15-18):

1. An **active phase**, in which motile bacteria increase the gastric pH by producing **ammonia** through the action of **urease.**

2. A **stationary phase**, consisting in the bacterial attachment to **fucose-containing receptors** on the surface of mucous surface cells of the pyloric region. *H. pylori* attachment results in the production of **cytotoxic proteases** that ensure the bacteria a supply of nutrients from surface mucous cells and also attract leukocytes. Both ammonia production and cytotoxic proteases correlate with the development of peptic ulcers of the pyloric mucosa.

3. During the **colonization phase**, *H. pylori* detach from the fucose-containing receptors of the surface mucus epithelium, increase in number by replication within the mucus blanket, and remain attached to glycoproteins containing sialic acid. Despite the rapid turnover of the gastric mucus-secreting cells, *H. pylori* avoids being flushed away with dead epithelial cells by producing urease and displaying high motility.

About 20% of the population is infected with *H. pylori* by age 20 years. The incidence of the infection increases to about 60% by age 60.

Most infected individuals do not have clinical symptoms. Increasing evidence for the infectious origin of acid peptic disease and chronic gastritis led to the implementation of antibiotic therapy for all ulcer patients shown to be infected with *H. pylori.* Intense, sudden, persistent stomach pain (relieved by eating and antacid medications), **hematemesis** (blood vomit), or **melena** (tarlike black stool) are clinical symptoms. Blood tests to detect antibodies to *H. pylori* and urea breath tests are effective diagnostic methods. Treatment usually consists in a combination of antibiotics, suppressors of H^+,K^+-dependent ATPase, and stomach protectors.

More recently, attention has been directed to adhesins and fucose-containing receptors as potential targets for drug action. The objective is to prevent binding of pathogenic bacteria without interfering with the endogenous bacterial flora by the use of antibiotics.

Gastroenteroendocrine cells

The function of the alimentary tube is regulated by **peptide hormones**, produced by gastroenteroendocrine cells, and **neuroendocrine mediators**, produced by neurons.

Peptide hormones are synthesized by gastroenteroendocrine cells dispersed throughout the mucosa from the stomach through the colon. The population of gastroenteroendocrine cells is so large that the gastrointestinal segment is regarded as the **largest endocrine organ in the body.**

Gastroenteroendocrine cells are members of the **APUD system**, so called because of the **amine precursor uptake and decarboxylation** property of amino acids (Figure 15-19). Because not all the cells accumulate amine precursors, the designation APUD has been replaced by **DNES** (for **diffuse neuroendocrine system**).

Neuroendocrine mediators are released from nerve terminals. **Acetylcholine** is released at the terminals of postganglionic cholinergic nerves. **Gastrin-releasing peptide** is released by postsynaptic neurons activated by stimulation of the vagus nerve (see Figure 15-19).

Peptide hormones produced by gastrointestinal endocrine cells have the following general functions: (1) regulation of water, electrolyte metabolism, and enzyme

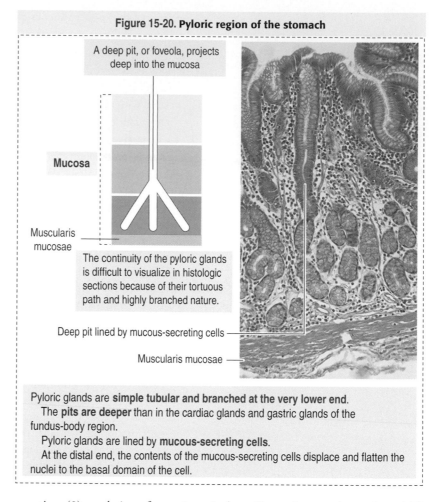

Figure 15-20. Pyloric region of the stomach

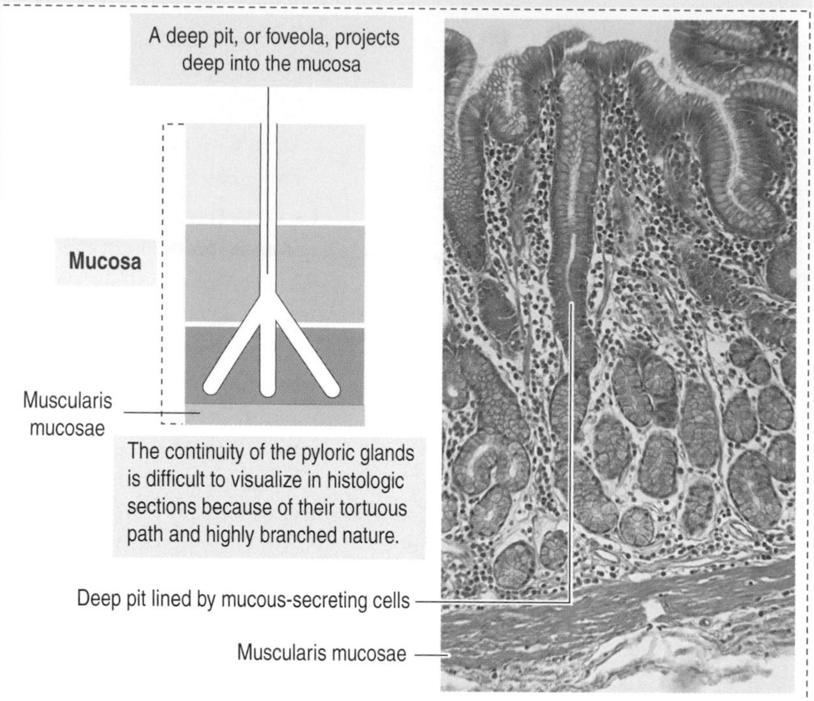
A deep pit, or foveola, projects deep into the mucosa
Mucosa
Muscularis mucosae
The continuity of the pyloric glands is difficult to visualize in histologic sections because of their tortuous path and highly branched nature.
Deep pit lined by mucous-secreting cells
Muscularis mucosae

Pyloric glands are **simple tubular and branched at the very lower end.**

The **pits are deeper** than in the cardiac glands and gastric glands of the fundus-body region.

Pyloric glands are lined by **mucous-secreting cells.**

At the distal end, the contents of the mucous-secreting cells displace and flatten the nuclei to the basal domain of the cell.

secretion; (2) regulation of gastrointestinal motility and mucosal growth; and (3) stimulation of the release of other peptide hormones.

We consider six major gastrointestinal peptide hormones: **secretin**, **gastrin**, **cholecystokinin** (**CCK**), **glucose-dependent insulinotropic peptide**, **motilin**, and **ghrelin**.

Secretin was the first peptide hormone to be discovered (in 1902). Secretin is released by cells in the **duodenal glands of Lieberkühn** when the gastric contents enter the duodenum. Secretin stimulates **pancreatic and duodenal (Brunner's glands) bicarbonate** and **fluid release to control the gastric acid secretion** (antacid effect) and regulate the pH of the duodenal contents. Secretin, together with CCK, stimulates the growth of the exocrine pancreas. In addition, **secretin** (and acetylcholine) **stimulates chief cells to secrete pepsinogen**, and **inhibits gastrin** release to reduce HCl secretion in the stomach.

Gastrin is produced by **G cells** located in the pyloric antrum. Three forms of gastrin have been described: **little gastrin**, or **G_{17}** (which contains 17 amino acids), **big gastrin**, or **G_{34}** (which contains 34 amino acids), and **minigastrin**, or **G_{14}** (which consists of 14 amino acids). G cells produce primarily G_{17}. The duodenal mucosa in humans contains G cells producing mainly G_{34}. The neuroendocrine mediator **gastrin-releasing peptide** regulates the release of gastrin. **Somatostatin,** produced by adjacent **D cells**, inhibits the release of gastrin (see Figure 15-19).

The main function of gastrin is to stimulate the production of hydrochloric acid by parietal cells. Gastrin can also activate CCK to stimulate gallbladder contraction. **Gastrin has a trophic effect on the mucosa** of the small and large intestine and the fundic region of the stomach.

Gastrin stimulates the growth of **ECL cells** of the stomach. Continued hypersecretion of gastrin results in hyperplasia of ECL cells. ECL cells produce histamine by decarboxylation of histidine. Histamine binds to the **histamine H_2 receptor** on **parietal cells** to **potentiate the effect of gastrin and acetylcholine on HCl secretion** (see Figure 15-19). Histamine H_2 receptor blocking drugs (such as cimetidine [Tagamet] and ranitidine [Zantac]) are effective inhibitors of acid secretion.

CCK is produced in the duodenum. CCK stimulates **gallbladder contraction** and **relaxation of the sphincter of Oddi** when protein- and fat-rich chyme enters the duodenum.

Glucose-dependent insulinotropic peptide (**GIP**), formerly called **gastric-inhibitory peptide,** is produced in the duodenum. GIP stimulates insulin release (**insulinotropic effect**) when glucose is detected in the small intestine.

Motilin is released cyclically (every 90 minutes) during fasting from the upper small intestine and stimulates gastrointestinal motility. A **neural control mechanism** regulates the release of motilin.

Ghrelin is produced in the stomach (fundus). Ghrelin binds to its receptor present in **growth hormone–secreting cells of the anterior hypophysis.** Ghrelin stimulates the secretion of growth hormone. Ghrelin plasma levels increase during fasting triggering hunger by acting on hypothalamic feeding centers.

Plasma levels of ghrelin are high in patients with **Prader-Willi syndrome** (caused by abnormal gene imprinting; see section on epigenetics in Chapter 20, Spermatogenesis). Severe hypotonia and feeding difficulties in early infancy, followed by obesity and uncontrollable appetite, hypogonadism, and infertility are characteristics of Prader-Willi syndrome.

Clinical significance: Zollinger-Ellison syndrome

Patients with gastrin-secreting tumors (**gastrinomas**, or **Zollinger-Ellison syndrome**) display hyperplasia and hypertrophy of the fundic region of the stomach and high acid secretion independent of feeding. The complications of gastrinomas are **fulminant stomach ulceration**, **diarrhea** (due to an inhibitory effect of water and electrolyte absorption by the intestine caused by gastrin), **steatorrhea** (caused by inactivation of pancreatic lipase determined by the low pH), and **hypokalemia.**

Pyloric glands

Pyloric glands differ from the cardiac and gastric glands in the following layers: (1) the gastric pits, or foveolae, are deeper and extend halfway through the depth of the mucosa; and (2) pyloric glands have a larger lumen and are highly branched (Figure 15-20).

The predominant epithelial cell type of the pyloric gland is a mucus-secreting cell that resembles the mucous neck cells of the gastric glands. Most of the cell contains large and pale secretory mucus and secretory granules containing **lysozyme**, a bacterial lytic enzyme. Occasionally, parietal cells can be found in the pyloric glands. Enteroendocrine cells, **gastrin-secreting G cells** in particular, are abundant in the antrum pyloric region. Lymphoid nodules can be seen in the lamina propria.

Mucosa, submucosa, and muscularis of the stomach

We complete this discussion by pointing out additional structural and functional details of the mucosa, submucosa, and muscularis of the stomach.

The **mucosa** consists of loose connective tissue, called the **lamina propria,** surrounding cardiac, gastric, and pyloric glands. Reticular and collagen fibers predominate in the lamina propria, and elastic fibers are rare. The cell components of the lamina propria include fibroblasts, lymphocytes, mast cells, eosinophils, and a few plasma cells. The muscularis mucosae can project thin strands of muscle cells into the mucosa to facilitate the release of secretions from the glands.

The **submucosa** consists of dense irregular connective tissue in which collagenous and elastic fibers are abundant. A large number of arterioles, venous plexuses, and lymphatics are present in the submucosa. Also present are the cell bodies and nerve fibers of the **submucosal plexus of Meissner**.

The **muscularis** (or **muscularis externa**) of the stomach consists of three poorly defined layers of smooth muscle oriented in circular, oblique, and longitudinal directions. At the level of the distal pyloric antrum, the circular muscle layer thickens to form the annular **pyloric sphincter**.

Contraction of the muscularis is under control of the autonomic nerve plexuses located between the muscle layers (myenteric plexus of Auerbach).

Based on motility functions, the stomach can be divided into two major regions: the **orad** (Latin *os* [plural *ora*], mouth; *ad*, to; toward the mouth) **portion**, consisting of the fundus and part of the body, and the **caudad** (Latin *cauda*, tail; *ad*, to; toward the tail) **portion**, comprising the distal body and the antrum (see Figure 15-11). During swallowing, the orad region of the stomach and the LES relax to accommodate the ingested material. The tonus of the muscularis adjusts to the volume of the organ without increasing the pressure in the lumen.

Contraction of the caudad portion of the stomach mixes and propels the gastric contents toward the gastroduodenal junction. Most solid contents are propelled back (**retropulsion**) into the main body of the stomach because of the closure of the distal antrum. Liquids empty more rapidly. Retropulsion determines both mixing and mechanical dissociation of solid particles. When the gastric juice empties into the duodenum, peristaltic waves from the orad to the caudad portion of the stomach propel the contents in coordination with the relaxation of the pyloric sphincter.

Essential concepts | **Upper Digestive Segment**

• Mouth or oral cavity. The mouth is the entry site to the digestive tube. Its functions are ingestion, partial digestion, and lubrication of the food, or bolus. The mouth includes the lips, gums (or gingivae), hard palate, soft palate, and uvula.

Lips consist of three regions: (1) The cutaneous region (thin skin; keratinized stratified squamous epithelium with hair follicles, and sebaceous and sweat glands). (2) The red region (lined by stratified squamous epithelium supported by a highly vascularized connective tissue and skeletal muscles). (3) The oral mucosal region, continuous with the mucosa of the cheeks and gums.

The epithelial lining of the gums is similar to the red region of the lips. The lamina propria binds to the periosteum of the alveolar processes of the maxilla and mandible. Submucosa or glands are not seen.

The hard palate is lined by a keratinizing stratified squamous epithelium. Collagenous fibers in the submucosa bind the mucosa to the periosteum of the hard palate.

The soft palate and uvula are lined by nonkeratinizing stratified squamous epithelium extending into the oropharynx.

• Tongue. The dorsal surface of the tongue is covered by nonkeratinizing stratified squamous epithelium supported by a lamina propria associated to a skeletal muscle core. The dorsal surface of the tongue contains lingual papillae. They are of four types: (1) Filiform papillae, the most abundant; the only type of papilla without taste buds. (2) Fungiform papillae. (3) Circumvallate papillae (associated with serous glands, or Ebner's glands). (4) Foliate papillae (poorly developed in humans).

Taste buds consist of taste receptor cells, supporting cells (immature taste cells), and precursor taste cells (basal cells). Tastants (sweet, sour, bitter, salty, and umami) enter through the taste pore and bind to taste receptors (present in apical microvilli of taste receptor cells) linked to G-protein. Ionic changes within taste cells cause either depolarization or hyperpolarization. An increase in intracellular Ca^{2+} triggers the release of neurotransmitters at afferent nerve terminals.

• Tooth. It consists of a crown, neck, and a single or multiple roots. Enamel and dentin are part of the crown. The outer surface of the root is covered by cementum. Cementum is associated with the periodontal ligament, firmly attached to the alveolar bone. A central chamber, the pulp, opens at the apical foramen, the site where blood vessels, nerves, and lymphatics enter and leave the pulp chamber.

Tooth development. The ectoderm (ameloblasts), cranial neural crest (odontoblasts), and mesenchyme (cementocytes) contribute to tooth development.

Odontoblasts are present at the periphery of the pulp. Odontoblasts produce predentin (nonmineralized material surrounding the apical processes of the odontoblast) and dentin (consisting of 20% organic material, primarily type I collagen; 70% inorganic material; and 10% water). Mineralized dentin (crystals of hydroxyapatite and fluoroapatite) forms the dentinal tubes containing the odontoblast apical processes.

Ameloblasts, present in the developing tooth only, face the dentin material and secrete enamel. The apical region of the ameloblast, Tomes' process, becomes surrounded by enamel, the hardest substance found in the body (95% crystals of hydroxyapatite and a decreasing content of protein during mineralization). Enamel consists of enamel rods separated by an interrod region. The major proteins of enamel are amelogenin and enamelin.

• General organization of the digestive tube (esophagus, stomach, small intestine, and large intestine). Digestive organs have four concentric layers: (1) Mucosa (epithelium, lamina propria, and muscularis mucosae). (2) Submucosa. (3) Muscularis (inner circular layer; outer longitudinal layer). (4) Adventitia, or serosa. The mucosa of the esophagus has folds. The mucosa of the stomach has gastric glands with opening pits. The mucosa of the small intestine (duodenum, jejunum, and ileum) displays evaginations (villi) of segment-specific shape and length. The mucosa of the large intestine has tubular glands with openings.

The digestive tube is innervated by the autonomic nervous system, consisting of an extrinsic component (parasympathetic and sympathetic innervation) and intrinsic components: the submucosal plexus of Meissner and the myenteric plexus of Auerbach.

Esophagus. The esophagus is a muscular tube lined by a mucosa consisting of stratified squamous epithelium. The mucosa and submucosa form longitudinal folds. Mucosal and submucosal glands lubricate the surface of the esophageal epithelium. The muscularis has segment-dependent variations: the upper region consists of skeletal muscle; the middle region has a combination of skeletal and smooth muscle; and the lower region has predominantly smooth muscle.

An anatomically upper esophageal sphincter ([UES]; cricopharyngeal muscle) is involved in the initiation of swallowing; a functional lower esophageal sphincter (LES) prevents reflux of gastric juice into the esophagus.

At the gastroesophageal junction (transformation zone), the esophageal epithelium changes from stratified squamous to a simple columnar type. Gastric juice reflux can produce an inflammatory reaction (**reflux esophagitis**) or ulceration and difficulty in swallowing (**dysphagia**). Persistent reflux replaces, at the gastroesophageal junction, the esophageal stratified columnar epithelium by a less resistant columnar epithelium. **Hiatus hernia**, caused by a failure of the diaphragm to close during development, enables a portion of the stomach to move into the thoracic cavity. A portion of the stomach can slide through the diaphragmatic hiatus causing a **sliding hiatus hernia**.

Stomach. The function of the stomach is to homogenize and chemically process the swallowed semisolid food. The stomach is divided into the cardia, fundus, body, and pyloric antrum. The glands of the cardia region are tubular with a coiled end. In the fundus and body, the gastric glands are simple tubular branched. In the pyloric antrum, glands have a deep pit and are simple tubular branched.

Characteristic features of the stomach are the ruga, a fold of the gastric mucosa and submucosa, and a gastric mucosal blanket.

The gastric gland (present in the fundus and body) has a pit, a neck, and a body. The cell types found in the gastric glands are (1) surface mucous cells (found in the pit); (2) mucous neck cells (located at the junction of the pit with the body); and (3) zymogen-producing chief cells and HCl-producing parietal cells seen in the body region of the gland. Two additional cell types are the stem cells (precursor cells of all glandular cells), and gastroenteroendocrine cells (enterochromaffin cells). Chief cells have a well-developed rough endoplasmic reticulum and apical secretory zymogen granules, and predominate in the lower third of the body of the gland. They produce pepsinogen, which upon release is converted to pepsin. Parietal cells predominate in the upper region of the body of the gland and produce HCl (following stimulation by acetylcholine, gastrin, and histamine) and intrinsic factor. Parietal cells have abundant mitochondria, an intracellular canaliculus, and H^+,K^+-dependent ATPase–rich tubulovesicular system. Autoantibodies to H^+,K^+-dependent ATPase and intrinsic factor cause **autoimmune gastritis**. Destruction of parietal cells reduces HCl in the gastric juice (**achlorhydria**) and intrinsic factor (required for the transport and uptake of vitamin B_{12} by enterocytes in the ileum). Vitamin B_{12} deficiency causes pernicious anemia characterized by a decrease in the production of red blood cells and the release into the blood circulation of large red blood cells (**megaloblastic anemia**).

Based on the motility pattern, the stomach can be divided into an orad area (consisting of the fundus and a portion of the body, which relax during swallowing), and a caudad area (consisting of the distal body and the antrum, which are involved in the regulation of gastric emptying).

Helicobacter pylori infection affects the integrity of the protective gastric mucus blanket, enables the aggressive action of pepsin and HCl, and of *H. pylori*–derived cytotoxic proteases on the unprotected gastric mucosa. **Gastritis** and **peptic ulcer disease** develop. **Hematemesis** (blood vomit) or **melena** (tarlike black stool) are typical findings in patients with bleeding gastric ulcers.

• Gastroenteroendocrine cells, present in the mucosa from the stomach to the colon, synthesize peptide hormones, which regulate several functions of the digestive system and associated glands. Originally, gastroenteroendocrine cells (called enterochromaffin cells) were regarded as members of the APUD system because of their property of amino precursor uptake and decarboxylation of amino acids. The designation diffuse neuroendocrine system (DNES) has replaced the APUD designation because not all cells accumulate amine precursors.

Secretin is produced by cells in the duodenal glands of Lieberkühn when the gastric content enters the duodenum. Secretin stimulates the production of pancreatic and Brunner's gland bicarbonate to regulate the duodenal pH by buffering the entering gastric acid secretion.

Gastrin stimulates the production of HCl by parietal cells. It is produced by G cells in the glands of the pyloric antrum. The release of gastrin is regulated by gastrin-releasing peptide, a neuroendocrine mediator. Somatostatin, produced by D cells (adjacent to G cells) inhibits the release of gastrin. Excessive production of gastrin is a characteristic of the **Zollinger-Ellison syndrome**. A gastrinoma, a gastrin-producing benign tumor of the pyloric antrum or the pancreas, causes excessive HCl production resulting in the development of multiple gastric and duodenal ulcers.

Cholecystokinin stimulates the contraction of the gallbladder and relaxes the sphincter of Oddi.

Glucose-dependent insulinotropic peptide, produced in the duodenum, stimulates insulin release (insulinotropic effect) when glucose is detected in the small intestine.

Motilin is released cyclically during fasting from the upper small intestine and stimulates gastrointestinal motility.

Ghrelin is produced in the stomach (fundus). Ghrelin stimulates the secretion of growth hormone. Ghrelin plasma levels increase during fasting, triggering hunger by acting on hypothalamic feeding centers. Plasma levels of ghrelin are high in patients with **Prader-Willi syndrome**. Severe hypotonia and feeding difficulties in early infancy, followed by obesity and uncontrollable appetite, are characteristics of Prader-Willi syndrome.

16. LOWER DIGESTIVE SEGMENT

Small intestine

The **main functions** of the small intestine are (1) **to continue in the duodenum the digestive process initiated in the stomach** and (2) **to absorb digested food after enzymes produced in the intestinal mucosa and the pancreas**, together with the emulsifying bile produced in the liver, enable uptake of protein, carbohydrate, and lipid components.

This section describes first the **main distinctive histologic features** of the three major segments of the small intestine. The structural and functional details of the cellular components of the intestinal mucosa are discussed afterward.

The 4- to 7-m-long small intestine is divided into three sequential segments: (1) **duodenum**, (2) **jejunum**, and (3) **ileum**.

The duodenum is about 25 cm in length, is mainly retroperitoneal, and surrounds the head of the pancreas. At its distal end, the duodenum is continuous with the jejunum, a movable intestinal segment suspended by a mesentery. The ileum is the continuation of the jejunum.

The wall of the small intestine consists of four layers (Figures 16-1 to 16-3): (1) the **mucosa**, (2) the **submucosa**, (3) the **muscularis**, and (4) the **serosa,** or **peritoneum**. As you will see, histologic differences are seen in the **mucosa** and **submucosa** of the three major portions of the small intestine. The **muscularis externa** and **serosa** layers are similar.

Intestinal wall

An increase in the total surface of the mucosa reflects the absorptive function of the small intestine. Four degrees of folding amplify the absorptive surface area of the mucosa (see Figure 16-2): (1) the **plicae circulares** (circular folds; also known as the **valves of Kerkring**), (2) the **intestinal villi**, (3) the **intestinal glands**, and (4) the **microvilli** on the apical surface of the lining epithelium of the intestinal cells (enterocytes).

Figure 16-1. Small intestine

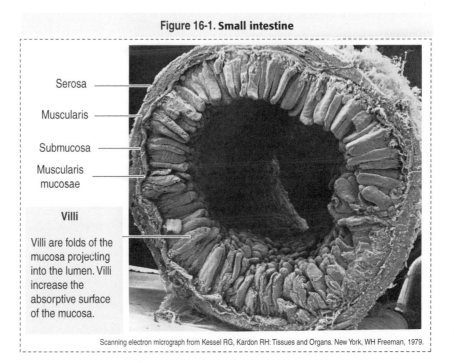

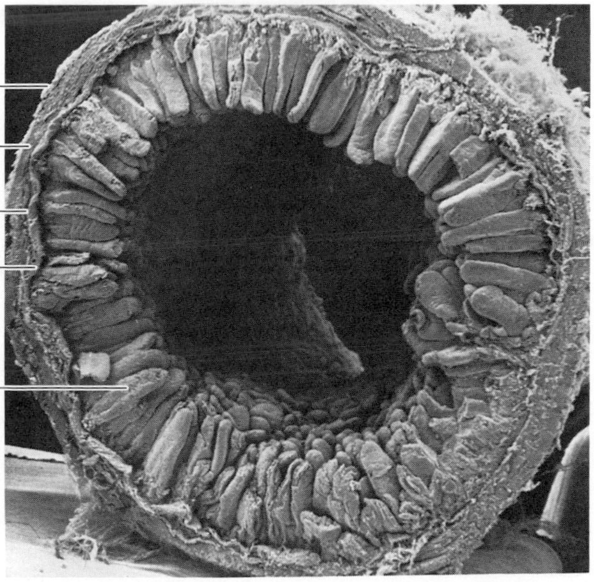
Serosa
Muscularis
Submucosa
Muscularis mucosae

Villi

Villi are folds of the mucosa projecting into the lumen. Villi increase the absorptive surface of the mucosa.

Scanning electron micrograph from Kessel RG, Kardon RH: Tissues and Organs. New York, WH Freeman, 1979.

Figure 16-2. Plica circularis, villi, glands of Lieberkühn, and microvilli

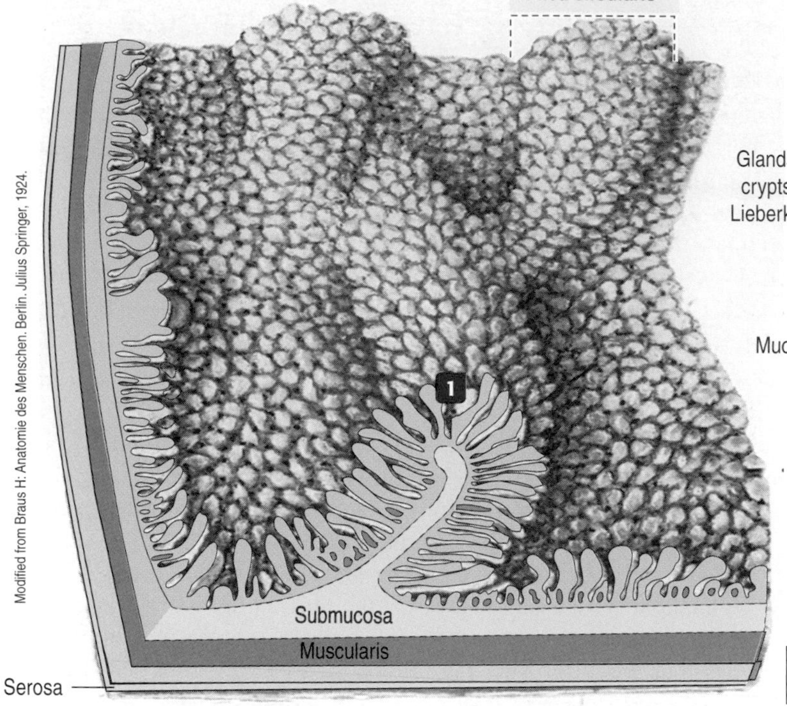

Plica circularis
1
Submucosa
Muscularis
Serosa

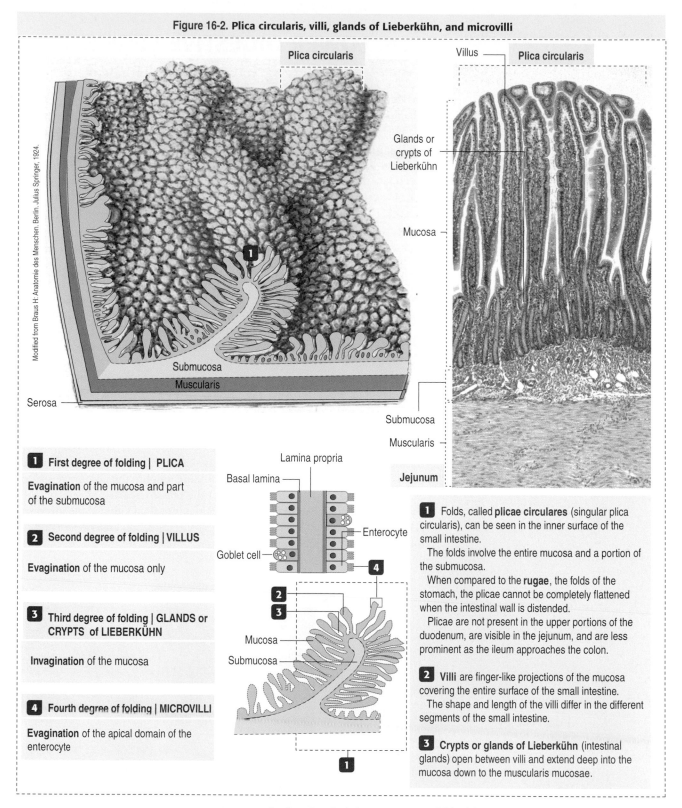

Modified from Braus H: Anatomie des Menschen. Berlin, Julius Springer, 1924.

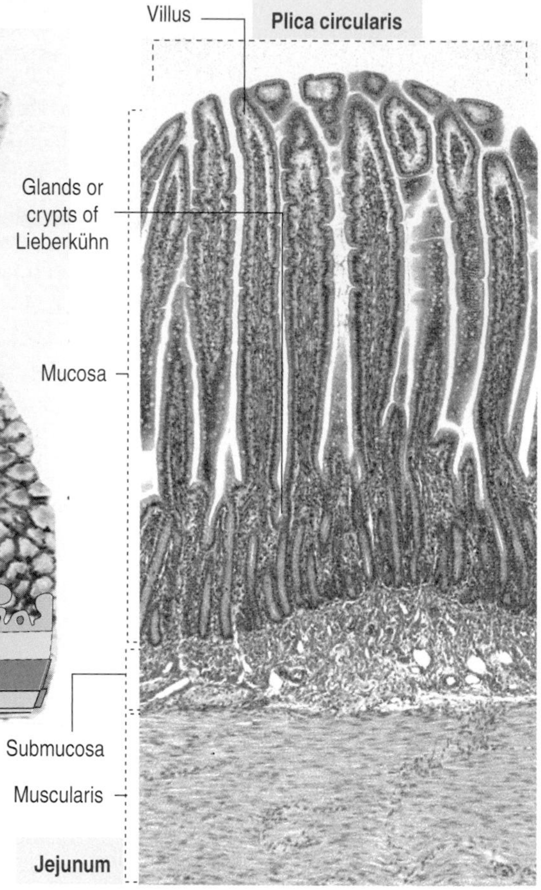

Villus
Plica circularis
Glands or crypts of Lieberkühn
Mucosa
Submucosa
Muscularis
Jejunum

1 First degree of folding | PLICA

Evagination of the mucosa and part of the submucosa

2 Second degree of folding | VILLUS

Evagination of the mucosa only

3 Third degree of folding | GLANDS or CRYPTS of LIEBERKÜHN

Invagination of the mucosa

4 Fourth degree of folding | MICROVILLI

Evagination of the apical domain of the enterocyte

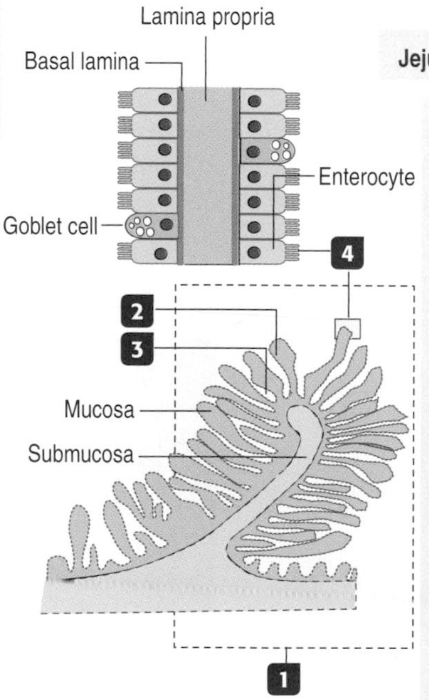

Lamina propria
Basal lamina
Enterocyte
Goblet cell
4
2
3
Mucosa
Submucosa
1

1 Folds, called **plicae circulares** (singular plica circularis), can be seen in the inner surface of the small intestine.

The folds involve the entire mucosa and a portion of the submucosa.

When compared to the **rugae**, the folds of the stomach, the plicae cannot be completely flattened when the intestinal wall is distended.

Plicae are not present in the upper portions of the duodenum, are visible in the jejunum, and are less prominent as the ileum approaches the colon.

2 Villi are finger-like projections of the mucosa covering the entire surface of the small intestine.

The shape and length of the villi differ in the different segments of the small intestine.

3 Crypts or glands of Lieberkühn (intestinal glands) open between villi and extend deep into the mucosa down to the muscularis mucosae.

A **plica circularis** is a permanent fold of the **mucosa** and **submucosa** encircling the intestinal lumen.

Plicae appear about 5 cm distal to the aborad outlet of the stomach, become distinct where the duodenum joins the jejunum, and diminish in size progressively to disappear halfway along the ileum.

The **intestinal villi** are finger-like projections of the **mucosa** covering the entire surface of the small intestine. Villi extend deep into the mucosa to form crypts

Figure 16-3. **Blood, lymphatic, and nerve supply to the small intestine**

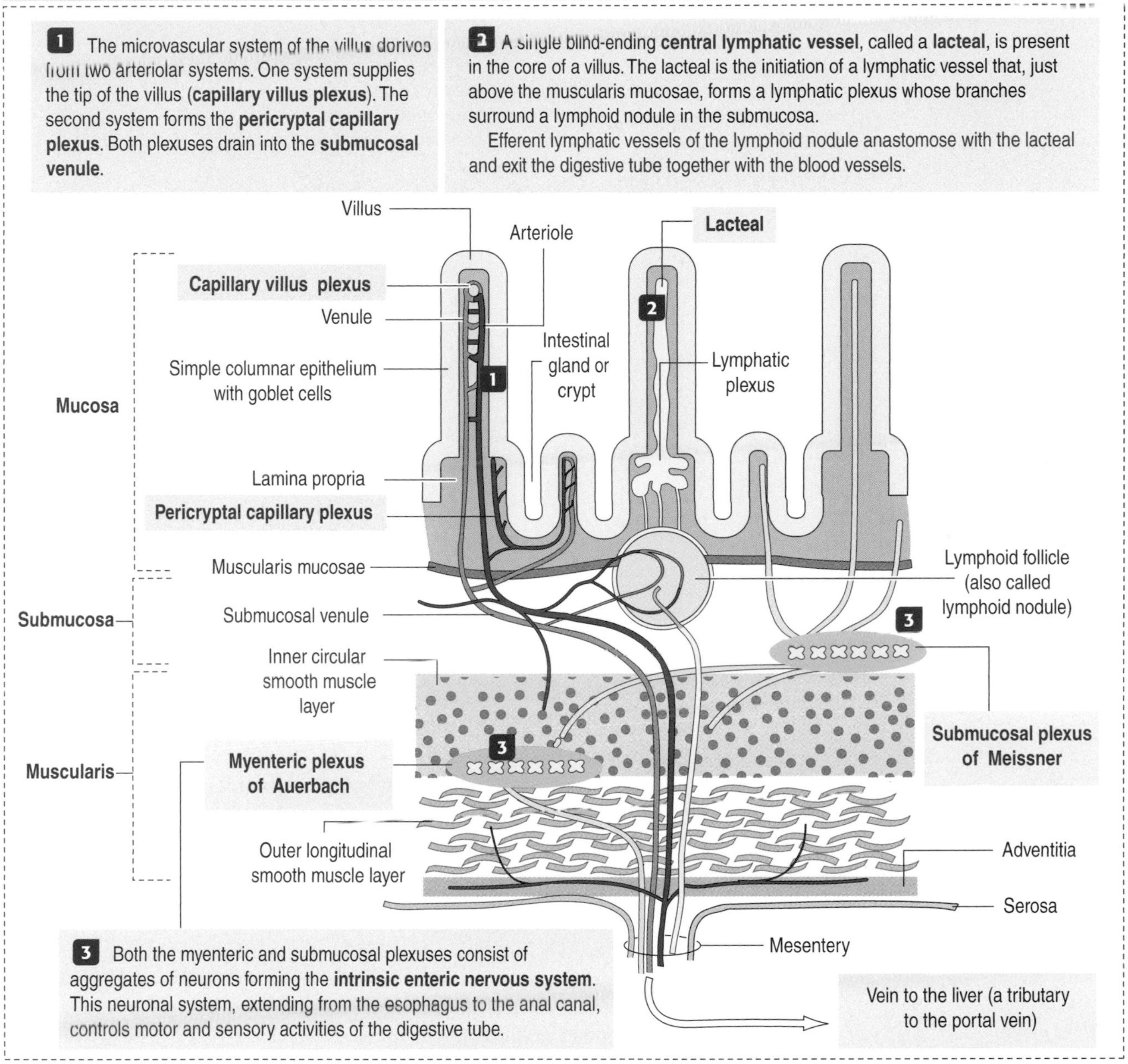
1 The microvascular system of the villus derives from two arteriolar systems. One system supplies the tip of the villus (capillary villus plexus). The second system forms the pericryptal capillary plexus. Both plexuses drain into the submucosal venule.
2 A single blind-ending central lymphatic vessel, called a lacteal, is present in the core of a villus. The lacteal is the initiation of a lymphatic vessel that, just above the muscularis mucosae, forms a lymphatic plexus whose branches surround a lymphoid nodule in the submucosa.
Efferent lymphatic vessels of the lymphoid nodule anastomose with the lacteal and exit the digestive tube together with the blood vessels.
Villus
Arteriole
Lacteal
Capillary villus plexus
Venule
Intestinal gland or crypt
Lymphatic plexus
Simple columnar epithelium with goblet cells
Mucosa
Lamina propria
Pericryptal capillary plexus
Muscularis mucosae
Lymphoid follicle (also called lymphoid nodule)
Submucosa
Submucosal venule
Inner circular smooth muscle layer
Submucosal plexus of Meissner
Muscularis
Myenteric plexus of Auerbach
Outer longitudinal smooth muscle layer
Adventitia
Serosa
Mesentery
3 Both the myenteric and submucosal plexuses consist of aggregates of neurons forming the intrinsic enteric nervous system. This neuronal system, extending from the esophagus to the anal canal, controls motor and sensory activities of the digestive tube.
Vein to the liver (a tributary to the portal vein)

ending at the muscularis mucosae. The length of the villi depends on the degree of distention of the intestinal wall and the contraction of smooth muscle fibers in the villus core.

Crypts of Lieberkühn, or **intestinal glands**, are **simple tubular glands** that increase the intestinal surface area. The crypts are formed by invaginations of the mucosa between adjacent intestinal villi.

The **muscularis mucosae** is the boundary between the mucosa and submucosa (see Figure 16-3). The **muscularis** consists of inner circular smooth muscle and outer longitudinal smooth muscle. The muscularis is responsible for **segmentation** and **peristaltic movement** of the contents of the small intestine (Figure 16-4). The **adventitia**, a thin layer of connective tissue, is covered by the **visceral peritoneum**, a serosal layer lined by a simple squamous epithelium, or **mesothelium**. The **parietal peritoneum** covers the inner surface of the abdominal wall.

Microcirculation of the small intestine

A difference from the microcirculation of the stomach (see Figure 15-8 in Chap-

Figure 16-4. **Intestinal motility: Muscular contraction patterns**

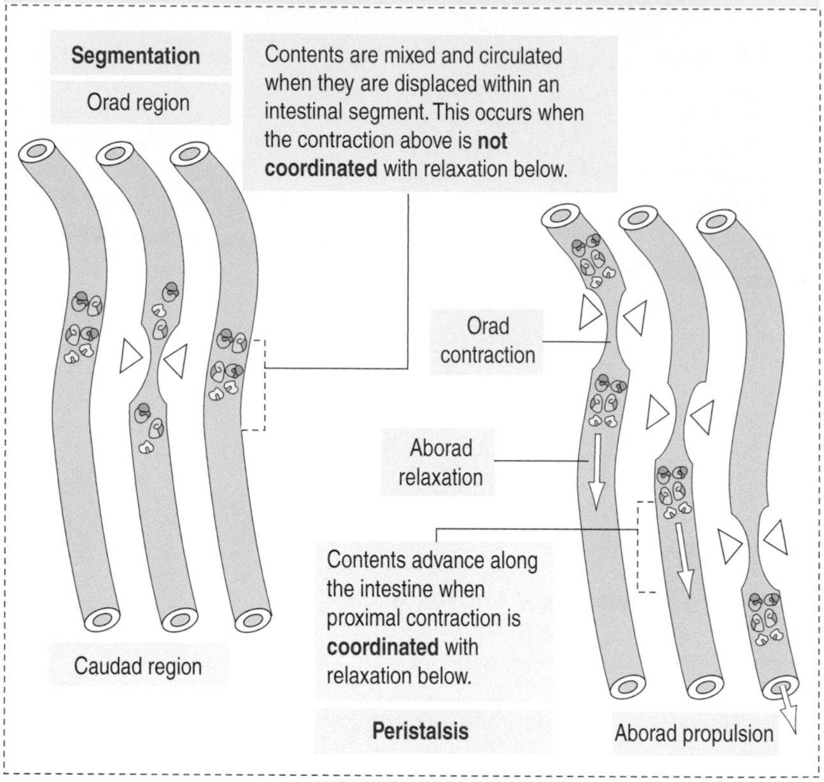

Segmentation
Orad region
Contents are mixed and circulated when they are displaced within an intestinal segment. This occurs when the contraction above is not coordinated with relaxation below.
Orad contraction
Aborad relaxation
Contents advance along the intestine when proximal contraction is coordinated with relaxation below.
Caudad region
Peristalsis
Aborad propulsion

ter 15, Upper Digestive Segment) is that **the intestinal submucosa is the main distribution site of blood and lymphatic flow** (see Figure 16-3).

Branches of the submucosal plexus supply capillaries to the muscularis and intestinal mucosa. Arterioles derived from the **submucosal plexus** enter the mucosa of the small intestine and give rise to two capillary networks: (1) the **villus capillary plexus** supplies the intestinal villus and upper portion of the crypts of Lieberkühn; and (2) the **pericryptal capillary plexus** supplies the lower half of the crypts of Lieberkühn.

A single blind-ending **central lymphatic vessel**, the **lacteal**, is present in the core of a villus. The lacteal is the initiation of a lymphatic vessel that, just above the muscularis mucosae, forms a **lymphatic plexus** whose branches surround a lymphoid nodule in the mucosa-submucosa. Efferent lymphatic vessels of the lymphoid nodule anastomose with the lacteal and leave the digestive tube through the mesentery, together with the blood vessels.

Innervation and motility of the small intestine

Motility of the small intestine is controlled by the autonomic nervous system. The intrinsic autonomic nervous system of the small intestine, consisting of the submucosal **plexus of Meissner** and **myenteric plexus of Auerbach**, is similar to that of the stomach (see Figure 15-9 in Chapter 15, Upper Digestive Segment).

Neurons of the plexuses receive **intrinsic input from the mucosa and muscle wall** of the small intestine and **extrinsic input from the central nervous system** through the **parasympathetic** (vagus nerve) **and sympathetic nerve trunks.**

Contraction of the muscularis is coordinated to achieve two objectives (see Figure 16-4): (1) To **mix and mobilize the contents within an intestinal segment.** This is accomplished when muscular contraction activity is not coordinated and the intestine becomes transiently divided into segments. This process is known as **segmentation.** (2) To **propel the intestinal contents** when there is a proximal (**orad**) contraction coordinated with a distal (**aborad**; Latin *ab*, from; *os*, mouth; away from the mouth) relaxation. When coordinated contraction-relaxation occurs

Figure 16-5. Histologic differences: Duodenum, jejunum, and ileum

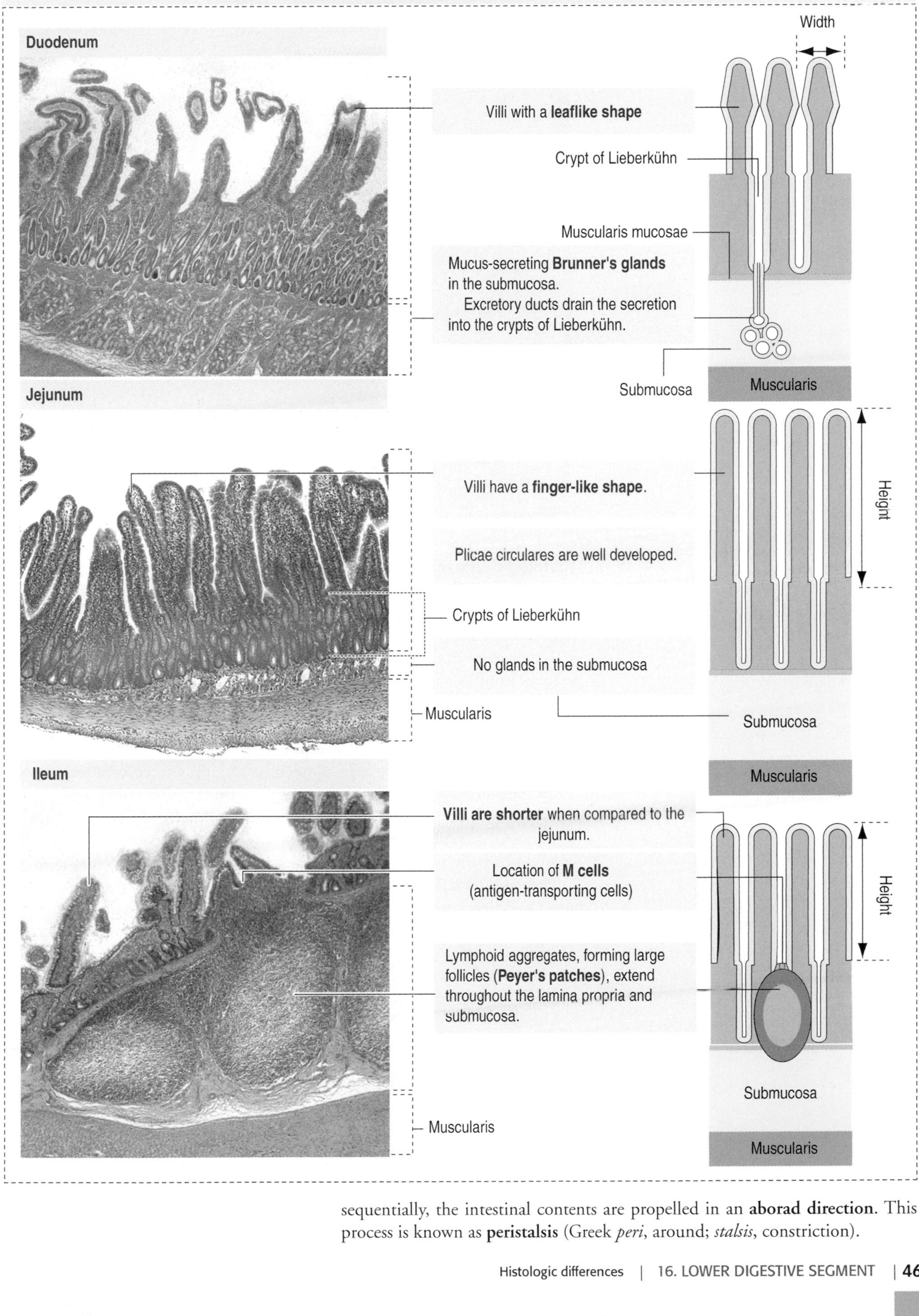

Duodenum
Width
Villi with a leaflike shape
Crypt of Lieberkühn
Muscularis mucosae
Mucus-secreting Brunner's glands in the submucosa.
Excretory ducts drain the secretion into the crypts of Lieberkühn.
Submucosa
Muscularis
Jejunum
Villi have a finger-like shape.
Height
Plicae circulares are well developed.
Crypts of Lieberkühn
No glands in the submucosa
Muscularis
Submucosa
Muscularis
Ileum
Villi are shorter when compared to the jejunum.
Location of M cells (antigen-transporting cells)
Height
Lymphoid aggregates, forming large follicles (Peyer's patches), extend throughout the lamina propria and submucosa.
Submucosa
Muscularis
Muscularis

sequentially, the intestinal contents are propelled in an **aborad direction**. This process is known as **peristalsis** (Greek *peri*, around; *stalsis*, constriction).

Figure 16-6. **Epithelial cells of the villus and crypt of Lieberkühn**

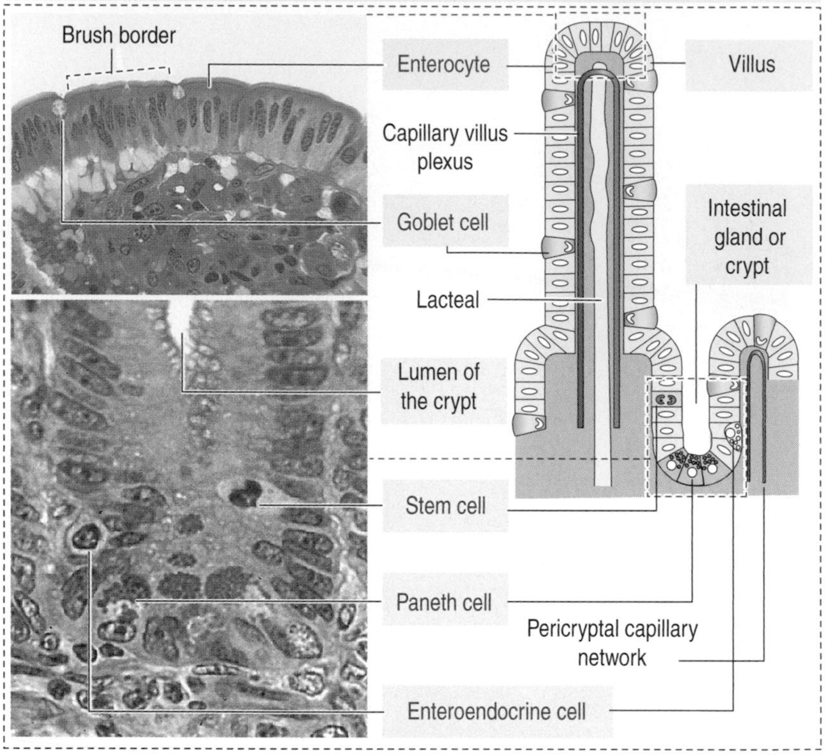
Brush border
Enterocyte
Villus
Capillary villus plexus
Goblet cell
Intestinal gland or crypt
Lacteal
Lumen of the crypt
Stem cell
Paneth cell
Pericryptal capillary network
Enteroendocrine cell

Histologic differences between the duodenum, jejunum, and ileum

Each of the three major anatomic portions of the small intestine—the duodenum, jejunum, and ileum—has **distinctive features that allow recognition under the light microscope** (Figure 16-5).

The **duodenum** extends from the pyloric region of the stomach to the junction with the jejunum and has the following characteristics: (1) It has **Brunner's glands in the submucosa**. Brunner's glands are **tubuloacinar mucous glands** producing an **alkaline secretion** (pH 8.8 to 9.3) that neutralizes the acidic chyme coming from the stomach. (2) The **villi are broad and short** (leaflike shape). (3) The duodenum is surrounded by an incomplete serosa and an extensive adventitia. (4) The duodenum collects bile and pancreatic secretions transported by the common bile duct and pancreatic duct, respectively. The **sphincter of Oddi** is present at the terminal ampullary portion of the two converging ducts. (5) The base of the crypts of Lieberkühn may contain **Paneth cells**.

The **jejunum** has the following characteristics: (1) It has long finger-like villi and a **well-developed lacteal in the core of the villus**. (2) The jejunum **does not contain Brunner's glands** in the submucosa. (3) Peyer's patches in the lamina propria may be present but they are not predominant in the jejunum. Peyer's patches are a characteristic feature of the ileum. (4) **Paneth cells** are found at the base of the crypts of Lieberkühn.

The **ileum** has a prominent diagnostic feature: **Peyer's patches**, lymphoid follicles (also called **nodules**) found in the mucosa and part of the submucosa. The lack of Brunner's glands and the presence of shorter finger-like villi—when compared with the jejunum—are additional landmarks of the ileum. As in the jejunum, **Paneth cells** are found at the base of the crypts of Lieberkühn.

Villi and crypts of Lieberkühn

The intestinal mucosa, including the crypts of Lieberkühn, are lined by a **simple columnar epithelium** containing four major cell types (Figure 16-6): (1) **absorptive cells**, or **enterocytes**, (2) **goblet cells**, (3) **Paneth cells**, and (4) **enteroendocrine**

Figure 16-7. Intestinal epithelium

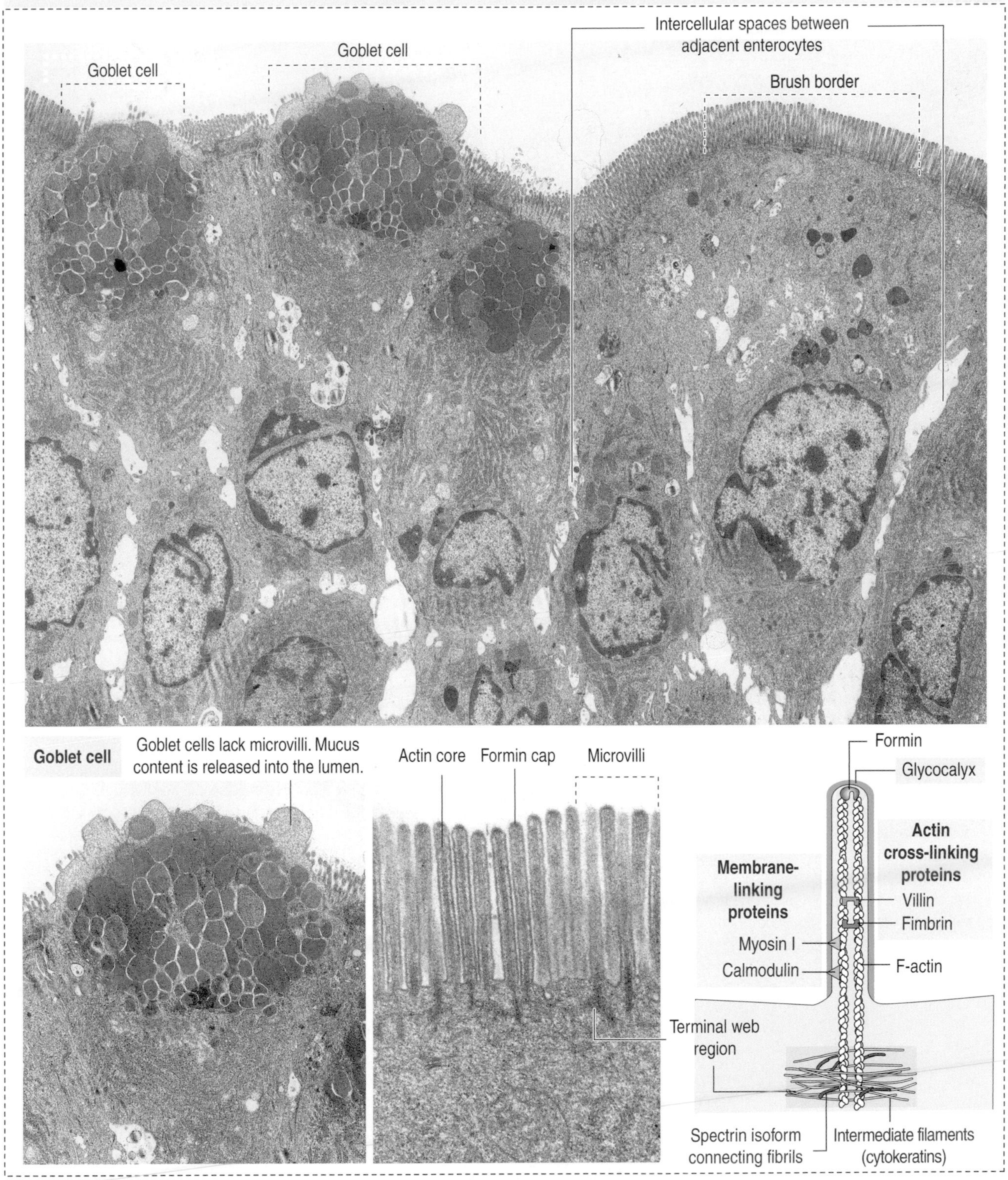

Goblet cell
Goblet cell
Intercellular spaces between adjacent enterocytes
Brush border
Goblet cell
Goblet cells lack microvilli. Mucus content is released into the lumen.
Actin core
Formin cap
Microvilli
Terminal web region
Formin
Glycocalyx
Actin cross-linking proteins
Villin
Fimbrin
F-actin
Membrane-linking proteins
Myosin I
Calmodulin
Spectrin isoform connecting fibrils
Intermediate filaments (cytokeratins)

cells. Stem cells, Paneth cells, and enteroendocrine cells are found in the crypts of Lieberkühn (see Figure 16-6).

Absorptive intestinal cells, or enterocytes

The **absorptive intestinal cell** or **enterocyte** has an apical domain with a prominent **brush border** (also called a **striated border**), ending on a clear zone, called the **terminal web**, which contains transverse cytoskeletal filaments. The brush

Figure 16-8. Digestion and absorption of proteins and carbohydrates

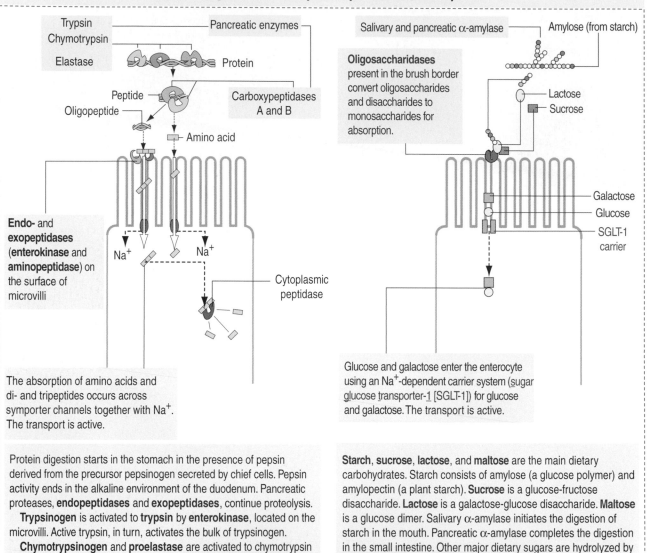

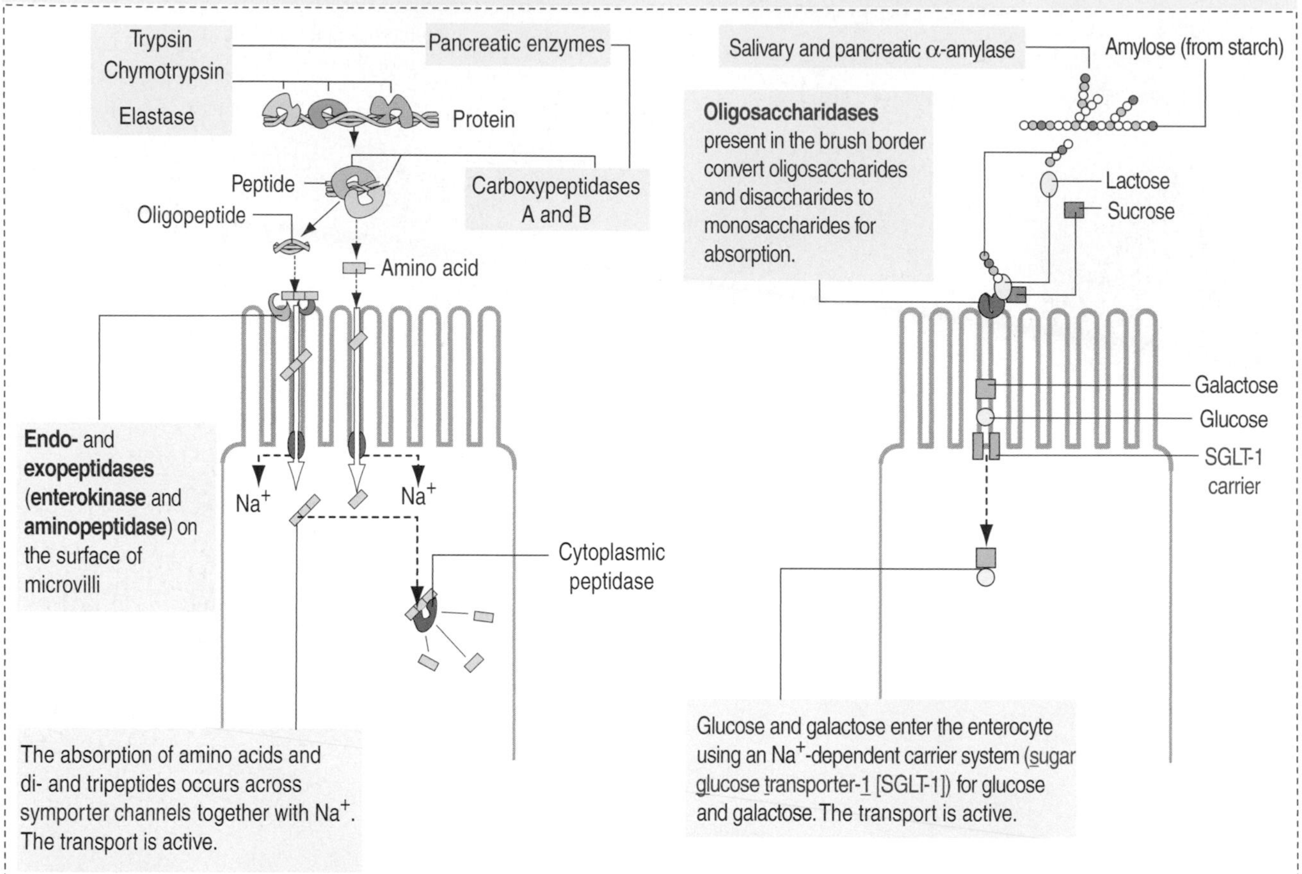
Trypsin
Chymotrypsin
Elastase
Pancreatic enzymes
Protein
Peptide
Oligopeptide
Carboxypeptidases A and B
Amino acid
Endo- and exopeptidases (enterokinase and aminopeptidase) on the surface of microvilli
Na+
Na+
Cytoplasmic peptidase
The absorption of amino acids and di- and tripeptides occurs across symporter channels together with Na+. The transport is active.
Salivary and pancreatic α-amylase
Amylose (from starch)
Oligosaccharidases present in the brush border convert oligosaccharides and disaccharides to monosaccharides for absorption.
Lactose
Sucrose
Galactose
Glucose
SGLT-1 carrier
Glucose and galactose enter the enterocyte using an Na+-dependent carrier system (sugar glucose transporter-1 [SGLT-1]) for glucose and galactose. The transport is active.

Protein digestion starts in the stomach in the presence of pepsin derived from the precursor pepsinogen secreted by chief cells. Pepsin activity ends in the alkaline environment of the duodenum. Pancreatic proteases, **endopeptidases** and **exopeptidases**, continue proteolysis.

Trypsinogen is activated to **trypsin** by **enterokinase**, located on the microvilli. Active trypsin, in turn, activates the bulk of trypsinogen.

Chymotrypsinogen and **proelastase** are activated to chymotrypsin and elastase, respectively. Carboxypeptidases A and B derive from procarboxypeptidase A and B precursors.

Trypsin plays a significant role in the activation and inactivation of pancreatic proenzymes. Tripeptides in the cytosol are digested by cytoplasmic peptidases into amino acids.

Starch, **sucrose**, **lactose**, and **maltose** are the main dietary carbohydrates. Starch consists of amylose (a glucose polymer) and amylopectin (a plant starch). **Sucrose** is a glucose-fructose disaccharide. **Lactose** is a galactose-glucose disaccharide. **Maltose** is a glucose dimer. Salivary α-amylase initiates the digestion of starch in the mouth. Pancreatic α-amylase completes the digestion in the small intestine. Other major dietary sugars are hydrolyzed by **oligosaccharidases** (sucrase, lactase, isomaltase) present in the plasma membrane of the microvilli.

Cellulose is not digested in the human small intestine because cellulase is not present. Cellulose accounts for the undigested dietary fiber.

border of each absorptive cell contains about 3000 closely packed **microvilli**, which increase the surface luminal area 30-fold.

The length of a microvillus ranges from 0.5 to 1.0 μm. The core of a microvillus (Figure 16-7) contains a bundle of 20 to 40 parallel **actin filaments** cross-linked by **fimbrin** and **villin**. The actin bundle core is anchored to the plasma membrane by **formin** (protein of the cap), **myosin I**, and the calcium-binding protein **calmodulin**. Each actin bundle projects into the apical portion of the cell as a **rootlet**, which is cross-linked by an **intestinal isoform of spectrin** to an adjacent rootlet. The end portion of the rootlet attaches to **cytokeratin-containing intermediate filaments**. Spectrin and cytokeratins form the **terminal web**. The terminal web is responsible for maintaining the upright position and shape of the microvillus and anchoring the actin rootlets.

A **surface coat** or **glycocalyx** consisting of glycoproteins as integral components of the plasma membrane covers each microvillus.

The **microvilli**, forming a **brush border**, contain intramembranous enzymes,

Figure 16-9. Digestion and absorption of lipids

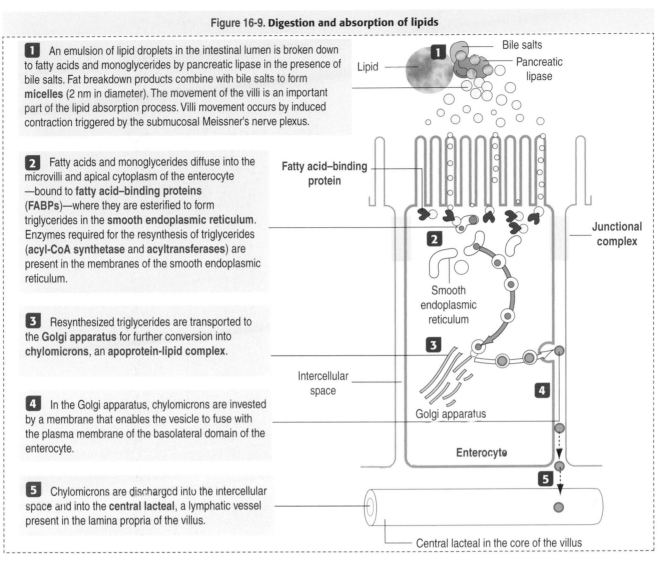

1 An emulsion of lipid droplets in the intestinal lumen is broken down to fatty acids and monoglycerides by pancreatic lipase in the presence of bile salts. Fat breakdown products combine with bile salts to form **micelles** (2 nm in diameter). The movement of the villi is an important part of the lipid absorption process. Villi movement occurs by induced contraction triggered by the submucosal Meissner's nerve plexus.

2 Fatty acids and monoglycerides diffuse into the microvilli and apical cytoplasm of the enterocyte —bound to **fatty acid–binding proteins (FABPs)**—where they are esterified to form triglycerides in the **smooth endoplasmic reticulum**. Enzymes required for the resynthesis of triglycerides (**acyl-CoA synthetase** and **acyltransferases**) are present in the membranes of the smooth endoplasmic reticulum.

3 Resynthesized triglycerides are transported to the **Golgi apparatus** for further conversion into **chylomicrons**, an **apoprotein-lipid complex**.

4 In the Golgi apparatus, chylomicrons are invested by a membrane that enables the vesicle to fuse with the plasma membrane of the basolateral domain of the enterocyte.

5 Chylomicrons are discharged into the intercellular space and into the **central lacteal**, a lymphatic vessel present in the lamina propria of the villus.

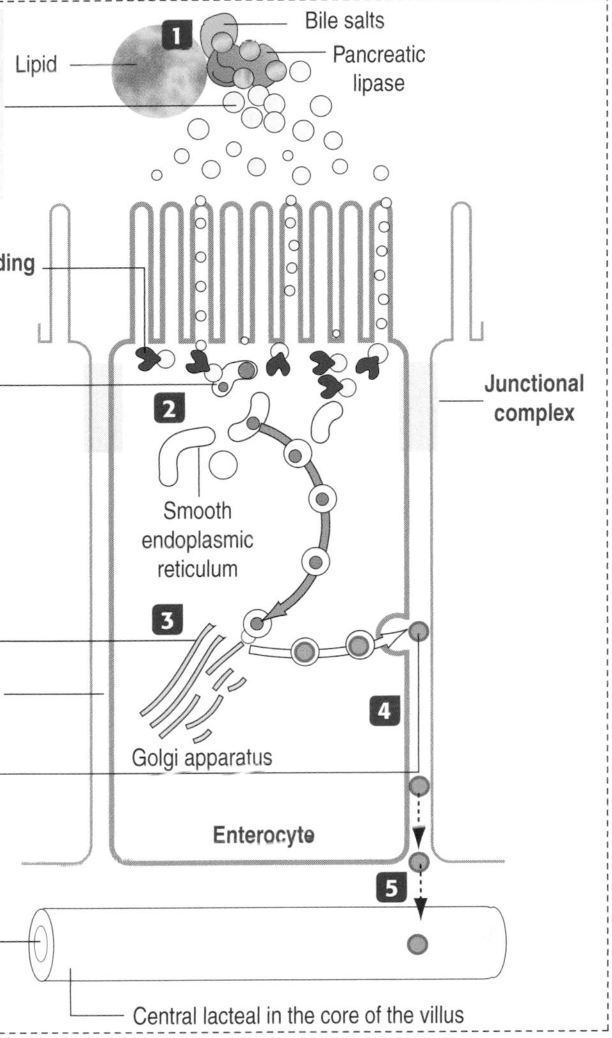

including **lactase**, **maltase**, and **sucrase** (Figure 16-8). These oligosaccharides reduce carbohydrates to hexoses, which can be transported into the enterocyte by **carrier proteins**. A **genetic defect in lactase** prevents the absorption of lactose-rich milk, leading to diarrhea (lactose intolerance). Therefore, the brush border not only increases the absorptive surface of enterocytes but is also the site where enzymes are involved in the terminal digestion of carbohydrates and proteins.

Final breakdown of oligopeptides, initiated by the action of gastric pepsin, is extended by pancreatic trypsin, chymotrypsin, elastase, and carboxypeptidases A and B. **Enterokinase** and **aminopeptidase**, localized in the microvilli, degrade oligopeptides into dipeptides, tripeptides, and amino acids before entering the enterocyte across symporter channels together with Na^+. **Cytoplasmic peptidases** degrade dipeptides and tripeptides into amino acids, which then diffuse or are transported by a carrier-mediated process across the basolateral plasma membrane into the blood.

The **absorption of lipids** involves the enzymatic breakdown of dietary lipids into **fatty acids** and **monoglycerides**, which can diffuse across the plasma membrane of the microvilli and the apical plasma membrane of the enterocyte. Details of the **process of fat absorption** are depicted in Figure 16-9.

Goblet cells

Goblet cells are columnar mucus-secreting cells scattered among enterocytes of the intestinal epithelium (see Figure 16-7).

Figure 16-10. **Roles of gastrin, secretin, and cholecystokinin in digestion**

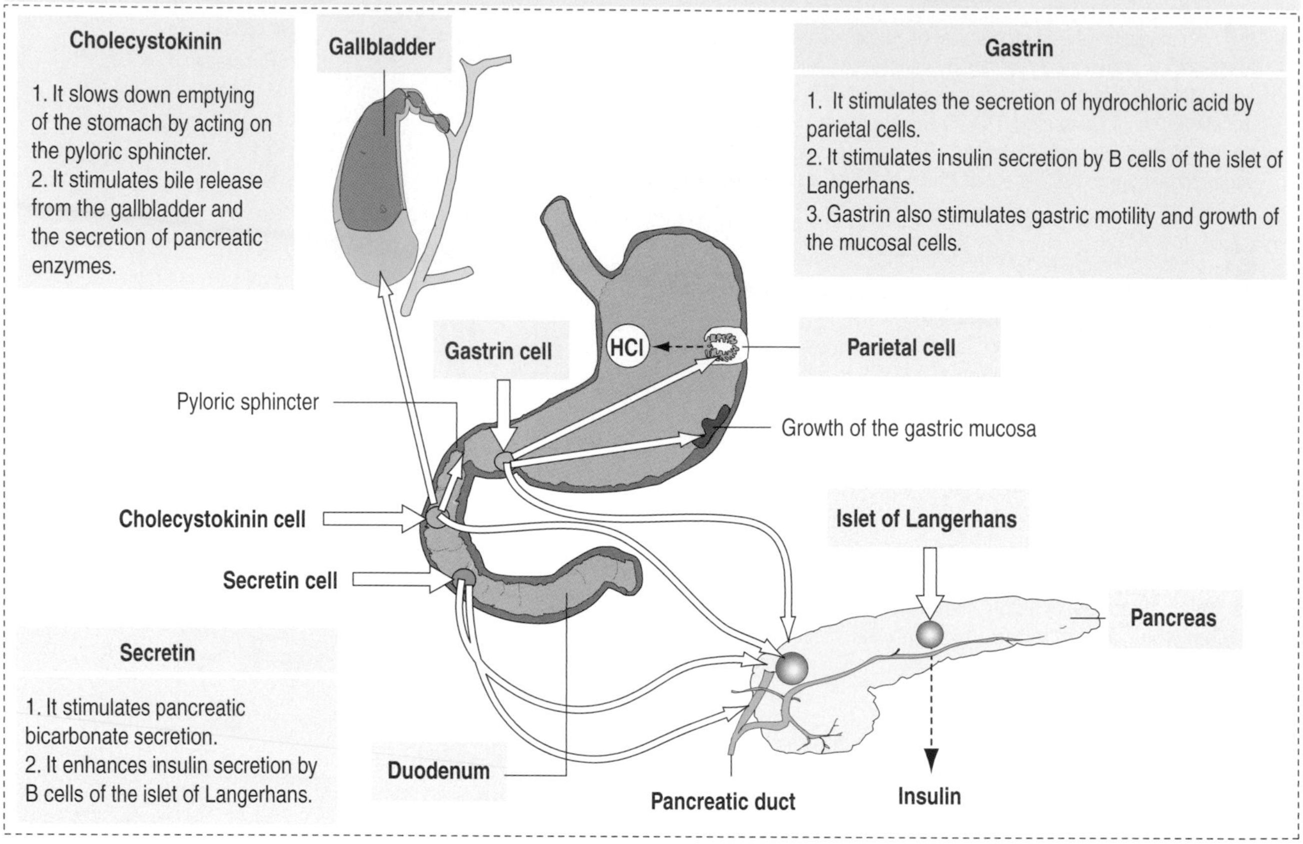

Cholecystokinin
1. It slows down emptying of the stomach by acting on the pyloric sphincter.
2. It stimulates bile release from the gallbladder and the secretion of pancreatic enzymes.
Gallbladder
Gastrin
1. It stimulates the secretion of hydrochloric acid by parietal cells.
2. It stimulates insulin secretion by B cells of the islet of Langerhans.
3. Gastrin also stimulates gastric motility and growth of the mucosal cells.
Gastrin cell
HCl
Parietal cell
Pyloric sphincter
Growth of the gastric mucosa
Cholecystokinin cell
Islet of Langerhans
Secretin cell
Pancreas
Secretin
1. It stimulates pancreatic bicarbonate secretion.
2. It enhances insulin secretion by B cells of the islet of Langerhans.
Duodenum
Pancreatic duct
Insulin

Goblet cells have two domains: (1) a cup- or goblet-shaped **apical domain** containing large mucus granules that are discharged on the surface of the epithelium and (2) a narrow **basal domain**, which attaches to the basal lamina and contains the rough endoplasmic reticulum in which the protein portion of mucus is produced. The **Golgi apparatus**, which adds oligosaccharide groups to mucus, is prominent and situated above the basally located nucleus.

The secretory product of goblet cells contains **glycoproteins** (80% carbohydrate and 20% protein) released by **exocytosis**. On the surface of the epithelium, **the mucus hydrates to form a protective gel coat to shield the epithelium from mechanical abrasion and bacterial invasion.**

Enteroendocrine cells

In addition to its digestive function, the gastrointestinal tract is the largest diffuse endocrine gland in the body.

We have already studied the structural and functional features of enteroendocrine cells in the stomach (see Chapter 15, Upper Digestive Segment). As in the stomach, enteroendocrine cells secrete peptide hormones controlling several functions of the gastrointestinal system. The location and function of **gastrin**-, **secretin**-, and **cholecystokinin**-secreting cells are summarized in Figure 16-10.

Protection of the small intestine

The large surface of the gastrointestinal tract is vulnerable to potentially invasive microorganisms and antigens. We discuss in Chapter 15, Upper Digestive Segment, the role of the mucus blanket in the protection of the surface of the stomach during *Helicobacter pylori* infection.

Several defensive mechanisms operate in the alimentary tube: (1) **Peyer's patches** and associated **M cells** perform the **cellular surveillance of antigens** present in the intestinal lumen; (2) **immunoglobulin A (IgA)**, a product of **plasma cells**

Figure 16-11. **Peyer's patch: A component of the gut-associated lymphoid tissue (GALT)**

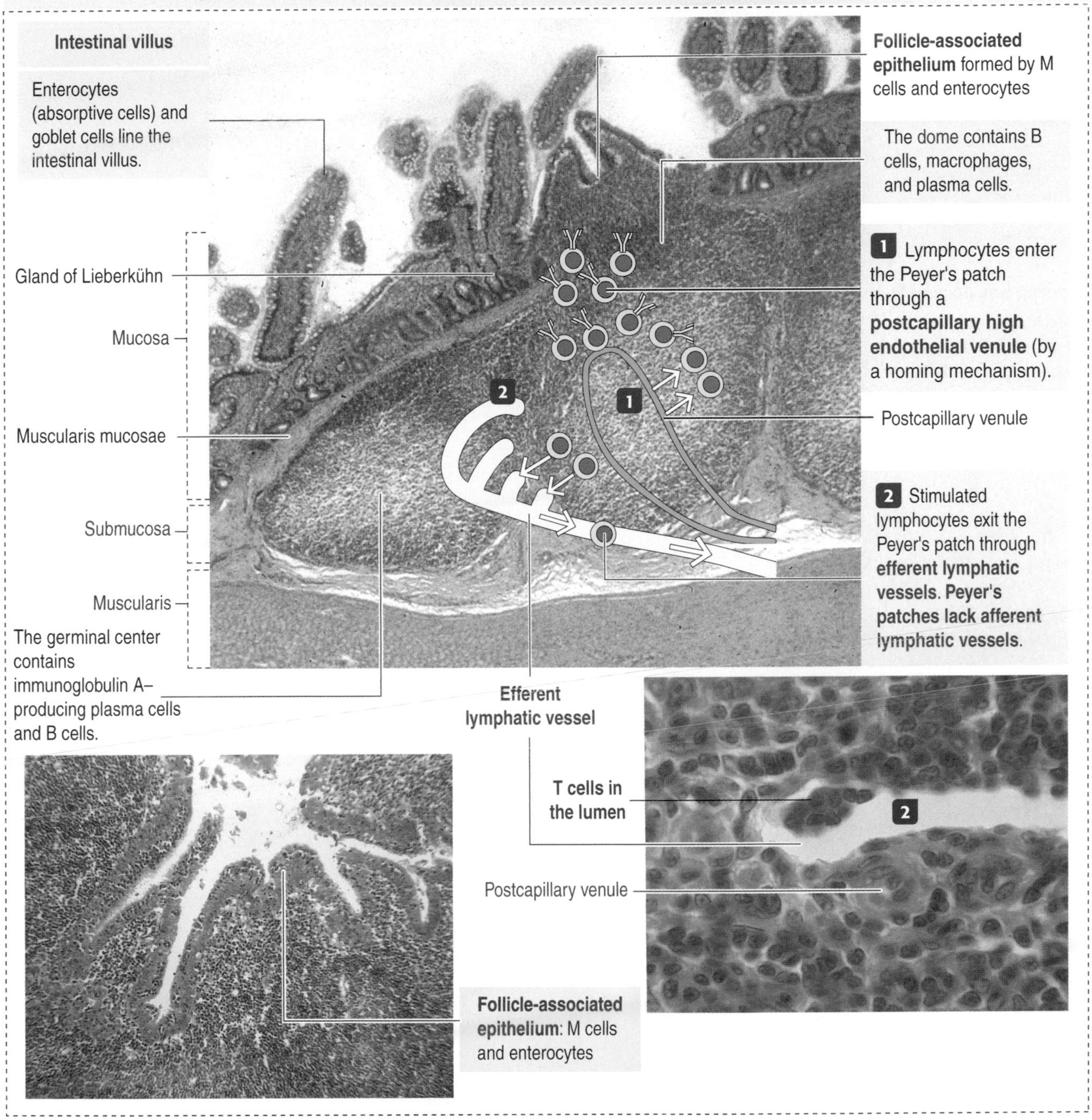

Intestinal villus
Enterocytes (absorptive cells) and goblet cells line the intestinal villus.
Gland of Lieberkühn
Mucosa
Muscularis mucosae
Submucosa
Muscularis
The germinal center contains immunoglobulin A–producing plasma cells and B cells.
Follicle-associated epithelium formed by M cells and enterocytes
The dome contains B cells, macrophages, and plasma cells.
1 Lymphocytes enter the Peyer's patch through a postcapillary high endothelial venule (by a homing mechanism).
Postcapillary venule
2 Stimulated lymphocytes exit the Peyer's patch through efferent lymphatic vessels. Peyer's patches lack afferent lymphatic vessels.
1
2
Efferent lymphatic vessel
T cells in the lumen
2
Postcapillary venule
Follicle-associated epithelium: M cells and enterocytes

secreted by the intestinal epithelium and in the bile, neutralizes antigens; and (3) the bacteriostatic **Paneth cells** contribute antimicrobial peptides (for example, defensins) to the control of the resident and pathogenic microbial flora. (4) The acidity of the **gastric juice** inactivates ingested microorganism and (5) the propulsive intestinal motility (peristalsis) prevents bacterial colonization.

Peyer's patches

Peyer's patches—the main component of the **gut-associated lymphoid tissue** (GALT)—are specialized lymphoid follicles found in the intestinal mucosa and part of the submucosa. A Peyer's patch displays two main components (Figure 16-11): (1) a **dome** and (2) a **germinal center**. Peyer's patches are lined by the **follicle-associated epithelium** (FAE), consisting of M cells and enterocytes—both derived from stem cells present in the intestinal glands.

Figure 16-12. **Peyer's patch: Cellular immune surveillance system of the intestinal tract**

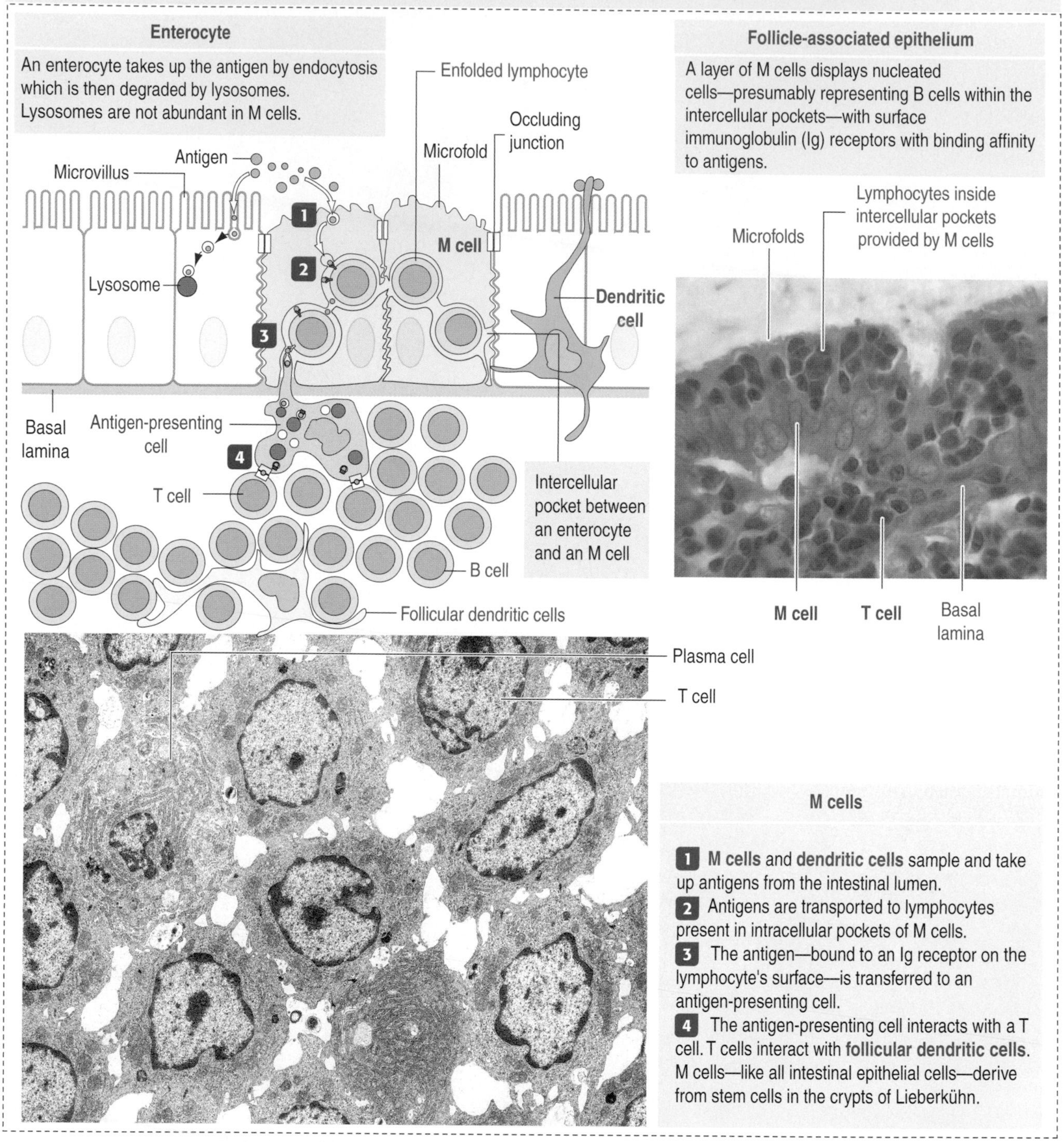

Enterocyte
An enterocyte takes up the antigen by endocytosis which is then degraded by lysosomes.
Lysosomes are not abundant in M cells.
Enfolded lymphocyte
Occluding junction
Microfold
Antigen
Microvillus
M cell
Lysosome
Dendritic cell
Basal lamina
Antigen-presenting cell
T cell
Intercellular pocket between an enterocyte and an M cell
B cell
Follicular dendritic cells
Follicle-associated epithelium
A layer of M cells displays nucleated cells—presumably representing B cells within the intercellular pockets—with surface immunoglobulin (Ig) receptors with binding affinity to antigens.
Microfolds
Lymphocytes inside intercellular pockets provided by M cells
M cell
T cell
Basal lamina
Plasma cell
T cell
M cells
1 **M cells** and **dendritic cells** sample and take up antigens from the intestinal lumen.
2 Antigens are transported to lymphocytes present in intracellular pockets of M cells.
3 The antigen—bound to an Ig receptor on the lymphocyte's surface—is transferred to an antigen-presenting cell.
4 The antigen-presenting cell interacts with a T cell. T cells interact with **follicular dendritic cells.**
M cells—like all intestinal epithelial cells—derive from stem cells in the crypts of Lieberkühn.

The **dome** separates the Peyer's patch from the overlying surface epithelium and contains **B cells** expressing all immunoglobulin isotypes, except immunoglobulin D (IgD).

The **germinal center** contains IgA-positive B cells, $CD4^+$ T cells, and antigen-presenting cells. A few plasma cells are present in the Peyer's patches.

The main components of the FAE are the **M cell** (Figure 16-12), a specialized epithelial cell that takes up antigens into **protease (cathepsin E)-containing vesicles**, and the **dendritic cell**, an antigen-binding cell extending **cytoplasmic processes across epithelial tight junctions**. Antigens are **transported by transcytosis to adjacent intercellular spaces and presented to immunocompetent cells (B cells)**.

Figure 16-13. IgA dimer: Molecular immune surveillance of the intestinal tract

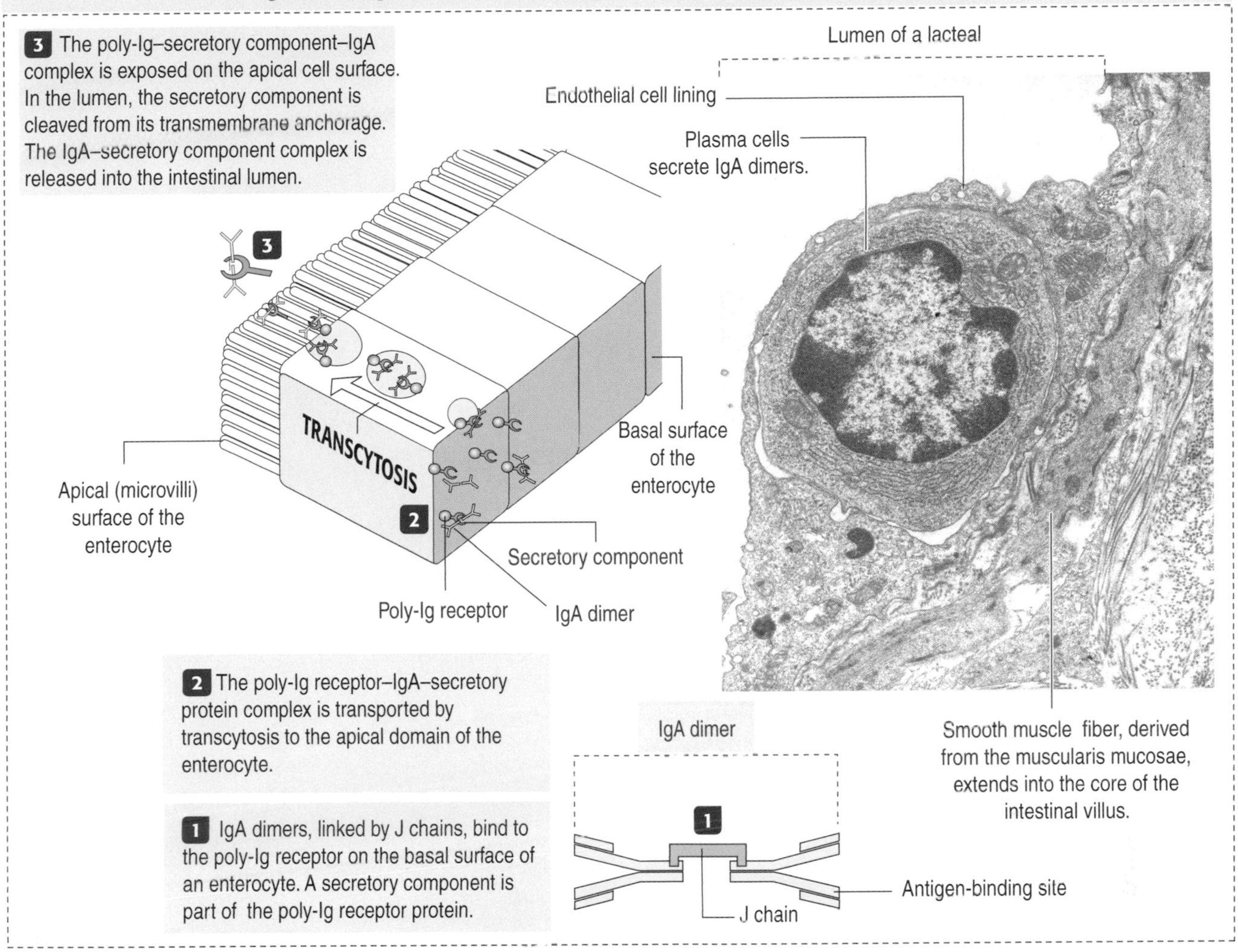

3 The poly-Ig–secretory component–IgA complex is exposed on the apical cell surface. In the lumen, the secretory component is cleaved from its transmembrane anchorage. The IgA–secretory component complex is released into the intestinal lumen.
3
TRANSCYTOSIS
2
Apical (microvilli) surface of the enterocyte
Basal surface of the enterocyte
Secretory component
Poly-Ig receptor
IgA dimer
Lumen of a lacteal
Endothelial cell lining
Plasma cells secrete IgA dimers.
Smooth muscle fiber, derived from the muscularis mucosae, extends into the core of the intestinal villus.
2 The poly-Ig receptor–IgA–secretory protein complex is transported by transcytosis to the apical domain of the enterocyte.
1 IgA dimers, linked by J chains, bind to the poly-Ig receptor on the basal surface of an enterocyte. A secretory component is part of the poly-Ig receptor protein.
IgA dimer
1
Antigen-binding site
J chain

The apical domain of M cells has short **microfolds** (hence the name M cell). The basolateral domain of M cells forms **intraepithelial pockets**, the home site for a subpopulation of intraepithelial B cells.

Intestinal antigens, bound to immunoglobulin receptors on the surface of B cells, interact with **antigen-presenting cells** at the dome region. Processed antigens are presented to **follicular dendritic cells** and $CD4^+$ T cells to initiate an immune reaction.

Clinical significance: Targeting mucosal vaccine vectors to M cells

M cells are unique among epithelial cells in that endocytosed antigens enter a transepithelial vesicular transport pathway and are released at pocket membrane sites to induce an immune response. This property has stimulated current interest in developing **mucosal vaccine vectors** to induce protective mucosal immune responses.

This host defense strategy can eventually lead to the production of secretory IgA dimer (Figure 16-13) and proteins from Paneth cells (Figure 16-14) to clear the mucosal surface of pathogens.

Plasma cells and secretory IgA dimer

Plasma cells secrete **IgA dimers** into the intestinal lumen, the respiratory epithelium, the lactating mammary gland, and salivary glands. Most plasma cells are present in the **lamina propria** of the intestinal villi, together with three types of inflammatory cells: (1) **eosinophils**, (2) **mast cells**, and (3) **macrophages**.

Figure 16-14. Paneth cells: Adaptive antimicrobial immunity

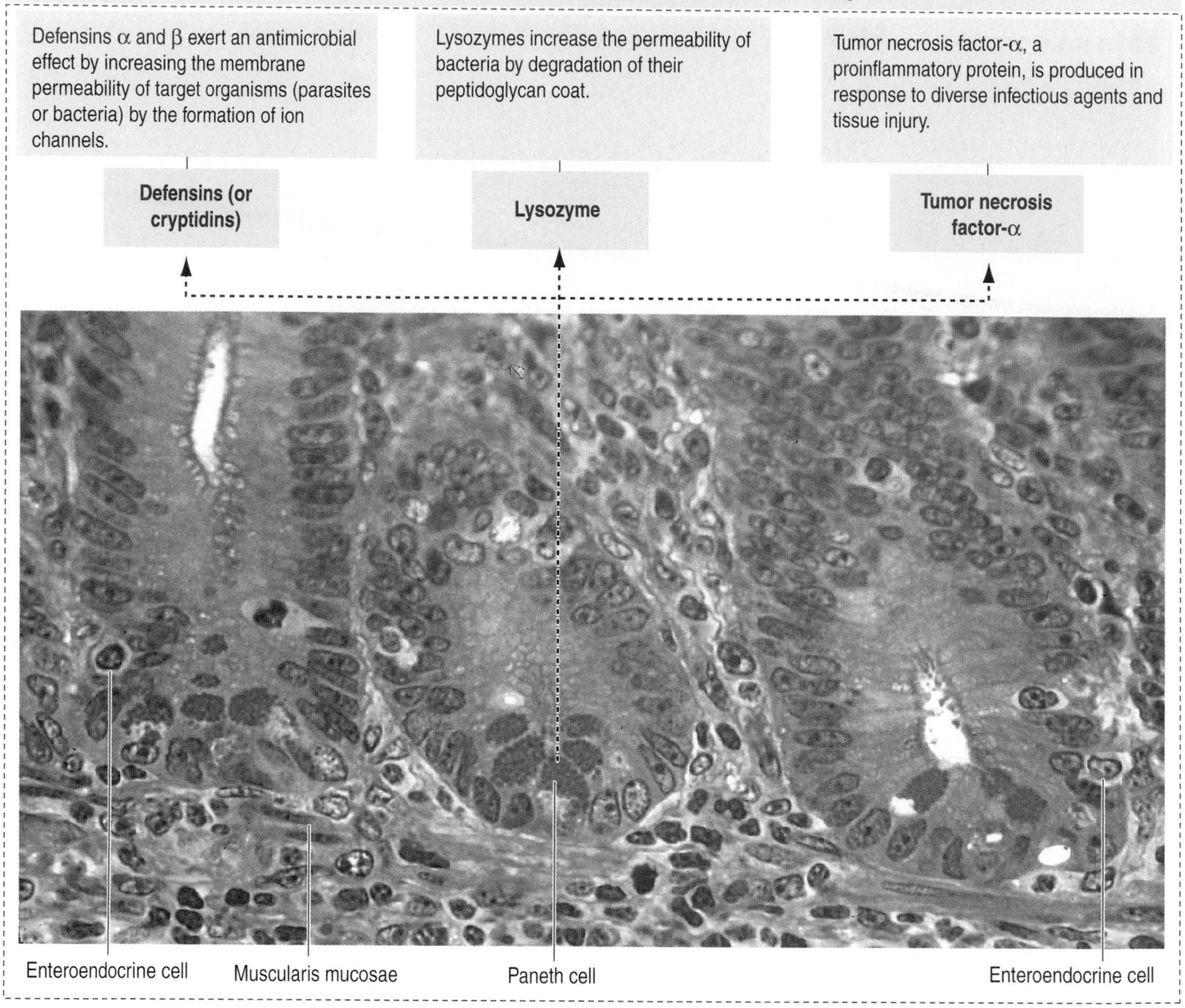
Defensins α and β exert an antimicrobial effect by increasing the membrane permeability of target organisms (parasites or bacteria) by the formation of ion channels.
Lysozymes increase the permeability of bacteria by degradation of their peptidoglycan coat.
Tumor necrosis factor-α, a proinflammatory protein, is produced in response to diverse infectious agents and tissue injury.
Defensins (or cryptidins)
Lysozyme
Tumor necrosis factor-α
Enteroendocrine cell
Muscularis mucosae
Paneth cell
Enteroendocrine cell

IgA molecules secreted by plasma cells are transported from the lamina propria to the intestinal lumen by a **transcytosis mechanism** consisting of the following steps (see Figure 16-13): (1) IgA is secreted into the lamina propria as a dimeric molecule associated with a joining peptide, called the **J chain**. (2) The IgA dimer binds to a specific receptor, called the **poly-immunoglobulin (poly-Ig) receptor**, expressed on the basolateral surfaces of the intestinal epithelial cell. The poly-Ig receptor has an attached extracellular **secretory component**. (3) The **IgA–poly-Ig receptor–secretory component complex is internalized and transported across the cell to the apical surface** of the epithelial cell (transcytosis). (4) At the apical surface, the complex is cleaved enzymatically and the **IgA-secretory component complex is released into the intestinal lumen**. The secretory component protects the dimeric IgA from proteolytic degradation. (5) IgA antibodies prevent the attachment of bacteria or toxins to epithelial cells. (6) Excess IgA dimers diffuse from the lamina propria into the bloodstream and are excreted into the intestinal lumen via the bile.

Patients with **obstructive jaundice**—in which the bile does not reach the duodenum—show an increase of secretory IgA in blood plasma.

Paneth cell

Paneth cells are present at the base of the crypts of Lieberkühn and have a lifetime

Figure 16-15. Lower half of an intestinal gland (crypt of Lieberkühn)

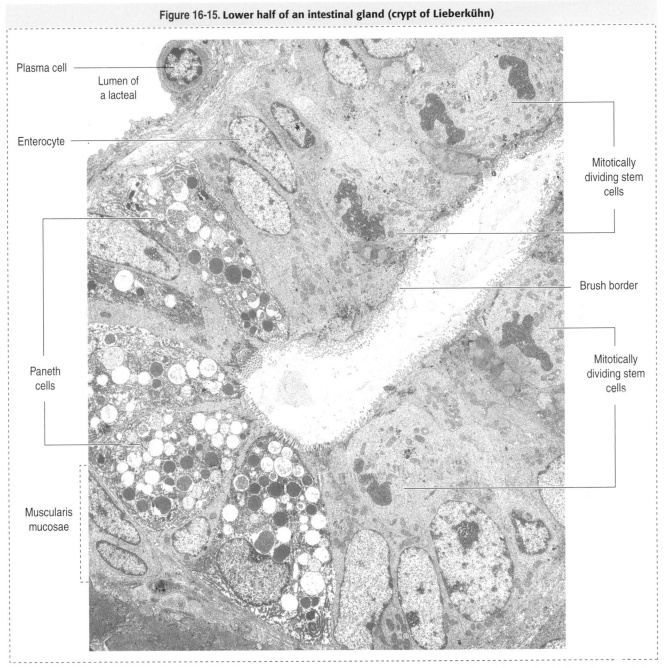

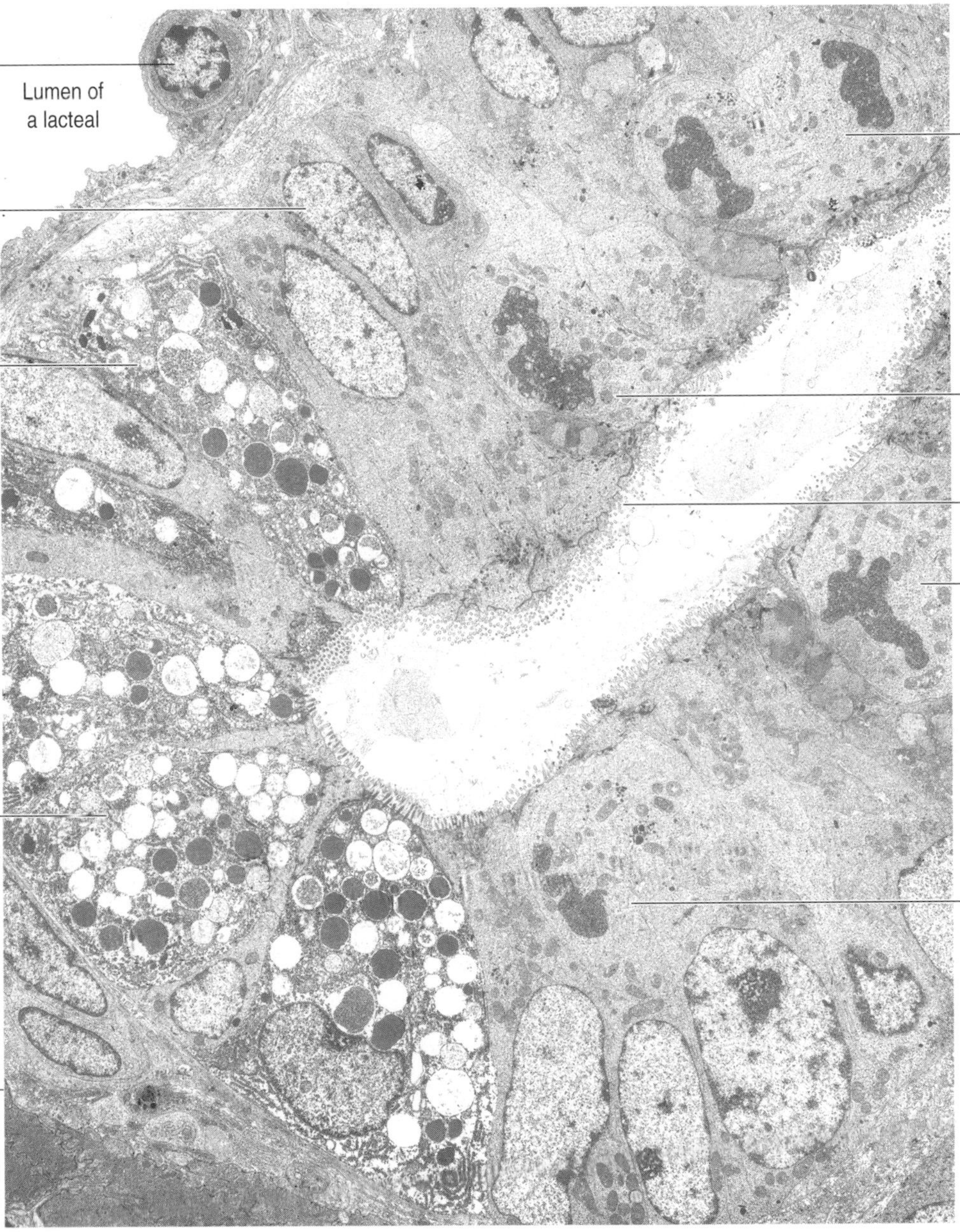
Plasma cell
Lumen of
a lacteal
Enterocyte
Paneth
cells
Muscularis
mucosae
Mitotically
dividing stem
cells
Brush border
Mitotically
dividing stem
cells

of about 20 days. The pyramid-shaped Paneth cells have a basal domain containing the rough endoplasmic reticulum. The apical region contains numerous protein granules (Figure 16-15; see also Figure 16-14).

Paneth cells secrete products that protect the luminal surface of the epithelium from pathogenic microorganisms. The three major products contained in the granules of Paneth cells are (1) **tumor necrosis factor-α (TNF-α)**, (2) **lysozyme**, and (3) a group of proteins known as **defensins** or **cryptidins**. Defensins are produced continuously or in response to microbial products or proinflammatory cytokines (for example, TNF-α). The cytocidal effect of defensins is based on the lack of cholesterol and abundance of negatively charged phospholipids of the membrane of microorganisms. Defensins disrupt the microbial membrane by inserting themselves within the phospholipid membranes. Defensins enhance the recruitment of dendritic cells to the site of infection and facilitate the uptake of antigens by forming defensin-antigen complexes.

TNF-α is a proinflammatory substance produced in response to diverse in-

Figure 16-16. Crohn's disease

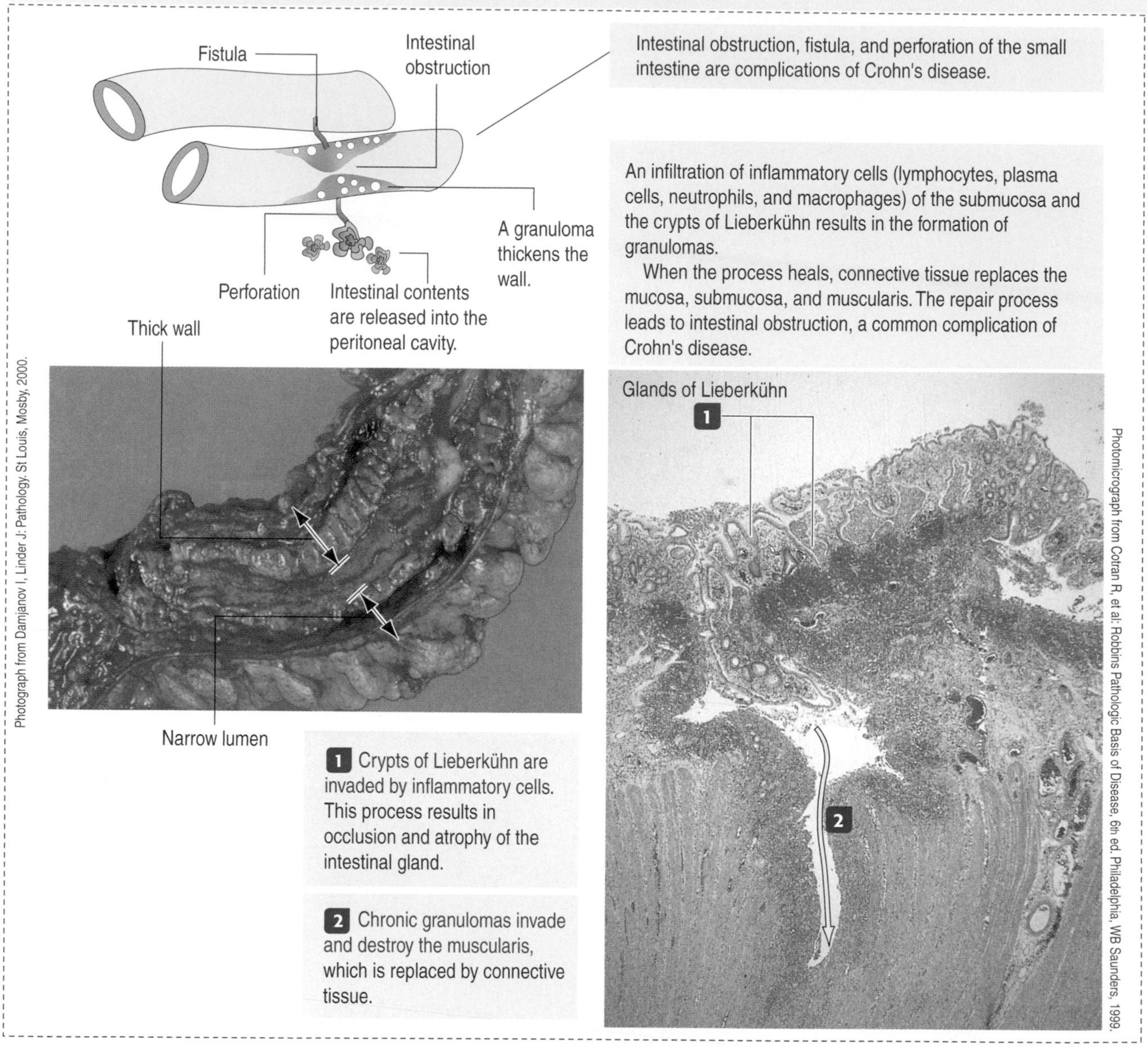

Fistula
Intestinal obstruction
A granuloma thickens the wall.
Perforation
Intestinal contents are released into the peritoneal cavity.
Thick wall
Narrow lumen
Glands of Lieberkühn
1
2

Intestinal obstruction, fistula, and perforation of the small intestine are complications of Crohn's disease.

An infiltration of inflammatory cells (lymphocytes, plasma cells, neutrophils, and macrophages) of the submucosa and the crypts of Lieberkühn results in the formation of granulomas.

When the process heals, connective tissue replaces the mucosa, submucosa, and muscularis. The repair process leads to intestinal obstruction, a common complication of Crohn's disease.

1 Crypts of Lieberkühn are invaded by inflammatory cells. This process results in occlusion and atrophy of the intestinal gland.

2 Chronic granulomas invade and destroy the muscularis, which is replaced by connective tissue.

Photograph from Damjanov I, Linder J: Pathology. St Louis, Mosby, 2000.

Photomicrograph from Cotran R, et al: Robbins Pathologic Basis of Disease, 6th ed. Philadelphia, WB Saunders, 1999.

fectious agents and tissue injury. Lysozyme is a proteolytic enzyme that cleaves peptidoglycan bonds. Peptidoglycan is present in bacteria but not in human cells. Lysozyme-treated bacteria swell and rupture as the result of the entrance of water into the cell. Defensins have an antimicrobial effect by increasing the membrane permeability of a target organism (parasites or bacteria) through the formation of ion channels.

Clinical significance: Inflammatory bowel disease and the enteric bacterial microflora

Inflammatory bowel disease includes **ulcerative colitis** and **Crohn's disease**. Both are clinically characterized by diarrhea, pain, and periodic relapses. **Ulcerative colitis can affect the mucosa of the large intestine. Crohn's disease affects any segment of the intestinal tract.**

Crohn's disease is a chronic inflammatory process involving the terminal ileum but is also observed in the large intestine. Inflammatory cells (neutrophils, lymphocytes, and macrophages) produce cytokines that cause damage to the intestinal mucosa (Figure 16-16).

The initial alteration of the intestinal mucosa consists in the infiltration of

Figure 16-17. **Cytokines and resident and pathogenic bacterial microflora**

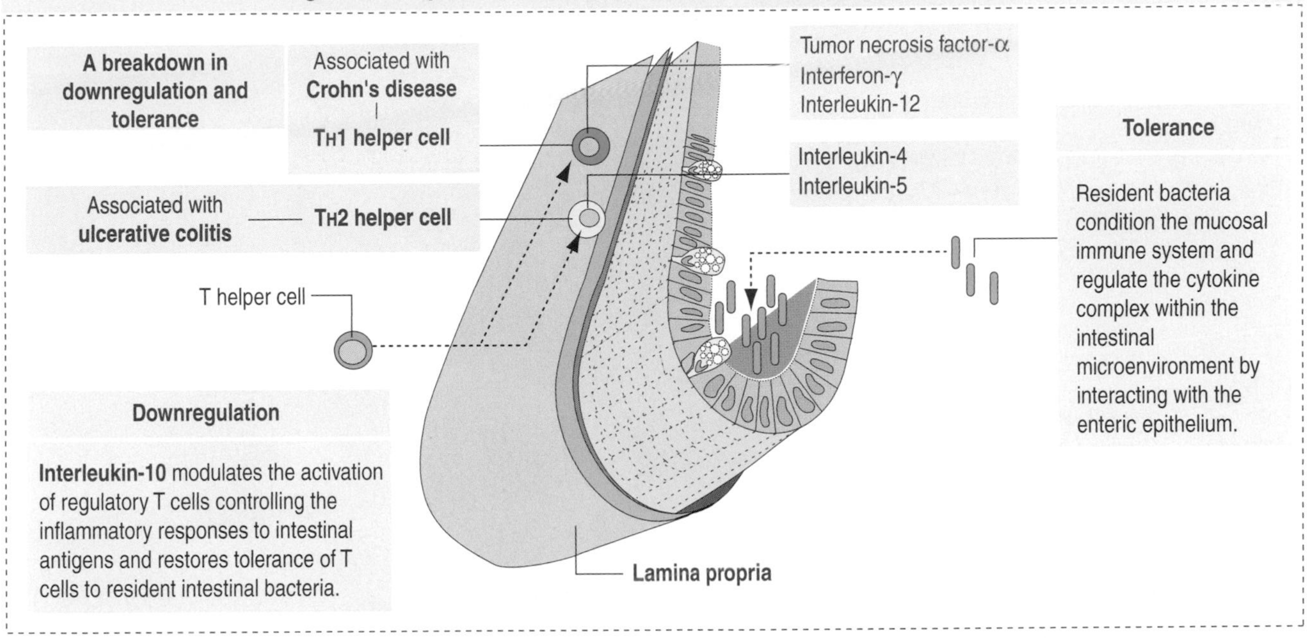
A breakdown in downregulation and tolerance
Associated with Crohn's disease
TH1 helper cell
Associated with ulcerative colitis
TH2 helper cell
T helper cell
Tumor necrosis factor-α
Interferon-γ
Interleukin-12
Interleukin-4
Interleukin-5
Tolerance
Resident bacteria condition the mucosal immune system and regulate the cytokine complex within the intestinal microenvironment by interacting with the enteric epithelium.
Downregulation
Interleukin-10 modulates the activation of regulatory T cells controlling the inflammatory responses to intestinal antigens and restores tolerance of T cells to resident intestinal bacteria.
Lamina propria

neutrophils into the crypts of Lieberkühn. This process results in the destruction of the intestinal glands by the formation of **crypt abscesses** and the progressive **atrophy** and **ulceration** of the mucosa.

The chronic inflammatory process infiltrates the submucosa and muscularis. Abundant accumulation of lymphocytes forms aggregates of cells, or **granulomas**, a typical feature of Crohn's disease.

Major complications of the disease are **occlusion of the intestinal lumen by fibrosis** and the **formation of fistulas** in other segments of the small intestine, and **intestinal perforation**. Segments affected by Crohn's disease are separated by normal stretches of intestinal segments.

The cause of Crohn's disease is unknown. The risk of intestinal cancer is threefold higher in patients with Crohn's disease.

The pathogenesis of inflammatory bowel disease is caused by three contributing factors: (1) **genetic susceptibility of the patient**, (2) **intestinal bacteria**, and (3) **the immune response of the intestinal mucosa**, determined by an abnormal signaling exchange with the resident bacterial microflora. In genetically susceptible individuals, inflammatory bowel disease occurs when the mucosal immune machinery regards the normal bacterial microflora as pathogenic and triggers an immune response. Cytokines produced by helper T cells within the intestinal mucosa cause the inflammatory process that characterizes inflammatory bowel disease.

In Crohn's disease, **type 1 helper cells** (TH1 cells) produce TNF-α, interferon-γ, and interleukin-12. Because TNF-α is both a regulatory and effector cytokine in TH1 responses, antibodies to this cytokine are being administered to patients with Crohn's disease. In ulcerative colitis, **type 2 helper cells** (TH2 cells) release interleukin-4 and interleukin-5 (Figure 16-17).

Interleukin-10, a regulatory cytokine of T cells, can restore tolerance of T cells to the resident intestinal bacterial flora in mice. Dietary administration of the genetically engineered enteric bacterium *Lactococcus lactis*—to overproduce interleukin-10 within the intestinal lumen—has been shown to be effective in the treatment of inflammatory bowel disease in mouse experimental models.

Clinical significance: Malabsorption syndromes

Malabsorption syndromes are characterized by a deficit in the absorption of fats, proteins, carbohydrates, salts, and water by the mucosa of the small intestine.

Figure 16-18. Large intestine

Large intestine

The layers of the large intestine are the same as in the small intestine: mucosa, submucosa, muscularis, and serosa.

The **main function of the mucosa** is the absorption of water, sodium, vitamins, and minerals. The transport of sodium is active (energy-dependent), causing water to move along an osmotic gradient. As a result, the fluid chyme entering the colon is concentrated into semisolid feces. Potassium and bicarbonate are secreted into the lumen of the colon.

The absorptive capacity of the colon favors the uptake of many substances, including sedatives, anesthetics, and steroids. This property is of considerable therapeutic importance when medication cannot be administered through the mouth (for example, because of vomiting).

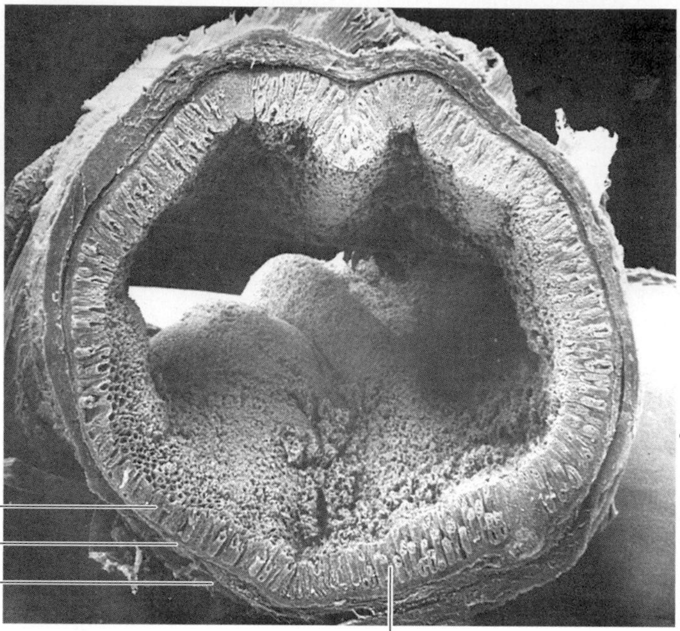

Scanning electron micrograph from: Kessel RG, Kardon RH: Tissues and Organs. New York, WH Freeman, 1979.

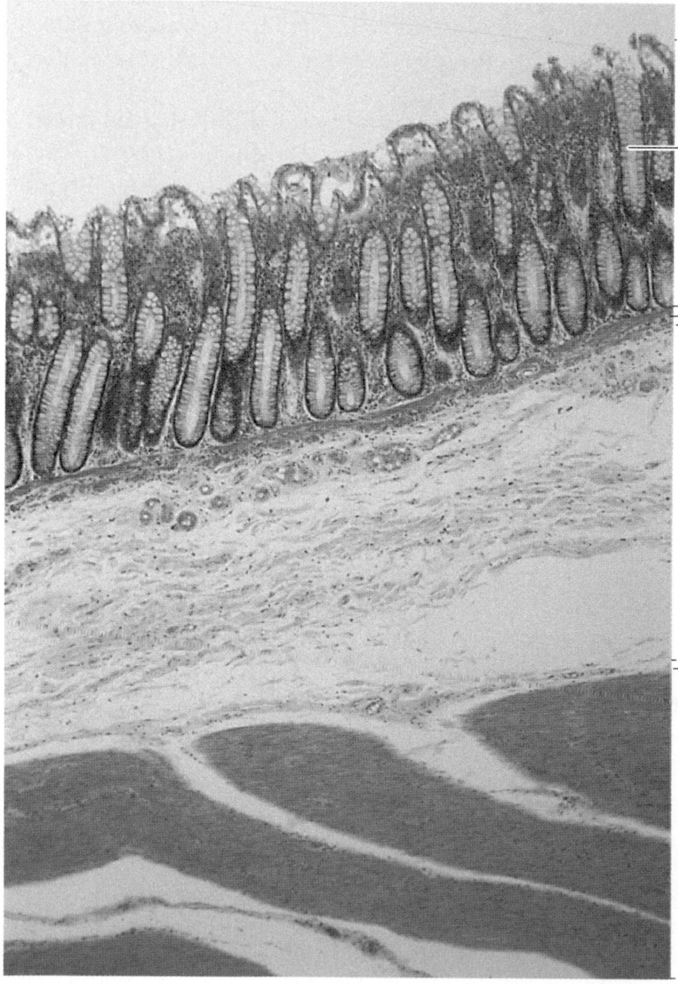

Tubular glands, or crypts of Lieberkühn, are oriented perpendicular to the long axis of the colon, are much deeper than in the small intestine, and have a higher proportion of goblet cells.

Mucosa of the large intestine

The mucosa of the colon is free of folds and villi.

Four cell types are present in the surface epithelium and tubular glands:

1. Simple columnar absorptive cells with apical microvilli (striated apical border).
2. Predominant goblet cells.
3. Stem cells at the base of the tubular glands of Lieberkühn, which give rise to absorptive and goblet cells.
4. Enteroendocrine cells.

The intestinal tubular glands are longer than in the small intestine (0.4 to 0.6 mm).

Lymphatic follicles can be seen in the lamina propria just under the muscularis mucosae, extending into the submucosa.

Figure 16-19. **Large intestine**

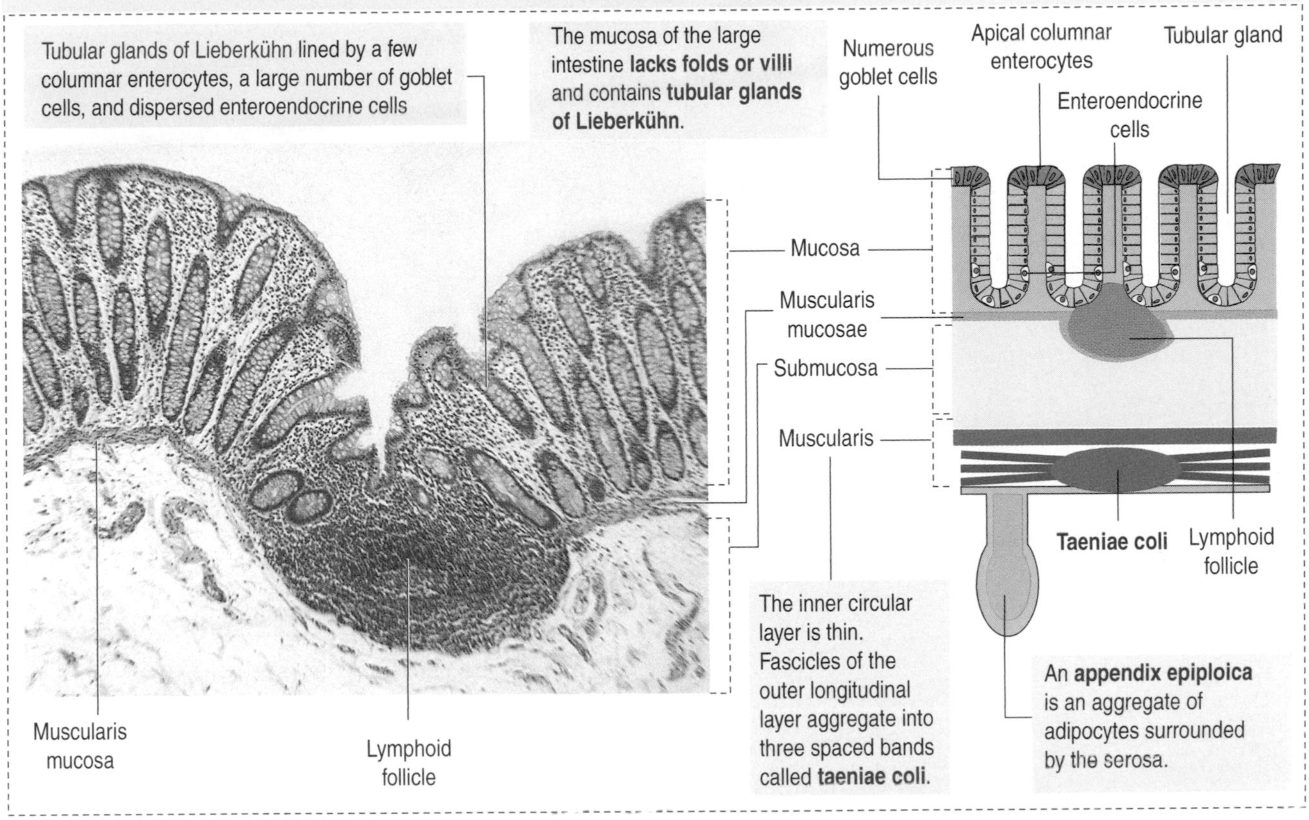

Tubular glands of Lieberkühn lined by a few columnar enterocytes, a large number of goblet cells, and dispersed enteroendocrine cells
The mucosa of the large intestine **lacks folds or villi** and contains **tubular glands of Lieberkühn.**
Numerous goblet cells
Apical columnar enterocytes
Tubular gland
Enteroendocrine cells
Mucosa
Muscularis mucosae
Submucosa
Muscularis
Taeniae coli
Lymphoid follicle
The inner circular layer is thin. Fascicles of the outer longitudinal layer aggregate into three spaced bands called **taeniae coli.**
An **appendix epiploica** is an aggregate of adipocytes surrounded by the serosa.
Muscularis mucosa
Lymphoid follicle

Malabsorption syndromes can be caused by (1) **abnormal digestion of fats and proteins** by pancreatic diseases (pancreatitis or cystic fibrosis) or **lack of solubilization of fats by defective bile secretion** (hepatic disease or obstruction of the flow of bile into the duodenum); (2) **enzymatic abnormalities at the brush border**, where disaccharidases and peptidases cannot hydrolyze carbohydrates (lactose intolerance) and proteins, respectively; and (3) a **defect in the transepithelial transport by enterocytes.**

Malabsorption syndromes affect many organ systems. **Anemia** occurs when vitamin B_{12}, iron, and other cofactors cannot be absorbed. Disturbances of the musculoskeletal system are observed when proteins, calcium, and vitamin D fail to be absorbed. A typical clinical feature of malabsorption syndromes is **diarrhea.**

Large intestine

The large intestine is formed by several successive segments: (1) the **cecum**, projecting from which is the **appendix**; (2) the **ascending**, **transverse**, and **descending colon**; (3) the **sigmoid colon**; (4) the **rectum**; and (5) the **anus**.

Plicae circulares and intestinal villi are not found beyond the ileocecal valve. Numerous openings of the straight **tubular glands** or **crypts of Lieberkühn** are characteristic of the mucosa of the colon (Figure 16-18).

The lining of the tubular glands of the colon consists of the following (Figures 16-19 and 16-20):

1. A **surface simple columnar epithelium** formed by absorptive **enterocytes** and **goblet cells**. Enterocytes have **short apical microvilli**, and the cells participate in the **transport of ions and water**. All regions of the colon absorb Na^+ and Cl^- ions facilitated by plasma membrane channels that are regulated by mineralocorticoids. Aldosterone increases the number of Na^+ channels and increases the absorption of Na^+. Na^+ ions entering the absorptive enterocytes are extruded by an Na^+ pump. Goblet cells secrete mucus to lubricate the mucosal surface and serve as a protective barrier.

Figure 16-20. **Cell types of the glands of the large intestine**

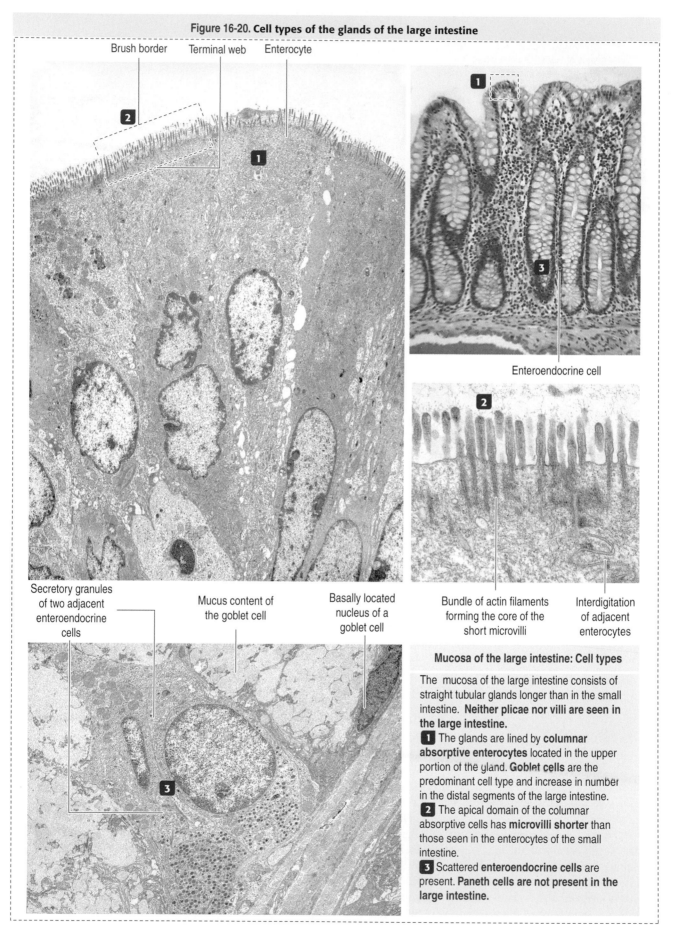

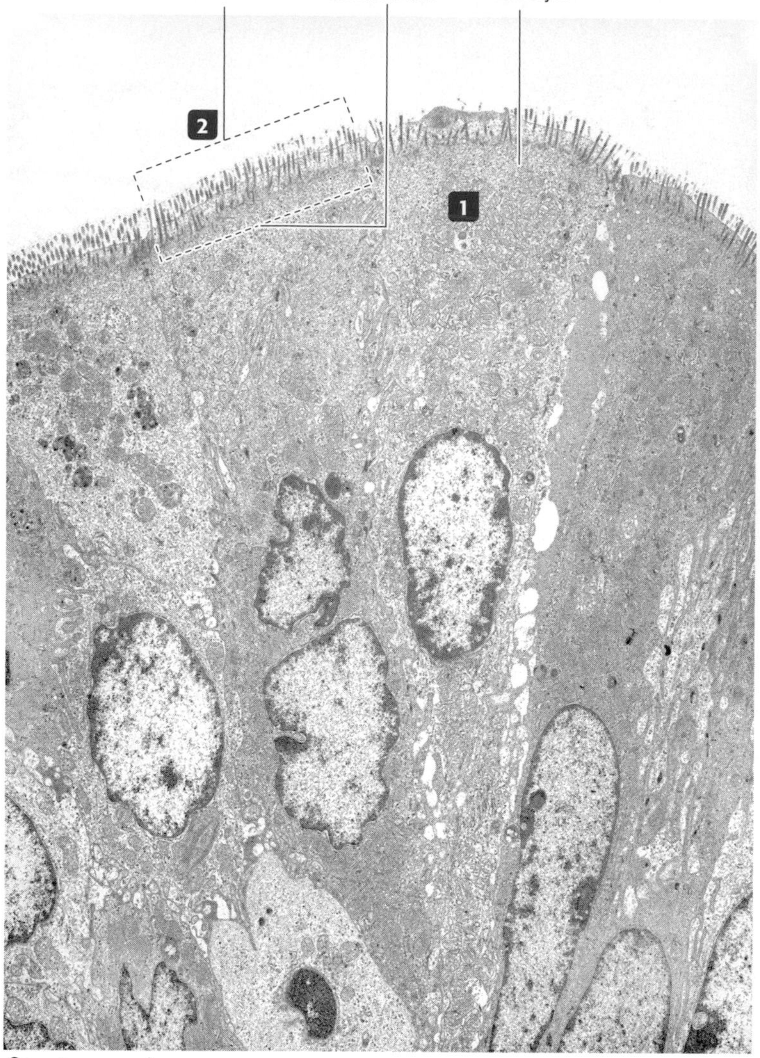
Brush border
Terminal web
Enterocyte
2
1

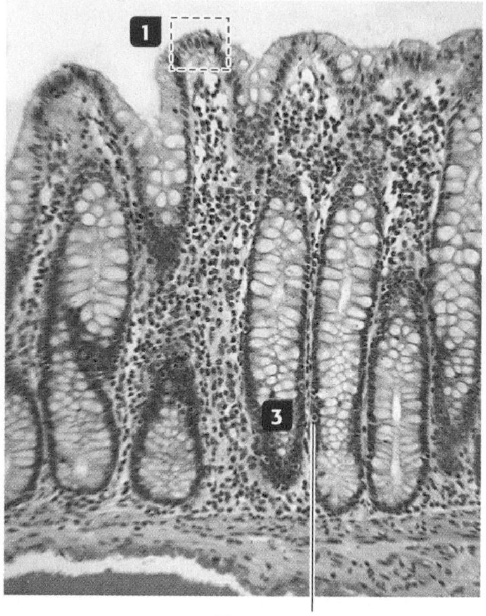
1
3
Enteroendocrine cell

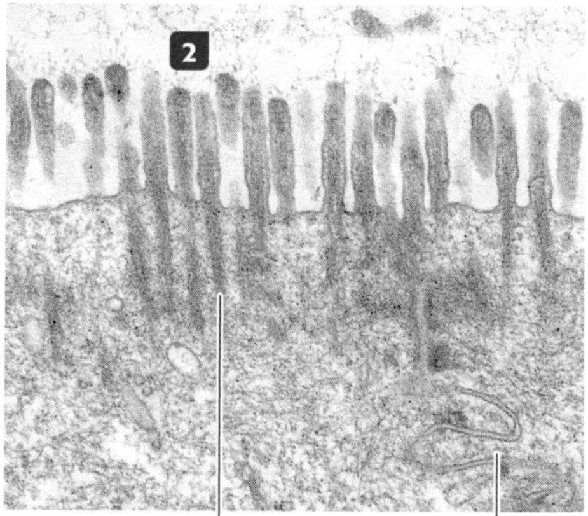
2
Bundle of actin filaments forming the core of the short microvilli
Interdigitation of adjacent enterocytes

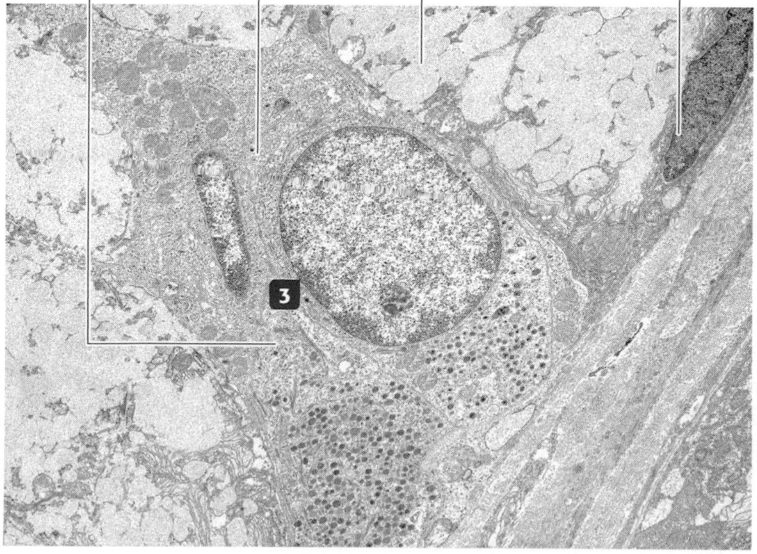
Secretory granules of two adjacent enteroendocrine cells
Mucus content of the goblet cell
Basally located nucleus of a goblet cell
3

Mucosa of the large intestine: Cell types

The mucosa of the large intestine consists of straight tubular glands longer than in the small intestine. **Neither plicae nor villi are seen in the large intestine.**

1 The glands are lined by **columnar absorptive enterocytes** located in the upper portion of the gland. **Goblet cells** are the predominant cell type and increase in number in the distal segments of the large intestine.

2 The apical domain of the columnar absorptive cells has **microvilli shorter** than those seen in the enterocytes of the small intestine.

3 Scattered **enteroendocrine cells** are present. **Paneth cells are not present in the large intestine.**

Figure 16-21. Appendix

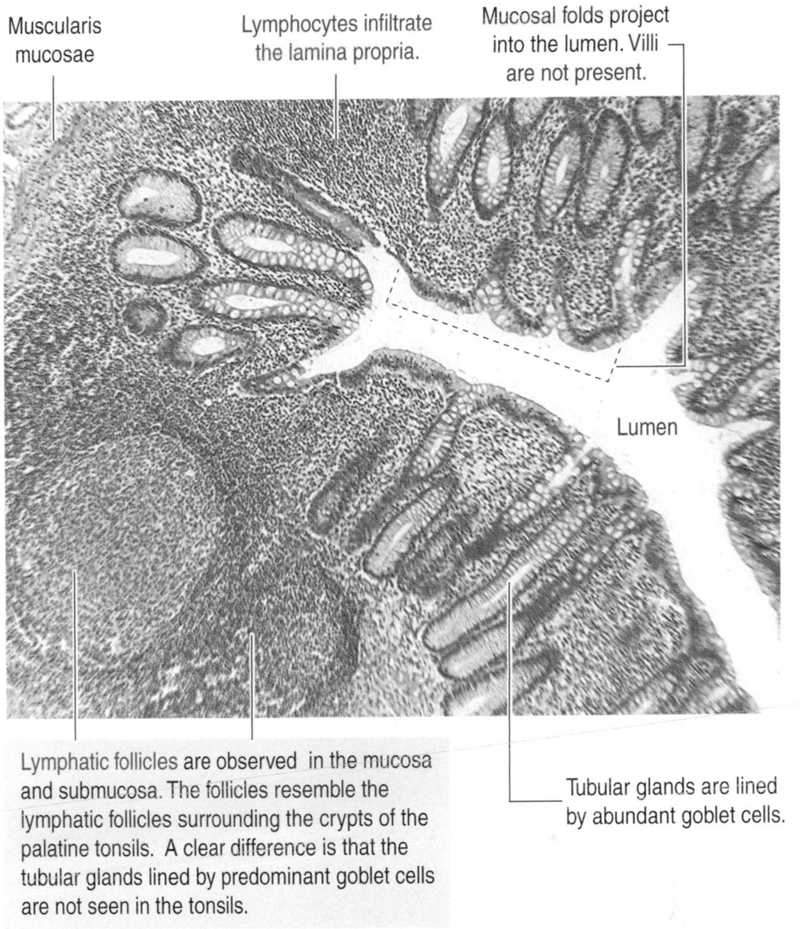
Muscularis mucosae
Lymphocytes infiltrate the lamina propria.
Mucosal folds project into the lumen. Villi are not present.
Lumen
Lymphatic follicles are observed in the mucosa and submucosa. The follicles resemble the lymphatic follicles surrounding the crypts of the palatine tonsils. A clear difference is that the tubular glands lined by predominant goblet cells are not seen in the tonsils.
Tubular glands are lined by abundant goblet cells.

2. A **glandular epithelium,** lining the glands or crypts of Lierberkühn, consists of enterocytes and predominant goblet cells, stem cells, and dispersed **enteroendocrine cells**. Paneth cells may be present in the cecum.

A lamina propria and a muscularis mucosae are present, as are **lymphoid follicles** penetrating the submucosa. Glands are not present in the submucosa.

The muscularis has a particular feature: The bundles of its outer longitudinal layer fuse to form the **taeniae coli**. The taeniae coli consist of three longitudinally oriented ribbon-like bands, each 1 cm wide. The contraction of the taeniae coli and circular muscle layer draws the colon into sacculations called **haustra**.

The serosa has scattered sacs of adipose tissue, the **appendices epiploicae**, which is a unique feature, together with the haustra, of the colon.

The **appendix** (Figure 16-21) is a diverticulum of the cecum and has layers similar to those of the large intestine. The characteristic features of the appendix are the **lymphoid tissue**, represented by multiple lymphatic follicles, and **lymphocytes** infiltrating the lamina propria.

Lymphatic follicles extend into the mucosa and submucosa and disrupt the continuity of the muscularis mucosae.

The **rectum**, the terminal portion of the intestinal tract, is a continuation of the sigmoid colon. The rectum consists of two parts: (1) the upper part, or rectum proper, and (2) the lower part, or anal canal.

In the rectum, the mucosa is thicker, with prominent veins, and the crypts of Lieberkühn are longer (0.7 mm) than in the small intestine and lined predominantly by goblet cells. At the level of the anal canal, the crypts gradually disappear and the serosa is replaced by an adventitia.

Figure 16-22. **Rectum, anal canal, and anus**

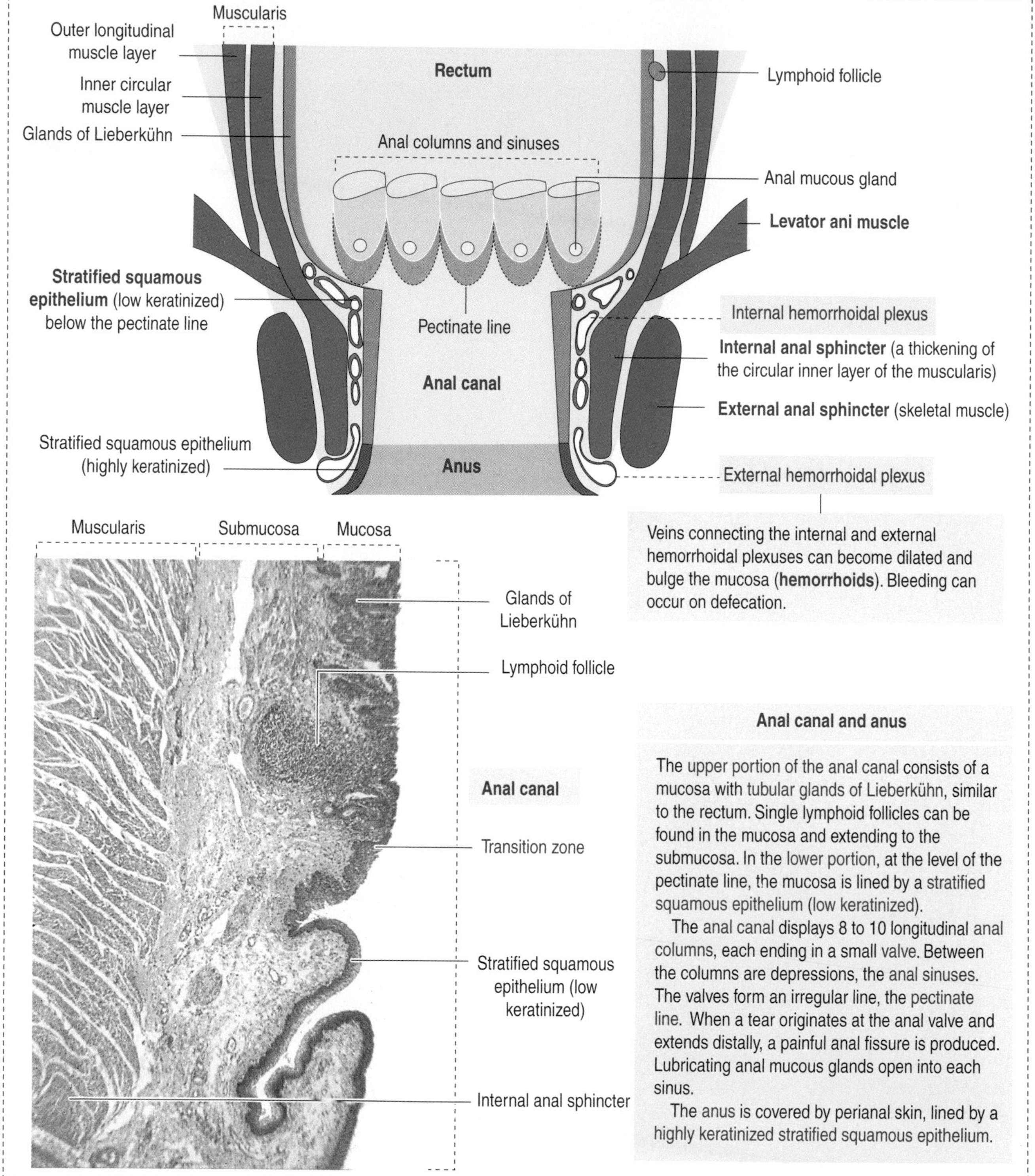
Muscularis
Outer longitudinal muscle layer
Inner circular muscle layer
Glands of Lieberkühn
Rectum
Lymphoid follicle
Anal columns and sinuses
Anal mucous gland
Levator ani muscle
Stratified squamous epithelium (low keratinized) below the pectinate line
Pectinate line
Internal hemorrhoidal plexus
Internal anal sphincter (a thickening of the circular inner layer of the muscularis)
Anal canal
External anal sphincter (skeletal muscle)
Stratified squamous epithelium (highly keratinized)
Anus
External hemorrhoidal plexus
Muscularis
Submucosa
Mucosa
Glands of Lieberkühn
Lymphoid follicle
Anal canal
Transition zone
Stratified squamous epithelium (low keratinized)
Internal anal sphincter

Veins connecting the internal and external hemorrhoidal plexuses can become dilated and bulge the mucosa (**hemorrhoids**). Bleeding can occur on defecation.

Anal canal and anus

The upper portion of the anal canal consists of a mucosa with tubular glands of Lieberkühn, similar to the rectum. Single lymphoid follicles can be found in the mucosa and extending to the submucosa. In the lower portion, at the level of the pectinate line, the mucosa is lined by a stratified squamous epithelium (low keratinized).

The anal canal displays 8 to 10 longitudinal anal columns, each ending in a small valve. Between the columns are depressions, the anal sinuses. The valves form an irregular line, the pectinate line. When a tear originates at the anal valve and extends distally, a painful anal fissure is produced. Lubricating anal mucous glands open into each sinus.

The anus is covered by perianal skin, lined by a highly keratinized stratified squamous epithelium.

The **anal canal** extends from the anorectal junction to the anus (Figure 16-22). A characteristic feature of the mucosa of the anal canal are 8 to 10 longitudinal **anal columns**. The base of the anal columns is the **pectinate line**. The anal columns are connected at their base by **valves**, corresponding to transverse folds of the mucosa. Small pockets, called **anal sinuses**, or crypts, are found behind the valves. **Anal mucous glands** open into each sinus.

The valves and sinuses prevent leakage from the anus. When the canal is dis-

Figure 16-23. **Hirschsprung's disease (congenital megacolon)**

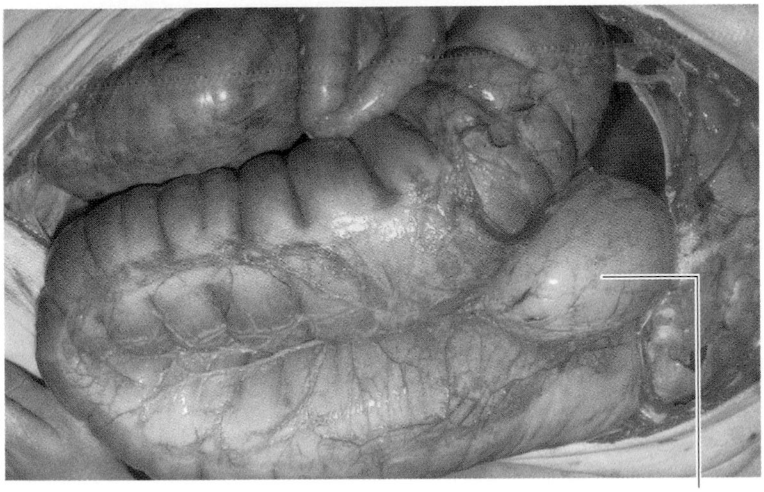

From Cooke RA, Stewart B: Anatomical Pathology. New York, Churchill Livingstone, 1995.

Defects of neural crest cell migration and development: Hirschsprung's disease

Hirschsprung's disease (congenital megacolon) is caused by mutations in one to four different genes that prevent the migration and differentiation of neural crest cells into neurons of the enteric nervous system.

The mutated genes encode cell membrane receptors **rearranged during transfection** (RET), and **endothelin B** (EDNRB), and the ligand for EDNRB, **endothelin 3** (EDN3).

Some individuals with mutations in either EDNRB or EDN3 have **melanocyte abnormalities** producing hypopigmented patches in skin and **hearing loss**. This disorder is called the **Waardenburg-Shah syndrome**.

tended with feces, the columns, sinuses, and valves flatten, and mucus is discharged from the sinuses to lubricate the passage of the feces.

Beyond the pectinate line, the simple columnar epithelium of the rectal mucosa is replaced by a **stratified squamous epithelium**. At the level of the anus, **the inner circular layer of smooth muscle thickens to form the internal anal sphincter.** The longitudinal smooth muscle layer extends over the sphincter and attaches to the connective tissue. Below this zone, the mucosa consists of stratified squamous epithelium with a few sebaceous and sweat glands in the submucosa (**circumanal glands** similar to the axillary sweat glands). The **external anal sphincter** is formed by **skeletal muscle** and lies inside the levator ani muscle, also with a sphincter function.

Clinical significance: Hirschsprung's disease (congenital megacolon)

We discuss in Chapter 8, Nervous Tissue, that during formation of the neural tube, neural crest cells migrate from the neuroepithelium along defined pathways to tissues where they differentiate into various cell types. One destination of neural crest cells is the alimentary tube, where they develop the **enteric nervous system**.

The enteric nervous system partially controls and coordinates the normal movements of the alimentary tube that facilitate digestion and transport of bowel contents. The large intestine, like the rest of the alimentary tube, is innervated by the enteric nervous system receiving impulses from extrinsic parasympathetic and sympathetic nerves and from receptors within the large intestine. The myenteric plexus is concentrated beneath the taeniae coli.

The transit of contents from the small intestine to the large intestine is intermittent and regulated at the ileocecal junction by a sphincter mechanism: When the sphincter relaxes, ileal contractions propel the contents into the large intestine.

Segmental contractions in an orad-to-aborad direction move the contents over short distances. The material changes from a liquid to a semisolid state when it reaches the descending and sigmoid colon. The rectum is usually empty. Contraction of the inner anal sphincter closes the anal canal. Defecation occurs when the sphincter relaxes as part of the **rectosphincteric reflex** stimulated by distention of the rectum.

Delayed transit through the colon leads to severe **constipation**. An abnormal form of constipation is seen in **Hirschsprung's disease** (**congenital megacolon**) caused by the **absence of the enteric nervous system in a segment of the distal colon** (Figure 16-23). This condition, called **aganglionosis**, is the result of an **arrest in the migration of cells from the neural crest**, the precursors of the intramural

Figure 16-24. **APC (adenomatous polyposis coli) and cancer of the colon**

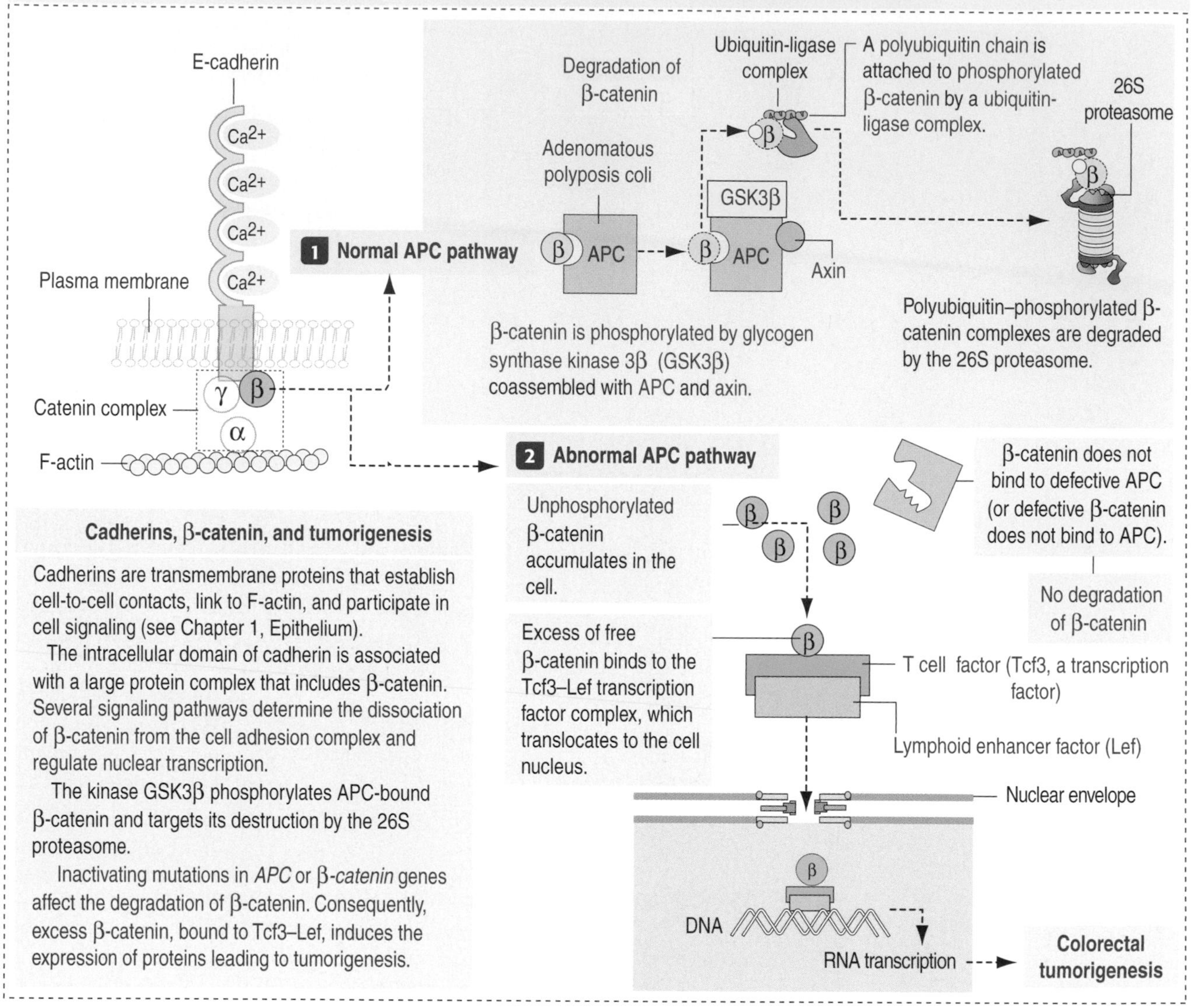

E-cadherin
Ca2+
Ca2+
Ca2+
Ca2+
Plasma membrane
Catenin complex
γ
β
α
F-actin
1 Normal APC pathway
Degradation of β-catenin
Ubiquitin-ligase complex
A polyubiquitin chain is attached to phosphorylated β-catenin by a ubiquitin-ligase complex.
26S proteasome
Adenomatous polyposis coli
GSK3β
APC
Axin
β-catenin is phosphorylated by glycogen synthase kinase 3β (GSK3β) coassembled with APC and axin.
Polyubiquitin–phosphorylated β-catenin complexes are degraded by the 26S proteasome.
2 Abnormal APC pathway
Unphosphorylated β-catenin accumulates in the cell.
β-catenin does not bind to defective APC (or defective β-catenin does not bind to APC).
No degradation of β-catenin
Excess of free β-catenin binds to the Tcf3–Lef transcription factor complex, which translocates to the cell nucleus.
T cell factor (Tcf3, a transcription factor)
Lymphoid enhancer factor (Lef)
Nuclear envelope
DNA
RNA transcription
Colorectal tumorigenesis
Cadherins, β-catenin, and tumorigenesis
Cadherins are transmembrane proteins that establish cell-to-cell contacts, link to F-actin, and participate in cell signaling (see Chapter 1, Epithelium).
The intracellular domain of cadherin is associated with a large protein complex that includes β-catenin. Several signaling pathways determine the dissociation of β-catenin from the cell adhesion complex and regulate nuclear transcription.
The kinase GSK3β phosphorylates APC-bound β-catenin and targets its destruction by the 26S proteasome.
Inactivating mutations in APC or β-catenin genes affect the degradation of β-catenin. Consequently, excess β-catenin, bound to Tcf3–Lef, induces the expression of proteins leading to tumorigenesis.

ganglion cells of the plexuses of Meissner and Auerbach.

Aganglionosis is caused by mutations affecting the **rearranged during transfection** ***(RET)*** gene as well as the cell membrane receptor **endothelin B** or its ligand, **endothelin 3** (see Figure 16-23). The *RET* gene encodes a **receptor tyrosine kinase** required for the migration of neural crest cells into the distal portions of the large intestine and for differentiation into neurons of the enteric nervous system.

The permanently contracted aganglionic segment does not allow the entry of the contents. An increase in muscular tone in the orad segment results in its dilation, thus generating a megacolon or megarectum. This condition is apparent shortly after birth when the abdomen of the infant becomes distended and little meconium is eliminated.

The diagnosis is confirmed by a biopsy of the mucosa and submucosa of the rectum showing thick and irregular nerve bundles and a lack of ganglion cells. Surgical removal of the affected colon segment is the treatment of choice.

Clinical significance: Familial polyposis gene and colorectal tumorigenesis

Colorectal tumors develop from a **polyp**, a tumoral mass that protrudes into the lumen of the intestine. Some polyps are non-neoplastic and are relatively common in persons 60 years or older. Polyps can be present in large number (100 or more) in **familial polyposis syndromes** such as **familial adenomatous polyposis** and the **Peutz-Jeghers syndrome.** Familial polyposis is determined by autosomal dominant mutations, in particular in the *APC* **(adenomatous polyposis coli) gene.** Mutations in the *APC* gene have been detected in 85% of colon tumors, indicating that, as with the retinoblastoma (*Rb*) gene, the inherited gene is also important in the development of the sporadic form of the cancer.

The *APC* gene encodes **APC protein** with binding affinity to microtubules and **β-catenin**, a molecule associated with a catenin complex linked to E-cadherin (discussed in Chapter 1, Epithelium) and also a component of nuclear transcription complexes.

When β-catenin is not part of the catenin α, β, γ complex, free β-catenin interacts with DNA binding proteins of a family of transcription factor proteins called **T cell factor–lymphoid enhancer factor** (**Tcf3-Lef**) to form a transactivator complex that stimulates transcription of immediate gene targets (Figure 16-24).

When free β-catenin binds to the **glycogen synthase kinase 3β** (GSK3β)–axin–APC complex, it is phosphorylated by GSK3β. **Phosphorylated β-catenin** is subsequently recognized by a **ubiquitin ligase complex** that catalyzes the attachment of polyubiquitin chains to phosphorylated β-catenin. Polyubiquitin conjugates of β-catenin are rapidly degraded by the **26S proteasome.** The lack of β-catenin inactivates the β-catenin–Tcf–Lef pathway. A mutation in the *APC* gene results in a defective protein that reduces cell-cell contact and increases the pool of available β-catenin. Essentially, *APC* is a tumor suppressor gene.

The *APC* gene is also a major regulator of the **Wnt pathway**, a signaling system expressed during early development and embryogenesis (see Chapter 3, Cell Signaling). The Wnt pathway has an important function in the development of neural crest–derived cells. Wnt proteins can inactivate GSK3β, prevent the phosphorylation of β-catenin, and abrogate its destruction by the 26S proteasome. Consequently, an excess of β-catenin translocates to the cell nucleus to affect gene transcription.

A defective β-catenin pathway can overexpress the **microphthalmia-associated transcription factor** (**MITF**). We discuss in Chapter 11, Integumentary System, the significance of MITF in the survival and proliferation of melanoma cells.

Hereditary nonpolyposis colon cancer (**HNPCC**) is an inherited form of colorectal cancer caused by mutations in genes involved in the repair of DNA mismatch. HNPCC is an example of a cancer syndrome caused by **mutations in DNA repair proteins.** Patients with the HNPCC syndrome do not show the very large number of colon polyps typical of the familial polyposis syndrome, but a small number of polyps occur frequently among gene carriers.

Essential concepts | Lower Digestive Segment

• Small intestine. The main functions of the small intestine are to continue in the duodenum the digestive process initiated in the stomach, and to absorb digested food after enzymatic breakdown.

The intestinal wall is constructed to perform absorptive functions and propel the intestinal contents to the next segment of the small intestine.

There are four degrees of folding to amplify the absorptive intestinal surface: (1) the plicae circulares (permanent evaginations or folds of the mucosa and part of the submucosa); (2) the intestinal villi (finger-like evaginations of the mucosa only; a typical feature of the small intestine); (3) the glands or crypts of Lieberkühn (invaginations of the mucosa between adjacent villi, extending down to the muscularis mucosae); and (4) microvilli (apical differentiation of the enterocyte, the absorptive cell of the small intestine).

The muscularis mucosae (a component of the mucosa, together with the lining epithelium of the villi and intestinal glands and the connective tissue lamina propria) is the boundary between the mucosa and submucosa. The muscularis, consisting of inner circular smooth muscle fibers and outer longitudinal smooth muscle fibers, is responsible for mixing the intestinal contents and for peristaltic movements from a proximal (orad) to a distal (aborad) direction. The adventitia is covered by the peritoneum, lined by a simple squamous epithelium (mesothelium).

The intestinal wall is supplied by a rich blood, lymphatic, and nerve supply (derived from the submucosal plexus of Meissner and myenteric plexus of Auerbach, components of the autonomic nervous system). A central lymphatic vessel (lacteal) is present in the lamina propria of the intestinal villus. A capillary villus plexus supplies the intestinal villus; a pericryptal capillary plexus supplies the glands of Lieberkühn.

• The three major sequential segments of the small intestine are (1) the duodenum, (2) the jejunum, and (3) the ileum.

The duodenum has Brunner's glands in the submucosa, and the villi are broad and short (leaflike). The jejunum has long villi (finger-like), each with a prominent lacteal. Brunner's glands are not present in the submucosa. The ileum has shorter finger-like villi. A relevant feature are the Peyer's patches. Paneth cells are found at the base of the glands of Lieberkühn in the duodenum, jejunum, and ileum.

• The intestinal villus and glands of Lieberkühn are lined by a simple columnar epithelium consisting of (1) absorptive enterocytes (columnar cells with apical microvilli, the brush border); (2) goblet cells (a mucus-secreting cell forming a protective gel coat to shield the epithelium from mechanical abrasion and bacterial invasion); (3) Paneth cells (producing the bacteriostatic proteins defensins and lysozyme); and (4) enteroendocrine cells. A stem cell gives rise to these cell types. The surface of the epithelium is coated by the glycocalyx, consisting of glycoproteins representing enzymes involved in the digestive process.

Enterocytes are involved in the absorption of proteins, carbohydrate, lipids, calcium, and other substances.

Pancreatic proteolytic enzymes break down proteins into peptides and amino acids. Once absorbed, peptides are broken down by cytoplasmic peptidases into amino acids.

Salivary and pancreatic amylase, and enzymes (oligosaccharidases) present in the plasma membrane of the intestinal villi convert sugars into monosaccharides (galactose and glucose), which are transported inside the enterocyte by an Na^+-dependent carrier system.

Lipids are emulsified in the intestinal lumen by bile salts and pancreatic lipase to form micelles (fatty acids and monoglycerides). Micelles diffuse into the cytoplasm of the enterocyte bound to fatty acid–binding protein, and esterified into triglycerides in the smooth endoplasmic reticulum. Tryglycerides are transported to the Golgi apparatus and converted into chylomicrons (apoprotein-lipid complex). Chylomicrons are released into the enterocyte intercellular space and into the central lacteal.

Malabsorption syndromes can be caused by abnormal digestion of fats and proteins by pancreatic diseases (pancreatitis or cystic fibrosis), or lack of solubilization of fats by defective bile secretion (hepatic disease or obstruction of bile flow to the duodenum). Enzymatic abnormalities in the brush border hamper protein and carbohydrate (lactose intolerance) absorption. An abnormal transport mechanism across enterocytes can cause malabsorption syndromes.

Anemia can occur when the **intrinsic factor–vitamin B_{12} complex**, iron, and other cofactors are not absorbed. **Functional alterations of the musculoskeletal system** occur when proteins, calcium, and vitamin D are not absorbed.

Enteroendocrine cells produce gastrin, secretin, and cholecystokinin. Their distribution and function of enteroendocrine cells are summarized in Essential Concepts in Chapter 15, Upper Digestive Segment.

• The small intestine is protected from pathogens by (1) Peyer's patches and associated M cells of the intestinal epithelium, participating in the cellular surveillance of antigens; (2) the neutralization of antigens by IgA, produced by plasma cells in the lamina propria of the intestinal villus and transported to the intestinal lumen across the enterocyte (by a mechanism called transcytosis); and (3) the inactivation of microbial pathogens by defensins, products of Paneth cells.

A defect in the protective system accounts for **ulcerative colitis** (large intestine) and **Crohn's disease** (involving the terminal ileum but also observed in the large intestine).

• The large intestine consists of (1) the cecum and associated appendix; (2) the ascending, transverse, and descending colon; (3) the sigmoid colon; (4) the rectum; and (5) the anus.

Plicae circulares and intestinal villi are not observed beyond the ileocecal valve. The mucosa of the large intestine is lined by a simple columnar epithelium formed by enterocytes and abundant goblet cells. Enterocytes have short apical microvilli. A major function of enterocytes in the large intestine is the transport of ions and water. Secretory products of goblet cells lubricate the mucosal surface.

Glands of Lieberkühn are observed. They contain enteroendocrine cells and stem cells. Paneth cells are not observed (they may be present in the cecum).

A characteristic feature of the large intestine is the taeniae coli, formed by fused bundles of the outer smooth muscle layer. Contraction of the taeniae coli and the inner circular smooth muscle layer produces periodic saccular structures called haustra.

The appendix is a diverticulum of the cecum. Prominent lymphoid follicles or nodules are seen in the mucosa and submucosa.

The rectum, the terminal portion of the large intestine and a continuation of the sigmoid colon, consists of two regions: (1) the upper region, or rectum proper, and (2) the lower region, or anal canal, which extends from the anorectal junction to the anus.

The mucosa of the rectum displays long glands of Lieberkühn; glands disappear at the level of the anal canal. Anal columns are present in the anal canal. They consist of valves, transverse fold of the mucosa, and sinuses, with mucous glandular crypts behind the valves secreting lubricating mucus. Anal columns prevent leakage from the anus. A tear originating at the anal valves and extending distally produces painful **anal fissures**.

The base of the anal columns forms the pectinate line. Beyond the pectinate line, the simple columnar epithelium of the rectal mucosa is replaced by a stratified squamous epithelium, and the inner circular layer of smooth muscle thickens to form the internal anal sphincter. Beyond this region, the anal mucosa is lined by a keratinizing stratified squamous epithelium and the submucosa contains sebaceous and sweat glands (circumanal glands). The external anal sphincter, formed by skeletal muscle, is present.

• **Hirschsprung's disease** (congenital megacolon) is caused by a defect in the migration and differentiation of neural crest cells, which give rise to neurons of the enteric nervous system.

Familial polyposis and **colorectal tumorigenesis** is determined by a defect in the protein adenomatous polyposis coli (APC), which prevents the normal disposal of β-catenin. Excess of this protein, bound to T cell factor–lymphoid enhancer factor (Tcf3 Lef) transactivator complex, activates genes leading to colorectal tumorigenesis.

17. DIGESTIVE GLANDS

Digestive glands have **lubricative**, **protective**, **digestive**, and **absorptive** functions mediated by their secretory products, which are released into the oral cavity and the duodenum.

The three major digestive glands are:

1. The **major salivary glands** (parotid, submandibular, and sublingual glands), associated with the oral cavity through independent excretory ducts. The **minor salivary glands** have short branching tubules and are located throughout the oral mucosa and tongue, where they contribute to **saliva**, the product of the salivary glands.

2. The **exocrine pancreas** secretes a combined aqueous and enzymatic product draining into the duodenum. The endocrine function of the pancreas (represented

Figure 17-1. Review of the general histologic organization of a compound gland

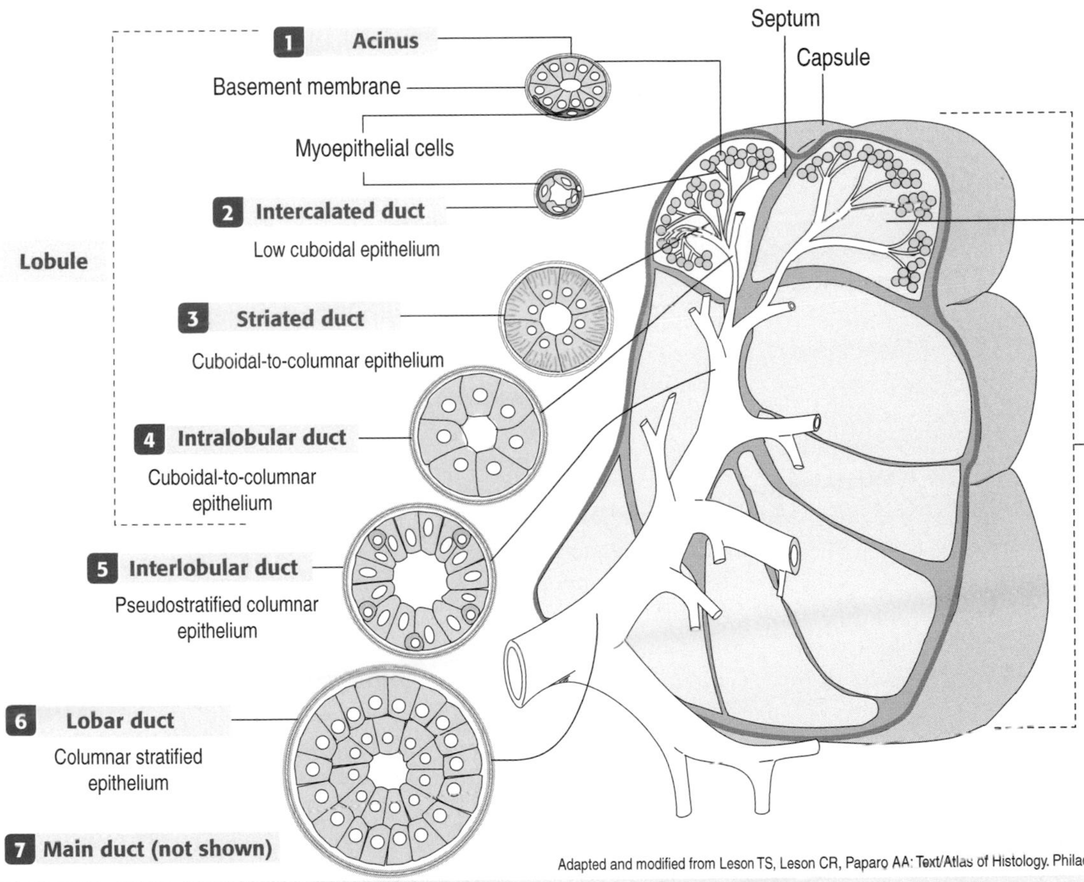

Adapted and modified from Leson TS, Leson CR, Paparo AA: Text/Atlas of Histology. Philadelphia, WB Saunders, 1988.

All **branched exocrine glands** contain epithelial components (secretory acini and ducts) called **parenchyma**, and supporting connective tissue, including blood vessels and nerves, the **stroma.**

The gland is enclosed by a connective tissue **capsule** that branches inside the gland forming **septa** (singular *septum*) that subdivide the parenchyma.

In large branched glands, the parenchyma is anatomically subdivided into **lobes**. Adjacent lobes are separated by an **interlobar septum.** A lobe is formed by **lobules**, separated from each other by a thin **interlobular septum.**

Septa support the major branches of the **excretory duct. Interlobular ducts** extend along **interlobular septa; interlobar ducts** extend along **interlobar septa.** However, **intralobular ducts** lie within lobules and are surrounded by little connective tissue.

Intralobular ducts are lined by a **simple cuboidal-to-columnar epithelium,** whereas the epithelial lining of **interlobular ducts** is pseudostratified columnar. **Lobar ducts** are lined by a **stratified columnar epithelium.**

> **Box 17-A | Classification of exocrine glands**
>
> • Depending on the **structure of the excretory duct**, glands can be divided into **simple** (unbranched duct) and **branched** or **compound** (branched duct).
> • According to the **structure of the secretory units**, glands can be classified as **tubular** or **alveolar** (acinar).
> • Considering the **secretory product**, glands are **serous** when they secrete a watery fluid, or **mucous** when the secretion is thick and rich in glycoproteins.
> • Taking into account the **secretory mechanism**, glands can be **merocrine** when the product is released by exocytosis (for example, the pancreas). In **holocrine** glands, the whole cell is the secretory product (for example, the sebaceous glands of the skin). An **apocrine** gland releases its product together with a small amount of the apical cytoplasm of the secretory cell (for example, the mammary gland).

by the **islet of Langerhans**) is described in Chapter 19, Endocrine System.

3. The **liver**, a combined endocrine and exocrine gland, has extensive access to the blood circulation and releases **bile** into the duodenum. Bile is a complex mixture of organic and inorganic components that enable the absorption of fats by the small intestine.

The structure and function of the **gallbladder** are included at the end of the liver section.

Branching duct system of a salivary gland

We initiate the discussion with the general organization of a salivary gland, in particular its branching ducts (see Box 17-A).

The secretory product of an acinus is drained sequentially by the following (Figures 17-1 and 17-2):

1. An **intercalated duct** (lined by **low squamous-to-cuboidal epithelium**). The intercalated duct is longest in the parotid gland.

2. A **striated duct** (a segment lined by **cuboidal-to-columnar epithelial cells** with **basal infoldings** containing numerous **mitochondria**). The striated duct is well developed in the submandibular gland. The epithelium of the striated duct participates in ion and water transport and secretes kallikrein. Both intercalated and striated ducts are modestly developed in the sublingual gland.

3. The intercalated, striated, and excretory intralobular segments are observed **within the lobule**, embedded in the connective tissue septa. An **excretory intralobular duct** is initially lined by **cuboidal-to-columnar epithelium**; it becomes pseudostratified columnar when it joins the interlobular duct.

4. Intralobular ducts join to form the **interlobular duct**, which is located **outside the lobule**, between adjacent lobules. An **interlobular duct** is lined by **pseudostratified columnar epithelium**.

5. Interlobular ducts converge to form a **lobar duct**. Lobar ducts (lined by **stratified columnar epithelium,** one of the few sites in the body lined by this type of epithelium) join the **main duct** (lined by **stratified squamous epithelium**) near the opening into the oral cavity.

The **parotid**, **submandibular** (or **submaxillary**), and **sublingual glands** are classified as **branched tubuloalveolar glands**. Their excretory ducts open into the oral cavity.

Saliva is the major product of salivary glands

Saliva, amounting to a half-liter daily, contains proteins, glycoproteins (mucus), ions, water, and immunoglobulin A (IgA) (Figure 17-3). The submandibular gland produces about 70% of the saliva. The parotid gland contributes 25% and secretes an amylase-rich saliva. The production of saliva is under the control of the autonomic nervous system. Upon stimulation, the parasympathetic system induces the secretion of a water-rich saliva; the sympathetic system stimulates the release of a protein-rich saliva.

The mucus and water in saliva **lubricate** the mucosa of the tongue, cheek, and lips during speech and swallowing, dissolve food for the function of the taste buds, and moisten food for easy swallowing. The **protective** function of the saliva depends on the antibacterial function of three constituents of saliva: (1) **lysozyme**, which attacks the walls of bacteria; (2) **lactoferrin**, which chelates iron necessary for bacterial growth; and (3) **IgA**, which neutralizes bacteria and viruses. The **digestive** function of saliva relies on (1) **amylase** (ptyalin), which initiates the digestion of carbohydrates (starch) in the oral cavity; and (2) **lingual lipase**, which participates in the hydrolysis of dietary lipids.

Parotid gland

The parotid gland is the largest salivary gland. It is a **branched tubuloalveolar gland** surrounded by a connective tissue capsule with **septa**—representing a component of the **stroma**, the supporting tissue of the gland. Adipose cells are

Figure 17-2. General organization of the salivary glands and pancreas

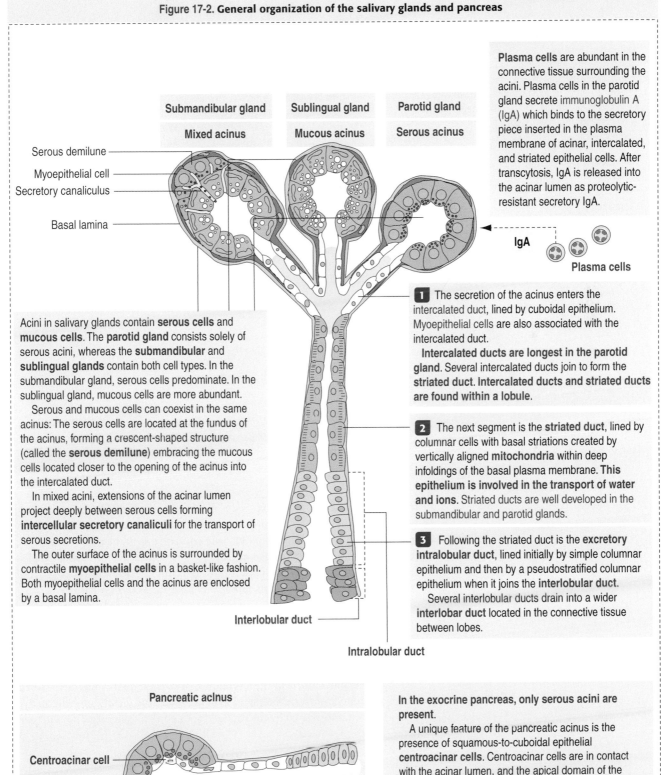

Plasma cells are abundant in the connective tissue surrounding the acini. Plasma cells in the parotid gland secrete immunoglobulin A (IgA) which binds to the secretory piece inserted in the plasma membrane of acinar, intercalated, and striated epithelial cells. After transcytosis, IgA is released into the acinar lumen as proteolytic-resistant secretory IgA.

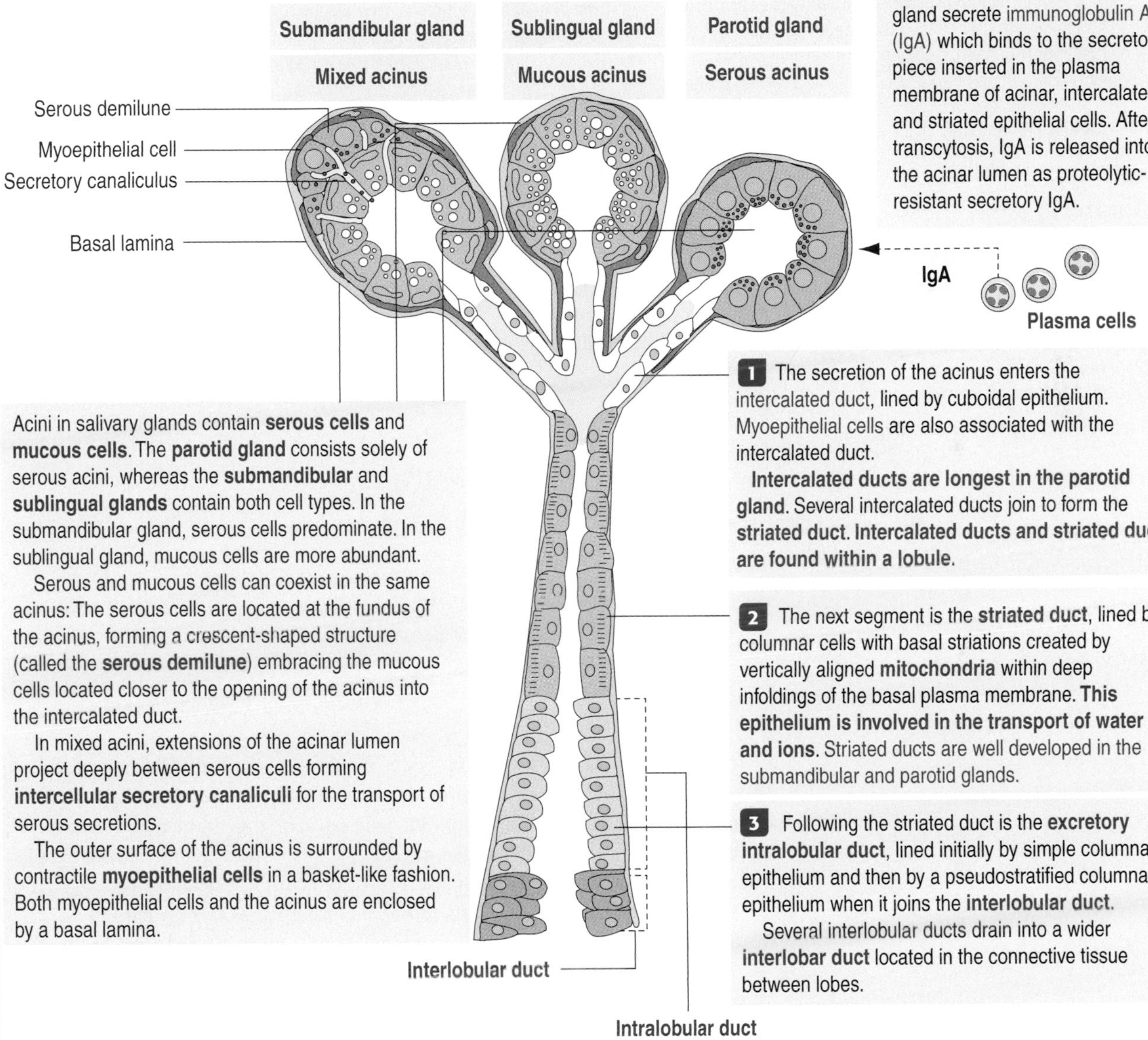
Submandibular gland
Mixed acinus
Sublingual gland
Mucous acinus
Parotid gland
Serous acinus
Serous demilune
Myoepithelial cell
Secretory canaliculus
Basal lamina
IgA
Plasma cells
Interlobular duct
Intralobular duct

Acini in salivary glands contain **serous cells** and **mucous cells**. The **parotid gland** consists solely of serous acini, whereas the **submandibular** and **sublingual glands** contain both cell types. In the submandibular gland, serous cells predominate. In the sublingual gland, mucous cells are more abundant.

Serous and mucous cells can coexist in the same acinus: The serous cells are located at the fundus of the acinus, forming a crescent-shaped structure (called the **serous demilune**) embracing the mucous cells located closer to the opening of the acinus into the intercalated duct.

In mixed acini, extensions of the acinar lumen project deeply between serous cells forming **intercellular secretory canaliculi** for the transport of serous secretions.

The outer surface of the acinus is surrounded by contractile **myoepithelial cells** in a basket-like fashion. Both myoepithelial cells and the acinus are enclosed by a basal lamina.

1 The secretion of the acinus enters the intercalated duct, lined by cuboidal epithelium. Myoepithelial cells are also associated with the intercalated duct.

Intercalated ducts are longest in the parotid gland. Several intercalated ducts join to form the **striated duct. Intercalated ducts and striated ducts are found within a lobule.**

2 The next segment is the **striated duct**, lined by columnar cells with basal striations created by vertically aligned **mitochondria** within deep infoldings of the basal plasma membrane. **This epithelium is involved in the transport of water and ions.** Striated ducts are well developed in the submandibular and parotid glands.

3 Following the striated duct is the **excretory intralobular duct**, lined initially by simple columnar epithelium and then by a pseudostratified columnar epithelium when it joins the **interlobular duct.**

Several interlobular ducts drain into a wider **interlobar duct** located in the connective tissue between lobes.

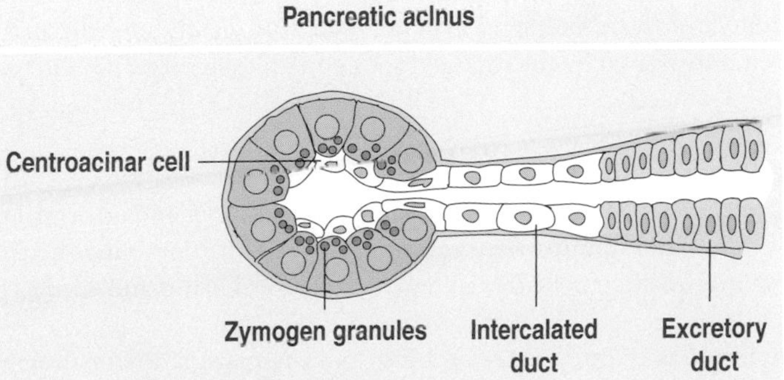
Pancreatic acinus
Centroacinar cell
Zymogen granules
Intercalated duct
Excretory duct

In the exocrine pancreas, only serous acini are present.

A unique feature of the pancreatic acinus is the presence of squamous-to-cuboidal epithelial **centroacinar cells.** Centroacinar cells are in contact with the acinar lumen, and the apical domain of the serous acinar cells is in continuity with the intercalated duct. Centroacinar cells can be regarded as the intra-acinar segment of the intercalated duct.

Striated ducts and myoepithelial cells are not present in the exocrine pancreas.

Figure 17-3. Functional aspects of a salivary gland

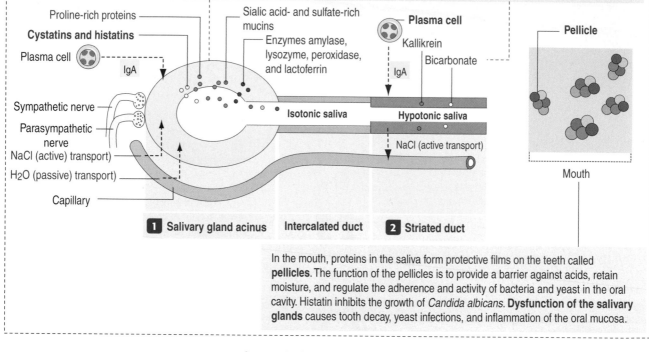

1 **Acinar cells** pump Na+ and Cl⁻ actively into the acinar lumen and allow free passage of water from the surrounding blood capillaries. This results in the formation of isotonic primary saliva. **Mucous cells** release mucins. **Serous cells** secrete several proteins, including proline-rich proteins (which are modified in the striated duct by the enzyme kallikrein), enzymes (amylases, peroxidases, lysozyme), lactoferrin, cystatins (cysteine-rich proteins), and histatins (histidine-rich proteins).

2 In the **striated duct**, Na+ and Cl⁻ are reabsorbed and the saliva becomes hypotonic. **Kallikrein**, a serine protease secreted by epithelial cells of the striated duct, processes the proline-rich proteins and cystatins in the saliva. In addition, plasma cells secrete immunoglobulin A (**IgA**) which reaches the lumen of the acinus and striated duct by transcytosis. The final saliva contains a complex of proteins with antimicrobial activity and with digestive function (amylase). **Bicarbonate**, the primary buffering agent of the saliva, is produced in the **striated duct**.

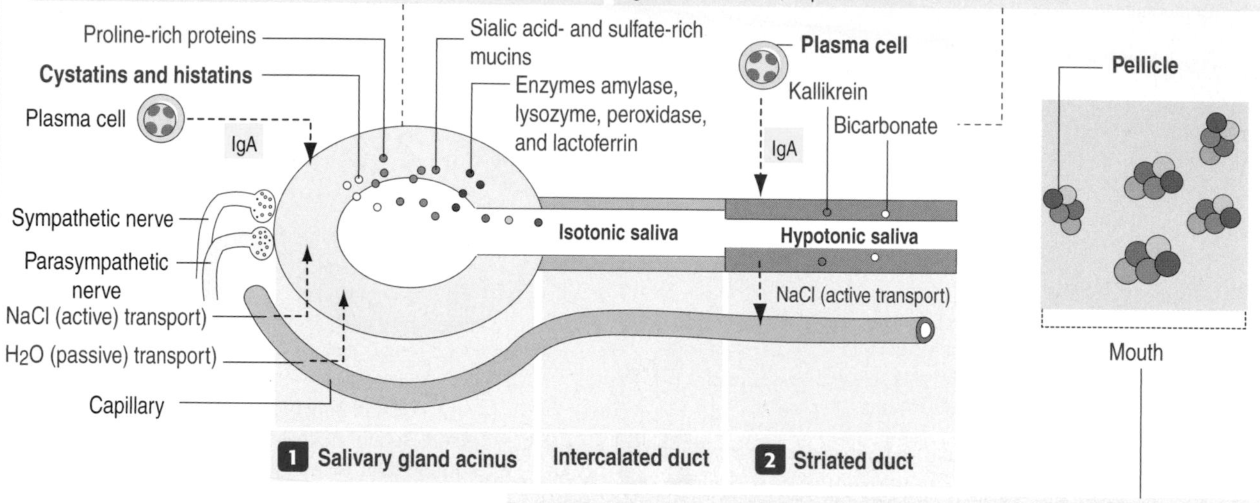

Proline-rich proteins
Cystatins and histatins
Plasma cell
IgA
Sialic acid- and sulfate-rich mucins
Enzymes amylase, lysozyme, peroxidase, and lactoferrin
Plasma cell
Kallikrein
Bicarbonate
IgA
Pellicle
Sympathetic nerve
Parasympathetic nerve
NaCl (active) transport)
H2O (passive) transport)
Capillary
Isotonic saliva
Hypotonic saliva
NaCl (active transport)
Mouth
1 Salivary gland acinus
Intercalated duct
2 Striated duct

In the mouth, proteins in the saliva form protective films on the teeth called **pellicles**. The function of the pellicles is to provide a barrier against acids, retain moisture, and regulate the adherence and activity of bacteria and yeast in the oral cavity. Histatin inhibits the growth of *Candida albicans*. **Dysfunction of the salivary glands** causes tooth decay, yeast infections, and inflammation of the oral mucosa.

frequently found in the stroma. Septa divide the gland into lobes and lobules (see Figure 17-1). Septa also provide support to blood vessels, lymphatics, and nerves gaining access to the acini, the main components of the **parenchyma**—the functional constituent of the gland. Acini are surrounded by reticular connective tissue, a rich capillary network, plasma cells, and lymphocytes. Acini consist mainly of **serous secretory cells** and, therefore, are classified as **serous acini**.

Each serous acinus is lined by pyramidal cells with a basally located nucleus. Similar to all protein-producing cells, a prominent rough endoplasmic reticulum system occupies the cell basal region. Secretory granules are visible in the apical region (Figure 17-4).

The lumen of the acinus collects the secretory products, which are transported by **long intercalated ducts to the less abundant striated ducts** (Figure 17-5). The secretory product of the serous acini is modified by the secretion of the striated duct and then transported by the oral cavity by a main excretory duct (Stensen's duct).

Clinical significance: Mumps, rabies, and tumors

In addition to its role in the production of saliva, the parotid gland is the primary target of the **rabies and mumps virus** transmitted in saliva containing the virus. The mumps virus causes transient swelling of the parotid gland and confers immunity.

Two complications of mumps are **orchitis** and **meningitis**. Bilateral orchitis caused by the mumps virus can result in sterility.

The parotid gland is the most frequent site for slow-growing **benign salivary gland tumors**. Its surgical removal is complicated by the need to protect the facial

Figure 17-4. **Histologic aspects of the major salivary glands**

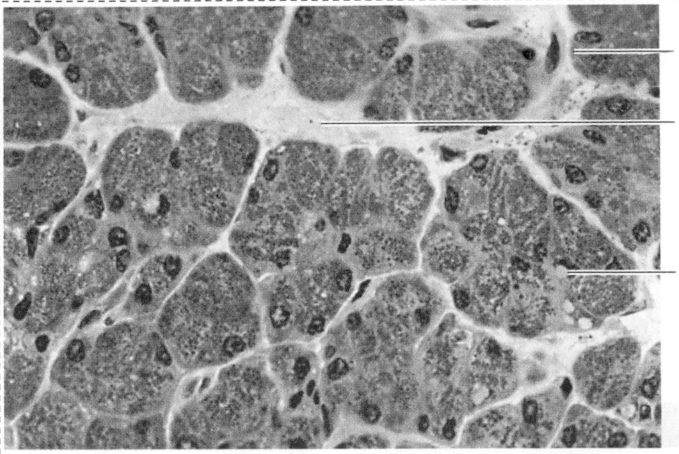

Myoepithelial cell
Connective tissue septum
Serous acinus
Parotid gland

The **parotid gland** is formed by acini containing exclusively serous cells with a basal nucleus and an apical cytoplasm with secretory granules. Granules are rich in proteins, including **proline-rich proteins, enzymes** (amylase, peroxidase, and lysozyme), and proteins with antimicrobial activity (**cystatins** and **histatins**). Although not visible in this image, **the parotid gland has the longest intercalated ducts.**

Connective tissue and blood vessels (not seen here) surround the serous acini.

Myoepithelial cells can be visualized at the periphery of each acinus.

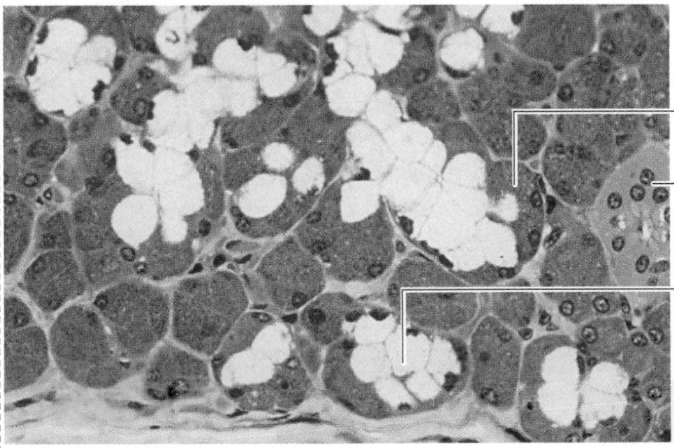

Serous demilune
Striated duct
Mucous cells in the mixed seromucous acinus
Submandibular gland

Submandibular glands are mixed serous and mucous tubuloacinar glands. **Mixed seromucous and serous acini are readily found. Pure mucous acini are uncommon in the submandibular gland.** Striated ducts lined by cuboid cells with basal infoldings, containing mitochondria, are observed within the lobule together with intercalated ducts (not seen here). Mucous cells secrete highly glycosylated mucins rich in sialic acid and sulfate that lubricate hard tissue surfaces, forming a thin protective film called a **pellicle**.

This film modulates the attachment of bacteria to oral surfaces and forms complexes with other proteins present in saliva.

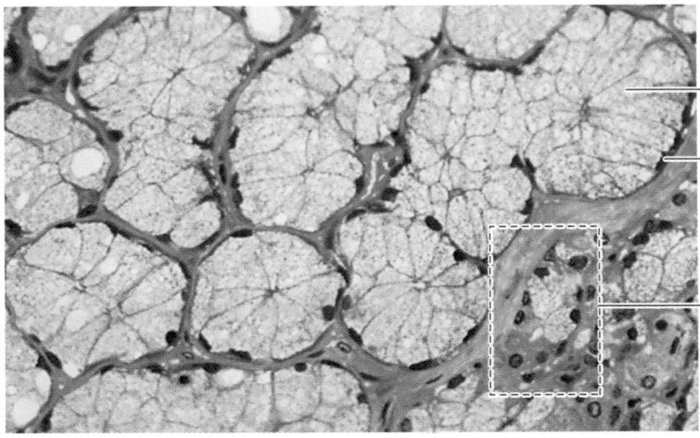

Mucous acinus
Basal nucleus of a mucous cell
Seromucous acinus
Sublingual gland

Sublingual glands are mixed serous and mucous tubuloacinar glands in which mucous cells predominate. A few seromucous acini can be found. **The intercalated and striated ducts are poorly developed in the sublingual gland.** Mucous cells resemble goblet cells of the intestinal epithelium. The nucleus is flattened against the basal plasma membrane. The apical region of the mucous cells is occupied by mucin-filled secretory vesicles (unstained). The cell boundaries are sharp. Mucous cells secrete highly glycosylated mucins that contribute to the formation of the protective pellicle film.

Serous acinar cell

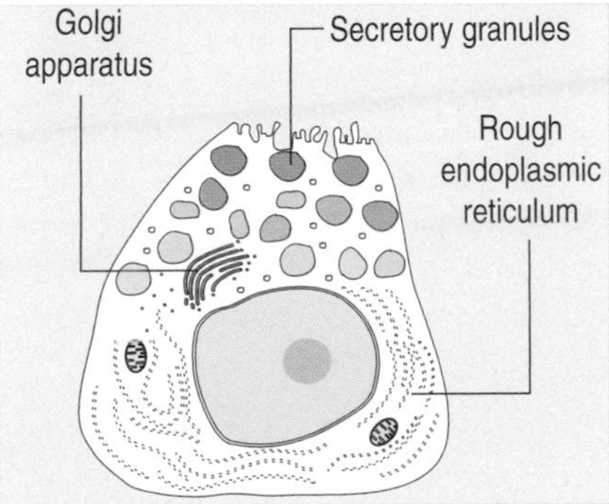

Golgi apparatus
Secretory granules
Rough endoplasmic reticulum

Mucous acinar cell

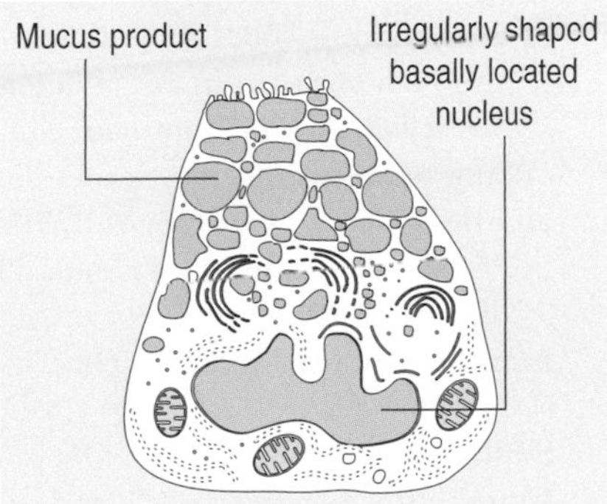

Mucus product
Irregularly shaped basally located nucleus

Striated duct cell

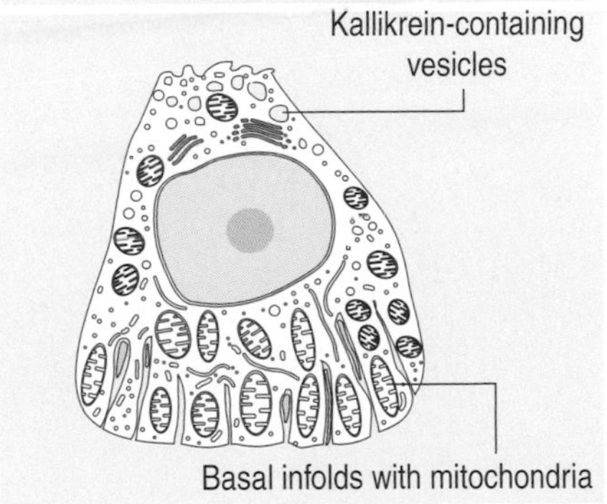

Kallikrein-containing vesicles
Basal infolds with mitochondria

Figure 17-5. **Structure of a mixed acinus and its striated duct**

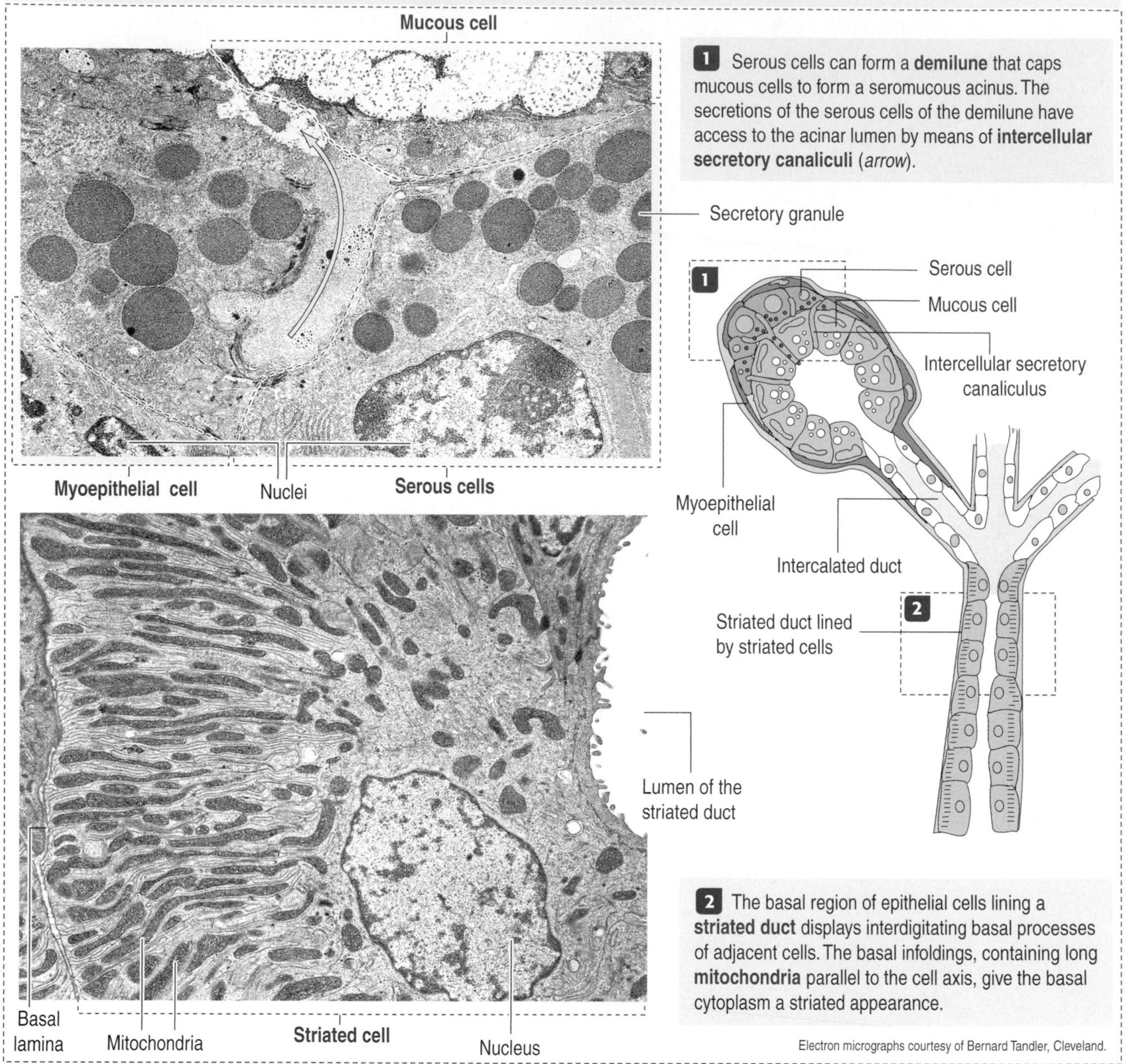
Mucous cell
1 Serous cells can form a **demilune** that caps mucous cells to form a seromucous acinus. The secretions of the serous cells of the demilune have access to the acinar lumen by means of **intercellular secretory canaliculi** (*arrow*).
Secretory granule
1
Serous cell
Mucous cell
Intercellular secretory canaliculus
Myoepithelial cell
Nuclei
Serous cells
Myoepithelial cell
Intercalated duct
2
Striated duct lined by striated cells
Lumen of the striated duct
2 The basal region of epithelial cells lining a **striated duct** displays interdigitating basal processes of adjacent cells. The basal infoldings, containing long **mitochondria** parallel to the cell axis, give the basal cytoplasm a striated appearance.
Basal lamina
Mitochondria
Striated cell
Nucleus
Electron micrographs courtesy of Bernard Tandler, Cleveland.

nerve running through the parotid gland.

Submandibular (submaxillary) gland

The submandibular gland is a branched tubuloalveolar gland surrounded by a connective tissue capsule. Septa derived from the capsule divide the parenchyma of the gland into lobes and lobules.

Although both serous and mucous cells are present in the secretory units, the **serous cells are the predominant component** (see Figure 17-4). Mucous cell–containing acini are capped by **serous demilunes. The intercalated ducts are shorter and the striated ducts longer than those in the parotid gland.** Adipocytes are not frequently seen in the submandibular gland.

The main excretory duct of the submandibular gland (Wharton's duct) opens near the frenulum of the tongue.

Sublingual gland

Contrasting with the parotid and submandibular glands, which are surrounded

Figure 17-6. **Exocrine pancreas**

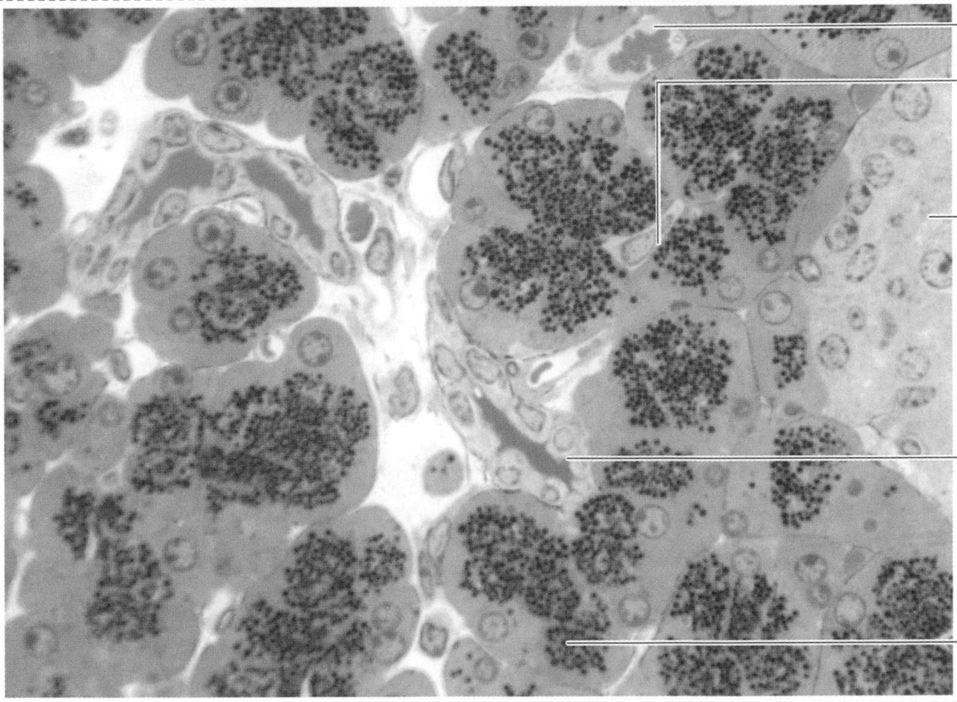

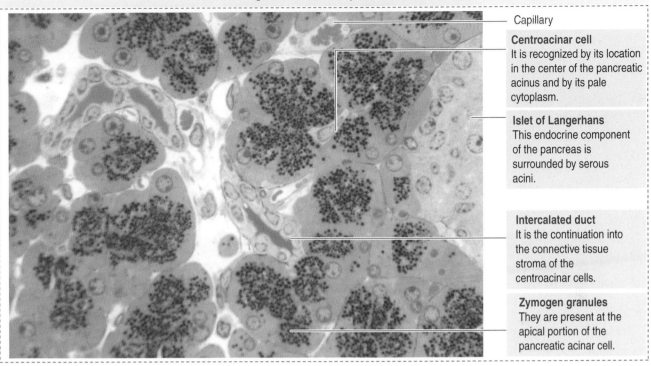

Capillary
Centroacinar cell
It is recognized by its location in the center of the pancreatic acinus and by its pale cytoplasm.
Islet of Langerhans
This endocrine component of the pancreas is surrounded by serous acini.
Intercalated duct
It is the continuation into the connective tissue stroma of the centroacinar cells.
Zymogen granules
They are present at the apical portion of the pancreatic acinar cell.

by a dense connective tissue capsule, the sublingual gland does not have a defined capsule. However, connective tissue septa divide the glandular parenchyma into small lobes. The sublingual gland is a branched **tubuloalveolar gland with both serous and mucous cells** (see Figure 17-4), although most of the secretory units contain mucous cells. **The intercalated and striated ducts are poorly developed.** Usually each lobe has its own excretory duct that opens beneath the tongue.

Exocrine pancreas

The pancreas is a combined **endocrine** and **exocrine gland**. The endocrine component is the **islet of Langerhans** and represents about 2% of the pancreas volume. The main function of the endocrine pancreas is the **regulation of glucose metabolism** by hormones secreted into the bloodstream (see discussion of the islet of Langerhans in Chapter 19, Endocrine System).

The exocrine pancreas is a **branched tubuloacinar gland** organized into four anatomic components: (1) a **head**, lying in the concavity of the second and third part of the duodenum; (2) a **neck**, in contact with the portal vein; (3) a **body**, placed anterior to the aorta; and (4) a **tail**, ending near the hilum of the spleen.

The pancreas lies close to the posterior abdominal wall in the upper abdomen, and therefore it is protected from severe trauma. Blood is provided by vessels derived from the celiac artery, the superior mesenteric artery, and the splenic artery. The venous drainage flows into the portal venous system and the splenic vein. Efferent innervation is through the vagus and splanchnic nerves.

The **main pancreatic duct (of Wirsung)** runs straight through the tail and the body, collecting secretions from ductal tributaries. It turns downward when it reaches the head of the pancreas and drains directly into the duodenum at the **ampulla of Vater**, after joining the **common bile duct**. A circular smooth **muscle sphincter (of Oddi)** is seen where the common pancreatic and bile duct cross the wall of the duodenum.

The pancreas has structural similarities to the salivary glands: (1) It is surrounded by connective tissue but does not have a capsule proper. (2) Lobules are separated by connective tissue septa containing blood vessels, lymphatics, nerves, and excretory ducts.

Figure 17-7. Pancreatic acinus

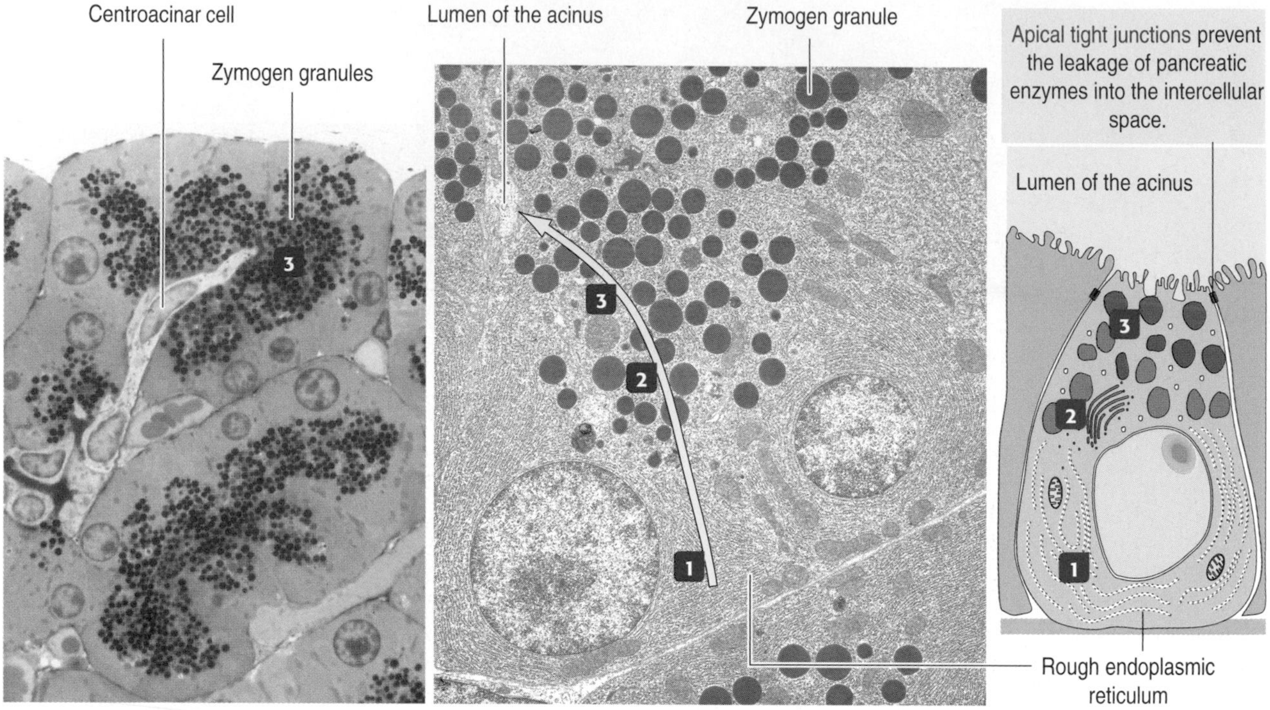

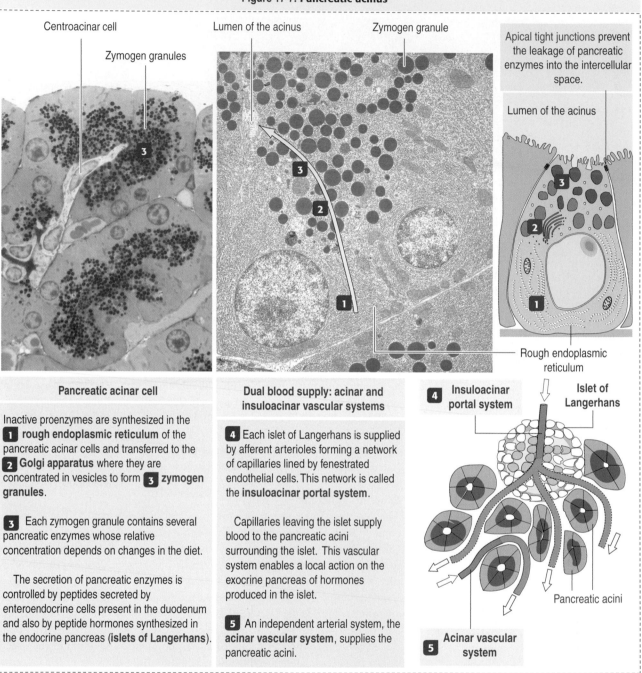

Centroacinar cell
Zymogen granules
Lumen of the acinus
Zymogen granule
Apical tight junctions prevent the leakage of pancreatic enzymes into the intercellular space.
Lumen of the acinus
Rough endoplasmic reticulum
1
2
3

Pancreatic acinar cell

Inactive proenzymes are synthesized in the **1 rough endoplasmic reticulum** of the pancreatic acinar cells and transferred to the **2 Golgi apparatus** where they are concentrated in vesicles to form **3 zymogen granules**.

3 Each zymogen granule contains several pancreatic enzymes whose relative concentration depends on changes in the diet.

The secretion of pancreatic enzymes is controlled by peptides secreted by enteroendocrine cells present in the duodenum and also by peptide hormones synthesized in the endocrine pancreas (**islets of Langerhans**).

Dual blood supply: acinar and insuloacinar vascular systems

4 Each islet of Langerhans is supplied by afferent arterioles forming a network of capillaries lined by fenestrated endothelial cells. This network is called the **insuloacinar portal system**.

Capillaries leaving the islet supply blood to the pancreatic acini surrounding the islet. This vascular system enables a local action on the exocrine pancreas of hormones produced in the islet.

5 An independent arterial system, the **acinar vascular system**, supplies the pancreatic acini.

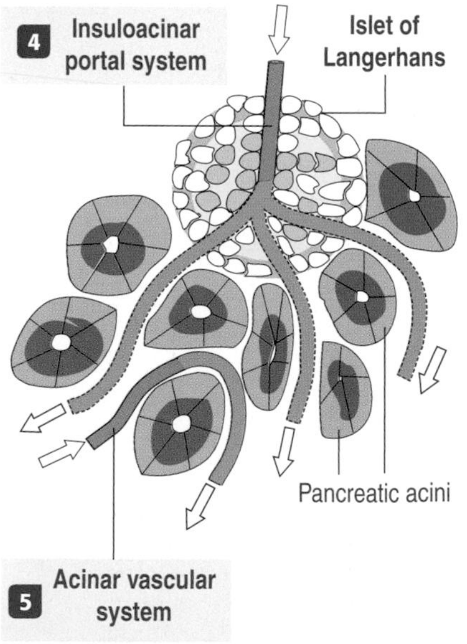

4 Insuloacinar portal system
Islet of Langerhans
Pancreatic acini
5 Acinar vascular system

The functional histologic unit of the exocrine pancreas is the **acinus** (Figures 17-6 to 17-8). The lumen of the acinus is the initiation of the secretory-excretory duct system and contains **centroacinar cells that are unique to the pancreas.** Centroacinar cells are continuous with the **low cuboidal epithelial** lining of the **intercalated duct. The exocrine pancreas lacks striated ducts and myoepithelial cells.** Intercalated ducts converge to form **interlobular ducts** lined by a **columnar epithelium** with a few goblet cells and occasional enteroendocrine cells. Interlobular ducts anastomose to form the **main pancreatic duct.**

Clinical significance: Carcinoma of the pancreas

The pancreatic duct–bile duct anatomic relationship is of clinical significance in **carcinoma of the pancreas** localized in the **head region**, because compression of the bile duct causes **obstructive jaundice**. The close association of the pancreas

Figure 17-8. Pancreatic acinus

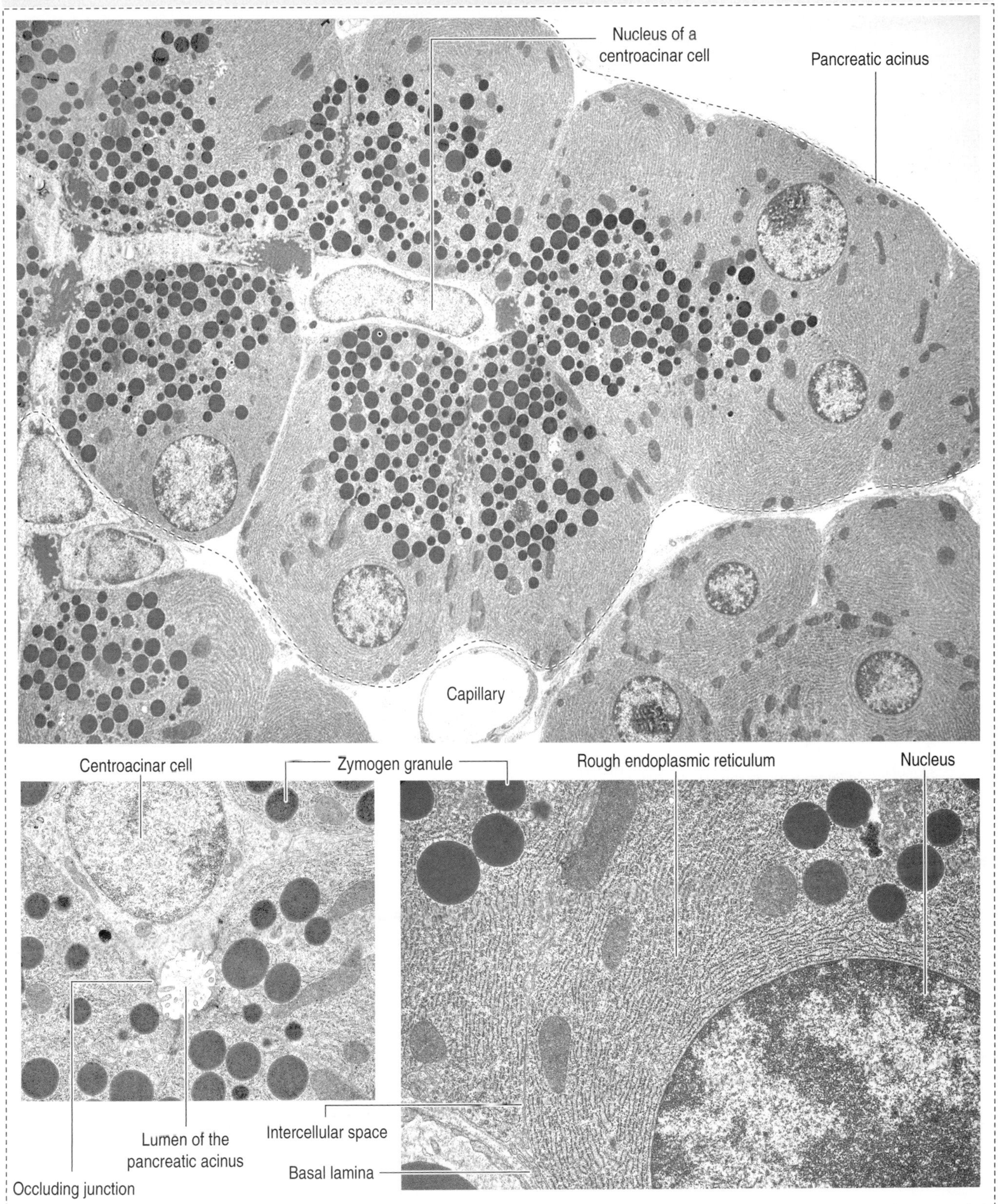

Nucleus of a centroacinar cell
Pancreatic acinus
Capillary
Centroacinar cell
Zymogen granule
Rough endoplasmic reticulum
Nucleus
Lumen of the pancreatic acinus
Intercellular space
Basal lamina
Occluding junction

with large blood vessels, the extensive and diffuse abdominal drainage to lymph nodes, and the frequent spread of carcinoma cells to the liver via the portal vein are factors contributing to the ineffectiveness of surgical removal of pancreatic tumors.

Figure 17-9. **Function of the exocrine pancreas**

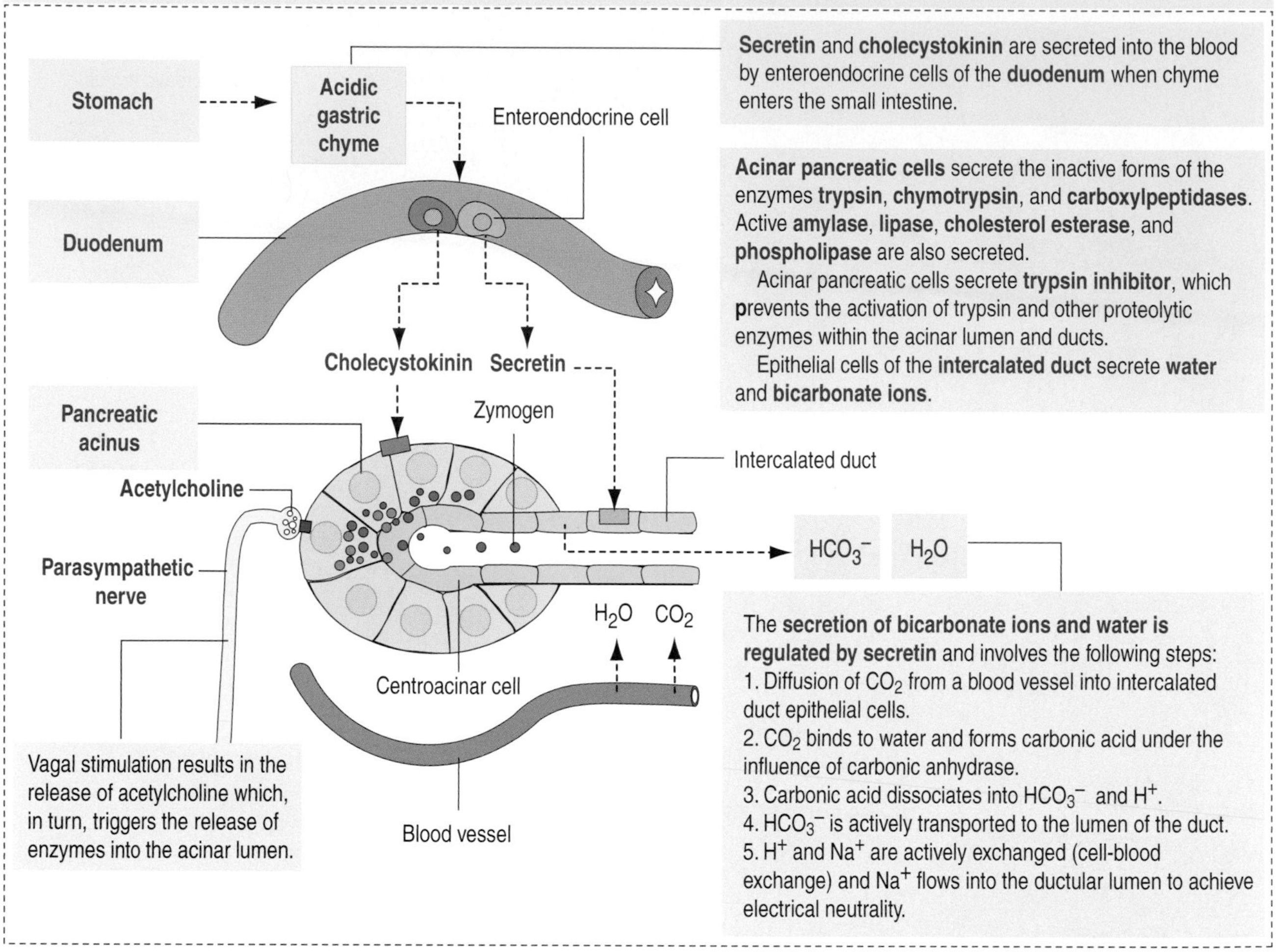

Secretin and cholecystokinin are secreted into the blood by enteroendocrine cells of the duodenum when chyme enters the small intestine.
Stomach
Acidic gastric chyme
Enteroendocrine cell
Duodenum
Acinar pancreatic cells secrete the inactive forms of the enzymes trypsin, chymotrypsin, and carboxylpeptidases. Active amylase, lipase, cholesterol esterase, and phospholipase are also secreted.
Acinar pancreatic cells secrete trypsin inhibitor, which prevents the activation of trypsin and other proteolytic enzymes within the acinar lumen and ducts.
Epithelial cells of the intercalated duct secrete water and bicarbonate ions.
Cholecystokinin
Secretin
Zymogen
Pancreatic acinus
Intercalated duct
Acetylcholine
HCO_3^-
H_2O
Parasympathetic nerve
H_2O
CO_2
Centroacinar cell
The secretion of bicarbonate ions and water is regulated by secretin and involves the following steps:
1. Diffusion of CO_2 from a blood vessel into intercalated duct epithelial cells.
2. CO_2 binds to water and forms carbonic acid under the influence of carbonic anhydrase.
3. Carbonic acid dissociates into HCO_3^- and H^+.
4. HCO_3^- is actively transported to the lumen of the duct.
5. H^+ and Na^+ are actively exchanged (cell-blood exchange) and Na^+ flows into the ductular lumen to achieve electrical neutrality.
Vagal stimulation results in the release of acetylcholine which, in turn, triggers the release of enzymes into the acinar lumen.
Blood vessel

Pancreatic acinus

The pancreatic acinus is lined by pyramidal cells joined to each other by apical junctional complexes (see Figure 17-8), which prevent the reflux of secreted products from the ducts into the intercellular spaces. The basal domain of an acinar pancreatic cell is associated with a basal lamina and contains the nucleus and a well-developed rough endoplasmic reticulum. The apical domain displays numerous **zymogen granules** (see Figure 17-8) and the Golgi apparatus.

The concentration of about 20 different pancreatic enzymes in the zymogen granules varies with the dietary intake. For example, an increase in the synthesis of **proteases** is associated with a **protein-rich diet**. A **carbohydrate-rich diet** results in the selective synthesis of **amylases** and a decrease in the synthesis of proteases. Amylase gene expression is regulated by insulin, an event that stresses the significance of the **insuloacinar portal system**.

The administration of a cholinergic drug or of the gastrointestinal hormones cholecystokinin and secretin increases the flow of pancreatic fluid (about 1.5 to 3.0 L/day).

The polypeptide hormone **cholecystokinin**, produced in enteroendocrine cells of the duodenal mucosa, binds to specific receptors of **acinar cells** and **stimulates the release of zymogen** (Figure 17-9).

Secretin is released when acid chyme enters the duodenum. Secretin is produced in the duodenum, binds to receptors on the surface of **intercalated ductal cells**, and **triggers the release of bicarbonate ions and water** into the pancreatic ducts. HCO_3^- ions and the alkaline secretion of Brunner's glands, present in the submucosa of the duodenum, neutralize the acidic gastric chyme in the duodenal

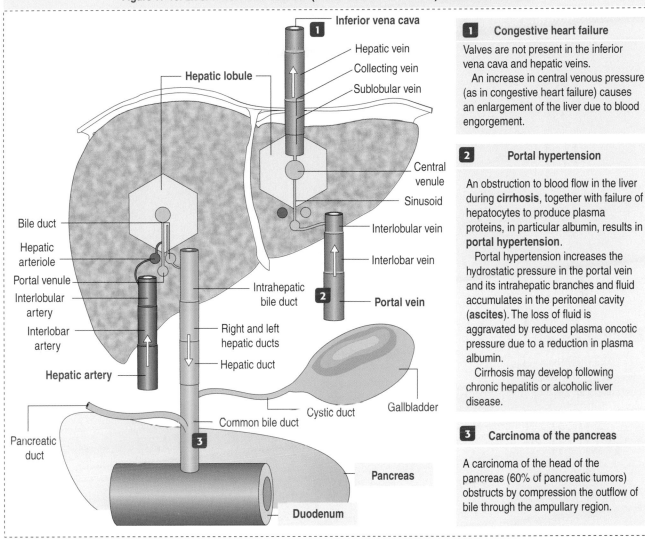

Figure 17-10. **Liver inflow and outflow (blood vessels and ducts) in clinical disease**

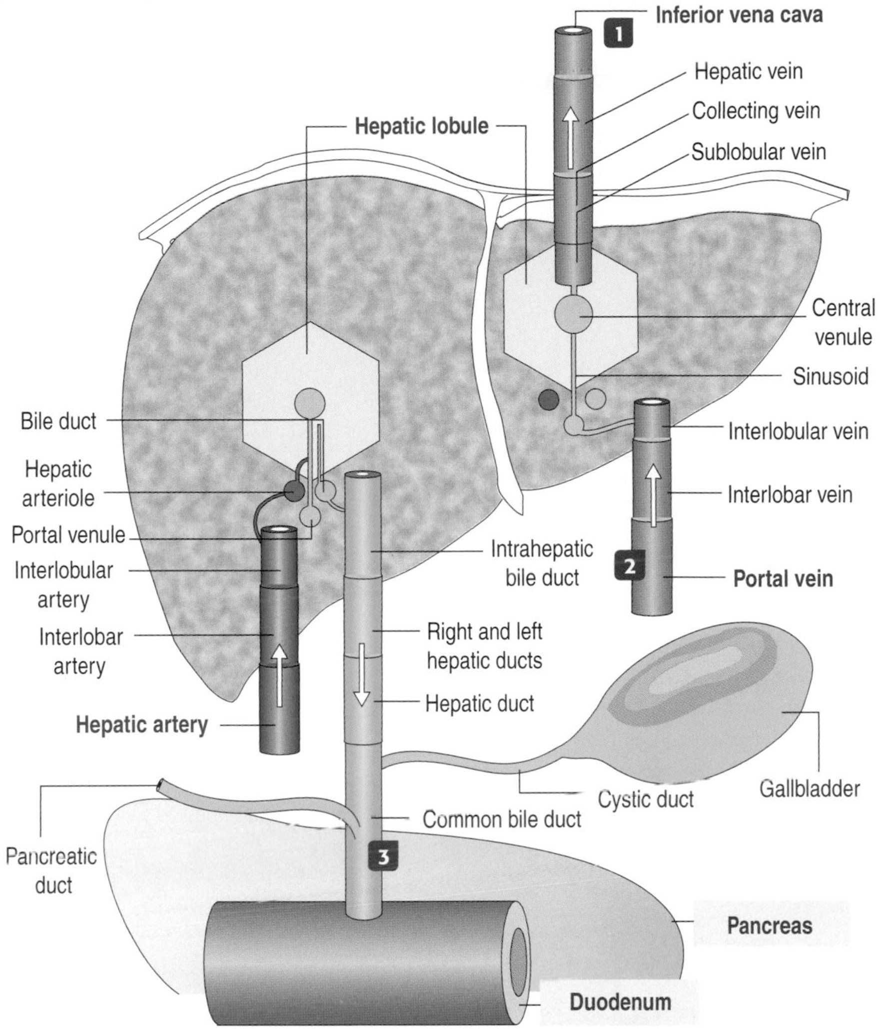

Inferior vena cava
Hepatic vein
Collecting vein
Sublobular vein
Hepatic lobule
Central venule
Sinusoid
Bile duct
Hepatic arteriole
Portal venule
Interlobular artery
Interlobar artery
Hepatic artery
Interlobular vein
Interlobar vein
Portal vein
Intrahepatic bile duct
Right and left hepatic ducts
Hepatic duct
Cystic duct
Gallbladder
Common bile duct
Pancreatic duct
Pancreas
Duodenum
1
2
3

1 Congestive heart failure

Valves are not present in the inferior vena cava and hepatic veins.

An increase in central venous pressure (as in congestive heart failure) causes an enlargement of the liver due to blood engorgement.

2 Portal hypertension

An obstruction to blood flow in the liver during **cirrhosis**, together with failure of hepatocytes to produce plasma proteins, in particular albumin, results in **portal hypertension**.

Portal hypertension increases the hydrostatic pressure in the portal vein and its intrahepatic branches and fluid accumulates in the peritoneal cavity (**ascites**). The loss of fluid is aggravated by reduced plasma oncotic pressure due to a reduction in plasma albumin.

Cirrhosis may develop following chronic hepatitis or alcoholic liver disease.

3 Carcinoma of the pancreas

A carcinoma of the head of the pancreas (60% of pancreatic tumors) obstructs by compression the outflow of bile through the ampullary region.

lumen and activate the pancreatic digestive enzymes.

Clinical significance: Acute pancreatitis and cystic fibrosis

Zymogen granules contain **inactive proenzymes** that are activated within the duodenal environment. A premature activation of pancreatic enzymes, in particular **trypsinogen** to **trypsin**, and the inactivation of **trypsin inhibitor** (tightly bound to the active site of trypsin), result in the autodigestion of pancreatic acini. This condition—known to occur in **acute hemorrhagic pancreatitis**—usually follows heavy meals or excessive alcohol ingestion. The clinical features of acute pancreatitis (severe abdominal pain, nausea, and vomiting) and rapid elevation of amylase and lipase in serum (within 24 to 72 hours) are typical diagnostic features.

Cystic fibrosis is an inherited, autosomal recessive disease affecting the function of mucus-secreting tissues of the respiratory (see Chapter 13, Respiratory System), intestinal, and reproductive systems; the sweat glands of the skin (see Chapter 11, Integumentary System); and the **exocrine pancreas** in children and young adults. A thick sticky mucus obstructs the duct passages of the airways, pancreatic and biliary ducts, and intestine, followed by bacterial infections and damage of the functional tissues. A large number of patients (85%) have **chronic pancreatitis** characterized by a loss of acini and dilation of the pancreatic excretory ducts into cysts surrounded by extensive fibrosis (hence the designation **cystic fibrosis of the pancreas**). Insufficient exocrine pancreatic secretions cause the malabsorption of

Figure 17-11. Histologic and functional classification of the hepatic lobule

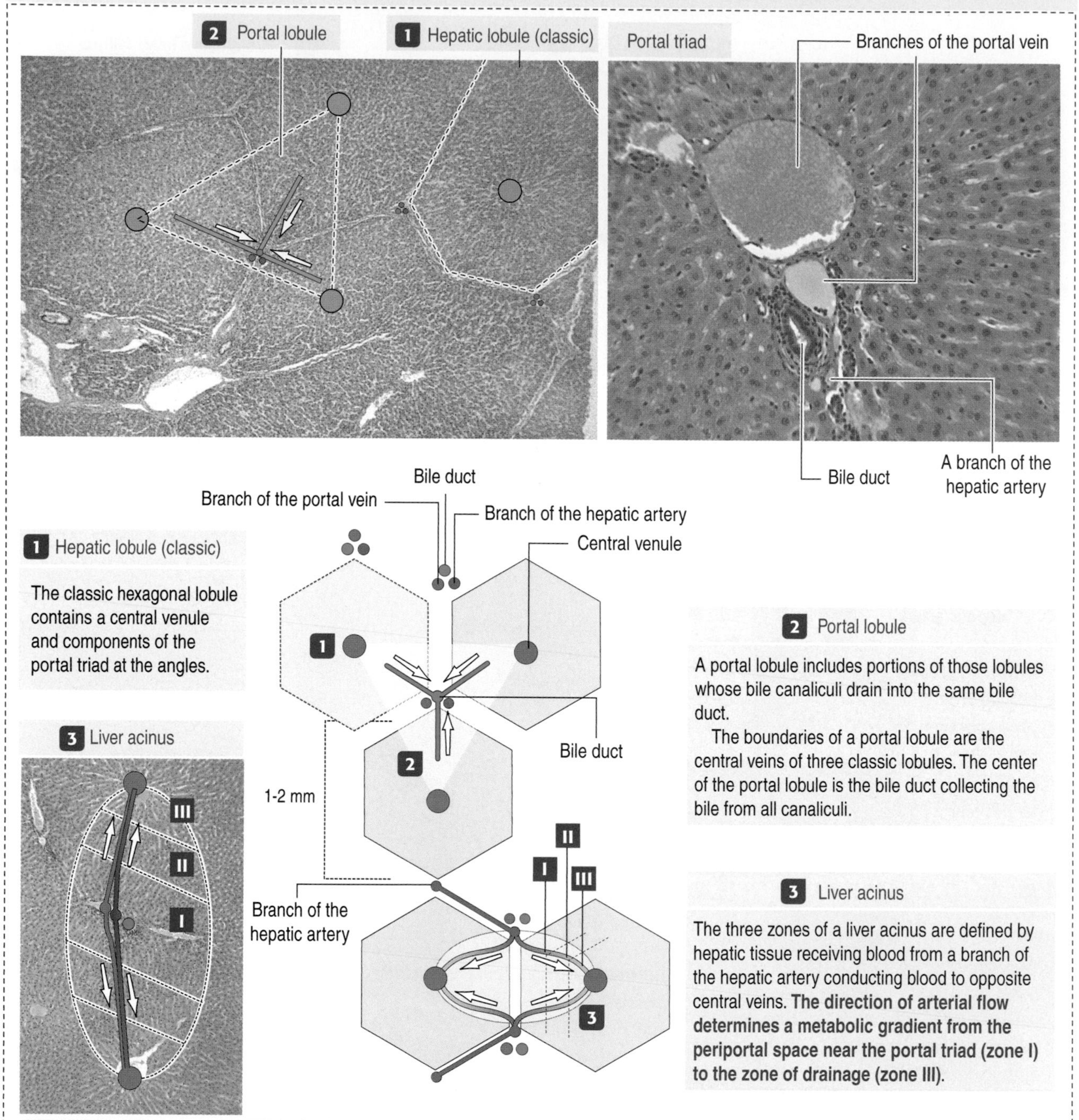

1 Hepatic lobule (classic)

The classic hexagonal lobule contains a central venule and components of the portal triad at the angles.

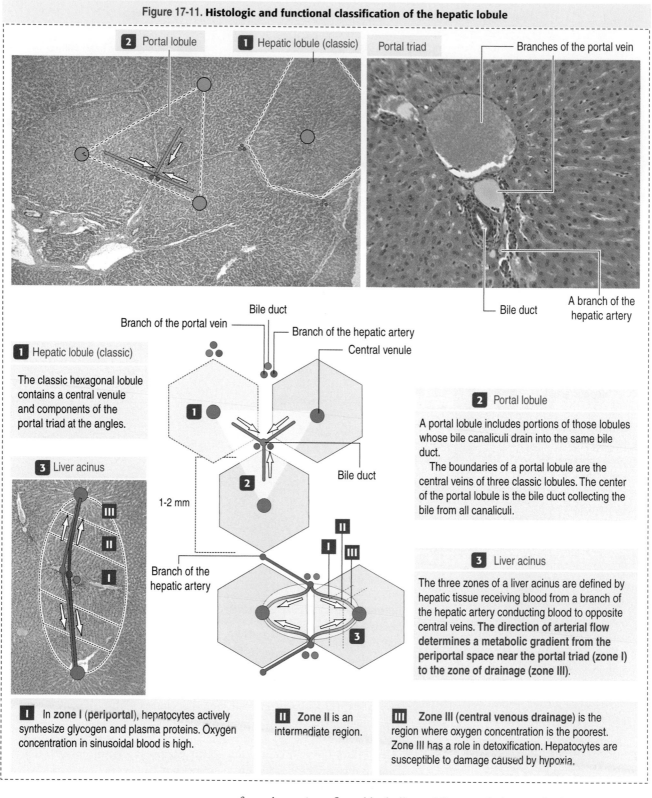

2 Portal lobule

A portal lobule includes portions of those lobules whose bile canaliculi drain into the same bile duct.

The boundaries of a portal lobule are the central veins of three classic lobules. The center of the portal lobule is the bile duct collecting the bile from all canaliculi.

3 Liver acinus

The three zones of a liver acinus are defined by hepatic tissue receiving blood from a branch of the hepatic artery conducting blood to opposite central veins. **The direction of arterial flow determines a metabolic gradient from the periportal space near the portal triad (zone I) to the zone of drainage (zone III).**

I In **zone I (periportal)**, hepatocytes actively synthesize glycogen and plasma proteins. Oxygen concentration in sinusoidal blood is high.

II **Zone II** is an intermediate region.

III **Zone III (central venous drainage)** is the region where oxygen concentration is the poorest. Zone III has a role in detoxification. Hepatocytes are susceptible to damage caused by hypoxia.

fat and protein, reflected by bulky and fatty stools (**steatorrhea**).

The lack of transport of Cl^- ions across epithelia is associated with a defective secretion of Na^+ ions and water. A genetic defect in the chloride channel protein called **cystic fibrosis transmembrane conductance regulator** (CFTR) is responsible for cystic fibrosis. The disease is detected by the demonstration of increased concentration of NaCl in sweat. Children with cystic fibrosis "taste salty" after copious sweating.

Figure 17-12. **Portal space and the bile ducts**

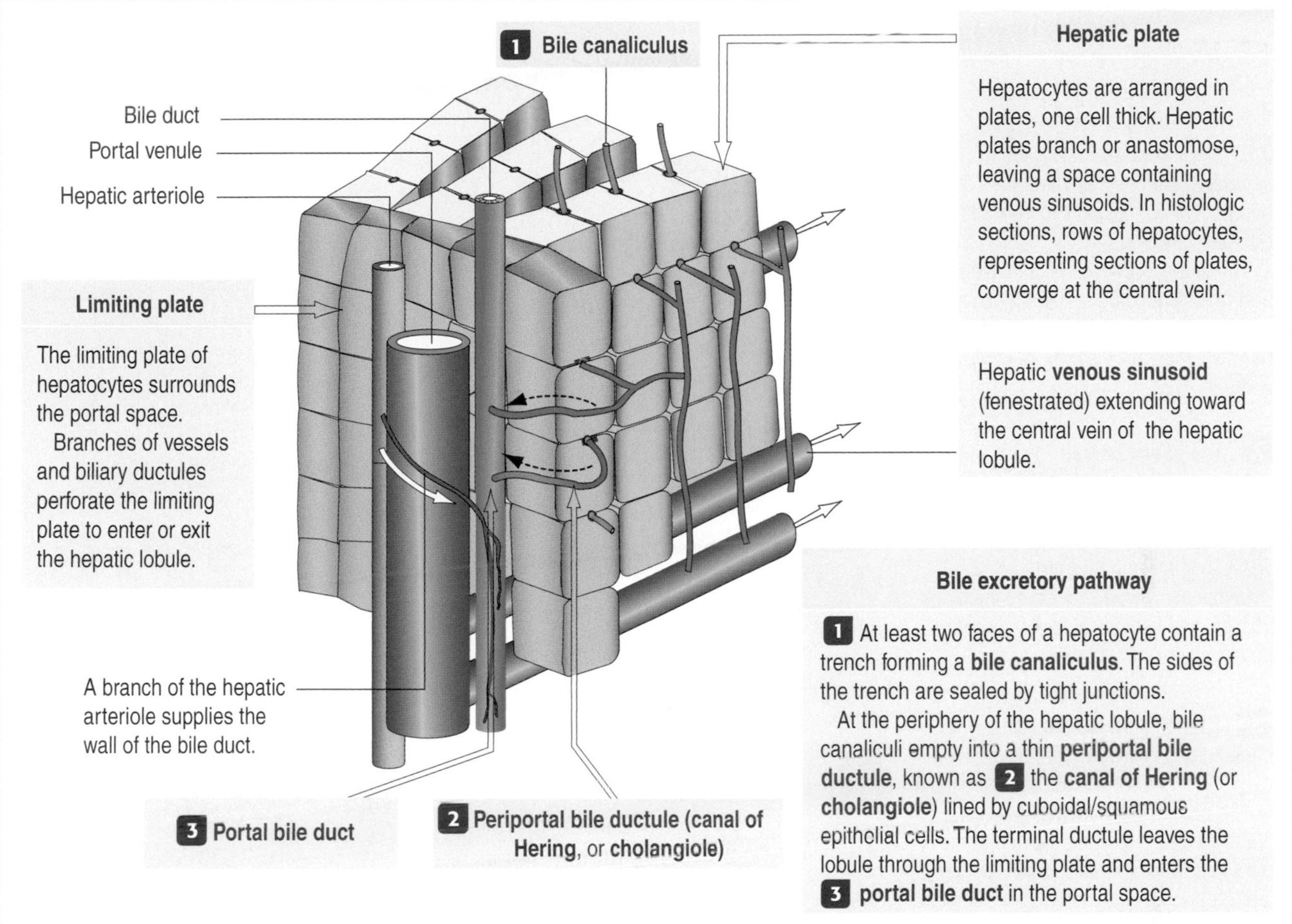
1 Bile canaliculus
Hepatic plate
Hepatocytes are arranged in plates, one cell thick. Hepatic plates branch or anastomose, leaving a space containing venous sinusoids. In histologic sections, rows of hepatocytes, representing sections of plates, converge at the central vein.
Bile duct
Portal venule
Hepatic arteriole
Limiting plate
The limiting plate of hepatocytes surrounds the portal space.
Branches of vessels and biliary ductules perforate the limiting plate to enter or exit the hepatic lobule.
Hepatic venous sinusoid (fenestrated) extending toward the central vein of the hepatic lobule.
A branch of the hepatic arteriole supplies the wall of the bile duct.
Bile excretory pathway
1 At least two faces of a hepatocyte contain a trench forming a bile canaliculus. The sides of the trench are sealed by tight junctions.
At the periphery of the hepatic lobule, bile canaliculi empty into a thin periportal bile ductule, known as 2 the canal of Hering (or cholangiole) lined by cuboidal/squamous epithelial cells. The terminal ductule leaves the lobule through the limiting plate and enters the 3 portal bile duct in the portal space.
3 Portal bile duct
2 Periportal bile ductule (canal of Hering, or cholangiole)

Liver

The liver, the largest gland of the human body, consists of four poorly defined **lobes**. The liver is surrounded by a collagen-elastic fiber–containing **capsule (of Glisson)** and is lined by the peritoneum.

Blood is supplied to the liver by two blood vessels (Figure 17-10): (1) The **portal vein** (75% to 80% of the afferent blood volume) transports blood from the digestive tract, spleen, and pancreas. (2) The **hepatic artery**, a branch of the celiac trunk, supplies 20% to 25% of oxygenated blood to the liver by the **interlobar artery** and **interlobular artery** pathway before reaching the **portal space**.

Blood from branches of the portal vein and the hepatic artery mixes in the **sinusoids** of the **liver lobules**, as we discuss in detail later. Sinusoidal blood converges at the **central venule** of the liver lobule. Central venules converge to form the **sublobular veins**, and blood returns to the **inferior vena cava** following the **collecting veins** and **hepatic veins** pathway.

The **right** and **left hepatic bile ducts** leave the liver and merge to form the **hepatic duct**. The hepatic duct becomes the **common bile duct** soon after giving rise to the **cystic duct**, a thin tube connecting the bile duct to the **gallbladder** (see Figure 17-10).

Hepatic lobule

The structural and functional unit of the liver is the **hepatic lobule**. The hepatic lobule consists of anastomosing **plates of hepatocytes** limiting blood **sinusoidal spaces** (see Figure 17-12). A **central venule** (or vein) in the core of the hepatic lobule collects the sinusoidal blood containing a mixture of blood supplied by branches of the portal vein and the hepatic artery.

Figure 17-13. **Organization of the hepatic lobule**

1 The perisinusoidal **space of Disse** separates the basolateral domain of the hepatocyte from blood circulating in the hepatic sinusoid.

The space of Disse contains type I, III, and IV collagen fibers. Protein absorption and secretion take place across the narrow space of Disse (0.2 to 0.5 μm wide).

2 The **space of Mall**—found at the periphery of the hepatic lobule—is continuous with the space of Disse. The space of Mall is drained by lymphatic vessels piercing the **limiting plate**.

Lymphatic vessels surround the blood vessels and bile ductules in the portal space.

3 The **canal of Hering** (or cholangiole) is the terminal point of the network of bile canalicular trenches found on the hepatocyte surfaces.

The canal of Hering is located at the periphery of the hepatic lobule (periportal site), is lined by a squamous-to-cuboidal simple epithelium, and connects with the bile ductules in the portal space after perforating the limiting plate.

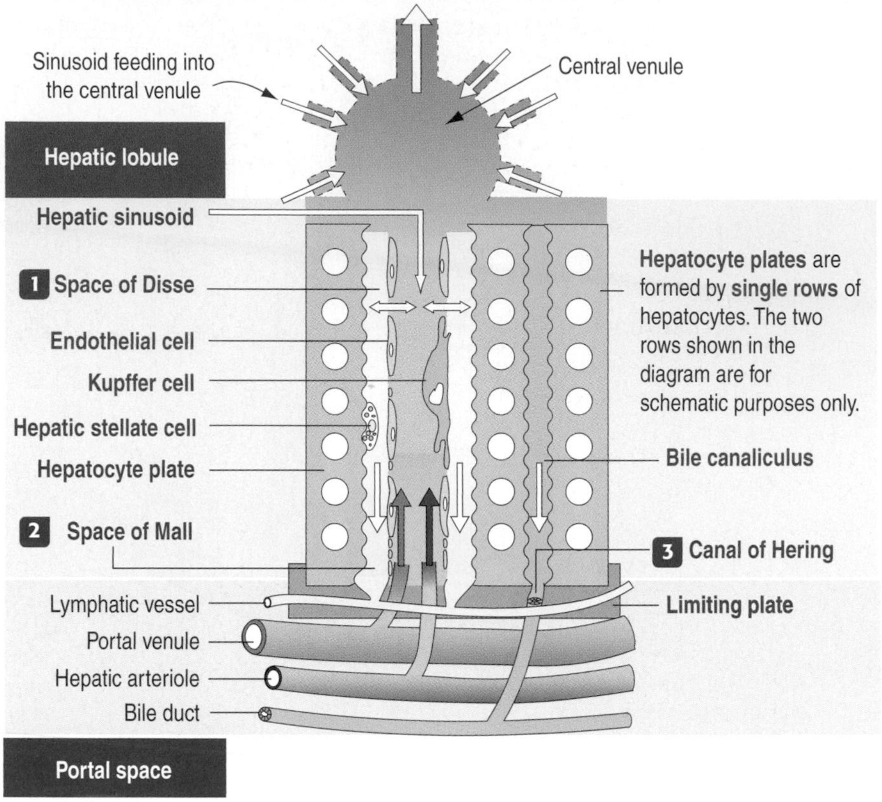

The connective tissue of the **portal space** provides support to the **portal triad** formed by branches of the **hepatic artery** (arteriole), **portal vein** (venule), and **bile duct** (ductule). In addition, lymphatic vessels and nerve fibers are present in the portal space (also designated portal canal, portal area, or portal tract).

Note that blood and bile and lymph flow in opposite directions

Branches of the hepatic artery and portal vein, together with a bile duct, form the classic **portal triad** found in the portal space surrounding the hexagonal-shaped hepatic lobule (Figure 17-11).

Bile produced in the hepatocytes is secreted into narrow intercellular spaces, the **bile canaliculi**, located between the apposed surfaces of adjacent hepatocytes.

Bile flows in the opposite direction to the blood. Bile flows from the **bile canaliculi** into **periportal bile ductules** (**cholangioles**, or **canals of Hering**), and then into the **bile ducts** (or ductules) of the portal space after crossing the **hepatic plate** at the periphery of the hepatic lobule (Figure 17-12). Bile ductules converge at the **intrahepatic bile ducts.**

Functional view of the hepatic lobule

There are three conceptual interpretations of the architecture of the liver lobule (see Figure 17-11): (1) the **classic concept** of the **hepatic lobule**, based on structural parameters; (2) the **portal lobule concept**, based on the bile drainage pathway from adjacent lobules toward the same bile duct; and (3) the **liver acinus concept**, based on the gradient distribution of oxygen along the venous sinusoids of adjacent lobules.

The **classic hepatic lobule** is customarily described as a polyhedral structure, usually depicted as a hexagon with a central venule to which blood sinusoids converge (see Figure 17-11).

Figure 17-14. Endoplasmic reticulum in hepatocytes

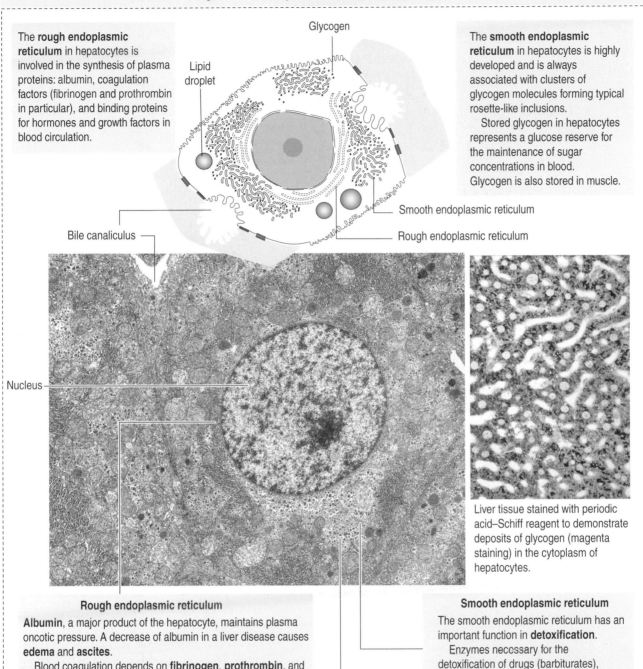

The **rough endoplasmic reticulum** in hepatocytes is involved in the synthesis of plasma proteins: albumin, coagulation factors (fibrinogen and prothrombin in particular), and binding proteins for hormones and growth factors in blood circulation.

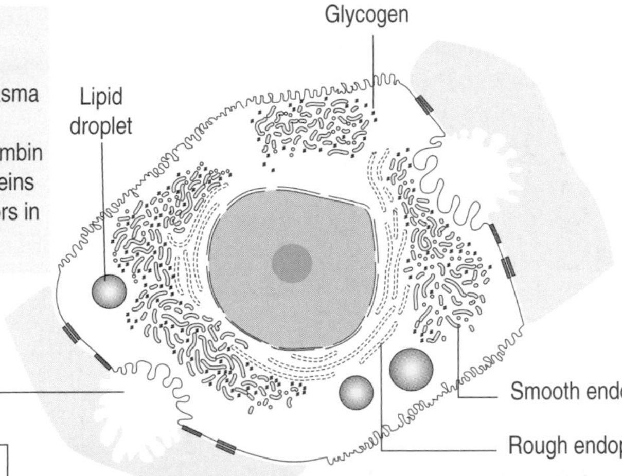

Glycogen
Lipid droplet
Smooth endoplasmic reticulum
Rough endoplasmic reticulum
Bile canaliculus

The **smooth endoplasmic reticulum** in hepatocytes is highly developed and is always associated with clusters of glycogen molecules forming typical rosette-like inclusions.

Stored glycogen in hepatocytes represents a glucose reserve for the maintenance of sugar concentrations in blood. Glycogen is also stored in muscle.

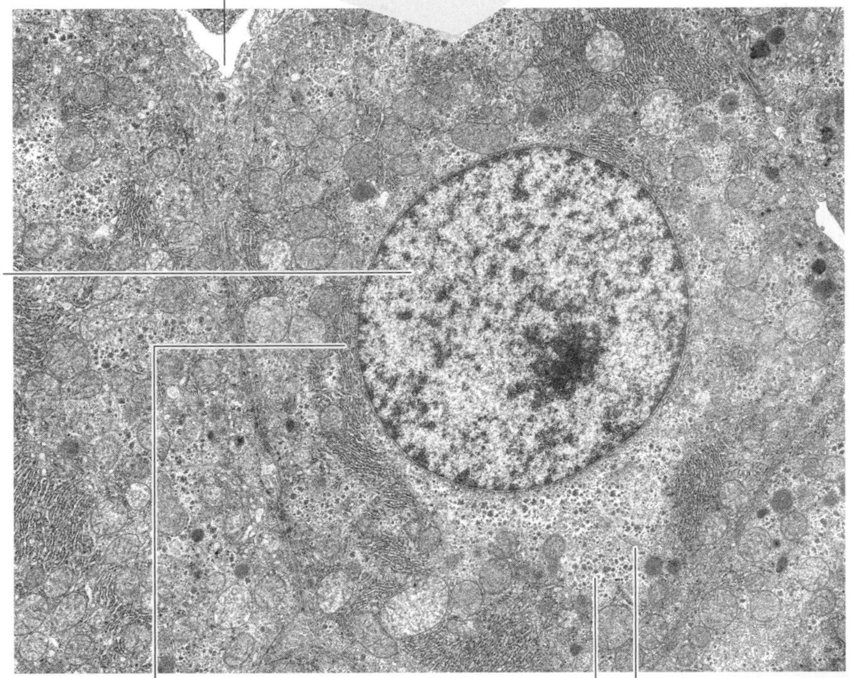

Nucleus
Glycogen

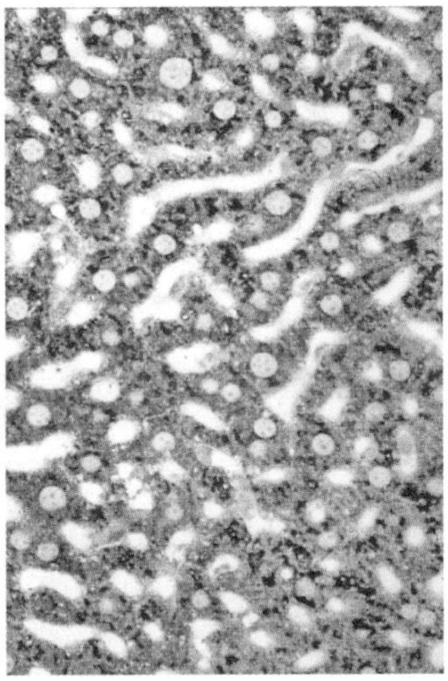

Liver tissue stained with periodic acid–Schiff reagent to demonstrate deposits of glycogen (magenta staining) in the cytoplasm of hepatocytes.

Rough endoplasmic reticulum

Albumin, a major product of the hepatocyte, maintains plasma oncotic pressure. A decrease of albumin in a liver disease causes **edema** and **ascites**.

Blood coagulation depends on **fibrinogen**, **prothrombin**, and **factor VIII** produced in the hepatocyte. **Bleeding** is associated with liver failure. **Complement proteins**, synthesized by hepatocytes, participate in the destruction of pathogens.

Smooth endoplasmic reticulum

The smooth endoplasmic reticulum has an important function in **detoxification**.

Enzymes necessary for the detoxification of drugs (barbiturates), steroids, alcohol, and other toxicants reside in the membrane of the smooth endoplasmic reticulum.

Components of the **portal triad**, constituting a branch of the portal vein and hepatic artery and a bile duct, are usually found at the angles of the hexagon. This geometric organization is poorly defined in humans because the limiting perilobular connective tissue is not abundant. However, recognition of the components of the portal triad is helpful in determining the boundaries of the human hepatic lobule.

In the **portal lobule**, the portal triad is the central axis, draining bile from the surrounding hepatic parenchyma.

Functional considerations have modified the classic view and a **liver acinus**

Figure 17-15. Apical and basolateral domains of hepatocytes

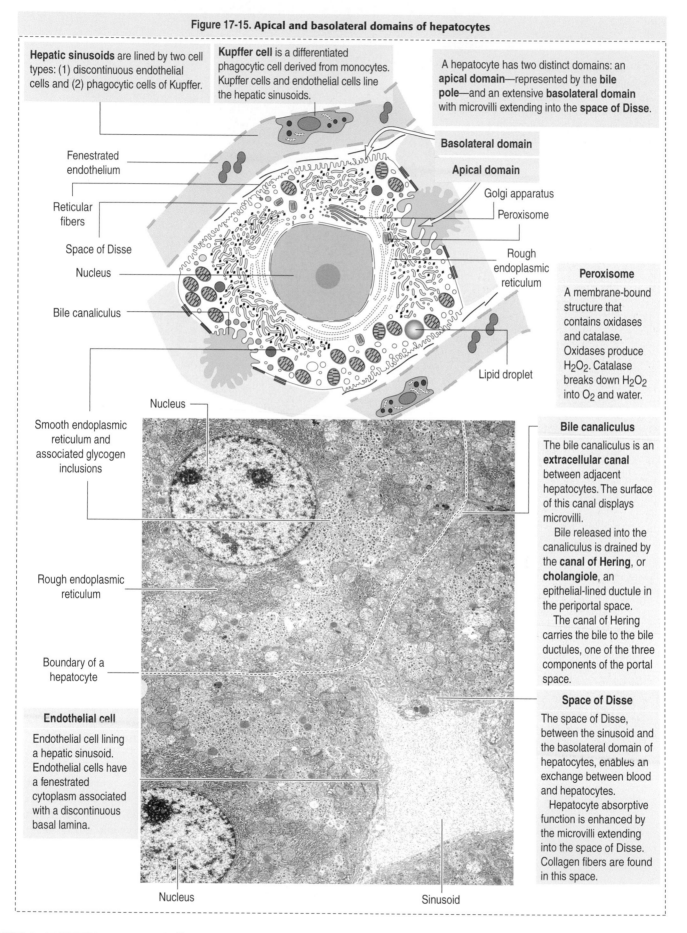

Hepatic sinusoids are lined by two cell types: (1) discontinuous endothelial cells and (2) phagocytic cells of Kupffer.

Kupffer cell is a differentiated phagocytic cell derived from monocytes. Kupffer cells and endothelial cells line the hepatic sinusoids.

A hepatocyte has two distinct domains: an **apical domain**—represented by the **bile pole**—and an extensive **basolateral domain** with microvilli extending into the **space of Disse**.

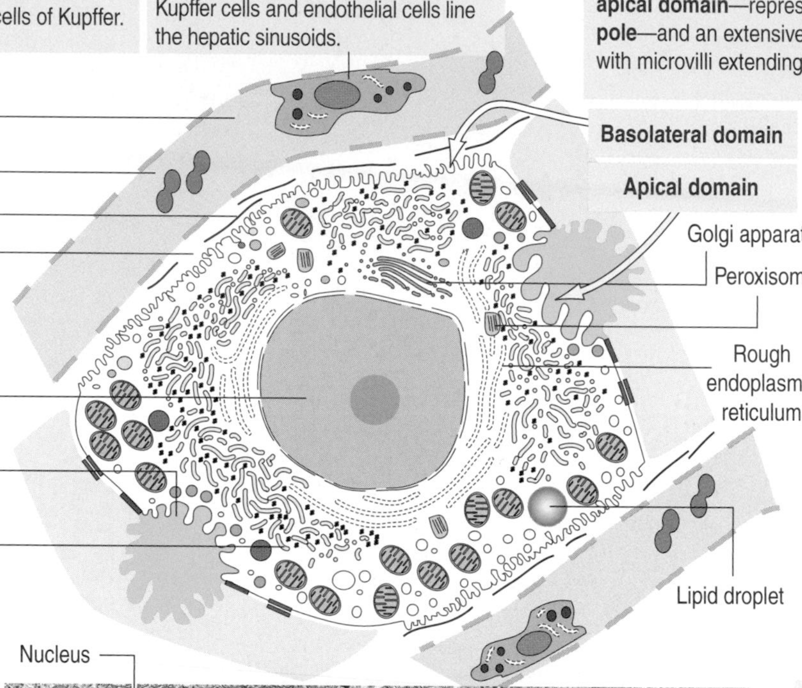

Fenestrated endothelium
Reticular fibers
Space of Disse
Nucleus
Bile canaliculus
Basolateral domain
Apical domain
Golgi apparatus
Peroxisome
Rough endoplasmic reticulum
Lipid droplet
Smooth endoplasmic reticulum and associated glycogen inclusions

Peroxisome

A membrane-bound structure that contains oxidases and catalase. Oxidases produce H_2O_2. Catalase breaks down H_2O_2 into O_2 and water.

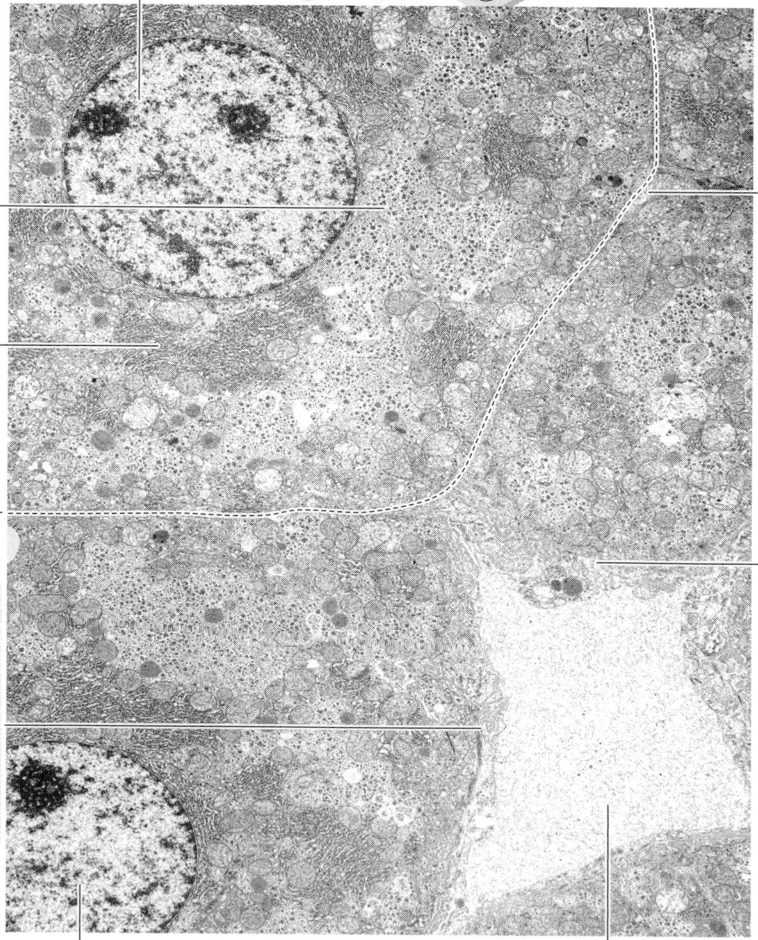

Nucleus
Smooth endoplasmic reticulum and associated glycogen inclusions
Rough endoplasmic reticulum
Boundary of a hepatocyte
Nucleus
Sinusoid

Bile canaliculus

The bile canaliculus is an **extracellular canal** between adjacent hepatocytes. The surface of this canal displays microvilli.

Bile released into the canaliculus is drained by the **canal of Hering**, or **cholangiole**, an epithelial-lined ductule in the periportal space.

The canal of Hering carries the bile to the bile ductules, one of the three components of the portal space.

Space of Disse

The space of Disse, between the sinusoid and the basolateral domain of hepatocytes, enables an exchange between blood and hepatocytes.

Hepatocyte absorptive function is enhanced by the microvilli extending into the space of Disse. Collagen fibers are found in this space.

Endothelial cell

Endothelial cell lining a hepatic sinusoid. Endothelial cells have a fenestrated cytoplasm associated with a discontinuous basal lamina.

Figure 17-16. Hepatic sinusoids and bile canaliculi

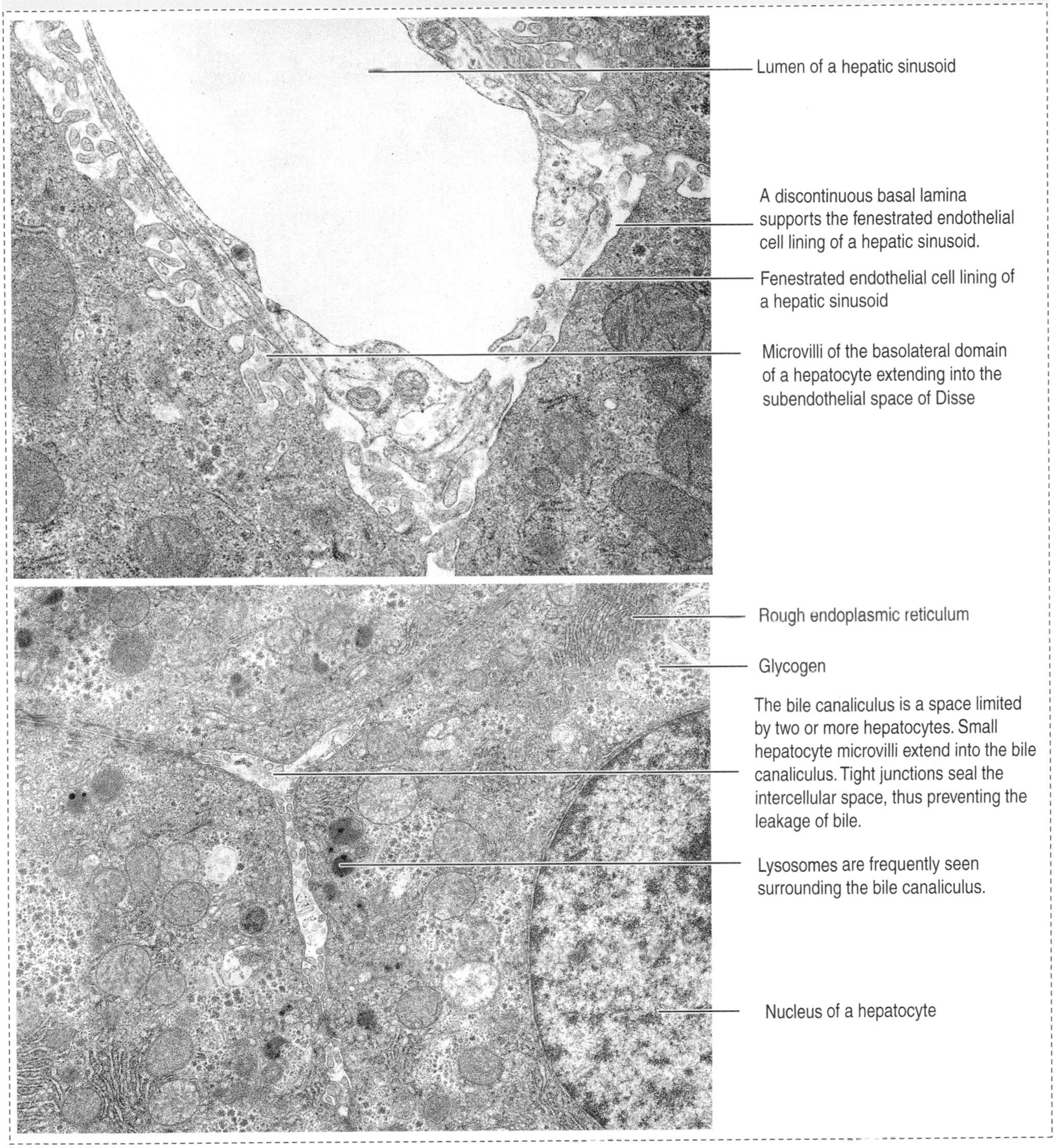

Lumen of a hepatic sinusoid
A discontinuous basal lamina supports the fenestrated endothelial cell lining of a hepatic sinusoid.
Fenestrated endothelial cell lining of a hepatic sinusoid
Microvilli of the basolateral domain of a hepatocyte extending into the subendothelial space of Disse
Rough endoplasmic reticulum
Glycogen
The bile canaliculus is a space limited by two or more hepatocytes. Small hepatocyte microvilli extend into the bile canaliculus. Tight junctions seal the intercellular space, thus preventing the leakage of bile.
Lysosomes are frequently seen surrounding the bile canaliculus.
Nucleus of a hepatocyte

concept has gained ground in pathophysiology. In the liver acinus, **the boundaries are determined by a terminal branch of the hepatic artery**. The flow of arterial blood within the venous sinusoids creates gradients of oxygen and nutrients classified as **zones I, II, and III**. Zone I is the richest in oxygen and nutrients. Zone III, closer to the central vein, is oxygen-poor. Zone II is intermediate in oxygen and nutrients (see Figure 17-11).

Although pathologic changes in the liver are usually described in relation to the classic lobule, the liver acinus concept is convenient for understanding liver regeneration patterns, liver metabolic activities, and the development of cirrhosis.

Hepatocyte

The hepatocyte is the functional **exocrine** and **endocrine** cell of the hepatic lobule. Hepatocytes form anastomosing **one-cell-thick plates** limiting the sinusoidal spaces. The perisinusoidal **space of Disse** separates the hepatocytes from the blood sinusoidal space (Figure 17-13).

The components of the portal triad, embedded in connective tissue, are separated from the hepatic lobule by a **limiting plate** of hepatocytes (see Figure 17-12). Blood from the portal vein and hepatic artery flows into the sinusoids and is drained by the central venule. Recall that bile flows in the opposite direction, from the hepatocytes to the bile duct in the portal space (see Figure 17-13).

A hepatocyte has two cellular domains: (1) a **basolateral domain** and (2) an **apical domain** (Figures 17-14 to 17-16):

The **basolateral domain** contains abundant **microvilli** and **faces the space of Disse**. Excess fluid in the space of Disse is collected in the **space of Mall**, located at the periphery of the hepatic lobule. Lymphatic vessels piercing the limiting plate drain the fluid of the space of Mall. **Gap junctions** on the lateral surfaces of adjacent hepatocytes enable intercellular functional coupling.

The basolateral domain participates in the **absorption of blood-borne substances** and in the **secretion of plasma proteins** (such as **albumin**, **fibrinogen**, **prothrombin**, and **coagulation factors** V, VII, and IX). Note that hepatocytes synthesize several plasma proteins required for blood clotting (see Chapter 6, Blood and Hematopoiesis). Blood coagulation disorders are associated with liver disease.

The **apical domain** borders the **bile canaliculus**, a trenchlike depression lined by microvilli and sealed at the sides by **occluding junctions** to prevent leakage of **bile**, the exocrine product of the hepatocyte (see Figure 17-15).

The hepatocyte contains a **rough endoplasmic reticulum** (see Figure 17-14), involved in the synthesis of plasma proteins, and a highly developed **smooth endoplasmic reticulum**, associated with synthesis of **glycogen**, **lipid**, and **detoxification mechanisms** (Figure 17-17).

Enzymes inserted in the membrane of the **smooth endoplasmic reticulum** are involved in the following **functions**: (1) the synthesis of cholesterol and bile salts; (2) the glucuronide conjugation of bilirubin, steroids, and drugs; (3) the breakdown of glycogen into glucose; (4) the esterification of free fatty acids to triglycerides; (5) the removal of iodine from the thyroid hormones triiodothyronine (T_3) and thyroxine (T_4); and (6) the **detoxification of lipid-soluble drugs** such as **phenobarbital**, during which the smooth endoplasmic reticulum is significantly developed.

The **Golgi apparatus** contributes to glycosylation of secretory proteins and the sorting of lysosomal enzymes. **Lysosomes** degrade aged plasma glycoproteins internalized at the basolateral domain by a hepatic lectin membrane receptor—the **asialoglycoprotein receptor**—with binding affinity to terminal galactose after the removal of sialic acid. Lysosomes in hepatocytes store iron, which can exist as **soluble ferritin** and **insoluble hemosiderin**, the degradation product of ferritin.

Peroxisomes

Peroxisomes are **membrane-bound organelles** with a high content of **oxidases** that generate **hydrogen peroxide** (Figure 17-18). Because hydrogen peroxide is a toxic metabolite, the enzyme **catalase** degrades this product into **oxygen** and **water**. This catalytic event occurs in hepatocytes and cells of the kidney.

Peroxisomes derive from preexisting peroxisomes by a budding process. Then, the organelle imports peroxisomal matrix proteins. A peroxisome contains about 50 enzymes involved in various metabolic pathways. The biogenesis of peroxisomes and their role in inherited disorders are outlined in Figure 17-18 and in Chapter 2, Epithelial Glands.

Figure 17-17. Ethanol metabolism in hepatocytes

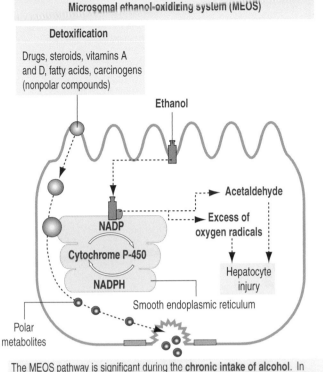

Alcohol dehydrogenase (ADH) pathway

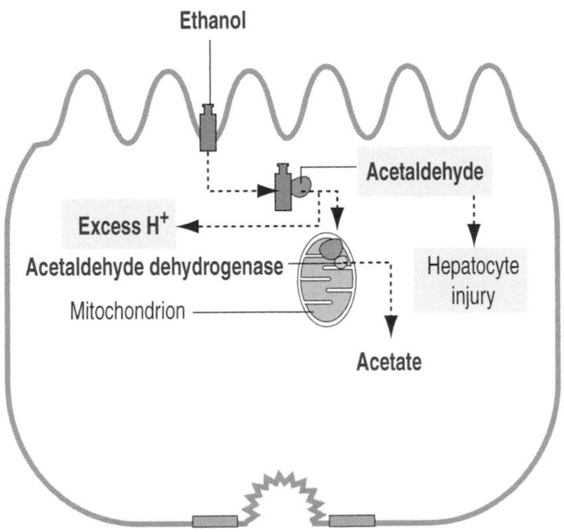

Ethanol
Acetaldehyde
Excess H+
Acetaldehyde dehydrogenase
Mitochondrion
Hepatocyte injury
Acetate

The ADH is the major pathway. **Alcohol is oxidized to acetaldehyde** in the cytoplasm and **acetaldehyde is converted to acetate** in mitochondria.

An excess of H^+ and acetaldehyde causes mitochondrial damage, disrupts microtubules, and alters proteins that can induce autoimmune responses leading to hepatocyte injury.

Microsomal ethanol-oxidizing system (MEOS)

Detoxification

Drugs, steroids, vitamins A and D, fatty acids, carcinogens (nonpolar compounds)

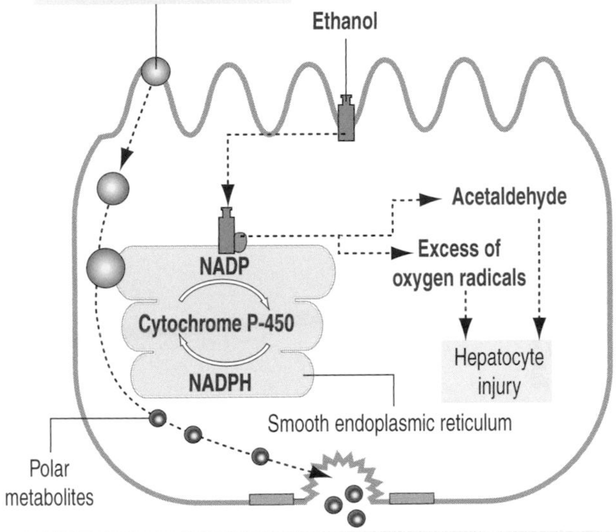

Ethanol
Acetaldehyde
Excess of oxygen radicals
NADP
Cytochrome P-450
NADPH
Hepatocyte injury
Smooth endoplasmic reticulum
Polar metabolites

The MEOS pathway is significant during the **chronic intake of alcohol**. In contrast to the ADH pathway that produces acetaldehyde and excess H^+, **the MEOS pathway produces acetaldehyde and an excess of oxygen radicals**.

Reactive oxygen produces injury to hepatocytes by causing lipid peroxidation, resulting in cell membrane damage. In addition, an upregulated MEOS affects detoxification activities of the hepatocyte that require cytochrome P-450 for the oxidation of various drugs, toxins, vitamins A and D, and potential carcinogens. The accumulation of these products is often toxic.

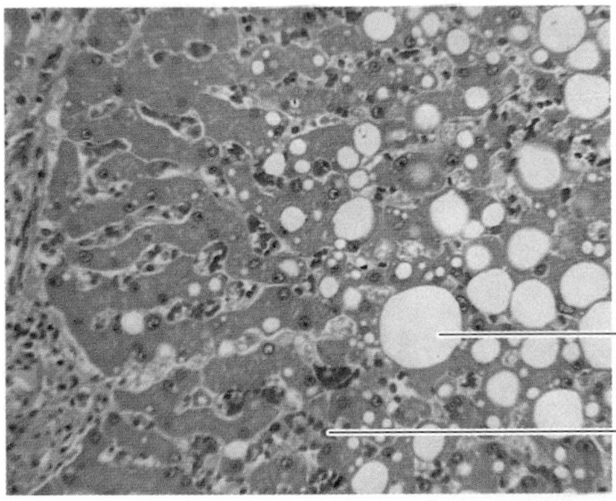

Large fat deposits in the cytoplasm of hepatocytes are observed in **fatty liver (steatosis)** following long-term consumption of alcohol.

Sinusoid

Clinical significance: Liver storage diseases

Severe liver diseases can result from the excessive storage of iron and copper. **Hereditary hemochromatosis** is an example of a disease characterized by increased **iron** absorption and accumulation in lysosomal hepatocytes. Cirrhosis and cancer of the liver are complications of hemochromatosis.

Wilson's disease (**hepatolenticular degeneration**) is a hereditary disorder of **copper** metabolism in which excessive deposits of copper in liver and brain lysosomes produce chronic hepatitis and cirrhosis.

Clinical significance: Alcoholism and fatty liver (alcoholic steatohepatitis)

After absorption in the stomach, most ethanol is transported to the liver, where it is metabolized to **acetaldehyde** and **acetate** in the hepatocytes. Ethanol is mainly oxidized by **alcohol dehydrogenase**, an NADH (reduced form of nicotinamide adenine dinucleotide)–dependent enzyme. This mechanism is known as the **alcohol dehydrogenase** (**ADH**) **pathway**. An additional metabolic pathway is the **microsomal ethanol-oxidizing system** (MEOS), present in the smooth en-

Figure 17-18. Peroxisome

1 Proteins for peroxisomes are synthesized by free cytosolic ribosomes and then transported into peroxisomes. Phospholipids and membrane proteins are also imported to peroxisomes from the endoplasmic reticulum.

2 Proteins are targeted to the interior of the peroxisome by targeting amino acid signals (mainly Ser-Lys-Leu at the C-terminal). Other amino acid signals target proteins to the peroxisome membrane. Targeting amino acid signals are not cleaved.

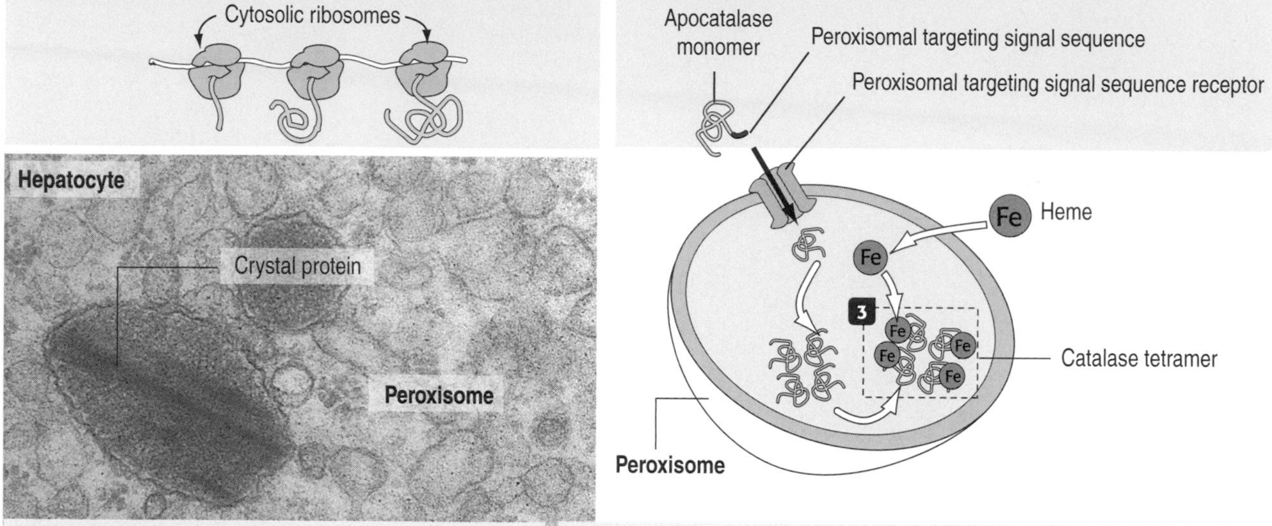

Cytosolic ribosomes
Hepatocyte
Crystal protein
Peroxisome
Apocatalase monomer
Peroxisomal targeting signal sequence
Peroxisomal targeting signal sequence receptor
Fe
Heme
3
Catalase tetramer
Peroxisome

4 **Zellweger syndrome** is a lethal condition caused by the defective assembly of peroxisomes due to the lack of transport of enzyme proteins (but not membrane proteins) into the peroxisome.

Newly synthesized peroxisomal enzymes remain in the cytosol and eventually are degraded. Cells in patients with Zellweger syndrome contain **empty peroxisomes**.

3 **Catalase**, the major protein of the peroxisome, decomposes H_2O_2 into H_2O.

Catalase is a tetramer of apocatalase molecules assembled within the peroxisome.

Heme is added to each monomer to prevent it from moving back into the cytosol across the peroxisomal membrane.

Peroxisomes are abundant in liver (hepatocytes).

doplasmic reticulum. The two pathways are summarized in Figure 17-17.

Long-term consumption of ethanol results in **fatty liver** (a reversible process if ethanol consumption is discontinued), **steatohepatitis** (fatty liver accompanied by an inflammatory reaction), **cirrhosis** (collagen proliferation or fibrosis), and **hepatocellular carcinoma** (malignant transformation of hepatocytes).

The production of **tumor necrosis factor-α** (TNF-α) is one of the initial events in liver injury. **TNF-α** triggers the production of other cytokines. **TNF-α**, regarded as a **proinflammatory cytokine,** recruits inflammatory cells that cause hepatocyte injury and promote the production of type I collagen fibers by **perisinusoidal cells of Ito** (a process known as **fibrogenesis**) as a healing response.

Injury of hepatocytes results in programmed cell death, or apoptosis, caused by the activation of caspases (see Chapter 3, Cell Signaling). **TNF-α** participates in a number of inflammatory processes such as in the articular joints (Chapter 5, Osteogenesis) and the extravasation of inflammatory cells (Chapter 10, Immune-Lymphatic System).

Ethanol, viruses, or toxins induce Kupffer cells to synthesize TNF-α as well as **transforming growth factor-β** (TGF-β) and **interleukin-6** (Figure 17-19). TGF-β stimulates the production of type I collagen by perisinusoidal cells of Ito, which increase in number. **TNF-α** acts on biliary ducts to interfere with the flow of bile (cholestasis).

Clinical significance: Perisinusoidal cell of Ito

Perisinusoidal cells of Ito are found in the space of Disse in proximity to the hepatic sinusoids. These cells are of mesenchymal origin, contain fat, and are involved in (1) the storage and release of retinoids; (2) production and turnover

Figure 17-19. **Cytokines in chronic liver disease**

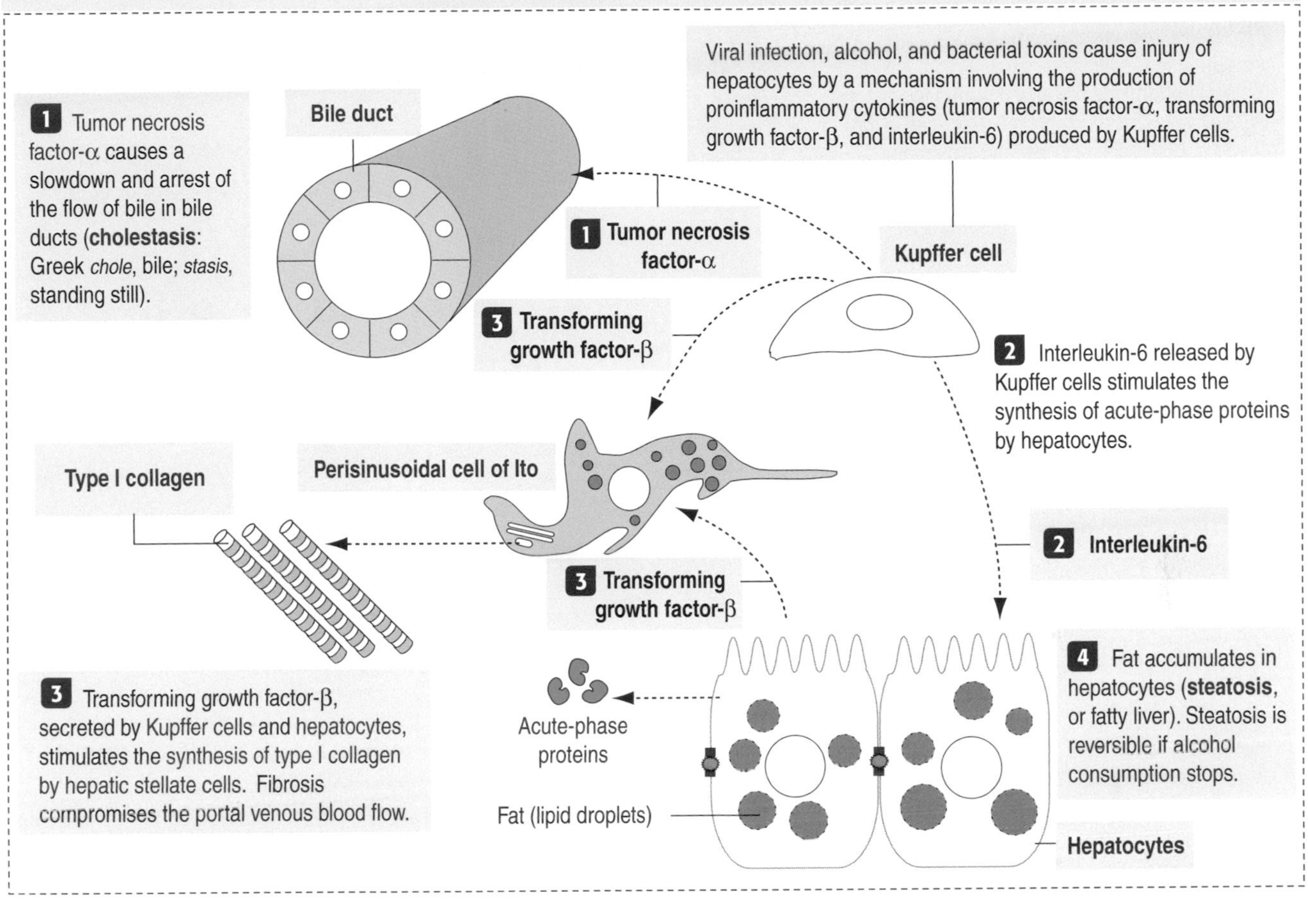

Viral infection, alcohol, and bacterial toxins cause injury of hepatocytes by a mechanism involving the production of proinflammatory cytokines (tumor necrosis factor-α, transforming growth factor-β, and interleukin-6) produced by Kupffer cells.
1 Tumor necrosis factor-α causes a slowdown and arrest of the flow of bile in bile ducts (cholestasis: Greek chole, bile; stasis, standing still).
Bile duct
1 Tumor necrosis factor-α
Kupffer cell
3 Transforming growth factor-β
2 Interleukin-6 released by Kupffer cells stimulates the synthesis of acute-phase proteins by hepatocytes.
Type I collagen
Perisinusoidal cell of Ito
2 Interleukin-6
3 Transforming growth factor-β
3 Transforming growth factor-β, secreted by Kupffer cells and hepatocytes, stimulates the synthesis of type I collagen by hepatic stellate cells. Fibrosis compromises the portal venous blood flow.
Acute-phase proteins
Fat (lipid droplets)
4 Fat accumulates in hepatocytes (steatosis, or fatty liver). Steatosis is reversible if alcohol consumption stops.
Hepatocytes

of extracellular matrix; and (3) regulation of blood flow in the sinusoids. Perisinusoidal cells remain in a quiescent, nonproliferative state, but can proliferate when activated by Kupffer cells and hepatocytes. Activation occurs after partial hepatectomy, focal hepatic lesions, and in different conditions that lead to fibrosis (Figure 17-20).

In pathologic conditions, perisinusoidal cells change into collagen-producing cells. In addition to the synthesis and secretion of type I collagen, perisinusoidal cells secrete **laminin**, **proteoglycans**, and **growth factors**. The deposit of collagen and extracellular matrix components increases, leading to a progressive fibrosis of the liver, which is typical of **cirrhosis**.

TGF-β, produced by Kupffer cells and hepatocytes (see Figures 17-19 and 17-20), stimulates collagen production by perisinusoidal cells. An increased deposit of collagen fibers and extracellular matrix within the space of Disse is followed by a **loss of fenestrations and gaps of sinusoidal endothelial cells.**

As the fibrotic process advances, perisinusoidal cells change into **myofibroblasts** constricting the lumen of the sinusoids and increasing vascular resistance. **An increase in resistance to the flow of portal venous blood in the hepatic sinusoids leads to portal hypertension in cirrhosis.**

Bile: Mechanism of secretion

Bile is a complex mixture of organic and inorganic substances produced by the hepatocyte, transported by the bile canaliculus, an extracellular canal between adjacent hepatocytes (Figure 17-21). The bile canaliculus defines the **apical domain** of the hepatocyte. The **basolateral domain** faces the sinusoidal space. **Tight junctions** between adjacent hepatocytes seal the biliary canalicular compartment.

The primary organic components of bile are conjugated bile acids (called bile salts), glycine, and taurine *N*-acyl amidated derivatives of bile acids derived from

Figure 17-20. Perisinusoidal cell of Ito

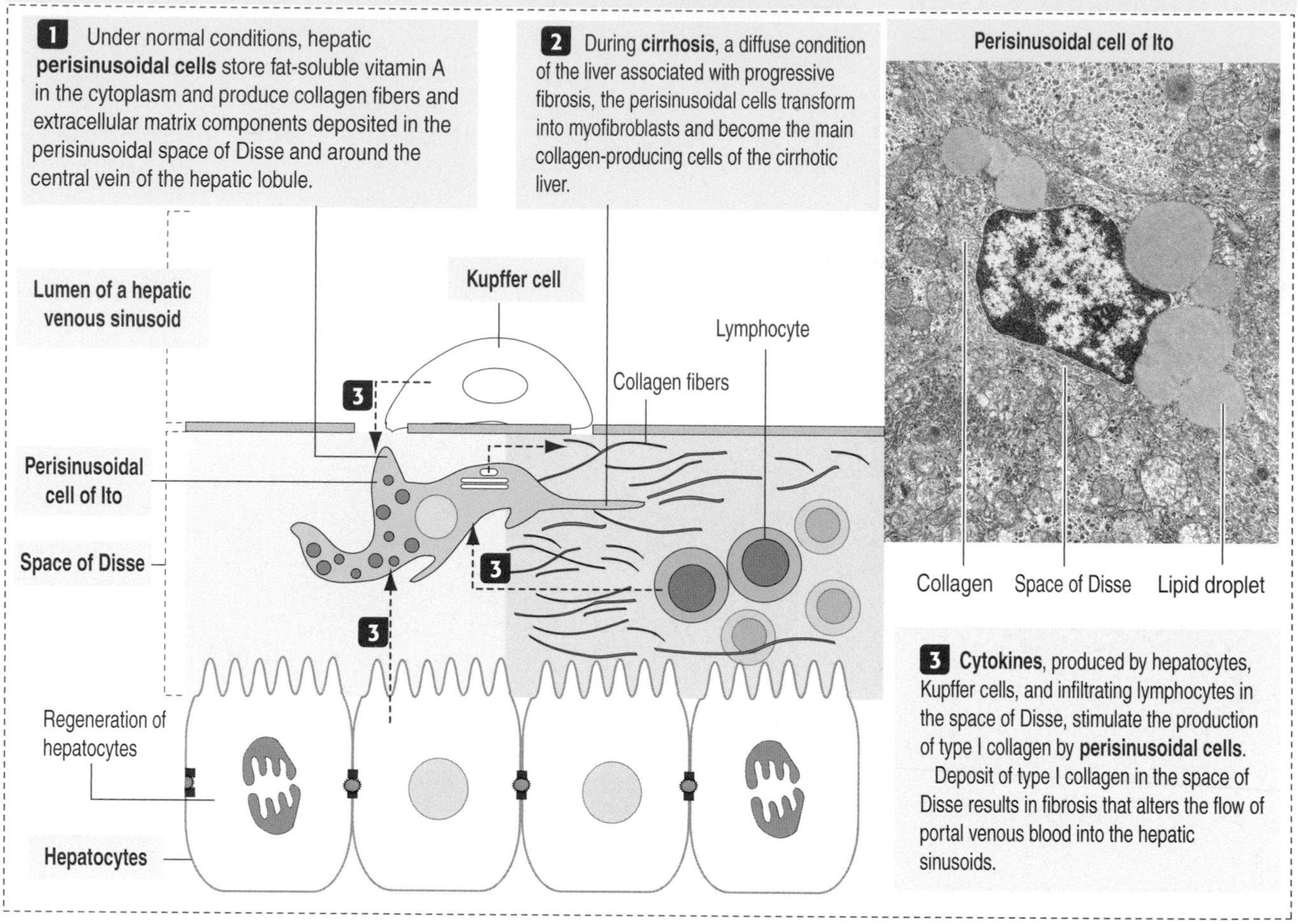
1 Under normal conditions, hepatic perisinusoidal cells store fat-soluble vitamin A in the cytoplasm and produce collagen fibers and extracellular matrix components deposited in the perisinusoidal space of Disse and around the central vein of the hepatic lobule.
2 During cirrhosis, a diffuse condition of the liver associated with progressive fibrosis, the perisinusoidal cells transform into myofibroblasts and become the main collagen-producing cells of the cirrhotic liver.
Perisinusoidal cell of Ito
Lumen of a hepatic venous sinusoid
Kupffer cell
Lymphocyte
Collagen fibers
Perisinusoidal cell of Ito
Space of Disse
Regeneration of hepatocytes
Hepatocytes
Collagen
Space of Disse
Lipid droplet
3 Cytokines, produced by hepatocytes, Kupffer cells, and infiltrating lymphocytes in the space of Disse, stimulate the production of type I collagen by perisinusoidal cells.
Deposit of type I collagen in the space of Disse results in fibrosis that alters the flow of portal venous blood into the hepatic sinusoids.

cholesterol.

Bile has five major functions:

1. The excretion of **cholesterol, phospholipids, bile salts, conjugated bilirubin**, and **electrolytes**.

2. Contributes to **fat absorption in the intestinal lumen** (see Chapter 16, Lower Digestive Segment).

3. Transports **IgA** to the intestinal mucosa by the enterohepatic circulation.

4. The excretion of metabolic products of drugs and heavy metals processed in the hepatocyte.

5. Conjugated bile acids inhibit the growth of bacteria in the small intestine.

The transport of bile and other organic substances from the hepatocyte to the lumen of the bile canaliculus is an adenosine triphosphate (ATP)–mediated process. Four ATP-dependent transporters, present in the canalicular plasma membrane, participate in transport mechanisms of the bile (Figure 17-22).

1. **Multidrug resistance 1** transporter (**MDR1**), which mobilizes cholesterol across the plasma membrane.

2. **Multidrug resistance 2** transporter (**MDR2**), which transports phospholipids.

3. **Multispecific organ anionic transporter** (**MOAT**), which exports bilirubin glucuronide and glutathione conjugates.

4. **Biliary acid transporter** (**BAT**), which transports bile salts.

These ATP transporters belong to the family of **ABC transporters** characterized by highly conserved ATP-binding domains, or ATP binding cassettes. The first ABC transporter was discovered as the product of the gene ***mdr*** (for multiple drug resistance). The *mdr* gene is highly expressed in cancer cells and the encoded product, MDR transporter, pumps drugs out of cells, making cancer cells resistant

Figure 17-21. **Bile canaliculus and the polarity of the hepatocyte**

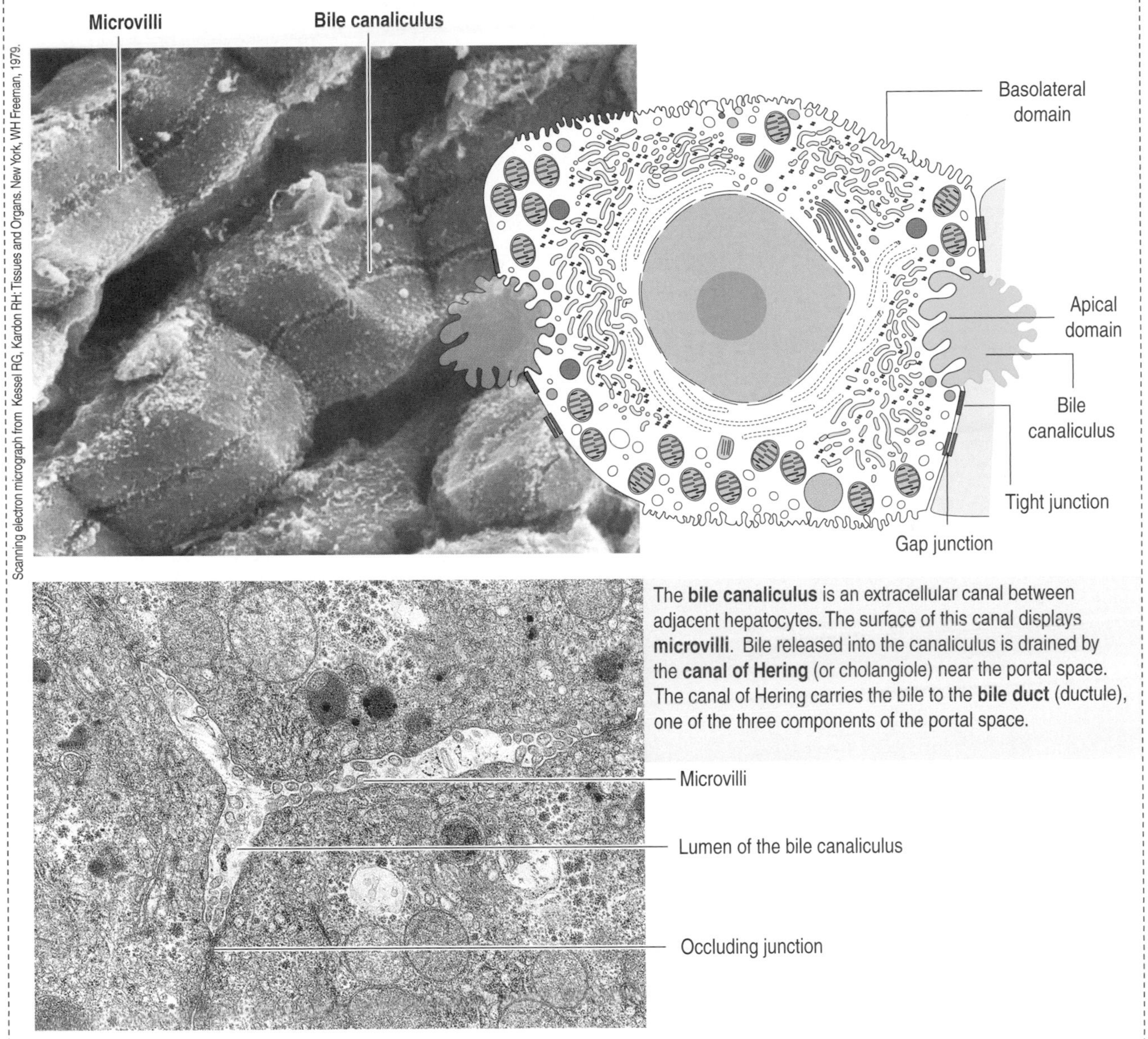
Microvilli
Bile canaliculus
Scanning electron micrograph from Kessel RG, Kardon RH: Tissues and Organs. New York, WH Freeman, 1979.
Basolateral domain
Apical domain
Bile canaliculus
Tight junction
Gap junction
Microvilli
Lumen of the bile canaliculus
Occluding junction

The **bile canaliculus** is an extracellular canal between adjacent hepatocytes. The surface of this canal displays **microvilli**. Bile released into the canaliculus is drained by the **canal of Hering** (or cholangiole) near the portal space. The canal of Hering carries the bile to the **bile duct** (ductule), one of the three components of the portal space.

to cancer treatment with chemotherapeutic agents (see Cell Nucleus in Chapter 1, Epithelium).

The secretion of bile acids generates the osmotic gradient necessary for osmotic water flow into the bile canaliculus. In addition, an **ion exchanger** enables the passage of HCO_3^- and Cl^- ions. Finally, hydrolytic enzymes associated with the plasma membrane (**ectoenzymes**) of the bile canaliculus and bile duct produce nucleoside and amino acid breakdown products, which are reabsorbed by ductular epithelial cells.

A genetic defect in MDR2 causes focal hepatocyte necrosis, proliferation of bile ductules, and an inflammatory reaction in the portal space. Very low levels of phospholipids are detected in the bile of MDR2 mutants.

Metabolism of bilirubin

Bilirubin is the end product of heme catabolism and about 85% originates from senescent red blood cells destroyed mainly in the spleen by macrophages (Figure 17-23).

Figure 17-22. Transport of bile into the bile canaliculus

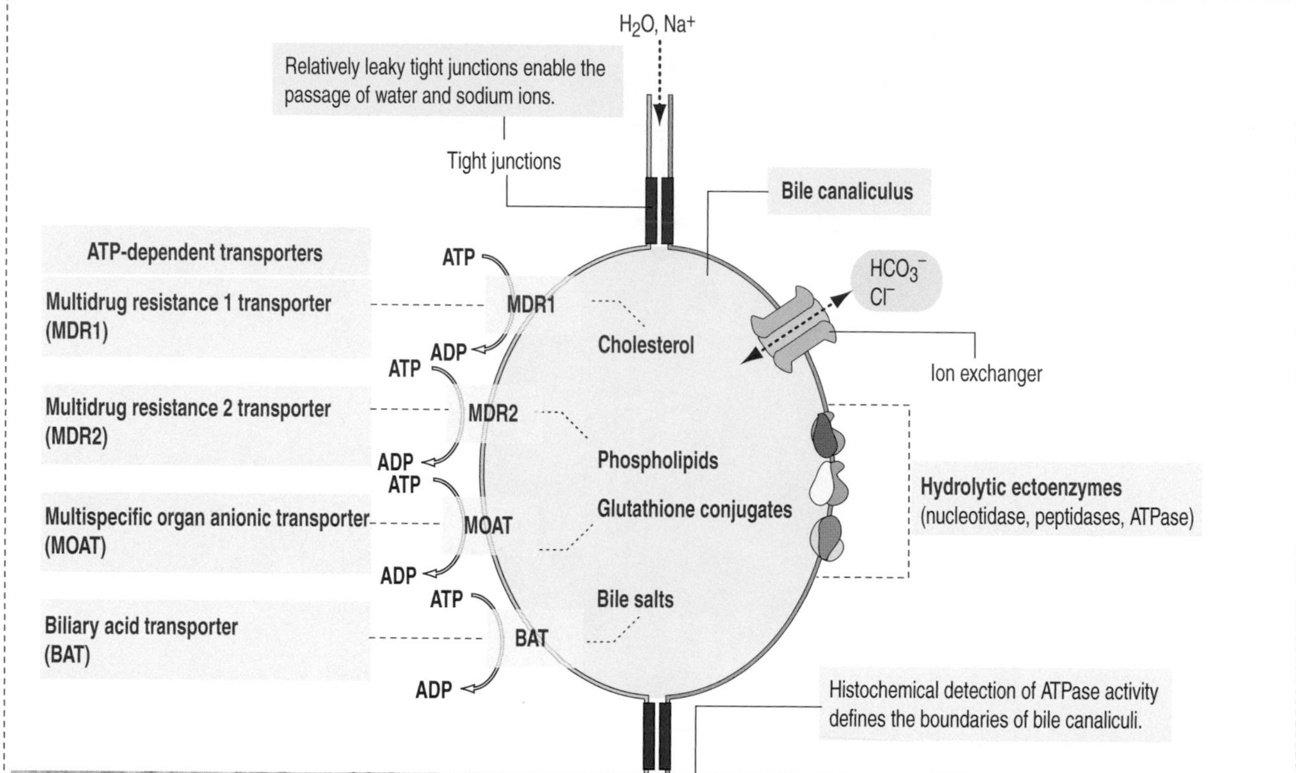

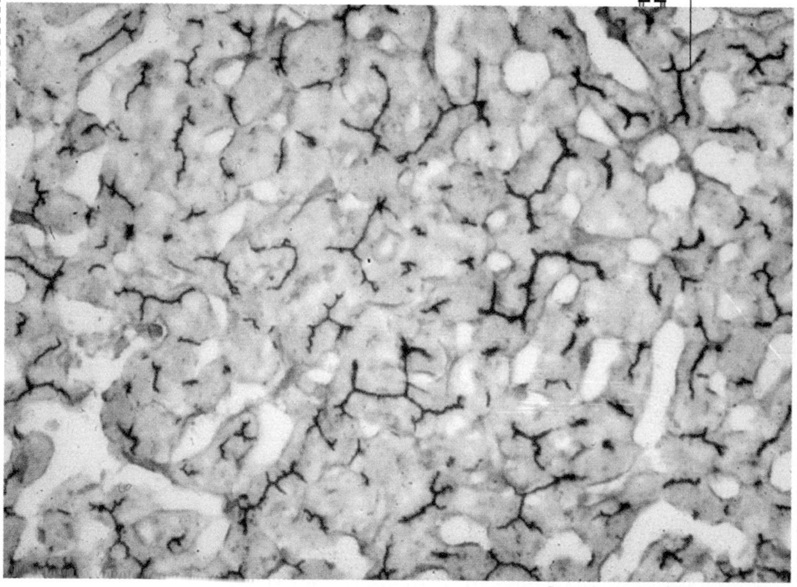

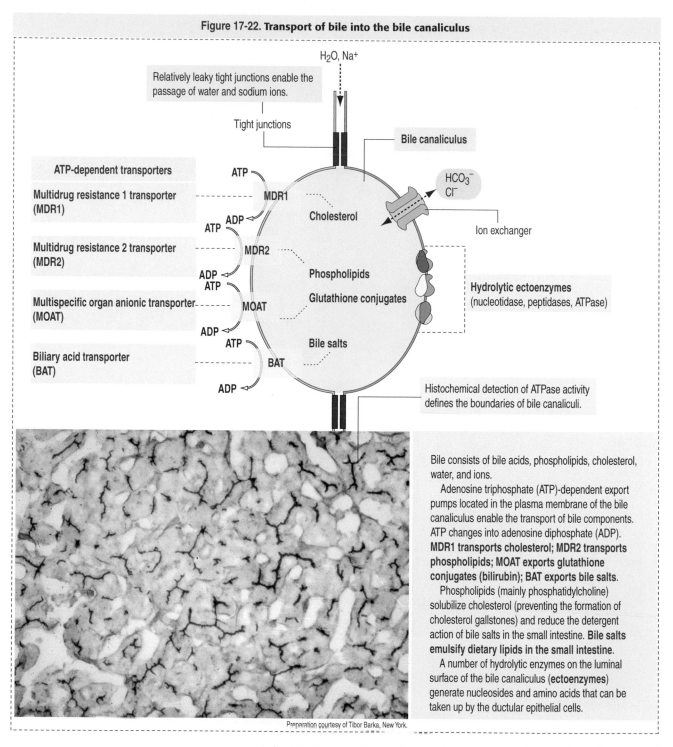

Bile consists of bile acids, phospholipids, cholesterol, water, and ions.

Adenosine triphosphate (ATP)-dependent export pumps located in the plasma membrane of the bile canaliculus enable the transport of bile components. ATP changes into adenosine diphosphate (ADP). **MDR1 transports cholesterol; MDR2 transports phospholipids; MOAT exports glutathione conjugates (bilirubin); BAT exports bile salts.**

Phospholipids (mainly phosphatidylcholine) solubilize cholesterol (preventing the formation of cholesterol gallstones) and reduce the detergent action of bile salts in the small intestine. **Bile salts emulsify dietary lipids in the small intestine.**

A number of hydrolytic enzymes on the luminal surface of the bile canaliculus (**ectoenzymes**) generate nucleosides and amino acids that can be taken up by the ductular epithelial cells.

Bilirubin is released into the circulation where it is bound to albumin and transported to the liver. **Unlike albumin-bound bilirubin, free bilirubin is toxic to the brain.** Recall from our discussion of **erythroblastosis fetalis** (see Chapter 6, Blood and Hematopoiesis) that an antibody-induced hemolytic disease in the newborn is caused by blood group incompatibility between mother and fetus. The hemolytic process results in hyperbilirubinemia caused by elevated amounts of **free bilirubin**, which causes irreversible damage to the central nervous system (**kernicterus**).

When albumin-conjugated bilirubin reaches the hepatic sinusoids, the **albumin-bilirubin complex** dissociates, and bilirubin is transported across the plasma membrane of hepatocytes after binding to a plasma membrane receptor. Inside

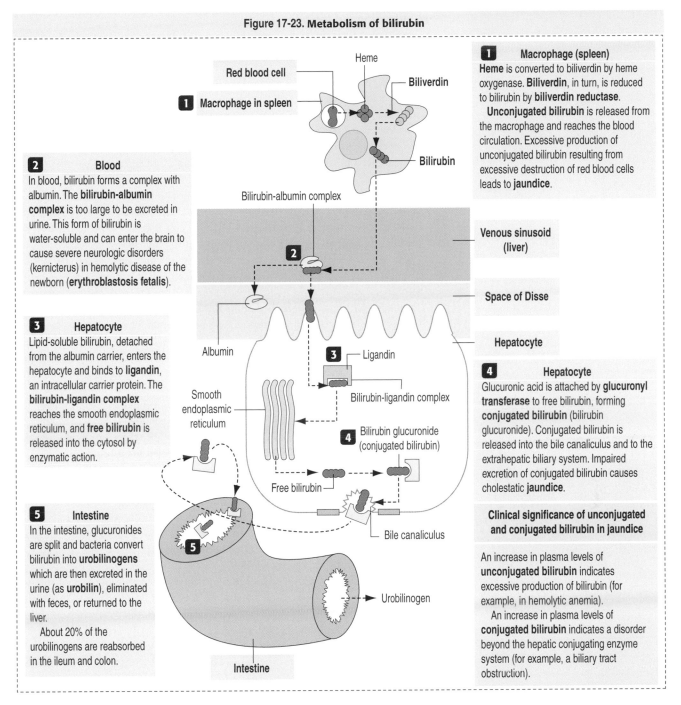

Figure 17-23. Metabolism of bilirubin

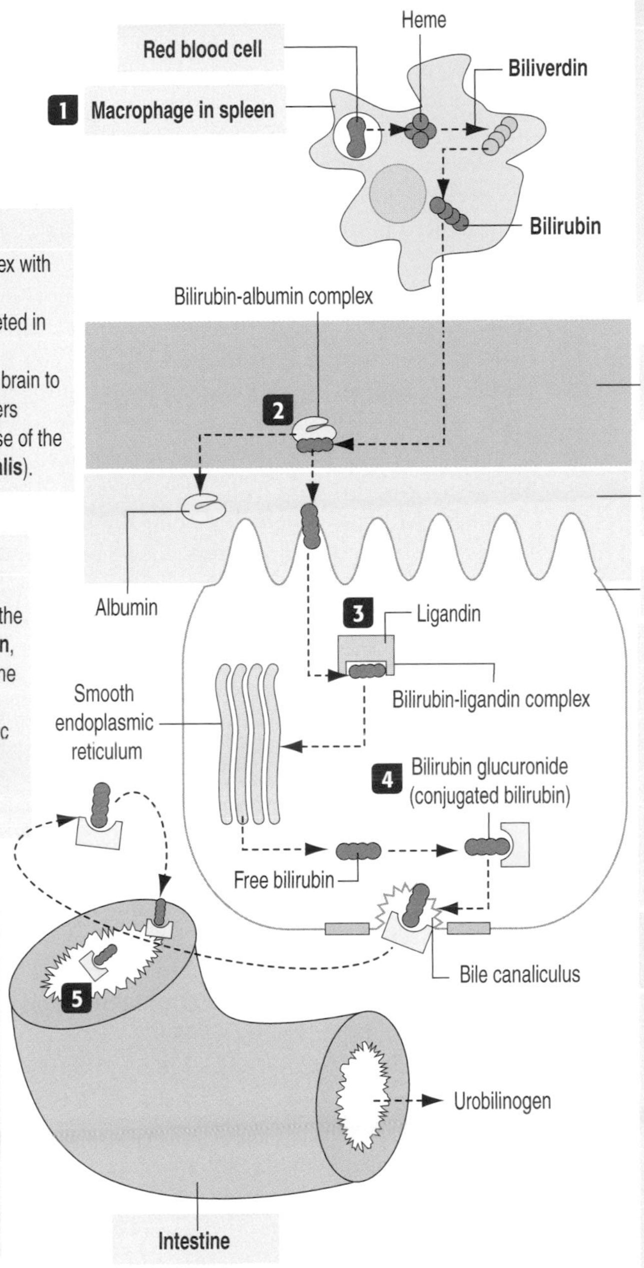

1 Macrophage (spleen)

Heme is converted to biliverdin by heme oxygenase. **Biliverdin**, in turn, is reduced to bilirubin by **biliverdin reductase**.

Unconjugated bilirubin is released from the macrophage and reaches the blood circulation. Excessive production of unconjugated bilirubin resulting from excessive destruction of red blood cells leads to **jaundice**.

2 Blood

In blood, bilirubin forms a complex with albumin. The **bilirubin-albumin complex** is too large to be excreted in urine. This form of bilirubin is water-soluble and can enter the brain to cause severe neurologic disorders (kernicterus) in hemolytic disease of the newborn (**erythroblastosis fetalis**).

3 Hepatocyte

Lipid-soluble bilirubin, detached from the albumin carrier, enters the hepatocyte and binds to **ligandin**, an intracellular carrier protein. The **bilirubin-ligandin complex** reaches the smooth endoplasmic reticulum, and **free bilirubin** is released into the cytosol by enzymatic action.

4 Hepatocyte

Glucuronic acid is attached by **glucuronyl transferase** to free bilirubin, forming **conjugated bilirubin** (bilirubin glucuronide). Conjugated bilirubin is released into the bile canaliculus and to the extrahepatic biliary system. Impaired excretion of conjugated bilirubin causes cholestatic **jaundice**.

5 Intestine

In the intestine, glucuronides are split and bacteria convert bilirubin into **urobilinogens** which are then excreted in the urine (as **urobilin**), eliminated with feces, or returned to the liver.

About 20% of the urobilinogens are reabsorbed in the ileum and colon.

Clinical significance of unconjugated and conjugated bilirubin in jaundice

An increase in plasma levels of **unconjugated bilirubin** indicates excessive production of bilirubin (for example, in hemolytic anemia).

An increase in plasma levels of **conjugated bilirubin** indicates a disorder beyond the hepatic conjugating enzyme system (for example, a biliary tract obstruction).

the hepatocyte, bilirubin binds to **ligandin**, a protein that prevents bilirubin reflux into the circulation. The **bilirubin-ligandin complex** is transported to the smooth endoplasmic reticulum, where **bilirubin is conjugated to glucuronic acid** by the uridine diphosphate (UDP)–**glucuronyl transferase system**. This reaction results in the formation of a **water-soluble bilirubin diglucuronide**, which diffuses through the cytosol into the bile canaliculus, where it is secreted into the bile.

In the small intestine, conjugated bilirubin in bile remains intact until it reaches the distal portion of the small intestine and colon, where **free bilirubin is generated by the intestinal bacterial flora**.

Unconjugated bilirubin is then reduced to **urobilinogen**. Most urobilinogen is excreted in the feces. A small portion returns to the liver following absorption by a process known as **enterohepatic bile circulation**. Another small fraction is excreted in the urine.

Composition of the bile

The human liver produces about 600 mL of bile per day. The bile consists of **organic components** (such as **bile acids**, the major component; **phospholipids**, mainly lecithins; **cholesterol**; and **bile pigments, bilirubin**) and **inorganic components** (predominantly Na^+ and Cl^- **ions**).

Bile acids (cholic acid, chenodeoxycholic acid, deoxycholic acid, and lithocholic acid) are synthesized by the hepatocytes. Cholic and chenodeoxycholic acids are synthesized from cholesterol as a precursor and are called **primary bile acids**. Deoxycholic and lithocholic acids are called **secondary bile acids** because they are produced in the intestinal lumen by the action of intestinal bacteria on the primary bile acids.

The synthetic bile acid pathway is the major mechanism of elimination of cholesterol from the body. **Micelles** are formed by the aggregation of bile acid molecules conjugated to taurine or glycine. Cholesterol is located inside the micelles. Bile pigments are not components of the micelles.

Bile secreted by the liver is stored in the gallbladder and released into the duodenum during a meal to facilitate the breakdown and absorption of fats (see Figure 16-9 in Chapter 16, Lower Digestive Segment). About 90% of both primary and secondary bile acids is absorbed from the intestinal lumen by enterocytes and transported back to the liver through the portal vein. This process is known as the **enterohepatic circulation**. The absorption of bile acids by the enterocyte is mediated at the apical plasma membrane by an Na^+-dependent transporter protein and released through the basolateral plasma membrane by an Na^+-independent anion exchanger.

Bilirubin is not absorbed in the intestine. Bilirubin is reduced to **urobilinogen** by bacteria in the distal small intestine and colon (see Figure 17-23). Urobilinogen is partially secreted in the feces, part returns to the liver through the portal vein, and some is excreted in urine as **urobilin**, the oxidized form of urobilinogen.

Bile acids establish an osmotic gradient that mobilizes water and electrolytes into the bile canaliculus. HCO_3^- ions, secreted by epithelial cells lining the bile ducts, are added to the bile, which becomes alkaline as Na^+ and Cl^- ions and water are absorbed. **Secretin** increases the active transport of HCO_3^- into the bile.

The flow of bile into the duodenum depends on (1) the secretory pressure generated by the actively bile-secreting hepatocytes and (2) the flow resistance in the bile duct and **sphincter of Oddi**.

The sphincter of Oddi is a thickening of the circular muscle layer of the bile duct at the duodenal junction. During fasting, the sphincter of Oddi is closed and bile flows into the gallbladder. The gallbladder's ability to concentrate bile 5 to 20 times compensates for the limited storage capacity of the gallbladder (20 to 50 mL of fluid) and the continuous production of bile by the liver.

Bile secretion during meal digestion is initiated by the **cholecystokinin**-induced contraction of the muscularis of the gallbladder in response to lipids in the intestinal lumen, assisted by the muscular activities of the common bile duct, the sphincter of Oddi, and the duodenum. Cholecystokinin stimulates the relaxation of the sphincter of Oddi, enabling bile to enter the duodenum. Note that **cholecystokinin has opposite effects**: it stimulates **muscle contraction** of the **gallbladder** and induces **muscle relaxation** of the **sphincter of Oddi**.

Clinical significance: Pathologic conditions affecting bile secretion

Because bile secretion involves hepatocytes, bile ducts, gallbladder, and intestine, any perturbation along this pathway can result in a pathologic condition. For example, destruction of hepatocytes by viral infection (**viral hepatitis**) and toxins can lead to a decrease in bile production as well as an increase in bilirubin in blood (**jaundice**).

Obstruction of the passages by **gallstones**, **infection**, or **tumors** can block the flow of bile, with bile reflux to the liver and then to the systemic circulation.

Figure 17-24. Gallbladder

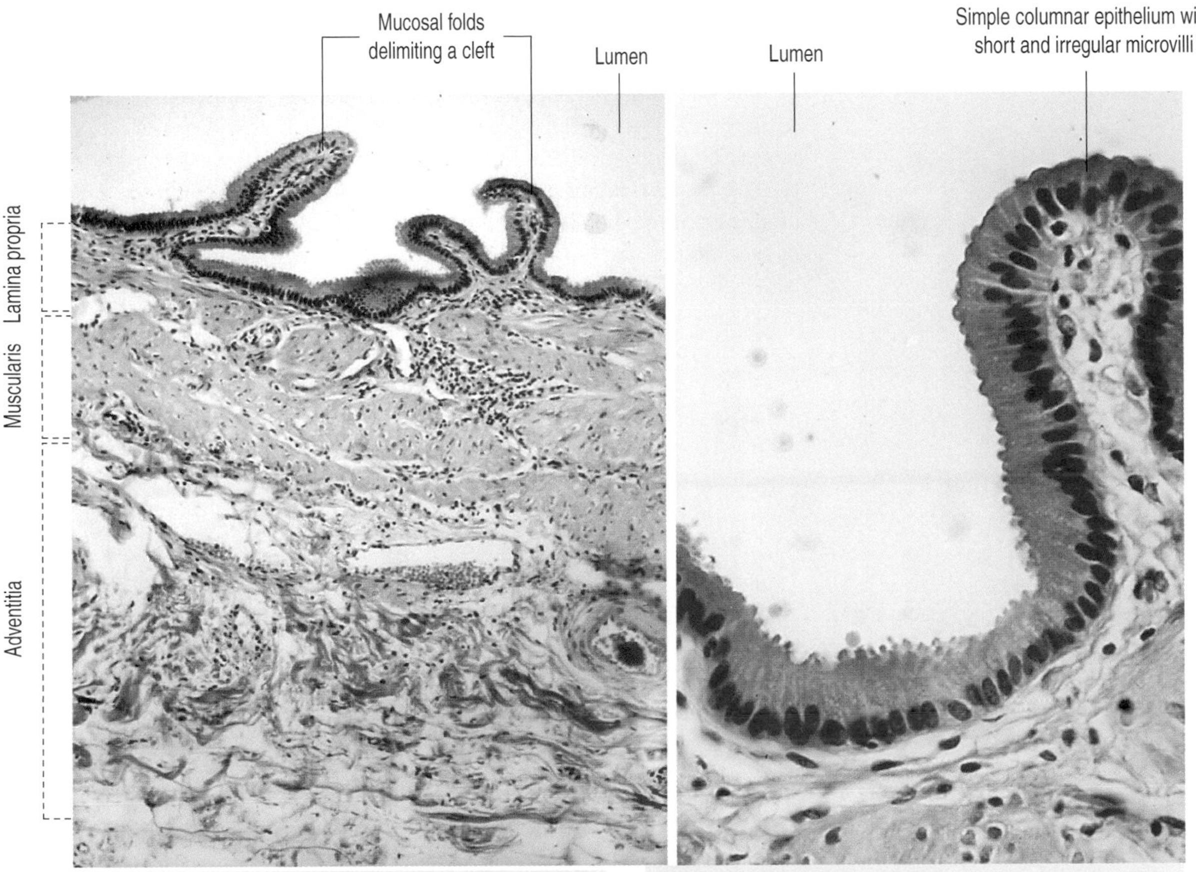

Mucosal folds delimiting a cleft
Lumen
Lumen
Simple columnar epithelium with short and irregular microvilli
Lamina propria
Muscularis
Adventitia

Gallbladder

The major functions of the gallbladder are:

1. Concentration (up to 10-fold) and storage of bile between meals.
2. Release of bile by contraction of the muscularis in response to **cholecystokinin** stimulation (produced by enteroendocrine cells in the duodenum) and **neural stimuli**, together with **relaxation of the sphincter of Oddi** (a muscular ring surrounding the opening of the bile duct in the wall of the duodenum).
3. Regulation of hydrostatic pressure within the biliary tract.

Clinical significance

Cholestasis defines the impaired formation and excretion of the bile at the level of the hepatocyte (**intrahepatic cholestasis**) or a structural (tumor of the pancreas or biliary tract—cholangiocarcinoma) or mechanical (**cholelithiasis**, produced by gallstones) perturbation in the excretion of bile (**extrahepatic cholestasis**).

Clinically, cholestasis is detected by (1) the presence in blood of **bilirubin** and bile acids, secreted into bile under normal conditions; (2) elevation in serum of **alkaline phosphatase** (an enzyme associated with the plasma membrane of the bile canaliculus); and (3) **radiologic examination** (many gallstones are radiopaque and can be detected on a plain radiograph).

Clinical significance: Hyperbilirubinemia

Several diseases occur when one or more of the metabolic steps of bilirubin formation are disrupted. A characteristic feature of these diseases is **hyperbilirubinemia**—an increase in the concentration of bilirubin in the blood (more than 0.1 mg/mL).

An inherited defect in the **UDP–glucuronyl transferase system**, known as **Crigler-Najjar disease**, results in failure to conjugate bilirubin in hepatocytes and the absence of conjugated bilirubin diglucuronide in bile. Infants with this disease develop **bilirubin encephalopathy**.

The **Dubin-Johnson syndrome** is a familial disease caused by a **defect in the transport of conjugated bilirubin to the bile canaliculus**. In addition to the transport of conjugated bilirubin, there is a general defect in the transport and excretion of organic anions in these patients.

Gallbladder

The main functions of the gallbladder are **storage**, **concentration**, and **release of bile.** Dilute bile from the hepatic ducts is transported through the cystic duct into the gallbladder. After concentration, bile is discharged into the common bile duct.

The wall of the gallbladder consists of a **mucosa**, a **muscularis**, and an **adventitia** (Figure 17-24). The portion of the gallbladder that does not face the liver is covered by the peritoneum.

The mucosa displays multiple **folds** lined by a **simple columnar epithelium** and is supported by a lamina propria that contains a **vascular plexus.** The mucosa creates deep clefts known as **Rokitansky-Aschoff sinuses.** In the **neck region** of the gallbladder, the lamina propria contains **tubuloacinar glands.**

There is no submucosa in the gallbladder. The **muscularis** is represented by smooth muscle bundles associated with collagen and elastic fibers.

Essential concepts | Digestive Glands

• The three major digestive glands are (1) the salivary glands: the parotid, submandibular, and sublingual glands; (2) the exocrine pancreas; and (3) the liver.

• Salivary glands consist of branched ducts and secretory portions, acini, producing a mucous, serous, or mucous-serous product. They are classified as branched (compound) tubuloalveolar glands.

Each acinus is drained sequentially by (1) an intercalated duct (lined by low squamous-to-cuboidal simple epithelium). The intercalated duct is longest in the parotid gland; (2) a striated duct (lined by a cuboidal-to-columnar simple epithelium with abundant basal mitochondria). The striated duct is well developed in the submandibular gland; and (3) an intralobular duct (lined initially by a cuboidal-to-columnar simple epithelium). Intercalated, striated, and excretory intralobular ducts are observed within a lobule.

Intralobular ducts converge to form an interlobular duct (found between lobules; lined by a pseudostratified columnar epithelium). Interlobular ducts converge to form lobar ducts (lined by stratified columnar epithelium). Lobar ducts join the main duct, which displays a stratified squamous epithelium near its opening in the oral cavity. Connective tissue septa provide support to the branching duct system. Blood vessels, lymphatics, and nerves are found along the ducts.

Saliva is the major product of salivary glands. Saliva contains protein, glycoproteins, ions, water, and immunoglobulin A. Submandibular glands produce 70% of the saliva; the parotid glands contribute 25% and the enzyme amylase. Proteins in saliva form pellicles, a protective film on the teeth.

The parotid gland consists of serous acini surrounded by myoepithelial cells. The parotid gland has the longest intercalated ducts.

The submandibular gland contains mixed seromucous and serous acini, also surrounded by myoepithelial cells. Serous cells form demilunes capping the mucous cells of the serous-mucous acinus. Secretion of the serous cells is transported to the acinar lumen along intercellular secretory canaliculi.

The sublingual gland has predominant mucous acini; a few seromucous acini can be found. Myoepithelial cells are present. The intercalated and striated ducts are poorly developed.

• Exocrine pancreas. The pancreas is a combined exocrine branched tubuloacinar gland and endocrine gland (islet of Langerhans). The pancreas is surrounded by a connective tissue but does not have a capsule proper. Lobules are separated by connective tissue partitions. The pancreatic acinus contains serous-secreting cells and centroacinar cells, unique to the pancreas. Intercalated ducts (lined by a low cuboidal epithelium) drain the acinus. Neither striated ducts nor myoepithelial cells are present in the exocrine pancreas. Intercalated ducts converge to form interlobular ducts lined by a simple columnar epithelium.

Secretin and cholecystokinin regulate the function of the pancreatic acinus and intercalated duct. Cholecystokinin and acetylcholine trigger the release of inactive forms of trypsin, chymotrypsin, and carboxylpeptidases produced by the pancreatic acinar cells. Lipase, amylase, cholesterol esterase, and phospholipase are also secreted. Secretin stimulates the secretion of water and bicarbonate ions by epithelial cells of the intercalated duct.

Acute hemorrhagic pancreatitis is the result of pancreatic tissue autodigestion by the premature activation of pancreatic enzymes. It occurs following a heavy meal or excessive alcohol ingestion.

Cystic fibrosis is an inherited disease affecting mucus-secreting tissues of the respiratory, digestive, reproductive, and integumentary systems. Chronic pancreatitis in cystic fibrosis is characterized by a loss of acini, dilation of the pancreatic excretory ducts, and extensive fibrosis (increase in connective tissue). A genetic defect in the cystic fibrosis transmembrane conductance regulator (CFTR) protein prevents the transport of chloride ions. Mucus becomes thick and prone to bacterial infections.

• Liver. The liver consists of poorly defined lobes surrounded by a collagen–elastic fiber capsule (of Glisson). Blood is supplied by two vessels: (1) the portal vein (75% to 80% of the afferent deoxygenated blood volume; transporting blood from the digestive tract, spleen, and pancreas); and (2) the hepatic artery (20% to 25% of oxygenated blood). Blood from the portal vein and hepatic artery mixes in the hepatic sinusoid of the liver lobules. Sinusoidal blood converges to the central venule (or vein), and is drained by the sublobular vein, collecting vein, and hepatic vein into the inferior vena cava.

Bile, the exocrine product of the liver, is collected by the intrahepatic bile duct, and drained by the right and left hepatic ducts. Bile is stored in the gallbladder and released in the duodenum through the common bile duct.

The hepatic lobule is the structural and functional unit of the liver. The hepatic lobule consists of anastomosing plates of hepatocytes limiting blood sinusoidal spaces lined by endothelial cells and Kupffer cells. The space of Disse is interposed between the sinusoidal space and the hepatocytes. Perisinusoidal cells of Ito (the storage site of retinoids) are present in the space of Disse. A central venule (or vein) collects the sinusoidal blood. Branches of the portal vein and hepatic artery, together with a bile duct, form the portal triad found in the connective tissue surrounding the hepatic lobule.

A limiting plate of hepatocytes is the boundary between the hepatocyte parenchyma and the connective tissue stroma.

Bile, produced by hepatocytes, flows in opposite direction to the blood. Bile is transported through bile canaliculi into the canal of Hering (or cholangiole), and then into the bile duct in the portal triad space.

• The liver lobule can be conceptualized as (1) the classic hepatic lobule (described above); (2) the portal lobule (based on the bile drainage pathway; the portal triad is the center of the portal lobule); and (3) the liver acinus (based on the zone gradient distribution of hepatic artery–derived oxygenated blood along the sinusoidal spaces).

• The hepatocyte is the functional endocrine and exocrine cell of the liver. The hepatocyte has a basolateral domain with abundant microvilli extending into the space of Disse. Excess of fluid in the space of Disse, not absorbed by the hepatocytes, is drained into the lymphatic circulation through the space of Mall located adjacent to the limiting plate. The basolateral domain participates in the absorption of blood-borne substances (for example, bilirubin, peptide and steroid hormones, vitamin B_{12}, and substances to be detoxified), and the secretion of plasma proteins (for example, albumin, fibrinogen, prothrombin, coagulation factors, and complement proteins).

The apical domain borders the bile canaliculus, a trenchlike depression lined by microvilli and sealed by tight junctions.

Hepatocytes contain smooth endoplasmic reticulum (SER) associated with glycogen inclusions. The functions of the SER include (1) synthesis of cholesterol and bile salts; (2) glucuronide conjugation of bilirubin, steroids, and drugs; (3) the breakdown of glycogen into glucose; and (4) the detoxification of lipid-soluble drugs (for example, phenobarbital). The rough endoplasmic reticulum and Golgi apparatus participate in the synthesis and glycosylation of the secretory proteins indicated above. Peroxisomes are prominent in hepatocytes.

• Alcoholism and fatty liver. Hepatocytes participate in the metabolism of ethanol. Long-term consumption of ethanol results in fatty liver, a reversible process if alcohol ingestion is discontinued; cirrhosis (collagen proliferation of fibrosis of the liver), and hepatocellular carcinoma (malignant transformation of hepatocytes).

Ethanol can be metabolized by the alcohol dehydrogenase (ADH) pathway, and the microsomal ethanol-oxidizing system (MEOS).

In the ADH pathway, ethanol is oxidized to acetaldehyde in the cytoplasm and acetaldehyde is converted to acetate in mitochondria. Excess of acetaldehyde and protons can cause hepatocyte injury. In the MEOS pathway, ethanol metabolized in the SER produces acetaldehyde and excess of oxygen radicals (instead of protons). Both produce hepatocyte injury.

• The perisinusoidal cell of Ito is found in the space of Disse, in the proximity of hepatic sinusoids. These cells (1) store and release retinoids; (2) produce and turn over extracellular matrix components; (3) regulate blood flow in the sinusoids; and (4) proliferate when activated by cytokines produced by Kupffer cells. Under pathologic conditions (for example, cirrhosis), perisinusoidal cells can become collagen-producing cells and transform into myofibroblasts constricting the sinusoidal lumen and leading to portal hypertension, a characteristic aspect of cirrhosis.

• Bile is a mixture of organic and inorganic substances produced by the hepatocyte. Bile participates in the excretion of cholesterol, phospholipids, bile salts, conjugated bilirubin, and electrolytes. Fat absorption in the intestinal lumen depends on the fat-emulsifying function of bile salts. Bile transports IgA to the intestinal mucosa (enterohepatic circulation), and inhibits bacterial growth in the small intestine.

The secretion of bile into the bile canaliculus is an adenosine triphosphate (ATP)-mediated process involving multidrug resistance 1 and 2 transporters (MDR1 and MDR2), multispecific organ anionic transporter (MOAT), and biliary acid transporter (BAT).

• Metabolism of bilirubin. Bilirubin is the end product of heme catabolism. About 85% of bilirubin originates from senescent red blood cells destroyed in the spleen by macrophages. Macrophages convert heme into biliverdin, which is transformed into unconjugated bilirubin released into the blood circulation. In the blood circulation, bilirubin forms a complex with albumin. When the bilirubin-albumin complex reaches the hepatic sinusoids, albumin detaches and bilirubin is internalized by the hepatocyte. Bilirubin binds to ligandin in the hepatocyte cytosol and is transported to the SER, which releases free bilirubin that becomes conjugated with glucuronic acid. Bilirubin glucuronide is released into the bile canaliculus and transported to the small intestine. Glucuronide separates from bilirubin in the small intestine and bilirubin is converted by intestinal bacteria into urobilinogen, which is excreted. Urobilin is eliminated by urine.

Hyperbilirubinemia (an increase in the concentration of bilirubin circulating in blood) can occur when bilirubin cannot be conjugated in the hepatocyte (**Crigler-Najjar disease**). Infants with this disease develop bilirubin encephalopathy. A defect in the transport of conjugated bilirubin to the bile canaliculus is the cause of the **Dubin-Johnson syndrome**.

• The gallbladder is the storage, concentration, and release site of bile. The wall of the gallbladder consists of a mucosa with folds and deep clefts, lined by a simple columnar epithelium. There is no submucosa. A muscularis and adventitia can be seen.

18. NEUROENDOCRINE SYSTEM

Highlights of the hypothalamohypophysial system

The hypothalamus and the hypophysis (also known as the **pituitary**) form an integrated neuroendocrine network known as the **hypothalamohypophysial system.**

The hypothalamohypophysial system consists of two components: (1) the **hypothalamic adenohypophysial system**, connecting the hypothalamus to the anterior hypophysis; and (2) the **hypothalamic neurohypophysial system**, linking the hypothalamus to the posterior hypophysis.

The **hypothalamus**, corresponding to the floor of the diencephalon and forming part of the walls of the third ventricle, consists of clusters of neurons, called **nuclei**, some of which secrete hormones. These **neuroendocrine cells** are located **behind** the blood-brain barrier, but their secretory products are released **outside** the blood-brain barrier.

The neuroendocrine cells of the hypothalamus exert **positive** and **negative** effects on the pituitary gland through peptides called **releasing** and **inhibitory hormones** or **factors**, have a **very short response time** (fractions of a second) to neurotransmitters, and send **axons** into the neurohypophysis.

Axon terminals of the neuroendocrine cells in the **neurohypophysis** have abundant storage granules containing peptide hormones bound to a **carrier protein**, called **neurophysin**. Both hormones and carrier proteins are released by exocytosis into adjacent fenestrated capillaries under the control of neural stimuli.

The **anterior hypophysis** is highly vascularized. It has a fenestrated capillary plexus (called the **primary plexus**) in the lower hypothalamus, or pituitary stalk. The primary plexus is connected to a **secondary plexus** in the anterior lobe of the hypophysis by **portal veins**, forming the **hypothalamohypophysial portal circulation.**

Hormones from the anterior hypophysis are produced by epithelial cells, stored in granules—without a carrier protein—and released in a **cyclic**, **rhythmic**, or **pulsatile** manner into the secondary capillary plexus by endocrine stimuli.

The effects of hormones derived from the epithelial cells of the anterior hypophysis have a **longer response time** (minutes or hours) and can persist for as long as a day or even a month.

Hypophysis

The hypophysis (Greek *hypo*, under; *physis*, growth) consists of two embryologically distinct tissues (Figure 18-1): (1) the **adenohypophysis**, the **glandular epithelial** portion; and (2) the **neurohypophysis**, the **neural** portion.

The **adenohypophysis** is formed by three subdivisions or parts. (1) The **pars distalis**, or **anterior lobe**, is the main part of the gland. (2) The **pars tuberalis** envelops, like a partial or total collar, the infundibular stem or stalk, a neural component. Together they make up the pituitary stalk. (3) The **pars intermedia**, or intermediate lobe, is rudimentary in the adult. It is a thin wedge separating the pars distalis from the neurohypophysis.

The **neurohypophysis** is formed by two subdivisions: the **pars nervosa**, or neural lobe, and the **infundibulum**. The infundibulum, in turn, consists of two components: the **infundibular process** and the **median eminence**, a funnel-like extension of the hypothalamus.

Embryologic origin of the hypophysis

The anterior hypophysis and neurohypophysis have different embryologic origins (Figure 18-2). The anterior hypophysis derives from an evagination (pouch

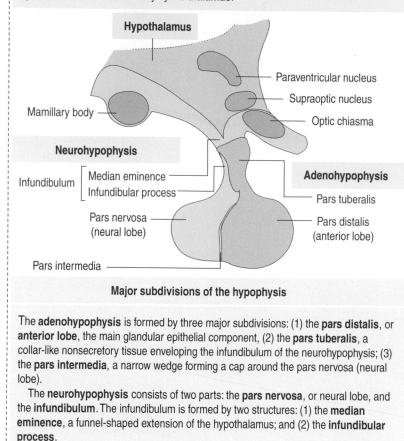

Figure 18-1. Regions of the hypophysis (pituitary gland)

The **hypothalamus** is divided into two symmetrical halves by the third ventricle. It is limited rostrally by the **optic chiasma**, caudally by the **mamillary bodies**, laterally by the **optic tracts**, and dorsolaterally by the **thalamus**.

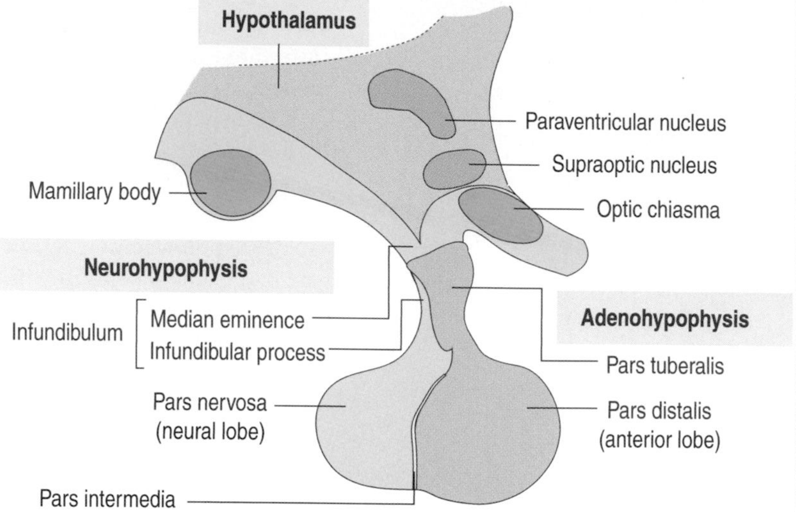

Hypothalamus
Paraventricular nucleus
Supraoptic nucleus
Mamillary body
Optic chiasma
Neurohypophysis
Infundibulum
Median eminence
Infundibular process
Adenohypophysis
Pars tuberalis
Pars nervosa
(neural lobe)
Pars distalis
(anterior lobe)
Pars intermedia

Major subdivisions of the hypophysis

The **adenohypophysis** is formed by three major subdivisions: (1) the **pars distalis**, or **anterior lobe**, the main glandular epithelial component, (2) the **pars tuberalis**, a collar-like nonsecretory tissue enveloping the infundibulum of the neurohypophysis; (3) the **pars intermedia**, a narrow wedge forming a cap around the pars nervosa (neural lobe).

The **neurohypophysis** consists of two parts: the **pars nervosa**, or neural lobe, and the **infundibulum**. The infundibulum is formed by two structures: (1) the **median eminence**, a funnel-shaped extension of the hypothalamus; and (2) the **infundibular process**.

of Rathke) of the ectodermal lining of the future oral cavity extending upward toward the developing neurohypophysis. The neurohypophysis develops from an **infundibular downgrowth from the floor of the diencephalon**. The connecting stem attached to the pouch of Rathke disappears. However, the connecting stem of the neurohypophysis remains as the core of the infundibular stem, or stalk.

The pouch of Rathke develops into three different regions: (1) cells of the anterior surface of the pouch give rise to the pars distalis (the bulk of the gland), (2) cells of the posterior surface invade the infundibular process, (3) superior extensions of the pouch surround the infundibular stem, forming the pars tuberalis.

Blood supply of the hypophysis: Hypothalamohypophysial portal circulation

The **superior hypophysial artery** (derived from the internal carotid arteries) (Figure 18-3) enters the median eminence and upper part of the infundibular stem and forms the **first sinusoidal capillary plexus (primary capillary plexus)**, which receives the secretion of the neuroendocrine cells grouped in the **hypothalamic hypophysiotropic nuclei** of the hypothalamus.

Capillaries arising from the primary capillary plexus project down the infundibulum and pars tuberalis to form the **portal veins. Capillaries arising from the portal veins form a secondary capillary plexus that supplies the anterior hypophysis and receives secretions from endocrine cells of the anterior hypophysis. There is no direct arterial blood supply to the anterior hypophysis.**

Figure 18-2. **Development of the hypophysis**

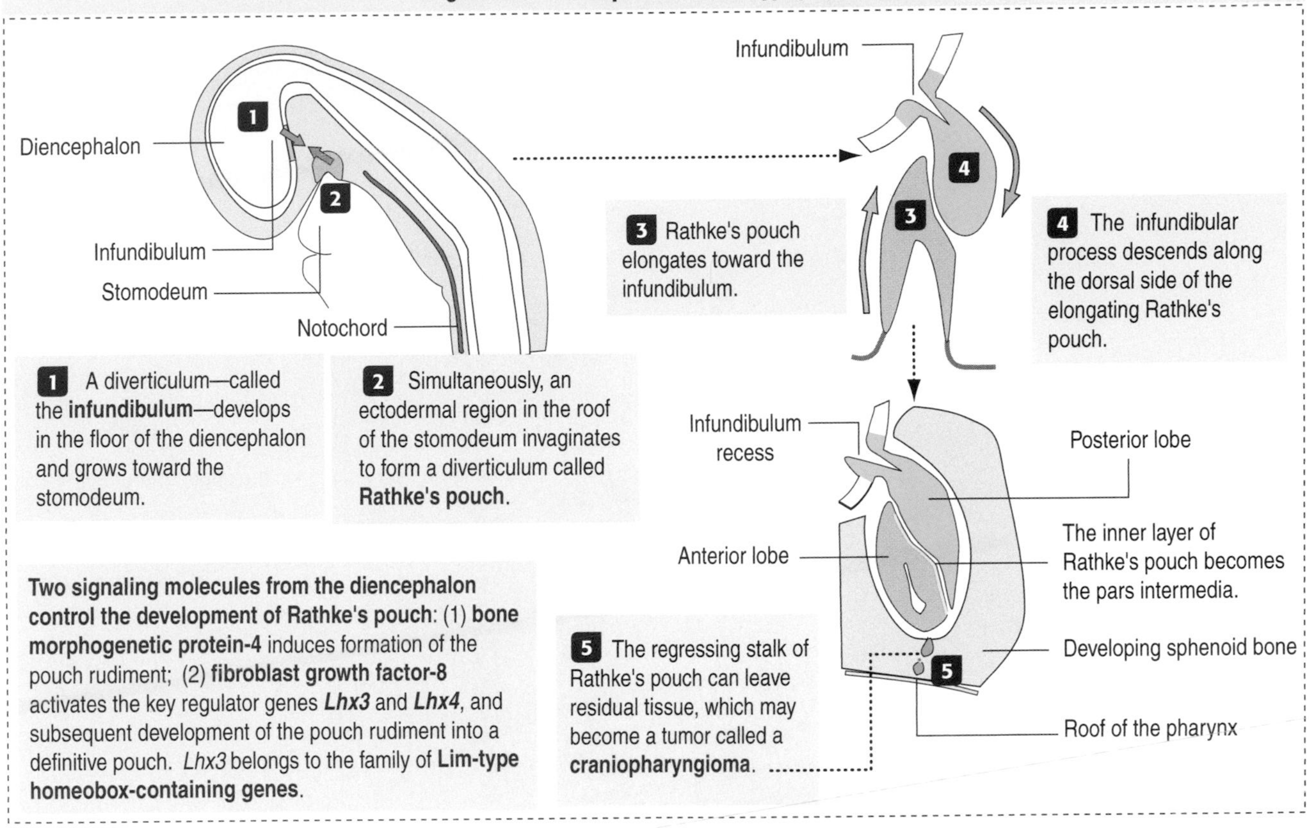

Diencephalon
Infundibulum
Stomodeum
Notochord
1 A diverticulum—called the **infundibulum**—develops in the floor of the diencephalon and grows toward the stomodeum.
2 Simultaneously, an ectodermal region in the roof of the stomodeum invaginates to form a diverticulum called **Rathke's pouch**.
Two signaling molecules from the diencephalon control the development of Rathke's pouch: (1) **bone morphogenetic protein-4** induces formation of the pouch rudiment; (2) **fibroblast growth factor-8** activates the key regulator genes ***Lhx3*** and ***Lhx4***, and subsequent development of the pouch rudiment into a definitive pouch. *Lhx3* belongs to the family of **Lim-type homeobox-containing genes**.
Infundibulum
3 Rathke's pouch elongates toward the infundibulum.
4 The infundibular process descends along the dorsal side of the elongating Rathke's pouch.
Infundibulum recess
Posterior lobe
Anterior lobe
The inner layer of Rathke's pouch becomes the pars intermedia.
Developing sphenoid bone
Roof of the pharynx
5 The regressing stalk of Rathke's pouch can leave residual tissue, which may become a tumor called a **craniopharyngioma**.

The hypothalamohypophysial portal system enables (1) the transport of hypothalamic releasing and inhibitory hormones from the primary capillary plexus to the hormone-producing epithelial cells of the anterior hypophysis; (2) the secretion of hormones from the anterior hypophysis into the secondary capillary plexus and to the general circulation; and (3) the functional integration of the hypothalamus with the anterior hypophysis, provided by the **portal veins.**

A **third capillary plexus**, derived from the inferior hypophysial artery, supplies the neurohypophysis. This third capillary plexus collects secretions from neuroendocrine cells present in the hypothalamus. The secretory products (vasopressin and oxytocin) are transported along the axons into the neurohypophysis.

Histology of the pars distalis (anterior lobe)

The pars distalis is formed by three components: (1) cords of **epithelial cells** (Figure 18-4), (2) minimal supporting **connective tissue stroma**; and (3) **fenestrated capillaries** (or **sinusoids**) (Figure 18-5), which are part of the secondary capillary plexus.

There is no blood-brain barrier in the anterior hypophysis.

The epithelial cells are arranged in cords surrounding fenestrated capillaries carrying blood from the hypothalamus. Secretory hormones diffuse into a network of capillaries, which drain into the hypophysial veins and from there into the venous sinuses.

There are three distinct types of endocrine cell in the anterior hypophysis (see Figure 18-4): (1) **acidophils** (cells that stain with an acidic dye), which are prevalent at the sides of the gland; (2) **basophils** (cells that stain with a basic dye and are periodic acid–Schiff [PAS]-positive), which are predominant in the middle of the gland; and (3) **chromophobes** (cells lacking cytoplasmic staining).

Acidophils secrete two major **peptide hormones: growth hormone** and **prolactin**. Basophils secrete **glycoprotein hormones: the gonadotropin follicle-stimulating hormone** (FSH), **luteinizing hormone** (LH), **thyroid-stimulating**

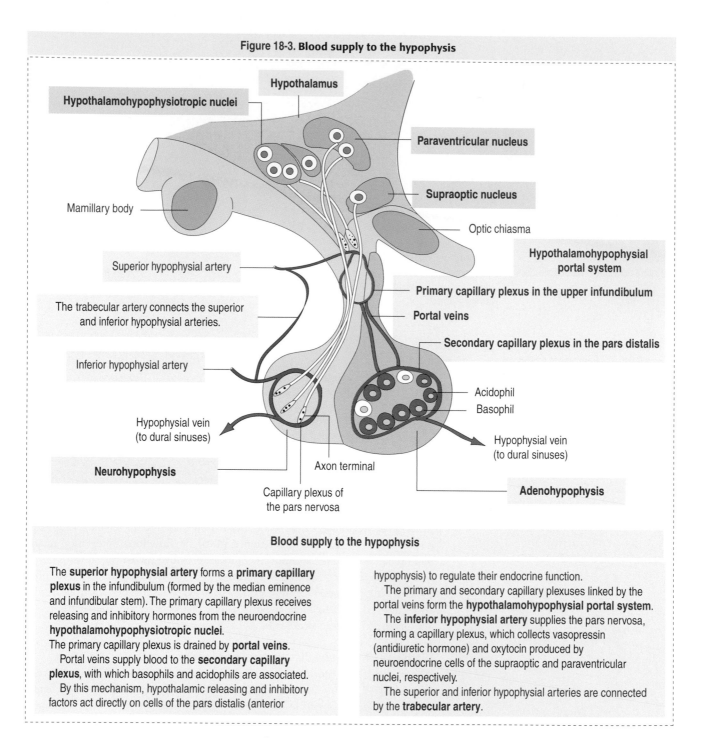

Figure 18-3. **Blood supply to the hypophysis**

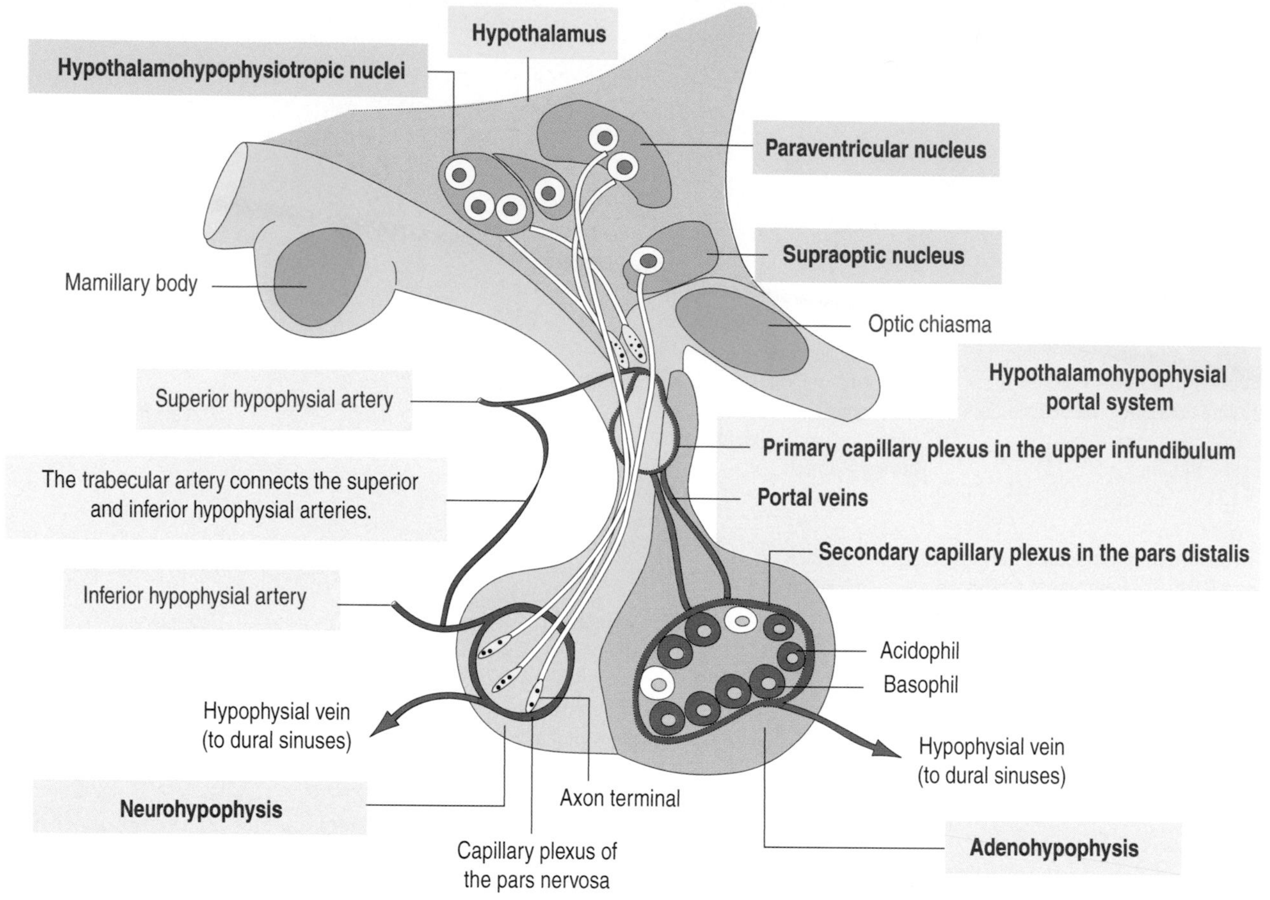

Hypothalamus
Hypothalamohypophysiotropic nuclei
Paraventricular nucleus
Supraoptic nucleus
Mamillary body
Optic chiasma
Hypothalamohypophysial portal system
Superior hypophysial artery
Primary capillary plexus in the upper infundibulum
The trabecular artery connects the superior and inferior hypophysial arteries.
Portal veins
Secondary capillary plexus in the pars distalis
Inferior hypophysial artery
Acidophil
Basophil
Hypophysial vein (to dural sinuses)
Hypophysial vein (to dural sinuses)
Neurohypophysis
Axon terminal
Capillary plexus of the pars nervosa
Adenohypophysis

Blood supply to the hypophysis

The **superior hypophysial artery** forms a **primary capillary plexus** in the infundibulum (formed by the median eminence and infundibular stem). The primary capillary plexus receives releasing and inhibitory hormones from the neuroendocrine **hypothalamohypophysiotropic nuclei**.

The primary capillary plexus is drained by **portal veins**.

Portal veins supply blood to the **secondary capillary plexus**, with which basophils and acidophils are associated.

By this mechanism, hypothalamic releasing and inhibitory factors act directly on cells of the pars distalis (anterior hypophysis) to regulate their endocrine function.

The primary and secondary capillary plexuses linked by the portal veins form the **hypothalamohypophysial portal system**.

The **inferior hypophysial artery** supplies the pars nervosa, forming a capillary plexus, which collects vasopressin (antidiuretic hormone) and oxytocin produced by neuroendocrine cells of the supraoptic and paraventricular nuclei, respectively.

The superior and inferior hypophysial arteries are connected by the **trabecular artery**.

hormone (TSH), and **adrenocorticotropic hormone** (ACTH), or corticotropin. Chromophobes include cells that have depleted their hormone content and lost the staining affinity typical of acidophils and basophils.

The precise identification of the endocrine cells of the anterior hypophysis is by **immunohistochemistry**, which demonstrates their hormone content using specific antibodies (see Figure 18-4).

Hormones secreted by acidophils: Growth hormone and prolactin

Acidophils secrete **growth hormone**, also called **somatotropin**. These acidophilic cells, called **somatotrophs**, represent a large proportion (40% to 50%) of the cell population of the anterior hypophysis. Prolactin-secreting cells, or **lactotrophs**, represent 15% to 20% of the cell population of the anterior hypophysis.

Figure 18-4. **Identification of basophil, acidophil, and chromophobe cells in the anterior hypophysis**

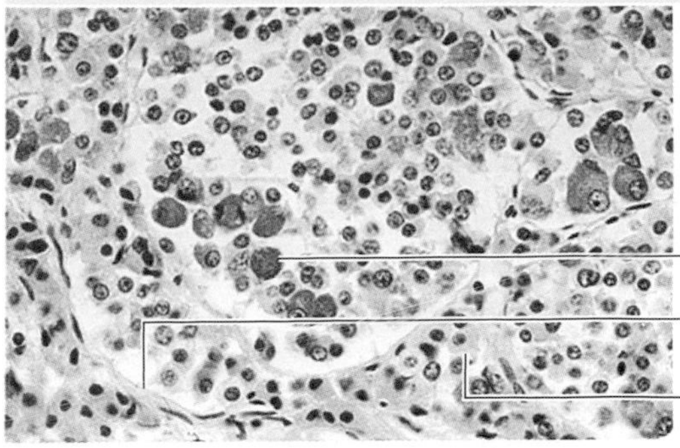
Basophil
Fenestrated capillary
Acidophil

Hematoxylin-eosin staining (H&E)
The anterior hypophysis consists of clusters of epithelial cells adjacent to fenestrated capillaries. With hematoxylin and eosin (H&E), the cytoplasm of **basophils** stains **blue-purple (glycoproteins)** and **acidophils** stain **light pink (proteins)**. Chromophobe cells display a very light pink cytoplasm.

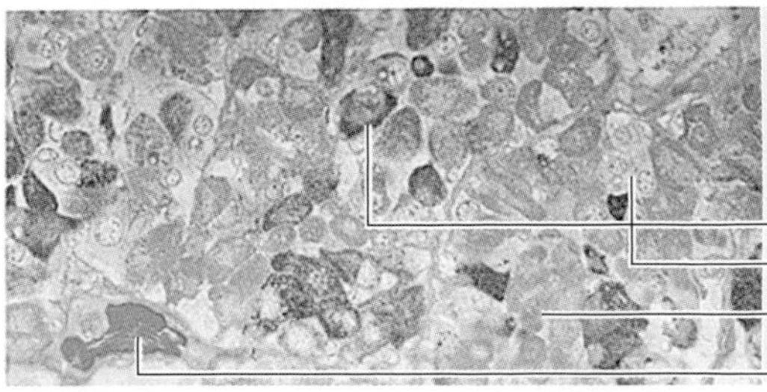
Basophil
Chromophobe
Acidophil
Red blood cells

Trichrome stain (aniline blue, orange G, and azocarmine)
With the trichrome stain, the cytoplasm of **basophils** stains **blue-purple** and **acidophils orange. Chromophobe cells** stain **light blue.** Red blood cells in the lumen of the capillaries stain **deep orange**.

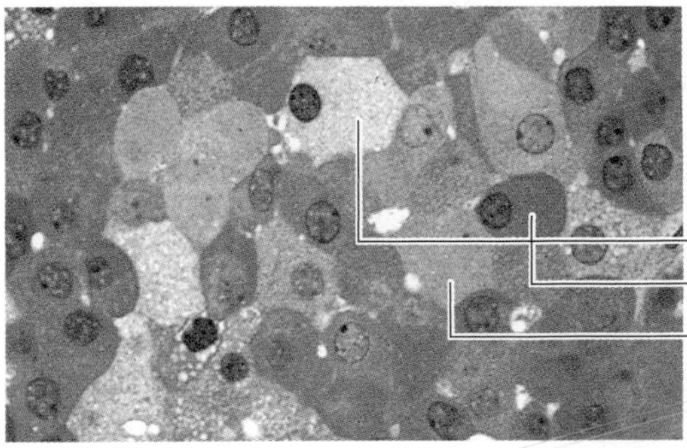
Chromophobe
Basophil
Acidophil

Plastic section stained with basic fuchsin and hematoxylin
The polygonal shape of the epithelial cells of the anterior hypophysis is well defined in this preparation. The cytoplasm of **basophils** stains **dark pink, acidophils** stain **light pink**, and **chromophobe cells** are **unstained**.

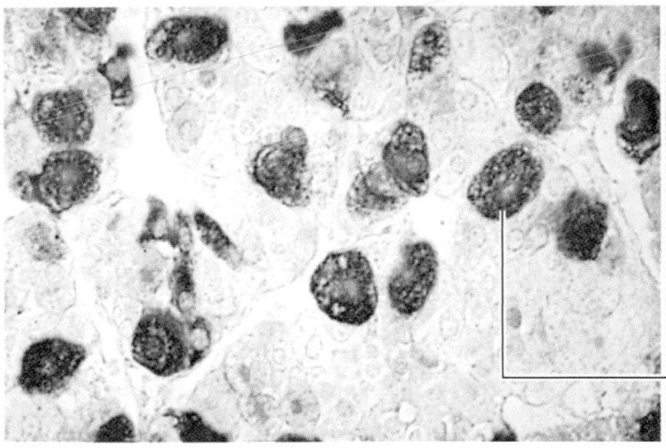
FSH-secreting cell (classified
as basophil by H&E staining)

Immunohistochemistry (immunoperoxidase)
An antibody against the β chain of follicle-stimulating hormone (FSH) has been used to identify gonadotrophs within the anterior hypophysis in this illustration.

The use of specific antibodies against hormones produced in the anterior hypophysis has enabled (1) the precise identification of all hormone-producing cells of the anterior hypophysis; (2) the identification of hormone-producing **adenomas**; and (3) the elucidation of the negative and positive feedback pathways regulating the secretion of hypophysial hormones.

Growth hormone

Growth hormone is a peptide of 191 amino acids in length (22 kd). It has the following characteristics (Figure 18-6): (1) Growth hormone has structural homology similar to prolactin and human placental lactogen. There is some overlap in the activity of these three hormones. (2) It is released into the blood circulation in the form of **pulses** throughout a 24-hour sleep-wake period, with **peak secretion occurring during the first two hours of sleep**. (3) Despite its name, growth hormone does not directly induce growth; rather, it acts by stimulating in hepatocytes the production of **insulin-like growth factor-1** (IGF-1), also known as **somatomedin** C. The cell receptor for IGF-1 is similar to that for insulin (formed by dimers of two glycoproteins with integral cytoplasmic protein tyrosine kinase domains). (4) The release of growth hormone is regulated by two neuropeptides.

A **stimulatory** effect is caused by **growth hormone–releasing hormone**

Figure 18-5. Vascular relationships and fine structure of the anterior hypophysis

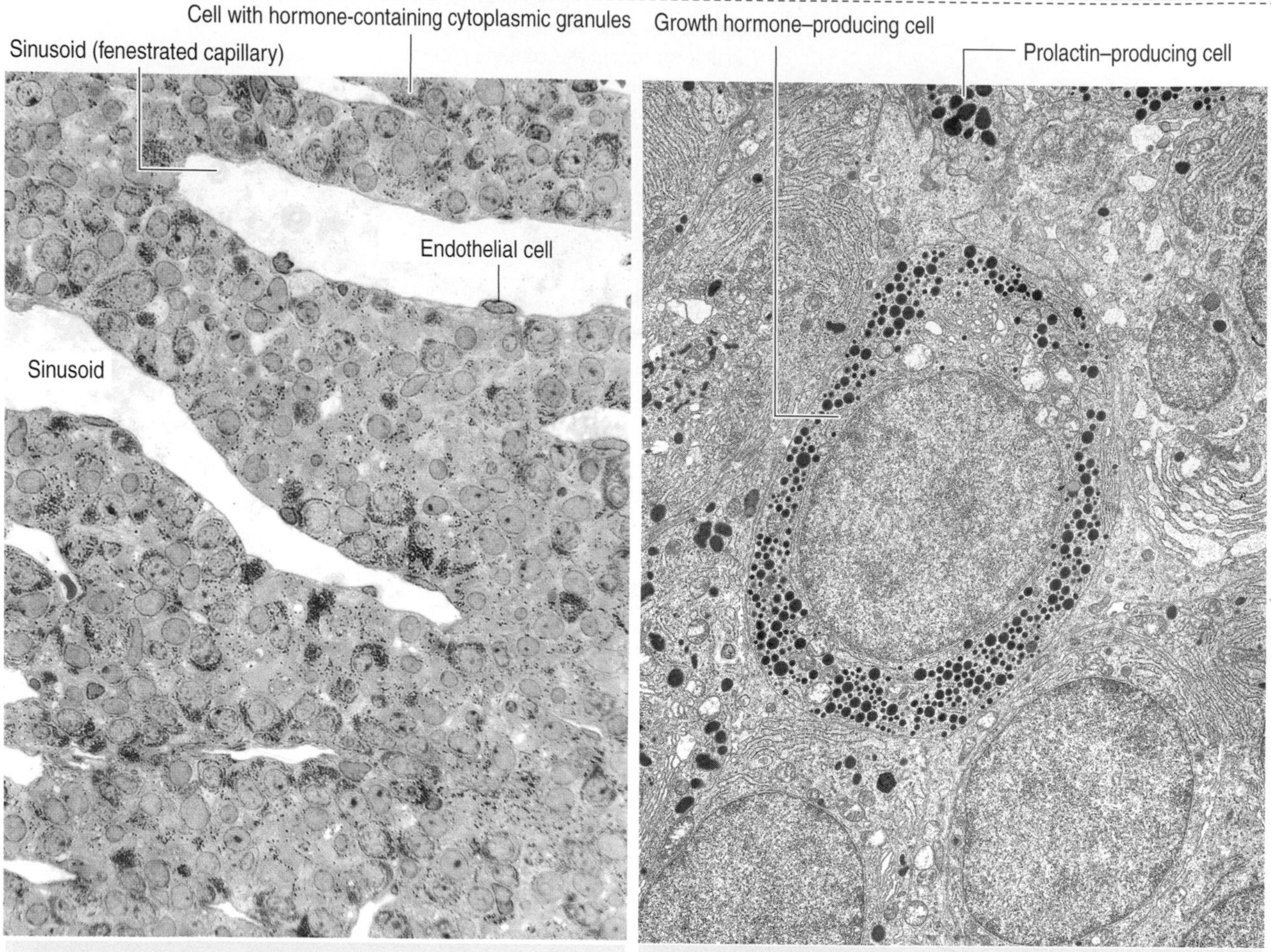

Cell with hormone-containing cytoplasmic granules
Sinusoid (fenestrated capillary)
Endothelial cell
Sinusoid
Growth hormone–producing cell
Prolactin–producing cell

Light microscopy (plastic section)
Cells of the pars distalis are surrounded by sinusoids (fenestrated capillaries) that receive the secreted hormones. Hormones are then transported in the bloodstream to regulate the function of target cells.

Electron microscopy
Electron microscopy has provided a powerful tool for examining the **size**, **distribution**, **content**, and **mode of synthesis** and **secretion** of the various hormones stored in secretory granules in the cytoplasm of endocrine cells of the anterior hypophysis.

(GHRH), a peptide of 44 amino acids. An **inhibitory** effect is produced by **somatostatin** (a peptide of 14 amino acids) and by **elevated blood glucose levels**. Both GHRH and somatostatin derive from the hypothalamus. Somatostatin is also produced in the islet of Langerhans (pancreas).

IGF-1 (7.5 kd) stimulates the overall growth of bone and soft tissues. In children, IGF-1 stimulates the growth of long bones at the epiphyseal plates. Clinicians measure IGF-1 in blood to determine growth hormone function. **A drop in IGF-1 serum levels stimulates the release of growth hormone**.

IGF target cells secrete several **IGF-binding proteins** and **proteases**. The latter can regulate the delivery and action of IGF on target cells by reducing available IGF-binding proteins.

Clinical significance: Gigantism (in children) and acromegaly (in adults)

Excessive secretion of growth hormone can occur in the presence of a benign tumor called an **adenoma**.

When the growth hormone–secreting tumor occurs during childhood and puberty, at a time when the epiphyseal plates are still active, **gigantism** (Greek *gigas*, giant; extremely tall stature) is observed. If excessive growth hormone secretion occurs in the adult, when the epiphyseal plates are inactive, **acromegaly** (Greek

Figure 18-6. **Growth hormone**

Growth hormone induces growth through **insulin-like growth factor-1** (IGF-1) produced by hepatocytes.

GHRH stimulates the release of growth hormone from acidophils.

Somatostatin and **high blood glucose levels** inhibit the release of growth hormone.

IGF-1 stimulates the growth of long bones by stimulating the hypertrophy of chondrocytes at the **epiphyseal plates**.

Excess of growth hormone causes **gigantism in children** and **acromegaly in adults**. In most cases, an adenoma of the anterior hypophysis is responsible for growth hormone hypersecretion.

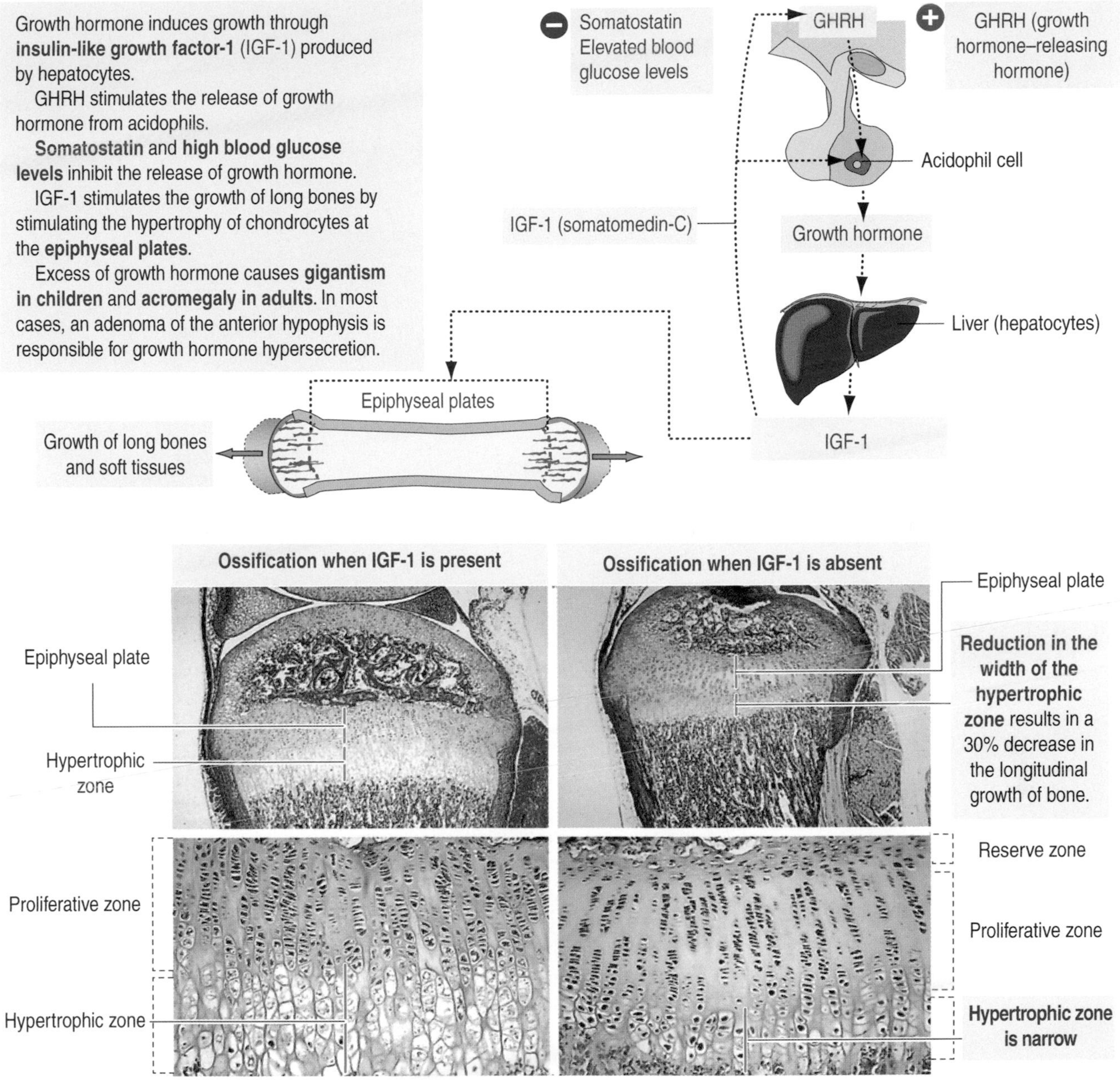

Somatostatin
Elevated blood glucose levels
GHRH
GHRH (growth hormone–releasing hormone)
Acidophil cell
IGF-1 (somatomedin-C)
Growth hormone
Liver (hepatocytes)
IGF-1
Epiphyseal plates
Growth of long bones and soft tissues
Ossification when IGF-1 is present
Ossification when IGF-1 is absent
Epiphyseal plate
Hypertrophic zone
Epiphyseal plate
Reduction in the width of the hypertrophic zone results in a 30% decrease in the longitudinal growth of bone.
Proliferative zone
Hypertrophic zone
Reserve zone
Proliferative zone
Hypertrophic zone is narrow

Micrographs from Wang J, Zhou J, Bondy CA: IGF-1 promotes longitudinal bone growth by insulin-like actions augmenting chondrocyte hypertrophy. FASEB J, 13:1985-1990,1999.

akron, end or extremity; *megas*, large) develops. In acromegaly, the hands, feet, jaw, and soft tissues become enlarged. Long bones do not grow in length, but cartilage (nose, ears) and membranous bones (mandible and calvarium) continue to grow, leading to gross deformities.

A growth hormone–secreting adenoma does not show the typical pulsatile secretory pattern of the hormone. Growth hormone secretion is not suppressed by glucose. A **decrease** in the secretion of growth hormone in children results in short stature (**dwarfism**).

Prolactin

Prolactin is a 199-amino-acid single-chain protein (22 kd). Prolactin, growth hormone, and human placental lactogen share some amino acid homology and overlapping activity,

The predominant action of prolactin is to stimulate the initiation and mainte-

Figure 18-7. Prolactin

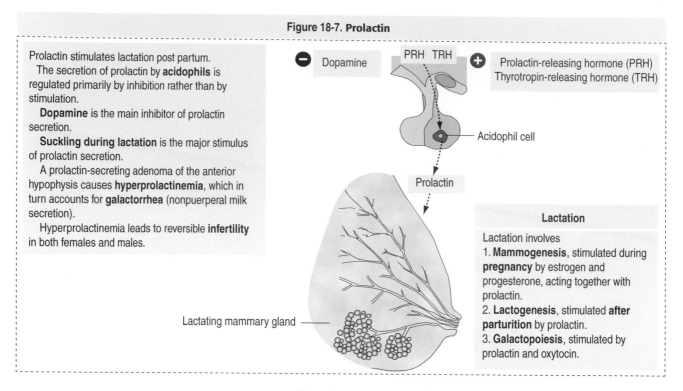

Prolactin stimulates lactation post partum.

The secretion of prolactin by **acidophils** is regulated primarily by inhibition rather than by stimulation.

Dopamine is the main inhibitor of prolactin secretion.

Suckling during lactation is the major stimulus of prolactin secretion.

A prolactin-secreting adenoma of the anterior hypophysis causes **hyperprolactinemia**, which in turn accounts for **galactorrhea** (nonpuerperal milk secretion).

Hyperprolactinemia leads to reversible **infertility** in both females and males.

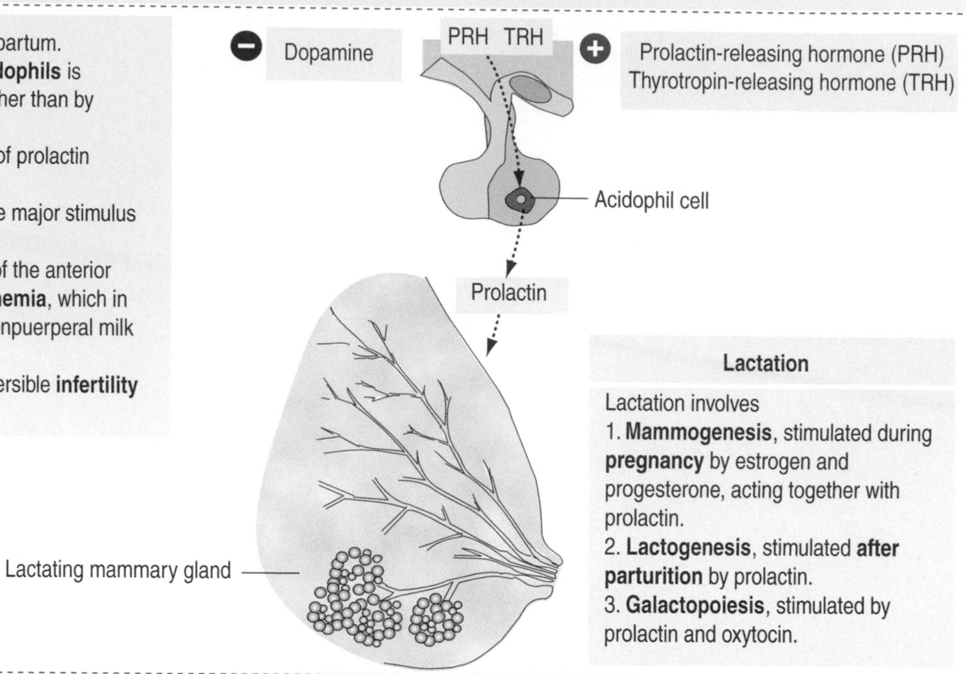

Lactation

Lactation involves
1. **Mammogenesis**, stimulated during **pregnancy** by estrogen and progesterone, acting together with prolactin.
2. **Lactogenesis**, stimulated **after parturition** by prolactin.
3. **Galactopoiesis**, stimulated by prolactin and oxytocin.

nance of **lactation** post partum (Figure 18-7). Lactation involves the following: (1) **Mammogenesis**, the growth and development of the mammary gland, is stimulated primarily by estrogen and progesterone in coordination with prolactin and human placental lactogen. (2) **Lactogenesis**, the initiation of lactation, is triggered by prolactin acting on the developed mammary gland by the actions of estrogens and progesterone. Lactation is inhibited during pregnancy by high levels of estrogen and progesterone, which decline at delivery. Either estradiol or prolactin antagonists are used clinically to stop lactation. (3) **Galactopoiesis**, the maintenance of milk production, requires both prolactin and oxytocin.

The effect of prolactin, placental lactogen, and steroids on the development of the lactating mammary gland is discussed in Chapter 23, Fertilization, Placentation, and Lactation.

Unlike other hormones of the anterior hypophysis, **the secretion of prolactin is regulated primarily by inhibition rather than by stimulation**. The main inhibitor is **dopamine**. Dopamine secretion is stimulated by prolactin to inhibit its own secretion.

A **stimulatory** effect on prolactin release is exerted by **prolactin-releasing hormone** (PRH) and **thyrotropin-releasing hormone** (TRH). Prolactin is released from **acidophils** in a pulsatile fashion, coinciding with and following each period of suckling. **Intermittent surges of prolactin stimulate milk synthesis.**

Clinical significance: Hyperprolactinemia

Prolactin-secreting tumors alter the hypothalamohypophysial-gonadal axis, leading to gonadotropin deficiency. Hypersecretion of prolactin in women can be associated with **infertility**, caused by the lack of **ovulation** and **oligomenorrhea** or **amenorrhea** (dysfunctional uterine bleeding).

A decrease in fertility and libido is found in males. These antifertility effects are found in both sexes and are usually reversible. **Galactorrhea** (nonpuerperal milk secretion) is a common problem in **hyperprolactinemia** and can also occur in males.

Hormones secreted by basophils: Gonadotropins, TSH, and ACTH

Gonadotropins (FSH and LH) and TSH have common features: (1) they are

Figure 18-8. Gonadotropins (FSH and LH)

Neurons in the **arcuate nucleus** of the hypothalamus secrete **GnRH** (gonadotropin-releasing hormone). GnRH is secreted in pulses at 60- to 90-minute intervals and stimulates the pulsatile secretion of **gonadotropins** by the basophilic gonadotrophs.

In the female, FSH stimulates **follicular cells** of the ovarian follicle to proliferate and secrete **estradiol**, **inhibin**, and **activin**. LH stimulates progesterone secretion by the **corpus luteum**.

In the male, FSH stimulates **Sertoli cell** function in the seminiferous epithelium (synthesis of **inhibin**, **activin**, and **androgen-binding protein**). LH stimulates the production of **testosterone** by **Leydig cells**.

A lack of FSH and LH in females and males leads to **infertility**.

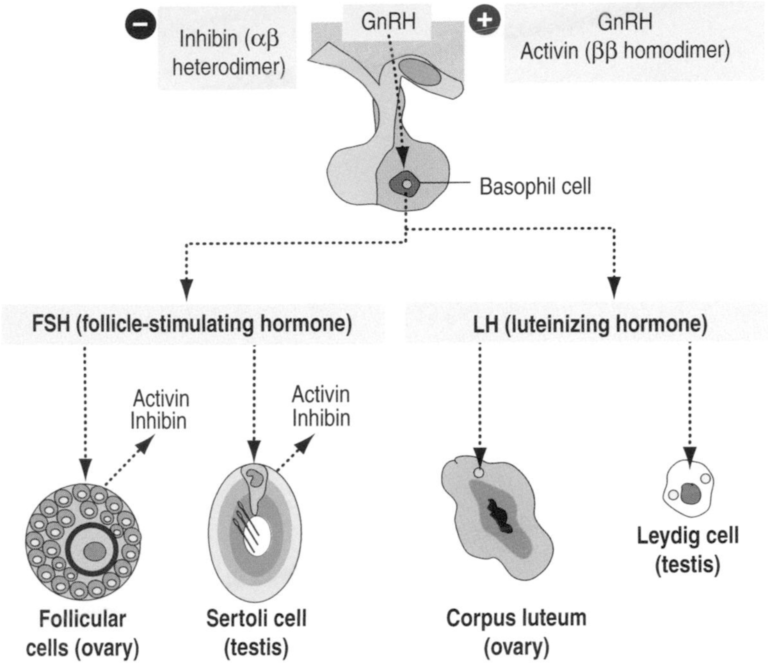

glycoproteins (hence the PAS-positive staining of basophils), and (2) they consist of **two chains**. The α chain is a glycoprotein common to FSH, LH, and TSH, but the β chain is specific for each hormone. Therefore, **the β chain confers specificity to the hormone**.

Gonadotropins: Follicle-stimulating hormone and luteinizing hormone

Gonadotrophs (gonadotropin-secreting cells) (Figure 18-8) secrete **both FSH and LH**. Gonadotrophs constitute about 10% of the total cell population of the anterior hypophysis.

The release of gonadotropins is stimulated by **gonadotropin-releasing hormone (GnRH;** also called **luteinizing hormone–releasing hormone [LHRH]**), a decapeptide produced in the **arcuate nucleus** of the hypothalamus. GnRH is secreted in pulses at 60- to 90-minute intervals into the portal vasculature. **A single basophil can synthesize and release both FSH and LH** in a pulsatile fashion.

In the female, **FSH** stimulates the development of the ovarian follicles by a process called **folliculogenesis**. In the male, FSH acts on **Sertoli cells** in the testis to stimulate the aromatization of estrogens from androgens and the production of **androgen-binding protein**, with binding affinity to testosterone.

In the female, **LH** stimulates **steroidogenesis** in the ovarian follicle and corpus luteum. In the male, LH controls the rate of **testosterone** synthesis by **Leydig cells** in the testis. The function of FSH and LH in the male is analyzed in Chapter 20, Spermatogenesis.

The release of FSH and GnRH is **inhibited** by (1) **inhibin**, a **heterodimer** protein formed by α- and β-peptide chains, secreted by the male and female target cells (Sertoli and follicular cells and cells of the anterior hypophysis), and (2) **estradiol**.

The release of FSH in both females and males is **enhanced** by a homodimer protein, called **activin**, secreted by Sertoli cells and follicular cells. It consists of two β chains. Little is known about what controls αβ (inhibin) and ββ (activin) dimerization.

We discuss in Chapter 20, Spermatogenesis, and Chapter 22, Follicle Development and Menstrual Cycle, the function of FSH and LH in spermatogenesis, Leydig cell function, folliculogenesis, and luteogenesis.

Figure 18-9. **Thyroid-stimulating hormone (TSH)**

Thyrotropin-releasing hormone (**TRH**), a tripeptide, modulates the synthesis and release of TSH (thyroid-stimulating hormone) from basophils.

TSH is a glycoprotein that binds to a receptor in the plasma membrane of thyroid follicular epithelial cells. The hormone-receptor complex stimulates the formation of cAMP. The production of the thyroid hormones T_3 (triiodothyronine) and T_4 (thyroxine) is stimulated by cAMP.

Some T_4 is converted to T_3 in peripheral tissues. **T_3 is more active than T_4 and has a negative feedback (inhibitory) action on TSH synthesis and release.**

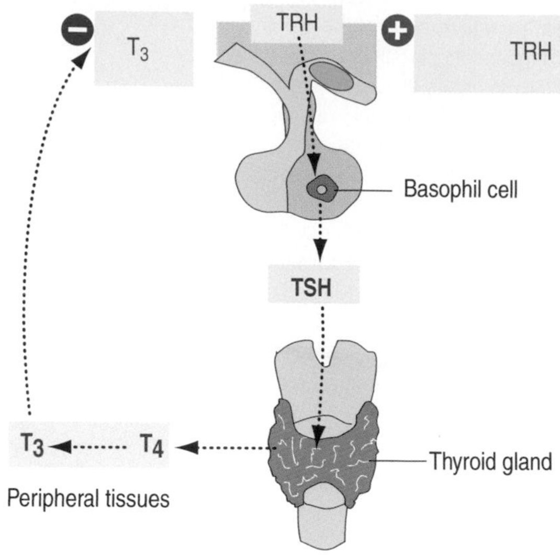

Clinical significance: Infertility

The secretion of FSH and LH can decrease when there is a deficient secretion of GnRH, caused by anorexia or a tumor of the hypophysis, which can destroy the gonadotrophs, thereby decreasing FSH and LH secretion.

A decrease in fertility and reproductive functions can be observed in females and males. Females can have menstrual disorders. Small testes and infertility can be seen in males (a condition known as **hypogonadotropic hypogonadism**) when GnRH secretion is deficient.

Castration (**ovariectomy** in the female and **orchidectomy** in the male) causes a significant **increase** in the synthesis of FSH and LH as a result of a **loss of feedback inhibition**. Hyperfunctional gonadotropic cells are large and vacuolated and are called **castration cells.**

Thyroid-stimulating hormone (thyrotropin)

Thyrotropic cells represent about 5% of the total population of the anterior hypophysis.

TSH is the regulatory hormone of **thyroid function** (Figure 18-9) and **growth**. The mechanism of action of TSH on thyroid cell function is discussed in the thyroid gland section of Chapter 19, Endocrine System. **Thyrotropin-releasing hormone** (**TRH**), a 3-amino-acid-peptide produced in the hypothalamus, **stimulates** the synthesis and release of TSH from **basophils**. TRH also stimulates the release of prolactin. The release of TSH is **inhibited** by increased concentrations of the thyroid hormones triiodothyronine (T_3) and thyroxine (T_4).

Clinical significance: Hypothyroidism

A deficiency in the secretion of TSH (observed in rare cases of congenital hypoplasia of the hypophysis) produces **hypothyroidism**, characterized by reduced cell metabolism and temperature and basal metabolic rate and mental lethargy. Hypothyroidism is also observed in the autoimmune disorder **Hashimoto's disease.** Hypothyroidism can also result from a disease of the thyroid gland or a deficiency in dietary iodine. We will discuss **hyperthyroidism** in the thyroid gland section of Chapter 19, Endocrine System when we describe **Graves' disease.**

Adrenocorticotropic hormone

ACTH, or **corticotropin,** is a **single-chain** protein, 39 amino acids in length (4.5 kd), with a short circulating time (7 to 12 minutes). Its primary action is **to**

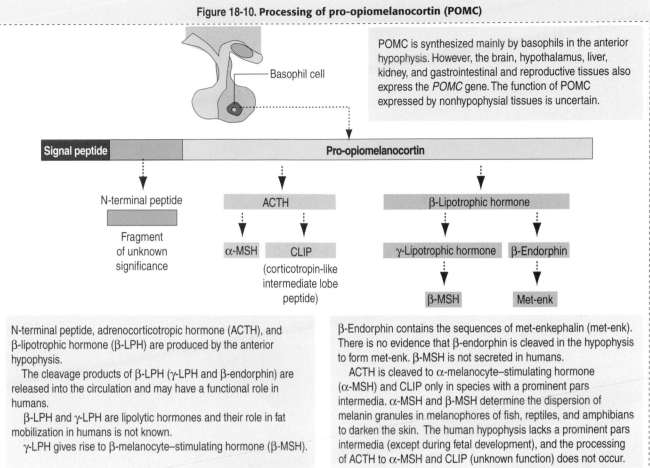

Figure 18-10. Processing of pro-opiomelanocortin (POMC)

POMC is synthesized mainly by basophils in the anterior hypophysis. However, the brain, hypothalamus, liver, kidney, and gastrointestinal and reproductive tissues also express the *POMC* gene. The function of POMC expressed by nonhypophysial tissues is uncertain.

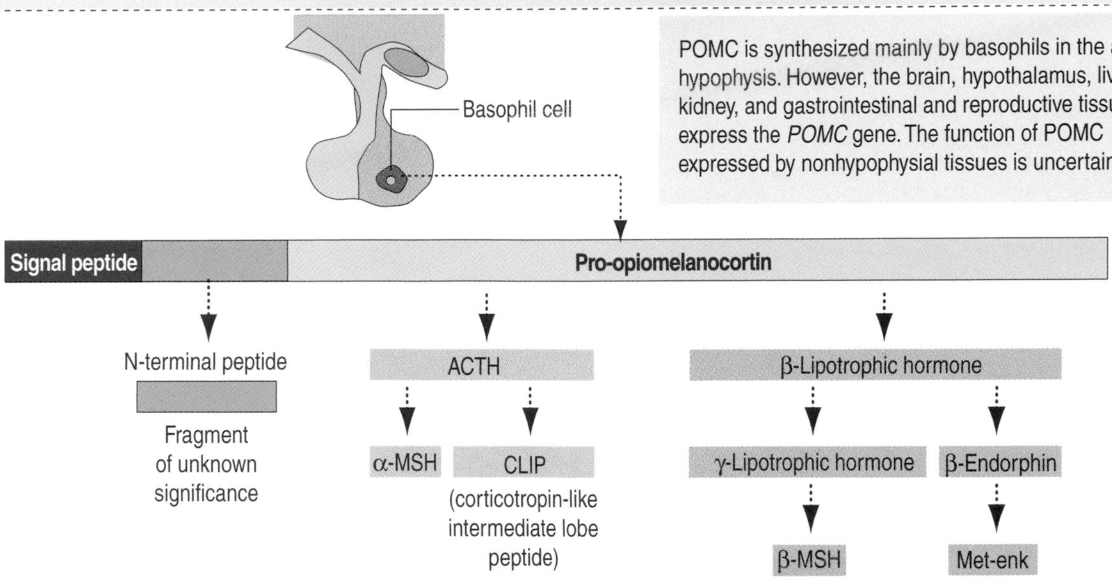
Basophil cell
Signal peptide
Pro-opiomelanocortin
N-terminal peptide
Fragment of unknown significance
ACTH
α-MSH
CLIP
(corticotropin-like intermediate lobe peptide)
β-Lipotrophic hormone
γ-Lipotrophic hormone
β-Endorphin
β-MSH
Met-enk

N-terminal peptide, adrenocorticotropic hormone (ACTH), and β-lipotrophic hormone (β-LPH) are produced by the anterior hypophysis.

The cleavage products of β-LPH (γ-LPH and β-endorphin) are released into the circulation and may have a functional role in humans.

β-LPH and γ-LPH are lipolytic hormones and their role in fat mobilization in humans is not known.

γ-LPH gives rise to β-melanocyte–stimulating hormone (β-MSH).

β-Endorphin contains the sequences of met-enkephalin (met-enk). There is no evidence that β-endorphin is cleaved in the hypophysis to form met-enk. β-MSH is not secreted in humans.

ACTH is cleaved to α-melanocyte–stimulating hormone (α-MSH) and CLIP only in species with a prominent pars intermedia. α-MSH and β-MSH determine the dispersion of melanin granules in melanophores of fish, reptiles, and amphibians to darken the skin. The human hypophysis lacks a prominent pars intermedia (except during fetal development), and the processing of ACTH to α-MSH and CLIP (unknown function) does not occur.

stimulate growth and **steroid synthesis** in the zonae fasciculata and reticularis of the **adrenal cortex**. The zona glomerulosa of the adrenal cortex is under the control of angiotensin II (see the adrenal gland section of Chapter 19, Endocrine System). The effects of ACTH on the adrenal cortex are mediated by cyclic adenosine monophosphate (cAMP). ACTH also acts beyond the adrenal gland by increasing skin pigmentation and lipolysis.

ACTH derives from a large glycosylated precursor of 31 kd called **pro-opiomelanocortin** (POMC), processed in the anterior hypophysis. The products of POMC are the following (Figure 18-10):

1. An **N-terminal peptide** of unknown function, **ACTH**, and **β-lipotrophic hormone** (β-LPH). These three POMC derivatives are secreted by the anterior hypophysis.

2. The cleavage products of **β-LPH**, **γ-LPH**, and **β-endorphin** are released into circulation. β-LPH and γ-lipotrophic hormone (γ-LPH) have **lipolytic action**, but their precise role in fat mobilization in humans is unknown.

3. γ-LPH contains the amino acid sequence of **β-melanocyte–stimulating hormone** (β-MSH; not secreted in humans). β-Endorphin contains the sequences of **met-enkephalin** (met-enk). There is no evidence that β-endorphin is cleaved in the hypophysis to form met-enk.

4. ACTH is cleaved to α-melanocyte–stimulating hormone (α-MSH) and **corticotropin-like intermediate peptide** (CLIP). α-MSH and CLIP hormones, found in species with a hypophysis with a prominent pars intermedia, cause dispersion of melanin granules in melanophores and darkening of the skin of many fish, amphibians, and reptiles.

The release of ACTH is controlled by the following (Figure 18-11):

1. A stimulatory effect determined by **corticotropin-releasing hormone** (CRH)

Figure 18-11. **Adrenocorticotropic hormone (ACTH)**

ACTH controls predominantly the function of two zones of the adrenal cortex (**zona fasciculata** and **zona reticularis**). The zona glomerulosa is regulated by **angiotensin II** derived from the processing of the liver protein angiotensinogen by the proteolytic action of renin (kidney) and converting enzyme (lung).

ACTH stimulates the synthesis of cortisol (a glucocorticoid) and androgens. Cortisol and other steroids are metabolized in liver.

Low levels of cortisol in blood, stress, and vasopressin (antidiuretic hormone [ADH]) stimulate ACTH secretion from basophils by stimulation of CRH release (positive feedback). **Cortisol is the dominating regulatory factor.**

ACTH increases the pigmentation of skin. Skin darkening in Addison's disease and Cushing's disease is not determined by melanocyte-stimulating hormone (MSH), which is not normally present in human serum.

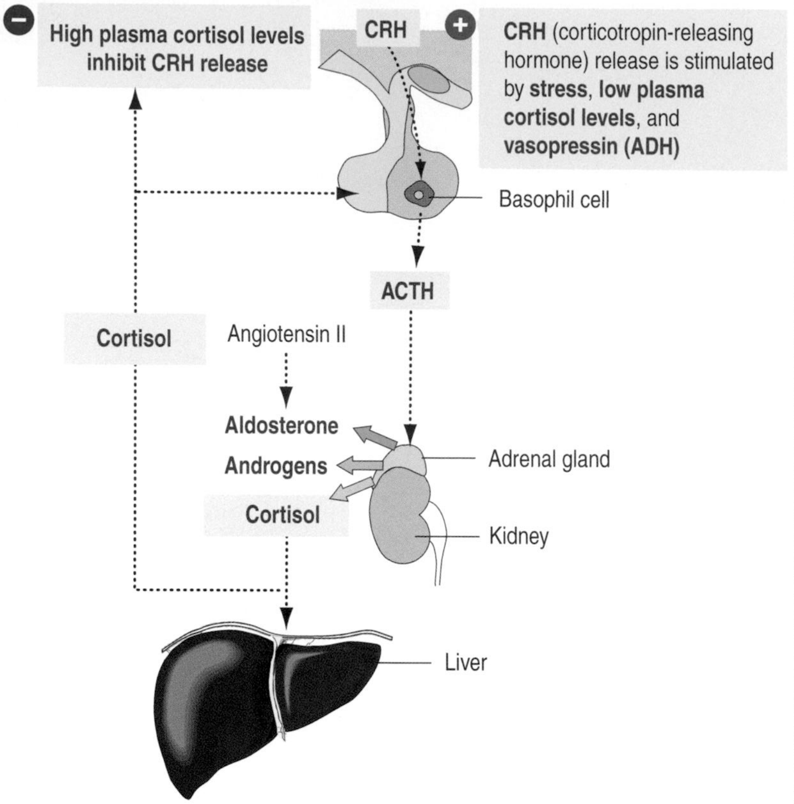
High plasma cortisol levels inhibit CRH release
CRH
CRH (corticotropin-releasing hormone) release is stimulated by stress, low plasma cortisol levels, and vasopressin (ADH)
Basophil cell
ACTH
Cortisol
Angiotensin II
Aldosterone
Androgens
Cortisol
Adrenal gland
Kidney
Liver

from the hypothalamus. CRH co-localizes with **antidiuretic hormone** (ADH; see later section, Neurohypophysis) in the paraventricular nuclei. Both ADH and angiotensin II potentiate the effect of CRH on the release of ACTH.

2. An **inhibitory** effect caused by high levels of **cortisol** in blood either by preventing the release of CRH or by blocking the release of ACTH by basophil **corticotropic cells** (ACTH-secreting cells).

ACTH is secreted in a circadian manner (morning peaks followed by a slow decline afterward).

Clinical significance: Cushing's disease

An ACTH-secreting adenoma of the hypophysis causes **Cushing's disease**. This disease is characterized by an increase in the production of cortisol by the zona fasciculata of the adrenal cortex (see the adrenal gland section in Chapter 19, Endocrine System), obesity, osteoporosis, and muscle wasting. A **reduction** in the secretion of ACTH results in diminished secretion of cortisol and in hypoglycemia.

A loss of ACTH decreases adrenal androgen secretion. In females, androgen deficiency causes loss of pubic and axillary hair. This effect is not observed in males because it is compensated for by testicular secretion of androgens.

Neurohypophysis

The neurohypophysis consists of three histologic components (Figures 18-12 and 18-13): (1) **Pituicytes**, resembling astrocytes, provide support to the axons. (2) **Unmyelinated axons**, derived from neuroendocrine cells (called **magnicellular neurons** because their cell bodies are large) of the **supraoptic** and **paraventricular nuclei**, make up the infundibulum and form the **hypothalamohypophysial tract.** Axons, with bulging intermittent segments and terminals (called **Herring bodies**) containing secretory products (the **neurophysin-hormone complex**), are found

Figure 18-12. Neurohypophysis

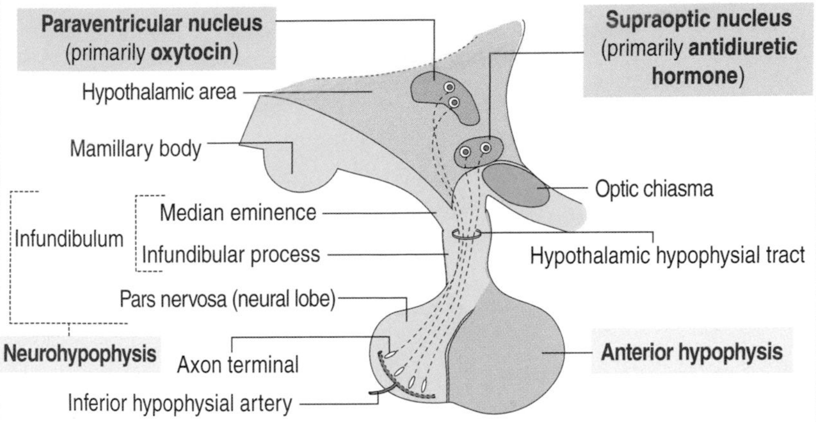

The hormones **antidiuretic hormone** (or **arginine vasopressin**) and **oxytocin** are synthesized in the neurons of the **supraoptic** and **paraventricular nuclei**, respectively.

The hormones are transported along the axons forming the **hypothalamic hypophysial tract**, together with the carrier protein **neurophysin**, and are released at the axon terminals. The hormones enter **fenestrated capillaries** derived from the inferior hypophysial artery.

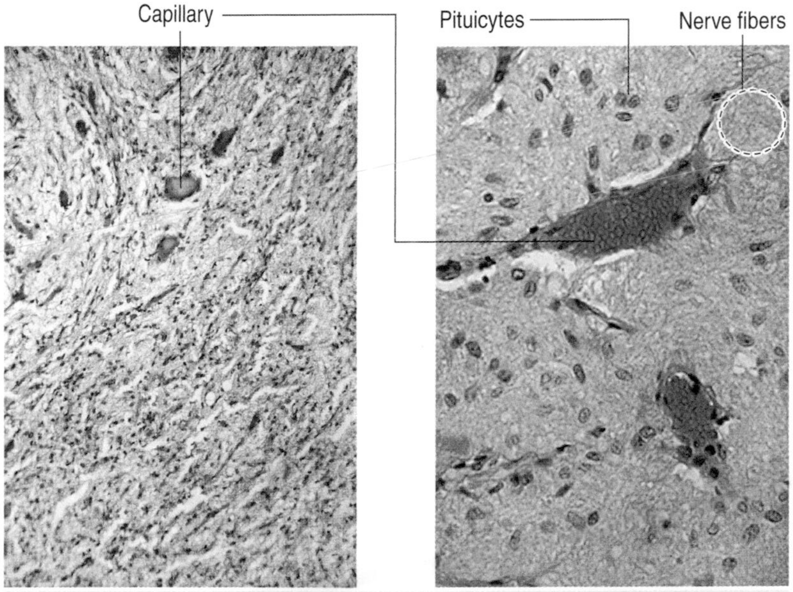

The neurohypophysis is formed by supporting neuroglial cells—the **pituicytes**—whose cytoplasmic processes surround the **unmyelinated nerve fibers** arising from neurons of the paraventricular and supraoptic nuclei. Abundant capillaries are visualized.

Antidiuretic hormone and oxytocin accumulate temporarily in axon dilations, forming the **Herring bodies** (not seen in these photomicrographs).

in the pars nervosa (neural lobe). Neurophysin is secreted with the hormone and does not have an apparent biological action other than serving as a hormone carrier during axonal transport. (3) **Fenestrated capillaries** are derived from the inferior hypophysial artery.

Pituicytes are astrocyte-like glial cells with abundant **glial fibrillary acidic proteins**, an intermediate filament protein, and a few **lipid droplets** in their cytoplasm. The cytoplasmic processes of pituicytes (Figure 18-14) (1) surround the axons derived from the neuroendocrine cells, (2) extend between the axon terminals and the basal lamina surrounding fenestrated capillaries, and (3) retract to enable the release into the blood of secretory granules stored in the axon

Figure 18-13. **Structure and function of the neuroendocrine cell**

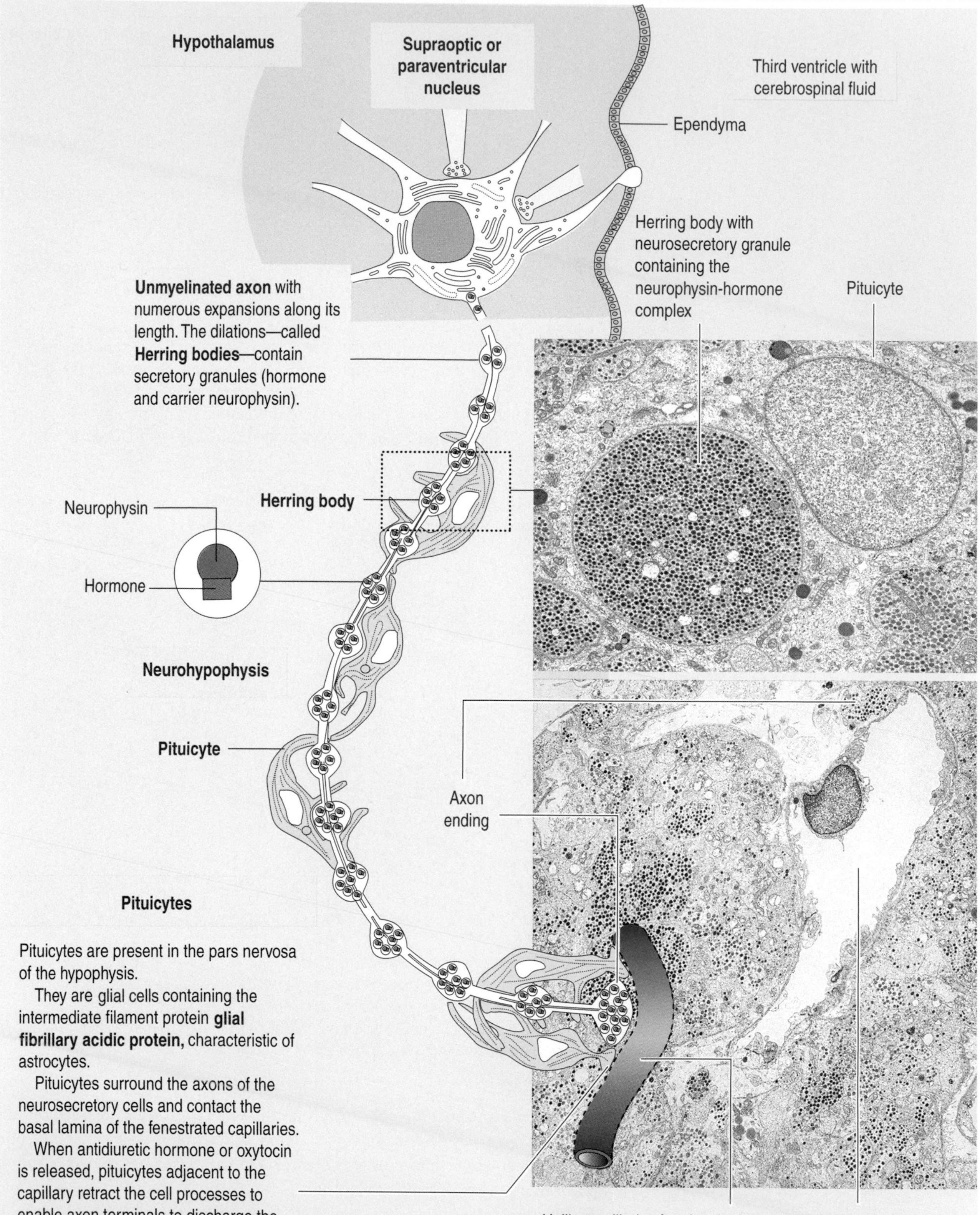

Hypothalamus
Supraoptic or paraventricular nucleus
Third ventricle with cerebrospinal fluid
Ependyma
Herring body with neurosecretory granule containing the neurophysin-hormone complex
Pituicyte
Unmyelinated axon with numerous expansions along its length. The dilations—called **Herring bodies**—contain secretory granules (hormone and carrier neurophysin).
Neurophysin
Herring body
Hormone
Neurohypophysis
Pituicyte
Axon ending
Pituicytes

Pituicytes are present in the pars nervosa of the hypophysis.

They are glial cells containing the intermediate filament protein **glial fibrillary acidic protein,** characteristic of astrocytes.

Pituicytes surround the axons of the neurosecretory cells and contact the basal lamina of the fenestrated capillaries.

When antidiuretic hormone or oxytocin is released, pituicytes adjacent to the capillary retract the cell processes to enable axon terminals to discharge the stored hormone into the circulation.

Unlike capillaries forming the blood-brain barrier, capillaries of the neurohypophysis are **fenestrated** to permit diffusion of secretions into the circulation.

Figure 18-14. Axon endings and pituicytes around fenestrated capillaries

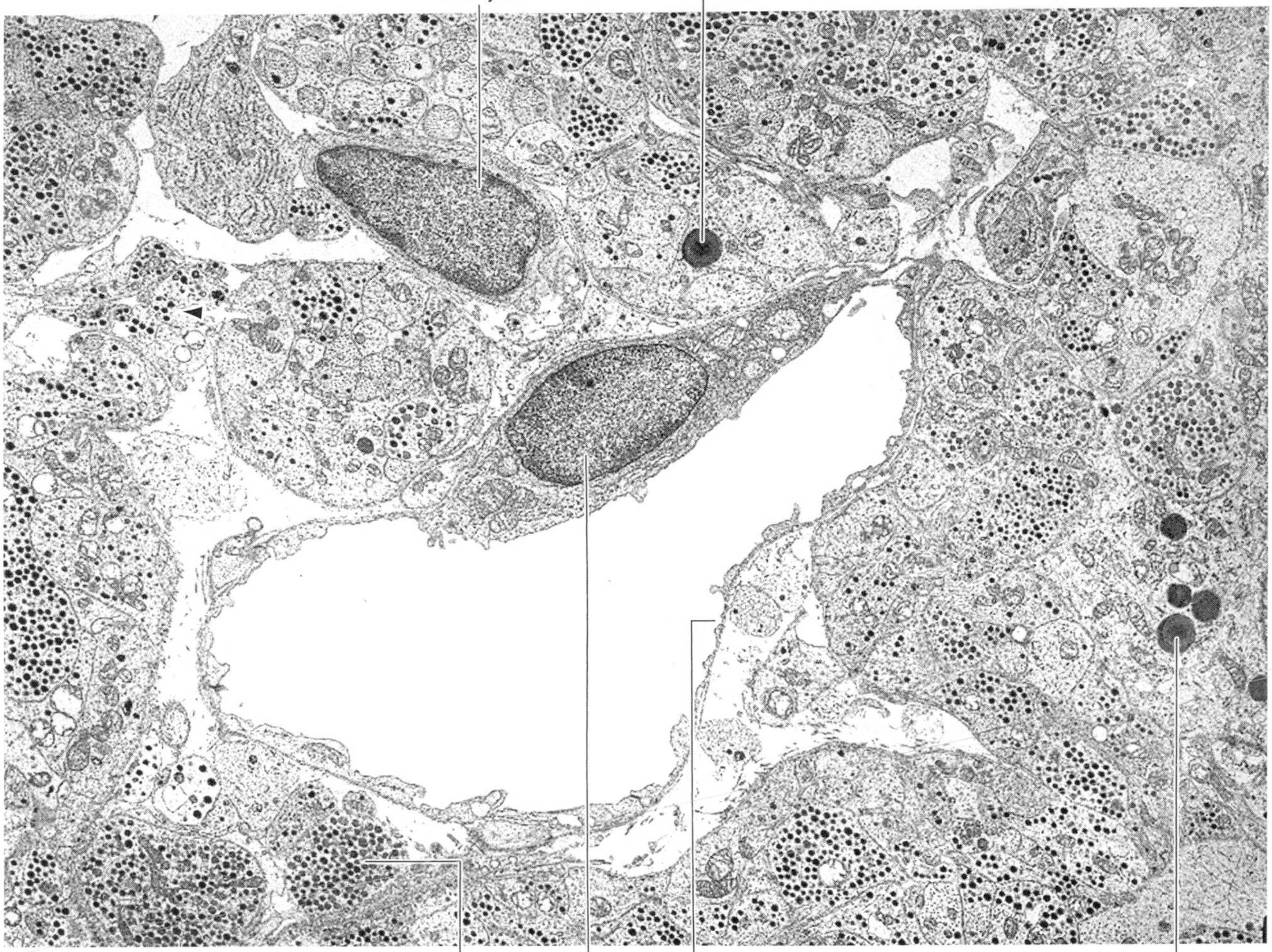
Pituicytes
Lipid droplet
A nerve terminal contains stored antidiuretic hormone or oxytocin in secretory granules
Fenestrated endothelial cell
Fenestrations
Lipid droplets in the cytoplasm of a pituicyte

terminals (see Figure 18-14).

Axons in the neurohypophysis derive from the **supraoptic nuclei** and the **paraventricular nuclei.**

Some neurons of the paraventricular nuclei are small and their axons project to the median eminence rather than to the pars nervosa. These neurons, called **parvicellular neurons** (Latin *parvus*, small), secrete ADH and oxytocin entering the hypophysial portal blood at the median eminence. Large neurons of the supraoptic and paraventricular nuclei, called **magnicellular neurons** (Latin *magnus*, large), give rise to axons forming the **hypothalamic hypophysial tract.** The terminals of these neurons are located in the pars nervosa. Both the supraoptic and paraventricular nuclei contain neurons synthesizing ADH and oxytocin. However, **neurons of the supraoptic nuclei produce primarily ADH and the paraventricular nuclei synthesize primarily oxytocin.**

In addition to these two nuclei, the hypothalamus has additional nuclei, **the hypothalamic hypophysiotropic nuclei**, with neurons producing releasing and inhibitory hormones to be discharged at the fenestrated capillaries of the primary plexus (see earlier, Blood supply of the hypophysis).

Although the neuroendocrine cells of the supraoptic and paraventricular nuclei are located **behind the blood-brain barrier**, their products are transported to nerve terminals and released **outside the blood-brain barrier** into fenestrated capillaries.

Figure 18-15. Antidiuretic hormone and oxytocin

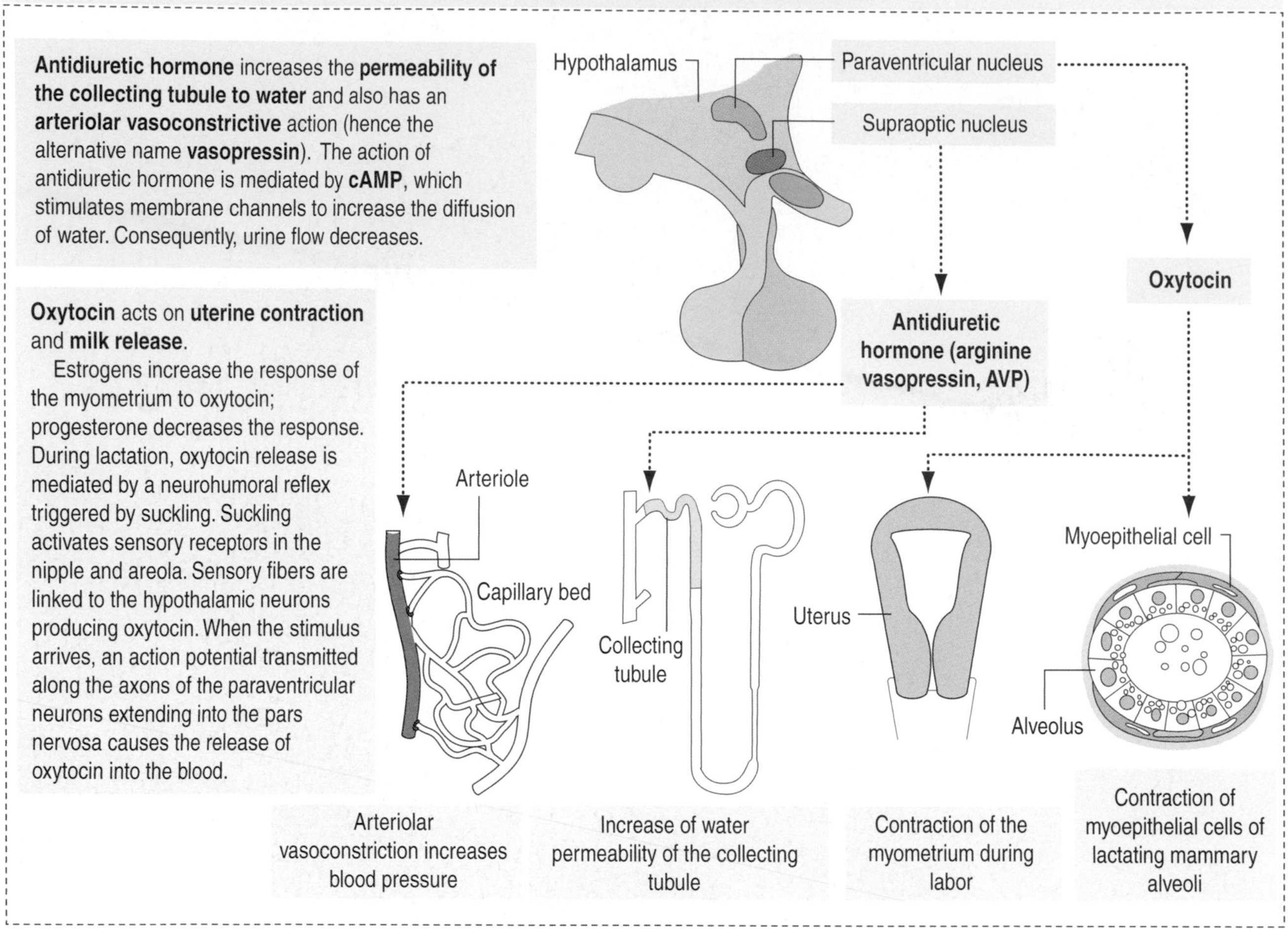

Antidiuretic hormone increases the **permeability of the collecting tubule to water** and also has an **arteriolar vasoconstrictive** action (hence the alternative name **vasopressin**). The action of antidiuretic hormone is mediated by **cAMP**, which stimulates membrane channels to increase the diffusion of water. Consequently, urine flow decreases.
Oxytocin acts on **uterine contraction** and **milk release**.
Estrogens increase the response of the myometrium to oxytocin; progesterone decreases the response. During lactation, oxytocin release is mediated by a neurohumoral reflex triggered by suckling. Suckling activates sensory receptors in the nipple and areola. Sensory fibers are linked to the hypothalamic neurons producing oxytocin. When the stimulus arrives, an action potential transmitted along the axons of the paraventricular neurons extending into the pars nervosa causes the release of oxytocin into the blood.
Hypothalamus
Paraventricular nucleus
Supraoptic nucleus
Oxytocin
Antidiuretic hormone (arginine vasopressin, AVP)
Arteriole
Capillary bed
Collecting tubule
Uterus
Myoepithelial cell
Alveolus
Arteriolar vasoconstriction increases blood pressure
Increase of water permeability of the collecting tubule
Contraction of the myometrium during labor
Contraction of myoepithelial cells of lactating mammary alveoli

Clinical significance: Diabetes insipidus

Oxytocin participates in the **contraction of smooth muscle**, in particular the **uterus during labor**, and **myoepithelial cells** lining the secretory acini and lactiferous ducts of the mammary gland to facilitate milk ejection (or **letdown of milk**) during lactation (Figure 18-15).

Antidiuretic hormone regulates water excretion in the kidney and is also a **potent vasoconstrictor at high doses** (see Figure 18-15). This is the basis for its alternative name, vasopressin (arginine vasopressin [AVP]). An increase in osmotic pressure in circulating blood or reduced blood volume triggers the release of ADH. Retention of water reduces plasma osmolality, which acts on hypothalamic osmoreceptors to suppress the secretion of ADH.

ADH and oxytocin are transported down the axons and stored in nerve terminals within secretory granules, packaged together with a carrier protein, **neurophysin**. A **common precursor** gives rise to ADH, oxytocin, and the carrier neurophysin. **ADH is bound to neurophysin II and oxytocin to neurophysin I**. The released hormones circulate in blood in an unbound form and have a half-life of 5 minutes.

Neurogenic diabetes insipidus occurs when the secretion of ADH is reduced or absent. **Polyuria** is a common clinical finding. Patients with diabetes insipidus can excrete up to 20 L of urine in 24 hours. Neurogenic diabetes insipidus is caused by a head injury, an invasive tumor damaging the hypothalamic hypophysial system, or autoimmune destruction of vasopressin-secreting neurons.

Nephrogenic diabetes insipidus occurs in certain chronic renal diseases that are **nonresponsive** to vasopressin or as a result of genetic defects in renal receptors for vasopressin.

Pineal gland

The pineal gland is an endocrine organ formed by cells with a neurosecretory function. The pineal gland is connected to the brain by a stalk, but **there are no direct nerve connections of the pineal gland with the brain**. Instead, **postganglionic sympathetic nerve fibers derived from the superior cervical ganglia** supply the pineal gland.

Preganglionic fibers to the superior cervical ganglia derive from the lateral column of the spinal cord. The function of the pineal gland is regulated by sympathetic nerves.

Development of the pineal gland

The pineal gland develops from a saccular outpocketing of the posterior diencephalic roof in the midline of the third ventricle (Figure 18-16).

Continued diverticulation and infolding result in a solid parenchymal mass of **cords** and **clusters of pinealocytes** and **glial-like interstitial cells** supported by a meninges-derived connective tissue that carries blood vessels and nerves to the pineal gland.

Histology of the pineal gland

Two cell types form the pineal gland (see Figure 18-16): (1) the **pinealocytes** and (2) the **glial-like interstitial cells**.

The **pinealocytes** are secretory cells organized into cords and clusters resting on a basal lamina and surrounded by connective tissue, blood vessels lined by fenestrated endothelial cells, and nerves. The pinealocyte has two or more cell processes ending in bulbous expansions. One of the processes ends near capillaries. The cytoplasm contains **abundant mitochondria** and **multiple synaptic ribbons that are randomly distributed** (Figure 18-17). **Single ribbon synapses** can be seen at the **synaptic end** of sensory cells of the **retina** (see Figure 9-18) and **inner ear** (see Figure 9-28).

Interstitial cells are found among pinealocytes. The glial-like interstitial cells and the connective tissue provide stromal support to the functional pinealocytes.

Like the anterior hypophysis, **the pineal gland lacks a blood-brain barrier.**

The function of pinealocytes is regulated by **β-adrenergic receptors**. The metabolic activity of pinealocytes is inhibited by β-adrenergic antagonists.

An important feature of the pineal gland is the presence of defined **areas of calcification**, called **corpora arenacea** ("brain sand"). Calcification starts early in childhood and becomes evident in the second decade of life. Pinealocytes secrete an extracellular matrix in which calcium phosphate crystals deposit. Calcification has no known effect on the function of the pineal gland. **A calcified pineal gland is an important radiographic marker of the midline of the brain.**

The pineal gland secretes melatonin, the "hormone of darkness"

Melatonin is the major biologically active substance secreted by the pineal gland. Melatonin is synthesized from **tryptophan** by pinealocytes and immediately secreted (Figure 18-18). During night (with complete darkness), the melatonin content of the pineal gland is highest.

Exposure to light or administration of β-adrenergic blocking agents causes a rapid decrease in ***N*-acetyltransferase** and a consequent decline in melatonin synthesis.

Melatonin is released into the general circulation (1) **to act on the hypothalamus and hypophysis, and, in many species, to inhibit gonadotropin** and **growth hormone secretion** and (2) to induce **sleepiness**. An unproven hypothesis is that melatonin contributes to drowsiness when lights are turned down.

Circadian clock, an endogenous oscillator controlling circadian rhythms

A 24-hour biological circadian (Latin *circa*, about; *dies*, day) clock regulates sleep and feeding patterns and is linked to the light-dark cycle or sleep-wake cycle.

Figure 18-16. Development of the pineal gland

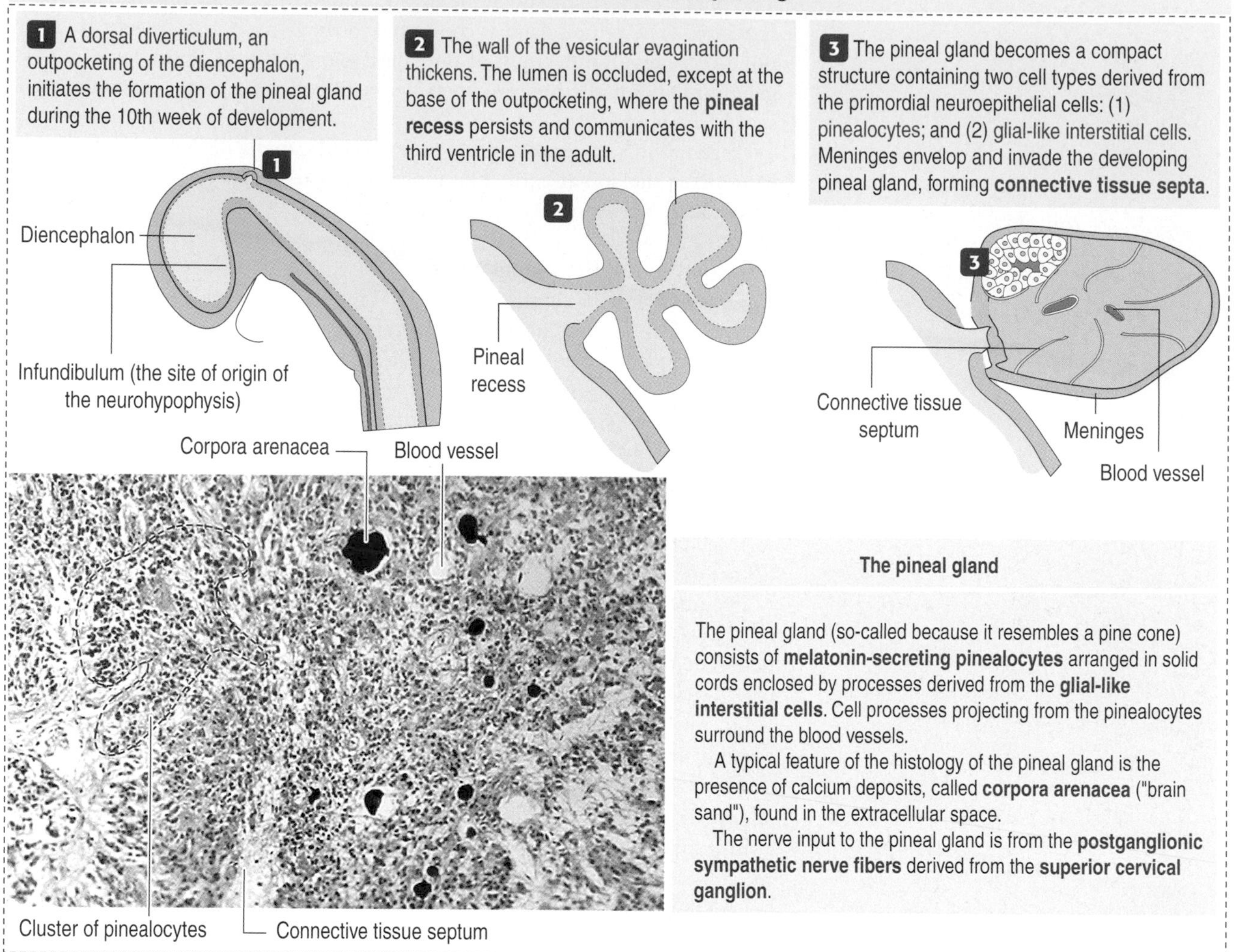

1 A dorsal diverticulum, an outpocketing of the diencephalon, initiates the formation of the pineal gland during the 10th week of development.
2 The wall of the vesicular evagination thickens. The lumen is occluded, except at the base of the outpocketing, where the **pineal recess** persists and communicates with the third ventricle in the adult.
3 The pineal gland becomes a compact structure containing two cell types derived from the primordial neuroepithelial cells: (1) pinealocytes; and (2) glial-like interstitial cells. Meninges envelop and invade the developing pineal gland, forming **connective tissue septa**.
Diencephalon
Infundibulum (the site of origin of the neurohypophysis)
Pineal recess
Connective tissue septum
Meninges
Blood vessel
Corpora arenacea
Blood vessel
Cluster of pinealocytes
Connective tissue septum

The pineal gland

The pineal gland (so-called because it resembles a pine cone) consists of **melatonin-secreting pinealocytes** arranged in solid cords enclosed by processes derived from the **glial-like interstitial cells**. Cell processes projecting from the pinealocytes surround the blood vessels.

A typical feature of the histology of the pineal gland is the presence of calcium deposits, called **corpora arenacea** ("brain sand"), found in the extracellular space.

The nerve input to the pineal gland is from the **postganglionic sympathetic nerve fibers** derived from the **superior cervical ganglion**.

The retinohypothalamic tract conducts light signals to the hypothalamic suprachiasmatic nucleus (the circadian "clock") as the initial step in the regulation of melatonin synthesis and secretion.

The **suprachiasmatic nucleus** is located adjacent to the optic chiasm and contains a network of neurons operating as **an endogenous pacemaker regulating circadian rhythmicity**. These neurons are **circadian oscillators** connected to specialized **melanopsin-producing ganglion cells** of the retina. Ganglion cells function as **luminance detectors** resetting the circadian oscillators. There is some evidence that the suprachiasmatic nucleus sends signals to the circadian pacemakers of the rest of the body through the proteins **transforming growth factor-α** and **prokineticin 2**.

When a suprachiasmatic nucleus is transplanted to a recipient with a damaged suprachiasmatic nucleus, it displays the circadian pacemaker properties of the donor rather than those of the host. The mechanism by which individual neurons of the suprachiasmatic nucleus are recruited to organize a pacemaker that oversees the circadian rhythms is not fully known.

In *Drosophila* and mice, a loss of the blue-light-absorbing photopigments **cryptochromes 1** and **2** (**Cry1** and **Cry2**) from still undetermined photoreceptors of the retina disables the circadian clock. Removal of the eyes abolishes the light-dark shifting responses of the circadian clock.

Jet lag, a condition associated with fatigue, insomnia, and disorientation experienced by many travelers, is caused by a disruption of the circadian rhythm. Bipolar disorder and sleep disorder are also linked to the abnormal functioning

Figure 18-17. Structure of the pinealocyte

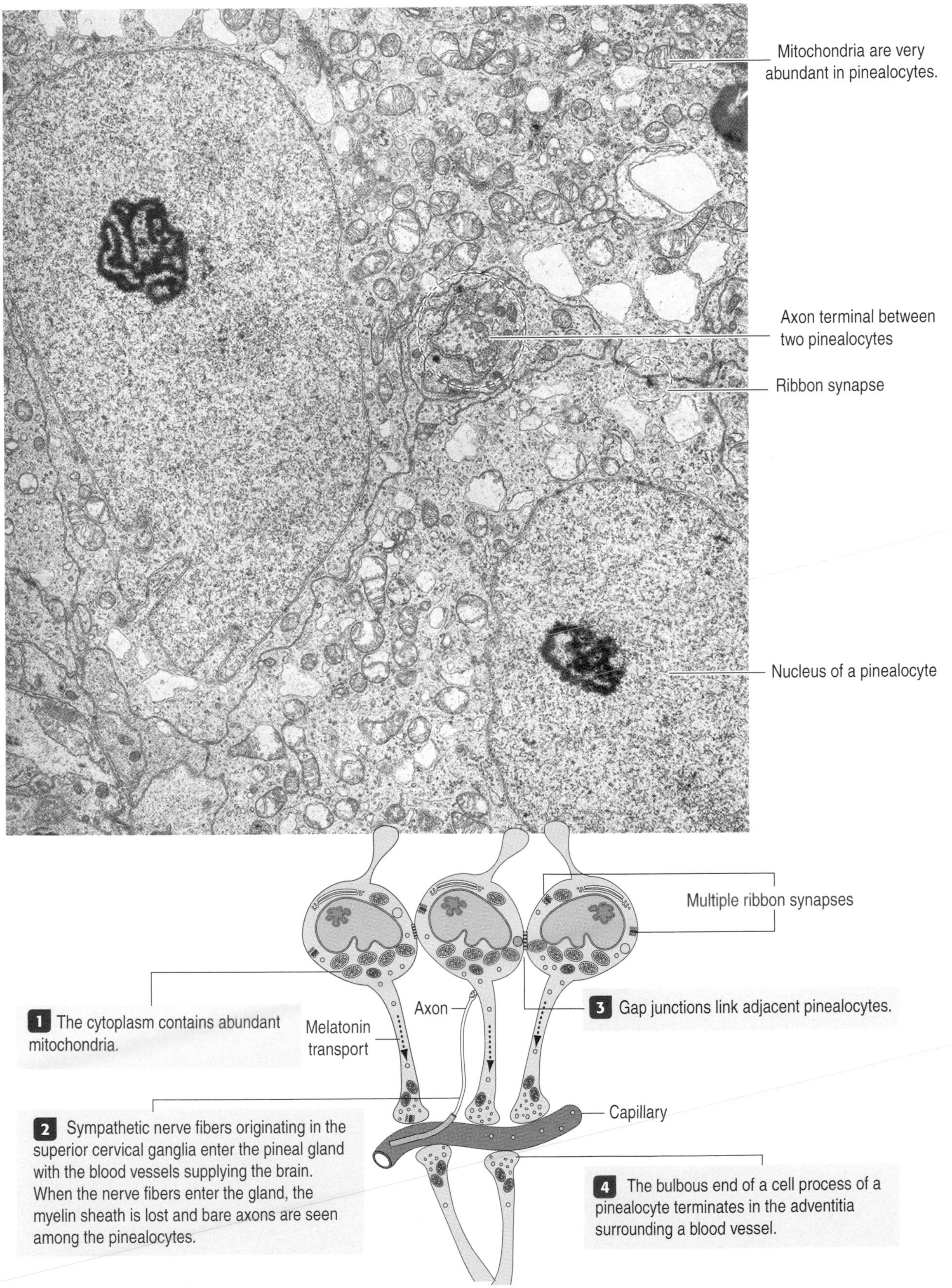

Mitochondria are very abundant in pinealocytes.
Axon terminal between two pinealocytes
Ribbon synapse
Nucleus of a pinealocyte
Multiple ribbon synapses
Axon
Melatonin transport
Capillary
1 The cytoplasm contains abundant mitochondria.
2 Sympathetic nerve fibers originating in the superior cervical ganglia enter the pineal gland with the blood vessels supplying the brain. When the nerve fibers enter the gland, the myelin sheath is lost and bare axons are seen among the pinealocytes.
3 Gap junctions link adjacent pinealocytes.
4 The bulbous end of a cell process of a pinealocyte terminates in the adventitia surrounding a blood vessel.

Figure 18-18. Synthesis and secretion of melatonin

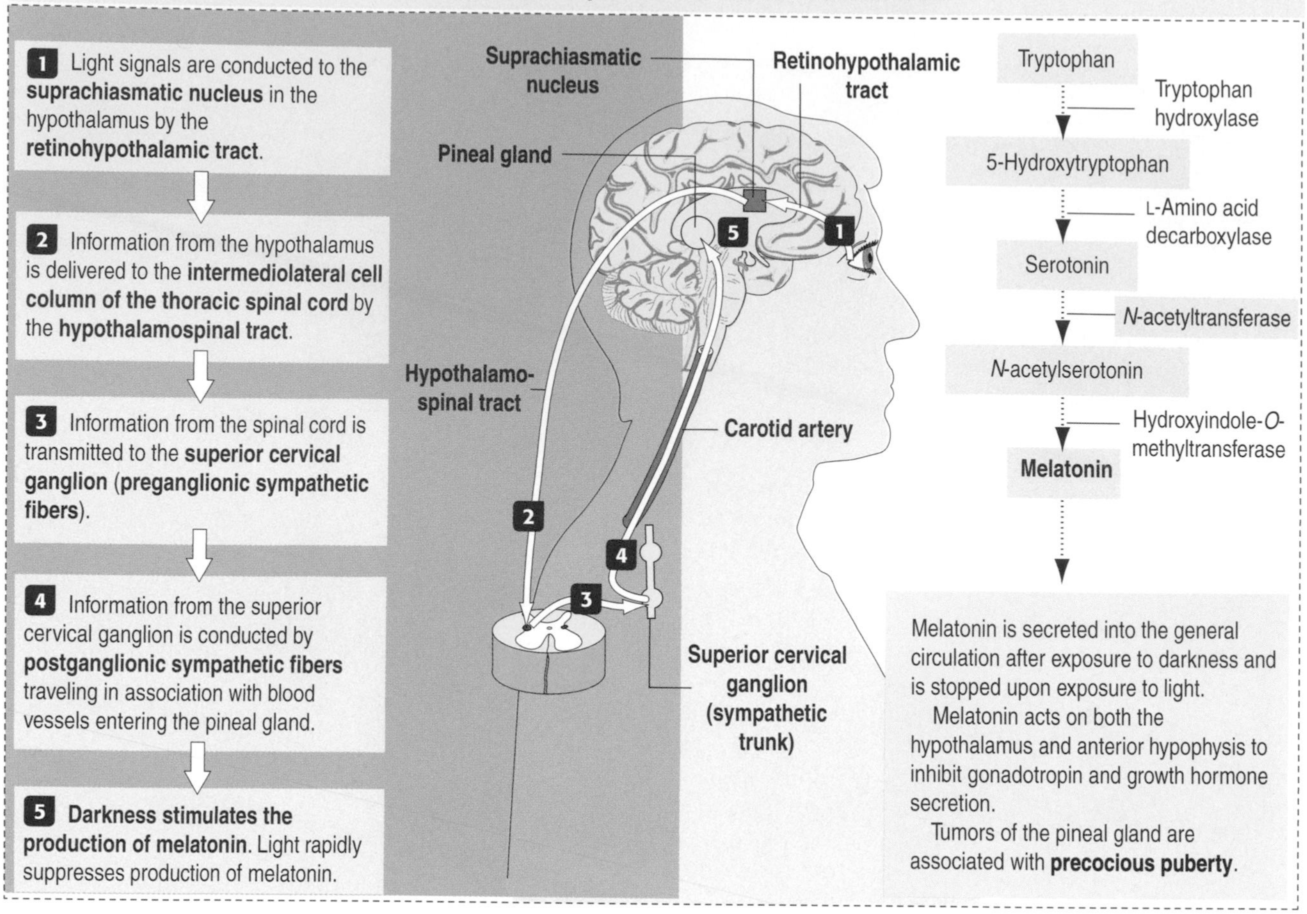
1 Light signals are conducted to the suprachiasmatic nucleus in the hypothalamus by the retinohypothalamic tract.
2 Information from the hypothalamus is delivered to the intermediolateral cell column of the thoracic spinal cord by the hypothalamospinal tract.
3 Information from the spinal cord is transmitted to the superior cervical ganglion (preganglionic sympathetic fibers).
4 Information from the superior cervical ganglion is conducted by postganglionic sympathetic fibers traveling in association with blood vessels entering the pineal gland.
5 Darkness stimulates the production of melatonin. Light rapidly suppresses production of melatonin.
Suprachiasmatic nucleus
Retinohypothalamic tract
Pineal gland
Hypothalamo-spinal tract
Carotid artery
Superior cervical ganglion (sympathetic trunk)
1
2
3
4
5
Tryptophan
Tryptophan hydroxylase
5-Hydroxytryptophan
L-Amino acid decarboxylase
Serotonin
N-acetyltransferase
N-acetylserotonin
Hydroxyindole-O-methyltransferase
Melatonin
Melatonin is secreted into the general circulation after exposure to darkness and is stopped upon exposure to light.
Melatonin acts on both the hypothalamus and anterior hypophysis to inhibit gonadotropin and growth hormone secretion.
Tumors of the pineal gland are associated with precocious puberty.

of the circadia rhythms.

Clinical significance: Precocious puberty

A tumor of the pineal gland (**pinealoma**) is associated with **precocious puberty**. Precocious puberty is characterized by the onset of androgen secretion and spermatogenesis in boys before the age of 9 or 10 years and the initiation of estrogen secretion and cyclic ovarian activity in girls before age 8. **Precocious puberty is probably caused by the effect of the tumor on the function of the hypothalamus rather than by a direct effect of pineal tumors on sexual function.**

Pinealomas cause a neurologic disorder known as **Parinaud's syndrome** (paralysis of upward gaze, looking steadily in one direction, pupillary areflexia to light, paralysis of convergence, and wide-based gait).

• General organization of the neuroendocrine system. The hypothalamus and the hypophysis (pituitary gland) form an integrated system known as the hypothalamohypophysial system consisting of two components: (1) the hypothalamic adenohypophysial system (linking the hypothalamus to the anterior hypophysis), and (2) the hypothalamic neurohypophysial system (connecting the hypothalamus to the neurohypophysis).

• Functional aspects of the neuroendocrine system. The hypothalamus contains clusters of neurons called nuclei. Some of the neurons are neuroendocrine cells exerting positive and negative effects on the two components of the hypophysis. These effects are mediated by releasing and inhibitory hormones or factors.

The transport of signaling molecules is mediated by the hypothalamohypophysial portal circulation consisting of a primary capillary plexus in the lower hypothalamus connected by portal veins to a secondary capillary plexus in the anterior lobe of the hypophysis. A third capillary plexus supplies the neurohypophysis.

The primary capillary plexus is supplied by the superior hypophysial artery; the third capillary plexus is supplied by the inferior hypophysial artery. The two arteries are connected by the trabecular artery. There is no connection between the secondary and third capillary plexuses. The hypophysial vein drains the second and third capillary plexuses to dural sinuses.

• The hypophysis consists of two embryologically distinct portions: (1) the adenohypophysis or glandular component, derived from Rathke's pouch, an invagination of the roof of the future oral cavity, and (2) the neurohypophysis or neural component, an infundibular downgrowth from the floor of the diencephalon.

The adenohypophysis consists of three subdivisions: (1) the pars distalis (anterior lobe), (2) the pars tuberalis, surrounding the neural infundibular stem or stalk, and (3) the pars intermedia (the rudimentary intermediate lobe). The neurohypophysis consists of two subdivisions: (1) the pars nervosa and (2) the median eminence.

The anterior lobe contains three components: (1) epithelial cell cords, (2) a connective tissue stroma, and (3) fenestrated capillaries (sinusoids) of the secondary capillary plexus.

There are three distinct cell populations: (1) acidophil cells (stain with an acidic dye), (2) basophil cells (stain with a basic dye), and (3) chromophobe cells (lacking cytoplasmic staining). Acidophil cells secrete peptide hormones (growth hormone and prolactin); basophils secrete glycoprotein hormones (gonadotropins FSH and LH, TSH, and ACTH). Chromophobe cells are cells that have depleted their cytoplasmic hormonal content.

• Growth hormone (also called somatotropin). It is secreted in a pulsatile pattern with peak secretion occurring during the first 2 hours of sleep. Growth hormone exerts its actions through insulin-like growth factor-1 (IGF-1) produced in hepatocytes after stimulation by growth hormone. The release of growth hormone is stimulated by growth hormone–releasing hormone produced in the hypothalamus and by high blood levels of IGF-1. Inhibition of growth hormone release is mediated by somatostatin (also produced in the hypothalamus and in the islets of Langerhans in the pancreas) and high blood levels of glucose.

Gigantism during childhood and puberty is caused by excessive secretion of growth hormone (usually produced by a benign tumor of the hypophysis called adenoma). **Acromegaly** (enlargement of hands, feet, jaw, and soft tissues) is seen in adults when growth hormone production is high.

• Prolactin has a main function: to stimulate the initiation and maintenance of lactation postpartum. Lactation involves (1) mammogenesis, the growth and development of the mammary gland, (2) lactogenesis, the initiation of lactation, and (3) galactopoiesis, the maintenance of milk production. A secondary function is to facilitate the steroidogenic action of LH in Leydig cells by upregulating the expression of the luteinizing hormone (LH) receptor. The pulsatile secretion of prolactin is regulated primarily by an inhibitory mechanism rather than by stimulation. The main inhibitor is dopamine. Prolactin-releasing hormone and thyrotropin-releasing hormone, both originating in the hypothalamus, stimulate prolactin release.

Excessive secretion of prolactin (hyperprolactinemia) by a benign tumor of the hypophysis in both sexes causes gonadotropin deficiency. In women, hyperprolactinemia is associated with infertility, anovulation, and oligomenorrhea or amenorrhea (dysfunctional uterine bleeding). A decrease in fertility and libido is seen in males. Galactorrhea (nonpuerperal milk secretion) caused by hyperprolactinemia is common in both sexes.

• Gonadotropins: FSH and LH. The release of gonadotropins is stimulated by gonadotropin-releasing hormone (GnRH; also called luteinizing hormone–releasing hormone or LHRH). GnRH is secreted in pulses at 60- to 90-minute intervals. A single basophil can produce both FSH and LH.

In the female, FSH stimulates folliculogenesis (the development of the ovarian follicle). In the male, FSH targets Sertoli cells in the testis to convert testosterone into estrogen (by aromatization) and produce androgen-binding protein (ABP).

In the female, LH stimulates steroidogenesis in the ovarian follicle and corpus luteum. In the male, LH controls the production of testosterone by Leydig cells.

The release of FSH and GnRH is inhibited by inhibin (an $\alpha\beta$ heterodimer) produced by the target cells (follicular cells and Sertoli cells), and estradiol. The release of FSH is enhanced by activin (a $\beta\beta$ homodimer).

A drop in the secretion of GnRH (caused by anorexia nervosa, a tumor of the hypophysis, or a condition known as **hypogonadotropic hypogonadism** in males) can abolish the secretion of FSH and LH. Castration (ovariectomy or orchidectomy) causes a significant increase in the synthesis of FSH and LH and the vacuolization of gonadotropin-secreting cells (castration cells).

• Thyroid-stimulating hormone (TSH; or thyrotropin) regulates thyroid function. Thyrotropin-releasing hormone stimulates the release of TSH (and prolactin). Thyroid hormones triiodothyronine (T_3) and thyroxine (T_4) inhibit the release of TSH.

Hy**pothyroidism**, characterized by reduced cell metabolism and temperature, is caused by deficient secretion of TSH and by the autoimmune disorder **Hashimoto's disease.** **Hyperthyroidism** is usually determined by an autoantibody directed against the TSH receptor in thyroid follicular cells (Graves' disease).

• Adrenocorticotropic hormone (ACTH; or corticotropin) stimulates growth and steroid synthesis in the zona fasciculata and zona reticularis of the adrenal cortex.

ACTH derives from the large precursor pro-opiomelanocortin (POMC) processed in the anterior hypophysis.

Corticotropin-releasing hormone (CRH) derived from neuroendocrine neurons of the paraventricular nuclei (which also produce antidiuretic hormone [ADH]), stimulates the release of ACTH. This CRH stimulatory effect is potentiated by ADH and angiotensin II. High levels of cortisol prevent the release of CRH or ACTH.

Cushing's disease, caused by an ACTH-producing adenoma of the hypophysis, results in the overproduction of cortisol by cells of the zona fasciculata of the adrenal cortex, obesity, osteoporosis, and muscle wasting.

• Neurohypophysis. Three histologic components are found in the neurohypophysis: (1) pituicytes, astrocyte-like cells containing the intermediate filament protein glial fibrillary acidic protein and providing support to axons, (2) unmyelinated axons derived from neuroendocrine cells of the hypothalamic supraoptic and paraventricular nuclei forming the hypothalamic hypophysial tract, and (3) fenestrated capillaries.

Axons display intermittent bulging segments called Herring bodies containing neuroendocrine secretory granules. Each secretory granule consists of two components: the carrier protein neurophysin and the associated hormone ADH (also called arginine vasopressin) or oxytocin.

Oxytocin participates in the contraction of uterine smooth muscle during labor, and of myoepithelial cells in the lactating mammary alveoli to facilitate milk ejection. ADH regulates water excretion in the kidney and, at a higher concentration, is also a potent vasoconstrictor.

Neurogenic diabetes insipidus occurs when the secretion of ADH is reduced. It is caused by severe head injury, an invasive tumor disrupting the hypothalamic hypophysial tract, or the autoimmune destruction of ADH-producing neurons. Polyuria is a common clinical finding. **Nephrogenic diabetes insipidus** occurs in certain chronic renal diseases that are not responsive to ADH.

• Pineal gland. The pineal gland is an endocrine organ containing cells with a neurosecretory function and without direct nerve connection with the brain. The pineal gland is supplied by postganglionic sympathetic nerve fibers derived from the superior cervical ganglia (SCG). Preganglionic fibers to the SCG derive from the lateral column of the spinal cord.

The pineal gland develops from a saccular outpocketing of the posterior diencephalic roof in the midline of the third ventricle. It contains cells called pinealocytes, arranged in cords and clusters, and supporting glial-like interstitial cells. The pinealocyte displays cytoplasmic extensions with bulbar endings. These cell processes end close to a capillary. Pinealocytes contain abundant mitochondria and characteristic multiple ribbon synapses. Remember that ribbon synapses are also seen in photoreceptor cells of the retina and in hair cells of the inner ear. An important landmark of the pineal gland are calcified deposits called corpora arenacea ("brain sand").

The major secretory product of the pineal gland is melatonin, synthesized from tryptophan by pinealocytes and immediately secreted. The concentration of melatonin in the pineal gland is high during the night.

The 24-hour circadian clock is an endogenous oscillator controlling circadian rhythms, including sleep and feeding patterns. The retinohypothalamic tract conducts light signals from the retina (in particular from melanopsin-producing ganglion cells that function as luminance detectors) to the hypothalamic suprachiasmatic nucleus (regarded as the circadian "clock"). This is the first regulatory step of melatonin synthesis and secretion.

Jet lag, a condition associated with fatigue, insomnia, and disorientation experienced by many travelers, is caused by a disruption of the circadian rhythm. Bipolar disorder and sleep disorder are also linked to the abnormal functioning of the circadian rhythms.

A tumor of the pineal gland (called **pinealoma**) is associated with **precocious puberty** and with a neurologic disorder known as **Parinaud's syndrome** (paralysis of upward gaze, looking steadily in one direction, pupillary areflexia to light, paralysis of convergence, and wide-based gait).

19. ENDOCRINE SYSTEM

Thyroid gland

Development of the thyroid gland

The thyroid gland (Greek *thyreos,* shield; *eidos,* form) develops as a median **endodermal** downgrowth at the base of the tongue. A transient structure, the **thyroglossal duct**, connects the developing gland to its point of origin, the **foramen cecum**, at the back of the tongue.

The thyroglossal duct disappears completely, leaving the thyroid to develop as a ductless gland. Persistent thyroglossal duct tissue remnants may give rise to **cysts**.

The thyroid gland responds to **thyroid-stimulating hormone** (**TSH**) at about week 22 in the fetus. The congenital absence of the thyroid gland causes irreversible neurologic damage in the infant (**cretinism**).

The thyroid gland consists of two lobes connected by a narrow band of thyroid tissue called the **isthmus**.

The thyroid gland is located below the larynx and the lobes rest on the sides of the trachea. The larynx provides a convenient landmark for locating the thyroid gland. The thyroid gland is surrounded by a double connective tissue capsule. Two pairs of parathyroid glands are located on the posterior surface of the thyroid gland, between or outside the two capsules.

Histologic organization of the thyroid gland

Each lobe of the thyroid gland consists of numerous **follicles**. The **thyroid follicle**, or acinus, is the structural and functional unit of the gland. It consists of a single layer of cuboidal epithelial cells, the **follicular epithelium** (Figures 19-1 and 19-2), enclosing a central lumen containing a **colloid** substance rich in **thyroglobulin**, an iodinated glycoprotein, yielding a periodic acid–Schiff (PAS)-positive reaction.

The follicular epithelium also contains about 10% of scattered **parafollicular cells**, also called **C cells**. C cells, derived from the **neural crest**, contain small cytoplasmic **granules** representing the stored hormone **calcitonin** (hence the designation C cells).

When the thyroid gland is **hypoactive**, as in **dietary iodide deficiency**, the follicle is enlarged with colloid. Because no triiodothyronine (T_3) or thyroxine (T_4) is made to exert a negative feedback, TSH synthesis and secretion increase. TSH stimulates growth and vascularization of the thyroid gland. Consequently, the gland enlarges.

When the thyroid gland is **active**, the follicular epithelium is columnar, and **colloid droplets** may be seen within the cells as well as large apical pseudopodia and microvilli (see Figure 19-2).

The thyroid epithelium is surrounded by a basal lamina and reticular fibers. A network of vasomotor and sympathetic nerve fibers and blood vessels, including fenestrated capillaries, can be observed in the connective tissue among thyroid follicles.

Function of the thyroid gland

In contrast to other endocrine organs, which have a limited storage capacity, the production of thyroid hormones depends on the follicular storage of the prohormone thyroglobulin in the colloid.

A characteristic feature of the thyroid follicular epithelium is its ability to concentrate iodide from the blood and synthesize the hormones **thyroxine** and **triiodothyronine**.

The synthesis and secretion of thyroid hormones involve two phases (Figure

Figure 19-1. **Histology of the thyroid gland**

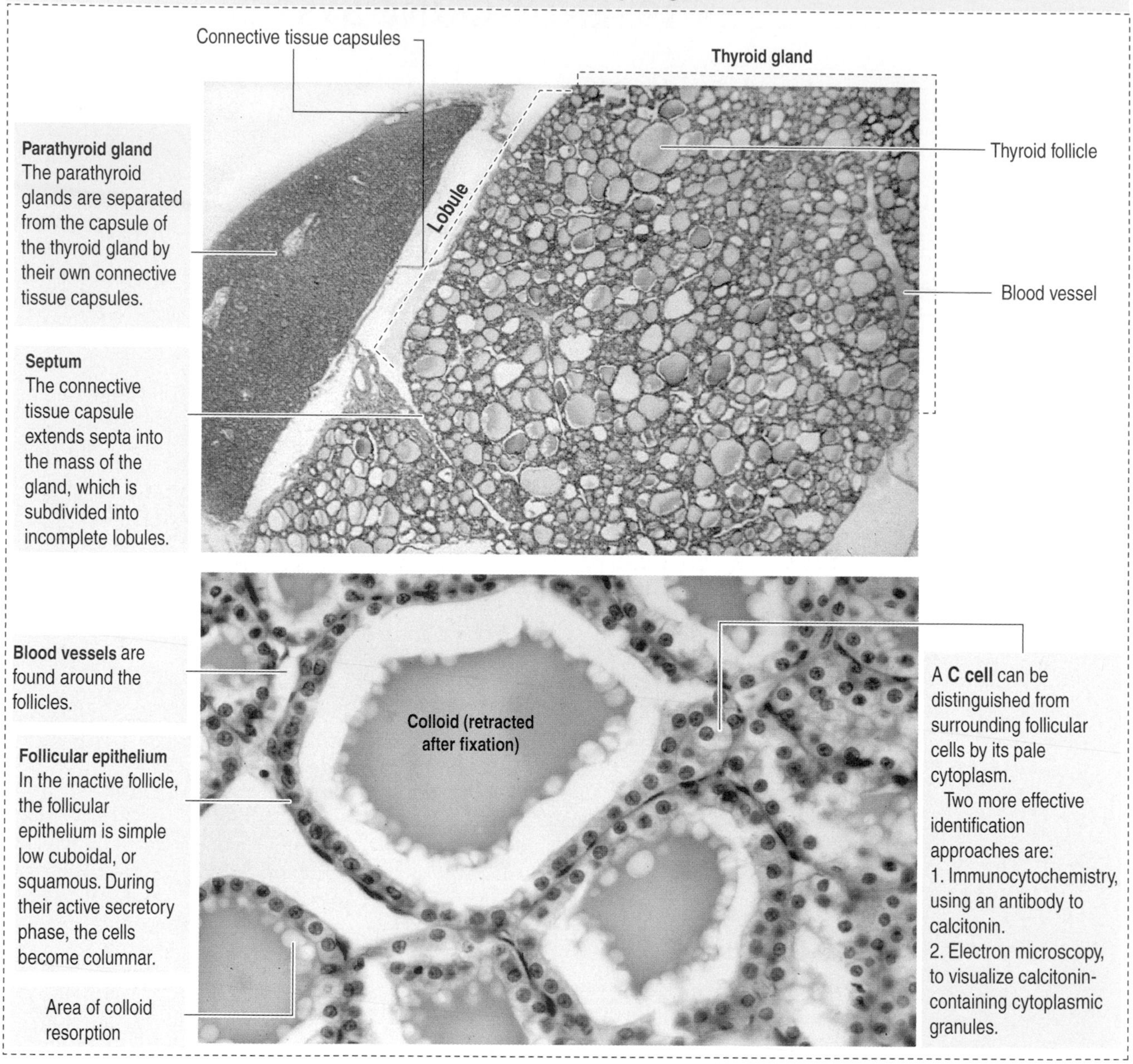

Connective tissue capsules
Thyroid gland
Parathyroid gland
The parathyroid glands are separated from the capsule of the thyroid gland by their own connective tissue capsules.
Lobule
Thyroid follicle
Blood vessel
Septum
The connective tissue capsule extends septa into the mass of the gland, which is subdivided into incomplete lobules.
Blood vessels are found around the follicles.
Colloid (retracted after fixation)
Follicular epithelium
In the inactive follicle, the follicular epithelium is simple low cuboidal, or squamous. During their active secretory phase, the cells become columnar.
Area of colloid resorption
A **C cell** can be distinguished from surrounding follicular cells by its pale cytoplasm.
Two more effective identification approaches are:
1. Immunocytochemistry, using an antibody to calcitonin.
2. Electron microscopy, to visualize calcitonin-containing cytoplasmic granules.

19-3): (1) an **exocrine phase** and (2) an **endocrine phase**.

Both phases are regulated by TSH by a mechanism that includes receptor binding and cyclic adenosine monophosphate (cAMP) production, as discussed in Chapter 3, Cell Signaling.

The **exocrine phase** (see Figure 19-3) consists of (1) the uptake of inorganic **iodide** from the blood, (2) the synthesis of **thyroglobulin**, and (3) the incorporation of **iodine** into tyrosyl residues of thyroglobulin by **thyroid peroxidase**.

The uptake of iodide requires an adenosine triphosphate (ATP)–driven iodide pump present in the basal plasma membrane of the follicular cells. This active transport system is referred to as the **iodide trap**. Intracellular iodide rapidly diffuses against both its concentration and electrical gradients to end up extracellularly in the colloid. Anions, such as **perchlorate** (ClO_4^-), are used clinically as a **competitive inhibitor of the iodide pump** to block iodide uptake by the thyroid follicular cell.

The rough endoplasmic reticulum and Golgi apparatus are sites involved in the synthesis and glycosylation of **thyroglobulin**, a 660-kd glycoprotein composed of

Figure 19-2. **Structure of the thyroid follicular cells**

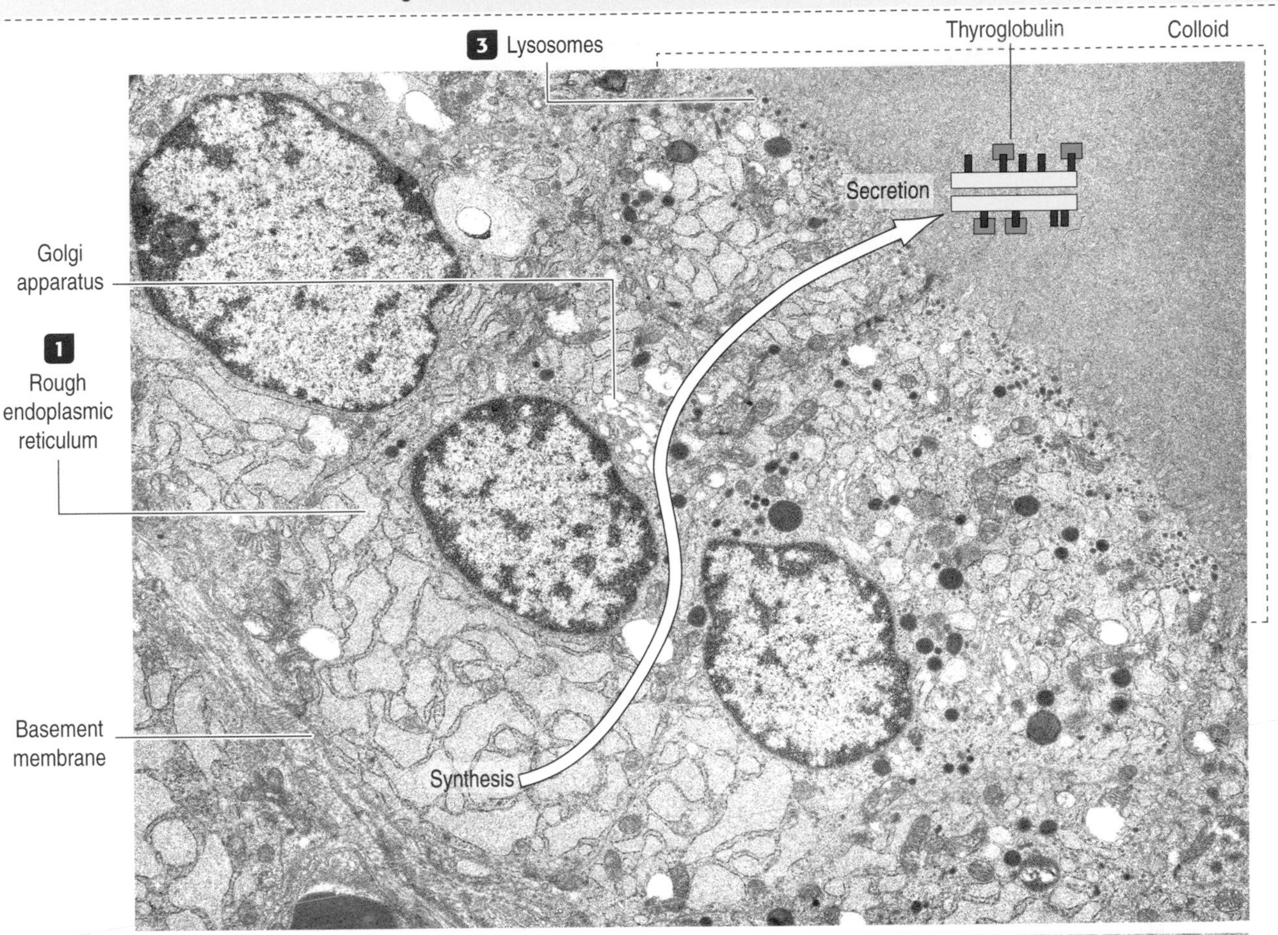
3 Lysosomes
Thyroglobulin
Colloid
Secretion
Golgi apparatus
1
Rough endoplasmic reticulum
Basement membrane
Synthesis

1 The synthesis of thyroglobulin, the precursor of triiodothyronine (T_3) and thyroxine (T_4), starts in the rough endoplasmic reticulum (RER). The cisternae of the RER are distended by the newly synthesized precursor and the cytoplasmic regions are reduced to very narrow areas. Thyroglobulin molecules are glycosylated in the Golgi apparatus.

2 Under the light microscope, thyroglobulin synthetic activity can be visualized in the cytoplasm of the follicular cells as optically clear vesicular spaces.

3 The apical domain of the follicular cells displays abundant lysosomes involved in the processing of the prohormone thyroglobulin into thyroid hormones.

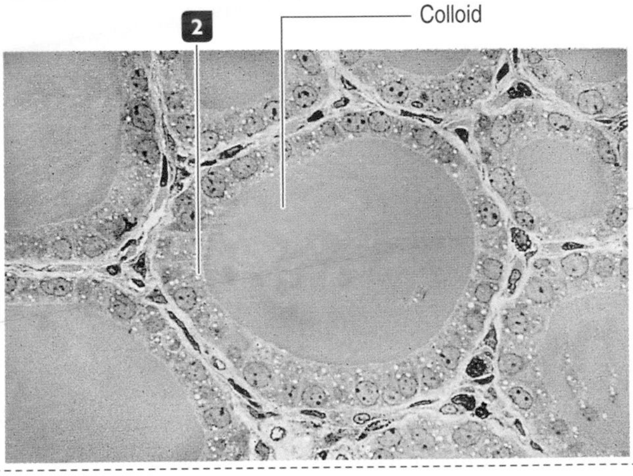
2
Colloid

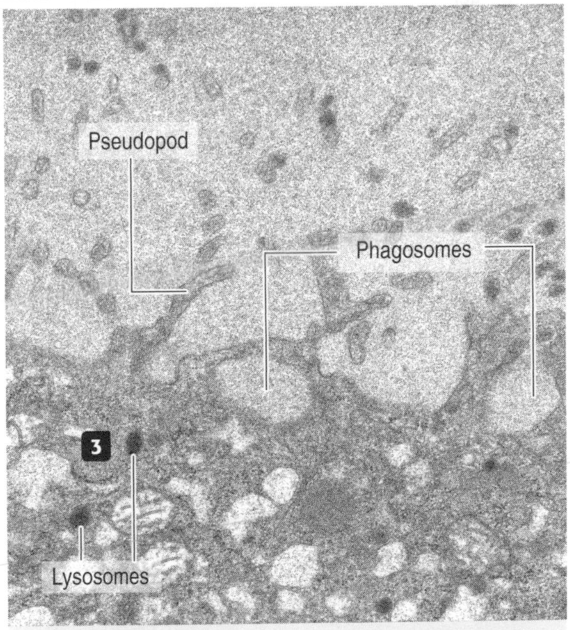
Pseudopod
Phagosomes
3
Lysosomes

Pseudopods extend from the apical domain of the thyroid follicular cells and, after surrounding a portion of the colloid (thyroglobulin), organize an intracellular phagosome. Lysosomes fuse with the phagosome and initiate the proteolytic breakdown of thyroglobulin while moving toward the basal domain of the follicular cell.

Figure 19-3. Synthesis and secretion of thyroid hormones T_3 and T_4

4 At the **apical plasma membrane, thyroid peroxidase** is activated and converts **iodide** into **iodine**. Two iodine atoms are linked to each tyrosyl residue. Iodination occurs within the lumen of the thyroid follicle.

After proteolytic processing, one monoiodotyrosine peptide combines with diiodotyrosine to form **T_3 (triiodothyronine).** Two diiodotyrosines combine to form **T_4** (thyroxine). One iodinated thyroglobulin molecule yields four molecules of T_3 and T_4.

Clinical significance: Propylthiouracil and **methyl mercaptoimidazole** (MMI) inhibit thyroid peroxidase–mediated iodination of tyrosine in thyroglobulin.

5 A droplet in the colloid of the thyroid follicle, containing iodinated thyroglobulin, is endocytosed by a pseudopod extension of the apical domain of a follicular epithelial cell. The **intracellular colloid droplet**, guided by cytoskeletal components, fuses with a **lysosome**. T_3 and T_4 molecules are released by the proteolytic action of lysosomal enzymes.

Clinical significance: Propylthiouracil can block the conversion of T_4 to T_3 in peripheral tissues (liver).

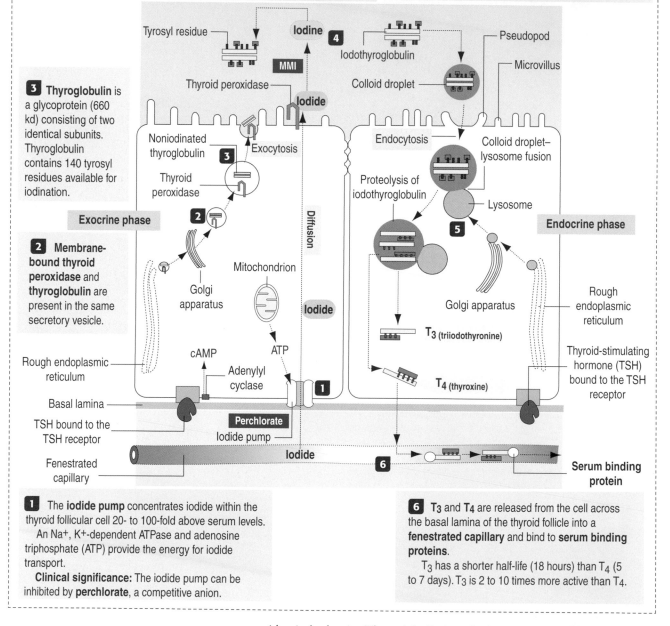

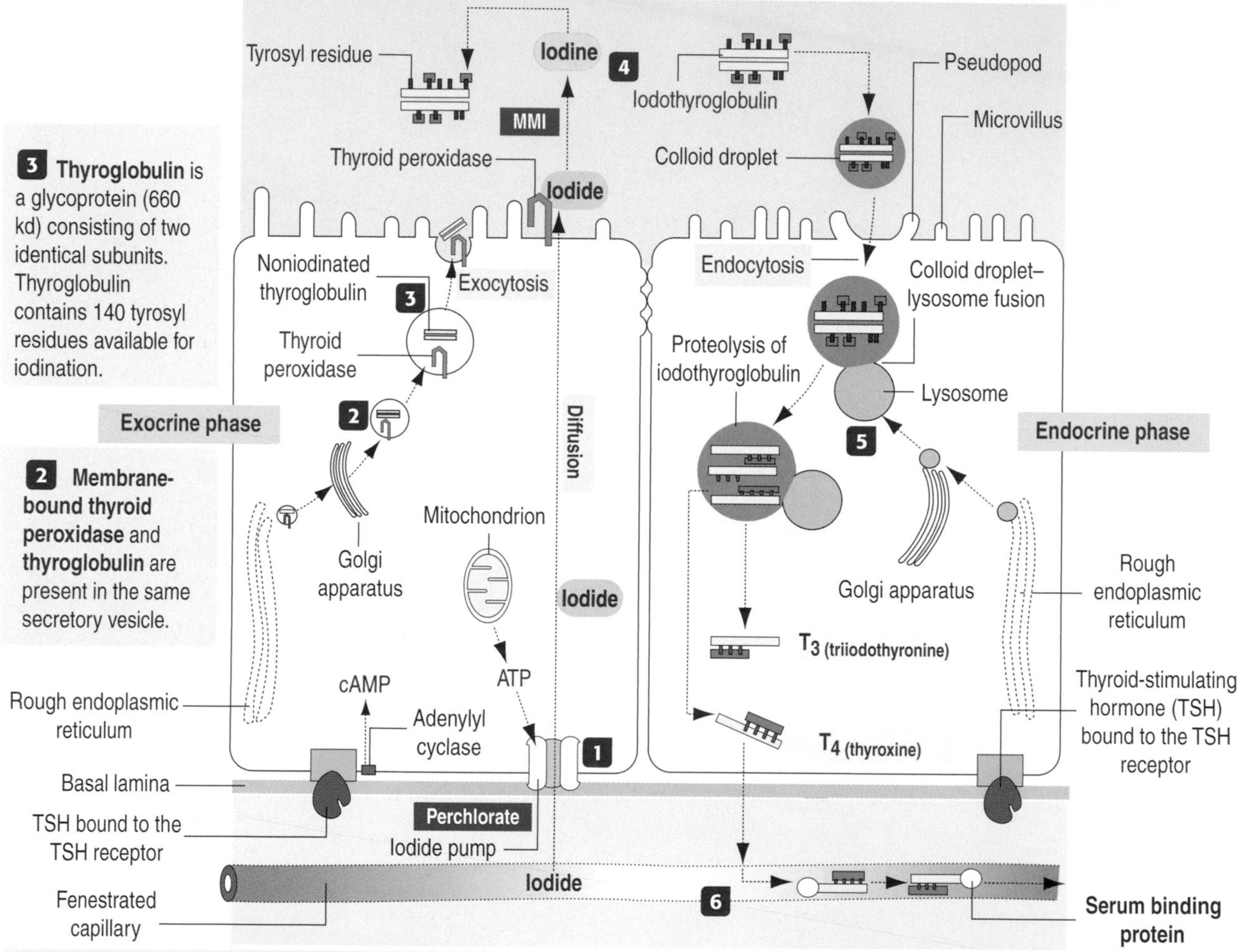

1 The **iodide pump** concentrates iodide within the thyroid follicular cell 20- to 100-fold above serum levels.

An Na^+, K^+-dependent ATPase and adenosine triphosphate (ATP) provide the energy for iodide transport.

Clinical significance: The iodide pump can be inhibited by **perchlorate**, a competitive anion.

6 T_3 and T_4 are released from the cell across the basal lamina of the thyroid follicle into a **fenestrated capillary** and bind to **serum binding proteins**.

T_3 has a shorter half-life (18 hours) than T_4 (5 to 7 days). T_3 is 2 to 10 times more active than T_4.

two identical subunits. Thyroglobulin is packed in secretory vesicles and released by exocytosis into the colloidal lumen. Thyroglobulin contains about 140 tyrosine residues available for iodination.

Thyroid peroxidase, the enzyme responsible for the iodination of thyroglobulin, is a heme-containing glycoprotein anchored in the membrane of the same secretory vesicle that contains thyroglobulin. After exocytosis, thyroid peroxidase is exposed at the luminal surface of the thyroid cell.

Figure 19-4. Graves' disease: Unregulated synthesis and secretion of thyroid hormones T_3 and T_4

Graves' disease: Pathogenesis

Excessive production of thyroid hormone is caused by the activation of thyroid receptors by an autoimmune response (antibodies produced against the thyroid stimulating hormone receptor). Inflammatory cells in the stroma of the thyroid gland produce cytokines (interleukin-1, tumor necrosis factor-α, and interferon-γ), that stimulate thyroid cells to produce cytokines, thus reinforcing the thyroidal autoimmune process. Antithyroid drugs reduce the production of cytokines (immunosuppressive effect), leading to remission in some patients.

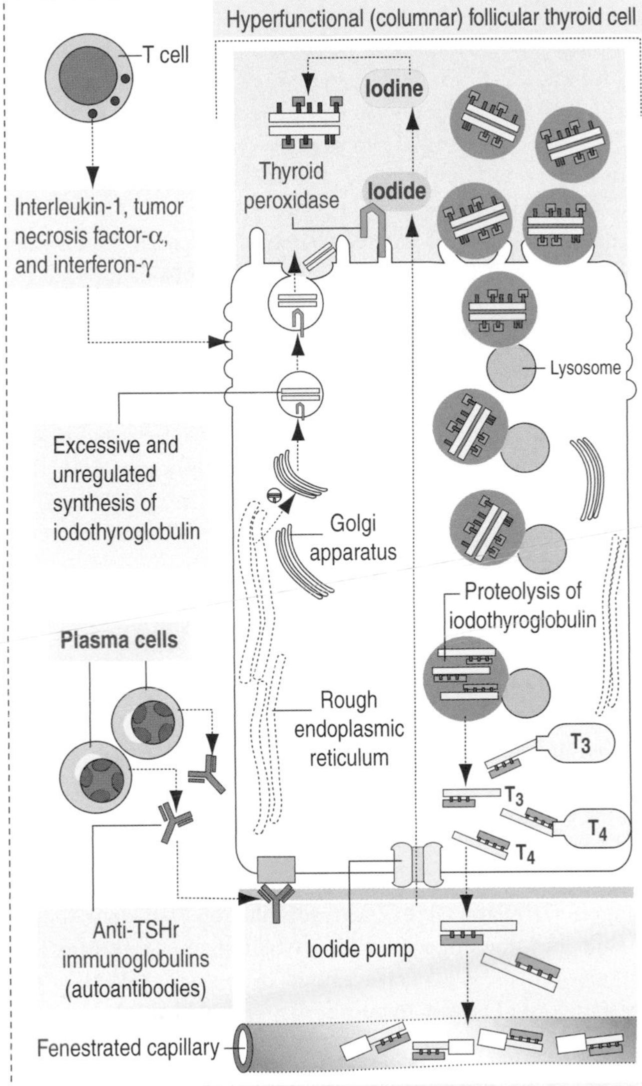

Graves' disease: Clinical characteristics

Two characteristics of Graves' disease are exophthalmos and cardiac manifestations (palpitations and tachycardia).

Exophthalmos consists in the presence of an inflammatory infiltrate (T cells, macrophages, and neutrophils) in the extraocular muscles and orbital tissue. Cytokines (produced by T cells) and anti–thyroid stimulating hormone receptor (anti-TSHr) immunoglobulins (Igs) (produced by extraocular plasma cells) stimulate the function of orbital fibroblasts and their differentiation into adipocytes.

Overproduction of fat and the hygroscopic nature of proteoglycans contribute to the development of exophthalmos.

Exophthalmos

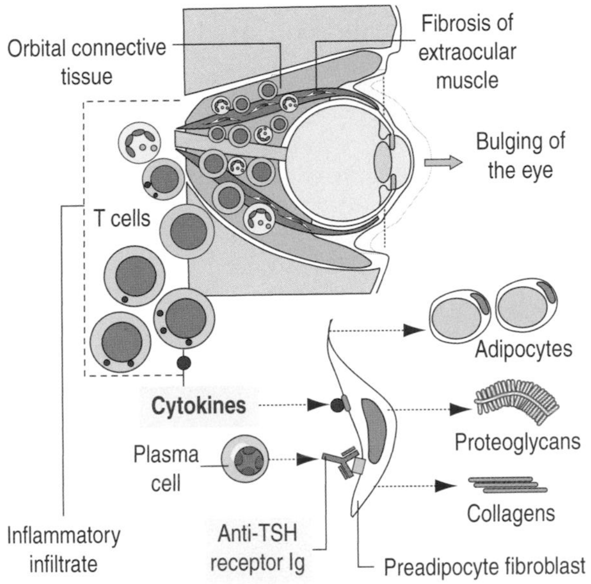

Graves' ophthalmopathy is characterized by inflammation of the extraocular muscles and an increase in orbital adipose and connective tissue. Circulating anti-TSHr Igs bind to the TSH receptor expressed by fibroblasts in the retrobulbar tissue.

Cytokines produced by T cells in the inflammatory infiltrate stimulate adipogenesis from preadipocyte fibroblasts.

Fibroblasts produce proteoglycans and collagen fibers leading to retrobulbar edema and fibrosis of the extraocular muscles.

Myocardial contractility

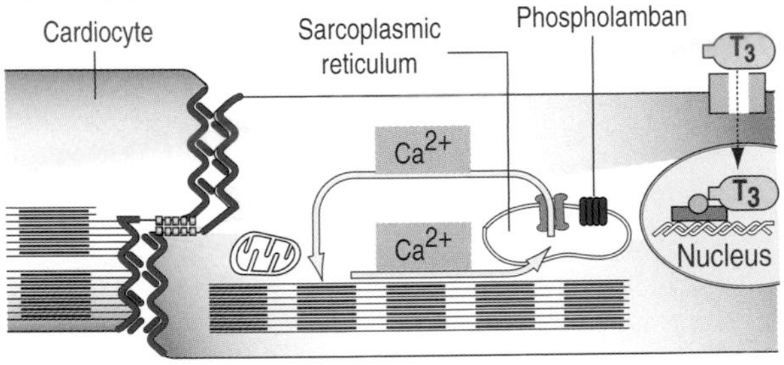

Triiodothyronine (T_3) enters the nucleus of a cardiocyte, binds to its nuclear receptors, and then binds to thyroid hormone response element in target genes.

T_3 stimulates phospholamban, a protein involved in the release and uptake of Ca^{2+} into the sarcoplasmic reticulum. This step is critical for systolic contraction and diastolic relaxation. The activity of phospholamban is regulated by its phosphorylation. Increased diastolic function in patients with hyperthyroidism is related to the role of phospholamban in thyroid hormone–mediated changes in the contractility of cardiac muscle.

Thyroid peroxidase is activated during exocytosis. **Activated thyroid peroxidase oxidizes iodide to iodine within the colloid**; the iodine is then transferred to acceptor tyrosyl residues of thyroglobulin. Thyroid peroxidase activity and the iodination process can be inhibited by **propylthiouracil** and **methyl mercapto-imidazole (MMI)**. These antithyroid drugs are used to inhibit the production of thyroid hormones by hyperactive glands.

The **endocrine phase** starts with the TSH-stimulated endocytosis of iodinated thyroglobulin into the follicular cell (see Figure 19-3):

1. **Colloid droplets** are enveloped by apical **pseudopods** and internalized to become colloid-containing vesicles.

2. Cytoskeletal components guide the colloid droplets to lysosomes, which fuse with the colloid droplets.

3. **Lysosomal enzymes degrade iodothyroglobulin to release T_3 (triiodothyronine, the active form of the hormone), T_4 (thyroxine)**, and other intermediate products. Iodotyrosines, amino acids, and sugars are recycled within the cell.

4. Thyroid hormones are then released across the basal lamina of the thyroid follicular epithelium—by a mechanism to be determined—and gain access to **serum carrier proteins** within the fenestrated capillaries.

T3 has a shorter half-life (18 hours), is **more potent**, and **less abundant than** T_4. The half-life of T_4 is 5 to 7 days and represents about 90% of the secreted thyroid hormones.

Thyroid hormones increase the basal metabolic rate. The primary site of action of T_3, and to a lesser extent T_4, is the **cell nucleus**. T_3 binds to thyroid hormone receptor bound to a specific DNA region, called **thyroid hormone–responsive element (TRE)**, to induce specific gene transcription. In cardiocytes (heart), thyroid hormone regulates the expression of genes encoding phospholamban in the sarcoplasmic reticulum, β-adrenergic receptors, Ca^{2+}-ATPase, and others. In the absence of T_3, unoccupied nuclear receptors bound to the TRE repress genes that are positively regulated by thyroid hormone.

Clinical significance: Hyperthyroidism (Graves' disease) and hypothyroidism

Graves' disease is an **autoimmune disease** in which the thyroid gland is hyperfunctional (Figure 19-4). **Autoantibodies** (called **thyroid-stimulating immunoglobulins** or **TSIs**), **produced by plasma cells derived from sensitized T cells against TSH receptors** present at the basal surface of thyroid follicular cells, bind to the receptor and mimic the effect of TSH, stimulating cAMP production.

As a result, thyroid follicular cells become columnar and secrete large amounts of thyroid hormones in the blood circulation in an unregulated fashion. Enlargement of the thyroid gland (**goiter**), bulging of the eyes (**exophthalmos**; see Figure 19-4), **tachycardia**, **warm skin**, and **fine finger tremors** are typical clinical features.

In the **adult**, hypothyroidism is generally caused by a thyroid disease, and a decrease in the **basal metabolic rate**, **hypothermia**, and **cold intolerance** are observed. Decreased sweating and cutaneous vasoconstriction make the skin dry and cool. Afflicted individuals tend to feel cold in a warm room. In the adult, hypothyroidism is manifested by coarse skin with a puffy appearance due to the accumulation of proteoglycans and retention of fluid in the dermis of the skin (**myxedema**) and muscle. Cardiac output is reduced, and the pulse rate slows down. Except for developmental disturbances, most symptoms are reversed when the thyroid disorder is corrected.

In the **fetus**, a lack of thyroid hormone causes **cretinism**. This condition is observed in iodide-deficient geographic areas. The symptoms of hypothyroidism in newborns can include respiratory distress syndrome, poor feeding, umbilical hernia, and retarded bone growth. Untreated hypothyroidism in children results in **mental retardation**.

Hashimoto's disease is an **autoimmune disease** associated with **hypothyroidism**.

It is caused by autoantibodies targeted to **thyroid peroxidase** and thyroglobulin. Antibodies to thyroid peroxidase are known as **antimicrosomal antibodies**. A progressive destruction of the thyroid follicles leads to a decrease in the function of the thyroid gland.

Calcium regulation

Ca^{2+} is found inside and outside cells, is a major component of the skeleton, is required for **muscle contraction, blood clotting**, nerve impulse transmission, and enzymatic activities. Ca^{2+} is an essential mediator in cell signaling (for example, through **calcium-binding calmodulin**).

The maintenance of Ca^{2+} homeostasis is regulated by (1) **parathyroid hormone**, (2) **calcitonin**, and (3) **vitamin D** (calcitriol, or 1,25-dihydroxycholecalciferol).

Parathyroid hormone acts on bone and kidney to raise Ca^{2+} levels in serum. Calcitonin, secreted by C cells in the thyroid follicle, lowers Ca^{2+} levels. Vitamin D is produced in the kidneys and increases the intestinal absorption of Ca^{2+} by stimulating synthesis of **Ca^{2+}-binding protein** by intestinal epithelial cells (enterocytes).

Parathyroid glands

Development of the parathyroid glands

The four parathyroid glands derive from the third and fourth branchial pouches. The third branchial pouch differentiates into the inferior parathyroid glands and the thymus. The fourth branchial pouch develops into the superior parathyroid glands and the ultimobranchial body.

Parathyroid glands are found on the posterior surface of the thyroid gland, between its capsule and the surrounding cervical connective tissue. In addition to the four parathyroid glands, accessory glands may be found in the mediastinum or in the neck.

The accidental removal of the normal parathyroid glands during thyroid surgery (thyroidectomy) causes **tetany**, characterized by spasms of the thoracic and laryngeal muscles, leading to asphyxia and death.

Histologic organization of the parathyroid glands

The parenchyma of the parathyroid glands consists of two cell populations supplied by sinusoidal capillaries (Figure 19-5): (1) the more numerous **chief** or **principal cell**, and (2) the **oxyphil** or **acidophilic cell.** Cells are arranged in cordlike or follicular-like clusters.

Chief or **principal cells** contain cytoplasmic granules with **parathyroid hormone**, an 84-amino-acid peptide derived from a large precursor of 115 amino acids (**preproparathyroid hormone**). This precursor gives rise to **proparathyroid hormone** (90 amino acids), which is processed by a proteolytic enzyme in the Golgi apparatus into **parathyroid hormone.** Parathyroid hormone is stored in **secretory granules. Glycogen inclusions** are also observed in chief cells.

The **Ca^{2+}-sensing receptor (CaSR)** is associated to G protein in the plasma membrane of chief cells. Serum Ca^{2+} binding to the extracellular region of the CaSR triggers the release of intracellular signals suppressing the secretion of parathyroid hormone, with the consequent decrease in the serum Ca^{2+} concentration. When the serum Ca^{2+} concentration decreases, the secretion of parathyroid hormone is stimulated, resulting in an increase in serum Ca^{2+}. In most cells Ca^{2+} enters a cell through a membrane-associated channel. Chief parathyroid cells are rather unusual because Ca^{2+} is a ligand for the CaSR resulting in the activation of G protein.

Oxyphil or **acidophilic cells** contain abundant mitochondria, which give this cell its typical stain. This cell type may represent transitional chief cells.

Figure 19-5. Structure and function of the parathyroid gland

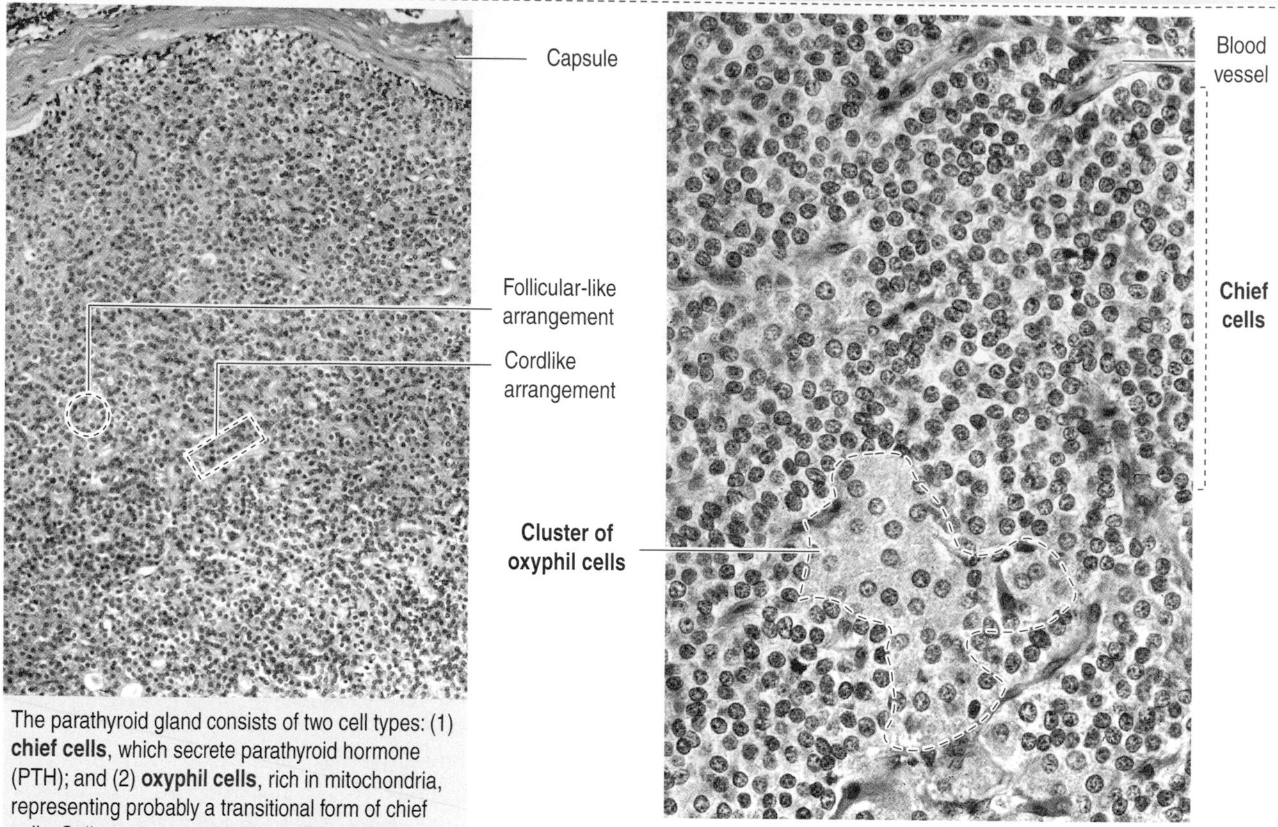

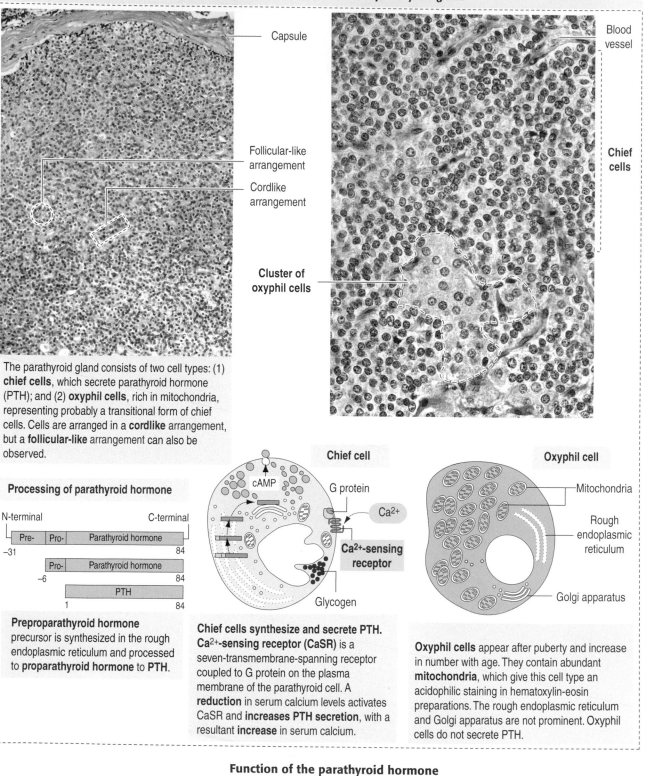

Capsule
Follicular-like arrangement
Cordlike arrangement
Cluster of oxyphil cells
Blood vessel
Chief cells

The parathyroid gland consists of two cell types: (1) **chief cells**, which secrete parathyroid hormone (PTH); and (2) **oxyphil cells**, rich in mitochondria, representing probably a transitional form of chief cells. Cells are arranged in a **cordlike** arrangement, but a **follicular-like** arrangement can also be observed.

Processing of parathyroid hormone

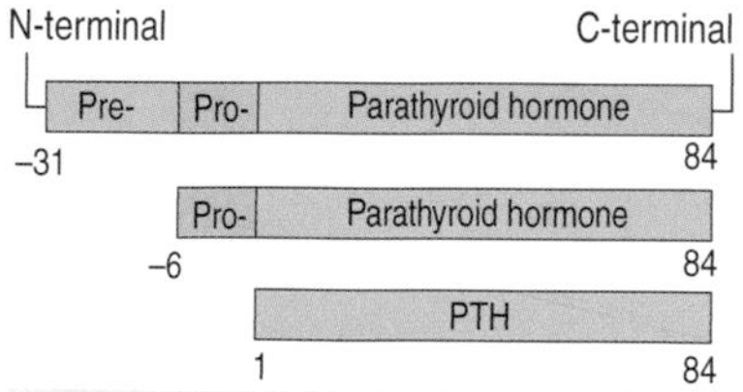

N-terminal
C-terminal
Pre-
Pro-
Parathyroid hormone
–31
84
Pro-
Parathyroid hormone
–6
84
PTH
1
84

Preproparathyroid hormone precursor is synthesized in the rough endoplasmic reticulum and processed to **proparathyroid hormone** to **PTH**.

Chief cell

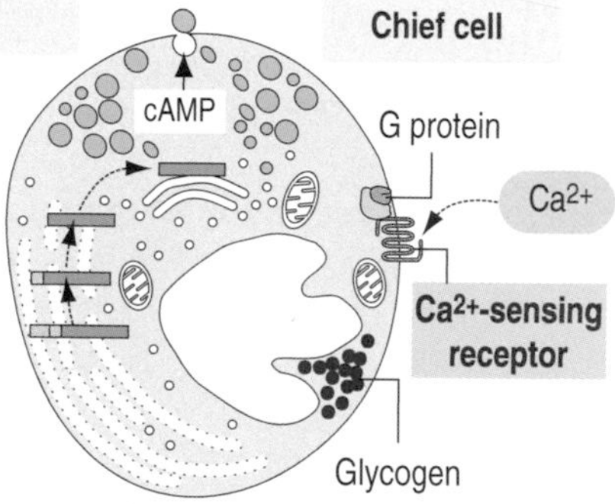

cAMP
G protein
Ca2+
Ca2+-sensing receptor
Glycogen

Chief cells synthesize and secrete PTH. Ca^{2+}-sensing receptor (CaSR) is a seven-transmembrane-spanning receptor coupled to G protein on the plasma membrane of the parathyroid cell. A **reduction** in serum calcium levels activates CaSR and **increases PTH secretion**, with a resultant **increase** in serum calcium.

Oxyphil cell

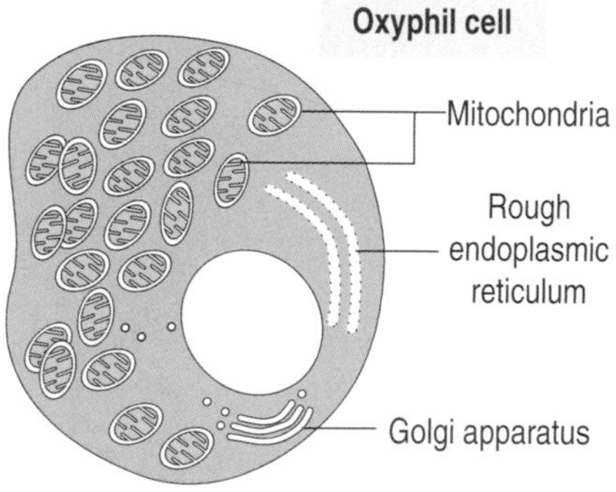

Mitochondria
Rough endoplasmic reticulum
Golgi apparatus

Oxyphil cells appear after puberty and increase in number with age. They contain abundant **mitochondria**, which give this cell type an acidophilic staining in hematoxylin-eosin preparations. The rough endoplasmic reticulum and Golgi apparatus are not prominent. Oxyphil cells do not secrete PTH.

Function of the parathyroid hormone

Parathyroid hormone regulates the Ca^{2+} and PO_4^{3-} balance in blood by acting on two main sites:

1. The **bone tissue**, where it stimulates the **resorption of mineralized bone by osteoclasts** and the release of Ca^{2+} into the blood. Serum Ca^{2+} levels normally average **9.5 mg/dL**.

2. The **uriniferous tubules**, where it stimulates the **resorption of Ca^{2+}** and activates the **production of active vitamin D**. Parathyroid hormone is secreted

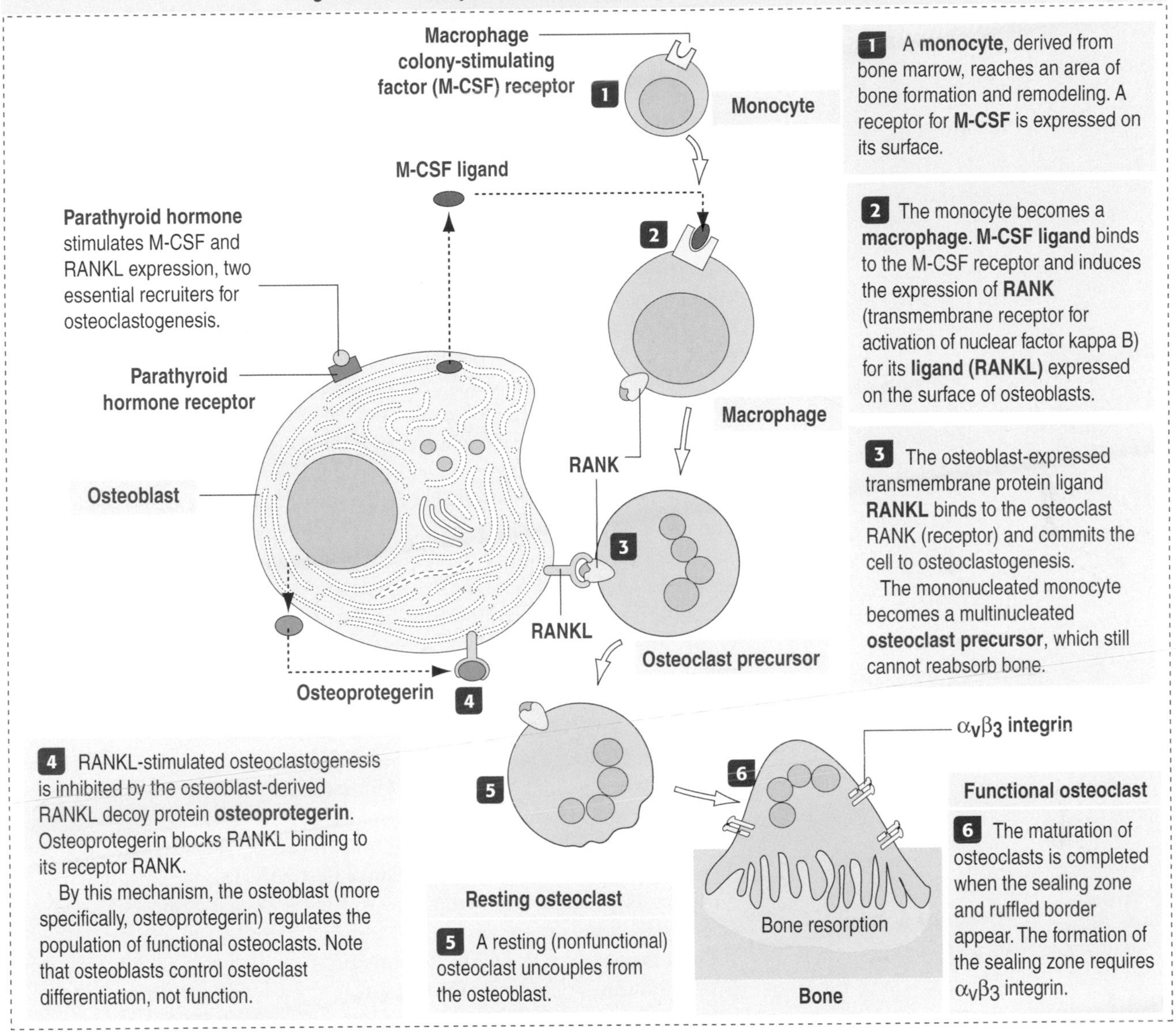

Macrophage colony-stimulating factor (M-CSF) receptor
1
Monocyte
1 A **monocyte**, derived from bone marrow, reaches an area of bone formation and remodeling. A receptor for **M-CSF** is expressed on its surface.
M-CSF ligand
Parathyroid hormone stimulates M-CSF and RANKL expression, two essential recruiters for osteoclastogenesis.
2
2 The monocyte becomes a **macrophage. M-CSF ligand** binds to the M-CSF receptor and induces the expression of **RANK** (transmembrane receptor for activation of nuclear factor kappa B) for its **ligand (RANKL)** expressed on the surface of osteoblasts.
Parathyroid hormone receptor
Macrophage
RANK
Osteoblast
3
3 The osteoblast-expressed transmembrane protein ligand **RANKL** binds to the osteoclast RANK (receptor) and commits the cell to osteoclastogenesis.
The mononucleated monocyte becomes a multinucleated **osteoclast precursor**, which still cannot reabsorb bone.
RANKL
Osteoclast precursor
Osteoprotegerin
4
$\alpha_V\beta_3$ integrin
4 RANKL-stimulated osteoclastogenesis is inhibited by the osteoblast-derived RANKL decoy protein **osteoprotegerin**. Osteoprotegerin blocks RANKL binding to its receptor RANK.
By this mechanism, the osteoblast (more specifically, osteoprotegerin) regulates the population of functional osteoclasts. Note that osteoblasts control osteoclast differentiation, not function.
5
6
Functional osteoclast
6 The maturation of osteoclasts is completed when the sealing zone and ruffled border appear. The formation of the sealing zone requires $\alpha_V\beta_3$ integrin.
Resting osteoclast
5 A resting (nonfunctional) osteoclast uncouples from the osteoblast.
Bone resorption
Bone

Figure 19-6. Parathyroid hormone regulates osteoclastogenesis

into the blood and has a half-life of about 5 minutes.

An **increase** in serum Ca^{2+} levels (**hypercalcemia**) **suppresses the release of parathyroid hormone** from chief cells. A **decrease** in Ca^{2+} levels (**hypocalcemia**) **stimulates parathyroid hormone release** by chief cells.

When Ca^{2+} levels are low, parathyroid hormone reestablishes homeostasis by acting on **osteoblasts**, which induce osteoclasts to reabsorb bone.

Parathyroid hormone binds to a cell surface receptor of the osteoblast to regulate the synthesis of three proteins essential for the differentiation and function of osteoclasts (Figure 19-6; see also the discussion of osteoclasts in Chapter 4, Connective Tissue):

1. **Macrophage colony-stimulating factor** (**M-CSF**) **ligand**, which induces the differentiation of monocytes into immature osteoclasts by activating the expression of the **receptor for activation of nuclear factor kappa B** (RANK).

2. **RANKL**, a cell membrane protein interacting as a ligand with RANK receptor present on the surface of the osteoclast precursor. RANK-RANKL interaction induces the differentiation of the osteoclast precursor into a resting osteoclast. RANKL is a member of the tumor necrosis factor superfamily of ligands and receptors.

3. **Osteoprotegerin**, a decoy protein that blocks binding of RANKL to the

RANK receptor to prevent completion of the final differentiation of functional osteoclasts. By this mechanism, osteoprotegerin regulates the population of functional osteoclasts.

You should be aware that RANKL not only regulates osteoclastogenesis but also is expressed by dendritic cells, T and B cells, components of the immune system. This is an important consideration in anti-RANKL treatment of some forms of osteoporosis, as discussed under Bone in Chapter 4, Connective Tissue.

Clinical significance: Hyperparathyroidism, hypoparathyroidism, and CaSR mutations

Hyperparathyroidism is caused by a functional benign tumor of the gland (**adenoma**). An abnormal increase in the secretion of parathyroid hormone causes:

1. **Hypercalcemia** and **phosphaturia** (increased urinary excretion of PO_4^{3-} anions).

2. **Hypercalciuria** (increased urinary excretion of Ca^{2+}) leading to the formation of **renal stones** in the calyces of the kidneys. When stones descend to the ureter, there is severe pain, caused by spasmodic contraction of the smooth muscle, **hematuria** (blood in urine), and infections of the renal tract (**pyelonephritis**).

3. **Hypercalcemia, the result of bone demineralization.** Extensive bone resorption results in the development of **cysts.**

4. **Accidental removal of parathyroid glands during surgery of the thyroid gland.** Within 24 to 48 hours of surgical removal of the parathyroid glands, hypocalcemia, increased excitability of nervous tissue, including paresthesia (sensation of pins and needles), and attacks of **tetany** or **epilepsy** occur. Administration of parathyroid hormone corrects these alterations.

Inactivating mutations of one allele of the **CaSR** prevent parathyroid chief cells to sense increases in serum Ca^{2+}, which results in an increase of parathyroid hormone secretion. This condition, called **familial benign hypercalcemia,** can be severe when two inactivated CaSR alleles exist. This condition, detected in newborns, requires immediate parathyroidectomy.

Idiopathic hypoparathyroidism results in a failure of tissues to respond to parathyroid hormone. An activating **mutation of the CaSR** leads the parathyroid gland into assuming that the Ca^{2+} serum level is elevated when it is not. This condition determines a reduction in serum Ca^{2+} and parathyroid hormone levels.

CaSR can also be a target of autoimmunity and either activate (causing hypoparathyroidism) or inactivate the CaSR (causing a syndrome similar to familial benign hypercalcemia). **Calcimimetic** drugs, which activate CaSR, reduce pathologic elevations of parathyroid hormone. CaSR-blocking drugs, called **calcilytics**, may be useful for the treatment of osteoporosis.

C cells (thyroid follicle) and calcitonin

C cells derive from neural crest cells and are associated with thyroid follicles. C cells (1) represent about 0.1% of the mass of thyroid tissue, (2) may be present within (or outside) the thyroid follicle but are not in contact with the colloid, and (3) produce **calcitonin**, encoded by a gene located on the short arm of chromosome 11 (Figure 19-7).

Calcitonin is a 32-amino-acid peptide derived from a 136-amino-acid precursor. It is stored in secretory granules.

The calcitonin gene is also expressed in other tissues (hypothalamus and hypophysis), giving rise to a **calcitonin gene–related peptide (CGRP)** consisting of 37 amino acids. CGRP has neurotransmitter and vasodilator properties.

The main function of calcitonin is **to antagonize the effects of parathyroid hormone. Calcitonin suppresses the mobilization of calcium from bone by osteoclasts** triggered by an increase in cAMP. Calcitonin secretion is stimulated by an **increase** in blood levels of calcium (hypercalcemia).

Figure 19-7. **Synthesis and mechanism of action of calcitonin**

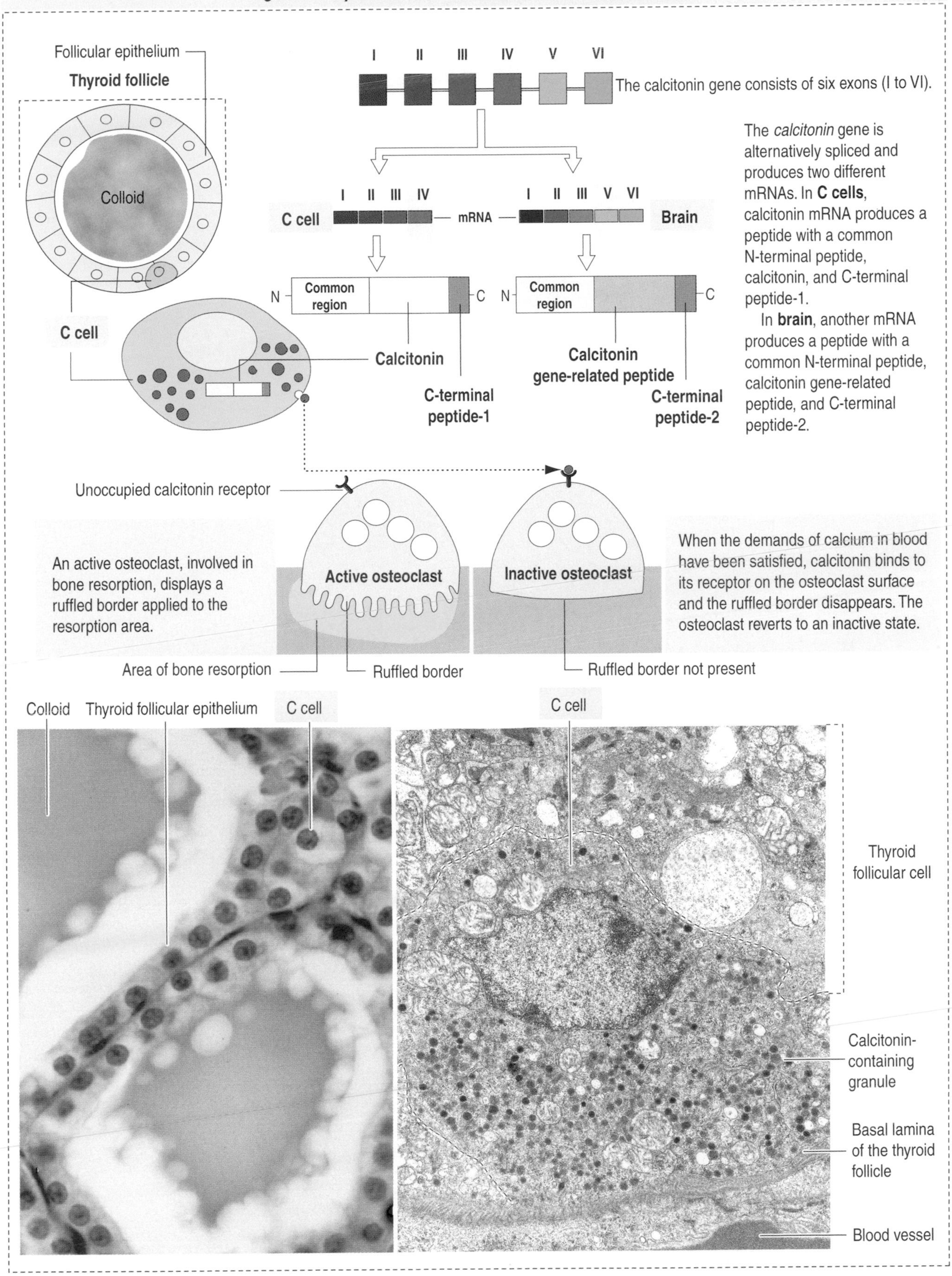

Follicular epithelium
Thyroid follicle
Colloid
C cell
I II III IV V VI
The calcitonin gene consists of six exons (I to VI).
I II III IV
C cell
mRNA
I II III V VI
Brain
N
Common region
C
Calcitonin
C-terminal peptide-1
Calcitonin gene-related peptide
C-terminal peptide-2
The *calcitonin* gene is alternatively spliced and produces two different mRNAs. In **C cells**, calcitonin mRNA produces a peptide with a common N-terminal peptide, calcitonin, and C-terminal peptide-1.
In **brain**, another mRNA produces a peptide with a common N-terminal peptide, calcitonin gene-related peptide, and C-terminal peptide-2.
Unoccupied calcitonin receptor
An active osteoclast, involved in bone resorption, displays a ruffled border applied to the resorption area.
Active osteoclast
Inactive osteoclast
When the demands of calcium in blood have been satisfied, calcitonin binds to its receptor on the osteoclast surface and the ruffled border disappears. The osteoclast reverts to an inactive state.
Area of bone resorption
Ruffled border
Ruffled border not present
Colloid
Thyroid follicular epithelium
C cell
C cell
Thyroid follicular cell
Calcitonin-containing granule
Basal lamina of the thyroid follicle
Blood vessel

Figure 19-8. **Metabolism of vitamin D and calcium absorption**

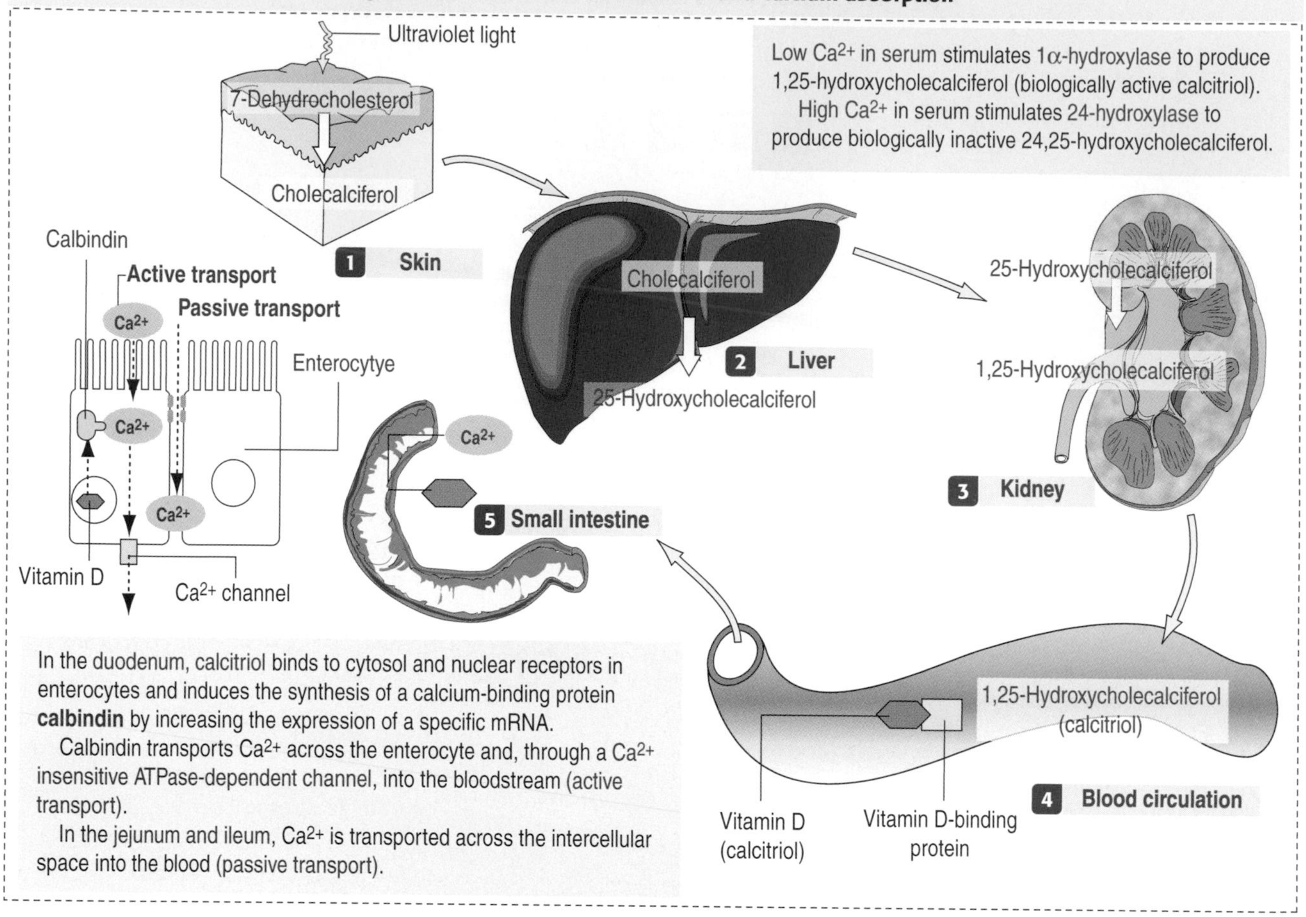
Ultraviolet light
7-Dehydrocholesterol
Cholecalciferol
1 Skin
Calbindin
Active transport
Passive transport
Ca2+
Enterocytye
Vitamin D
Ca2+ channel
Cholecalciferol
2 Liver
25-Hydroxycholecalciferol
Ca2+
5 Small intestine
Low Ca2+ in serum stimulates 1α-hydroxylase to produce 1,25-hydroxycholecalciferol (biologically active calcitriol).
High Ca2+ in serum stimulates 24-hydroxylase to produce biologically inactive 24,25-hydroxycholecalciferol.
25-Hydroxycholecalciferol
1,25-Hydroxycholecalciferol
3 Kidney
1,25-Hydroxycholecalciferol (calcitriol)
4 Blood circulation
Vitamin D (calcitriol)
Vitamin D-binding protein
In the duodenum, calcitriol binds to cytosol and nuclear receptors in enterocytes and induces the synthesis of a calcium-binding protein calbindin by increasing the expression of a specific mRNA.
Calbindin transports Ca2+ across the enterocyte and, through a Ca2+ insensitive ATPase-dependent channel, into the bloodstream (active transport).
In the jejunum and ileum, Ca2+ is transported across the intercellular space into the blood (passive transport).

Clinical significance: Multiple endocrine neoplasia syndrome

Tumors of C cells (medullary carcinoma of the thyroid gland) result in excessive production of calcitonin. However, calcium levels in serum are normal, with no apparent bone damage.

The presence of a calcitonin-producing tumor of the thyroid gland may be associated with pheochromocytoma, a tumor of the adrenal medulla (**multiple endocrine neoplasia** [MEN] **syndrome**).

Vitamin D

Vitamin D_2 is formed in the **skin** by the conversion of 7-dehydrocholesterol to **cholecalciferol** following exposure to ultraviolet light (Figure 19-8). Cholecalciferol is then absorbed into the blood circulation and transported to the **liver** where it is converted to **25-hydroxycholecalciferol** by the addition of a hydroxyl group to the side chain.

In the **nephron**, two events can occur:

1. **Low calcium levels** can stimulate the enzymatic activity of mitochondrial **1α-hydroxylase** to add another hydroxyl group to 25-hydroxycholecalciferol to form **1,25-dihydroxycholecalciferol** (**calcitriol**), the active form of vitamin D.
2. **High calcium levels** can stimulate the enzymatic activity of **24-hydroxylase** to convert 25-hydroxycholecalciferol to biologically inactive 24,25-hydroxycholecalciferol. In addition, parathyroid hormone and calcitonin suppress 1α-hydroxylase activity.

Calcitriol (active form) and 24,25-hydroxycholecalciferol (inactive form) circulate in blood bound to a **vitamin D–binding protein**.

The main function of vitamin D is to stimulate calcium absorption by the intestinal mucosa. Calcium is absorbed by (1) **transcellular absorption** (**active**

mechanism) in the duodenum, an active process that involves the import of calcium by enterocytes through **voltage-insensitive channels**, its transport across the cell—assisted by the carrier protein **calbindin**—and its release from the cell by a calcium-ATPase–mediated mechanism; and (2) **paracellular absorption (passive mechanism)** in the jejunum and ileum, through tight junctions into the intercellular spaces, and into blood. A small fraction (about 10%) of calcium absorption takes place in the large intestine by active and passive mechanisms.

Vitamin D, like all steroids, is transported to the **nucleus** of the intestinal cell to induce the synthesis of a calcium-binding protein, calbindin.

Clinical significance: Rickets and osteomalacia

In children, a deficiency of vitamin D causes **rickets.** In adults, the corresponding clinical condition is **osteomalacia.** The calcification of the bone matrix osteoid is deficient in both conditions.

In **rickets**, bone remodeling is defective. The ends of the bones bulge (rachitic rosary at the costochondral junctions), and poor calcification of the long bones causes bending (bowlegs or knock-knees).

In **osteomalacia**, pain, partial bone fractures, and muscular weaknesses are typical in the adult.

Chronic renal failure or a congenital disorder—resulting in the lack of 1α-hydroxylase—can also cause rickets or osteomalacia.

Hypercalcemia is frequently found in patients with metastasis causing bone destruction or in patients with tumors secreting a **parathyroid hormone–related peptide.**

The adrenal gland

Development of the adrenal gland

During the fifth week of fetal development, proliferating mesothelium-derived cells infiltrate the retroperitoneal mesenchyme at the cranial end of the mesonephros and give rise to the **primitive adrenal cortex.** A second proliferation of mesothelial-derived cells surrounds the primitive cortex and forms the cortex of the future adult gland.

At the seventh week of development, the mesothelial cellular mass is invaded at its medial region by **neural crest–derived chromaffinoblast cells**, which differentiate into the two classes of **chromaffin cells** of the **adrenal medulla. The adrenal medulla is homologous to a diffuse sympathetic ganglion without postganglionic processes.**

Mesenchymal cells surrounding the fetal cortex differentiate into fibroblasts and form the capsule of the adrenal gland. At this time, blood vessels and nerves of the adrenal gland develop.

At the end of fetal life, the adrenal glands are relatively larger than they are in the adult. At birth, the zonae glomerulosa and fasciculata are developed under the control of adrenocorticotropic hormone (ACTH) secreted by the fetal pituitary gland. **The fetal cortex regresses, disappears within the first year of life, and is replaced by the definitive cortex.**

Ectopic adrenocortical or medullary tissue may be found retroperitoneally, inferior to the kidney, along the aorta, and in the pelvis. Aggregates of ectopic chromaffin cells, called **paraganglia**, can be a site of tumor growth (**pheochromocytoma**).

Functions of the fetal adrenal cortex

During the early stage of gestation, the adrenal cortex synthesizes **dehydroepiandrosterone**, a precursor of the synthesis of estrogen by the placenta. A lack of 3β-hydroxysteroid dehydrogenase activity prevents the synthesis of progesterone, glucocorticoids, and androstenedione. The interaction between the fetal adrenal cortex and the placenta is known as the **fetoplacental unit** (see Chapter 23, Fer-

Figure 19-9. Histologic organization of the adrenal gland

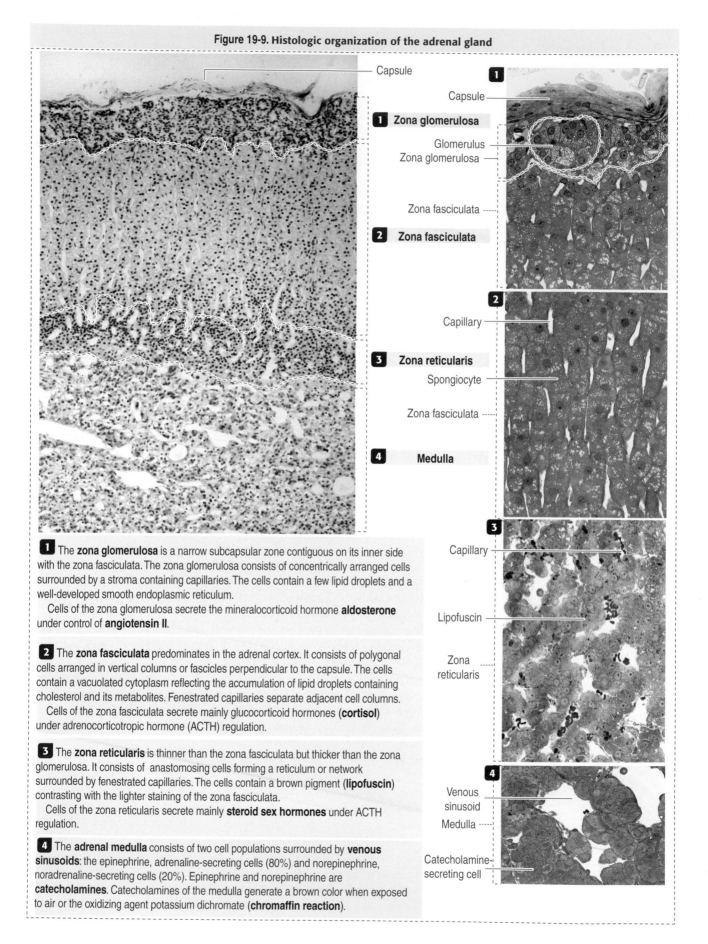

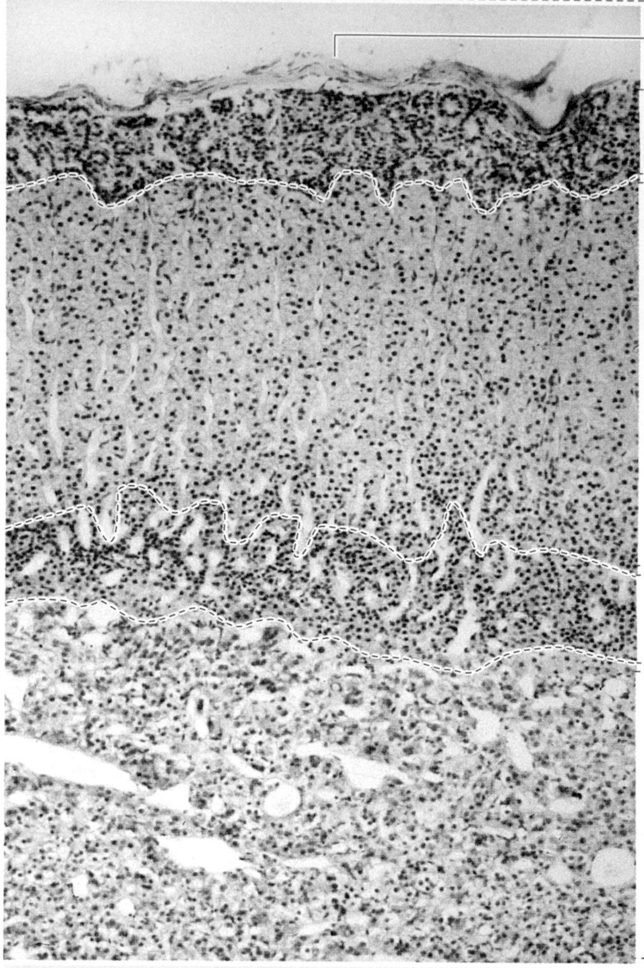

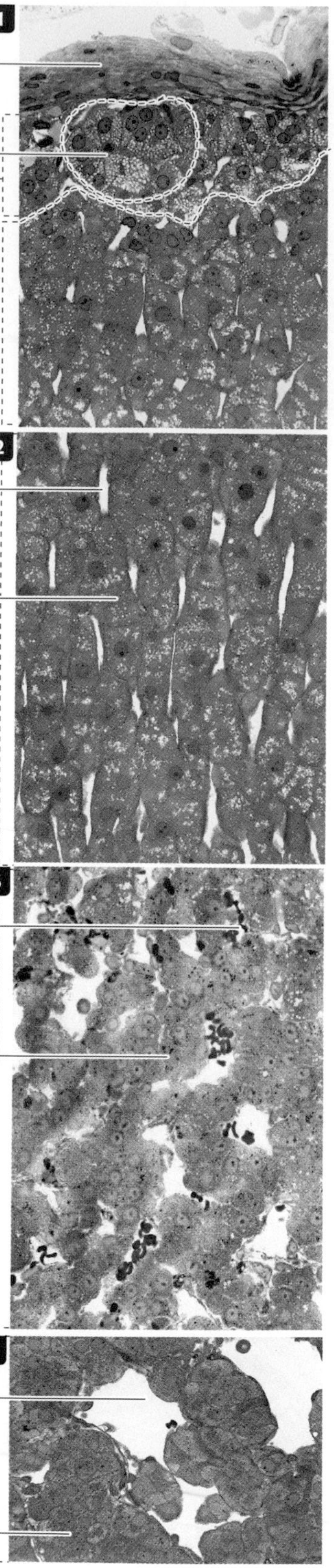

1 The **zona glomerulosa** is a narrow subcapsular zone contiguous on its inner side with the zona fasciculata. The zona glomerulosa consists of concentrically arranged cells surrounded by a stroma containing capillaries. The cells contain a few lipid droplets and a well-developed smooth endoplasmic reticulum.

Cells of the zona glomerulosa secrete the mineralocorticoid hormone **aldosterone** under control of **angiotensin II**.

2 The **zona fasciculata** predominates in the adrenal cortex. It consists of polygonal cells arranged in vertical columns or fascicles perpendicular to the capsule. The cells contain a vacuolated cytoplasm reflecting the accumulation of lipid droplets containing cholesterol and its metabolites. Fenestrated capillaries separate adjacent cell columns.

Cells of the zona fasciculata secrete mainly glucocorticoid hormones (**cortisol**) under adrenocorticotropic hormone (ACTH) regulation.

3 The **zona reticularis** is thinner than the zona fasciculata but thicker than the zona glomerulosa. It consists of anastomosing cells forming a reticulum or network surrounded by fenestrated capillaries. The cells contain a brown pigment (**lipofuscin**) contrasting with the lighter staining of the zona fasciculata.

Cells of the zona reticularis secrete mainly **steroid sex hormones** under ACTH regulation.

4 The **adrenal medulla** consists of two cell populations surrounded by **venous sinusoids**: the epinephrine, adrenaline-secreting cells (80%) and norepinephrine, noradrenaline-secreting cells (20%). Epinephrine and norepinephrine are **catecholamines**. Catecholamines of the medulla generate a brown color when exposed to air or the oxidizing agent potassium dichromate (**chromaffin reaction**).

tilization, Placentation, and Lactation).

Glucocorticoids, either of maternal origin or synthesized from placental progesterone by the fetus, are essential for three main developmental events: (1) **the production of surfactant by type II alveolar cells after the eighth month of fetal life**; (2) **the development of a functional hypothalamopituitary axis**; and (3) **the induction of thymic involution.**

Histologic organization of the adrenal cortex

The adrenal glands (Latin *ad*, near; *ren*, kidney) are associated with the superior poles of the kidneys. Each gland consists of a yellowish outer cortex (80% to 90% of the gland) and a reddish inner medulla (10% to 20%). The adrenal **cortex** is of **mesodermal** origin and produces **steroid hormones**. The adrenal **medulla** is of **neuroectodermic** origin and produces **catecholamines**.

The **adrenal cortex** consists of three concentric zones (Figures 19-9 and 19-10). (1) The **outermost layer of the cortex is the zona glomerulosa**. (2) The **middle layer of the cortex is the zona fasciculata**. (3) The **innermost layer of the cortex is the zona reticularis.**

Cells of the zona glomerulosa produce the mineralocorticoid **aldosterone** (Figures 19-11 and 19-12). Although the zona fasciculata is often associated with glucocorticoid production—mainly **cortisol**—and the zona reticularis with androgen production, the functional distinctions between the two layers are not precise and they appear as a functional unit. In addition, these two layers are stimulated by corticotropin (ACTH), whereas the zona glomerulosa is primarily **angiotensin II-dependent**. Angiotensin II stimulates both the growth of the zona glomerulosa and the synthesis of aldosterone (see Figure 19-12).

Angiotensin II is an octapeptide derived from the conversion of the **angiotensin I decapeptide** in the pulmonary circulation by **angiotensin-converting enzyme** (see Chapter 14, Urinary System). Aldosterone has a half-life of 20 to 30 minutes and acts directly on the distal convoluted tubule and collecting tubule, where it increases Na^+ reabsorption and excretion of K^+.

The **zona glomerulosa** (Latin *glomus,* ball) has the following characteristics (see Figure 19-9): (1) it lies under the capsule; (2) it represents 10% to 15% of the cortex; (3) its cells aggregate into a glomerulus-like arrangement and have a **moderate amount of lipid droplets** in the cytoplasm; and (4) it lacks the enzyme **17α-hydroxylase** and, therefore, cannot produce cortisol or sex steroids.

During aldosterone action, aldosterone binds to **intracellular receptor proteins** to activate transcription factors that enhance the expression of specific genes. Aldosterone-responsive cells do not respond to the glucocorticoid cortisol because cortisol is converted to **cortisone** by the enzyme 11β-hydroxysteroid dehydrogenase and cortisone does not bind to the aldosterone receptor.

Aldosterone stimulates the retention of Na^+ in the kidney, the retention of water (as a consequence of Na^+ reabsorption), and renal secretion of K^+ and H^+.

The **zona fasciculata** (Latin *fascis,* bundle) makes up 75% of the cortex. It is formed by cuboid cells, with the structural features of steroid-producing cells (see Figure 19-10), arranged in longitudinal cords separated by cortical fenestrated capillaries, or sinusoids (see Figure 19-11).

The cytoplasm of zona fasciculata cells shows three components that characterize their steroidogenic function: (1) the steroid hormone precursor cholesterol stored in abundant **lipid droplets** (see Figure 19-11); when lipids are extracted during histologic preparation or are unstained by the standard hematoxylin-eosin (H&E) procedures, the cells of the zona fasciculata display a foamy appearance and are called **spongiocytes**; (2) **mitochondria with tubular cristae** containing steroidogenic enzymes; and (3) well-developed **smooth endoplasmic reticulum**, also with enzymes involved in the synthesis of steroid hormones (see Figure 19-11).

Cells of the zona fasciculata and zona reticularis cannot produce aldosterone but

Figure 19-10. **Fine structure of steroid-producing cells of the adrenal cortex (zona fasciculata)**

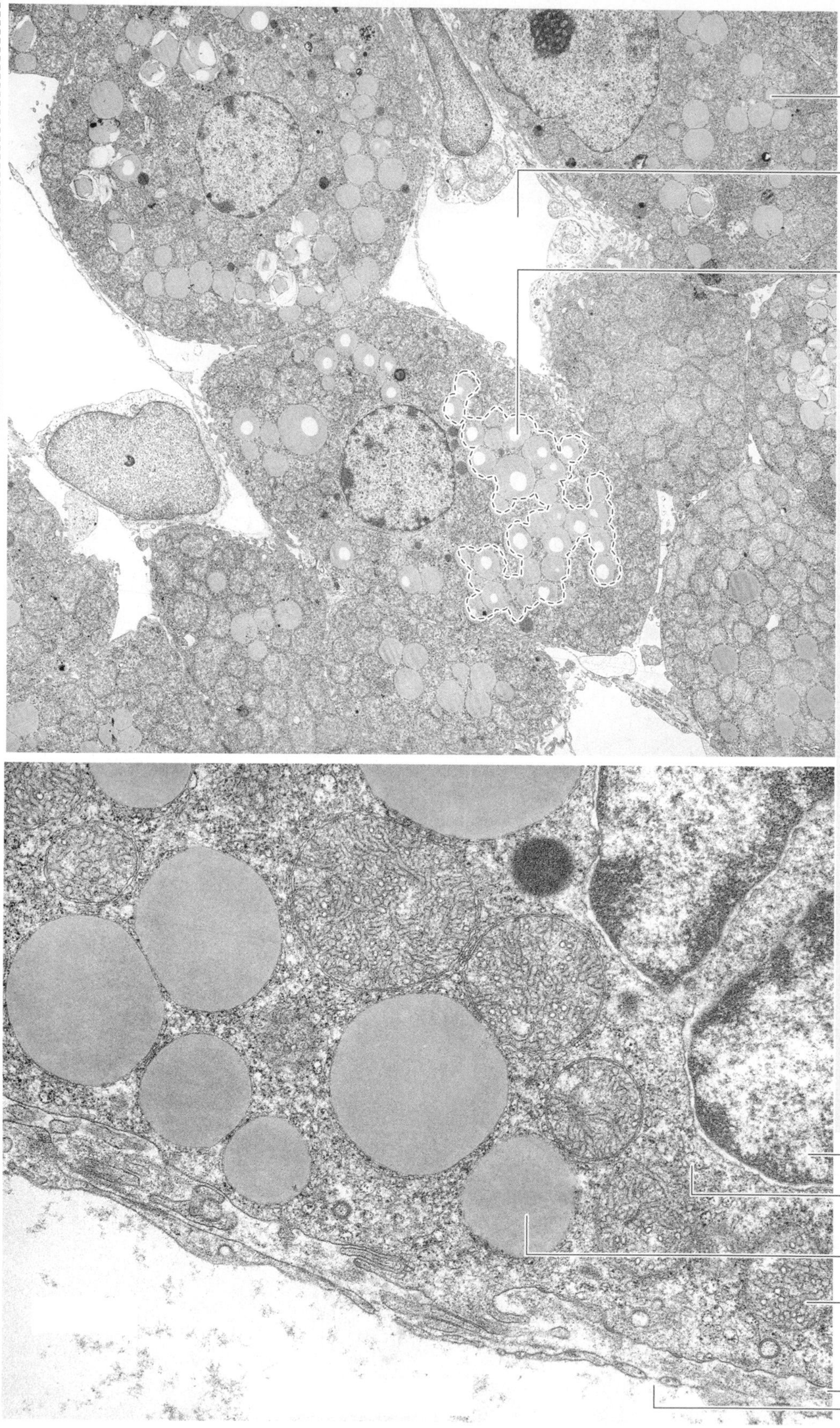
Spongiocyte of the zona fasciculata
Fenestrated capillary
Cluster of lipid droplets
Nucleus
Smooth endoplasmic reticulum
Lipid droplet
Mitochondria with tubular cristae
Basal lamina
Fenestrated endothelial cell

Spongiocytes

The ultrastructure of cells of the zona fasciculata and their close relationship with capillaries lined by fenestrated endothelial cells demonstrate their participation in the synthesis of steroid hormones released into the blood vascular system. Like steroid-producing cells of the theca interna and corpus luteum of the ovary and Leydig cells of the testis, cells of the zona fasciculata display three characteristic structural features representative of steroidogenesis: (1) **lipid droplets** containing cholesterol; (2) **mitochondria with tubular cristae** housing the enzymes involved in steroidogenesis; and (3) **smooth endoplasmic reticulum**, also containing membrane-associated enzymes involved in the production of steroids.

Figure 19-11. **Fine structure of steroid-producing cells of the adrenal cortex (zona reticularis)**

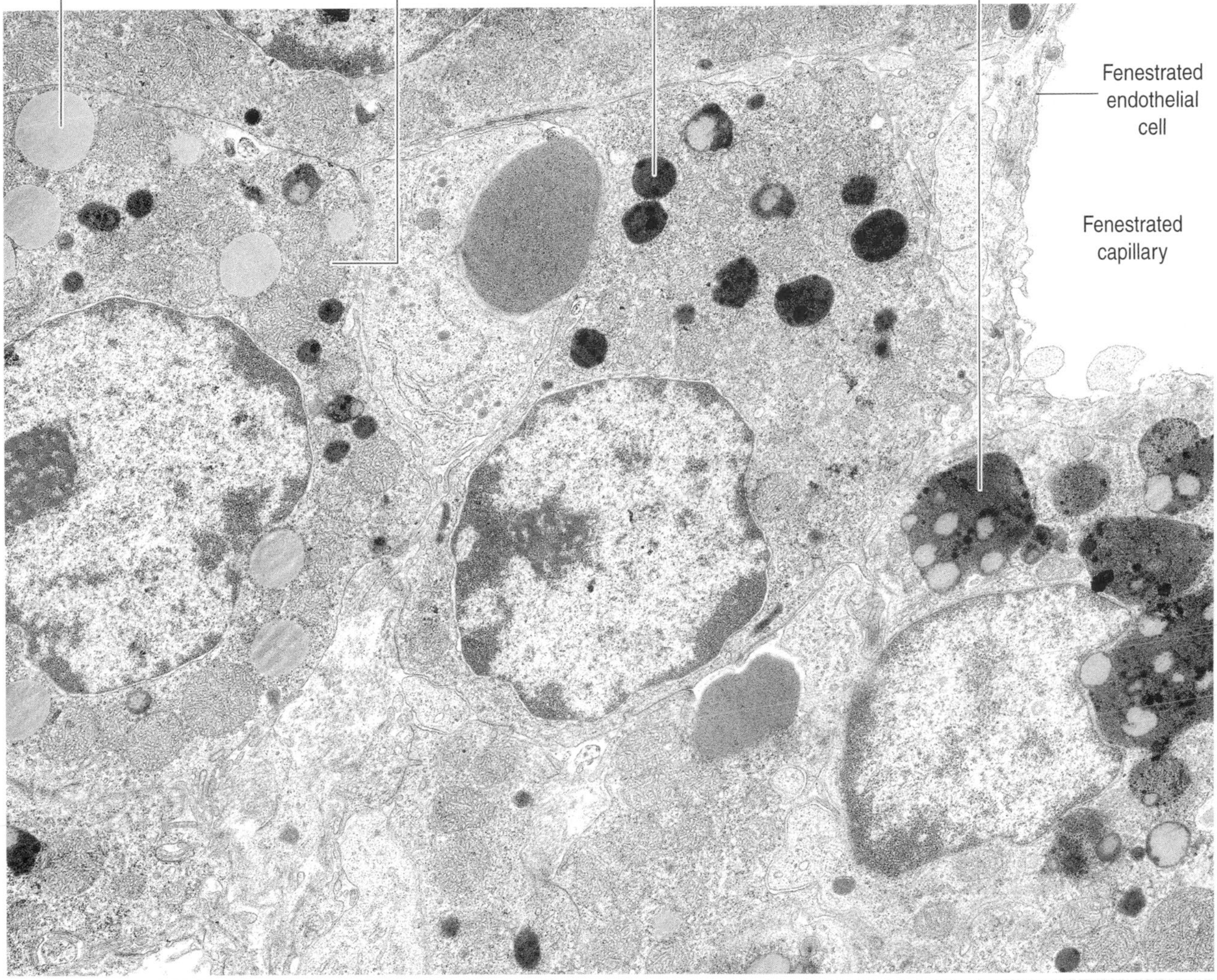

Cells of the **zona reticularis** are smaller than the cells of the zonae glomerulosa and fasciculata and contain fewer lipid droplets and mitochondria. However, mitochondria still display the characteristic tubular cristae. A structural feature not prominent in the cells of the other cortical zones is the presence of **lysosomes** and deposits of **lipofuscin**.

Lipofuscin is a remnant of lipid oxidative metabolism reflecting degradation within the adrenal cortex.

There are other relevant characteristics of the zona reticularis. (1) It receives steroid-enriched blood from the zonae glomerulosa (mineralocorticoids) and fasciculata (mainly cortisol). (2) It is in close proximity to the catecholamine-producing cells of the adrenal medulla. (3) In response to adrenocorticoptropic hormone (ACTH) stimulation, cells of **the zonae reticularis and fasciculata produce androgens** (dehydroepiandrosterone and androstenedione). **Cells of the zona reticularis synthesize dehydroepiandrosterone sulfate**.

Clinical significance: Adrenogenital syndrome

Although dehydroepiandrosterone, androstenedione, and dehydroepiandrosterone sulfate are weak androgens, they can be converted outside the adrenal cortex into more potent androgens and also estrogens.

This androgen conversion property has clinical significance in pathologic conditions such as the **adrenogenital syndrome**.

An excessive production of androgens in the adrenogenital syndrome in women leads to masculinization (abnormal sexual hair development—**hirsutism**—and enlargement of the clitoris).

Adrenal androgens in the male do not replace testicular androgens produced by Leydig cells, but, in women, adrenal androgens are responsible for the growth of axillary and pubic hair.

contain **17α-hydroxylase** necessary for the production of glucocorticoids—cortisol—and the enzyme **17,20-hydroxylase**, required for the production of sex hormones.

Cortisol is not stored in cells and new synthesis, stimulated by ACTH, is required for achieving a hormonal increase in blood circulation. Cortisol is converted in hepatocytes to cortisone.

Figure 19-12. Steroidogenic pathway

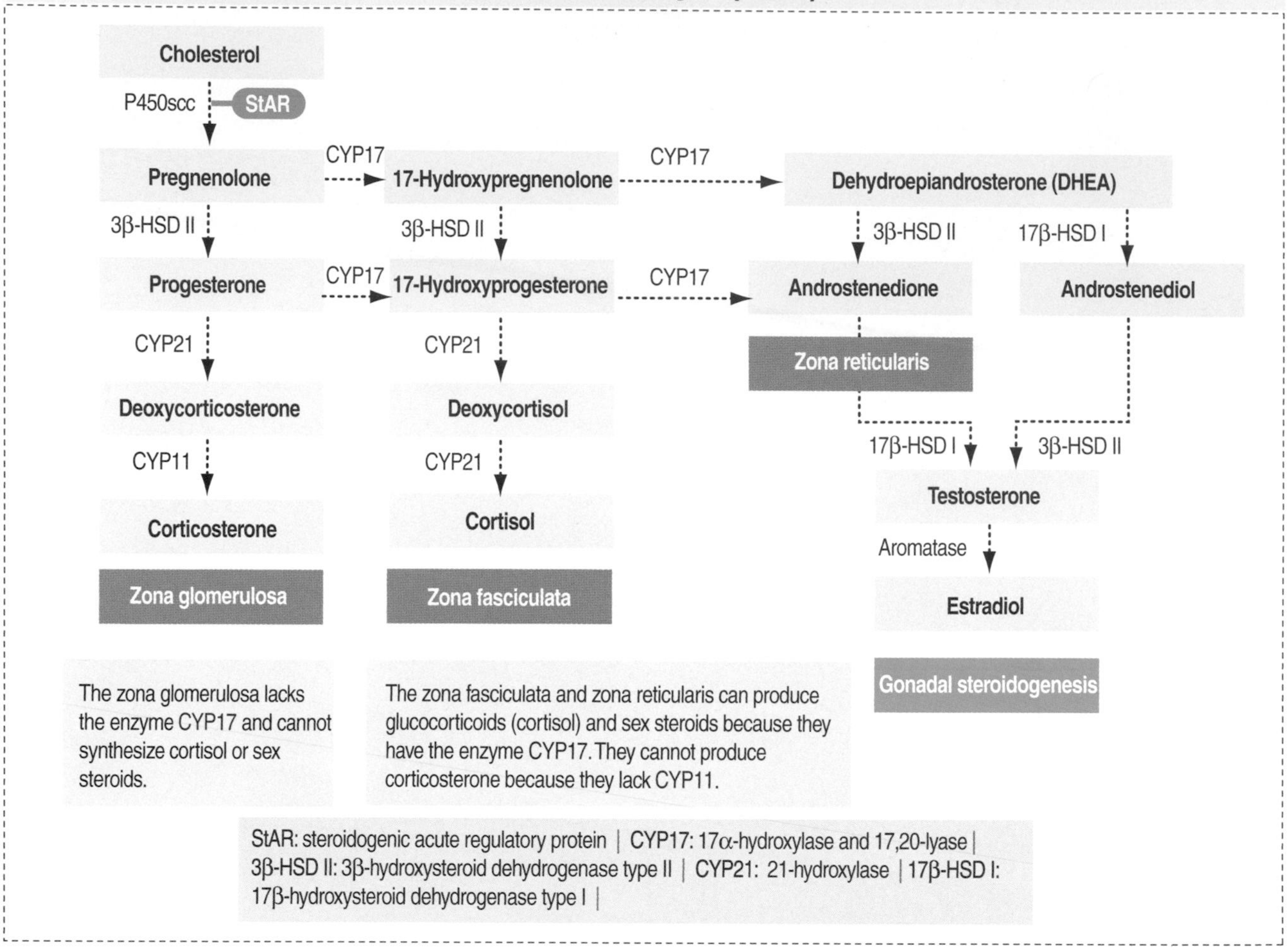

Cholesterol
P450scc
StAR
Pregnenolone
CYP17
17-Hydroxypregnenolone
CYP17
Dehydroepiandrosterone (DHEA)
3β-HSD II
3β-HSD II
3β-HSD II
17β-HSD I
Progesterone
CYP17
17-Hydroxyprogesterone
CYP17
Androstenedione
Androstenediol
CYP21
CYP21
Zona reticularis
Deoxycorticosterone
Deoxycortisol
17β-HSD I
3β-HSD II
CYP11
CYP21
Testosterone
Corticosterone
Cortisol
Aromatase
Estradiol
Zona glomerulosa
Zona fasciculata
Gonadal steroidogenesis
The zona glomerulosa lacks the enzyme CYP17 and cannot synthesize cortisol or sex steroids.
The zona fasciculata and zona reticularis can produce glucocorticoids (cortisol) and sex steroids because they have the enzyme CYP17. They cannot produce corticosterone because they lack CYP11.
StAR: steroidogenic acute regulatory protein | CYP17: 17α-hydroxylase and 17,20-lyase | 3β-HSD II: 3β-hydroxysteroid dehydrogenase type II | CYP21: 21-hydroxylase | 17β-HSD I: 17β-hydroxysteroid dehydrogenase type I |

Cortisol has two major effects: (1) **A metabolic effect**: Cortisol's effects are opposite to those of insulin. In the liver, cortisol stimulates gluconeogenesis to increase the concentration of glucose in blood. (2) **An anti-inflammatory effect**: Cortisol suppresses tissue responses to injury and decreases cellular and humoral immunity.

The **zona reticularis** (Latin *rete,* net) makes up 5% to 10% of the cortex. Cells of the zona reticularis form an anastomosing network of short cellular cords separated by fenestrated capillaries.

The cells of this zone are acidophilic, due to abundant **lysosomes**, large **lipofuscin granules**, and **fewer lipid droplets** (see Figure 19-11). Although cells of the zona fasciculata can synthesize androgens, the primary site of adrenal sex hormone production is the zona reticularis. **Dehydroepiandrosterone** (DHEA) and **androstenedione** are the predominant androgens produced by the cortex of the adrenal gland (see Figures 19-12 and 19-13). DHEA sulfate is synthesized in the zona reticularis.

Although DHEA and androstenedione are weak androgens, they can be converted to testosterone and even to estrogen in peripheral tissues. The adrenal gland is the major source of androgens in women; these androgens stimulate the growth of pubic and axillary hair during puberty.

The adrenal medulla

The adrenal medulla contains **chromaffin cells**, so named because of their ability to acquire a **brown coloration** when exposed to an aqueous solution of **potassium dichromate**. This reaction is due to the **oxidation of catecholamines** by chrome salts to produce a brown pigment.

Figure 19-13. Synthesis of steroids in the adrenal cortex

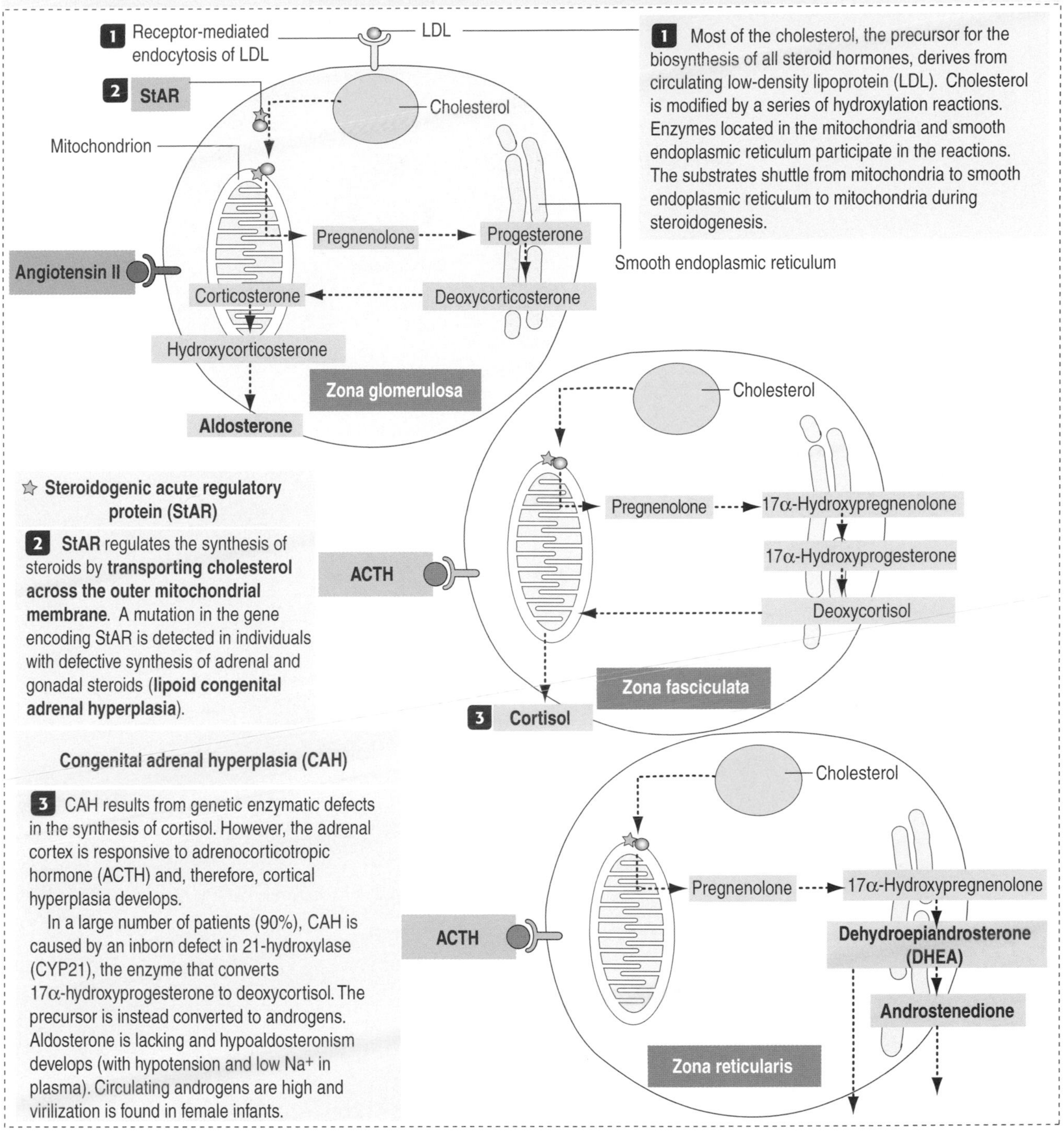
1 Receptor-mediated endocytosis of LDL
LDL
2 StAR
Cholesterol
Mitochondrion
Pregnenolone
Progesterone
Smooth endoplasmic reticulum
Angiotensin II
Corticosterone
Deoxycorticosterone
Hydroxycorticosterone
Zona glomerulosa
Aldosterone
1 Most of the cholesterol, the precursor for the biosynthesis of all steroid hormones, derives from circulating low-density lipoprotein (LDL). Cholesterol is modified by a series of hydroxylation reactions. Enzymes located in the mitochondria and smooth endoplasmic reticulum participate in the reactions. The substrates shuttle from mitochondria to smooth endoplasmic reticulum to mitochondria during steroidogenesis.
Steroidogenic acute regulatory protein (StAR)
2 StAR regulates the synthesis of steroids by transporting cholesterol across the outer mitochondrial membrane. A mutation in the gene encoding StAR is detected in individuals with defective synthesis of adrenal and gonadal steroids (lipoid congenital adrenal hyperplasia).
Cholesterol
ACTH
Pregnenolone
17α-Hydroxypregnenolone
17α-Hydroxyprogesterone
Deoxycortisol
Zona fasciculata
3 Cortisol
Congenital adrenal hyperplasia (CAH)
3 CAH results from genetic enzymatic defects in the synthesis of cortisol. However, the adrenal cortex is responsive to adrenocorticotropic hormone (ACTH) and, therefore, cortical hyperplasia develops.
In a large number of patients (90%), CAH is caused by an inborn defect in 21-hydroxylase (CYP21), the enzyme that converts 17α-hydroxyprogesterone to deoxycortisol. The precursor is instead converted to androgens. Aldosterone is lacking and hypoaldosteronism develops (with hypotension and low Na+ in plasma). Circulating androgens are high and virilization is found in female infants.
Cholesterol
ACTH
Pregnenolone
17α-Hydroxypregnenolone
Dehydroepiandrosterone (DHEA)
Androstenedione
Zona reticularis

Chromaffin cells (Figure 19-14) are **modified sympathetic postganglionic** neurons—without postganglionic processes—derived from the **neural crest** and forming epithelioid cords surrounded by **fenestrated capillaries**. The cytoplasm of chromaffin cells contains membrane-bound **dense granules** consisting in part of matrix proteins, called **chromogranins**, and one class of **catecholamine**, either **epinephrine** or **norepinephrine** (adrenaline or noradrenaline). Some granules contain both epinephrine and norepinephrine. Minimal secretion of **dopamine** also occurs, but the role of adrenal dopamine is not known.

Catecholamines are secreted into the blood instead of being secreted into a synapse, as in postganglionic terminals. The adrenal medulla is innervated by **sympathetic preganglionic fibers** that release **acetylcholine**.

Figure 19-14. Synthesis of catecholamines

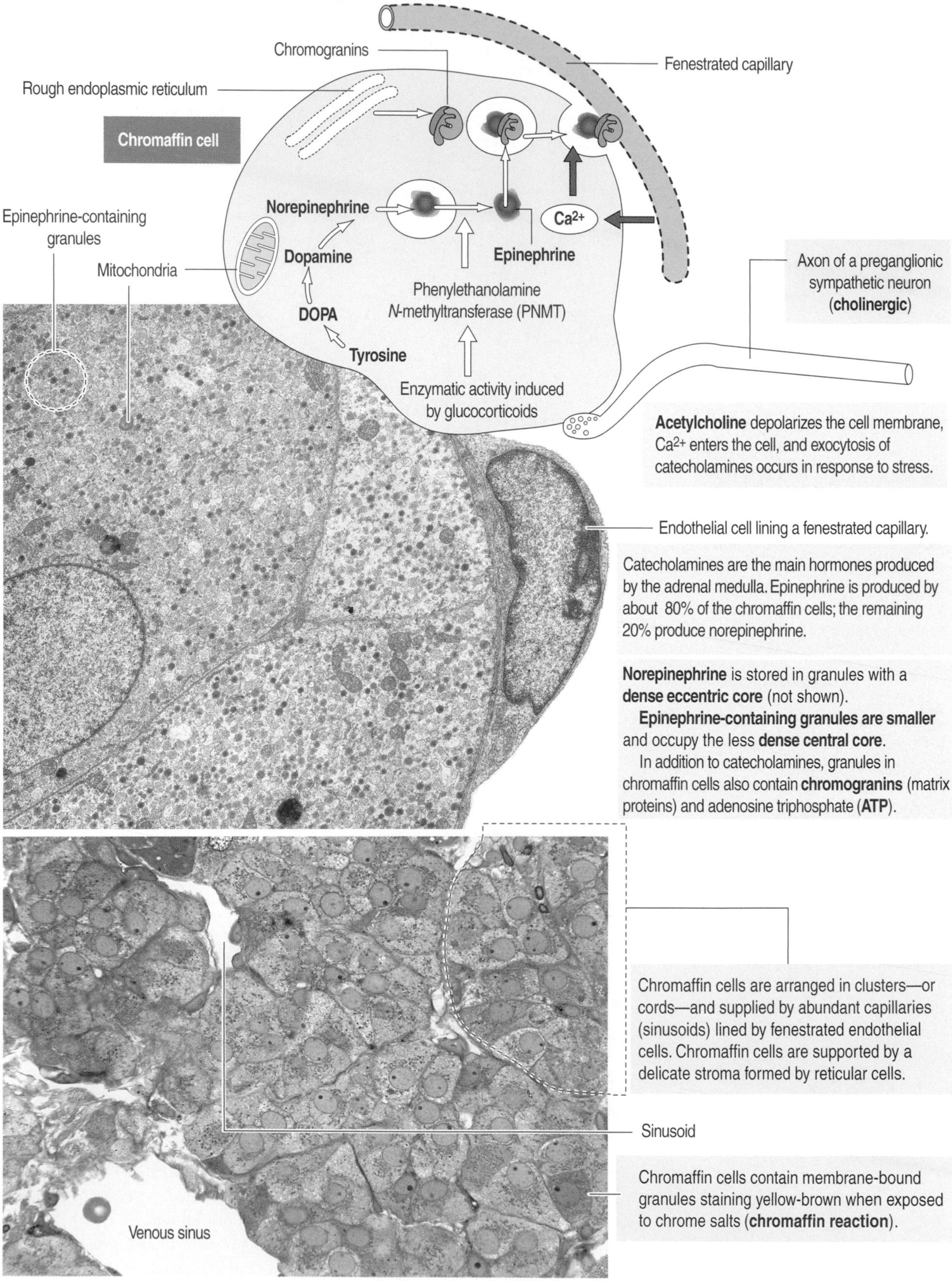

Chromogranins
Fenestrated capillary
Rough endoplasmic reticulum
Chromaffin cell
Norepinephrine
Ca2+
Epinephrine-containing granules
Dopamine
Epinephrine
Mitochondria
Phenylethanolamine N-methyltransferase (PNMT)
DOPA
Tyrosine
Enzymatic activity induced by glucocorticoids
Axon of a preganglionic sympathetic neuron (cholinergic)
Endothelial cell lining a fenestrated capillary.
Sinusoid
Venous sinus

Acetylcholine depolarizes the cell membrane, Ca^{2+} enters the cell, and exocytosis of catecholamines occurs in response to stress.

Catecholamines are the main hormones produced by the adrenal medulla. Epinephrine is produced by about 80% of the chromaffin cells; the remaining 20% produce norepinephrine.

Norepinephrine is stored in granules with a **dense eccentric core** (not shown).

Epinephrine-containing granules are smaller and occupy the less **dense central core**.

In addition to catecholamines, granules in chromaffin cells also contain **chromogranins** (matrix proteins) and adenosine triphosphate (**ATP**).

Chromaffin cells are arranged in clusters—or cords—and supplied by abundant capillaries (sinusoids) lined by fenestrated endothelial cells. Chromaffin cells are supported by a delicate stroma formed by reticular cells.

Chromaffin cells contain membrane-bound granules staining yellow-brown when exposed to chrome salts (**chromaffin reaction**).

Two different chromaffin cell types are present. About **80% of the cells produce epinephrine** and **20% synthesize norepinephrine.** These two cell populations can be distinguished at the electron microscope level by the morphology of the membrane-bound granules. Norepinephrine is stored in granules with a dense **eccentric core.** Epinephrine-containing granules are smaller and occupy the less dense **central core.** Note an important difference with cells of the adrenal cortex: **cells from the adrenal cortex do not store their steroid hormones in granules.**

Catecholamines are synthesized from **tyrosine** to **DOPA** (3,4-dihydroxyphenylalanine) in the presence of **tyrosine hydroxylase** (see Figure 19-14). DOPA is converted to **dopamine** by **DOPA decarboxylase.** Dopamine is transported into existing granules and converted inside them by **dopamine β-hydroxylase** to **norepinephrine.** The **membrane of the granules** contains the enzymes required for catecholamine synthesis and ATP-driven pumps for the transport of substrates.

Once synthesized, norepinephrine leaves the granule **to enter the cytosol,** where it is converted to epinephrine in a reaction driven by the enzyme **phenylethanolamine *N*-methyltransferase** (PNMT). The synthesis of PNMT is induced by **glucocorticoids** transported from the cortex to the medulla by the adrenocortical capillary system. When the conversion step to epinephrine is completed, epinephrine **moves back to the membrane-bound granule** for storage.

The degradation of catecholamines in the presence of the enzymes **monoamine oxidase** (MAO) and **catechol *O*-methyltransferase** (COMT) yields the main degradation products **vanillylmandelic acid** (VMA) and **metanephrine,** which are eliminated in urine. Urinary VMA and metanephrine are used clinically to determine the level of catecholamine production in a patient.

Actions of catecholamines are mediated by adrenergic receptors α and β

Catecholamines bind to α- and **β-adrenergic receptors** in target cells. There are α_1-, α_2-, β_1-, and β_2-adrenergic receptors. **Epinephrine has greater binding affinity for β_2-adrenergic receptors than norepinephrine.** Both hormones have similar binding affinity for β_1-, α_1-, and α_2-adrenergic receptors.

The stimulation of α-adrenergic receptors of blood vessels causes **vasoconstriction.** In blood vessels of **skeletal muscle,** activation of β_2-adrenergic receptors causes **vasodilation.** Epinephrine acting through α-adrenergic receptors causes **vasoconstriction,** but when it activates β-adrenergic receptors in skeletal muscle it causes **vasodilation.** The adrenergic receptors of the cardiac muscle are β_1-adrenergic receptors, and both epinephrine and norepinephrine have comparable effects.

Blood supply to the adrenal gland

Similar to all endocrine organs, the adrenal glands are highly vascularized. Arterial blood derives from three different sources (Figure 19-15): (1) the **inferior phrenic artery,** which gives rise to the **superior adrenal artery;** (2) the **aorta,** from which the **middle adrenal artery** branches out; and (3) the **renal artery,** which gives rise to the **inferior adrenal artery.**

All three adrenal arteries enter the adrenal gland capsule and form an **arterial plexus.** Three sets of branches emerge from the plexus: (1) One set supplies the **capsule.** (2) The second set enters the cortex forming **straight fenestrated capillaries** (also called **sinusoids**), percolating between the zonae glomerulosa and fasciculata, and forming a capillary network in the zona reticularis before entering the medulla. (3) The third set generates **medullary arteries** traveling along connective tissue trabeculae of the cortex **without branching** and **supplying blood only to the medulla.**

This blood vessel distribution results in (1) **dual blood supply to the adrenal medulla;** (2) the **transport of cortisol to the medulla,** necessary for the synthesis of PNMT and required for the conversion of norepinephrine to epinephrine; and (3) the **supply of fresh blood to the adrenal medulla,** required for rapid responses to stress.

Figure 19-15. **Blood supply to the adrenal gland**

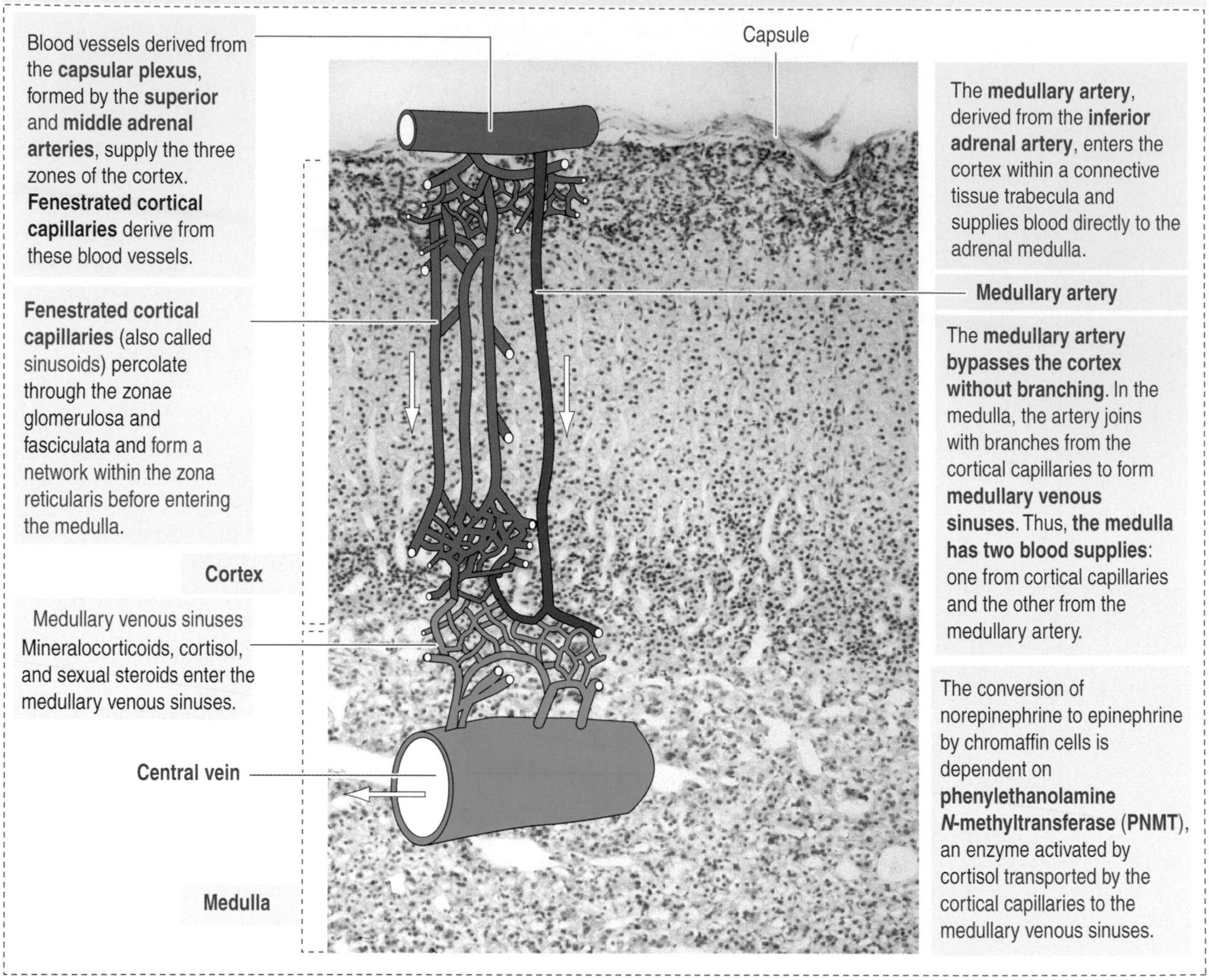
Blood vessels derived from the capsular plexus, formed by the superior and middle adrenal arteries, supply the three zones of the cortex. Fenestrated cortical capillaries derive from these blood vessels.
Fenestrated cortical capillaries (also called sinusoids) percolate through the zonae glomerulosa and fasciculata and form a network within the zona reticularis before entering the medulla.
Cortex
Medullary venous sinuses
Mineralocorticoids, cortisol, and sexual steroids enter the medullary venous sinuses.
Central vein
Medulla
Capsule
The medullary artery, derived from the inferior adrenal artery, enters the cortex within a connective tissue trabecula and supplies blood directly to the adrenal medulla.
Medullary artery
The medullary artery bypasses the cortex without branching. In the medulla, the artery joins with branches from the cortical capillaries to form medullary venous sinuses. Thus, the medulla has two blood supplies: one from cortical capillaries and the other from the medullary artery.
The conversion of norepinephrine to epinephrine by chromaffin cells is dependent on phenylethanolamine N-methyltransferase (PNMT), an enzyme activated by cortisol transported by the cortical capillaries to the medullary venous sinuses.

There are no veins or lymphatics in the adrenal cortex. The adrenal cortex and medulla are drained by the **central vein**, present in the adrenal medulla.

Clinical significance: Abnormal secretory activity of the adrenal cortex

Zona glomerulosa: A tumor localized in the zona glomerulosa can cause excessive secretion of aldosterone. This rare condition is known as **primary aldosteronism**, or **Conn's syndrome.** A more common cause of hyperaldosteronism is an increase in renin secretion (**secondary hyperaldosteronism**).

Zona fasciculata: An increase in aldosterone, cortisol, and adrenal androgen production—secondary to ACTH production—occurs in **Cushing's** ***disease***. Cushing's disease is caused by an **ACTH-producing tumor of the anterior hypophysis.** A **functional tumor of the adrenal cortex** can also result in overproduction of cortisol, as well as of aldosterone and adrenal androgens. This clinical condition is described as **Cushing's** ***syndrome*** (as opposed to Cushing's *disease*). The symptoms of Cushing's syndrome reflect the multiple actions of glucocorticoids, in particular, on the carbohydrate metabolism. Cortisol's effects are opposite to those of insulin.

Zona reticularis: When compared with the gonads, the zona reticularis secretes insignificant amounts of androgens. Androgen hypersecretion becomes important when there is an adrenal disorder resulting in reproductive abnormalities.

An **acute destruction** of the adrenal gland by meningococcal septicemia in infants is the cause of **Waterhouse-Friderichsen syndrome.** A **chronic destruc-**

tion of the adrenal cortex by an autoimmune process or tuberculosis results in the classic **Addison's disease.** In Addison's disease, ACTH secretion increases because of the cortisol deficiency. ACTH can cause an increase in skin pigmentation, in particular in the skin folds and gums. The loss of mineralocorticoids leads to hypotension and circulatory shock. A loss of cortisol decreases vasopressive responses to catecholamines and leads to an eventual drop in peripheral resistance, thereby contributing to hypotension. A deficiency in cortisol causes muscle weakness (asthenia).

Clinical significance: Hypersecretory activity of the adrenal medulla

Tumors of the adrenal medulla (**pheochromocytomas**) cause sustained or episodic **hypertension**. When pheochromocytomas are associated with other endocrine tumors, they are a component of the **multiple endocrine neoplasia (MEN) syndrome**. The presence of large amounts of VMA in urine has diagnostic relevance.

Clinical significance: Congenital adrenal hyperplasia

Congenital adrenal hyperplasia is a familial inherited condition in which a mutation in the gene encoding **steroidogenic acute regulatory protein (StAR)**, causes a deficiency in adrenocortical and gonadal steroidogenesis. StAR regulates the synthesis of steroids **by transporting cholesterol across the outer mitochondrial membrane. A steroidogenic deficiency increases ACTH secretion, leading to adrenal hyperplasia.**

Adrenal hyperplasia is seen in individuals with a deficiency of the enzyme **21-hydroxylase** who cannot produce cortisol or mineralocorticoids. These individuals are hypotensive because of a difficulty in retaining salt and maintaining extracellular volume. A deficiency in the enzyme **11-hydroxylase** (CYP11) results in the synthesis and accumulation of the mineralocorticoid deoxycorticosterone (DOC). Patients with this deficiency retain salt and water and become hypertensive.

See Figure 19-12 for the role of 21-hydroxylase (CYP21) and 11-hydroxylase (CYP11) in the synthesis of cortisol and mineralocorticoids.

Endocrine pancreas

Development of the pancreas

By week 4, two outpocketings from the endodermal lining of the duodenum develop as the ventral and dorsal pancreas, each with its own duct. The ventral pancreas forms the head of the pancreas and associates with the common bile duct. The dorsal pancreas forms part of the head, body, and tail of the pancreas. By week 12, pancreatic acini develop from the ducts. The endocrine pancreas develops at the same time as the exocrine pancreas. Endocrine cells are first observed along the base of the differentiating exocrine acini by weeks 12 to 16.

Histology of the islets of Langerhans

The pancreas has two portions (Figures 19-16 and 19-17):

1. The **exocrine pancreas**, consisting of acini involved in the synthesis and secretion of several digestive enzymes transported by a duct system into the duodenum.
2. The **endocrine pancreas** (2% of the pancreatic mass), formed by the **islets of Langerhans** scattered throughout the pancreas.

Each islet of Langerhans is formed by two components:

1. **Anastomosing cords** of **endocrine cells**—A (α cells), B (β cells), D (δ cells), and F cells—each secreting a single hormone.
2. A **vascular component**, the **insuloacinar portal system** (see Figure 19-16), which consists of an afferent arteriole giving rise to a capillary network lined by fenestrated endothelial cells. Venules leaving the islets of Langerhans supply blood to adjacent pancreatic acini. This portal system enables the local action of insular

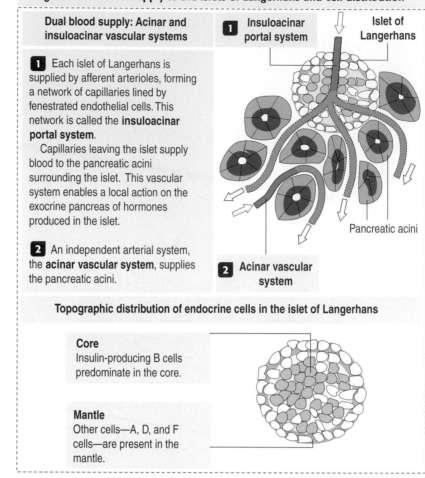

Figure 19-16. Blood supply to the islets of Langerhans and cell distribution

Dual blood supply: Acinar and insuloacinar vascular systems

1 Each islet of Langerhans is supplied by afferent arterioles, forming a network of capillaries lined by fenestrated endothelial cells. This network is called the **insuloacinar portal system**.

Capillaries leaving the islet supply blood to the pancreatic acini surrounding the islet. This vascular system enables a local action on the exocrine pancreas of hormones produced in the islet.

2 An independent arterial system, the **acinar vascular system**, supplies the pancreatic acini.

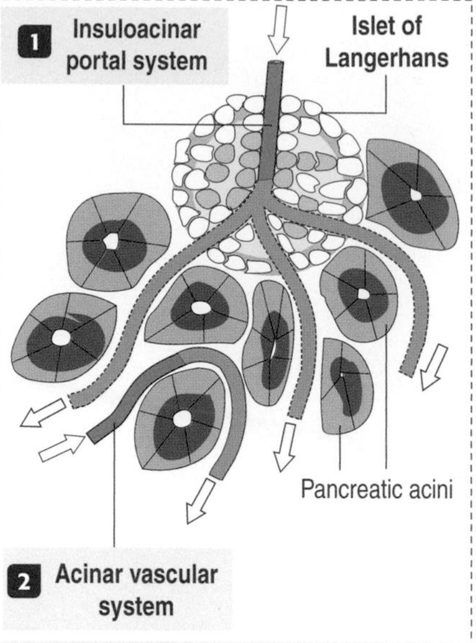

Topographic distribution of endocrine cells in the islet of Langerhans

Core
Insulin-producing B cells predominate in the core.

Mantle
Other cells—A, D, and F cells—are present in the mantle.

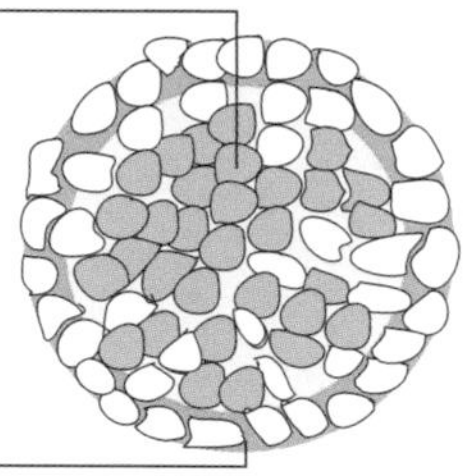

hormones on the exocrine pancreas.

An independent vascular system, the **acinar vascular system**, supplies blood directly to the exocrine pancreatic acini.

A cells (**α cells**) produce **glucagon**, **beta cells** synthesize **insulin**, **delta cells** secrete **gastrin** and **somatostatin**, and **F cells** produce **pancreatic polypeptide**.

Glucagon, a 29-amino-acid peptide, is stored in granules that are released by exocytosis when there is a **decrease** in the plasma levels of **glucose**. Glucagon increases glucose blood levels by increasing **hepatic glycogenolysis**. Glucagon binds to a specific membrane-bound receptor and this binding results in the synthesis of cAMP.

B cells (**β cells**) **produce** insulin, a 6-kd polypeptide consisting of two chains (Figure 19-18): (1) **chain A**, with 21 amino acids; and (2) **chain B**, with 30 amino acids. Chains A and B are linked by disulfide bonds.

Insulin derives from a large single-chain precursor, **preproinsulin**, encoded by a gene located on the short arm of chromosome 11. Preproinsulin is synthesized in the rough endoplasmic reticulum and is processed in the Golgi apparatus.

The large precursor gives rise to **proinsulin** (9 kd; 86 amino acids) in which **C peptide** connects A and B chains. Removal of C peptide by specific proteases results in (1) the separation of chains A and B and (2) the organization of a crystalline core consisting of a hexamer and zinc atoms. C peptide surrounds the crystalline core.

An **increase in blood glucose stimulates the release of both insulin and C peptide stored in secretory granules.** Glucose is taken up by B cells by an **insulin-independent, glucose transporter protein-2** (GLUT-2), and stored insulin is released in a Ca^{2+}–dependent manner.

Figure 19-17. **Islet of Langerhans**

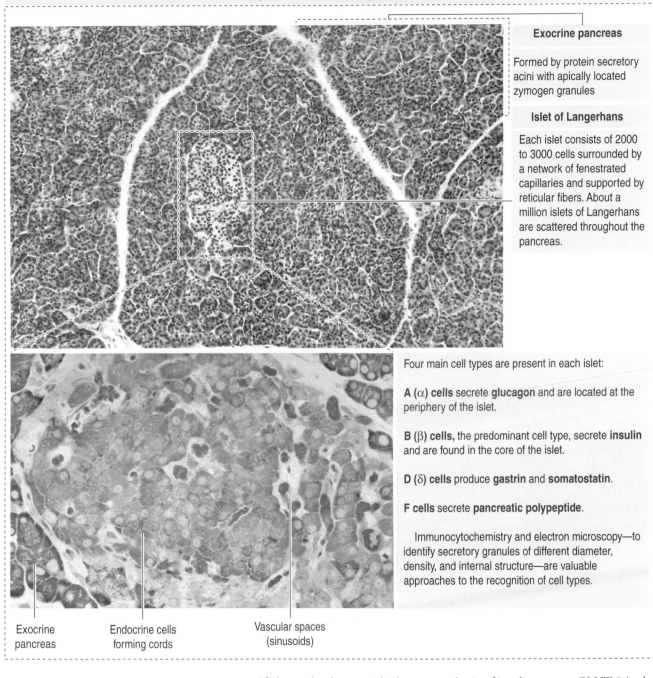

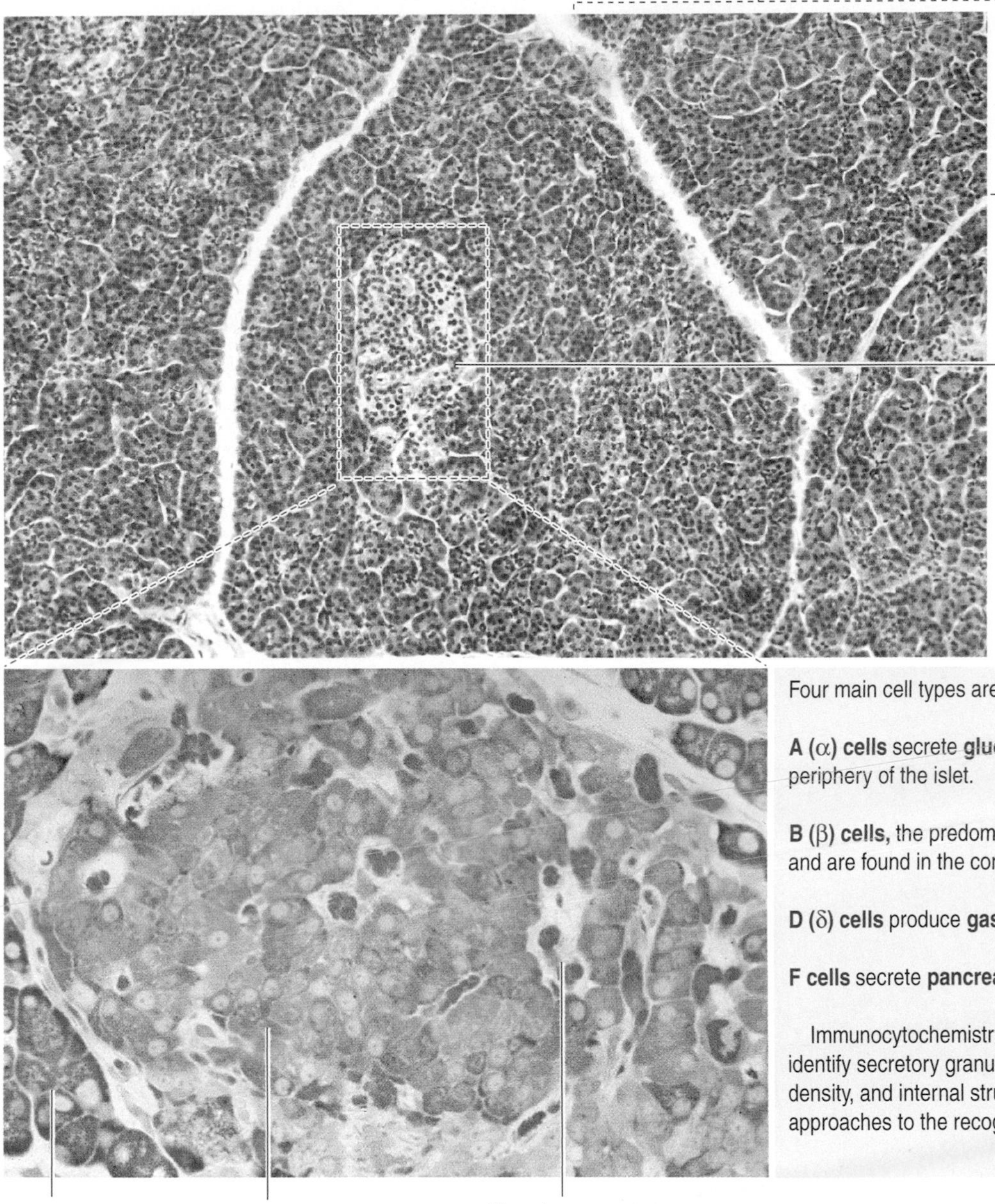

Exocrine pancreas
Endocrine cells forming cords
Vascular spaces (sinusoids)

Exocrine pancreas

Formed by protein secretory acini with apically located zymogen granules

Islet of Langerhans

Each islet consists of 2000 to 3000 cells surrounded by a network of fenestrated capillaries and supported by reticular fibers. About a million islets of Langerhans are scattered throughout the pancreas.

Four main cell types are present in each islet:

A (α) cells secrete **glucagon** and are located at the periphery of the islet.

B (β) cells, the predominant cell type, secrete **insulin** and are found in the core of the islet.

D (δ) cells produce **gastrin** and **somatostatin.**

F cells secrete **pancreatic polypeptide.**

Immunocytochemistry and electron microscopy—to identify secretory granules of different diameter, density, and internal structure—are valuable approaches to the recognition of cell types.

If glucose levels remain high, new synthesis of insulin occurs. GLUT-2 is also present in hepatocytes. Insulin is required for increasing the transport of glucose in cells (predominantly in hepatocytes, skeletal and cardiac muscle, fibroblasts, and adipocytes). This is accomplished by (1) the transmembrane transport of glucose and amino acids, (2) the formation of glycogen in hepatocytes and skeletal and cardiac muscle cells, and (3) the conversion of glucose to triglycerides in adipose cells (Figure 19-19).

Insulin initiates its effect by binding to the α subunit of its receptor. The **insulin receptor** consists of two subunits, α and β. The intracellular domain of the **β subunit** has **tyrosine kinase activity**, which autophosphorylates and triggers a number of intracellular responses. One of these responses is the translocation of **glucose transporter protein-4** (GLUT-4) from the Golgi apparatus to the plasma membrane to facilitate the uptake of glucose. **GLUT-4 is insulin-dependent** and

Figure 19-18. Synthesis and secretion of insulin by B cells of an islet of Langerhans

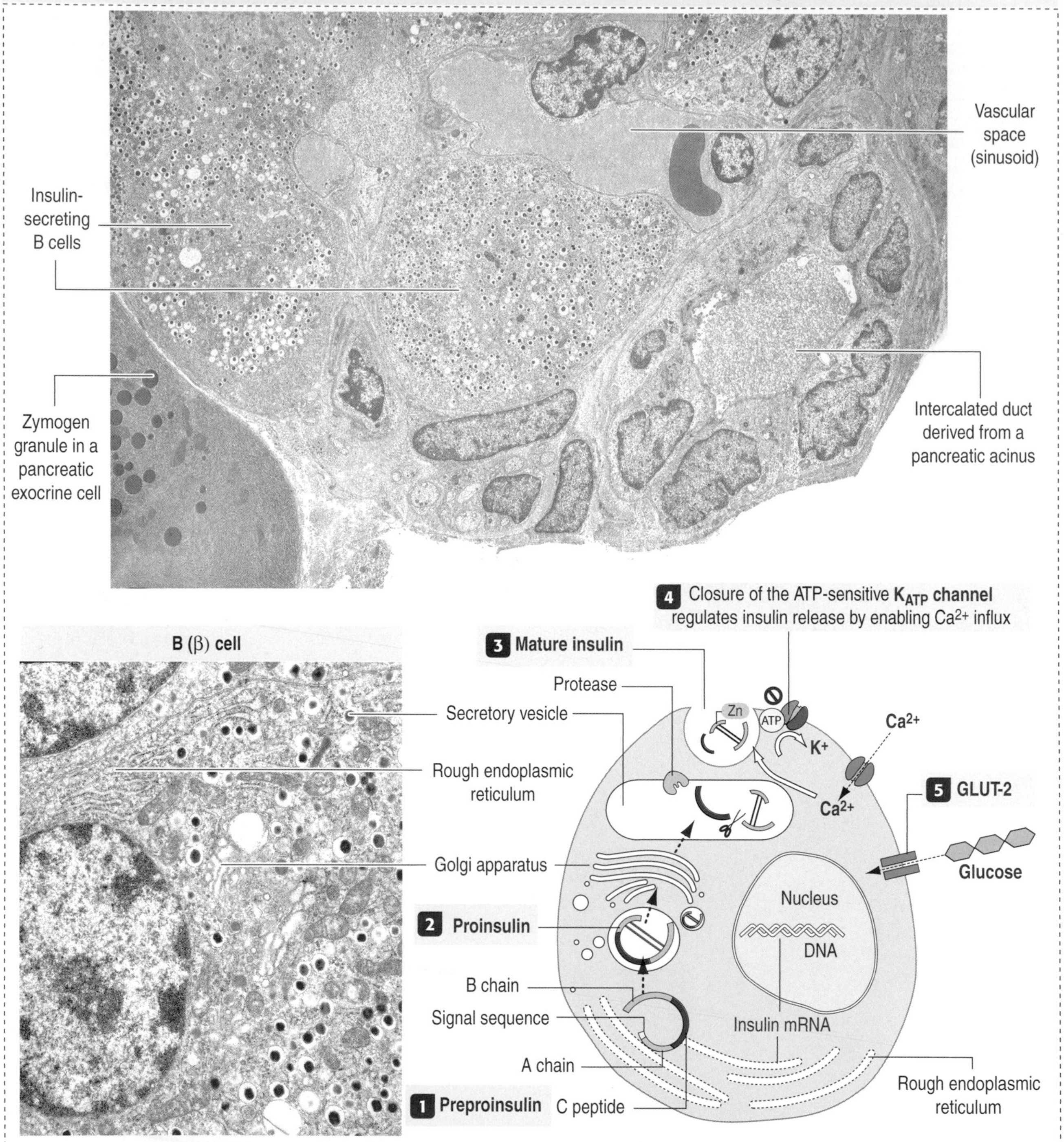

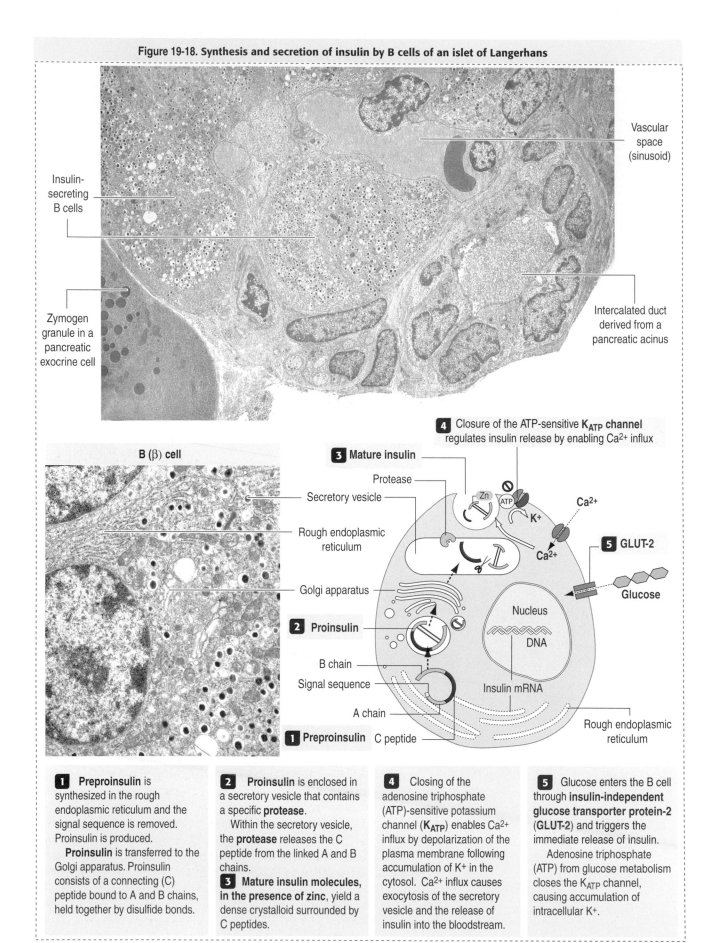

Vascular space (sinusoid)
Insulin-secreting B cells
Zymogen granule in a pancreatic exocrine cell
Intercalated duct derived from a pancreatic acinus
B (β) cell
4 Closure of the ATP-sensitive K_{ATP} channel regulates insulin release by enabling Ca^{2+} influx
3 Mature insulin
Protease
Secretory vesicle
Zn
ATP
K^+
Ca^{2+}
Rough endoplasmic reticulum
Ca^{2+}
5 GLUT-2
Golgi apparatus
Glucose
Nucleus
2 Proinsulin
DNA
B chain
Signal sequence
Insulin mRNA
A chain
1 Preproinsulin
C peptide
Rough endoplasmic reticulum

1 **Preproinsulin** is synthesized in the rough endoplasmic reticulum and the signal sequence is removed. Proinsulin is produced.

Proinsulin is transferred to the Golgi apparatus. Proinsulin consists of a connecting (C) peptide bound to A and B chains, held together by disulfide bonds.

2 **Proinsulin** is enclosed in a secretory vesicle that contains a specific **protease**.

Within the secretory vesicle, the **protease** releases the C peptide from the linked A and B chains.

3 **Mature insulin molecules, in the presence of zinc,** yield a dense crystalloid surrounded by C peptides.

4 Closing of the adenosine triphosphate (ATP)-sensitive potassium channel (**K_{ATP}**) enables Ca^{2+} influx by depolarization of the plasma membrane following accumulation of K^+ in the cytosol. Ca^{2+} influx causes exocytosis of the secretory vesicle and the release of insulin into the bloodstream.

5 Glucose enters the B cell through **insulin-independent glucose transporter protein-2** (**GLUT-2**) and triggers the immediate release of insulin.

Adenosine triphosphate (ATP) from glucose metabolism closes the K_{ATP} channel, causing accumulation of intracellular K^+.

Figure 19-19. **Adipose cell, lipid storage, and insulin**

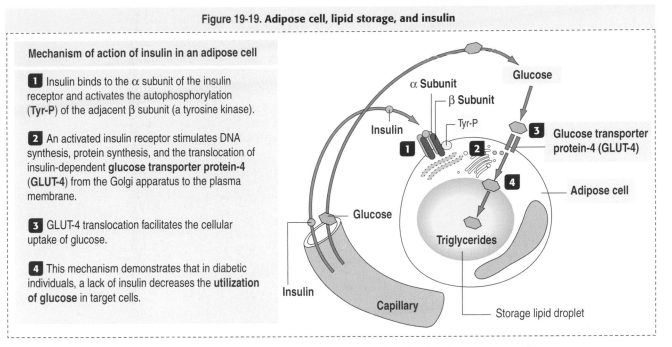

Mechanism of action of insulin in an adipose cell

1 Insulin binds to the α subunit of the insulin receptor and activates the autophosphorylation (**Tyr-P**) of the adjacent β subunit (a tyrosine kinase).

2 An activated insulin receptor stimulates DNA synthesis, protein synthesis, and the translocation of insulin-dependent **glucose transporter protein-4** (**GLUT-4**) from the Golgi apparatus to the plasma membrane.

3 GLUT-4 translocation facilitates the cellular uptake of glucose.

4 This mechanism demonstrates that in diabetic individuals, a lack of insulin decreases the **utilization of glucose** in target cells.

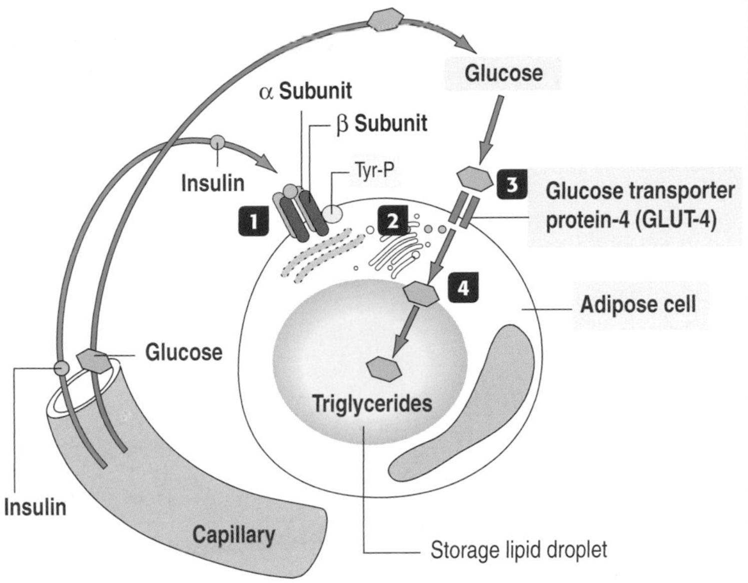

Glucose
α Subunit
β Subunit
Tyr-P
Insulin
1
2
3
Glucose transporter protein-4 (GLUT-4)
4
Adipose cell
Glucose
Triglycerides
Insulin
Capillary
Storage lipid droplet

is present in adipocytes and skeletal and cardiac muscle.

Note the functional difference between GLUT-2 and GLUT-4: (1) **GLUT-2 is insulin-independent and serves to transport glucose to insular B cells and hepatocytes**; (2) **GLUT-4 is insulin-dependent and serves to remove glucose from blood.**

A (α) cells produce **glucagon**, a 29-amino-acid peptide (3.5 kd) derived from a large precursor, **preproglucagon**, encoded by a gene present on chromosome 2. In addition to the pancreas, glucagon can be found in the gastrointestinal tract (enteroglucagon) and brain. About 30% to 40% of glucagon in blood derives from the pancreas; the remainder comes from the gastrointestinal tract. Circulating glucagon, of pancreatic and gastrointestinal origin, is transported to the liver and about 80% is degraded before reaching the systemic circulation. The liver is the primary target site of glucagon. Glucagon induces hyperglycemia by its glycogenolytic activity in hepatocytes.

Neither C peptide nor zinc are present in glucagon-containing secretory granules.

The actions of glucagon are antagonistic to those of insulin. The secretion of glucagon is stimulated by (1) a fall in the concentration of glucose in blood, (2) an increase of arginine and alanine in serum, and (3) stimulation of the sympathetic nervous system.

D (δ) cells produce **gastrin** (see discussion of enteroendocrine cells in Chapter 15, Upper Digestive Segment) and **somatostatin. Somatostatin** is a 14 amino-acid peptide identical to somatostatin produced in the hypothalamus. Somatostatin **inhibits the release of insulin and glucagon** in a paracrine manner.

Somatostatin also **inhibits the** secretion of HCl by parietal cells of the fundic stomach, the release of gastrin from enteroendocrine cells, the secretion of pancreatic bicarbonate and enzymes, and the contraction of the gallbladder. Somatostatin is also produced in the hypothalamus and inhibits the secretion of growth hormone from the anterior hypophysis.

Pancreatic polypeptide is a 36-amino-acid peptide that **inhibits the secretion of somatostatin.** Pancreatic polypeptide also inhibits the secretion of pancreatic enzymes and blocks the secretion of bile by inhibiting contraction of the gallbladder. Its function is to conserve digestive enzymes and bile between meals. Cholecystokinin stimulates the release of pancreatic polypeptide.

Cell types in the islets of Langerhans can be identified by (1) **immunocyto-**

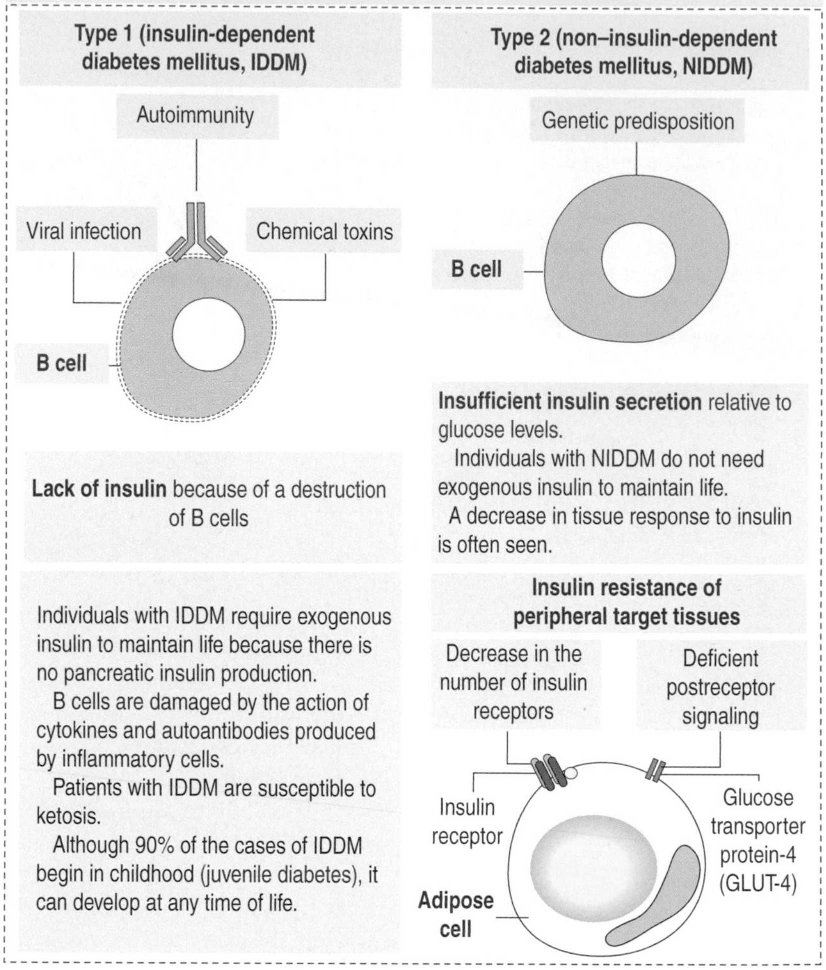
Type 1 (insulin-dependent diabetes mellitus, IDDM)
Autoimmunity
Viral infection
Chemical toxins
B cell
Lack of insulin because of a destruction of B cells
Individuals with IDDM require exogenous insulin to maintain life because there is no pancreatic insulin production.
B cells are damaged by the action of cytokines and autoantibodies produced by inflammatory cells.
Patients with IDDM are susceptible to ketosis.
Although 90% of the cases of IDDM begin in childhood (juvenile diabetes), it can develop at any time of life.
Type 2 (non–insulin-dependent diabetes mellitus, NIDDM)
Genetic predisposition
B cell
Insufficient insulin secretion relative to glucose levels.
Individuals with NIDDM do not need exogenous insulin to maintain life.
A decrease in tissue response to insulin is often seen.
Insulin resistance of peripheral target tissues
Decrease in the number of insulin receptors
Deficient postreceptor signaling
Insulin receptor
Glucose transporter protein-4 (GLUT-4)
Adipose cell

Figure 19-20. Diabetes mellitus: Clinical forms

chemistry, using antibodies specific for each cell product; (2) **electron microscopy**, to distinguish the size and structure of the secretory granules; and (3) the **cell distribution** in the islet. B cells are centrally located (core distribution) and surrounded by the other cell types (mantle distribution; see Figure 19-16).

Clinical significance: ATP-sensitive K^+ channel and insulin secretion

The **ATP-sensitive potassium (K_{ATP}) channel**, a complex of the **sulfonylurea receptor 1** (**SUR1**) and the **inward-rectifying K^+ channel** (**Kir6.2**) **subunits**, is the key regulator of insulin release. SUR1 is encoded by the *KCNJ11* (potassium channel J member 11) gene. Kir6.2 is encoded by the *ABCC8* (ATP-binding cassette, subfamily C, member 8) gene.

K_{ATP} channel modulates the influx of Ca^{2+} through voltage-gated Ca^{2+} channels. In the normal resting state, the K_{ATP} channel is open and the voltage-gated Ca^{2+} channel remains closed. No insulin is secreted. When glucose is taken up by B cells by GLUT-2, the K_{ATP} channel closes utilizing ATP derived from glucose metabolism. K^+ accumulates in the cell, the Ca^{2+} channel opens by membrane depolarization, and the influx of Ca^{2+} triggers insulin exocytosis (see Figure 19-18).

The clinical significance of this mechanism is highlighted by mutations in *SUR1* and *Kir6.2* genes. **Gain-of-function mutations** of SUR1 and Kir6.2 cause K_{ATP} channels to remain **open**, thereby decreasing insulin secretion and leading to **neonatal diabetes mellitus. Loss-of-function mutations** of *SUR1* and *Kir6.2* genes cause K_{ATP} channels to remain **closed**, thereby causing unregulated secretion of insulin leading to **neonatal hyperinsulinemic hypoglycemia.**

Figure 19-21. Clinical aspects of types 1 and 2 diabetes: Late complications

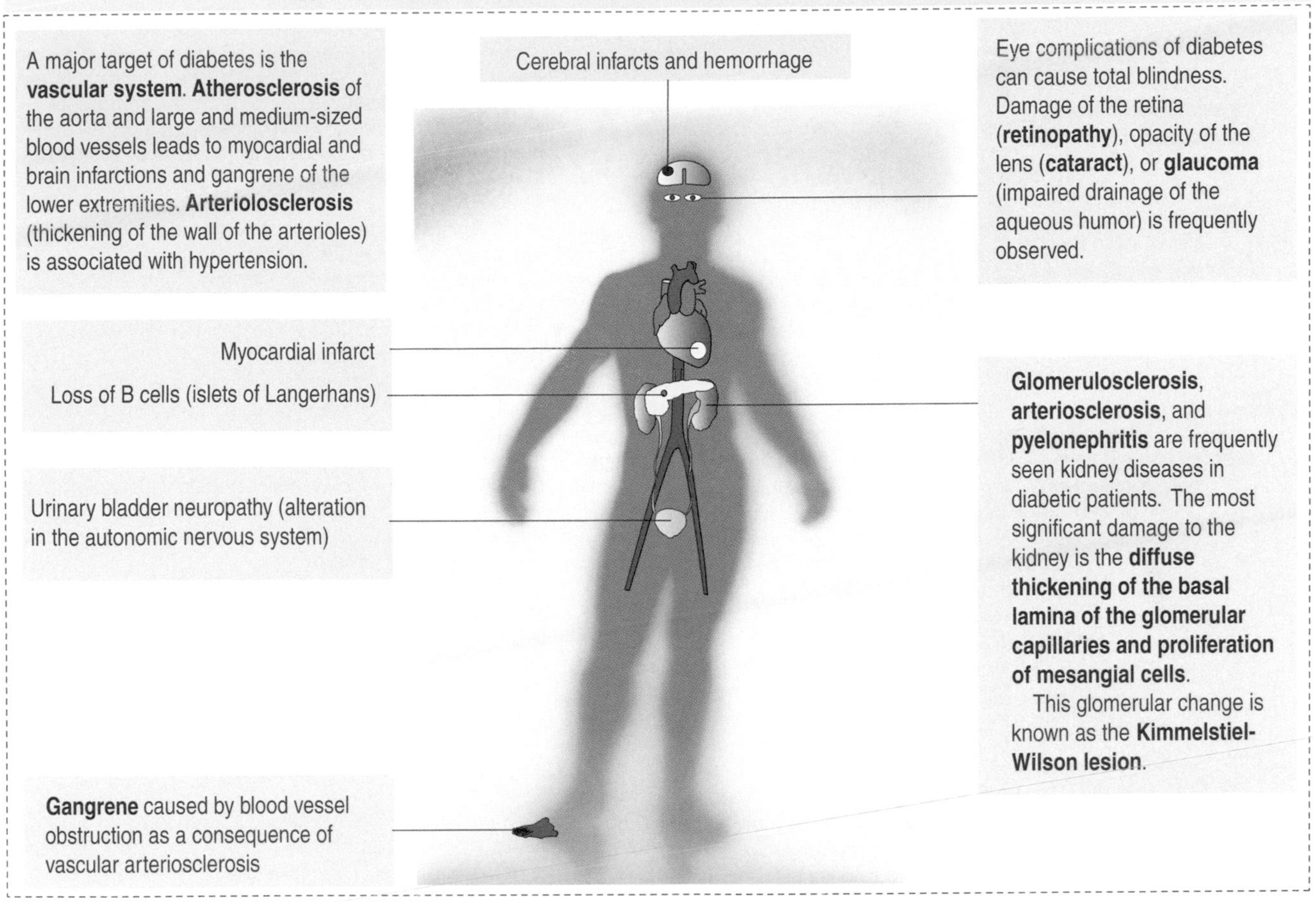
A major target of diabetes is the **vascular system**. **Atherosclerosis** of the aorta and large and medium-sized blood vessels leads to myocardial and brain infarctions and gangrene of the lower extremities. **Arteriolosclerosis** (thickening of the wall of the arterioles) is associated with hypertension.
Cerebral infarcts and hemorrhage
Eye complications of diabetes can cause total blindness. Damage of the retina (**retinopathy**), opacity of the lens (**cataract**), or **glaucoma** (impaired drainage of the aqueous humor) is frequently observed.
Myocardial infarct
Loss of B cells (islets of Langerhans)
Urinary bladder neuropathy (alteration in the autonomic nervous system)
Glomerulosclerosis, **arteriosclerosis**, and **pyelonephritis** are frequently seen kidney diseases in diabetic patients. The most significant damage to the kidney is the **diffuse thickening of the basal lamina of the glomerular capillaries and proliferation of mesangial cells.**
This glomerular change is known as the **Kimmelstiel-Wilson lesion.**
Gangrene caused by blood vessel obstruction as a consequence of vascular arteriosclerosis

Clinical significance: Insulin and diabetes

When blood glucose levels rise in a normal person, the immediate release of insulin ensures a return to normal levels within 1 hour. In a diabetic individual, increased blood glucose levels (**hyperglycemia**) remain high for a prolonged period of time.

Hyperglycemia can be the result of the following (Figure 19-20):

1. A **lack of insulin**, caused by autoimmune, toxic, or viral damage to B cells (**type 1 diabetes mellitus; insulin-dependent diabetes mellitus** [**IDDM**]). Insulinitis with an infiltration of lymphocytes is characteristic of the early stages of IDDM. This type of diabetes, also known as **juvenile diabetes**, accounts for about 90% of cases and often occurs before the age of 25 years (between 10 and 14). However, IDDM can occur at any age.

2. **Insufficient insulin secretion** relative to glucose levels and **resistance of peripheral target tissues to insulin** (**type 2 diabetes mellitus; non–insulin-dependent diabetes mellitus** [NIDDM]). The lack of responsiveness to insulin by target cells can be caused by a decrease in the number of available insulin receptors in the target cells and deficiency in postreceptor signaling (for example, the translocation of GLUT-4 from the Golgi apparatus to the plasma membrane to facilitate glucose uptake). This latter type of defect is most frequent (80%) and is observed in the adult.

The symptoms and consequences of type 1 and type 2 diabetes are generally similar. **Hyperglycemia**, **polyuria** (increased frequency of micturition and urine volume), and **polydipsia** (sensation of thirst and increased fluid intake) are the three characteristic symptoms. The clinical forms of diabetes mellitus are summarized in Figure 19-20. The late complications of diabetes mellitus are summarized in Figure 19-21.

• Thyroid gland. The thyroid gland develops from an endodermal downgrowth at the base of the tongue, connected by the thyroglossal duct. C cells, derived from the neural crest, are present in the thyroid gland.

The thyroid gland consists of thyroid follicles lined by a simple cuboidal epithelium, whose height varies with functional activity. The lumen contains a colloid substance rich in thyroglobulin, the precursor of the thyroid hormones triiodothyronine (T_3) and thyroxine (T_4). The main function of thyroid hormones is the regulation of the body's basal metabolism.

The synthesis and secretion of thyroid hormones involves two phases: (1) an excretory phase, and (2) an endocrine phase. Both phases can occur in the same thyroid cell and are regulated by thyroid stimulating hormone (TSH), produced by basophil cells in the anterior hypophysis.

The exocrine phase consists in the synthesis and secretion of thyroglobulin into the colloid-containing lumen and the uptake of inorganic iodide from blood through an ATP-dependent iodide pump. The enzyme thyroid peroxidase, present in the membrane of the secretory vesicle, which also contains thyroglobulin, converts iodide into iodine. Iodine atoms are attached to tyrosil residues on thyroglobulin, which become iodothyroglobulin.

The endocrine phase consists in the reuptake and processing of iodothyroglobulin. Colloid droplets, containing iodothyroglobulin, are enveloped by pseudopods and internalized to become colloid-containing vesicles. Lysosomes fuse with the internalized vesicles and iodothyroglobulin is processed to release T_3 and T_4 across the basal domain of the thyroid cell into the bloodstream. T_3 and T_4 are transported in the blood by serum carrier proteins. Thyroid hormones enter the cell nucleus of a target cell, and bind to the thyroid hormone–responsive element to activate specific gene expression.

• **Graves' disease** is an autoimmune disease that causes hyperfunction of the thyroid gland (hyperthyroidism). Autoantibodies (called thyroid-stimulating immunoglobulins) against the TSH receptor stimulate the unregulated function of the thyroid gland. Patients have an enlargement of the thyroid gland (goiter), bulging eyes (exophthalmos), and accelerated heart beat (tachycardia).

Hashimoto's disease is an autoimmune disease associated with hypofunction of the thyroid gland (hypothyroidism). It is caused by autoantibodies (known as antimicrosomal antibodies) to thyroid peroxidase and thyroglobulin.

• Ca^{2+} regulation. The maintenance of Ca^{2+} levels in blood is regulated by (1) parathyroid hormone, (2) calcitonin, and (3) vitamin D.

Parathyroid gland. The four parathyroid glands derive from the third and fourth branchial pouches. The parathyroid gland consists of two cell populations arranged in cords or clusters: (1) chief or principal cells, producing parathyroid hormone, and (2) oxyphil cells, presumably a transitional chief cell. Chief cells secrete parathyroid hormone. A Ca^{2+}-sensing receptor (CaSR) in the plasma membrane of chief cells detects Ca^{2+} concentration in serum. When Ca^{2+} levels go down, the secretion of parathyroid hormone is stimulated.

Parathyroid hormone regulates the Ca^{2+} and PO_4^{3-} balance by acting on: (1) the bone tissue, stimulating the function of osteoclasts and (2) the uriniferous tubule, by stimulating the resorption of Ca^{2+} by osteoclasts and activating the production of vitamin D. Parathyroid hormone induces the production of proteins in osteoblasts, which stimulate osteoclastogenesis. Proteins produced by osteoblasts and involved in osteoclastogenesis are macrophage-colony stimulating factor, RANKL, and osteoprotegerin.

Hyperparathyroidism is caused by an adenoma (benign tumor) of the partathyroid gland. Excessive secretion of parathyroid hormone causes hypercalcemia, phosphaturia, and hypercalciuria. Complications include the formation of renal stones and bone cysts caused by excessive removal of mineralized bone. Inactivating mutations of CaSR cause **familial benign hypercalcemia**. Activating mutations of CaSR result in **idiopathic hypoparathyroidism**.

C cells (present in the thyroid follicle) produce calcitonin, which antagonizes the effects of parathyroid hormone.

Vitamin D. Cholecalciferol is formed in the skin from 7-dehydrocholesterol. Before reaching its active form, cholecalciferol undergoes two hydroxylation steps, first in the liver (25-hydroxycholecalciferol) and the second in the kidney. Low Ca^{2+} levels stimulate 1α-hydroxylase to convert 25-hydroxycholecalciferol into calcitriol, the active form of vitamin D. The main function of vitamin D (calcitriol) is to stimulate the absorption of calcium by the intestinal mucosa.

Calcitriol is transported to the small intestine through the bloodstream, bound to vitamin D–binding protein. In the duodenum, calcitriol is taken up by enterocytes, which are stimulated by vitamin D to produce calbindin, a calcium-binding protein.

Calcium is absorbed in the duodenum by transcellular absorption, an active process that requires calbindin (for transcellular transport), and a voltage-insensitive channel controlled by calcium-ATPase (for export to the bloodstream). Calcium is absorbed in the jejunum and ileum by a passive paracellular absorption mechanism.

In children, a deficiency of vitamin D causes **rickets**. In adults, it causes **osteomalacia**.

• Adrenal gland. The adrenal gland consists of two components: (1) the adrenal cortex (derived from the mesoderm) and (2) the adrenal medulla (derived from neural crest cells).

The fetal adrenal cortex plays an important role during early gestation: it synthesizes dehydroepiandrosterone (DHEA), a precursor for the synthesis of estrogen by the placenta. This interaction is known as the fetoplacental unit. After the eighth month of gestation, glucocorticoids are essential for the production of surfactant by type II alveolar cells.

The adrenal cortex consists of three zones: (1) the outermost zona glomerulosa (which produces the mineralocorticoid aldosterone), (2) the middle layer of the zona fasciculata (which produces glucocorticoids, mainly cortisol), and (3) the inner layer of the zona reticularis (which synthesizes the androgens DHEA and androstenedione). The function of the zona glomerulosa is controlled by angiotensin II, and the functions of the zona fasciculata and zona reticularis are regulated by adrenocorticotropic hormone (ACTH).

The significant characteristics of steroid-producing cells are lipid droplets (containing cholesterol), mitochondria with tubular cristae (housing the enzymes involved in steroidogenesis), and smooth endoplasmic reticulum cisternae (also containing membrane-associated enzymes involved in the production of steroids).

Congenital adrenal hyperplasia results from a genetic enzymatic defect in the synthesis of cortisol. The adrenal cortex is responsive to ACTH and the adrenal cortex enlarges (adrenal hyperplasia).

Lipoid congenital adrenal hyperplasia is caused by a mutation in the gene encoding steroidogenic acute regulatory protein (StAR), a protein that transports cholesterol across the outer mitochondrial membrane. The synthesis of adrenal and gonadal steroids is affected.

Primary aldosteronism or **Conn's syndrome** is caused by a tumor in the zona glomerulosa that produces excessive aldosterone.

Cushing's *disease* is caused by an ACTH-producing tumor of the anterior hypophysis, resulting in an increased production of cortical steroids. **Cushing's *syndrome*** is caused by a functional tumor of the adrenal cortex, resulting in the overproduction of aldosterone, glucocorticoids, and androgens.

Waterhouse-Friderichsen syndrome, seen in infants, is the acute destruction of the adrenal gland by meningococcal septicemia.

Addison's disease is the chronic destruction of the adrenal cortex by an autoimmune process or tuberculosis.

• The adrenal medulla consists of two cell populations of chromaffin, catecholamine-producing cells or modified sympathetic postganglionic neurons: (1) Epinephrine-producing cells (80%), and (2) norepinephrine-producing cells (20%).

Epinephrine is stored in granules with a dense eccentric core; norepinephrine-containing granules are smaller and occupy a less dense central core than epinephrine-containing granules.

The synthesis of catecholamines includes the following steps: Tyrosine is converted to DOPA; DOPA is converted to dopamine, which changes into norepinephrine stored in a vesicle in the form of an eccentric granule. Norepinephrine leaves the granule, enters the cytosol, and becomes epinephrine under the influence of phenylethanolamine *N*-methyltransferase (PNMT). The synthesis of PNMT is stimulated by glucocorticoids arriving in the adrenal medulla from the zona fasciculata.

Epinephrine enters a vesicle and forms a complex with chromogranins, and is released into fenestrated capillaries following stimulation by a cholinergic axon from a preganglionic sympathetic neuron in the presence of calcium. In contrast to the adrenal medulla, cells of the adrenal cortex do not store steroid hormones in granules. Vanillylmandelic acid and metanephrine are metabolic products of catecholamines. They are used clinically to determine the production level of catecholamines.

• The adrenal medulla has a dual blood supply: (1) Blood vessels from the capsular plexus supply the three zones of the cortex. Fenestrated capillaries (called sinusoids) percolate between cells of the zona glomerulosa and zona fasciculata, and form a capillary network in the zona reticularis before entering the medulla. Medullary sinuses collect aldosterone, cortisol, and sexual steroids, which are drained by the central vein of the medulla. (2) The medullary artery (derived from the inferior adrenal artery) enters the cortex and supplies blood only to the medulla without branching in the adrenal cortex. There are no veins or lymphatics in the adrenal cortex.

• Endocrine pancreas. The pancreas has two portions: (1) The exocrine pancreas, consisting of acini involved in the production of enzymes transported to the duodenum; (2) the endocrine pancreas or islets of Langerhans.

The islets of Langerhans are formed by two components: (1) The endocrine cells A (α cells), B (β cells), D (δ cells), and F cells, each secreting a single hormone; and (2) a vascular component, the insuloacinar portal system, which enables a local action of insular hormone on the exocrine pancreas.

A cells secrete glucagon (which increases glucose blood levels), B cells secrete insulin (which increases the transport of glucose into cells; such as hepatocytes and skeletal and cardiac muscle cells), D cells secrete gastrin (which stimulates production of HCl by parietal cells in the stomach) and somatostatin (which inhibits the release of insulin and glucagon, and the secretion of HCl by parietal cells), and F cells produce pancreatic polypeptide (which inhibits the secretion of somatostatin and the secretion of pancreatic enzymes).

The secretion of insulin is stimulated by an influx of Ca^{2+} into B cells through voltage-gated Ca^{2+} channels. Ca^{2+} influx occurs when the adenosine triphosphate (ATP)-sensitive K^+ channel (K_{ATP}) closes and K^+ accumulates in the cytosol. Mutations in the *sulfonyurea receptor* (*Sur1*) gene and the *inward rectifying K+ channel* (*Kir6.2*) gene, components of the K_{ATP} channel are seen in patients with **neonatal diabetes mellitus**.

Diabetes is characterized by hyperglycemia, polyuria, and polydipsia.

Type 1 diabetes (also known as juvenile diabetes) is determined by autoimmunity, viral infection, and chemical toxins affecting insulin-producing B cells. There is a lack of insulin in type I diabetes.

Type 2 diabetes is caused by a genetic predisposition. The levels of insulin are insufficient relative to glucose levels. In addition, tissues decrease responsiveness to insulin (insulin resistance). Chronic diabetes affects the vascular system. Atherosclerosis of the aorta and large and medium-sized blood vessels leads to myocardial and brain infarctions and gangrene of the lower extremities. Capillaries are also affected. Retinopathy, cataract, and glaucoma can cause total blindness. Glomerulopathy (**Kimmelstiel-Wilson lesion**), consists in thickening of the glomerular basal lamina of glomerular capillaries, and proliferation of mesangial cells that affects glomerular filtration of the kidneys.

20. SPERMATOGENESIS

The male reproductive system is responsible for (1) the continuous production, nourishment, and temporary storage of the haploid male gamete (**spermatozoa** [sing. spermatozoon], or **sperm**); and (2) the synthesis and secretion of male sex hormones (**androgens**).

The male reproductive system consists of (1) the **testes**, which produce sperm and synthesize and secrete androgens; (2) the **epididymis, vas deferens, ejaculatory duct**, and a segment of the **male urethra**, which form the excurrent duct system responsible for the transport of spermatozoa to the exterior; (3) accessory glands, the **seminal vesicle**, the **prostate gland**, and the **bulbourethral glands** of Cowper, whose secretions form the bulk of the semen and provide nutrients to ejaculated spermatozoa; and (4) the **penis**, the copulatory organ, formed of erectile tissue.

The testis, epididymis, and the initial part of the vas deferens are located in the **scrotal sac**, a skin-covered pouch enclosing a mesothelium-lined cavity—the **tunica vaginalis**.

The testes

The testes are paired organs located in the scrotum, outside the abdominal cavity. This location enables maintenance of the testes at a temperature 2°C to 3°C below body temperature. A temperature of 34°C to 35°C is essential for normal **spermatogenesis**.

The posterior surface of the mature testis is associated with the epididymis. Both testis and epididymis are suspended in the scrotal sac by the **spermatic cord**, which contains the **vas deferens**, the **spermatic artery**, and the **venous** and **lymphatic plexuses**.

The testis is enclosed by the **tunica albuginea**, which is thickened to form the **mediastinum** where the **rete testis** is located (Figure 20-1). Fibrous septa from the mediastinum project into the testicular mass, dividing the tissue into 250 to 300 **lobules**. Each lobule contains one to four **seminiferous tubules**.

Each seminiferous tubule is about 150 µm in diameter and 80 cm long; it is

Figure 20-1. Testis, epididymis, and vas deferens

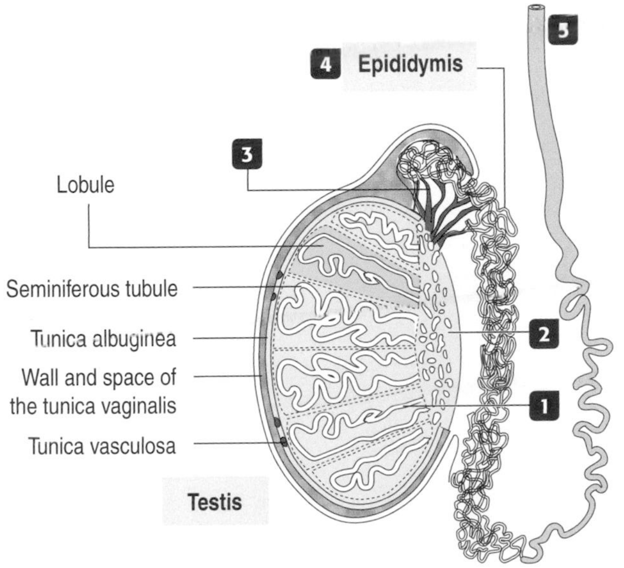
4 Epididymis
5
3
Lobule
Seminiferous tubule
Tunica albuginea
Wall and space of the tunica vaginalis
Tunica vasculosa
Testis
2
1

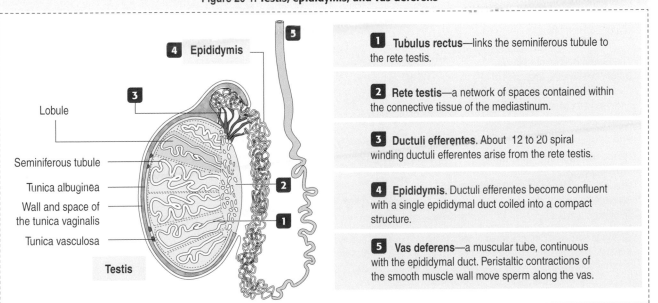

1 Tubulus rectus—links the seminiferous tubule to the rete testis.

2 Rete testis—a network of spaces contained within the connective tissue of the mediastinum.

3 Ductuli efferentes. About 12 to 20 spiral winding ductuli efferentes arise from the rete testis.

4 Epididymis. Ductuli efferentes become confluent with a single epididymal duct coiled into a compact structure.

5 Vas deferens—a muscular tube, continuous with the epididymal duct. Peristaltic contractions of the smooth muscle wall move sperm along the vas.

Figure 20-2. General organization of the seminiferous tubules

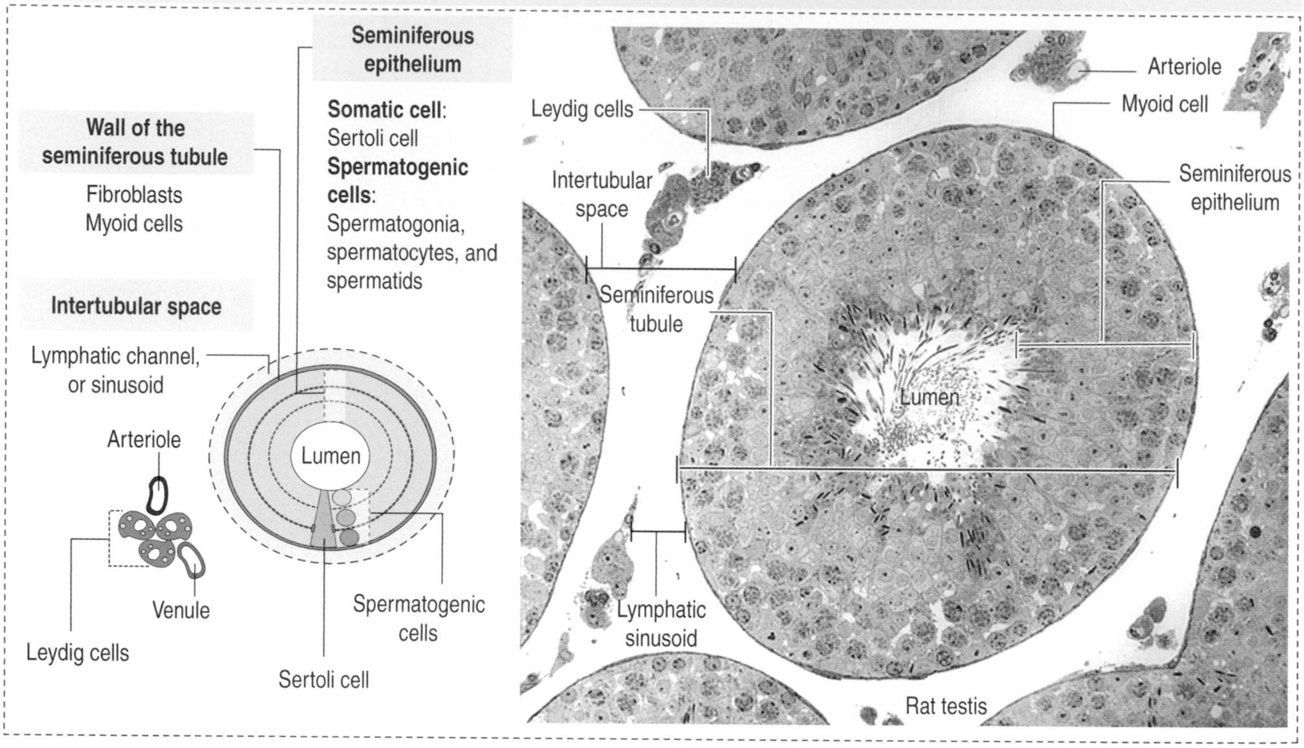

Figure 20-3. General histologic structure of the testis

Clusters of **Leydig cells** are present in the intertubular space. Leydig cells are in close contact with blood vessels and lymphatic channels. The major product of Leydig cells is testosterone.

The **wall of the seminiferous tubule** consists of peritubular myoid cells separated from the seminiferous epithelium by a basement membrane.

The **lumen of a seminiferous tubule** displays the free ends of the tails of developing spermatids. Fluid and secretory proteins from Sertoli cells are also found in the lumen.

Periodic acid–Schiff staining detects glycoproteins in the developing acrosome of spermatids adjacent to the lumen of the seminiferous tubule.

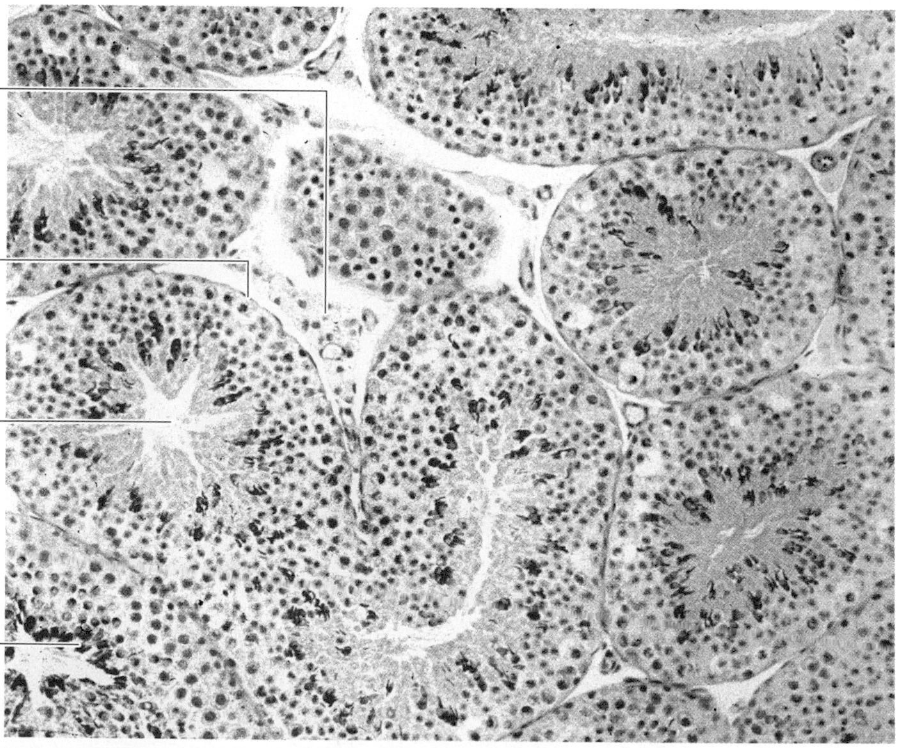

Although variations are observed in the cellular composition of the seminiferous epithelium—reflecting both synchrony and overlap of spermatogenic cell progenies during their development—Sertoli cells are the permanent somatic components of the epithelium.

Sertoli cells:
1. Maintain a close relationship with spermatogonia, primary and secondary spermatocytes, and spermatids.
2. Are postmitotic in the adult testis.

U-shaped with the two ends opening in the **rete testis.** The rete testis is a network of channels that collects the products of the **seminiferous epithelium** (testicular sperm, secretory proteins, and ions).

The seminiferous tubule (Figure 20-2) consists of a central lumen lined by a specialized seminiferous epithelium containing **two distinct cell populations:** (1) the **somatic Sertoli cells** and (2) the **spermatogenic cells** (spermatogonia, spermatocytes, and spermatids).

The seminiferous epithelium is encircled by a **basement membrane** and a wall formed by **collagenous fibers, fibroblasts,** and **contractile myoid cells.** Myoid cells are responsible for the **rhythmic contractile activity** that propels the **nonmotile sperm** to the rete testis. Sperm acquire forward motility after they have passed through the epididymal duct.

The space in between the seminiferous tubules is occupied by blood vessels and lymphatic channels or sinusoids, and aggregates of the androgen-producing **Leydig cells** (see Figure 20-2). The general histologic structure of the testis is shown in Figure 20-3.

Seminiferous epithelium

The seminiferous epithelium can be classified as a stratified epithelium with rather unusual characteristics not found in any stratified epithelium of the body. In this stratified epithelium, somatic columnar Sertoli cells interact with mitotically dividing spermatogonia, meiotically dividing spermatocytes, and a haploid population of spermatids undergoing a differentiation process called **spermiogenesis.**

Figure 20-4 illustrates relevant aspects of a mammalian spermatogenic cycle.

1. A **prespermatogonium** (also called **gonocyte**), derived from a primordial germinal cell in the fetal testis, divides by mitosis at puberty to generate two daughter cells. **One daughter cell initiates a spermatogenic cycle. The other cell becomes a stem cell with self-renewal capacity and able to initiate soon another spermatogenic cycle.** We have seen in Chapter 3, Cell Signaling, that stem cells can self-renew and give rise to either another stem cell or a cell entering a terminal differentiation pathway. The same rule applies to prespermatogonia.

2. After cell division, all **spermatogenic cells remain interconnected by intercellular bridges** because cytokinesis is incomplete.

3. Spermatogonia, spermatocytes, and spermatids complete their proliferation and differentiation sequence in a timely manner. **The spermatogenic cell cohorts proliferate and differentiate synchronously.**

4. Stem cells periodically initiate spermatogenic cell cycles to ensure the continuous production of sperm. We will study later how spermatogenic cell cycles overlap in a segment of a seminiferous tubule and generate constant combinations of spermatogenic cells called **cellular associations.**

5. Sertoli cells represent a stable somatic cell population. They facilitate the displacement of differentiating spermatogenic cells farther away from the periphery of the seminiferous tubule and closer to the lumen.

Sertoli cells

Sertoli cells are the predominant cell type of the seminiferous epithelium until **puberty.** After puberty, they represent about 10% of the cells lining the seminiferous tubules. In elderly men, when the population of spermatogenic cells decreases, Sertoli cells again become the major component of the epithelium.

Sertoli cells are columnar cells extending from the basal lamina to the lumen of the seminiferous tubule (Figure 20-5). They act as **bridge cells** between the intertubular space and the lumen of the seminiferous tubule.

The apical and lateral plasma membranes of Sertoli cells have an irregular outline because they provide **crypts** to house the developing spermatogenic cells.

The **nucleus** displays **indentations** and a **large nucleolus** with associated **heterochromatin masses.** The cytoplasm contains smooth and rough endoplasmic

Figure 20-4. Outline of the spermatogenic cycle

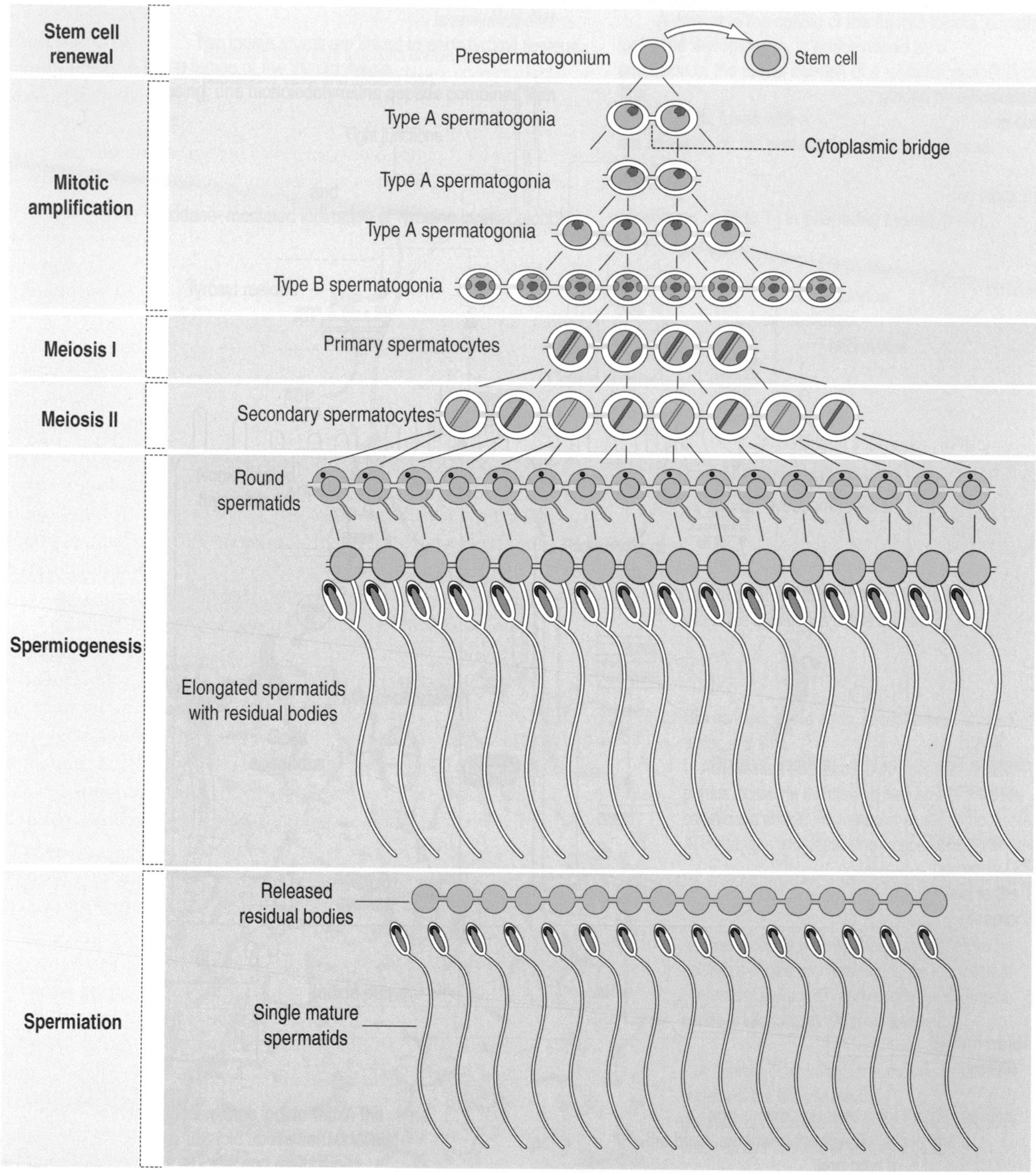
Stem cell renewal
Prespermatogonium
Stem cell
Mitotic amplification
Type A spermatogonia
Cytoplasmic bridge
Type A spermatogonia
Type A spermatogonia
Type B spermatogonia
Meiosis I
Primary spermatocytes
Meiosis II
Secondary spermatocytes
Round spermatids
Spermiogenesis
Elongated spermatids with residual bodies
Released residual bodies
Spermiation
Single mature spermatids

Spermatogenesis starts at puberty when a prespermatogonium undergoes mitotic cell division to produce two daughter cells. One daughter cell remains as a stem cell; the other initiates a mitotic amplification sequence giving rise to morphologically distinct spermatogonia type A and type B.

Type B spermatogonia complete the S phase (DNA synthesis) of their cell cycle and advance to G_2. Instead of undergoing mitotic cell division, they translocate to the adluminal compartment and initiate meiosis I.

A characteristic feature of spermatogenesis is incomplete cytokinesis. Cells are conjoined to each other by cytoplasmic bridges, a condition that persists until the completion of spermatogenesis.

Another typical aspect of spermatogenesis is cell cycle synchrony. All the cells initiate, progress, and complete a differentiation sequence in a coordinated manner.

The conjoined condition terminates when mature spermatids are released at the end of spermiogenesis by the process of spermiation. Residual bodies, linked by cytoplasmic bridges, separate from the spermatids and are phagocytosed by Sertoli cells. Mature spermatids become single cells transported to the rete testis.

reticulum, mitochondria, lysosomes, lipid droplets, an extensive Golgi apparatus, and a rich cytoskeleton (vimentin, actin, and microtubules).

At their **basolateral** domain, Sertoli cells form **tight junctions** with adjoining Sertoli cells.

Basolateral tight junctions (1) subdivide the seminiferous epithelium into a **basal compartment** and an **adluminal compartment** (see Figure 20-5) and (2) are the determining components of the so-called **blood-testis barrier**, which protects developing spermatocytes and spermatids from autoimmune reactions.

The **functions** of Sertoli cells are (1) to support, protect, and nourish developing spermatogenic cells; (2) to eliminate by **phagocytosis** excess cell portions, called **residual bodies**, discarded by spermatids at the end of **spermiogenesis**; (3) to facilitate the release of mature spermatids into the lumen of the seminiferous tubule by actin-mediated contraction, a process called **spermiation**; and (4) to secrete a fluid rich in proteins and ions into the seminiferous tubular lumen.

Sertoli cells respond to **follicle-stimulating hormone** (**FSH**) stimulation. FSH regulates the synthesis and secretion of **androgen-binding protein** (**ABP**).

ABP is a secretory protein with high binding affinity for the androgens **testosterone** and **dihydrotestosterone**. The androgen-ABP complex, whose function is unknown at present, is transported to the proximal segments of the epididymis (see Figure 20-16).

Note that although both ABP and the androgen receptor have binding affinity for androgens, they are distinct proteins. ABP is a secretory protein, whereas the androgen receptor is a cytoplasmic and nuclear protein.

Sertoli cells secrete **inhibin** and **activin** subunits (α and β subunits). Inhibin (an **$\alpha\beta$ heterodimer**) exerts a **negative feedback** on gonadotropin-releasing factor and FSH release by the hypothalamus and anterior hypophysis. **Activin** (an $\alpha\alpha$ or $\beta\beta$ **homodimer**) exerts a **positive feedback** on the release of FSH (see Chapter 18, Neuroendocrine System).

Sertoli cells are postmitotic **after puberty**. No mitotic cell division is observed in the adult testis.

Spermatogonia

Spermatogonia are diploid spermatogenic cells **directly in contact with the basal lamina** in the basal compartment (Figures 20-5 to 20-7). They are located below the inter–Sertoli cell occluding junctions and therefore **outside** the blood-testis barrier.

Spermatogonia derive from **spermatogonial stem cell**s and undergo successive rounds of mitotic cell divisions starting at **puberty**.

Two major morphologic spermatogonial cell types can be observed:

1. **Type A spermatogonia** display an oval euchromatic nucleus and a nucleolus attached to the nuclear envelope (see Figures 20-5 and 20-7). Subclasses of type A spermatogonia (with a dark nucleus, called **A dark spermatogonium,** and with a lighter nucleus, called **A pale spermatogonium**) are observed in human testes.
2. **Type B spermatogonia** have a round nucleus, masses of heterochromatin attached to the nuclear envelope, and a central nucleolus (see Figure 20-5).

Spermatogonial stem cells have important implications for male fertility. They are relatively quiescent and therefore resistant to radiation and cancer chemotherapy. Mitotically dividing spermatogonia, meiotically dividing spermatocytes, and differentiating spermatids are sensitive to radiation and cancer chemotherapy. After cessation of radiotherapy or anticancer chemotherapy, spermatogonial stem cells can reestablish the spermatogenic process. Postmitotic Sertoli cells are highly resistant to these therapies.

Spermatocytes

Type B spermatogonia enter meiotic prophase **immediately after completing the last S phase (DNA synthesis).** This last round of major DNA synthetic activity

Figure 20-5. Two compartments of the seminiferous epithelium

The **Sertoli cell** spans from the seminiferous tubular wall to the lumen and has cell-cell contacts with all proliferating and differentiating spermatogenic cells.

The cytoplasm of Sertoli cells encloses (1) spermatogonia in the basal compartment—between themselves and the basal lamina; (2) spermatocytes and early spermatids—in adluminal **niches** between adjacent Sertoli cells; and (3) late spermatids—in **crypts** at the luminal surfaces of Sertoli cells.

Basal tight junctions between adjacent Sertoli cells form the **blood-testis barrier**. The barrier prevents proteins, including antibodies, from reaching developing spermatogenic cells.

In an opposite direction, the barrier prevents proteins in developing spermatogenic cells from leaking and triggering an immune response.

Tight junctions divide the seminiferous epithelium into a **basal compartment**—below the junctions—and an **adluminal compartment**—above the junctions. Spermatogonia are located in the basal compartment and spermatocytes and spermatids occupy the adluminal compartment.

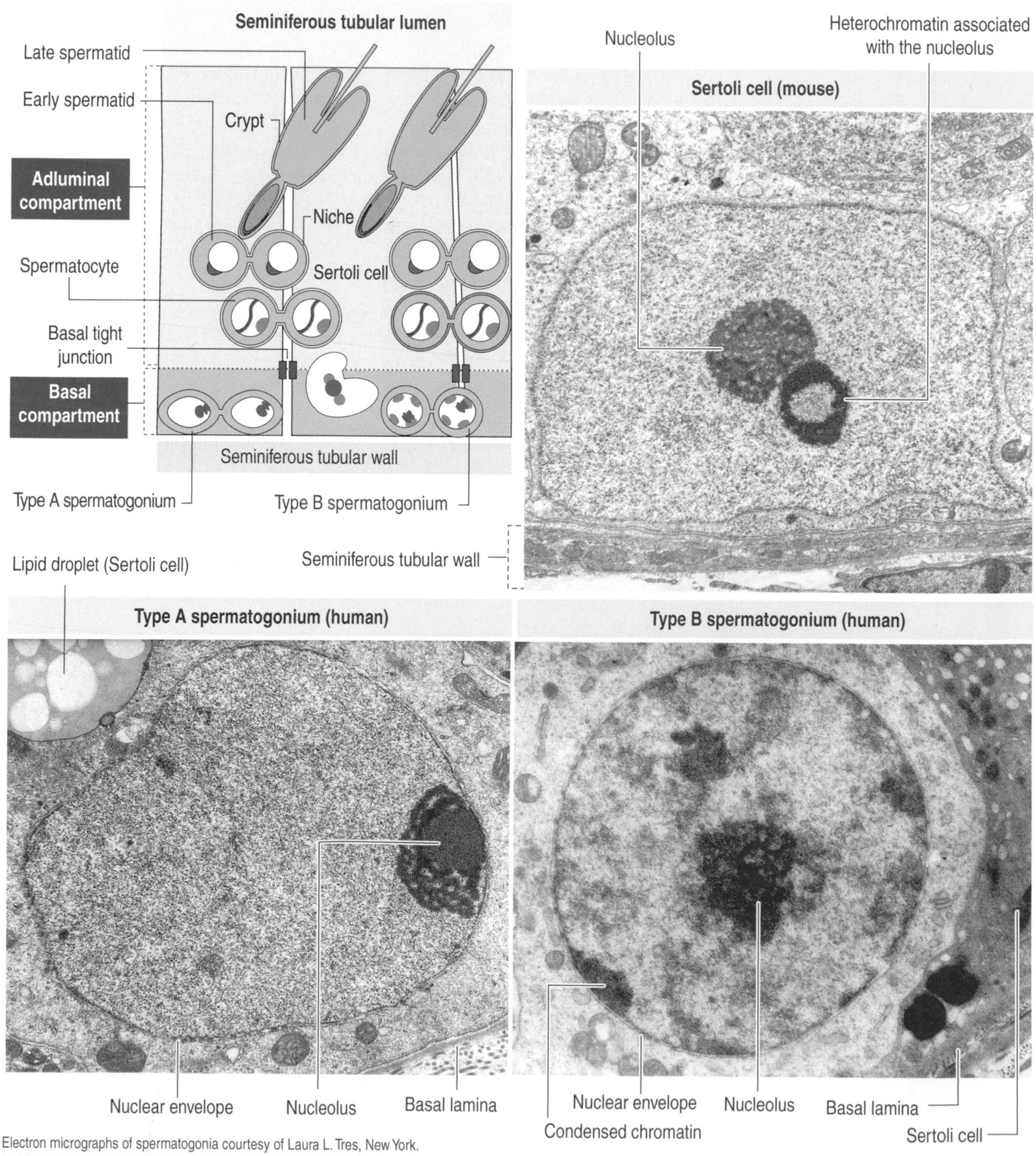

Seminiferous tubular lumen
Late spermatid
Early spermatid
Crypt
Adluminal compartment
Niche
Spermatocyte
Sertoli cell
Basal tight junction
Basal compartment
Seminiferous tubular wall
Type A spermatogonium
Type B spermatogonium
Nucleolus
Heterochromatin associated with the nucleolus
Sertoli cell (mouse)
Seminiferous tubular wall
Lipid droplet (Sertoli cell)
Type A spermatogonium (human)
Type B spermatogonium (human)
Nuclear envelope
Nucleolus
Basal lamina
Nuclear envelope
Nucleolus
Basal lamina
Condensed chromatin
Sertoli cell

Electron micrographs of spermatogonia courtesy of Laura L. Tres, New York.

Figure 20-6. Identification of seminiferous epithelial cells

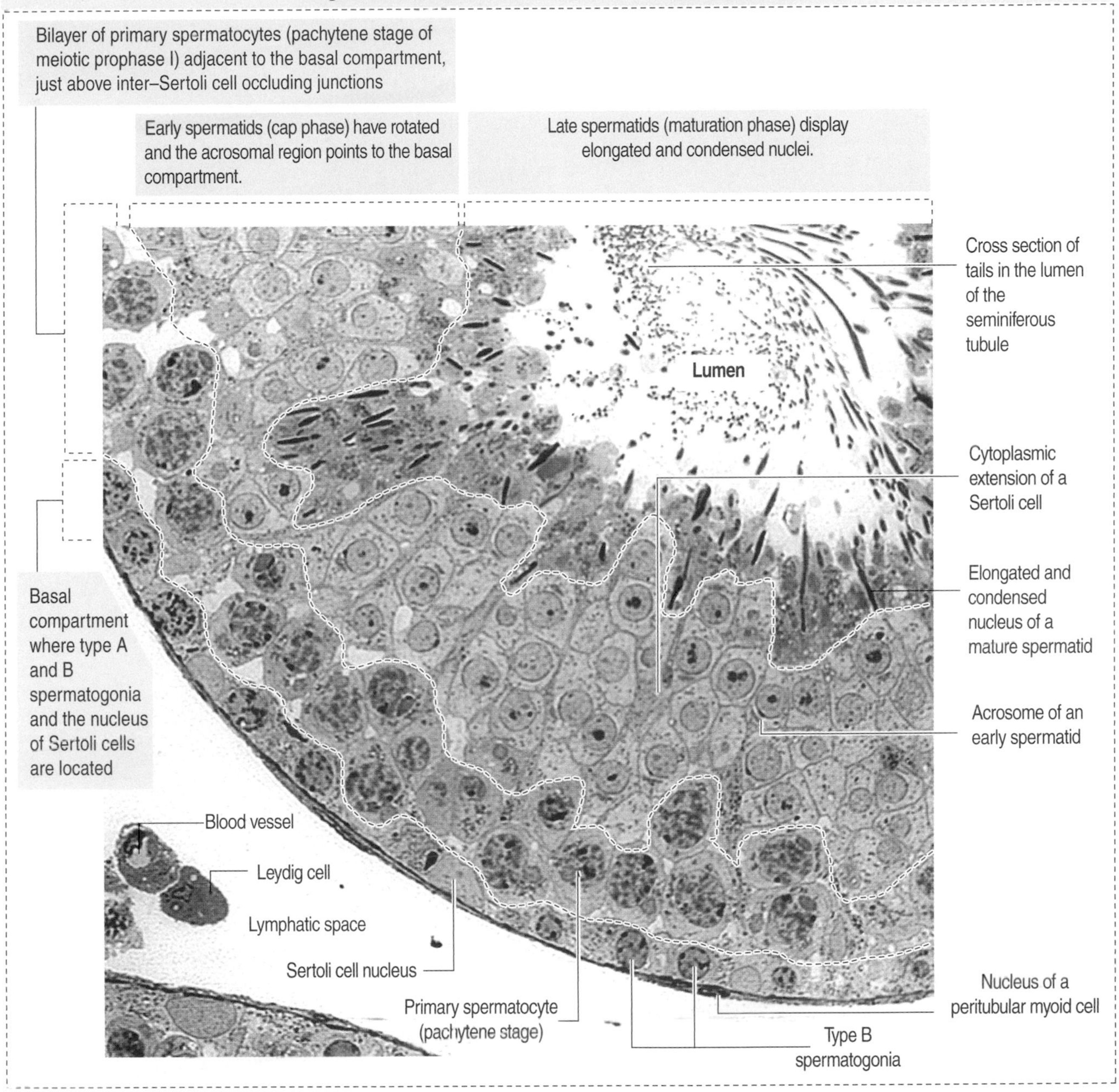

Bilayer of primary spermatocytes (pachytene stage of meiotic prophase I) adjacent to the basal compartment, just above inter–Sertoli cell occluding junctions
Early spermatids (cap phase) have rotated and the acrosomal region points to the basal compartment.
Late spermatids (maturation phase) display elongated and condensed nuclei.
Cross section of tails in the lumen of the seminiferous tubule
Lumen
Cytoplasmic extension of a Sertoli cell
Elongated and condensed nucleus of a mature spermatid
Acrosome of an early spermatid
Basal compartment where type A and B spermatogonia and the nucleus of Sertoli cells are located
Blood vessel
Leydig cell
Lymphatic space
Sertoli cell nucleus
Primary spermatocyte (pachytene stage)
Type B spermatogonia
Nucleus of a peritubular myoid cell

in the lifetime of spermatogenic cells determines that a primary spermatocyte starting meiotic prophase I will have **two times the amount of DNA of a spermatogonium.** The primary spermatocyte has a 4C DNA value, where 1C equals about 1.5 pg of DNA per cell.

Spermatocytes divide by **two successive meiotic cell divisions** (Figure 20-8) and are located in the **adluminal compartment** of the seminiferous epithelium, just above the inter–Sertoli cell occluding junctions. Therefore, meiosis occurs **inside** the blood-testis barrier.

A **primary spermatocyte** undergoes the first meiotic division (or **reductional division**) without significant DNA synthesis (only repair DNA synthesis occurs) to produce two **secondary spermatocytes.** The secondary spermatocytes rapidly undergo the second meiotic division (or **equational division**). Each secondary spermatocyte forms two spermatids that mature without further cell division into sperm.

Figure 20-7. Human seminiferous epithelium

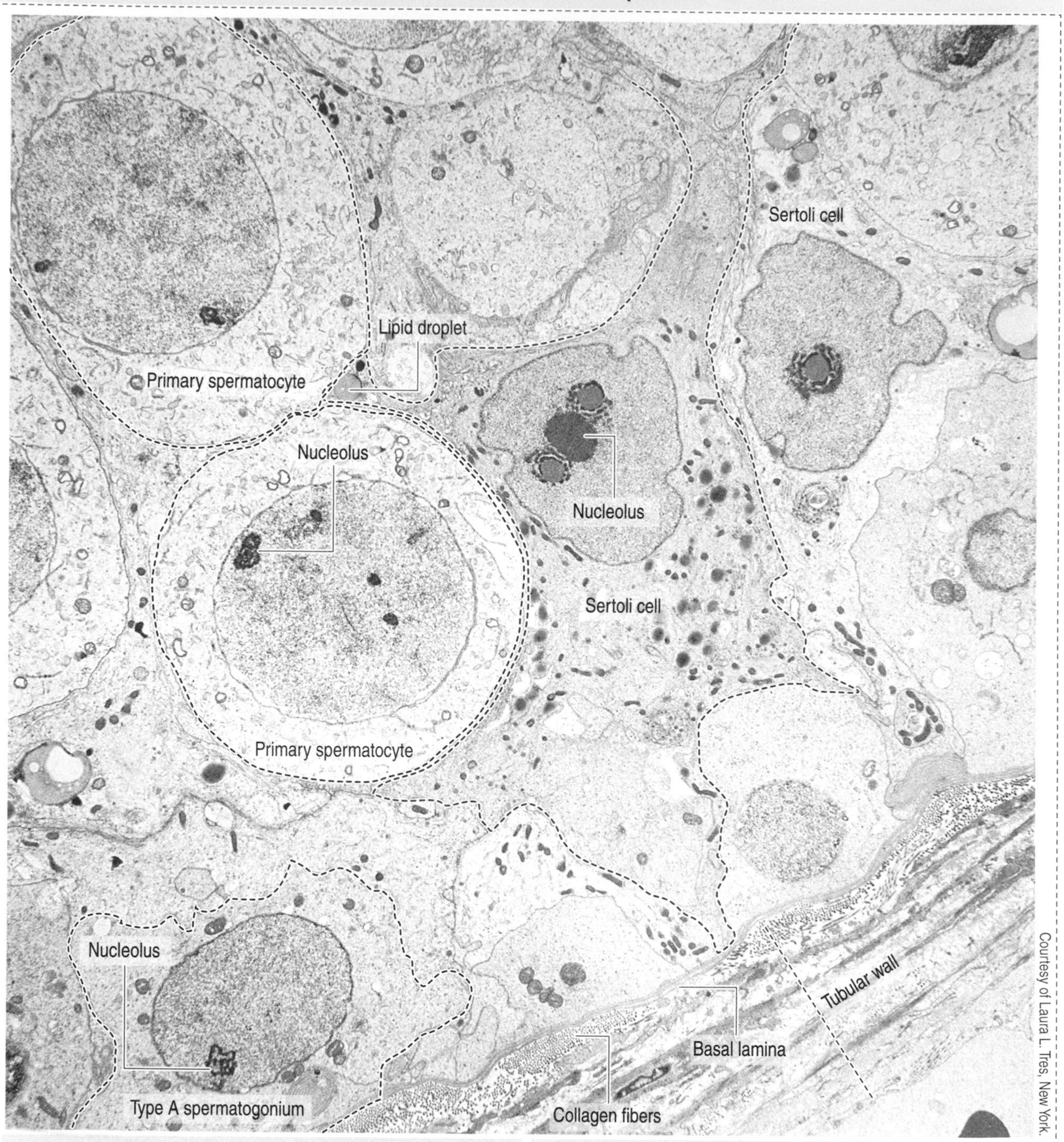

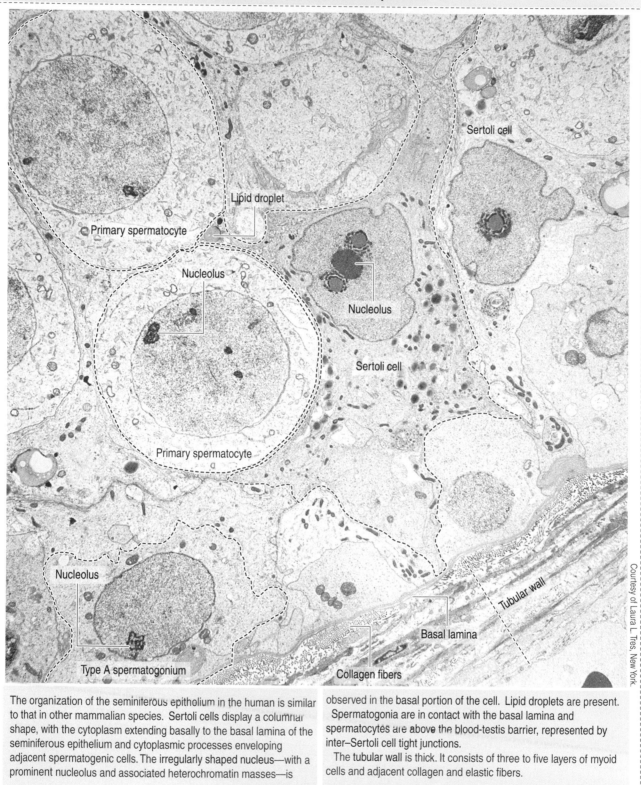

Sertoli cell
Lipid droplet
Primary spermatocyte
Nucleolus
Nucleolus
Sertoli cell
Primary spermatocyte
Nucleolus
Type A spermatogonium
Tubular wall
Basal lamina
Collagen fibers
Courtesy of Laura L. Tres, New York.

The organization of the seminiferous epithelium in the human is similar to that in other mammalian species. Sertoli cells display a columnar shape, with the cytoplasm extending basally to the basal lamina of the seminiferous epithelium and cytoplasmic processes enveloping adjacent spermatogenic cells. The irregularly shaped nucleus—with a prominent nucleolus and associated heterochromatin masses—is observed in the basal portion of the cell. Lipid droplets are present.

Spermatogonia are in contact with the basal lamina and spermatocytes are above the blood-testis barrier, represented by inter–Sertoli cell tight junctions.

The tubular wall is thick. It consists of three to five layers of myoid cells and adjacent collagen and elastic fibers.

By the end of the first meiotic division, the original 4C DNA content of a primary spermatocyte is reduced to 2C in a secondary spermatocyte. By the end of the second meiotic division, the 2C DNA content is reduced to 1C. The resulting spermatids are the haploid spermatids and initiate a complex differentiation

Figure 20-8. Meiosis in the male

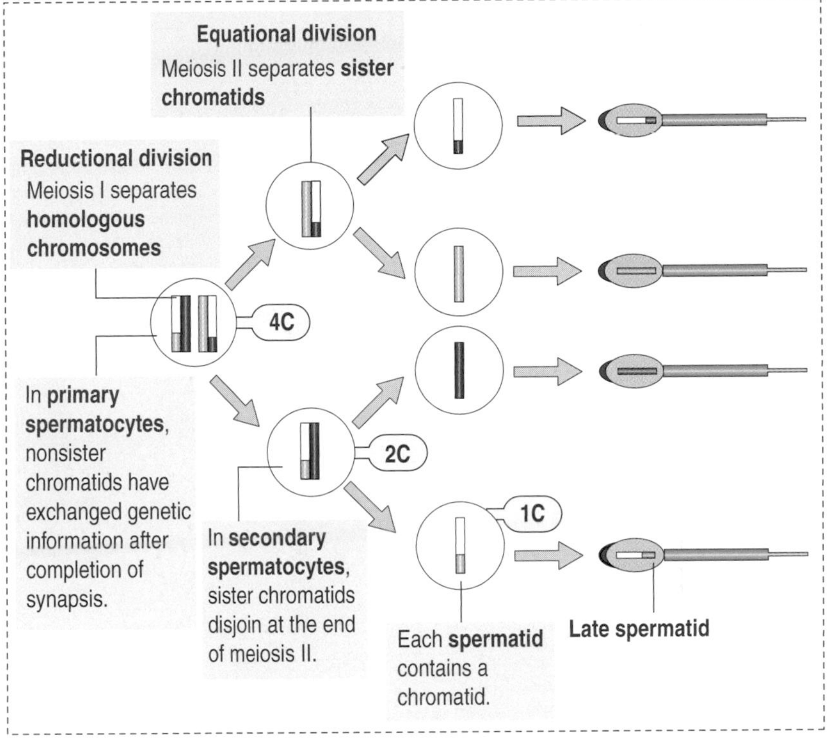

Equational division
Meiosis II separates sister chromatids
Reductional division
Meiosis I separates homologous chromosomes
4C
In primary spermatocytes, nonsister chromatids have exchanged genetic information after completion of synapsis.
2C
In secondary spermatocytes, sister chromatids disjoin at the end of meiosis II.
1C
Each spermatid contains a chromatid.
Late spermatid

process called **spermiogenesis**.

Because the first meiotic division is a long process (days) and the second meiotic division is very short (minutes), primary spermatocytes are the most abundant cells observed in the seminiferous epithelium. For comparison, Figure 20-9 illustrates

Figure 20-9. Meiosis in the female

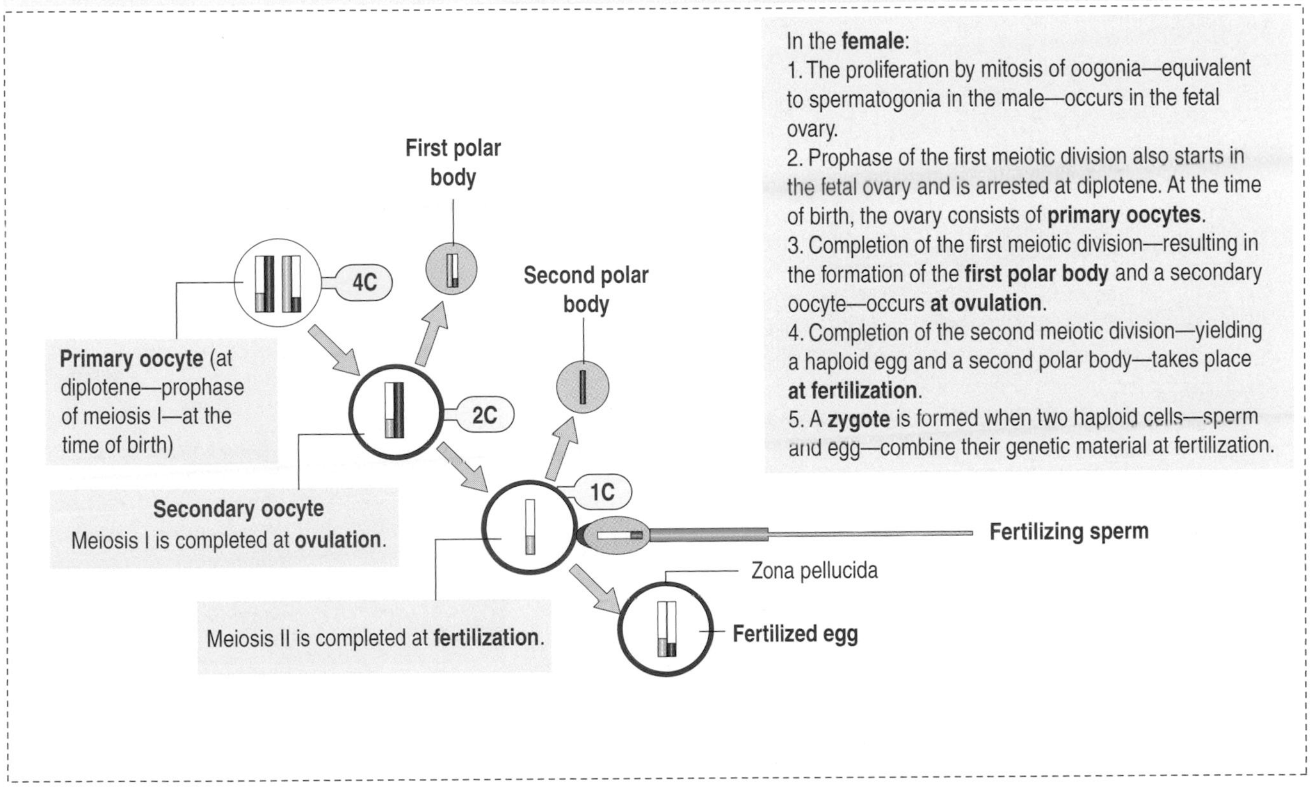

In the female:
1. The proliferation by mitosis of oogonia—equivalent to spermatogonia in the male—occurs in the fetal ovary.
2. Prophase of the first meiotic division also starts in the fetal ovary and is arrested at diplotene. At the time of birth, the ovary consists of primary oocytes.
3. Completion of the first meiotic division—resulting in the formation of the first polar body and a secondary oocyte—occurs at ovulation.
4. Completion of the second meiotic division—yielding a haploid egg and a second polar body—takes place at fertilization.
5. A zygote is formed when two haploid cells—sperm and egg—combine their genetic material at fertilization.
First polar body
4C
Second polar body
Primary oocyte (at diplotene—prophase of meiosis I—at the time of birth)
2C
Secondary oocyte
Meiosis I is completed at ovulation.
1C
Fertilizing sperm
Zona pellucida
Meiosis II is completed at fertilization.
Fertilized egg

Figure 20-10. First meiotic division (prophase stage): From leptotene to pachytene

A Leptotene

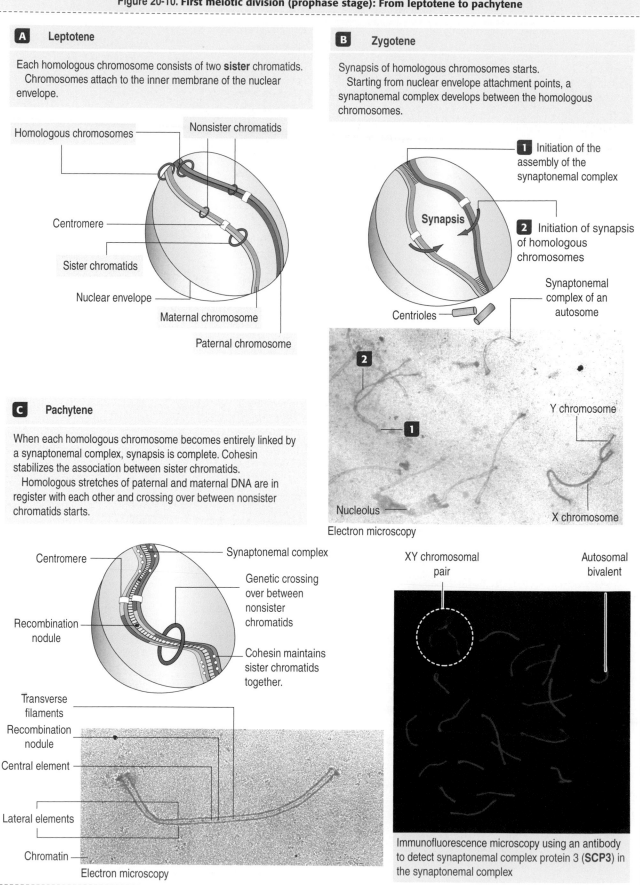

Each homologous chromosome consists of two **sister** chromatids.
Chromosomes attach to the inner membrane of the nuclear envelope.

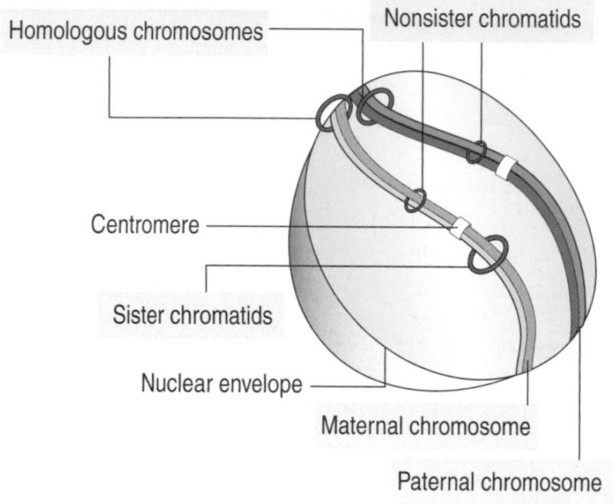
Homologous chromosomes
Nonsister chromatids
Centromere
Sister chromatids
Nuclear envelope
Maternal chromosome
Paternal chromosome

B Zygotene

Synapsis of homologous chromosomes starts.
Starting from nuclear envelope attachment points, a synaptonemal complex develops between the homologous chromosomes.

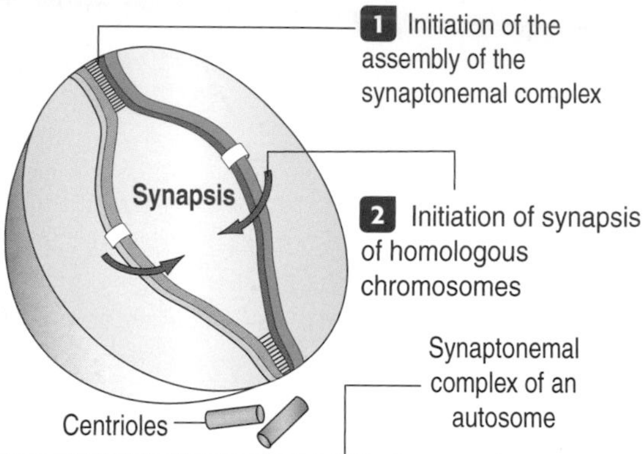
1 Initiation of the assembly of the synaptonemal complex
Synapsis
2 Initiation of synapsis of homologous chromosomes
Centrioles

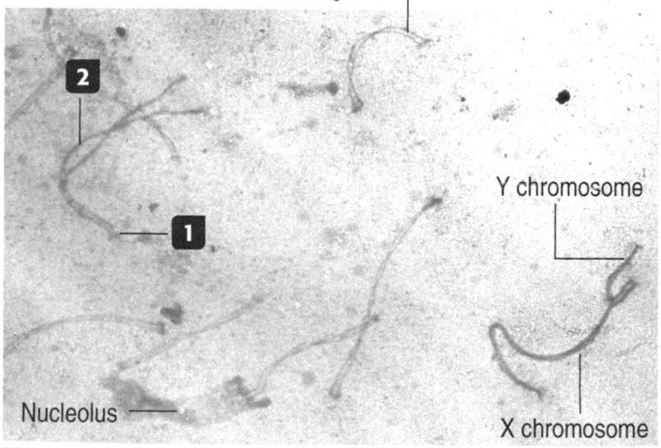
Synaptonemal complex of an autosome
2
1
Y chromosome
Nucleolus
X chromosome

Electron microscopy

C Pachytene

When each homologous chromosome becomes entirely linked by a synaptonemal complex, synapsis is complete. Cohesin stabilizes the association between sister chromatids.
Homologous stretches of paternal and maternal DNA are in register with each other and crossing over between nonsister chromatids starts.

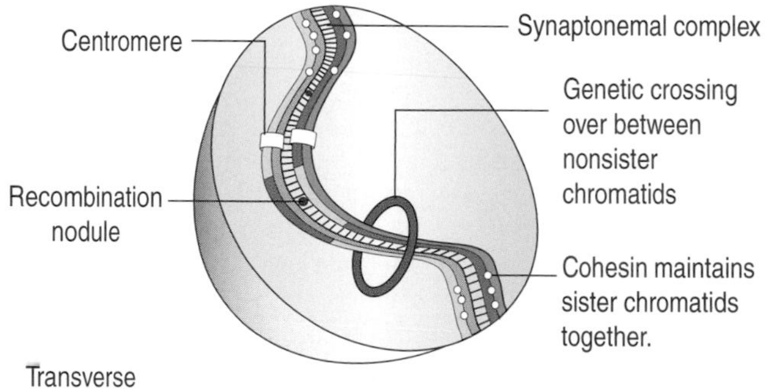
Centromere
Synaptonemal complex
Genetic crossing over between nonsister chromatids
Recombination nodule
Cohesin maintains sister chromatids together.

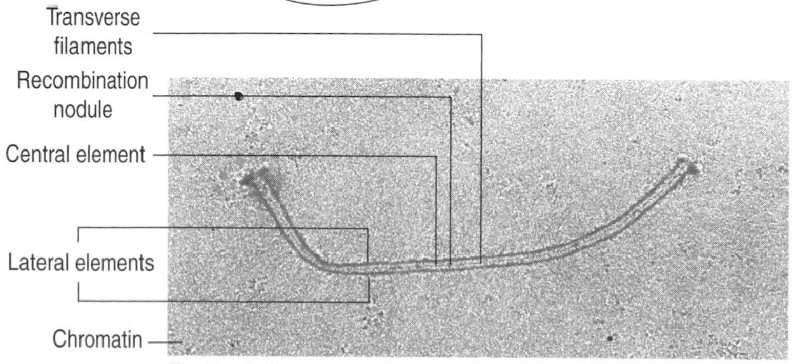
Transverse filaments
Recombination nodule
Central element
Lateral elements
Chromatin

Electron microscopy

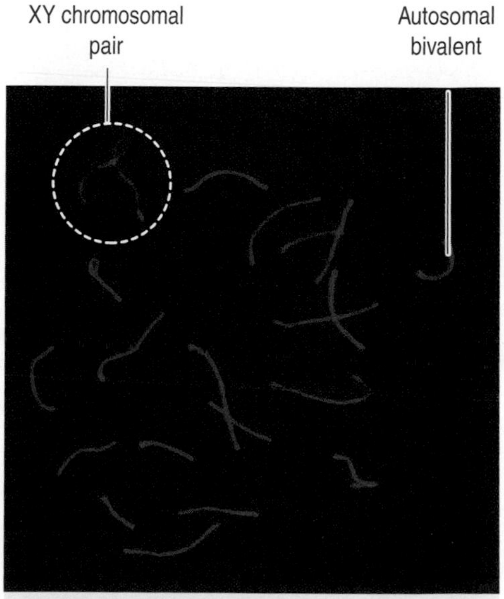
XY chromosomal pair
Autosomal bivalent

Immunofluorescence microscopy using an antibody to detect synaptonemal complex protein 3 (**SCP3**) in the synaptonemal complex

Figure 20-11. First meiotic division (prophase stage): From diplotene to diakinesis

D Diplotene

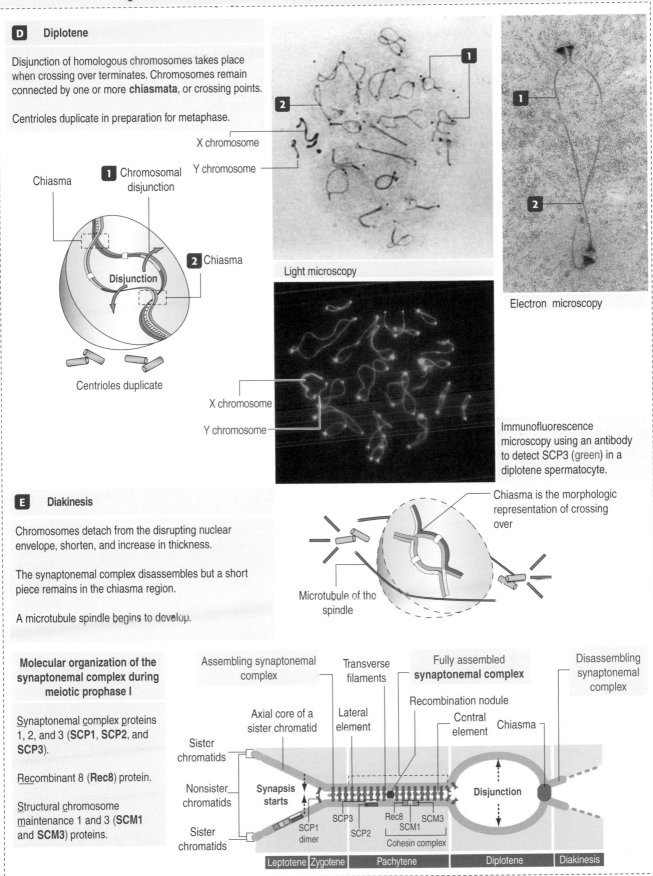

Disjunction of homologous chromosomes takes place when crossing over terminates. Chromosomes remain connected by one or more **chiasmata**, or crossing points.

Centrioles duplicate in preparation for metaphase.

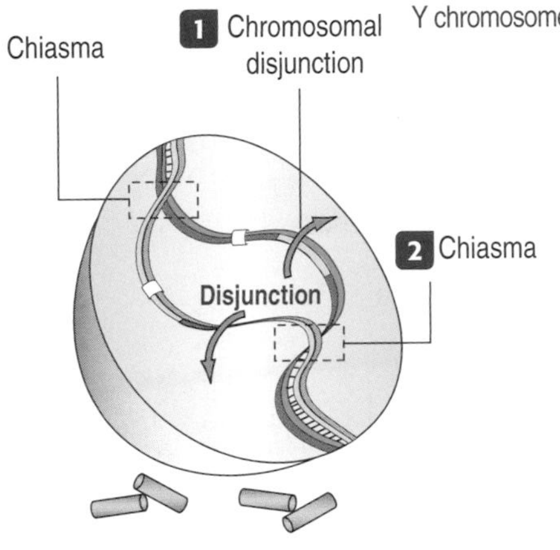

Chiasma
1 Chromosomal disjunction
2 Chiasma
Disjunction
Centrioles duplicate

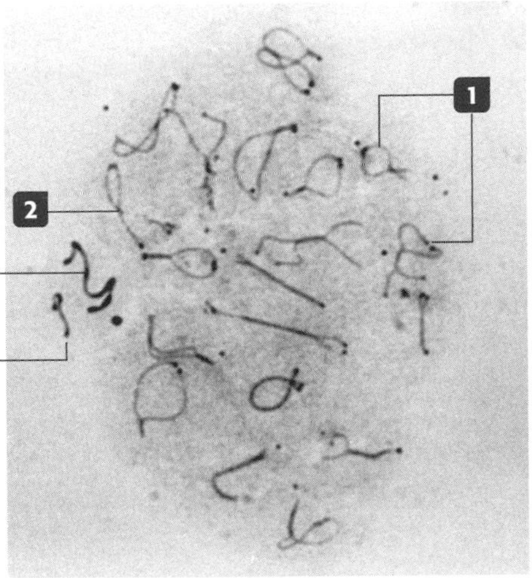

1
2
X chromosome
Y chromosome

Light microscopy

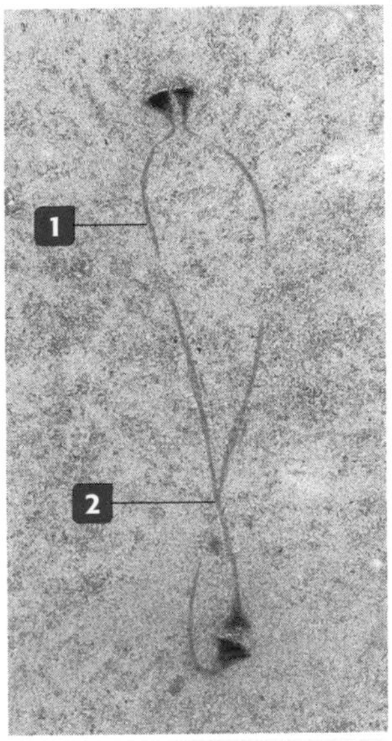

1
2

Electron microscopy

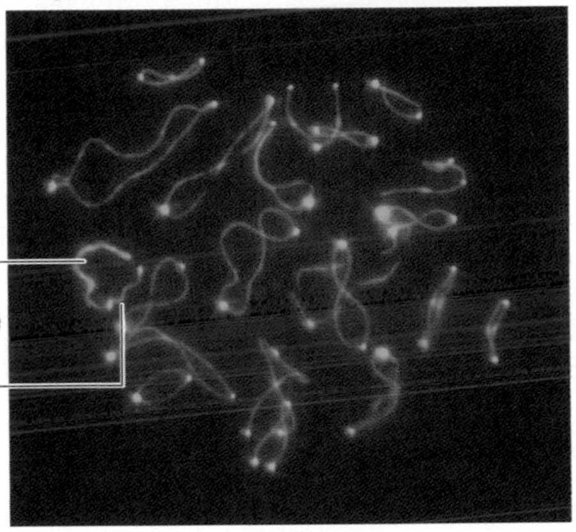

X chromosome
Y chromosome

Immunofluorescence microscopy using an antibody to detect SCP3 (green) in a diplotene spermatocyte.

E Diakinesis

Chromosomes detach from the disrupting nuclear envelope, shorten, and increase in thickness.

The synaptonemal complex disassembles but a short piece remains in the chiasma region.

A microtubule spindle begins to develop.

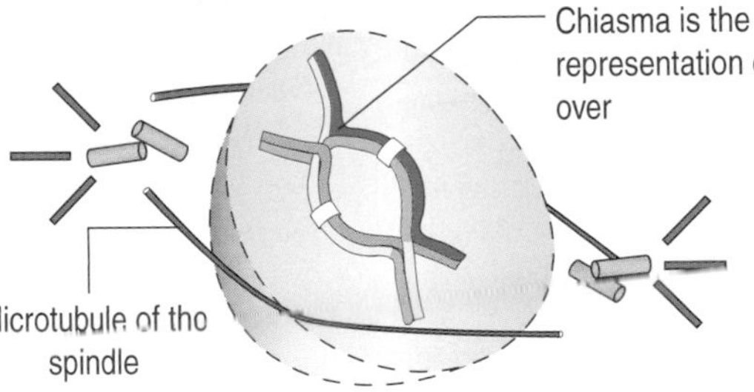

Chiasma is the morphologic representation of crossing over
Microtubule of the spindle

Molecular organization of the synaptonemal complex during meiotic prophase I

Synaptonemal complex proteins 1, 2, and 3 (**SCP1**, **SCP2**, and **SCP3**).

Recombinant 8 (**Rec8**) protein.

Structural chromosome maintenance 1 and 3 (**SCM1** and **SCM3**) proteins.

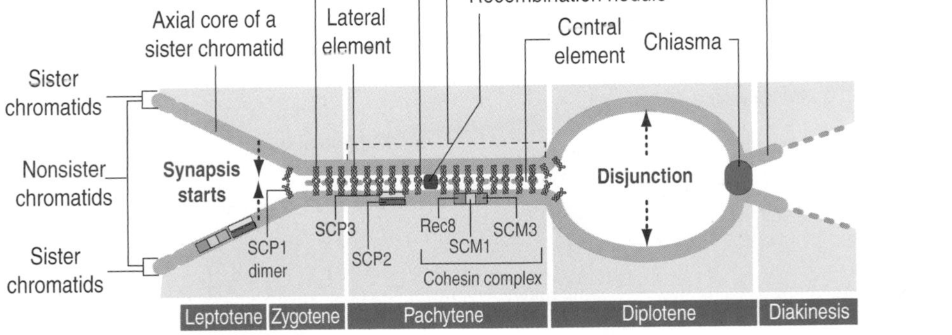

Assembling synaptonemal complex
Transverse filaments
Fully assembled synaptonemal complex
Disassembling synaptonemal complex
Recombination nodule
Axial core of a sister chromatid
Lateral element
Central element
Chiasma
Sister chromatids
Nonsister chromatids
Sister chromatids
Synapsis starts
Disjunction
SCP1 dimer
SCP3
SCP2
Rec8
SCM1
SCM3
Cohesin complex
Leptotene
Zygotene
Pachytene
Diplotene
Diakinesis

Box 20-A | **Synaptonemal complex**

- The function of the synaptonemal complex is to facilitate the **synapsis** of homologous chromosomes by stabilizing their axial alignment and association.
- Sister chromatids are maintained in close contact by the **cohesin protein complex**.
- The separation between synapsed homologous chromosomes is 100 nm.
- A synaptonemal complex consists of **two lateral elements** (closely associated to chromosomal chromatin loops) and a **central element**.
- The **lateral elements** are formed by the **cohesin protein complex** (Rec8, SCM1, and SCM3 proteins), SCP2, and SCP3 (**SCP** stands for synaptonemal complex protein).
- The lateral elements are bridged by transverse fibrous **SCP1 dimers**, whose terminal globular regions overlap in the center of the synaptonemal complex to form the **central element**.
- **Recombination nodules** are present along the synaptonemal complex during pachytene. They represent sites where genetic recombination between nonsister chromatids (called **reciprocal exchange**) will occur.

Box 20-B | **Intramanchette transport**

- The manchette is a **transient microtubular structure** that occupies a perinuclear position during the elongation and condensation of the spermatid nucleus.
- Microtubules are the major component of the manchette. They are formed by the polymerization of tubulin dimers with post-translational modifications (such as acetylation). F-actin microfilaments, aligned along microtubules, are present to a lesser extent.
- Molecules involved in **nucleocytoplasmatic transport** (such as Ran GTPase; see Chapter 1, Epithelium, Figure 1-39), 26S proteasome, and **microtubule- and F-actin–based molecular motors** are present in the manchette.
- Molecules targeted to the spermatid centriolar region and the developing tail are associated with microtubules of the manchette. Intramanchette transport appears essential for molecular delivery during spermiogenesis.
- **Tg737 mutant mice** have a defect in the gene expressing **Polaris/IFT88**, a component of the protein raft mobilized by a molecular motor along microtubules. This protein is present in the manchette of normal mice but absent in **Tg737 mutants, which have defective bronchial cilia and abortive sperm tail development**.

the meiotic process of the female gamete that is initiated in the ovary during fetal development (see Chapter 23, Fertilization, Placentation, and Lactation).

Meiosis

After the last mitotic division of type B spermatogonia, the resulting daughter cells synthesize DNA (S phase), advance into the G_2 phase, and start the first meiotic division with a 4C DNA content. The first meiotic division is characterized by a **long prophase**, lasting about 10 days.

The **prophase substages** of the **first meiotic division** are the **leptotene** (threadlike), **zygotene** (pairing), **pachytene** (thickening), **diplotene** (appearing double), and **diakinesis** (moving apart) stages (Figures 20-10 and 20-11).

These substages are characterized by four major events: (1) the formation of a **synaptonemal complex** (see Box 20-A) during zygotene-pachytene to facilitate the pairing or **synapsis** of homologous chromosomes (autosomes and sex chromosomes X and Y); (2) the pairing of homologous chromosomes (**synapsis**); (3) **crossing over** (the exchange of genetic information between **non-sister chromatids** of homologous chromosomes); and (4) **disjunction** (the separation of paired homologous chromosomes).

After this prolonged prophase, **pairs of sister chromatids** pass through metaphase, anaphase, and telophase and are separated into daughter cells—the **secondary spermatocytes.**

During the second meiotic division, prophase, metaphase, anaphase, and telophase separate **sister chromatids** into daughter cells—the **spermatids.**

In the female (see Figure 20-9), a **primary oocyte** (with a 4C DNA content) completes the first meiotic division **at ovulation** to produce a **secondary oocyte** (2C DNA content) and the **first polar body. When fertilization occurs**, the secondary oocyte completes the second meiotic division to reach the haploid state (1C DNA content), and a **second polar body** is generated.

The three most important **consequences of meiosis** are (1) Sperm and oocytes contain only one representative of each homologous pair of chromosomes. (2) Maternal and paternal chromosomes are randomly assorted. (3) Crossing over increases genetic variation.

Spermatids

Haploid spermatids are located in the **adluminal compartment**, in proximity to the seminiferous tubular lumen. There are two major types of spermatids: (1) **round** or **early spermatids,** housed in **niches** in the cytoplasm of Sertoli cells, and (2) **elongated** or **late spermatids,** housed in **crypts,** deep invaginations in Sertoli cell apical cytoplasm.

Spermatids are engaged in a highly differentiated cell process designated **spermiogenesis. Spermiogenesis is the last phase of spermatogenesis.** Mature spermatids are released into the seminiferous tubular lumen by a process called **spermiation.** Spermiation involves cytoskeletal contractile forces generated at the apical cytoplasmic region of Sertoli cells.

Four major events characterize spermiogenesis (Figures 20-12 and 20-13):

1. The **development of the flagellum.** The flagellum develops from the **distal centriole.** The **proximal centriole and pericentriolar matrix** give rise to a structure, called the **connecting piece**, linking the sperm head to the tail.

The sperm flagellum is a complex structure. It is formed by the **axoneme** (9 + 2 microtubule doublets in a concentric arrangement) surrounded by **mitochondria** forming a helicoidal sheath around the **proximal segment of the tail** (called the **middle piece**), and **outer dense fibers.** The **distal segment of the tail,** called the **principal piece,** consists of the axoneme surrounded by **outer dense fibers**, a pair of **ribs,** and a **fibrous sheath.** An **annulus,** which contains the protein **septin** 4, demarcates the middle-to-principal segment transition of the sperm tail (Figure 20-14). A lack of septin 4 causes male sterility.

Figure 20-12. Spermiogenesis

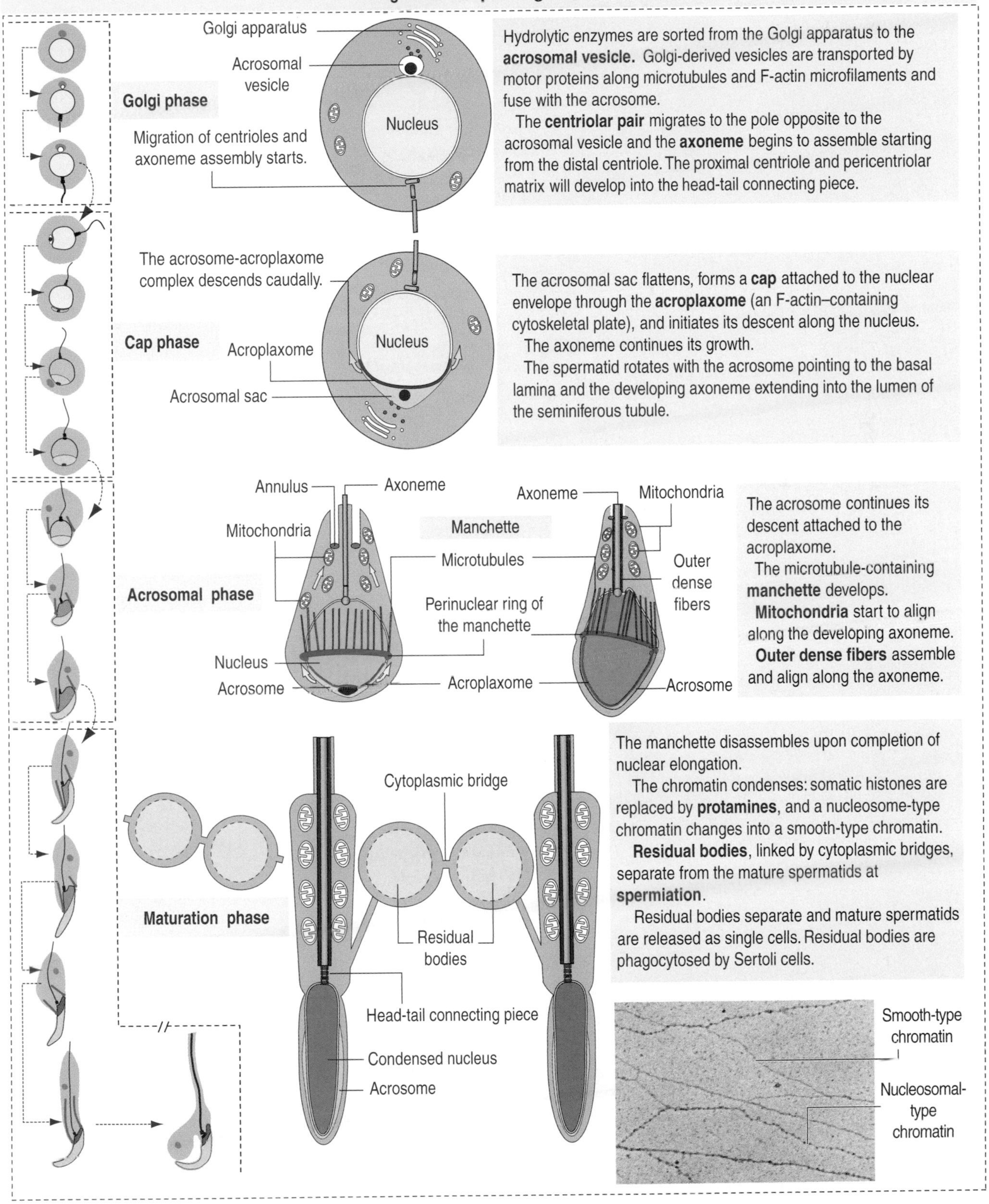

Golgi phase
Golgi apparatus
Acrosomal vesicle
Nucleus
Migration of centrioles and axoneme assembly starts.
Hydrolytic enzymes are sorted from the Golgi apparatus to the **acrosomal vesicle.** Golgi-derived vesicles are transported by motor proteins along microtubules and F-actin microfilaments and fuse with the acrosome.
The **centriolar pair** migrates to the pole opposite to the acrosomal vesicle and the **axoneme** begins to assemble starting from the distal centriole. The proximal centriole and pericentriolar matrix will develop into the head-tail connecting piece.
Cap phase
The acrosome-acroplaxome complex descends caudally.
Acroplaxome
Acrosomal sac
Nucleus
The acrosomal sac flattens, forms a **cap** attached to the nuclear envelope through the **acroplaxome** (an F-actin–containing cytoskeletal plate), and initiates its descent along the nucleus.
The axoneme continues its growth.
The spermatid rotates with the acrosome pointing to the basal lamina and the developing axoneme extending into the lumen of the seminiferous tubule.
Acrosomal phase
Annulus
Axoneme
Mitochondria
Manchette
Microtubules
Perinuclear ring of the manchette
Nucleus
Acrosome
Acroplaxome
Axoneme
Mitochondria
Outer dense fibers
Acrosome
The acrosome continues its descent attached to the acroplaxome.
The microtubule-containing **manchette** develops.
Mitochondria start to align along the developing axoneme.
Outer dense fibers assemble and align along the axoneme.
Maturation phase
Cytoplasmic bridge
Residual bodies
Head-tail connecting piece
Condensed nucleus
Acrosome
The manchette disassembles upon completion of nuclear elongation.
The chromatin condenses: somatic histones are replaced by **protamines**, and a nucleosome-type chromatin changes into a smooth-type chromatin.
Residual bodies, linked by cytoplasmic bridges, separate from the mature spermatids at **spermiation**.
Residual bodies separate and mature spermatids are released as single cells. Residual bodies are phagocytosed by Sertoli cells.
Smooth-type chromatin
Nucleosomal-type chromatin

2. **Development of the acrosome.** It consists in the progressive synthesis and storage of hydrolytic enzymes in the **acrosomal sac.** The acrosomal sac is attached to the nuclear envelope by the **acroplaxome,** a cytoskeletal plate that contains F-actin and the intermediate filament keratin 5.

The development of the acrosome consists of four sequential phases: the **Golgi**

Figure 20-13. **Spermiogenesis**

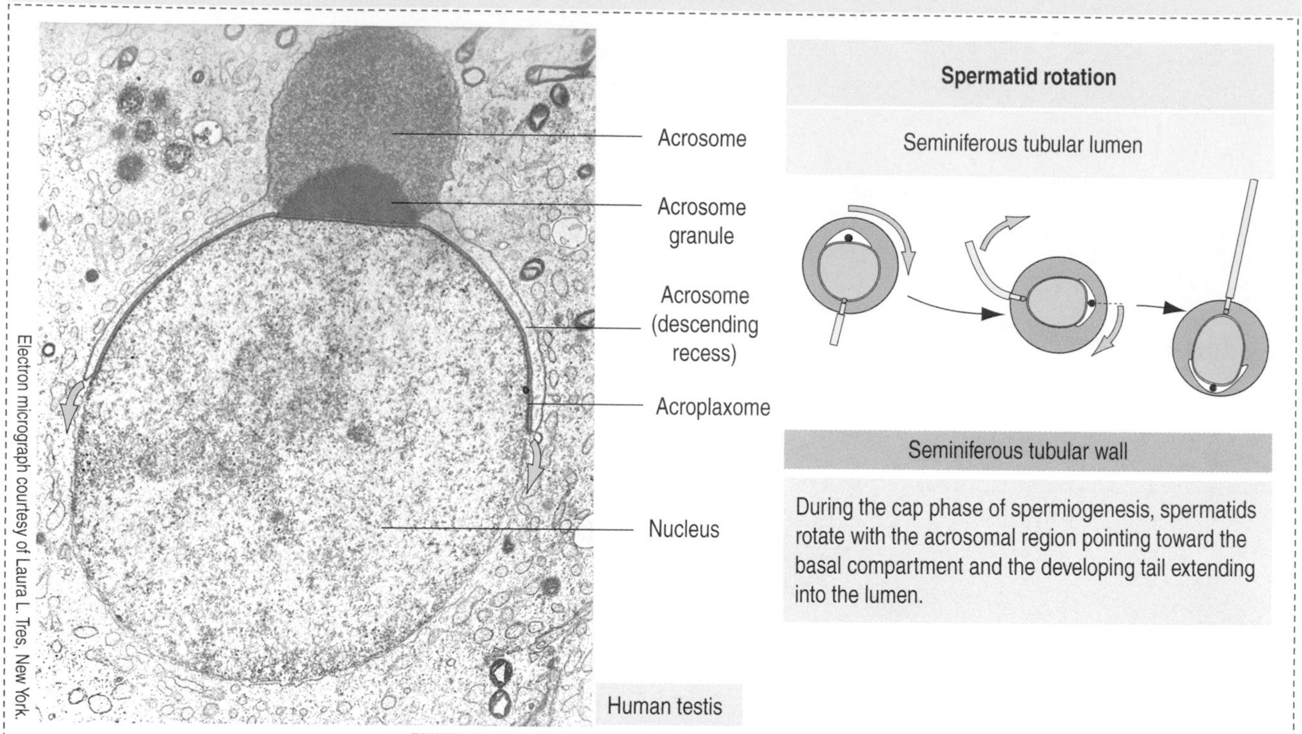
Acrosome
Acrosome granule
Acrosome (descending recess)
Acroplaxome
Nucleus
Electron micrograph courtesy of Laura L. Tres, New York.
Human testis
Spermatid rotation
Seminiferous tubular lumen
Seminiferous tubular wall
During the cap phase of spermiogenesis, spermatids rotate with the acrosomal region pointing toward the basal compartment and the developing tail extending into the lumen.

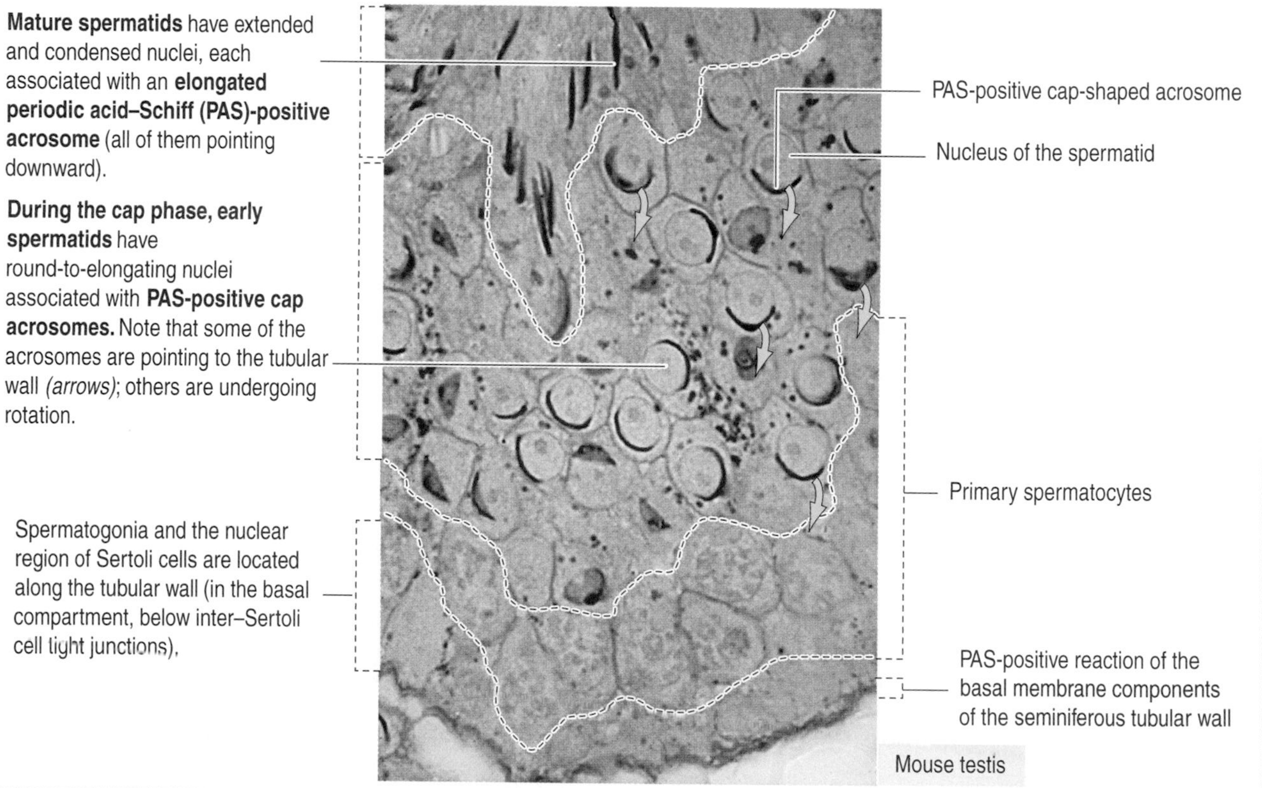
Mature spermatids have extended and condensed nuclei, each associated with an **elongated periodic acid–Schiff (PAS)-positive acrosome** (all of them pointing downward).
During the cap phase, early spermatids have round-to-elongating nuclei associated with **PAS-positive cap acrosomes.** Note that some of the acrosomes are pointing to the tubular wall *(arrows)*; others are undergoing rotation.
Spermatogonia and the nuclear region of Sertoli cells are located along the tubular wall (in the basal compartment, below inter–Sertoli cell tight junctions).
PAS-positive cap-shaped acrosome
Nucleus of the spermatid
Primary spermatocytes
PAS-positive reaction of the basal membrane components of the seminiferous tubular wall
Mouse testis

phase, **cap phase**, **acrosomal phase**, and **maturation phase** (see Figures 20-12 and 20-13). The acrosome is required for fertilization.

3. Development of the manchette. The manchette consists of a perinuclear ring and microtubules (see Figures 20-12 and 20-14 and Box 20-B). The perinuclear ring is adjacent to the acroplaxome. The manchette assembles soon after the initiation of axonemal development and disassembles when the elongation and condensation of the spermatid nucleus is near completion.

Figure 20-14. Manchette and intramanchette transport

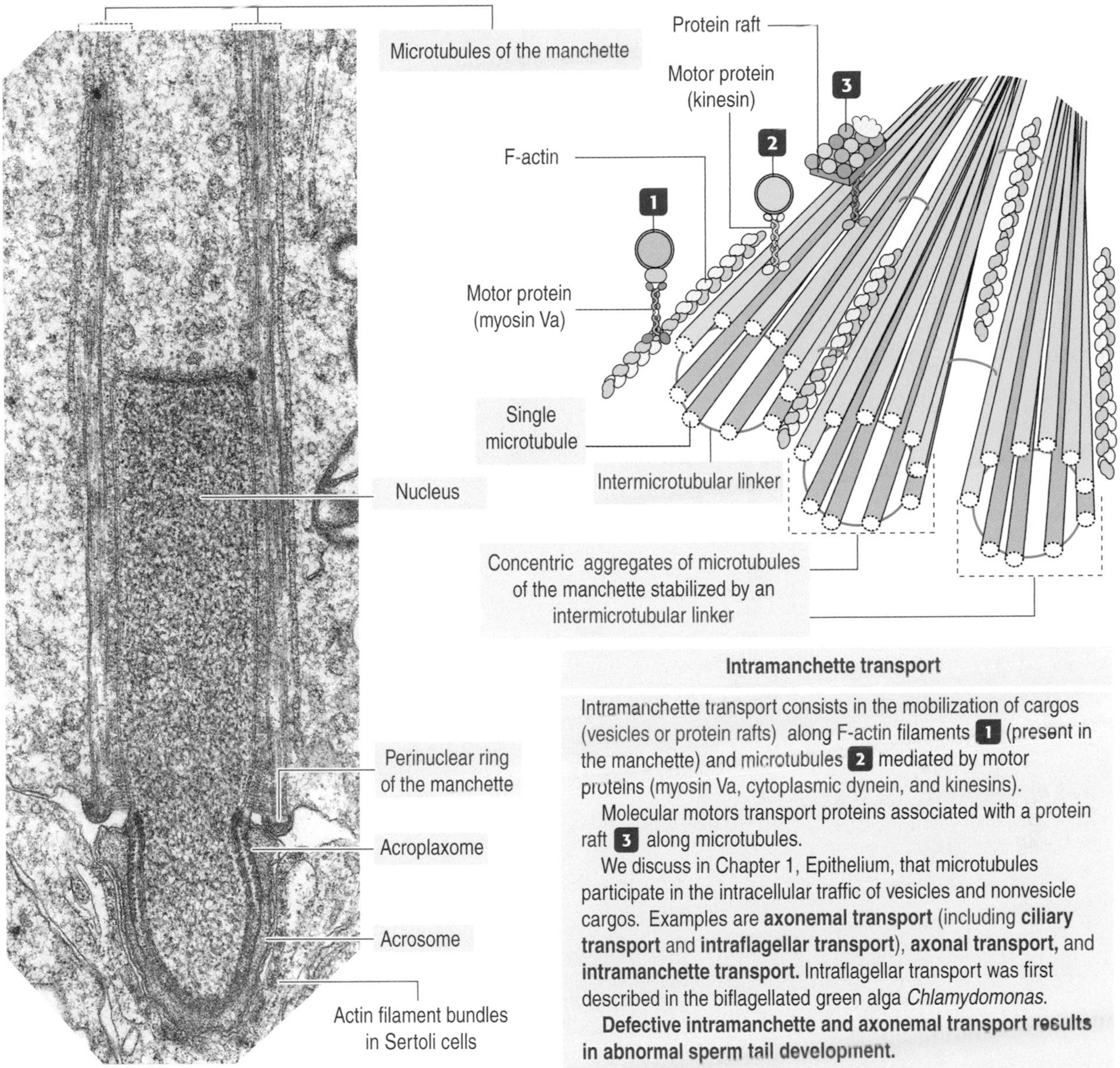

Microtubules of the manchette
Nucleus
Perinuclear ring of the manchette
Acroplaxome
Acrosome
Actin filament bundles in Sertoli cells
Protein raft
Motor protein (kinesin)
F-actin
Motor protein (myosin Va)
Single microtubule
Intermicrotubular linker
Concentric aggregates of microtubules of the manchette stabilized by an intermicrotubular linker

Intramanchette transport

Intramanchette transport consists in the mobilization of cargos (vesicles or protein rafts) along F-actin filaments 1 (present in the manchette) and microtubules 2 mediated by motor proteins (myosin Va, cytoplasmic dynein, and kinesins).

Molecular motors transport proteins associated with a protein raft 3 along microtubules.

We discuss in Chapter 1, Epithelium, that microtubules participate in the intracellular traffic of vesicles and nonvesicle cargos. Examples are **axonemal transport** (including **ciliary transport** and **intraflagellar transport**), **axonal transport,** and **intramanchette transport.** Intraflagellar transport was first described in the biflagellated green alga *Chlamydomonas*.

Defective intramanchette and axonemal transport results in abnormal sperm tail development.

4. **Nuclear condensation**. Nuclear condensation occurs when somatic histones are replaced by **arginine- and lysine-rich protamines**. After the somatic histone-to-protamine shift, nucleosomes disappear and smooth chromatin fibers associate side-by-side to condense the nuclear material. There is no significant RNA transcription after the maturation phase of spermiogenesis.

Events at the completion of spermiogenesis

During the final spermatid maturation phase (see Figure 20-12) **mitochondria** complete their alignment along the developing flagellum. The **nucleus** elongates and condenses, and the **manchette** migrates caudally and disassembles. The maturation process is completed when the nucleus acquires its final elongated condensed shape.

The **residual body**, an excess of cytoplasm from the mature spermatid, is phagocytosed by Sertoli cells at the end of spermiogenesis when **spermiation** (release of mature spermatids into the lumen of the seminiferous tubule) occurs. **Nuclear condensation**, consisting in the replacement of **somatic histones** by arginine- and lysine-rich **protamines**, defines the final step of spermiogenesis. This replacement

Figure 20-15. Sperm structure: Head and tail components

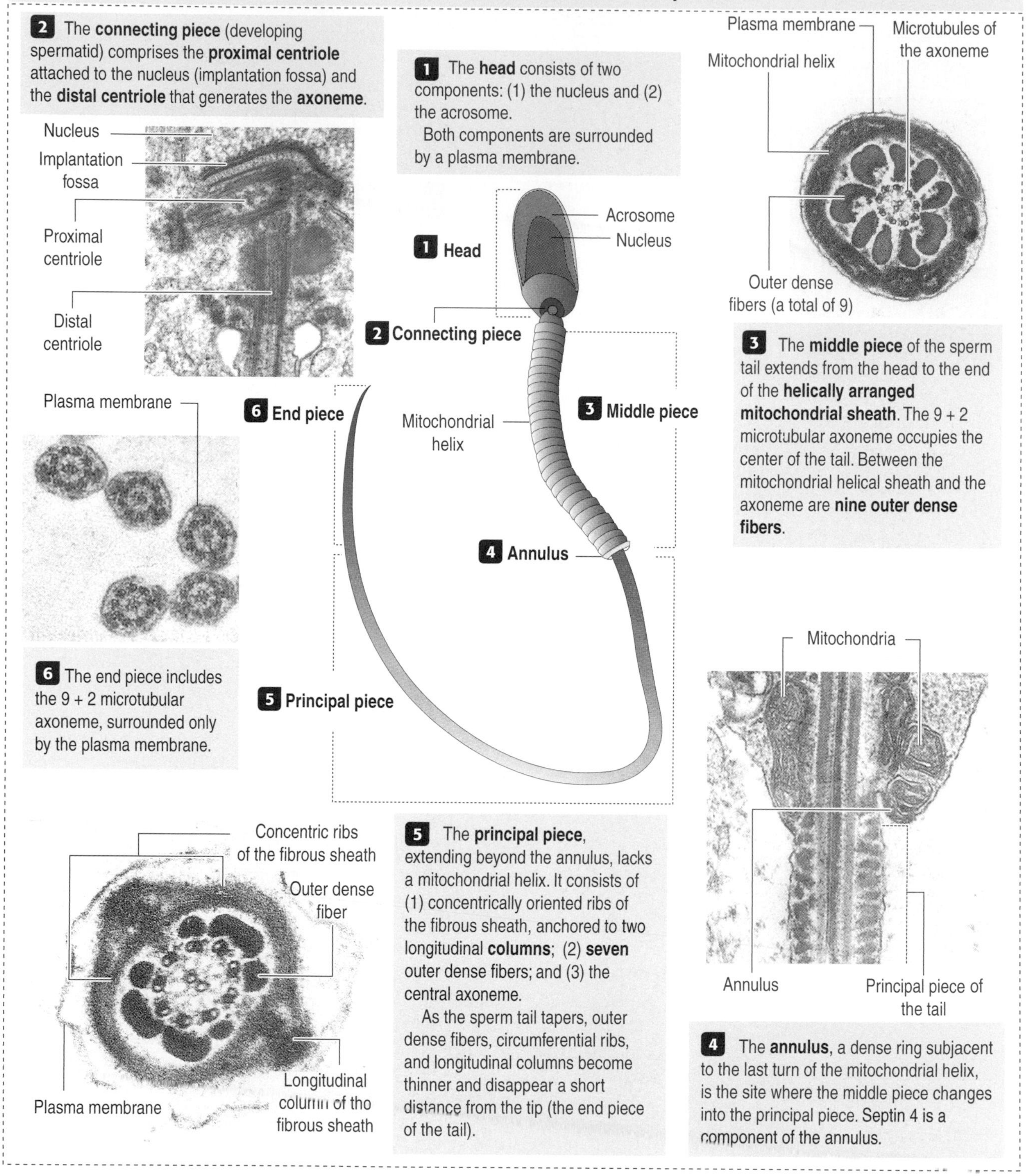

1 The **head** consists of two components: (1) the nucleus and (2) the acrosome.
Both components are surrounded by a plasma membrane.

2 The **connecting piece** (developing spermatid) comprises the **proximal centriole** attached to the nucleus (implantation fossa) and the **distal centriole** that generates the **axoneme**.

3 The **middle piece** of the sperm tail extends from the head to the end of the **helically arranged mitochondrial sheath**. The 9 + 2 microtubular axoneme occupies the center of the tail. Between the mitochondrial helical sheath and the axoneme are **nine outer dense fibers**.

4 The **annulus**, a dense ring subjacent to the last turn of the mitochondrial helix, is the site where the middle piece changes into the principal piece. Septin 4 is a component of the annulus.

5 The **principal piece**, extending beyond the annulus, lacks a mitochondrial helix. It consists of (1) concentrically oriented ribs of the fibrous sheath, anchored to two longitudinal **columns**; (2) **seven** outer dense fibers; and (3) the central axoneme.
As the sperm tail tapers, outer dense fibers, circumferential ribs, and longitudinal columns become thinner and disappear a short distance from the tip (the end piece of the tail).

6 The end piece includes the 9 + 2 microtubular axoneme, surrounded only by the plasma membrane.

stabilizes and protects the sperm genomic DNA.

Structure of the sperm

The mature sperm consists of two components (Figure 20-15): the **head** and the **tail**. A **connecting piece** links the head to the tail.

The tail is subdivided into three segments: the **middle piece**, the **principal piece**, and the **end piece**. A plasma membrane surrounds the head and tail regions of the sperm.

The **head** is composed of the **nucleus** covered by the **acrosome**. The **acroplaxome**, an F-actin–containing cytoskeletal plate, fastens the acrosome to the nuclear envelope. The nucleus is a flattened condensed structure. The acrosome covers the anterior half of the nucleus and contains **hydrolytic enzymes** (proteases, acid phosphatase, hyaluronidase, and neuraminidase, among others) usually found in lysosomes. The acrosome is generally regarded as a special type of lysosome.

Acrosomal enzymes are released at the time of **fertilization** (see Chapter 23, Fertilization, Placentation, and Lactation) to facilitate sperm penetration of the **corona radiata** and the **zona pellucida** surrounding the ovum (see Chapter 22, Follicle Development and Menstrual Cycle).

The **connecting piece**, joining the head to the tail, is a narrow segment containing a **pair of centrioles**. As we have already indicated, the **distal centriole** gives rise to the **axoneme** and the proximal centriole contributes to the assembly of the connecting piece.

The **middle piece** of the tail consists of a helically arranged mitochondrial sheath, the **axoneme**, and **nine longitudinal columns**, called **outer dense fibers,** projecting down the tail from the connecting piece at the neck of the sperm. The lower limit of the middle piece is marked by the termination of the mitochondrial helical sheath at the **annulus**.

The **principal piece** is the longest segment of the tail. It consists of the central axoneme surrounded by **seven outer dense fibers** (instead of nine, as in the middle piece) and a **fibrous sheath**.

The fibrous sheath is formed by **concentric ribs** projecting from equidistant **longitudinal columns**. Both outer dense fibers and the fibrous sheath contain fibrous proteins, which provide a rigid scaffold during microtubular sliding and bending of the tail during **forward motility of the sperm**.

The **end piece** is a very short segment of the tail in which only the axoneme is present because of an early termination of the outer dense fibers and fibrous sheath.

Clinical significance: Pathologic conditions affecting spermatogenesis

Temperature

A temperature of 35°C is critical for spermatogenesis. This temperature is achieved in the scrotum by the **pampiniform plexus** of veins surrounding the spermatic artery and functions as a **countercurrent heat exchanger** to dissipate heat. When the temperature is below 35°C, contraction of the **cremaster muscle** in the spermatic cord and of the **dartos muscle** in the scrotal sac brings the testis close to the body wall to increase the temperature.

Cryptorchidism

In cryptorchidism (or **undescended testis**), the testis fails to reach the scrotal sac during development and remains in the abdominal cavity or inguinal canal. Under these conditions, the normal body temperature (37°C to 38°C) inhibits spermatogenesis and sterility occurs if the condition is bilateral.

Testicular descent occurs in two phases: (1) **transabdominal descent**, presumably controlled by **müllerian inhibiting substance** (MIS) produced by fetal Sertoli cells and (2) **inguinal-scrotal descent**, probably controlled by **androgen secretion** induced by **calcitonin gene-related peptide** carried by the genitofemoral nerve. Recent research has shown that mutations of two genes, ***insulin-like factor 3*** and ***Hoxa-10***, are associated with bilateral cryptorchidism.

Defects in the transabdominal descent are not common. In most children, the undescended testis can be detected in the inguinal canal. Testes in the inguinal canal are subject to trauma and compression by local ligaments and bone.

A high incidence of **testicular tumors** is associated with the untreated cryptorchid testis. Cryptorchidism is an asymptomatic condition that is detected by physical examination of the scrotal sac after birth and before puberty. Hormonal treatment (administration of chorionic gonadotropin) may induce testicular descent. If that is unsuccessful, **surgery** is the next step, in which the testis is attached to the wall of the scrotal sac (a process called **orchiopexy**).

Cancer chemotherapy

Young male patients treated with antitumoral drugs may become transiently aspermatogenic because spermatogonial mitosis and spermatocyte meiosis can be affected. However, dormant **stem cells**—not involved in DNA synthesis and cell division—can repopulate the seminiferous epithelium once anticancer chemotherapy is discontinued.

Mumps

Mumps is a systemic viral infection with a 20% to 30% incidence of **acute orchitis** (sudden inflammation of the testis) in postpubertal males. In general, no alterations in spermatogenic function can be expected following mumps-caused orchitis.

Spermatic cord torsion

Twisting of the spermatic cord may disrupt the arterial blood supply to, and venous drainage from, the testis. This condition is generally caused by physical trauma or an abnormally mobile testis within the tunica vaginalis. If torsion is not treated immediately, hemorrhagic infarction and necrosis of the whole testis occur.

Varicocele

This condition is caused by the abnormal dilation of the veins of the spermatic cord. A consequence of varicocele is a decrease in sperm production (**oligospermia**). Recall that veins in the spermatic cord play a significant role in maintaining testicular temperature at 35°C by a countercurrent exchange mechanism with the spermatic artery.

Leydig cells

Aggregates of Leydig cells are present in the intertubular space in proximity to blood vessels and lymphatic channels or sinusoids (Figure 20-16). Like most steroid-producing cells, Leydig cells contain **lipid droplets**, **mitochondria with characteristic tubular cristae**, and a well-developed **smooth endoplasmic reticulum**.

After puberty and upon stimulation with **luteinizing hormone** (**LH**) by a cyclic adenosine monophosphate (cAMP)-mediated mechanism, Leydig cells produce **testosterone**, which can be converted to **dihydrotestosterone** by the enzyme **5α-reductase**. About 95% of the testosterone found in serum (bound to **sex hormone–binding globulin** [SHBG] and other proteins) is synthesized by Leydig cells; the remaining testosterone is produced by the adrenal cortex.

Testosterone can also be aromatized to estrogens in many tissues, in particular adipose tissue. ABP produced by Sertoli cells after stimulation by FSH, maintains a high concentration of testosterone in the proximity of developing spermatogenic cells.

Clinical significance: Steroidogenic acute regulatory protein

Fetal Leydig cells are steroidogenically active between 8 and 18 weeks of gestation. By week 18 of gestation, the Leydig cell population predominates in the testis. The androgens produced by fetal Leydig cells at this time are critical for the development of the male reproductive tract (see the development of the testis in Chapter 21, Sperm Transport and Maturation). In the neonate, testicular steroidogenesis reaches high levels at 2 to 3 months post partum and then decreases. Androgen levels remain low until puberty, when an increase in LH activates androgen synthesis.

Figure 20-16. Leydig cell: The androgen-producing cell of the testis

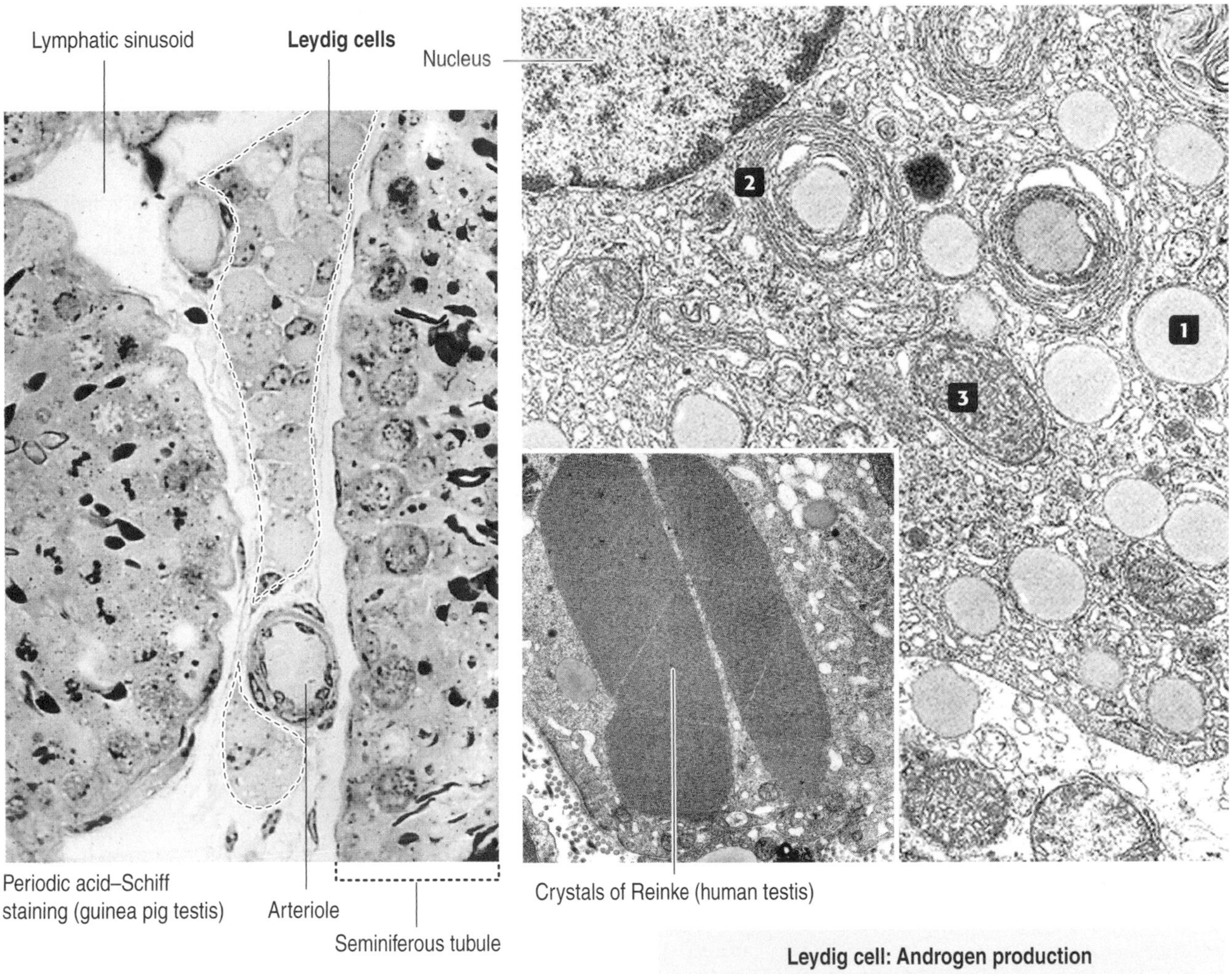

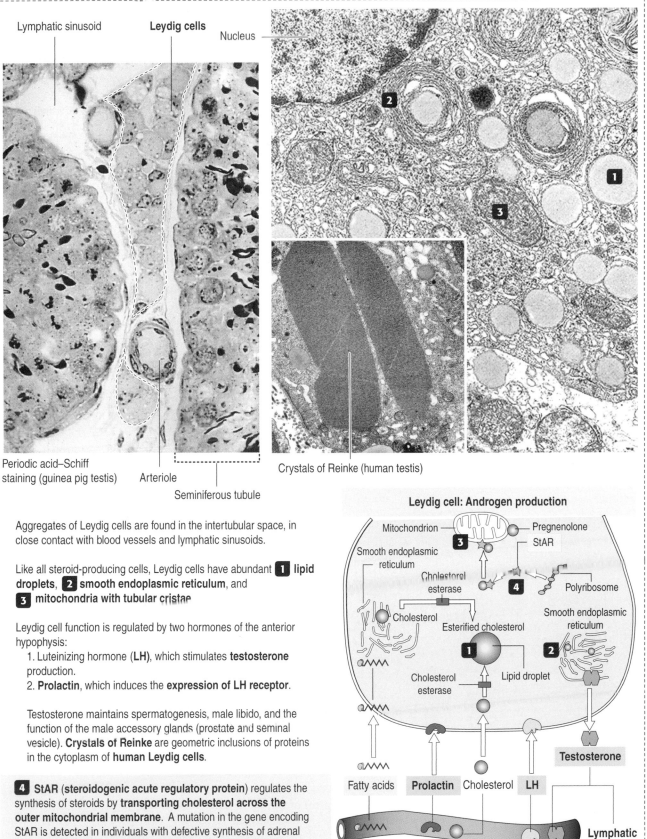

Lymphatic sinusoid
Leydig cells
Nucleus
2
1
3
Periodic acid–Schiff staining (guinea pig testis)
Arteriole
Seminiferous tubule
Crystals of Reinke (human testis)

Aggregates of Leydig cells are found in the intertubular space, in close contact with blood vessels and lymphatic sinusoids.

Like all steroid-producing cells, Leydig cells have abundant 1 **lipid droplets**, 2 **smooth endoplasmic reticulum**, and 3 **mitochondria with tubular cristae**

Leydig cell function is regulated by two hormones of the anterior hypophysis:

1. Luteinizing hormone (**LH**), which stimulates **testosterone** production.
2. **Prolactin**, which induces the **expression of LH receptor**.

Testosterone maintains spermatogenesis, male libido, and the function of the male accessory glands (prostate and seminal vesicle). **Crystals of Reinke** are geometric inclusions of proteins in the cytoplasm of **human Leydig cells**.

4 **StAR** (**steroidogenic acute regulatory protein**) regulates the synthesis of steroids by **transporting cholesterol across the outer mitochondrial membrane**. A mutation in the gene encoding StAR is detected in individuals with defective synthesis of adrenal and gonadal steroids (**lipoid congenital adrenal hyperplasia**).

Leydig cell: Androgen production

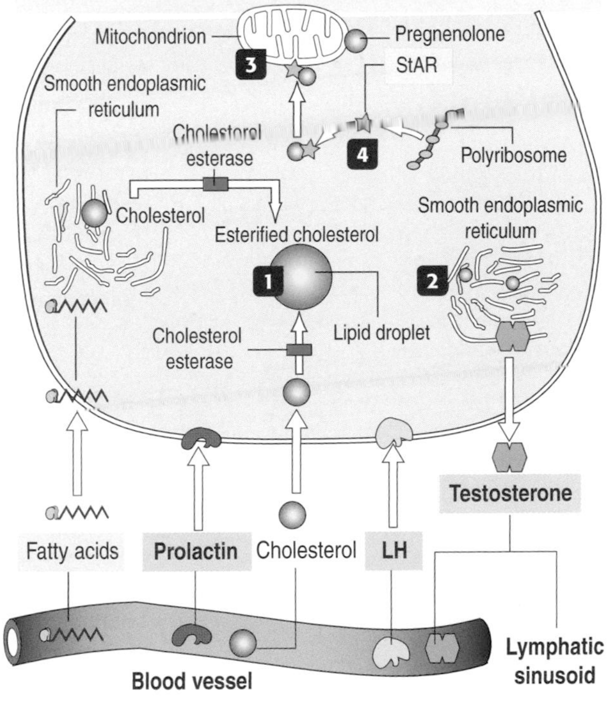

Mitochondrion
Pregnenolone
3
StAR
Smooth endoplasmic reticulum
Cholesterol esterase
4
Polyribosome
Cholesterol
Esterified cholesterol
Smooth endoplasmic reticulum
1
2
Cholesterol esterase
Lipid droplet
Testosterone
Fatty acids
Prolactin
Cholesterol
LH
Blood vessel
Lymphatic sinusoid

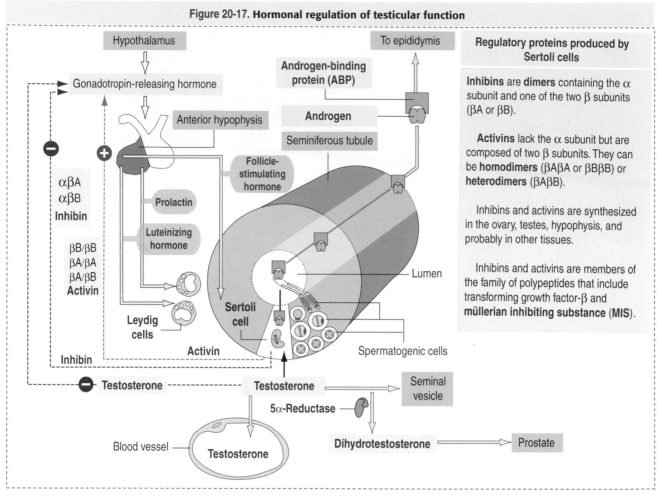

Figure 20-17. **Hormonal regulation of testicular function**

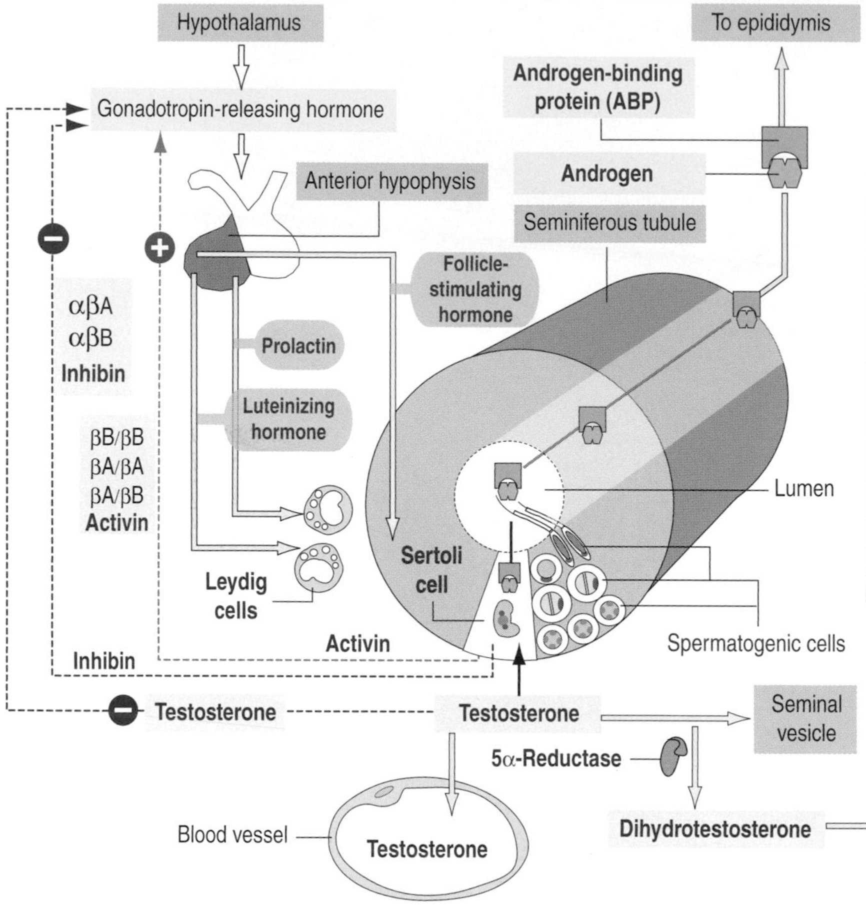

Regulatory proteins produced by Sertoli cells

Inhibins are **dimers** containing the α subunit and one of the two β subunits (βA or βB).

Activins lack the α subunit but are composed of two β subunits. They can be **homodimers** (βAβA or βBβB) or **heterodimers** (βAβB).

Inhibins and activins are synthesized in the ovary, testes, hypophysis, and probably in other tissues.

Inhibins and activins are members of the family of polypeptides that include transforming growth factor-β and **müllerian inhibiting substance (MIS)**.

LH and prolactin regulate the function of Leydig cells (Figure 20-17; see also Figures 20-16). Prolactin regulates the gene expression of the LH receptor. LH is responsible for the production of testosterone. **Hyperprolactinemia** inhibits male reproductive function by decreasing gonadotropin secretion and action on the testis. Excessive prolactin can decrease the production of androgens by Leydig cells, diminish spermatogenesis, and lead to erectile dysfunction and infertility.

During the synthesis of testosterone, plasma **cholesterol** enters the cell, is esterified by **acetyl coenzyme A** (acetyl CoA) and is stored in the cytoplasm as lipid droplets. **Fatty acids** are processed to cholesterol in the smooth endoplasmic reticulum.

Cholesterol is transported from the lipid droplet to mitochondria by **steroidogenic acute regulatory protein** (**StAR**) (synthesized in the cytosol by polyribosomes), and pregnenolone is produced.

Enzymes in the smooth endoplasmic reticulum convert pregnenolone to progesterone to testosterone. Two other less potent androgens produced by Leydig cells are **dehydroepiandrosterone** (**DHEA**) and **androstenedione**.

In the human testis, the cytoplasm of Leydig cells contains **crystals of Reinke,** inclusions of proteins in a geometric array, which become more apparent with age.

Hormonal control of the male reproductive tract

FSH and LH regulate the function of Sertoli and Leydig cells, respectively (see Figure 20-17). **FSH stimulates the production of inhibin and activin by Sertoli cells**. Inhibin exerts a **negative feedback** on the hypothalamic and hypophysial release of FSH. Activin has an opposite effect.

Box 20-C | **Androgen actions**

In the male fetus
- Regulation of the differentiation of the male internal and external genitalia.
- Stimulation of the growth, development, and function of male internal and external genitalia.

In the adult male
- Stimulation of sexual hair development.
- Stimulation of the secretion of sebaceous glands of the skin.
- Binding to androgen-binding protein produced by Sertoli cells after FSH stimulation.
- Initiation and maintenance of spermatogenesis.
- Maintenance of the secretory function of sex glands (seminal vesicle and prostate).

Figure 20-18. Arrangement of cellular associations in seminiferous tubules

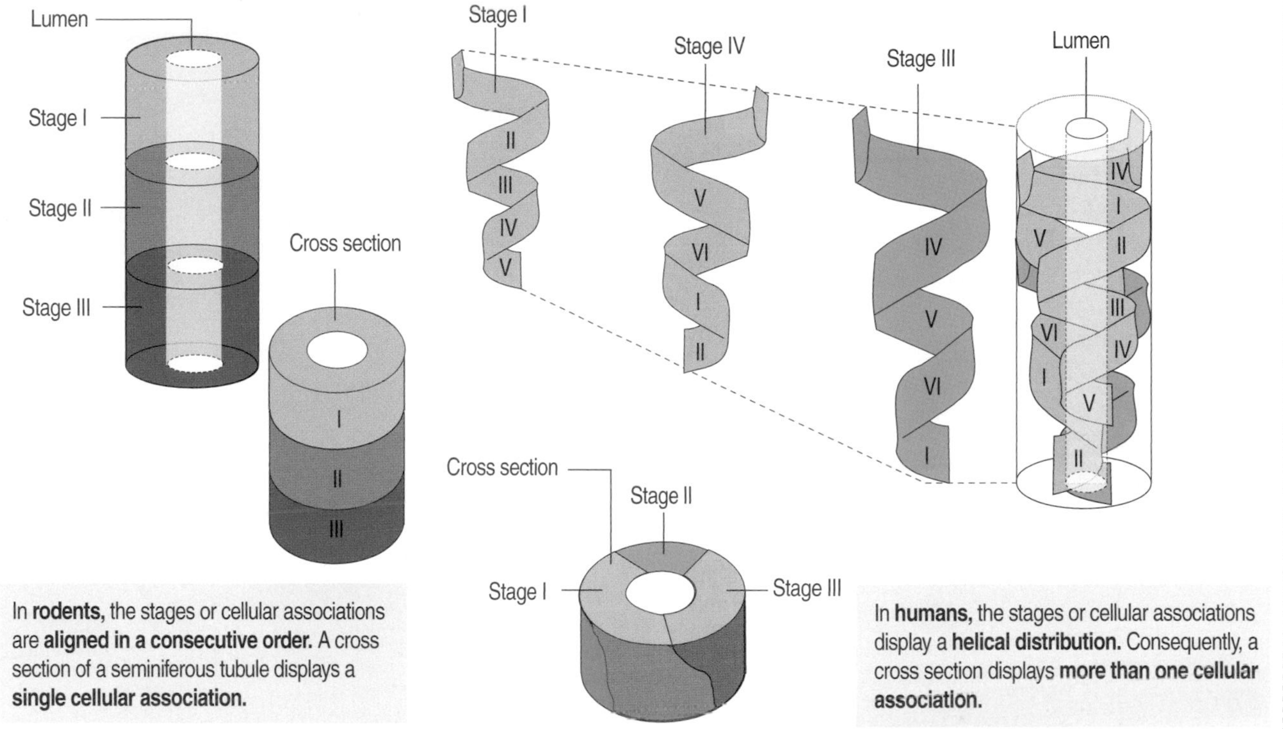
Arrangement of stages in rodents
Helical arrangement of stages in human
Lumen
Stage I
Stage II
Stage III
Cross section
I
II
III
Stage I
Stage IV
Stage III
Lumen
II
III
IV
V
VI
I
Cross section
Stage II
Stage I
Stage III

In **rodents,** the stages or cellular associations are **aligned in a consecutive order.** A cross section of a seminiferous tubule displays a **single cellular association.**

In **humans,** the stages or cellular associations display a **helical distribution.** Consequently, a cross section displays **more than one cellular association.**

FSH and LH are mandatory regulators of the spermatogenic process, as demonstrated by the arrest of spermatogenesis following experimental removal of the hypophysis (**hypophysectomy**).

The synthesis and secretion of **ABP** by Sertoli cells is stimulated by FSH. ABP binds androgens (testosterone or dihydrotestosterone) and the ABP-androgen complex maintains high levels of androgens in the proximity of developing spermatogenic cells. In addition, the complex is transported to the epididymis, where it keeps high concentration of androgens.

Sertoli cells in the **adult testis** produce three major secretory proteins: (1) **inhibin,** (2) **activin, and** (3) **ABP. Fetal Sertoli cells** synthesize and secrete **müllerian inhibiting substance.**

As we have already discussed, LH stimulates the synthesis of testosterone by Leydig cells (see Box 20-C). Both testosterone and dihydrotestosterone, the latter a metabolite of testosterone after reduction by **5α-reductase**, bind to the same **androgen receptor** (unrelated to ABP).

The **androgen receptor** is a member of the **steroid–thyroid–retinoic acid superfamily** of receptors and as such it has three domains: (1) a **DNA binding domain** that recognizes the **androgen-responsive element**, (2) a **transcription factors–binding domain**, and (3) an **androgen-binding domain.**

Recall that a defective androgen receptor—encoded by a gene in the X chromosome—determines the **androgen insensitivity syndrome** (**AIS**) also known as **testicular feminization**. The magnitude of symptoms in individuals with this genetic defect is variable depending on the partial to complete inability of the androgen receptor to bind to androgens.

Testosterone has a **negative feedback** effect on the release of LH. An excess of testosterone in circulating blood prevents the release of LH from the anterior hypophysis. Testosterone stimulates the function of the **seminal vesicles**, whereas dihydrotestosterone acts on the **prostate gland**.

Figure 20-19. Spermatogenic cycle

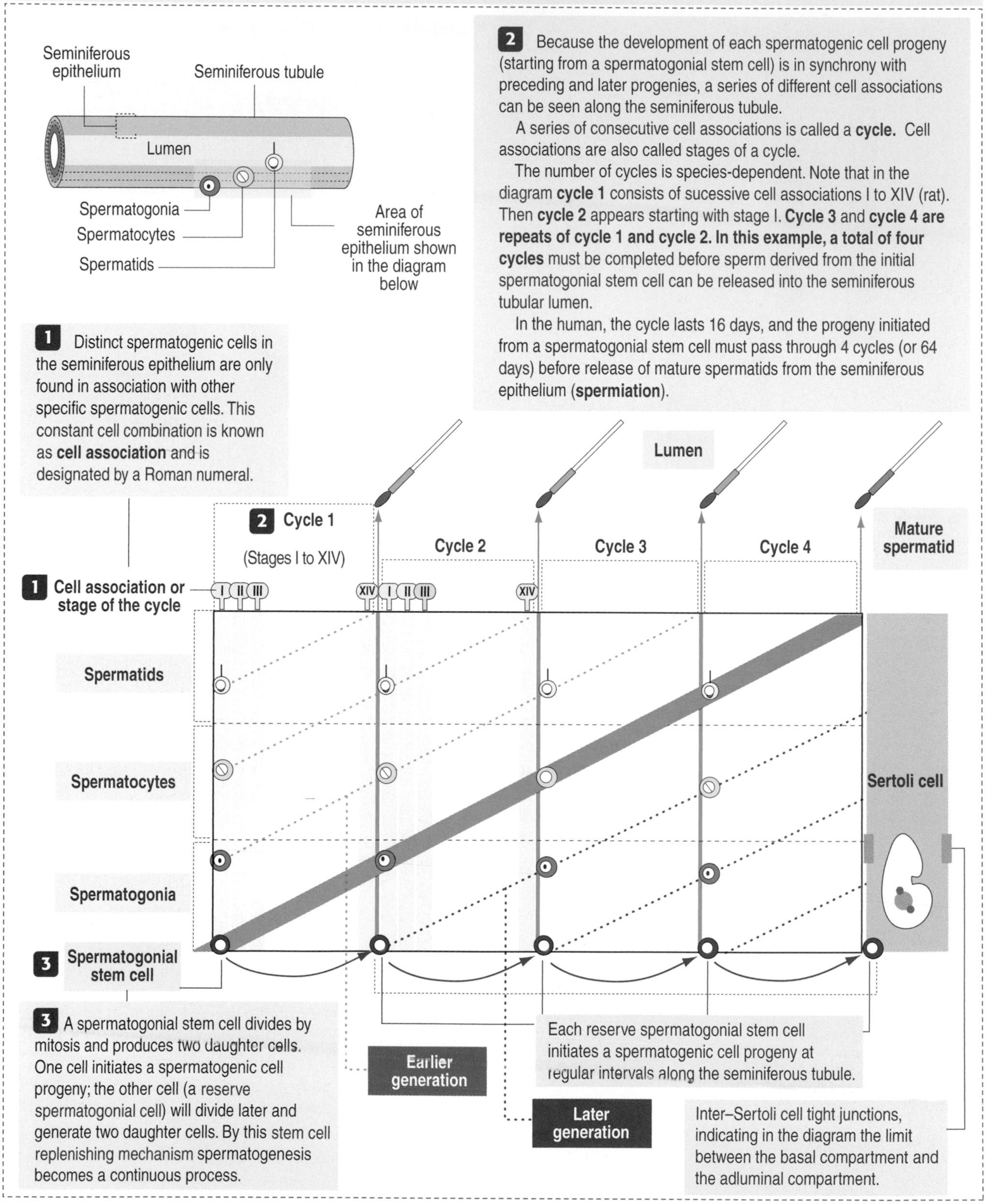

Seminiferous epithelium
Seminiferous tubule
Lumen
Spermatogonia
Spermatocytes
Spermatids
Area of seminiferous epithelium shown in the diagram below
2 Because the development of each spermatogenic cell progeny (starting from a spermatogonial stem cell) is in synchrony with preceding and later progenies, a series of different cell associations can be seen along the seminiferous tubule.
A series of consecutive cell associations is called a **cycle.** Cell associations are also called stages of a cycle.
The number of cycles is species-dependent. Note that in the diagram **cycle 1** consists of sucessive cell associations I to XIV (rat). Then **cycle 2** appears starting with stage I. **Cycle 3** and **cycle 4 are repeats of cycle 1 and cycle 2. In this example, a total of four cycles** must be completed before sperm derived from the initial spermatogonial stem cell can be released into the seminiferous tubular lumen.
In the human, the cycle lasts 16 days, and the progeny initiated from a spermatogonial stem cell must pass through 4 cycles (or 64 days) before release of mature spermatids from the seminiferous epithelium (**spermiation**).
1 Distinct spermatogenic cells in the seminiferous epithelium are only found in association with other specific spermatogenic cells. This constant cell combination is known as **cell association** and is designated by a Roman numeral.
Lumen
2 Cycle 1
(Stages I to XIV)
Cycle 2
Cycle 3
Cycle 4
Mature spermatid
1 Cell association or stage of the cycle
I II III
XIV I II III
XIV
Spermatids
Spermatocytes
Spermatogonia
Sertoli cell
3 Spermatogonial stem cell
3 A spermatogonial stem cell divides by mitosis and produces two daughter cells. One cell initiates a spermatogenic cell progeny; the other cell (a reserve spermatogonial cell) will divide later and generate two daughter cells. By this stem cell replenishing mechanism spermatogenesis becomes a continuous process.
Earlier generation
Each reserve spermatogonial stem cell initiates a spermatogenic cell progeny at regular intervals along the seminiferous tubule.
Later generation
Inter–Sertoli cell tight junctions, indicating in the diagram the limit between the basal compartment and the adluminal compartment.

Spermatogenic cycle

When you examine a number of seminiferous tubules under the light microscope, you will see a variable combination of spermatogenic cells. Spermatogenic cells are not arranged at random but are organized into well-defined combinations called **cellular associations** (Figures 20-18 to 20-20).

Figure 20-20. Spermatogenic cycle: Waves and cycles

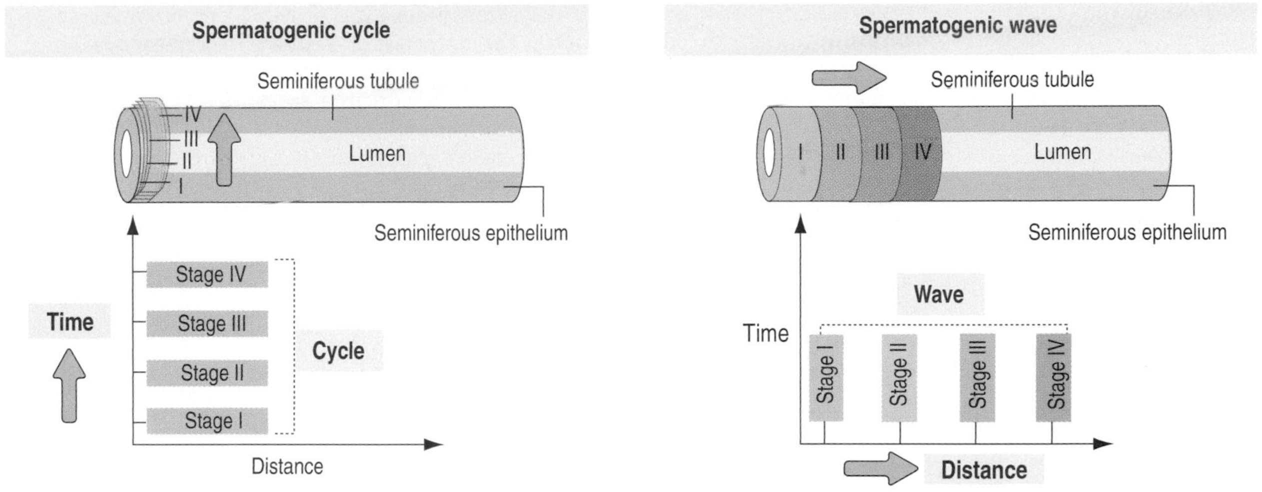

A **spermatogenic cycle** involves cellular association changes **with time** at one particular point of the seminiferous tubule. These changes occur as overlapping spermatogenic cell progenies advance in their development.

Imagine that you can monitor changes in the cellular associations or stages of a cycle using a time-lapse camera placed at that given point of the seminiferous tubule.

A **spermatogenic wave** involves changes **along a seminiferous tubule (distance)**.

Imagine that you can visualize a wave by "traveling" along the length of a seminiferous tubule.

A wave is not distinct in the human testis because of the **helical progression** of spermatogenic cell progenies.

For example, in a particular region of the seminiferous epithelium, spermatids, completing their differentiation, can be seen only in specific combination with early spermatids, spermatocytes, and spermatogonia at their respective developmental stages. These cellular associations (designated by Roman numerals) succeed one another at a given site of the seminiferous tubule and this sequence repeats itself cyclically. You should realize that it takes several cycles, each consisting of precise cellular associations that repeat themselves (at least four times in Figure 20-19), to produce mature spermatids that will be released into the tubular lumen.

How do these combinations of spermatogenic cells occur? Let us examine Figure 20-19. Note that all generations of spermatogenic cells coexist in a given segment of a seminiferous epithelium. The development of any single generation takes place concomitantly with the development of the earlier and later generations.

Each defined cell association or combination represents a **stage** in the cyclic process of spermatogenesis initiated by a spermatogonial stem cell. Because several spermatogonial stem cells give rise to a spermatogenic cell progeny at regular intervals along the seminiferous tubule and the progenies overlap, it is possible to understand that cellular associations derive from overlapping progenies at a given point in the seminiferous tubule.

Now, we need to discuss the difference between **spermatogenic cycle** and **spermatogenic wave** (see Figure 20-20). You realize that at a given point in the seminiferous tubule, the combination of spermatogenic cells will change with time as early and late progenies continue their development. It is just a question of time (hours and days) for the stages of the cycle (represented by cellular associations) to change. A **spermatogenic cycle is defined by the time it takes for a sequence of cellular associations (or stages of the cycle) at a particular point of the seminiferous tubule to change.**

We now want to determine the alignment of cell associations **along the length of the seminiferous tubule.** You realize that we have changed our parameter from time to distance. We isolate a seminiferous tubule, prepare serial histologic sections along its length, and use already available tables to verify whether cellular

Figure 20-21. Epigenetics reprogramming

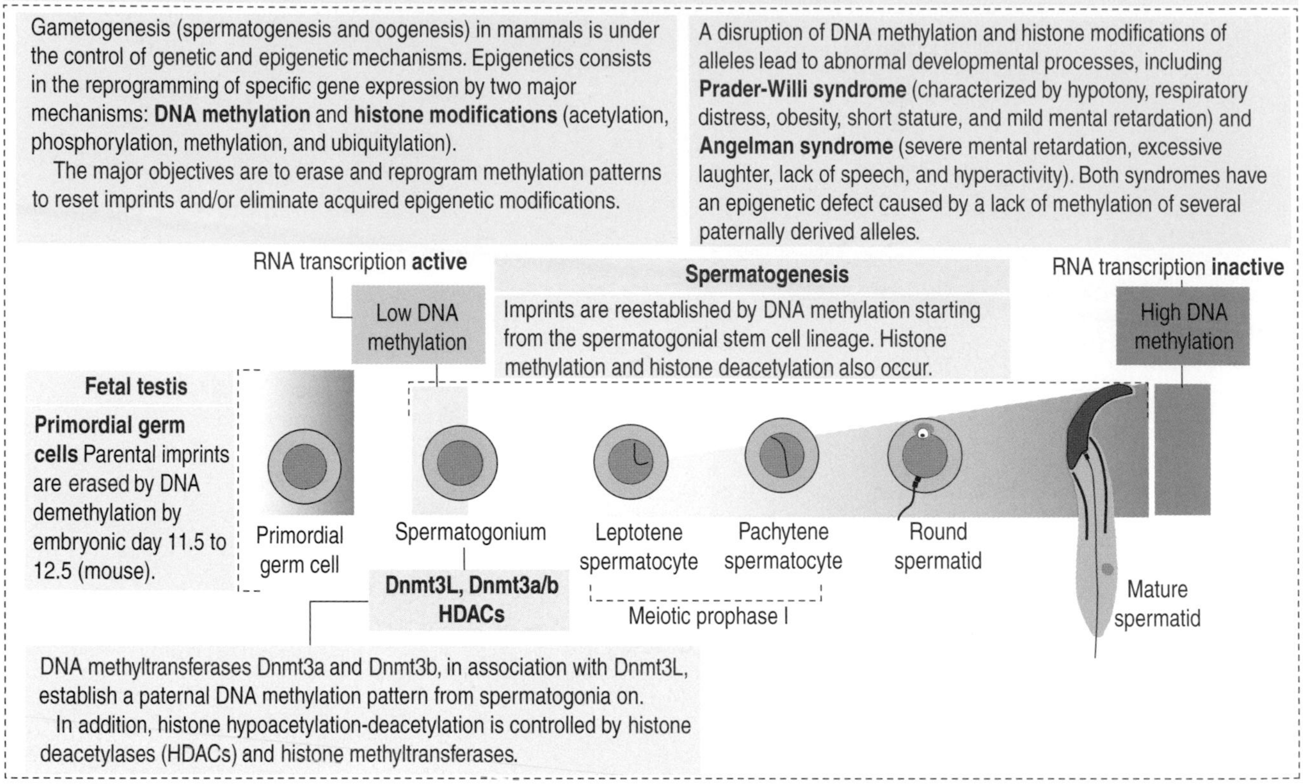

Gametogenesis (spermatogenesis and oogenesis) in mammals is under the control of genetic and epigenetic mechanisms. Epigenetics consists in the reprogramming of specific gene expression by two major mechanisms: DNA methylation and histone modifications (acetylation, phosphorylation, methylation, and ubiquitylation).
The major objectives are to erase and reprogram methylation patterns to reset imprints and/or eliminate acquired epigenetic modifications.
A disruption of DNA methylation and histone modifications of alleles lead to abnormal developmental processes, including Prader-Willi syndrome (characterized by hypotony, respiratory distress, obesity, short stature, and mild mental retardation) and Angelman syndrome (severe mental retardation, excessive laughter, lack of speech, and hyperactivity). Both syndromes have an epigenetic defect caused by a lack of methylation of several paternally derived alleles.
RNA transcription active
Low DNA methylation
Spermatogenesis
Imprints are reestablished by DNA methylation starting from the spermatogonial stem cell lineage. Histone methylation and histone deacetylation also occur.
RNA transcription inactive
High DNA methylation
Fetal testis
Primordial germ cells Parental imprints are erased by DNA demethylation by embryonic day 11.5 to 12.5 (mouse).
Primordial germ cell
Spermatogonium
Leptotene spermatocyte
Pachytene spermatocyte
Round spermatid
Mature spermatid
Dnmt3L, Dnmt3a/b HDACs
Meiotic prophase I
DNA methyltransferases Dnmt3a and Dnmt3b, in association with Dnmt3L, establish a paternal DNA methylation pattern from spermatogonia on.
In addition, histone hypoacetylation-deacetylation is controlled by histone deacetylases (HDACs) and histone methyltransferases.

associations are present. After examining a number of serial sections covering a distance of a few millimeters or centimeters, we realize **the presence of successive cellular associations (or stages of a cycle) along the length of the seminiferous tubule.** We realize that **all 14 cellular associations or stages (equivalent to one cycle) occur in a wavelike succession along a stretch of a seminiferous tubule** (as illustrated in Figure 20-19). The series of cycles, each formed by 14 consecutive stages, repeat themselves again and again. We measure the distance between two consecutive cycles (each represented by 14 consecutive cellular associations or stages of a cycle) and define what a **spermatogenic wave** is.

The number of cellular associations or stages in a cycle is constant for any given species (14 stages in the rat, **6 stages in man**, 12 in the monkey). In human testes, spermatogenic cell generations are organized in a helical fashion (see Figure 20-18). Consequently, a cross section of a seminiferous tubule will display three or four cellular associations instead of the single one observed in the rat testis. In man, the duration of one cycle is 16 days. It takes four cycles (64 days) to develop spermatogonia into testicular sperm.

Clinical significance: Epigenetics reprogramming

We have seen that somatic histones are removed from spermatids and replaced by arginine-, lysine-rich protamines. This histone-protamine shift results in (1) RNA transcriptional inactivation (called **gene silencing**) and (2) changes in chromatin structure from a nucleosomal-type to a smooth-type of chromatin in late spermatids (see Figure 20-12).

During gametogenesis (spermatogenesis and oogenesis), **genetic imprints are differentially erased to allow epigenetic reprogramming** to be transmitted to embryos by the gametes. Reprogramming during gametogenesis is required for the resetting of imprints or eliminating acquired epigenetic modifications.

Changes in DNA and histones can modify gene activity without changing DNA sequence. Such modifications are epigenetic, "outside conventional genetics." There is a close relationship between gene imprinting, chromatin structure,

Figure 20-22. DNA methylation and histone deacetylation

1 Transcriptionally active chromatin consists of transcription factors and RNA polymerase bound to the gene promoter region. Histones in the nucleosomal core are acetylated.

2 Transcriptional silencing starts when DNA methyltransferases methylate CpG islands on DNA. Methylated DNA binding proteins (MBD), including histone deacetylase, are recruited to the methylated CpG islands. Histone deacetylase relocates to the histone core and removes acetyl groups from histones.

3 Histone deacetylation enables histone methyltransferase to attach methyl groups to histones and heterochromatin protein-1 (HP1) is recruited to histone methylated sites.
Chromatin is condensed and transcription stops.

A mutation on the ***DNMT3b*** gene is observed in patients with the rare disease called **ICF** (immunodeficiency, centromeric instability, and facial anomalies syndrome).

A mutation in the ***MeCP2*** gene, encoding one of the MBD proteins, is the cause of the **Rett syndrome** in young girls (mental retardation).

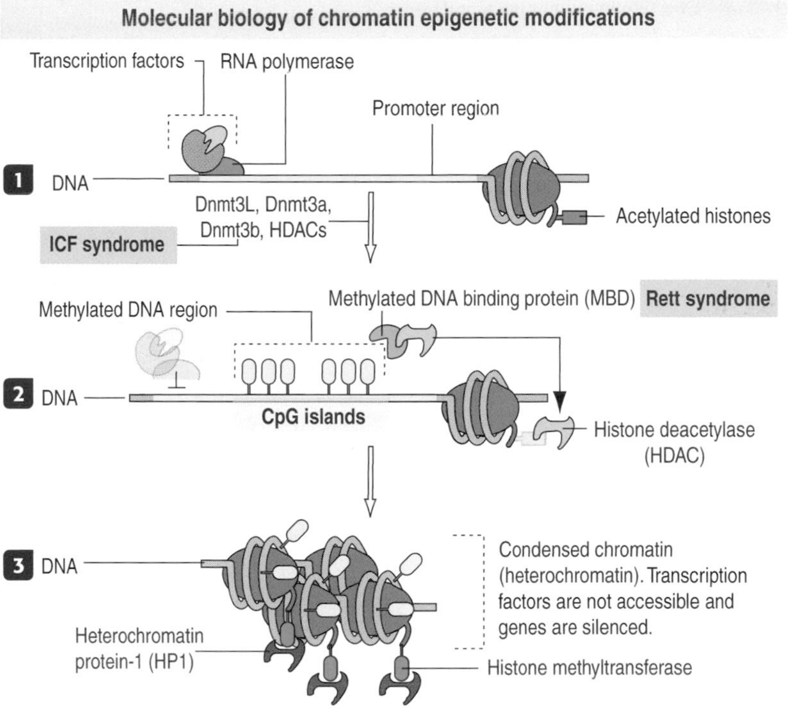

and DNA methylation. As we will see, DNA methylation can initiate a cascade of events silencing RNA transcription.

During gametogenesis, the differential expression of **alleles** (Greek *allos,* another) can be inhibited in paternal and maternal gametes. Genes come in pairs, one copy or allele inherited from each parent. During spermatogenesis and oogenesis one copy of the imprinted gene is selectively silenced. Imprinting disorders are seen when the alternative maternal or paternal copy (allele) does not appear.

Defects in parental imprinting include **Prader-Willi syndrome** and **Angelman syndrome** (Figure 20-21). Prader-Willi syndrome is characterized by hypotony, respiratory distress, obesity, short stature, and mild mental retardation. It is caused by the deletion of a paternal allele or the retention of two maternal copies. Angelman syndrome includes severe mental retardation, excessive inappropriate laughter, lack of speech, and hyperactivity. In contrast to Prader-Willi syndrome, the maternal allele has been lost or two paternal copies are retained. Although two alleles are available (one inherited from each parent), the affected individuals have mutations in the DNA regions controlling gene imprinting of the two alleles.

We now address with this background the molecular aspects of epigenetics reprogramming (Figure 20-22). Epigenetics is the study of differences in gene expression patterns that are not determined by heritable changes in DNA sequence. The basis of epigenetics are DNA methylation of normally unmethylated CpG (cytosine-phospho-guanosine) dinucleotide islands on the DNA; and histone modifications, in particular histone deacetylation. A large number of CpG islands are present in transcription initiation sites and in promoters of active genes.

Chromatin of an actively transcribing gene (euchromatin) has acetylated histones and the CpG islands are unmethylated. This "open" chromatin organization enables transcription factors and RNA polymerase to transcribe a gene. Chromatin can be condensed (heterochromatin) to become transcriptionally inactive. Two events take place to accomplish this task: (1) DNA methyltransferases methylate CpG islands and (2) histone deacetylases remove acetyl groups from the N-terminal tail of the nucleosomal histones.

Methylation consists of the attachment of a methyl group to a biological molecule by methyltransferases. **DNA methyltransferases** (Dnmt1, Dnmt3a, and Dnmt3b, with the participation of Dnmt3L) attach methyl groups to CpG dinucleotides. **Histone methyltransferases** attach methyl groups to histones after they have become deacetylated by **histone deacetylases.**

How do histone deacetylases know when to remove acetyl groups from histones? **Methylated DNA-binding protein** (MBD) and **histone deacetylase** (which removes acetyl groups) are recruited to the CpG island when they become methylated. Histone deacetylation is a prerequisite for histone methylation, which involves **histone methyltransferase** targeting histone 3 (H3). H3 methylation results in the recruitment of the effector **heterochromatin protein-1** (HP1). Chromatin condenses and transcription is inactivated ("closed" chromatin).

The clinical significance of DNA and histone methylation, coupled with histone deacetylation, points to the therapeutic reactivation of abnormally silenced tumor-suppressor genes. DNA methylation inhibitors and histone deacetylase inhibitors are promising agents in cancer treatment.

Essential concepts | **Spermatogenesis**

• Components of the male reproductive system. It consists of the testes (the site of production of sperm and androgens), the epididymis (the site of sperm maturation), the excurrent duct system (vas deferens, ejaculatory ducts, and urethra), the accessory glands (seminal vesicles, prostate gland, and bulbourethral glands of Cowper), and the penis (the copulatory organ).

• The testes are located in the scrotal sac. Each testis is surrounded by the tunica albuginea (dense connective tissue) concentrated in the mediastinum, where the rete testis is located. The network of blood vessels under the tunica albuginea is called tunica vasculosa. Septa or partitions derived from the mediastinum divide the testis into 250 to 300 lobules. Each lobule contains 1 to 4 seminiferous tubules.

• The seminiferous tubule consists of a wall (seminiferous tubular wall) and an epithelium (seminiferous epithelium) surrounding a central lumen. The wall consists of collagen-producing fibroblasts and contractile myoid cells. A basement membrane (consisting of a basal lamina and reticular lamina) separates the wall from the seminiferous epithelium.

The two ends of the tubule open in the rete testis, a network of channels collecting testicular sperm, secretory proteins, and fluid produced by the seminiferous epithelium. The space between seminiferous tubules is called the intertubular space. It contains blood vessels, lymphatic channels, and clusters of the androgen-producing Leydig cells.

• The seminiferous epithelium consists of somatic Sertoli cells and spermatogenic cells. The stratified cellular arrangement of spermatogenic cells (spermatogonia, primary and secondary spermatocytes, and spermatids) enables the classification of the seminiferous epithelium as being stratified with structural and functional characteristics not found in other stratified epithelia. For example, a postmitotic cell population of somatic Sertoli cells interacts with mitotically dividing spermatogonia, meiotically dividing spermatocytes, and differentiating haploid spermatids. The only permanent member of the epithelium is the Sertoli cell.

• The mammalian spermatogenic cycle starts at puberty from a prespermatogonial stem cell (derived from the primordial germ cells colonizing the gonadal ridges). Prespermatogonial stem cells (also called gonocyte) divide by mitosis to produce two daughter cells. One daughter cell initiates a spermatogenic cycle. The other daughter cell, a reserve stem cell that retains self-renewal capacity, will initiate a separate spermatogenic cycle at a later time. Reserve spermatogonial stem cells are resistant to radiation and cancer chemotherapy. This is an important consideration regarding the fertility of young patients undergoing one or both treatments.

There are two significant characteristics to remember: (1) All spermatogenic cells remain connected by cytoplasmic bridges after cell division. (2) Spermatogenic cell cohorts proliferate and differentiate synchronously.

• Sertoli cells. It is the predominant mitotically dividing cell type in the postnatal testis. After puberty, Sertoli cells become postmitotic. Sertoli cells are columnar cells extending from the tubular wall to the lumen. Sertoli cells are linked to each other by basally located tight junctions. Tight junctions, the basis for the blood-testis barrier, divide the seminiferous epithelium into a basal compartment (housing spermatogonia) and an adluminal compartment (where spermatocytes and spermatids are located). The nucleus of the Sertoli cells is usually found close to the seminiferous wall. It has an irregular outline with euchromatin and a large nucleolus flanked by two masses of heterochromatin.

After puberty, Sertoli cell function is regulated by follicle-stimulating hormone (FSH). Sertoli cells secrete the $\alpha\beta$ heterodimer inhibin, which exerts a negative feedback on the mechanism of release of FSH, and the $\alpha\alpha$ or $\beta\beta$ homodimer activin, which has positive feedback action on FSH release. FSH stimulates the production of androgen-binding protein (ABP), a secretory protein. In the fetal testis, Sertoli cells secrete müllerian inhibiting substance (MIS), a glycoprotein that prevents the development of the müllerian duct. Sertoli cells take up by phagocytosis residual bodies left behind by mature spermatids upon their release from Sertoli cell crypts at spermiation.

• Spermatogonia. Spermatogonial cells are diploid cells. They derive from the prespermatogonial stem cell progenitor and divide by mitosis several times while retaining cytoplasmic bridges. They are in direct contact with the tubular wall. There are two major types: (1) type A spermatogonia, with an oval euchromatic nucleus and eccentric nucleolus; and (2) type B spermatogonia, with round nuclei displaying clumps of chromatin near the nuclear envelope and a central nucleolus. In the human testis, type A spermatogonia can be subdivided into a pale and a dark type based on the nuclear characteristics.

• Spermatocytes. There are primary spermatocytes, derived from type B spermatogonia committed to meiosis (instead of mitosis) after duplicating their DNA content, and secondary spermatocytes, derived from the first meiotic division of primary spermatocytes.

Meiosis has two major objectives: (1) the exchange of genetic information between nonsister chromatids (called reciprocal exchange) of paired homologous chromosomes and (2) to achieve a haploid status at the end of meiosis II.

It is important to remember that oogenesis in the female starts in the fetal ovary, in contrast to the male, which starts spermatogenesis after puberty. In the fetal ovary, oogonia, the spermatogonia-equivalent in the male, divide by mitosis a number of times, enter meiosis I as primary oocytes and do not advance beyond the last phase of meiotic prophase I until after puberty. Primary oocytes, but not oogonia, are present in the ovary at the time of birth. It is also relevant that the completion of meiosis I of a primary oocyte (which occurs at ovulation) yields a secondary oocyte and a cell rudiment called a first polar body. If the secondary oocyte is fertilized, meiosis II is completed and a second polar body is produced. The objective here is to have the secondary oocyte pronucleus reach a haploid state at the time when the haploid male pronucleus penetrates the egg.

Meiosis consists of two steps: meiosis I, reductional division (when homologous chromosomes, each consisting of two sister chromatids, separate) and meiosis II, equational division (when sister chromatids separate). Meiosis I is prolonged (days) because it has a long prophase; meiosis II is shorter (minutes) and is not preceded by DNA synthesis.

Meiotic prophase I consists of well-defined substages: (1) leptotene, in which each chromosome consists of two sister chromatids; (2) zygotene, when homologous chromosomes (autosomes and sex chromosomes) start to pair (a process called synapsis) at the time when the synaptonemal complex starts to assemble; (3) pachytene, the longest substage of meiotic prophase I in which a synaptonemal complex is fully assembled and crossing over between nonsister chromatids of the paired chromosomes begins; (4) diplotene, a substage when disjunction (separation) of paired chromosomes occurs; and (5) diakinesis, represented by chiasmata (crossing points) and the disassembly of the synaptonemal complex.

The synaptonemal complex is a protein-containing structure. It consists of two lateral elements and a central element. Each lateral element, representing the remnant of the axial chromosomal core of each paired chromosome, contains a cohesin protein complex and proteins SCP3 and SCP2 (SCP stands for synaptonemal complex protein).

• Spermatids. There are two major types of spermatid: (1) round or early spermatids and (2) elongated or late spermatids. Spermatids are haploid cells derived from the division of secondary spermatocytes. They are involved in a process called spermiogenesis, the last phase of spermatogenesis, consisting of the development of the acrosome and the tail, and the elongation and condensation of the nucleus. Spermiogenesis consists of four phases: (1) Golgi phase, (2) cap phase, (3) acrosomal phase, and (4) maturation phase. These four phases describe the morphogenesis of the acrosome and the spermatid nucleus. In addition, spermiogenesis includes the development of the tail, a structure that contains the axoneme surrounded by outer dense fibers and a fibrous sheath.

The acrosome is a sac consisting of an outer acrosomal membrane and an inner acrosomal membrane and contains hydrolytic enzymes to be released following the acrosome reaction during fertilization. The inner acrosomal membrane is attached to the spermatid nuclear envelope and subjacent nuclear lamina by a cytoskeletal plate called the acroplaxome. The acroplaxome consists of F-actin, actin-polymerizing proteins, and keratin 5.

The manchette is a transient microtubular structure positioned caudally with respect to the acrosome-acroplaxome complex. The manchette participates in nucleocytoplasmic transport (an important event during the somatic histone-protamine shift during nuclear condensation) and intramanchette transport of cargos required for tail development.

• Sperm. Nonmotile mature spermatids are released into the seminiferous tubular lumen and transported to the rete testis. Transport depends on fluid flowing along the lumen of the seminiferous tubules and the contractile activity of myoid cells present in the seminiferous peritubular wall.

The sperm consists of a head and a tail connected to each other at the neck region by a connecting piece derived from the centrosome. The head contains the acrosome and the condensed nucleus. The tail is formed by three segments: (1) The middle piece contains the axoneme, outer dense fibers, and a mitochondrial sheath. Mitochondria provide adenosine triphosphate (ATP) as a source of energy for the sliding of axonemal microtubules during tail beating. (2) The principal piece consists of the axoneme, outer dense fibers, a pair of concentric ribs, and the fibrous sheath. (3) The end piece is a short segment containing the terminal portion of the axoneme. An annulus, containing the protein septin 4, represents the border between the middle piece and the principal piece.

• **Conditions affecting spermatogenesis.** A **temperature** of 35°C is essential for spermatogenesis. This temperature is achieved in the scrotum by the pampiniform plexus and spermatid artery participating in countercurrent heat exchange. **Varicocele** (dilation of the veins of the pampiniform plexus) hampers heat exchange and may lead to a decrease in sperm production.

Cryptorchidism (or undescended testis) is the failure of one or both testes to reach the scrotal sac. Testicular descent occurs in two phases: (1) transabdominal descent (probably under the control of MIS produced by fetal Sertoli cells) and (2) inguinal-scrotal descent (controlled by androgens). Mutations in *insulin-like factor 3* and *Hoxa-10* genes have been associated with bilateral cryptorchidism.

• Leydig cells. Clusters of Leydig cells are observed in the intertubular space associated with blood vessels and lymphatic channels. Leydig cells produce testosterone when stimulated by luteinizing hormone (LH) and prolactin. As in all steroid-producing cells (for example, in the adrenal cortex and the corpus luteum of the ovary), cholesterol is esterified by acetyl coenzyme A and stored as cytoplasmic lipid droplets. Cholesterol is transported to mitochondria by steroidogenic acute regulatory protein (StAR) to produce pregnenolone. Enzymes of the smooth endoplasmic reticulum convert pregnenolone to progesterone to testosterone.

• Hormonal regulation of spermatogenesis. Sertoli cell activities are dependent on the FSH-activin-inhibin complex. The production of testosterone by Leydig cells is under control of LH. Therefore, FSH and LH are mandatory regulators of spermatogenesis as demonstrated by the collapse of spermatogenesis following hypophysectomy (surgical removal of the hypophysis). Testosterone binds to ABP, produced by Sertoli cells following FSH stimulation. The ABP-testosterone complex is transported to the epididymis together with mature spermatids. Recall the importance of cytosol and nuclear androgen receptor in mediating androgen effects. As we have seen, the gene encoding androgen receptor is located in the X chromosome and patients with androgen insensitivity syndrome (testicular feminization) have a defective androgen receptor gene.

• The spermatogenic cycle. A few concepts need to be reviewed.

1. A prespermatogonial stem cell gives rise by mitosis to a daughter cell that initiates a spermatogenic cell progeny, and another daughter cell that becomes a reserve spermatogonial stem cell. The reserve cell will divide again and continue the same self-renewal cycle of its progenitor. This event starts at puberty.

2. At a given developmental time, several progenies will coexist: early and late progenies. A section of a seminiferous tubule represents the coexistence of two or more spermatogenic cell progenies started by different spermatogonial stem cells.

3. The progression of spermatogenesis is a precise timely process coordinated by the existence of cytoplasmic bridges within a spermatogonial, spermatocyte, and spermatid cohort. As a result, it is possible to determine with great precision a series of cellular combinations in sections of seminiferous tubules (except in man). Each cellular combination is called a cellular association.

4. It was noted that the cellular association sequence repeats a number of times. Each repeat of cellular associations is known as a cycle. Therefore, a cycle consists of cellular associations, each representing a stage of the cycle.

5. If you can trace a progeny starting from a radiolabeled spermatogonial stem cell, you will realize that no radiolabeled mature spermatids are ready for release at the end of the first cycle. It takes three additional cycles to accomplish this goal. By following day-by-day the radiolabeled progeny, it is possible to determine the duration of a cycle. If the completion of one cycle occurs within 16 days and four cycles are needed for mature spermatids to be ready for release, we can say that it takes 64 days to produce mature spermatids from a starting spermatogonial stem cell.

6. You should be able to distinguish the difference between a spermatogenic cycle and a spermatogenic wave. A spermatogenic cycle is defined by changes in cellular associations that occur with time. A spermatogenic wave is defined by the sequence of cellular associations that occurs along the length of a seminiferous tubule.

7. Although the concept of a spermatogenic cycle applies to human spermatogenesis, the concept of a spermatogenic wave is not as precise as in rodents. It will take 16 days for each of the four cycles (each consisting of 6 cellular associations) to result in the release, after 64 days, of mature spermatids from the human seminiferous epithelium. There is, however, a complication concerning the spermatogenic wave: the progression of the spermatogenic cell progenies, started by a spermatogonial stem cell, is helicoidal (instead of linear as in rodents). The turns of at least three helices, each with a different cellular association, can be visualized in a cross section of a human seminiferous tubule.

• **Epigenetics**. During spermatogenesis and oogenesis, genetic imprints are erased to allow epigenetic reprogramming to be transmitted to embryos by the gametes. Reprogramming determines the differential expression of a number of alleles in the paternal and maternal gametes. One copy of an imprinted gene is silenced during gametogenesis. A defect in parental imprinting can give rise to **Prader-Willi syndrome** and **Angelman syndrome.**

Epigenetics is the study of differences in gene expression patterns that are not determined by heritable changes in DNA sequence. The basis of epigenetics is the methylation of cytosine-phospho-guanosine (CpG) islands seen predominantly in actively transcribing genes. When DNA methylation occurs, with the participation of DNA methyltransferases, transcription factors and RNA polymerase fail to transcribe a gene "silenced" by methylation. Methylated CpG islands recruit methylated DNA-binding proteins. One of them is histone deacetylase. For transcription to occur, the N-terminal tail of histones must be acetylated. Histone deacetylation enables histone methyltransferases to methylate histone 3 and recruit heterochromatin protein-1 to trigger chromatin condensation. As you already know, heterochromatin (condensed chromatin) is transcriptionally inactive.

21. SPERM TRANSPORT AND MATURATION

Development of the testis

We start Chapter 21 by reviewing the major developmental steps of the gonads and excurrent (efferent) ducts. This review will lead us to an understanding of the histology, function, and clinical significance of the pathway followed by male and female gametes in the pursuit of fertilization.

An important aspect to keep in mind is that the cell precursors of both gametes have an **extra-embryonic origin**. Primordial germinal cells (**PGCs**) appear first in the endoderm of the **yolk sac** wall in the 4-week fetus (Figure 21-1).

Between 4 and 6 weeks, about 10 to 100 primordial germ cells migrate by **ameboid movements** from the yolk sac to the gut tube and from there to the right

Figure 21-1. Migration of primordial germinal cells from the yolk sac to the gonadal ridges

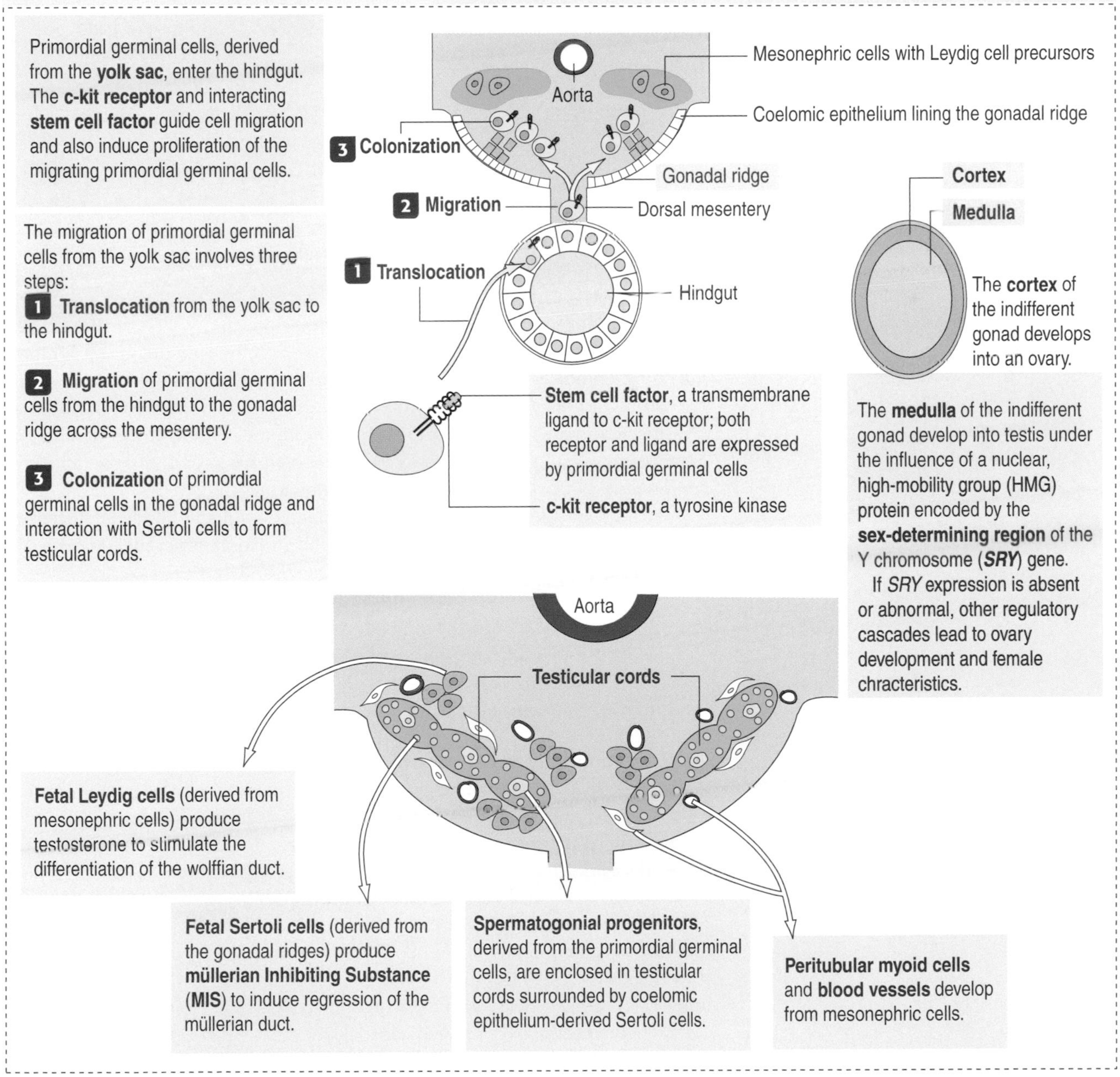

Primordial germinal cells, derived from the **yolk sac**, enter the hindgut. The **c-kit receptor** and interacting **stem cell factor** guide cell migration and also induce proliferation of the migrating primordial germinal cells.
The migration of primordial germinal cells from the yolk sac involves three steps:
1 **Translocation** from the yolk sac to the hindgut.
2 **Migration** of primordial germinal cells from the hindgut to the gonadal ridge across the mesentery.
3 **Colonization** of primordial germinal cells in the gonadal ridge and interaction with Sertoli cells to form testicular cords.
Aorta
Mesonephric cells with Leydig cell precursors
Coelomic epithelium lining the gonadal ridge
3 Colonization
Gonadal ridge
2 Migration
Dorsal mesentery
1 Translocation
Hindgut
Stem cell factor, a transmembrane ligand to c-kit receptor; both receptor and ligand are expressed by primordial germinal cells
c-kit receptor, a tyrosine kinase
Cortex
Medulla
The **cortex** of the indifferent gonad develops into an ovary.
The **medulla** of the indifferent gonad develop into testis under the influence of a nuclear, high-mobility group (HMG) protein encoded by the **sex-determining region** of the Y chromosome (***SRY***) gene.
If *SRY* expression is absent or abnormal, other regulatory cascades lead to ovary development and female characteristics.
Aorta
Testicular cords
Fetal Leydig cells (derived from mesonephric cells) produce testosterone to stimulate the differentiation of the wolffian duct.
Fetal Sertoli cells (derived from the gonadal ridges) produce **müllerian Inhibiting Substance** (**MIS**) to induce regression of the müllerian duct.
Spermatogonial progenitors, derived from the primordial germinal cells, are enclosed in testicular cords surrounded by coelomic epithelium-derived Sertoli cells.
Peritubular myoid cells and **blood vessels** develop from mesonephric cells.

Figure 21-2. Transformation of the indifferent gonad into the testis

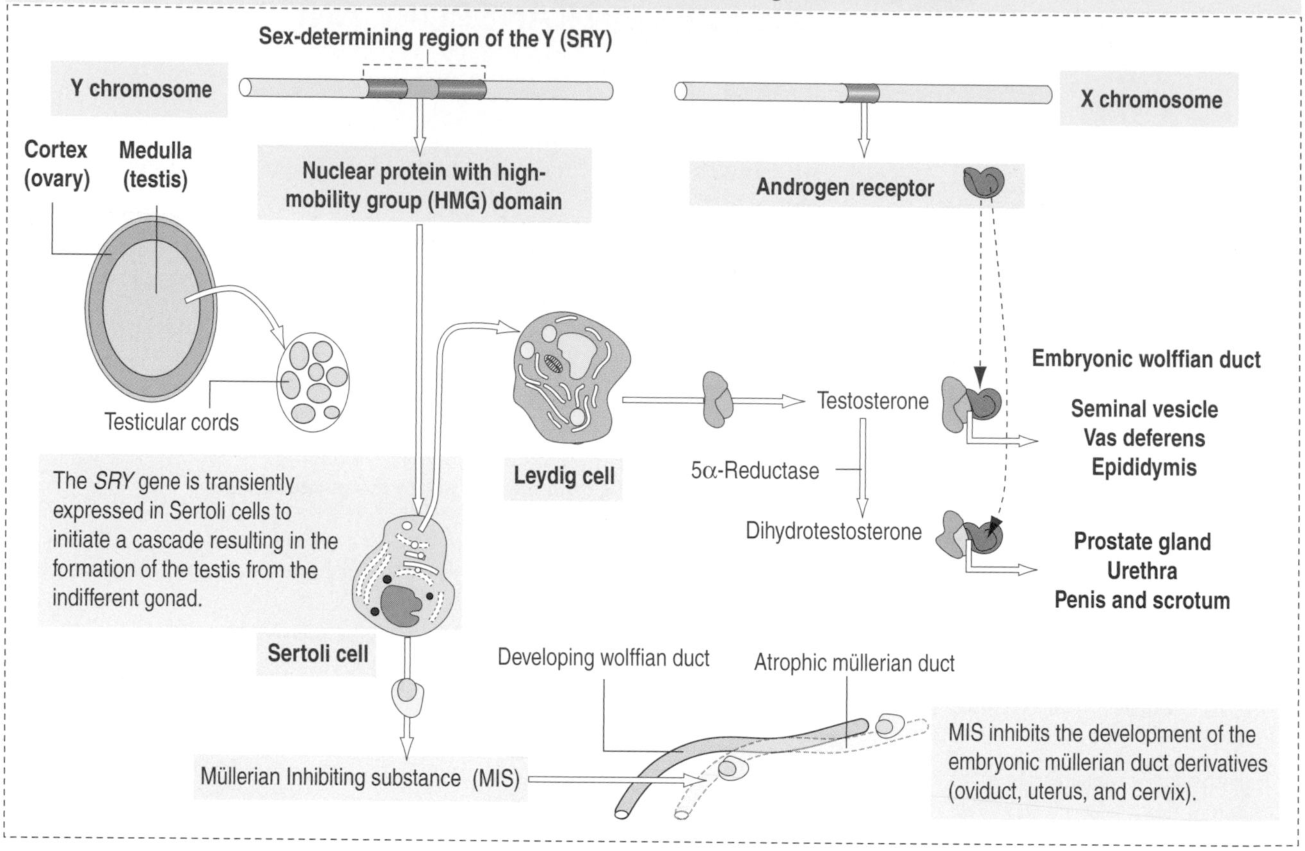
Sex-determining region of the Y (SRY)
Y chromosome
X chromosome
Cortex (ovary)
Medulla (testis)
Nuclear protein with high-mobility group (HMG) domain
Androgen receptor
Testicular cords
Embryonic wolffian duct
Testosterone
Seminal vesicle
Vas deferens
Epididymis
The SRY gene is transiently expressed in Sertoli cells to initiate a cascade resulting in the formation of the testis from the indifferent gonad.
Leydig cell
5α-Reductase
Dihydrotestosterone
Prostate gland
Urethra
Penis and scrotum
Sertoli cell
Developing wolffian duct
Atrophic müllerian duct
MIS inhibits the development of the embryonic müllerian duct derivatives (oviduct, uterus, and cervix).
Müllerian Inhibiting substance (MIS)

and left sides of the dorsal body wall through the mesentery. This movement can be followed by cytochemistry, since the plasma membrane of migrating and proliferating primordial germinal cells is rich in the enzyme **alkaline phosphatase**.

The migration and proliferation of primordial germinal cells are dependent on the interaction of the **c-kit receptor**, a **tyrosine kinase,** with its corresponding cell membrane ligand, **stem cell factor**. Both the c-kit receptor and stem cell factor are produced by primordial germinal cells along their migration route.

A lack of the c-kit receptor or stem cell factor results in gonads deficient in primordial germ cells. Hematopoiesis and the development of melanocytes and mast cells depend on the c-kit receptor and its ligand.

In the dorsal body wall, about 2500 to 5000 primordial germinal cells lodge in the mesenchyme at the level of the 10th thoracic vertebra and induce cells of the mesonephros and lining coelomic epithelium to proliferate, forming a pair of **gonadal ridges**. Coelomic epithelial cords grow into the mesenchyme of the gonadal ridge to form an **outer cortex** and **inner medulla** of the indifferent gonad.

Testis-determining factor controls the development of the testis

Until the seventh week of fetal development, there is one type of gonad common to both sexes. This is the "**indifferent**" stage of gonadal development. Thereafter, **in the female, the cortex develops into the ovary, and the medulla regresses. In the male, the cortex regresses and the medulla forms the testis.** The development of the testis is controlled by a **nuclear, high-mobility group** (HMG) **domain protein** encoded by the **sex-determining region of the Y chromosome** (***SRY***) **gene**. SRY protein binds and bends DNA. No target genes for SRY protein have been identified. **Sox9** (for SRY-box containing gene 9) is a possible candidate for a direct SRY target gene. Loss of Sox9 function results in **XY gonadal dysgenesis** in which patients have undeveloped gonadal structures (streak gonads) and absence of virilization (persistence of müllerian-derived structures).

Development of male and female internal genitalia: Role of müllerian-inhibiting substance and testosterone

The fetal testis is formed by **testicular cords** connected to the rete testis by tubuli recti. The cords are formed by **Sertoli cells**, derived from the coelomic epithelium, and **prespermatogonia** (also called **gonocytes**), derived from primordial germinal cells. **Leydig cells**, derived from the mesonephric mesenchyme, are present between the testicular cords.

Fetal Sertoli cells secrete **müllerian inhibiting substance** (MIS), which prevents müllerian ducts (also called paramesonephric ducts) from developing into the uterovaginal primordium (Figure 21-2). In the absence of MIS, the müllerian ducts persist and become the female internal genitalia.

By 8 weeks of gestation, fetal Leydig cells produce testosterone, which is regulated by placental human chorionic gonadotropin (hCG), since the fetal hypophysis is not secreting luteinizing hormone (LH).

The cephalic end of the wolffian ducts (also called mesonephric ducts) forms the epididymis, vas deferens, and ejaculatory duct. A diverticulum of the vas deferens forms the seminal vesicles.

The prostate gland and urethra develop from the urogenital sinus. The prostate gland has a dual origin: the glandular epithelium forms from outgrowths of the prostatic urethral endoderm; the stroma and smooth muscle derive from the surrounding mesoderm.

In the absence of androgen, the wolffian duct regresses and the prostate fails to develop. If high levels of androgen are present in the **female fetus**, both müllerian and wolffian ducts can persist (see Box 21-A).

Testicular descent

The **gubernaculum** forms on the lower pole of the testis, crosses obliquely through the abdominal wall, and attaches to the scrotal swelling. By week 28, the testis moves deep into the inguinal ring. The gubernaculum grows and the testis descends into the scrotum. For additional details, see Cryptorchidism (or undescended testis) in Chapter 20, Spermatogenesis.

Clinical significance: Klinefelter's syndrome

Klinefelter's syndrome is observed in males with an **extra X chromosome** (47,XXY). Individuals with this syndrome (1) are phenotypically males (presence of the Y chromosome); (2) have small testes and few spermatogenic cells are present; (3) have high follicle-stimulating hormone (FSH) levels because the function of Sertoli cells is abnormal (failure to produce inhibin); (4) have low testosterone levels, but **high estradiol levels**.

The excess of estradiol can lead to phenotypic feminization, including **gynecomastia**.

Clinical significance: Androgen insensitivity syndrome (testicular feminization)

Androgen insensitivity syndrome (AIS) results from a complete or partial defect in the gene controlling the expression of the androgen receptor. This gene is located on the X chromosome.

Although the karyotype is 46,XY, a deficiency in the action of androgen results in the lack of development of the wolffian duct and the regression of the müllerian duct because testes, and therefore Sertoli cell–derived MIS, are present.

No functional **internal genitalia** are present in patients with AIS: the testes remain in the abdomen (recall that androgens stimulate testicular descent).

The **external genitalia** develop as female. Individuals with complete AIS have labia, a clitoris, and a short vagina (these structures are not müllerian duct derivatives). Pubic and axillary hair is absent (sexual hair development is androgen-dependent).

At puberty, the production of both androgen and estradiol increases (the latter

Box 21-A | **Development of internal genitalia**

- When **Sertoli cell–derived MIS is not present**, the müllerian ducts become the fallopian tubes (oviducts), uterus, cervix, and upper one third of the vagina.
- When **Leydig cell–derived testosterone is present**, the wolffian ducts become the epididymis, vas deferens, seminal vesicles, and ejaculatory ducts.
- When **5-α reductase is present, testosterone is converted into dihydrotestosterone (DHT).** DHT induces the genital tubercle, genital fold, genital swelling, and urogenital sinus to become the penis, scrotum, and prostate.
- When **DHT is not present**, the genital tubercle, genital fold, genital swelling, and urogenital sinus become the labia majora, labia minora, clitoris, and lower two thirds of the vagina.

Figure 21-3. Sperm transport from testis to rete testis via straight tubules

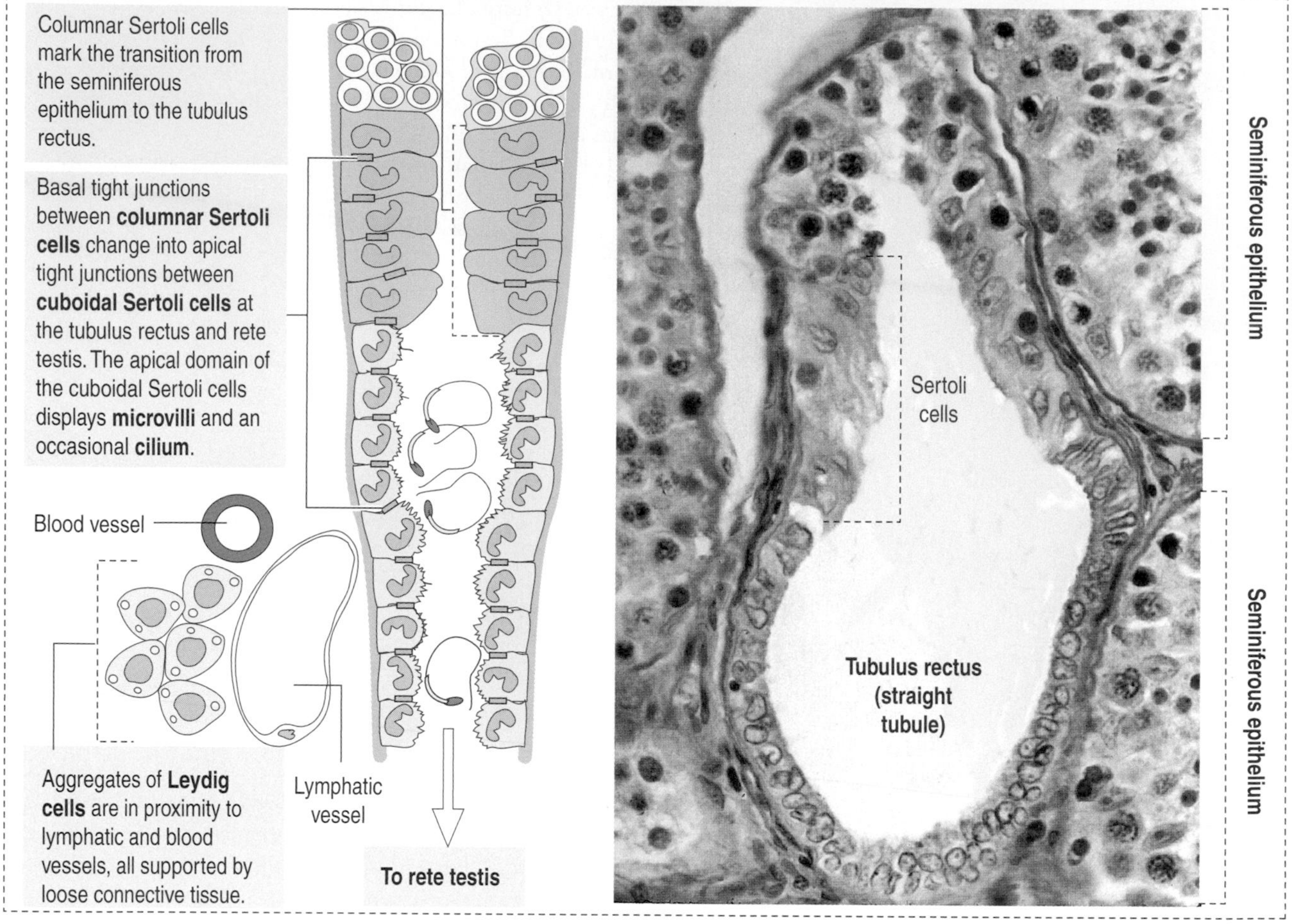
Columnar Sertoli cells mark the transition from the seminiferous epithelium to the tubulus rectus.
Basal tight junctions between **columnar Sertoli cells** change into apical tight junctions between **cuboidal Sertoli cells** at the tubulus rectus and rete testis. The apical domain of the cuboidal Sertoli cells displays **microvilli** and an occasional **cilium**.
Blood vessel
Aggregates of **Leydig cells** are in proximity to lymphatic and blood vessels, all supported by loose connective tissue.
Lymphatic vessel
To rete testis
Sertoli cells
Tubulus rectus (straight tubule)
Seminiferous epithelium
Seminiferous epithelium

from peripheral aromatization of androgens). Androgens cannot inhibit LH secretion (because a defective androgen receptor prevents LH feedback inhibition), and plasma levels of androgens remain high.

Clinical significance: 5α-Reductase deficiency

A defect in the activity of the enzyme 5α-reductase results in decreased formation of dihydrotestosterone (DHT). These individuals have normal internal genitalia (whose development from the wolffian duct is androgen-dependent) but nonmasculinized external genitalia. They are often mistaken for females at birth.

Sperm maturation pathway

After transport to the **rete testis** through a connecting **tubulus rectus** (Figure 21-3), sperm enter the **ductuli efferentes**. Ductuli efferentes link the rete testis to the initial segment of the epididymal duct, an irregularly coiled duct extending to the **ductus**, or **vas deferens**

Tubuli recti (**straight tubules**) are located in the mediastinum of the testis. They are lined by a **simple cuboidal epithelium** with structural features similar to those of Sertoli cells except that occluding junctions are now at the **apical domain**, instead of at the basal domain. Spermatogenic cells are not present.

The **rete testis** consists of irregularly anastomosing channels within the mediastinum of the testis (Figure 21-4). These channels are lined by a **simple cuboidal epithelium**. The wall, formed by fibroblasts and myoid cells, is surrounded by large lymphatic channels and blood vessels associated with large clusters of Leydig cells.

About 12 to 20 **ductuli efferentes** (**efferent ductules**) link the rete testis to the

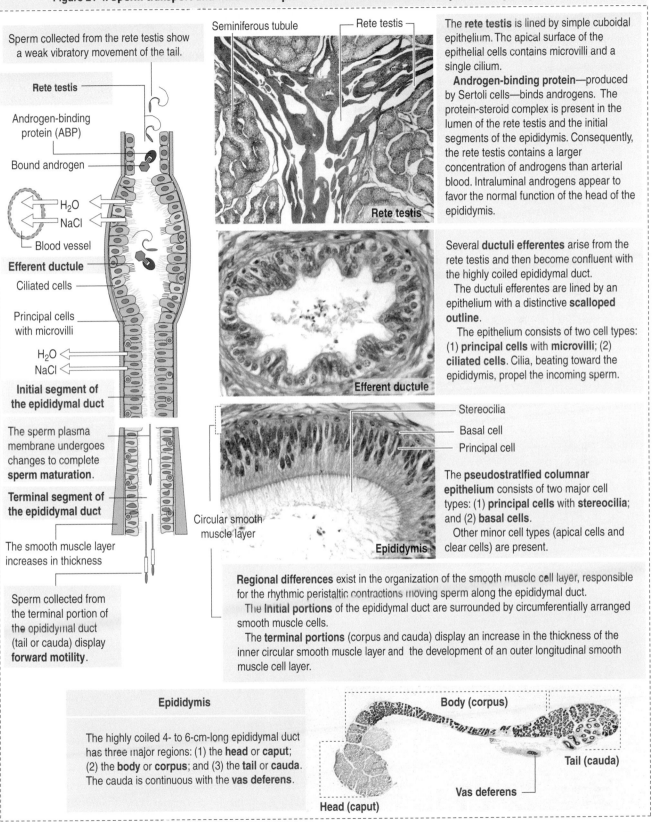

Figure 21-4. Sperm transport and fluid reabsorption in the efferent ductule and proximal epididymis

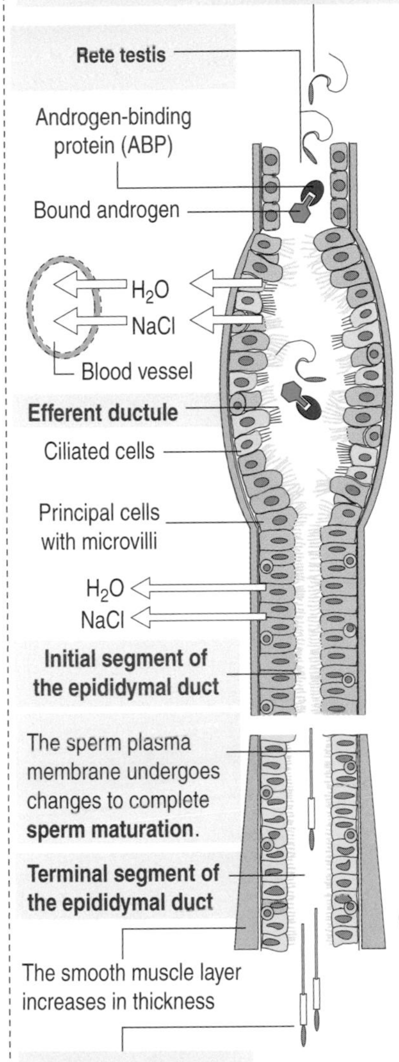
Sperm collected from the rete testis show a weak vibratory movement of the tail.
Rete testis
Androgen-binding protein (ABP)
Bound androgen
H_2O
NaCl
Blood vessel
Efferent ductule
Ciliated cells
Principal cells with microvilli
H_2O
NaCl
Initial segment of the epididymal duct
The sperm plasma membrane undergoes changes to complete **sperm maturation**.
Terminal segment of the epididymal duct
The smooth muscle layer increases in thickness
Sperm collected from the terminal portion of the epididymal duct (tail or cauda) display **forward motility**.

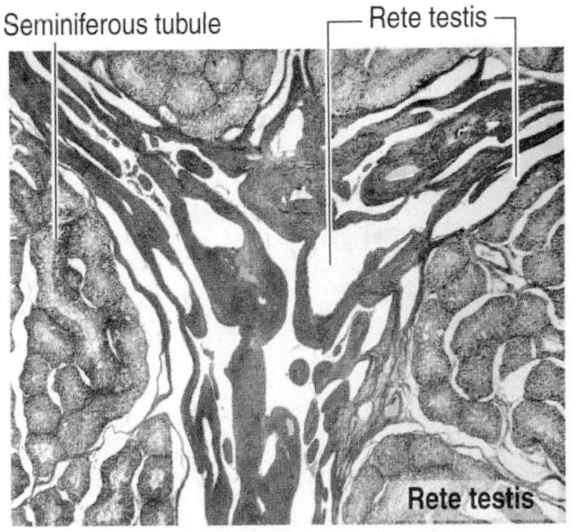
Seminiferous tubule
Rete testis
Rete testis

The **rete testis** is lined by simple cuboidal epithelium. The apical surface of the epithelial cells contains microvilli and a single cilium.

Androgen-binding protein—produced by Sertoli cells—binds androgens. The protein-steroid complex is present in the lumen of the rete testis and the initial segments of the epididymis. Consequently, the rete testis contains a larger concentration of androgens than arterial blood. Intraluminal androgens appear to favor the normal function of the head of the epididymis.

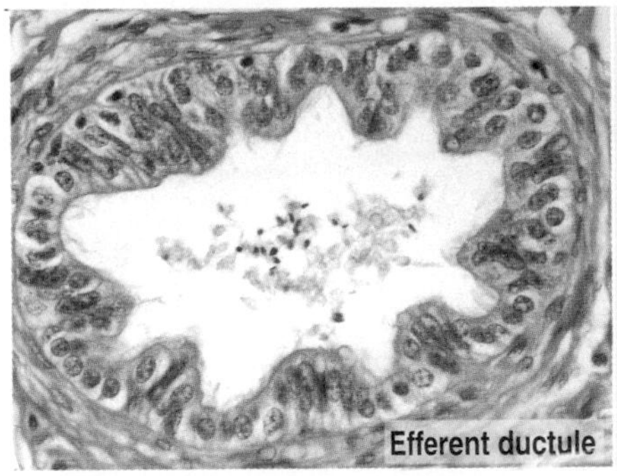
Efferent ductule

Several **ductuli efferentes** arise from the rete testis and then become confluent with the highly coiled epididymal duct.

The ductuli efferentes are lined by an epithelium with a distinctive **scalloped outline**.

The epithelium consists of two cell types: (1) **principal cells** with **microvilli**; (2) **ciliated cells**. Cilia, beating toward the epididymis, propel the incoming sperm.

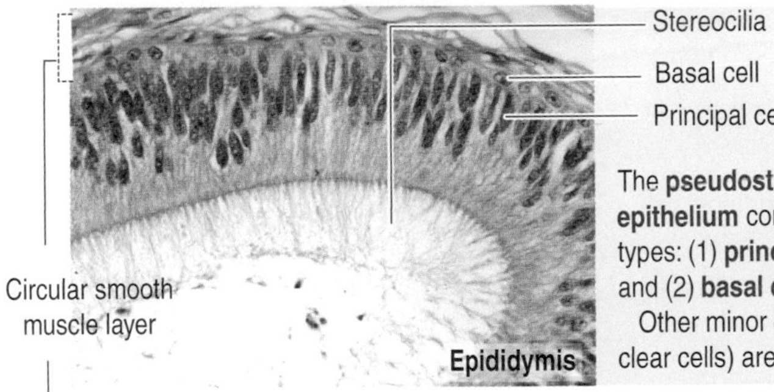
Stereocilia
Basal cell
Principal cell
Circular smooth muscle layer
Epididymis

The **pseudostratified columnar epithelium** consists of two major cell types: (1) **principal cells** with **stereocilia**; and (2) **basal cells**.

Other minor cell types (apical cells and clear cells) are present.

Regional differences exist in the organization of the smooth muscle cell layer, responsible for the rhythmic peristaltic contractions moving sperm along the epididymal duct.

The **initial portions** of the epididymal duct are surrounded by circumferentially arranged smooth muscle cells.

The **terminal portions** (corpus and cauda) display an increase in the thickness of the inner circular smooth muscle layer and the development of an outer longitudinal smooth muscle cell layer.

Epididymis

The highly coiled 4- to 6-cm-long epididymal duct has three major regions: (1) the **head** or **caput**; (2) the **body** or **corpus**; and (3) the **tail** or **cauda**. The cauda is continuous with the **vas deferens**.

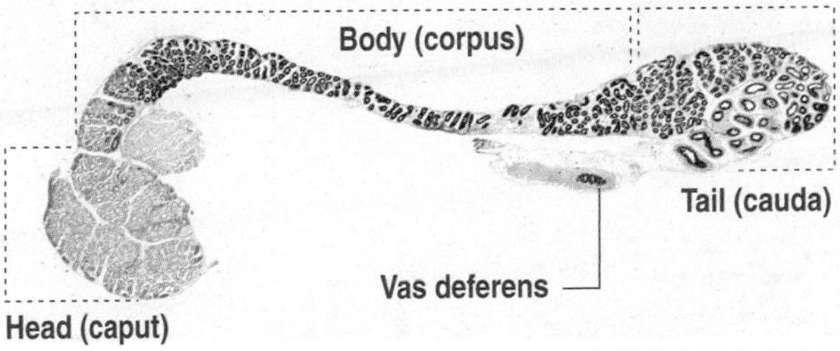
Body (corpus)
Tail (cauda)
Vas deferens
Head (caput)

epididymis after piercing the testicular tunica albuginea. Each ductule is lined by a **columnar epithelium** with **principal cells with microvilli**—with a role in the reabsorption of fluid from the lumen—and **ciliated cells,** which contribute

Figure 21-5. Epididymis

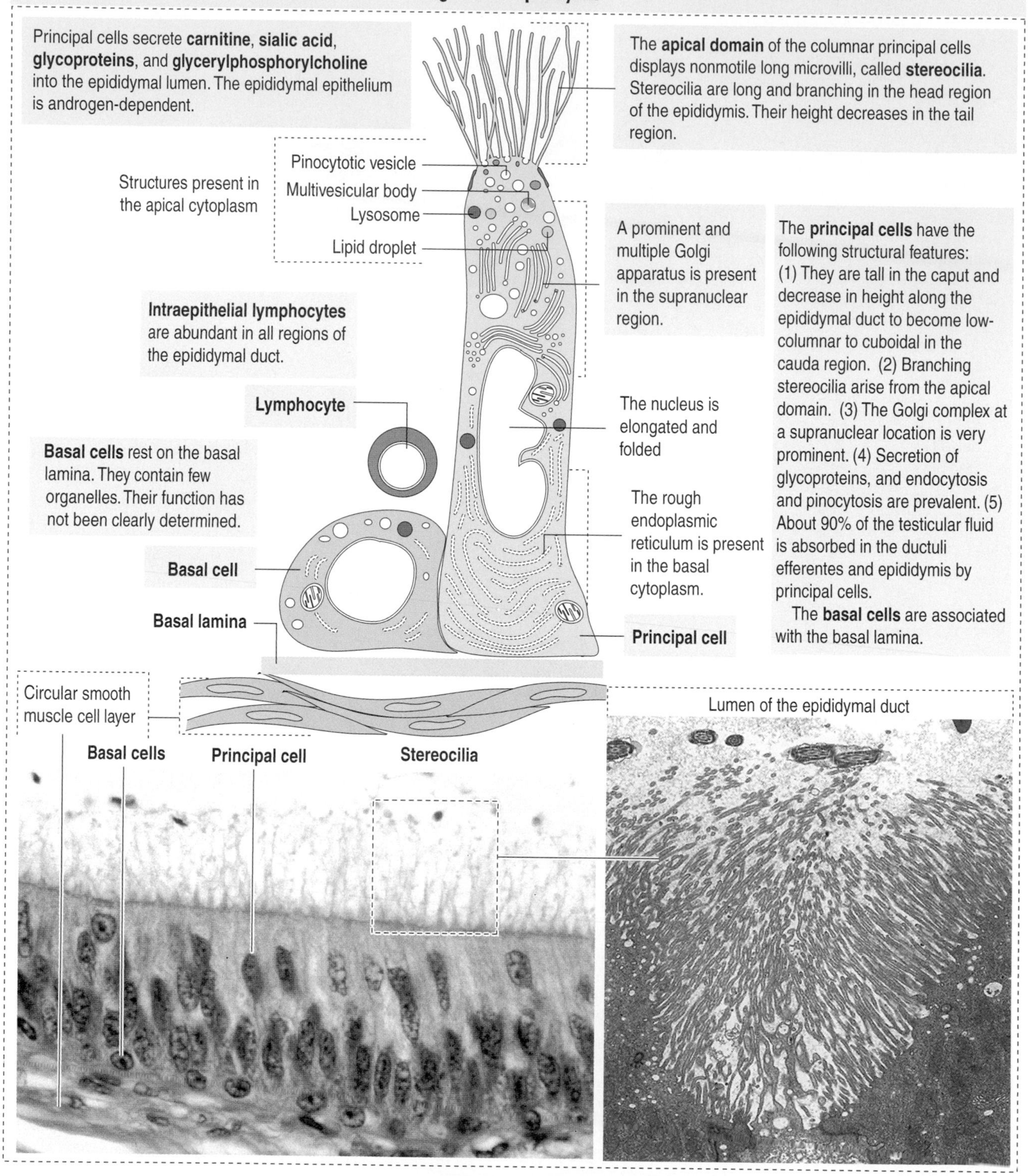

Principal cells secrete **carnitine**, **sialic acid**, **glycoproteins**, and **glycerylphosphorylcholine** into the epididymal lumen. The epididymal epithelium is androgen-dependent.
The **apical domain** of the columnar principal cells displays nonmotile long microvilli, called **stereocilia**. Stereocilia are long and branching in the head region of the epididymis. Their height decreases in the tail region.
Structures present in the apical cytoplasm
Pinocytotic vesicle
Multivesicular body
Lysosome
Lipid droplet
A prominent and multiple Golgi apparatus is present in the supranuclear region.
The **principal cells** have the following structural features: (1) They are tall in the caput and decrease in height along the epididymal duct to become low-columnar to cuboidal in the cauda region. (2) Branching stereocilia arise from the apical domain. (3) The Golgi complex at a supranuclear location is very prominent. (4) Secretion of glycoproteins, and endocytosis and pinocytosis are prevalent. (5) About 90% of the testicular fluid is absorbed in the ductuli efferentes and epididymis by principal cells.
The **basal cells** are associated with the basal lamina.
Intraepithelial lymphocytes are abundant in all regions of the epididymal duct.
Lymphocyte
The nucleus is elongated and folded
Basal cells rest on the basal lamina. They contain few organelles. Their function has not been clearly determined.
The rough endoplasmic reticulum is present in the basal cytoplasm.
Basal cell
Basal lamina
Principal cell
Circular smooth muscle cell layer
Lumen of the epididymal duct
Basal cells
Principal cell
Stereocilia

to the transport of **nonmotile sperm** toward the epididymis. **The epithelium has a characteristic scalloped outline that enables identification of the ductuli efferentes** (see Figure 21-4). A thin inner circular layer of **smooth muscle cells** underlies the epithelium and its basal lamina.

The **epididymis** is a highly coiled tubule (4 to 6 cm long) where spermatozoa mature (acquire a **forward motility pattern** essential to their **fertilizing ability**).

The epididymal duct is subdivided into three major segments: (1) the **head** or **caput**; (2) the **body** or **corpus**; and (3) the **tail** or **cauda** (see Figure 21-4).

Figure 21-6. **Spermatic cord**

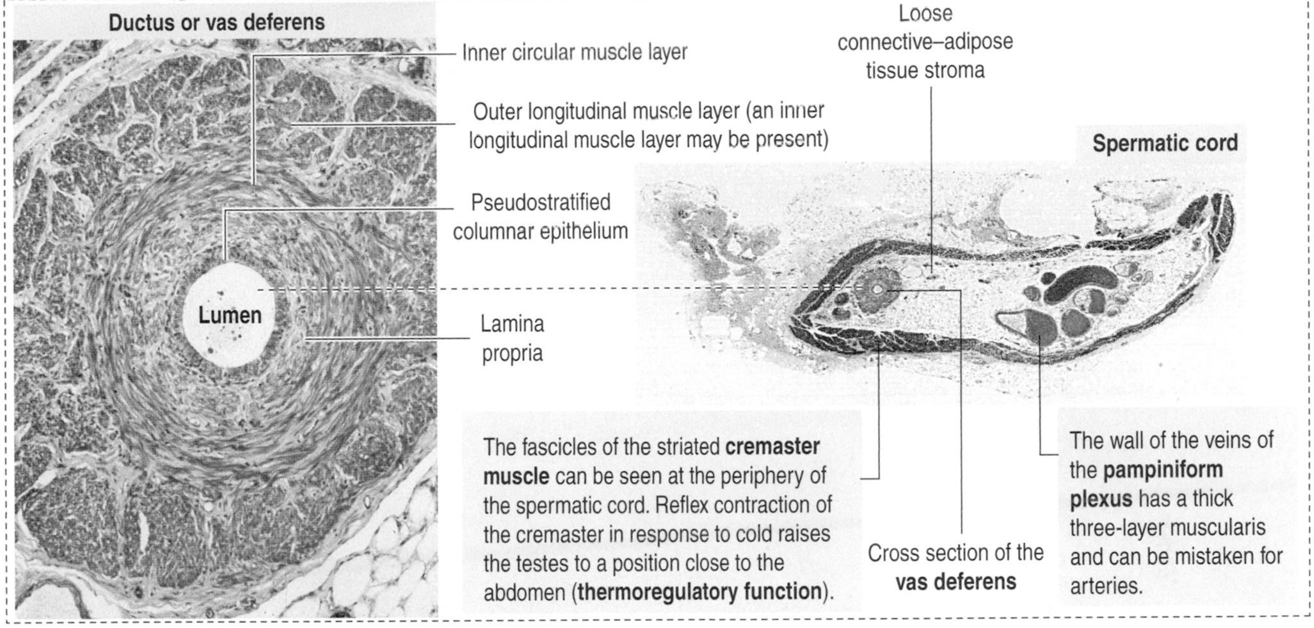

Ductus or vas deferens
Inner circular muscle layer
Outer longitudinal muscle layer (an inner longitudinal muscle layer may be present)
Pseudostratified columnar epithelium
Lumen
Lamina propria
Loose connective–adipose tissue stroma
Spermatic cord
The fascicles of the striated **cremaster muscle** can be seen at the periphery of the spermatic cord. Reflex contraction of the cremaster in response to cold raises the testes to a position close to the abdomen (**thermoregulatory function**).
Cross section of the **vas deferens**
The wall of the veins of the **pampiniform plexus** has a thick three-layer muscularis and can be mistaken for arteries.

The epithelium is **pseudostratified columnar** with long and branched **stereocilia**. The epithelium consists of **two major cell types** (Figure 21-5):

1. Columnar **principal cells**, extending from the lumen to the basal lamina. The apical domain of principal cells displays **branched stereocilia** and a well-developed Golgi apparatus, lysosomes, and vesicles.

2. **Basal cells** with a **pyramidal** shape associated with the basal lamina. Basal cells are regarded as the undifferentiated precursors of principal cells.

Other cell types are the **apical cells**, rich in mitochondria and predominant in the head of the epididymis, and the **clear cells**, predominant in the tail of the epididymis. **Intraepithelial lymphocytes** are distributed throughout the epididymis. They may be an important component of the epididymal immunologic barrier.

The **height of the epithelium** varies with respect to the segment of the epididymal duct. The epithelium is **taller in the head region** and **shorter in the tail region**. In an opposite fashion, the lumen of the epididymal duct is narrow in the head region and wider in the tail region.

An **inner smooth muscle circular layer**, of increasing thickness from head to tail, and an **outer longitudinal layer**, visible from the body on, surround the epithelium and basal lamina. The muscle layer displays **peristaltic movements** to facilitate sperm transport along the epididymal duct (Box 21-B).

The **vas deferens** (ductus deferens) is a 45-cm-long muscular tube with the following features: (1) the lining epithelium is **pseudostratified columnar with stereocilia** similar to that of the epididymis, and is supported by a connective tissue lamina propria with elastic fibers; (2) the muscular wall consists of **inner** and **outer layers** of longitudinally oriented muscle separated by a **middle circular layer**; and (3) the external layer consists of loose connective tissue and adipose cells.

In addition to the vas deferens, the **spermatic cord** contains the following components (Figure 21-6): (1) the **cremaster muscle**, (2) **arteries** (spermatic artery, cremasteric artery, and artery to the vas deferens), (3) **veins of the pampiniform plexus**, and (4) **nerves** (genital branch of the genitofemoral nerve, cremasteric nerve, and sympathetic branches of the testicular plexus). All these structures are surrounded by **loose connective tissue**.

An **ampulla**, the dilated portion of the vas deferens, leads directly into the prostate gland. The distal end receives the ducts of the seminal vesicle, forming the **ejaculatory ducts**, which pass through the prostate gland to empty secretion into the prostatic urethra at the seminal colliculus.

Box 21-B | **Epididymal duct**

The epididymis has three main functions:

- **Sperm transport** by peristalsis to the storage region, the tail of the epididymis. The time of sperm epididymal maturation is from 2 to 12 days.
- **Sperm storage** until ejaculation.
- **Sperm maturation**. Sperm collected from the head region of the epididymis are unable to fertilize. The fertilizing ability is acquired from the body to the tail of the epididymis.

  Sperm maturation includes:
  Stabilization of condensed chromatin.
  Changes in plasma membrane surface charge.
  Acquisition by sperm of new surface proteins.
  Acquisition of sperm forward motility.
- The development of the epididymal ducts, derived from the wolffian ducts, requires normal expression of *Homeobox A10 (Hoxa10)* and *Hoxa11* genes. Mutations in the genes encoding bone morphogenetic protein (Bmp) 4, Bmp7, and Bmp8 results in the defective differentiation of specific segments of the epididymal duct.

Figure 21-7. Seminal vesicle

Seminal vesicle

Highly folded mucosal layer. Primary epithelial folds branch into secondary and tertiary folds.

Epithelial folds are supported by loose connective tissue (lamina propria of the mucosa).

At high magnification, the epithelium of the seminal vesicle is **simple columnar** to **pseudostratified**.

The apical cytoplasm is vacuolated. It contains secretory granules.

The seminal vesicle contributes more than half of the volume of the semen. Sperm are not stored in the seminal vesicles.

The secretion consists of **fructose**, **prostaglandins**, and **seminal vesicle-specific proteins (coagulating proteins)**.

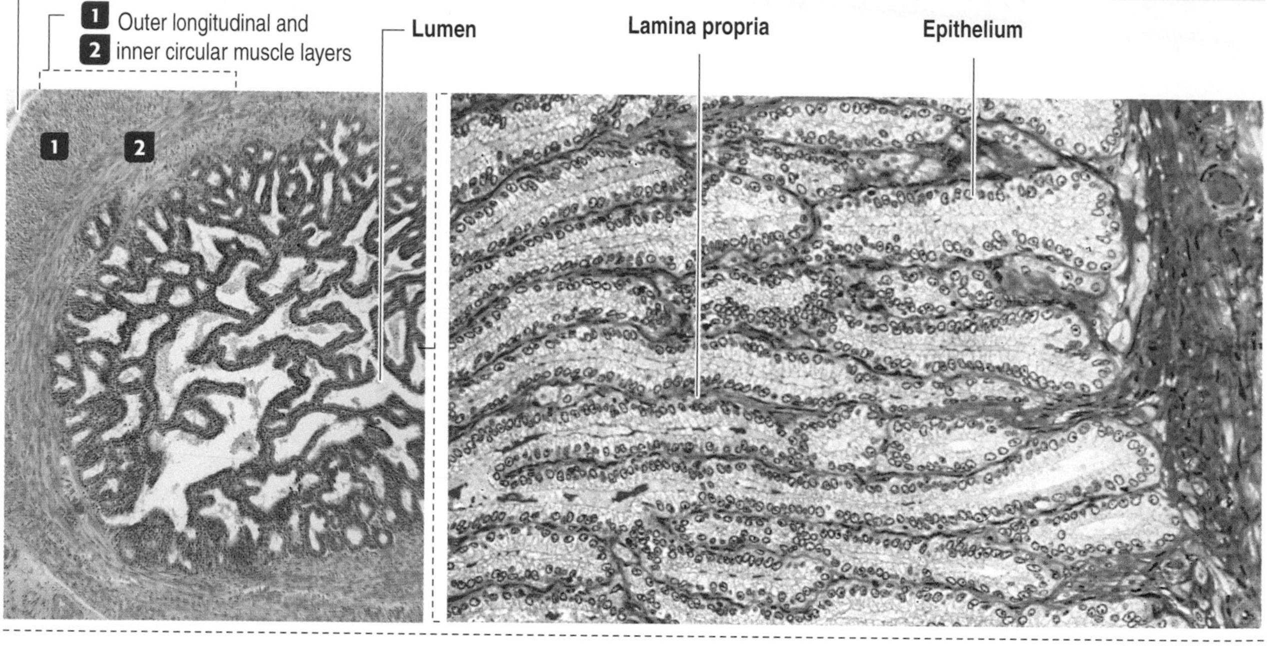

Connective tissue capsule
1 Outer longitudinal and
2 inner circular muscle layers
Lumen
Lamina propria
Epithelium
1
2

Figure 21-8. Ejaculatory ducts

The ducts of the seminal vesicles pierce the capsule of the prostate gland and join the vas deferens of the same side to form the **ejaculatory duct**.

The ejaculatory duct opens onto the posterior wall of the prostatic urethra. The wall of the ejaculatory ducts is folded and lined by **simple columnar epithelium** surrounded by connective tissue and bundles of smooth muscle.

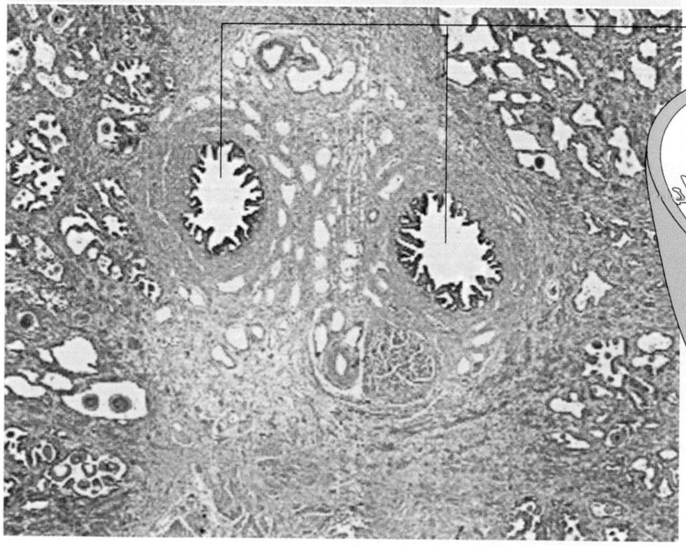

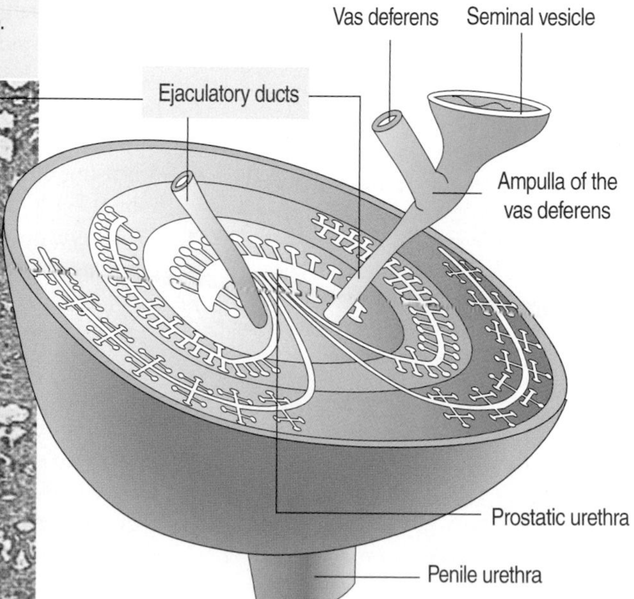

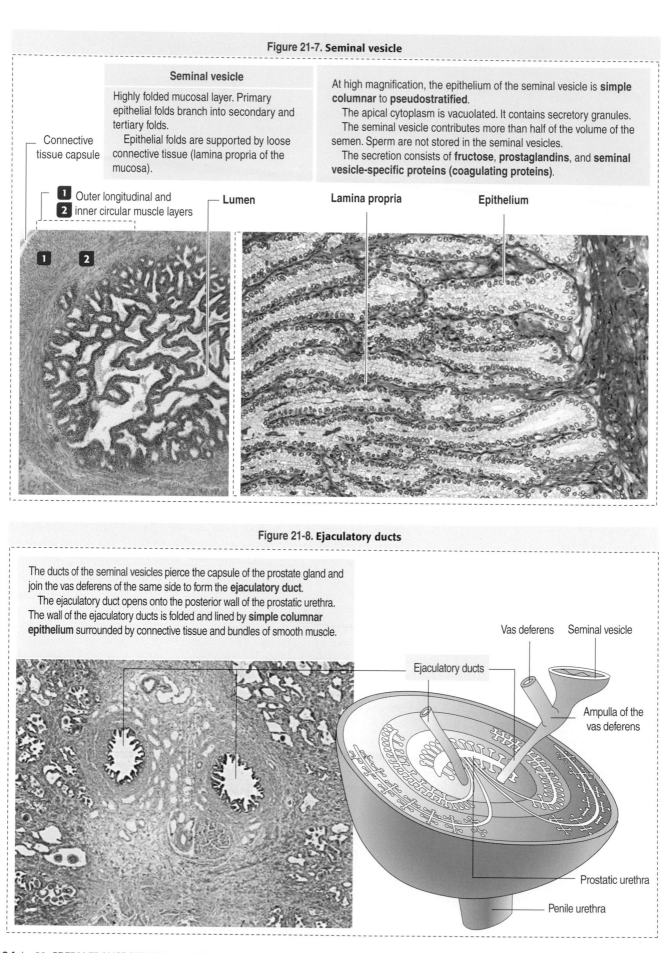

Vas deferens
Seminal vesicle
Ejaculatory ducts
Ampulla of the vas deferens
Prostatic urethra
Penile urethra

Accessory genital glands

The accessory glands of the male reproductive tract include two **seminal vesicles**, the **prostate gland**, and two **bulbourethral glands** of Cowper. The seminal vesicles and the prostate produce most of the seminal fluid, and their function is regulated by androgens (testosterone and DHT).

Seminal vesicles

The seminal vesicles are androgen-dependent organs. Each seminal vesicle consists of three components (Figure 21-7): (1) an **external connective tissue capsule**; (2) a **middle smooth muscle layer** (inner circular and outer longitudinal layers), and (3) an **internal highly folded mucosa** lined by a **simple cuboidal-to-pseudostratified columnar epithelium**.

The epithelial cells display a large Golgi apparatus with vesicles containing **secretory granules**. Seminal vesicles secrete an alkaline viscous fluid rich in **seminal coagulating proteins, fructose,** and **prostaglandins.** The fluid contributes about 70% to 85% of the human ejaculate.

Fructose is the major source of energy of the ejaculated sperm. Seminal vesicles do not store sperm. They contract during ejaculation. The excretory duct of each seminal vesicle penetrates the prostate after joining the vas deferens to form the ejaculatory duct (Figure 21-8).

Prostate gland

The prostate is the largest accessory genital gland surrounded by a capsule. It consists of 30 to 50 branched **tubuloalveolar glands** that empty their contents into the **prostatic urethra** via long excretory ducts.

The prostatic glands are arranged in three regions (Figure 21-9): (1) **periurethral mucosal glands**, (2) **periurethral submucosal glands**, and (3) **peripheral branched (compound) glands, called main glands**.

The glands are lined by **simple** or **pseudostratified columnar epithelium** (Figure 21-10). The lumen contains **prostatic concretions (corpora amylacea)** rich in glycoproteins and, sometimes, a site of **calcium deposition**. Cells contain abundant rough endoplasmic reticulum and Golgi apparatus.

The prostate produces an alkaline fluid that neutralizes the acidic vaginal content, provides nutrients and transports sperm, and liquefies semen.

Protein products include **prostate-specific acid phosphatase, prostate-specific antigen** (**PSA**, a valuable marker for early detection of prostatic cancer), **amylase**, and **fibrinolysin**.

Clinical significance: Benign prostatic hyperplasia and prostate cancer

Benign prostatic hyperplasia (or **BPH**) is a noncancerous enlargement of the prostate gland that can restrict the flow of urine through the prostatic urethra.

The periurethral mucosal and submucosal prostatic glands and the stroma undergo **nodular hyperplasia** (see Figure 21-9) in older men.

Nodular hyperplasia produces:

1. Difficulty in urination and urinary obstruction caused by compression of the prostatic urethra by the nodular growth.

2. Retention of urine in the bladder or inability to empty the urinary bladder completely. The possibility of infection leads to inflammation of the urinary bladder (**cystitis**) and renal infection (**pyelonephritis**). Acute and persistent urinary retention requires emergency catheterization.

BPH is caused by **DHT**, a metabolite of testosterone (Figure 21-11). The enzyme **5α-reductase**, present mainly in prostatic **stromal cells**, converts testosterone to DHT.

DHT binds to cytosol and nuclear androgen receptors to induce the expression of **growth factors** mitogenic to prostatic epithelial and stromal cells. Inhibitors of 5α-reductase reduce the production of DHT, decrease the periurethral nodular hyperplasia, and alleviate urinary obstruction.

Figure 21-9. Prostate gland

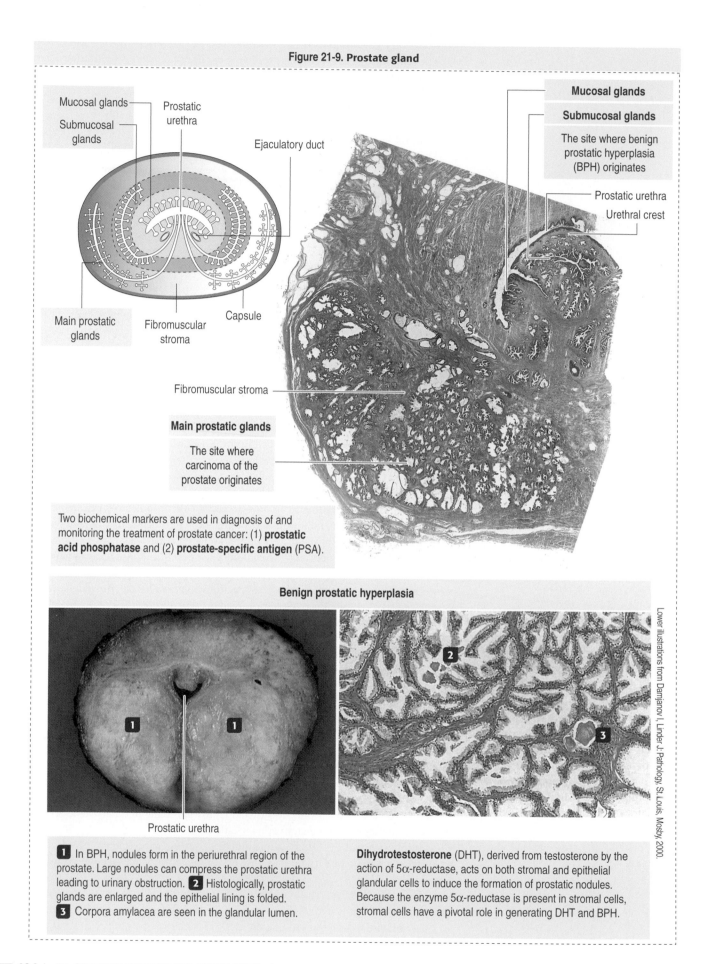

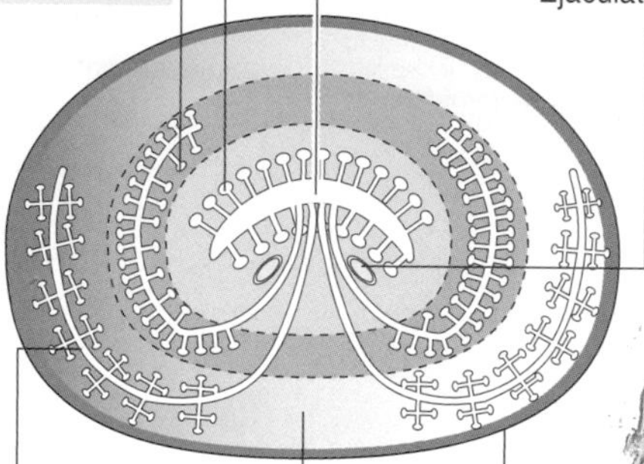

Mucosal glands
Submucosal glands
Prostatic urethra
Ejaculatory duct
Main prostatic glands
Fibromuscular stroma
Capsule

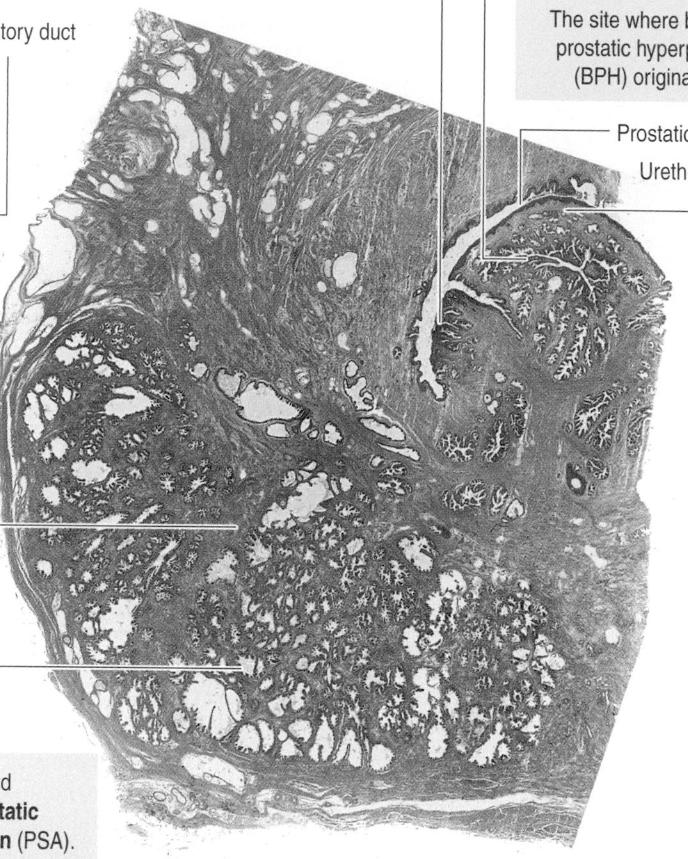

Mucosal glands
Submucosal glands
The site where benign prostatic hyperplasia (BPH) originates
Prostatic urethra
Urethral crest
Fibromuscular stroma
Main prostatic glands
The site where carcinoma of the prostate originates

Two biochemical markers are used in diagnosis of and monitoring the treatment of prostate cancer: (1) **prostatic acid phosphatase** and (2) **prostate-specific antigen** (PSA).

Benign prostatic hyperplasia

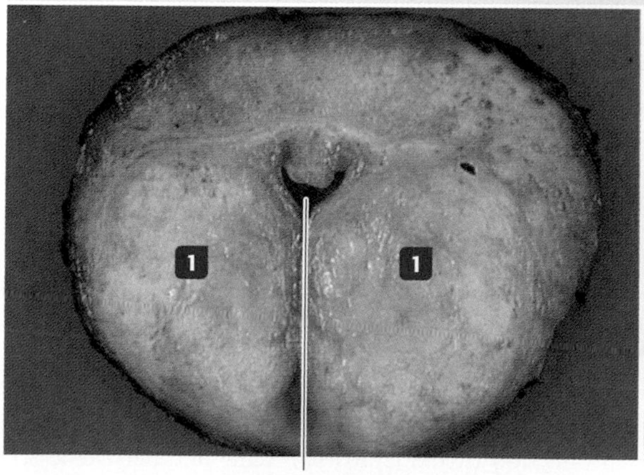

1
1
Prostatic urethra

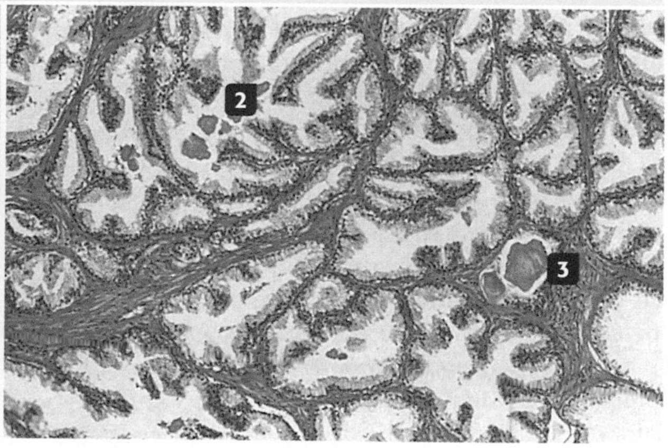

2
3

Lower illustrations from Damjanov I, Linder J: Pathology. St. Louis, Mosby, 2000.

1 In BPH, nodules form in the periurethral region of the prostate. Large nodules can compress the prostatic urethra leading to urinary obstruction. **2** Histologically, prostatic glands are enlarged and the epithelial lining is folded. **3** Corpora amylacea are seen in the glandular lumen.

Dihydrotestosterone (DHT), derived from testosterone by the action of 5α-reductase, acts on both stromal and epithelial glandular cells to induce the formation of prostatic nodules. Because the enzyme 5α-reductase is present in stromal cells, stromal cells have a pivotal role in generating DHT and BPH.

Figure 21-10. Main prostatic tubuloalveolar glands

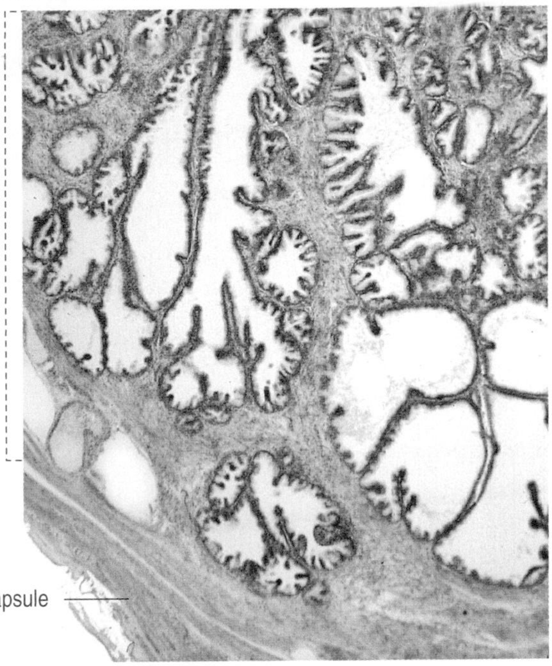
Main prostatic tubuloalveolar glands
Capsule

Main prostatic glands

The prostate is a muscular and glandular organ. It consists of three groups of glands: (1) **periurethral mucosal glands**; (2) **periurethral submucosal glands, linked to the urethra by short ducts**; and (3) **main prostatic glands**. About 30 to 50 tubuloalveolar glands open directly into the prostatic urethra through 15 to 30 long ducts ending at the sides of the urethral crest.

The epithelium of the main prostatic glands is **simple columnar** or **pseudostratified** and arranged into folds supported by a lamina propria. The lumen may contain **corpora amylacea**, a condensed structure rich in glycoproteins and cell fragments, with a tendency to calcify in older men.

The secretion of the prostate contains **fibrinolysin**, with a role in the liquefaction of semen. **Citric acid**, **zinc, amylase, prostate-specific antigen**, and **acid phosphatase** are present in high concentrations in prostatic fluid secreted in the semen.

The prostatic epithelium is androgen-dependent.

Carcinoma of the prostate originates from the main prostatic glands, farthest from the urethra. Urinary symptoms are not present at the early stage and tumor growth is often detected by digital palpation of the prostate, by elevated serum levels of **PSA**, or by back pain caused by vertebral **metastasis**. Transperineal or transrectal **biopsy**, if required, confirm a clinical diagnosis.

As in BPH, androgens also play a role in the development of prostate carcinoma. Tumor growth can be controlled by reducing androgen production (for example, using luteinizing hormone–releasing hormone [LH-RH] agonists and antiandrogens) or, in hormone-resistant prostate cancer, by **orchidectomy** (surgical removal of the testes, the major source of androgens) and chemotherapy.

Figure 21-11. Stromal-prostatic epithelial cell interaction

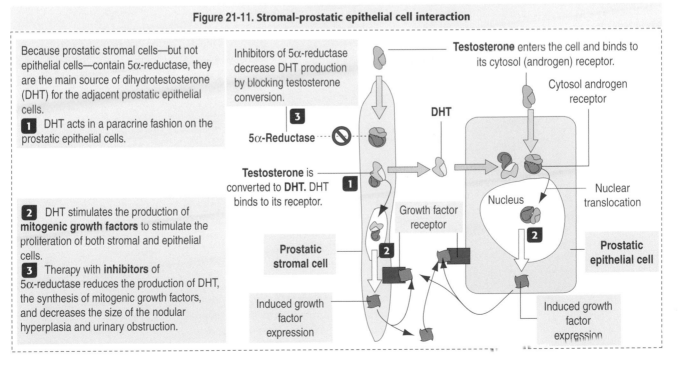

Because prostatic stromal cells—but not epithelial cells—contain 5α-reductase, they are the main source of dihydrotestosterone (DHT) for the adjacent prostatic epithelial cells.

1 DHT acts in a paracrine fashion on the prostatic epithelial cells.

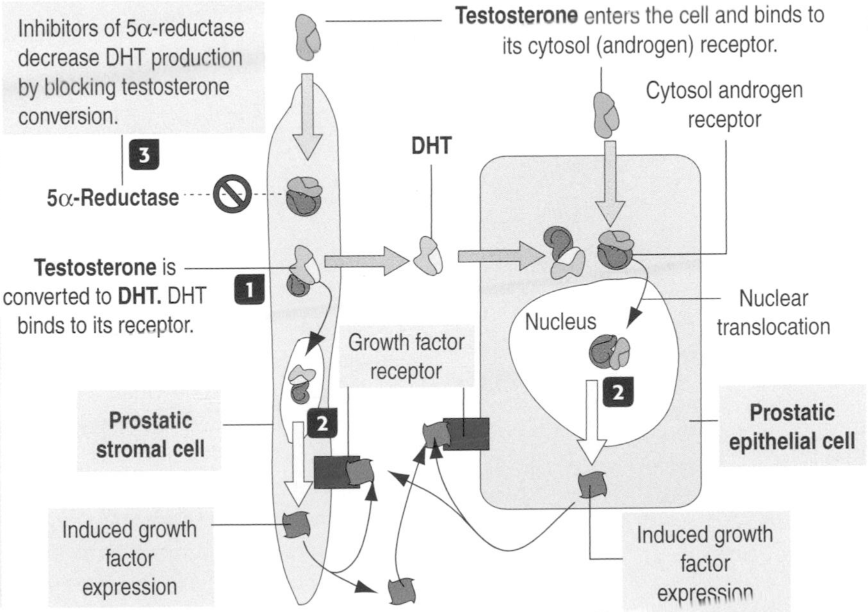
Inhibitors of 5α-reductase decrease DHT production by blocking testosterone conversion.
3
5α-Reductase
Testosterone enters the cell and binds to its cytosol (androgen) receptor.
Cytosol androgen receptor
DHT
Testosterone is converted to **DHT.** DHT binds to its receptor.
1
Nucleus
Nuclear translocation
Growth factor receptor
2
2
Prostatic stromal cell
Prostatic epithelial cell
Induced growth factor expression
Induced growth factor expression

2 DHT stimulates the production of **mitogenic growth factors** to stimulate the proliferation of both stromal and epithelial cells.

3 Therapy with **inhibitors** of 5α-reductase reduces the production of DHT, the synthesis of mitogenic growth factors, and decreases the size of the nodular hyperplasia and urinary obstruction.

Figure 21-12. **Female and male urethra**

Penis

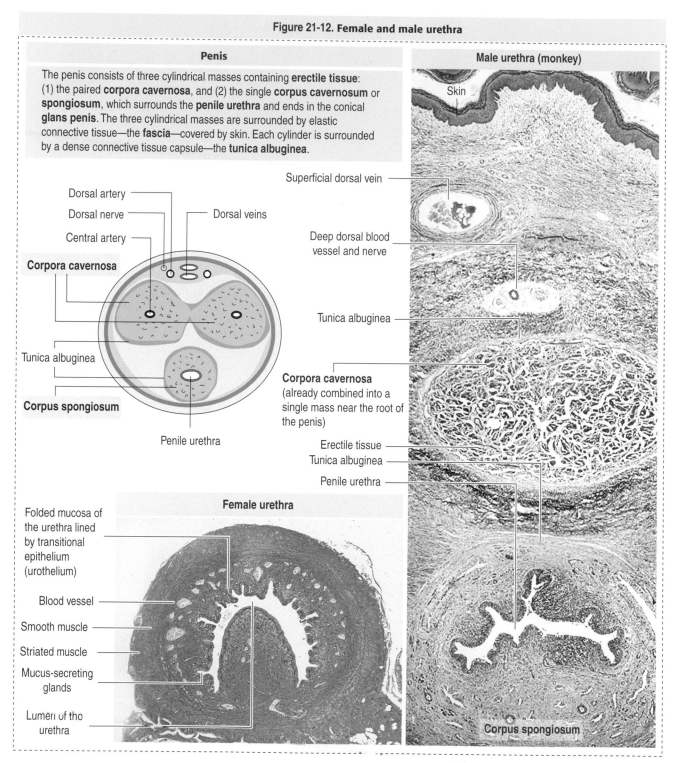

The penis consists of three cylindrical masses containing **erectile tissue**: (1) the paired **corpora cavernosa**, and (2) the single **corpus cavernosum** or **spongiosum**, which surrounds the **penile urethra** and ends in the conical **glans penis**. The three cylindrical masses are surrounded by elastic connective tissue—the **fascia**—covered by skin. Each cylinder is surrounded by a dense connective tissue capsule—the **tunica albuginea**.

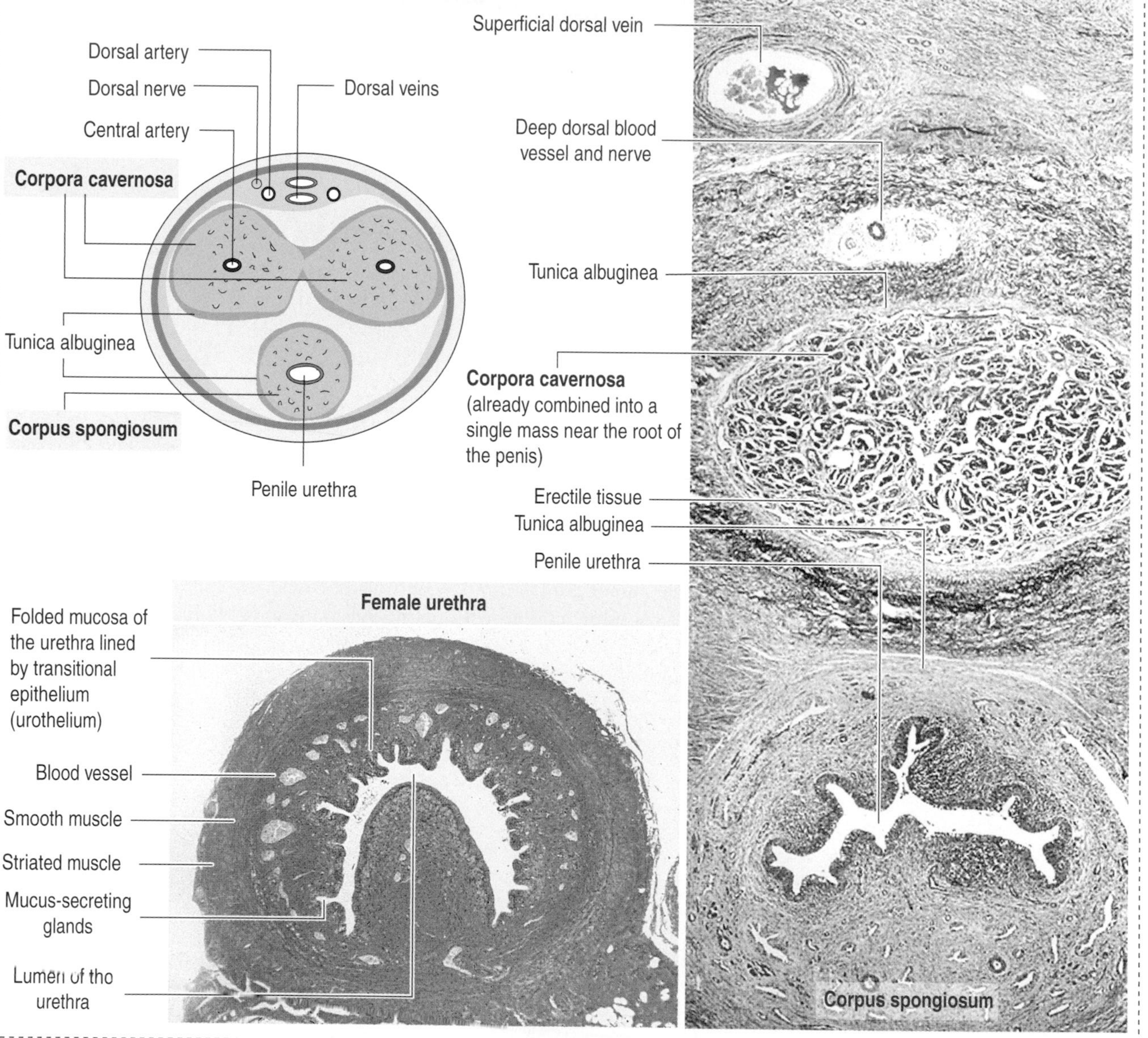

Dorsal artery
Dorsal nerve
Dorsal veins
Central artery
Corpora cavernosa
Tunica albuginea
Corpus spongiosum
Penile urethra
Male urethra (monkey)
Skin
Superficial dorsal vein
Deep dorsal blood vessel and nerve
Tunica albuginea
Corpora cavernosa (already combined into a single mass near the root of the penis)
Erectile tissue
Tunica albuginea
Penile urethra
Corpus spongiosum
Female urethra
Folded mucosa of the urethra lined by transitional epithelium (urothelium)
Blood vessel
Smooth muscle
Striated muscle
Mucus-secreting glands
Lumen of the urethra

Surgery (radical prostatectomy by retropubic or perineal surgery) and radiotherapy (external beam radiation therapy or radioactive seed implants in the prostate) are suitable when the tumor is localized as determined by computer imaging techniques.

Male and female urethra

The urethra in the **male** is 20 cm long and has three segments:

1. The **prostatic urethra**, which receives products transported by the ejaculatory ducts and the ducts of the prostatic glands.
2. The **membranous urethra**, the shortest segment.

Figure 21-13. Mechanism of penile erection

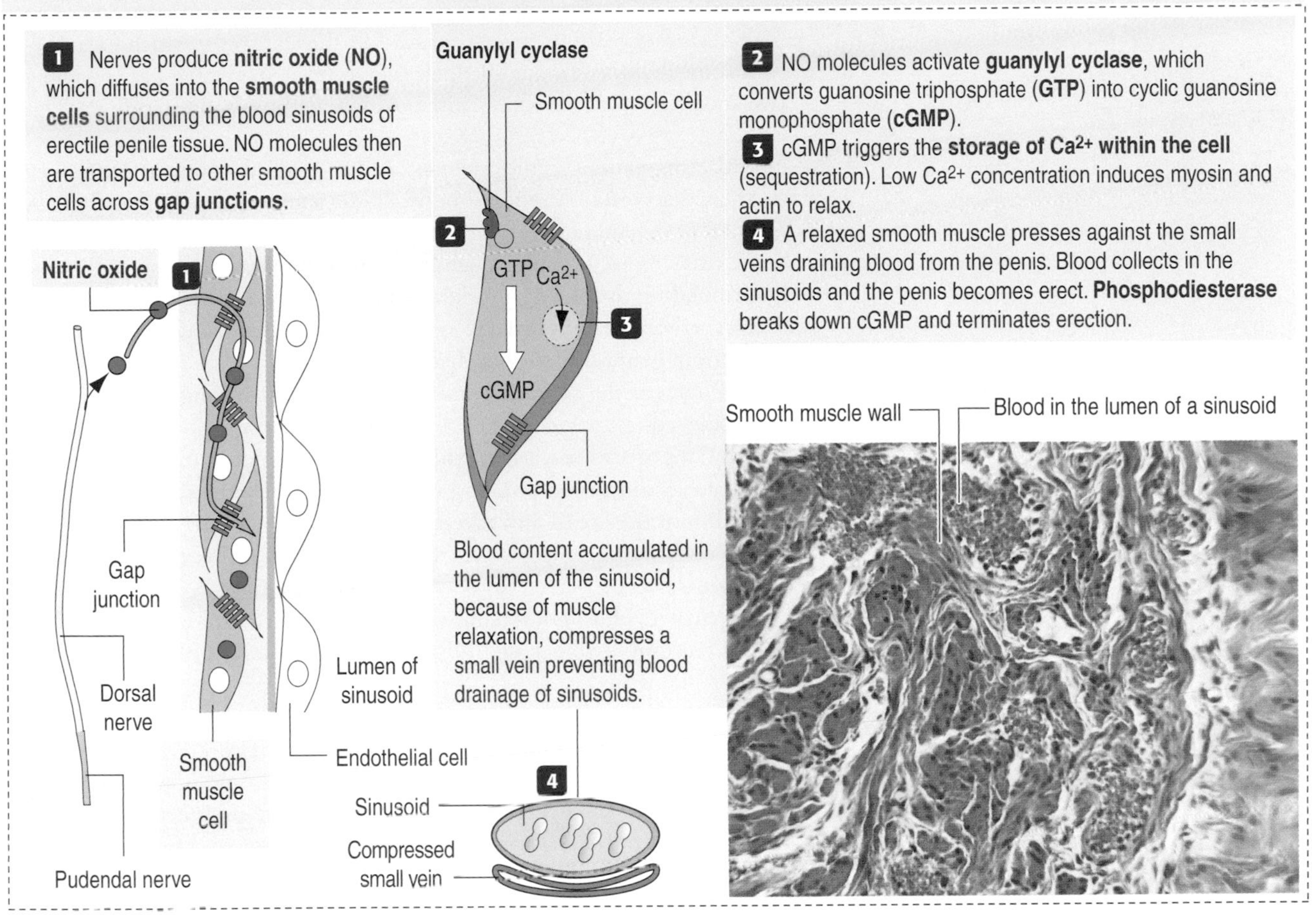
1 Nerves produce nitric oxide (NO), which diffuses into the smooth muscle cells surrounding the blood sinusoids of erectile penile tissue. NO molecules then are transported to other smooth muscle cells across gap junctions.
Guanylyl cyclase
Smooth muscle cell
2 NO molecules activate guanylyl cyclase, which converts guanosine triphosphate (GTP) into cyclic guanosine monophosphate (cGMP).
3 cGMP triggers the storage of Ca2+ within the cell (sequestration). Low Ca2+ concentration induces myosin and actin to relax.
4 A relaxed smooth muscle presses against the small veins draining blood from the penis. Blood collects in the sinusoids and the penis becomes erect. Phosphodiesterase breaks down cGMP and terminates erection.
Nitric oxide
1
2
GTP
Ca2+
3
cGMP
Gap junction
Smooth muscle wall
Blood in the lumen of a sinusoid
Gap junction
Dorsal nerve
Smooth muscle cell
Pudendal nerve
Lumen of sinusoid
Endothelial cell
Blood content accumulated in the lumen of the sinusoid, because of muscle relaxation, compresses a small vein preventing blood drainage of sinusoids.
4
Sinusoid
Compressed small vein

3. The **penile urethra**, which receives the ducts of the bulbourethral glands (Figure 21-12).

The epithelium of the prostatic urethra is **transitional (urothelium)**. It changes to a pseudostratified-to-stratified columnar epithelium in the membranous and penile urethra. The **muscle layer** in the membranous urethra consists of a smooth muscle sphincter (involuntary) and a striated muscle sphincter (voluntary). It controls the passage of urine or semen.

The urethra in the **female** is 4 cm long and is lined by **transitional epithelium** changing to pseudostratified columnar and stratified squamous nonkeratinized epithelium near the urethral meatus. The mucosa contains mucus-secreting glands (see Figure 21-12). An inner layer of smooth muscle is surrounded by a circular layer of striated muscle that closes the urethra when contracted.

Bulbourethral glands

The bulbourethral glands consist of several lobules containing tubuloalveolar secretory units and a main excretory duct lined by a stratified columnar epithelium. The lining epithelium of the secretory units is columnar and secretes a mucus product. The secretion, containing abundant **galactose** and a moderate amount of **sialic acid**, is discharged into the **penile urethra**. This secretion has a **lubrication function** and precedes the emission of semen along the penile urethra.

Penis

The penis consists of three cylindrical columnar masses of **erectile tissue** (see Figure 21-12): the right and left **corpora cavernosa**, and the ventral **corpus spongiosum**, transversed by the penile urethra. The three columns converge to form the shaft of the penis. The distal tip of the corpus spongiosum is the **glans penis**.

The corpora cavernosa and corpus spongiosum contain irregular and communicating blood spaces, or sinusoids, supplied by an artery and drained by venous channels. During erection, arterial blood fills the sinusoids, which enlarge and compress the draining venous channels (Figure 21-13).

Two chemicals control erection: **nitric oxide** and **phosphodiesterase** (see Figure 21-13).

1. Sexual stimulation, via the cerebral cortex and hypothalamus and transported down the spinal cord to autonomic nerves in the penis, causes the branches of the **dorsal nerve**, the end point of the pudendal nerve, to produce **nitric oxide.**

Nitric oxide molecules spread rapidly across **gap junctions** of **smooth muscle cells** surrounding the blood sinusoids. Within smooth muscle cells, nitric oxide molecules activate **guanylyl cyclase** to produce **cyclic guanosine monophosphate (cGMP) from guanosine triphosphate** (GTP).

cGMP **relaxes the smooth muscle cell wall** surrounding the sinusoids by inducing the **sequestration of Ca^{2+}** within intracellular storage sites. The lowered concentrations of Ca^{2+} determine the relaxation of smooth muscle cells, which leads to the accumulation of blood in the sinusoids by the rapid flow of arterial blood from the dorsal and cavernous arteries (see Figure 21-13). Sinusoids engorged with blood compress the small veins that drain blood from the penis and the penis becomes erect.

2. The enzyme **phosphodiesterase** (PDE) is produced to destroy cGMP and terminate erection. By blocking PDE activity, cGMP levels remain elevated and the penis remains erect.

Clinical significance: Erectile dysfunction

Factors that affect the cerebral cortex–hypothalamus–spinal cord–autonomic nerve pathway and vascular diseases can cause erectile dysfunction. Traumatic head and spinal cord injuries, stroke, Parkinson's disease, and systemic diseases, such as diabetes and multiple sclerosis, reduce nerve function and lead to erectile dysfunction. In addition, anxiety disorders can be a primary cause of erectile dysfunction.

Sildenafil (Viagra) was originally tested as a treatment for heart failure. During clinical trials, it was noticed that a significant number of patients were getting erections after taking the drug. This observation initiated an independent clinical study to evaluate the effect of sildenafil in the treatment of impotence.

In the penis, sildenafil blocks a specific phosphodiesterase found in smooth muscle cells, and, by this mechanism, inhibits the degradation of cGMP. High levels of cGMP induce Ca^{2+} to enter storage areas in the cell and induce the perisinusoidal smooth muscle cells to relax.

Sildenafil can cause dose-dependent side effects such as facial flushing, gastrointestinal distress, headaches, and a blue tinge to vision.

• Primordial germinal cells (PGCs), the precursors of the female and male gametes, have an extra-embryonic origin. They appear first in the wall of the yolk sac in the 4-week fetus.

Between 4 and 6 weeks, PGCs migrate to the gonadal ridges by translocation from the yolk sac to the hindgut, migration from the hindgut to the gonadal ridges across the mesentery, and colonization in the gonadal ridges. The migration step involves the participation of the c-kit receptor, a tyrosine kinase, and stem cell factor, the c-kit ligand. A lack of c-kit receptor or its ligand causes the gonadal ridges and gonads to be deficient in PGCs.

In the gonadal ridges, XX chromosome-containing PGCs occupy the cortex, and XY chromosome-containing PGCs localize in the medulla, the central portion of the gonadal ridges. After 7 weeks, the indifferent gonad contains a cortex, which develops into an ovary, and a medulla, which develops into a testis.

The development of the testis is controlled by testis-determining factor, a product of a gene on the sex-determining region of the Y chromosome (*SRY*).

The initial components of the fetal testis are the testicular cords. A testicular cord contains Sertoli cells and prespermatogonia (also called gonocytes) derived from PGCs. Leydig cells are present between the testicular cords. Fetal Sertoli cells secrete müllerian inhibiting substance (MIS), which induces regression by apoptosis of the müllerian duct (paramesonephric duct). Leydig cells, stimulated by human chorionic gonadotropin, secrete testosterone. Testosterone is converted to dihydrotestosterone (DHT) by 5α-reductase. Tetosterone stimulates the cephalic end of the wolffian duct (mesonephric duct) to develop the epididymis, vas deferens, and seminal vesicle. DHT stimulates the development of the prostate gland and urethra from the urogenital sinus. Testosterone and DHT bind to androgen receptor, a cytosol-nuclear protein encoded by a gene on the X chromosome.

Klinefelter's syndrome (47,XXY) is observed in males with an extra X chromosome. Individials are phenotypically males, have atrophic testes, and the blood levels of testosterone are low but the levels of estradiol are high. Excess of estradiol causes gynecomastia.

Androgen insensitivity syndrome (AIS, also called testicular feminization) is determined by a complete or partial defect in the expression of androgen receptor. A lack of development of the wolffian duct and regression of the müllerian duct are observed. Testes remain in the abdomen, and external genitalia develop as female. Blood levels of androgens and estradiol are high.

5α-Reductase deficiency determines a decrease in the conversion of testosterone to DHT. Individuals have normal internal genitalia but female external genitalia.

• Sperm maturation pathway. After leaving the seminiferous tubule, immature sperm follow this sequential pathway:

1. Tubuli recti (straight tubules): Narrow tubular structures lined by a simple cuboidal epithelium. Tight junctions occupy an apical position, in contrast to the basally located inter–Sertoli cell tight junctions.

2. Rete testis: A network of anastomosing channels lined by simple cuboidal epithelium. The wall consists of myoid cells and fibroblasts.

3. Ductuli efferentes (efferent ductules): They connect the rete testis to the initial region of the epididymal duct. The epithelial lining consists of principal cells with microvilli (instead of stereocilia) and ciliated cells, involved in the transport of nonmotile sperm toward the epididymis. Clusters of these two cell types, differing in height, give the epithelium a characteristic scalloped outline.

4. Epididymis: A highly coiled duct (4 to 6 cm long) with three typical anatomic regions: Head or caput, body or corpus, and tail or cauda. The lining epithelium is pseudostratified columnar with stereocilia. The wall contains smooth muscle cells. The two major epithelial cell types are the columnar principal cells with apical stereocilia, and basal cells, associated to the basal lamina. Intraepithelial lymphocytes are frequently seen. The height of the principal cells decreases towards the tail region. Consequently, the lumen becomes progressively wider. The thickness of the muscle wall increases toward the epididymal tail region.

5. Vas deferens (ductus deferens): A muscular tube with a length of 45 cm. It can be seen in the spermatic cord. The vas deferens is lined by pseudostratified columnar epithelium with stereocilia. The smooth muscle cell layer consists of a middle circular layer surrounded by inner and outer longitudinal layers. Additional components of the spermatic cord include the cremaster muscle, arteries (spermatic, cremasteric, and vas deferens arteries), veins of the pampiniform plexus (important for spermatic artery—pampiniform plexus heat transfer to maintain testicular temperature 2°C to 3°C below body temperature for normal spermatogenesis), and nerves. The vas deferens ends in a dilated ampulla receiving the duct of the seminal vesicle to form the ejaculatory duct passing through the prostate gland.

• Accessory genital glands. The accessory glands of the male reproductive system are the seminal vesicles, the prostate gland, and the bulbourethral glands of Cowper.

Each seminal vesicle consists of three components: (1) an external connective tissue capsule, (2) a middle smooth muscle layer, and (3) an internal highly folded mucosa lined by a simple cuboidal-to-pseudostratified columnar epithelium supported by a lamina propria. Under the influence of androgens, the seminal vesicle epithelium contributes 70% to 85% of an alkaline fluid to the human ejaculate. The fluid contains seminal coagulating proteins, fructose, and prostaglandins.

The prostate gland is a branched (compound) tubuloalveolar gland. The prostatic glands are distributed in three regions: (1) periurethral mucosal glands, (2) periurethral submucosal glands, and (3) peripheral branched glands, called main glands. Glands are lined by simple or pseudostratified columnar epithelium. The lumen contains corpora amylacea, rich in glycoproteins. The alkaline fluid produced by the prostate gland contains acid phosphatase and prostate-specific antigen (PSA). The alkaline nature of the semen neutralizes the acidic vaginal environment produced by vaginal lactic acid.

A combined enlargement of the periurethral mucosal and submucosal glands and surrounding stroma accounts for **benign prostatic hyperplasia (BPH).** BPH is determined by growth factors with mitogenic action produced by both stromal and glandular epithelial cells stimulated by dihydrotestosterone (DHT). Testosterone is converted to DHT by the enzyme 5α-reductase. Blocking agents of 5α-reductase activity and antiandrogens are used in the nonsurgical treatment of BPH. **Cancer of the prostate** is the result of the malignant transformation of the main prostatic glands. Blood levels of PSA are elevated in patients with prostatic cancer.

Bulbourethral glands secrete a lubricating mucus product into the penile urethra.

• Male and female urethra. The male urethra has a length of 20 cm and consists of three segments: (1) the prostatic urethra, whose lumen receives fluid transported by the ejaculatory ducts and products from the prostatic glands, (2) the membranous urethra, and (3) the penile urethra, which receives a lubricating fluid from the bulbourethral glands. The epithelium of the prostatic urethra is transitional (urothelium) with regional variations. Smooth muscle and striated muscle sphincters are present in the membranous urethra. The female urethra is shorter (4 cm long) and is lined by transitional epithelium, also with regional variations. The mucosa contains mucus-secreting glands. Inner smooth and outer striated muscle cell layers are observed.

• Penis. The penis consists of three cylindrical structures of erectile tissue: a pair of corpora cavernosa and a single corpus spongiosum. The three cylindrical structures converge to form the shaft of the penis. The tip of the corpus spongiosum is the glans penis. The erectile tissue contains vascular spaces, called sinusoids, supplied by arterial blood and drained by venous channels. During erection, arterial blood fills the sinusoids, which compress the adjacent venous channels preventing draining.

Nitric oxide, produced by branches of the dorsal nerve, spreads across gap junctions between smooth muscle cells surrounding the sinusoids. Within smooth muscle cells, nitric oxide activates guanylyl cyclase to produce cyclic guanosine monophosphate (cGMP) from guanosine triphosphate (GTP). cGMP relaxes the smooth muscle by sequestering calcium into intracellular storage sites, and arterial blood accumulates in the distended sinusoids and the penis becomes erect. The enzyme phosphodiesterase degrades cGMP, thus terminating erection. Sildenafil, a phosphodiesterase inhibitor, is used to prevent rapid cGMP degradation in cases of **erectile dysfunction.**

22. FOLLICLE DEVELOPMENT AND MENSTRUAL CYCLE

Development of the female reproductive tract

An important feature of the development of the female and male reproductive tracts is the initial **indifferent stage.** Knowledge of the developmental sequence from the indifferent stage to the fully developed stage is helpful in understanding the structural anomalies that can sometimes be observed. The female reproductive system is composed of the **ovaries**, the **ducts** (**oviduct**, **uterus**, and **vagina**), and the **external genitalia** (**labia majora**, **labia minora**, and **clitoris**). The development of these components is summarized in the next section.

Development of the ovary

As discussed in Chapter 21, Sperm Transport and Maturation, the **cortical region** of the primitive gonad develops into an ovary. The cortical region of the **indifferent gonad** initially contains the **primary sex cords**, extending into the mesenchyme from the **coelomic epithelium** (fifth week of development).

One week later, cells of the primary cell cords degenerate and are replaced by **secondary sex cords** that surround individual **oogonia** (Figure 22-1).

Oogonia result from the mitotic division of migrating **primordial germinal cells** derived from the yolk sac. Primordial germinal cells contain two X chromosomes. The **testis-determining factor** (TDF), encoded by the gene ***SRY*, on the sex-determining region of the Y chromosome**, is obviously not present.

In the fetal ovary, oogonia enter meiotic prophase I to become **primary oocytes** that become arrested after completion of crossing over (exchange of genetic information between nonsister chromatids of homologous chromosomes). **Meiotic prophase arrest continues until puberty**, when one or more follicles are stimulated to develop.

Figure 22-1. **From the indifferent gonad to the ovary and testis**

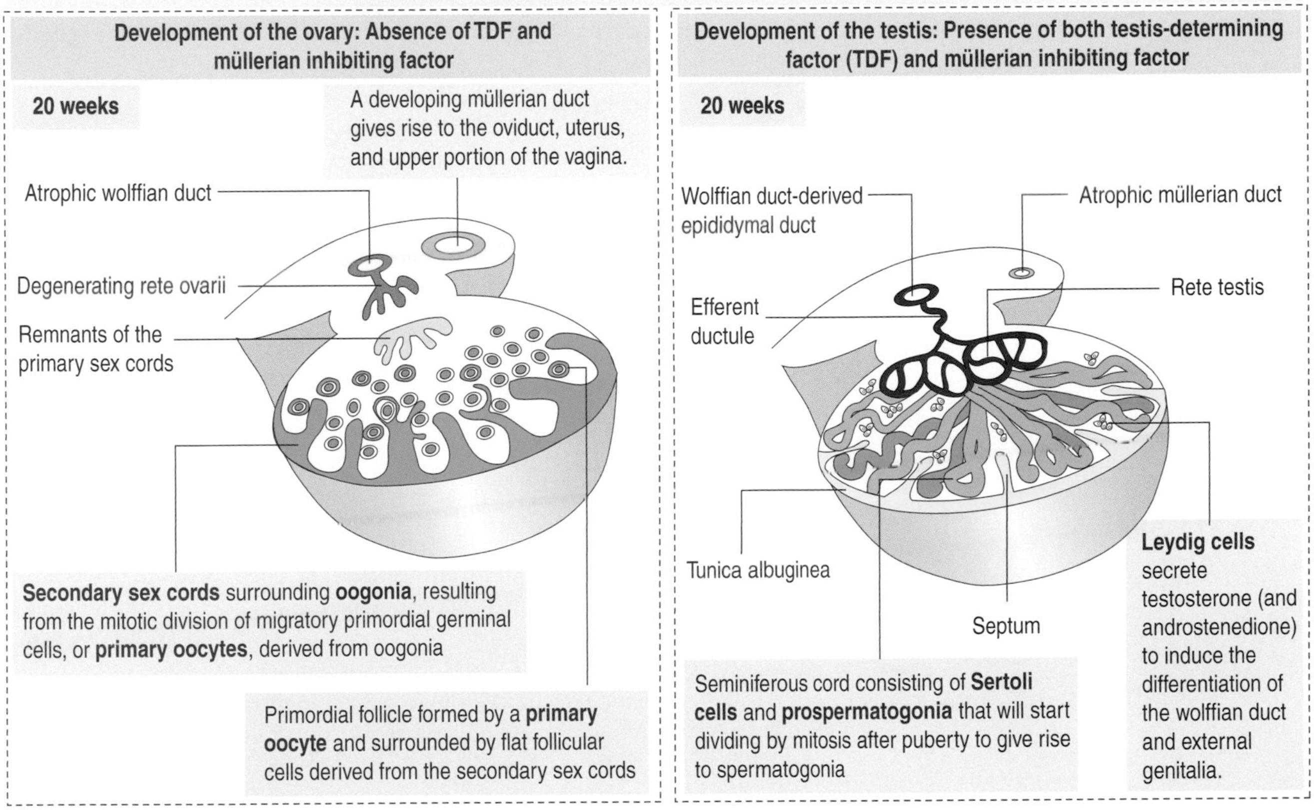
Development of the ovary: Absence of TDF and müllerian inhibiting factor
20 weeks
A developing müllerian duct gives rise to the oviduct, uterus, and upper portion of the vagina.
Atrophic wolffian duct
Degenerating rete ovarii
Remnants of the primary sex cords
Secondary sex cords surrounding oogonia, resulting from the mitotic division of migratory primordial germinal cells, or primary oocytes, derived from oogonia
Primordial follicle formed by a primary oocyte and surrounded by flat follicular cells derived from the secondary sex cords
Development of the testis: Presence of both testis-determining factor (TDF) and müllerian inhibiting factor
20 weeks
Wolffian duct-derived epididymal duct
Atrophic müllerian duct
Rete testis
Efferent ductule
Tunica albuginea
Septum
Seminiferous cord consisting of Sertoli cells and prospermatogonia that will start dividing by mitosis after puberty to give rise to spermatogonia
Leydig cells secrete testosterone (and androstenedione) to induce the differentiation of the wolffian duct and external genitalia.

Development of the female genital ducts

During development, the **cranial ends of the müllerian ducts** remain separated to form the **oviducts**, which open into the coelomic cavity (the future peritoneal cavity). The **caudal segments of the müllerian ducts** fuse to develop into the **uterovaginal primordium** that becomes the **uterus** and **upper part of the vagina**. The **broad ligaments** of the uterus, derived from two peritoneal folds, approach each other when the müllerian ducts fuse.

The **primitive cloaca** is divided by the **urorectal septum** into two regions: (1) the **ventral urogenital sinus** and (2) the **dorsal anorectal canal**.

The urorectal septum fuses with the cloacal membrane (the future site of the perineal body), which is divided into the **dorsal anal membrane** and the larger **ventral urogenital membrane**. By week 7, the membranes rupture.

The contact of the uterovaginal primordium with the urogenital sinus results in the formation of the **vaginal plate**. The **canalization of the vaginal plate** results in the development of the middle and lower portions of the vagina:

1. The solid mass of cells of the vaginal plate extends from the urogenital sinus into the uterovaginal primordium.
2. The central cells of the vaginal plate disappear, forming the lumen of the vagina.
3. The peripheral cells persist and form the vaginal epithelium.

The urogenital sinus also gives rise to the urinary bladder, urethra, vestibular glands, and hymen.

Development of the external genitalia

By week 4, the **genital tubercle**, or **phallus**, develops at the cranial end of the **cloacal membrane**. Then, **labioscrotal swellings** and **urogenital folds** develop at either side of the cloacal membrane.

The genital tubercle enlarges in both the female and male. In the absence of androgens, the external genitalia are feminized: the **phallus** develops into the **clitoris**. The **urogenital folds** form the **labia minora**, and the **labioscrotal swellings** develop into the **labia majora**.

Clinical significance: Developmental anomalies of the female genital tract

Imperforate hymen results from the **incomplete canalization of the vaginal plate**. This condition obstructs the passage of menstrual blood when menarche occurs and is accompanied by pain in the lower abdomen and bulging of the vaginal introitus. Hymenotomy is the definitive treatment.

In **müllerian agenesis (Rokitansky-Küster-Hauser syndrome)**, the uterus, cervix, and upper vagina are absent. Although **normal ovulation occurs**, there is **no menstruation**. In addition to agenesis of the müllerian duct, renal anomalies (unilateral kidney agenesis) occur in 25% to 30% of cases.

Clinical significance: Developmental anomalies of the ovary: Turner's syndrome

The fundamental genetic defect recognized in prepubertal and pubertal girls with **Turner's syndrome** is the **absence of all or part of a second X chromosome** (45,X) and **no Barr bodies**.

Both the short arm and the long arm of the X chromosome contain genes important for ovarian function. At birth, the ovaries are represented by **streaks**. Loss of the short arm (Xp, p for petite) results in **short stature and the typical skeletal changes**. A deletion on the Xp regions (Xp11.4) causes **lymphedema**, another typical feature of Turner's syndrome.

Ovarian failure is characterized by decreased or absent production of estrogens in association with elevated levels of gonadotropins, resulting in a failure to establish secondary sexual development (lack of estrogens).

Recombinant growth hormone administration is recommended when there is

Figure 22-2. Ovary

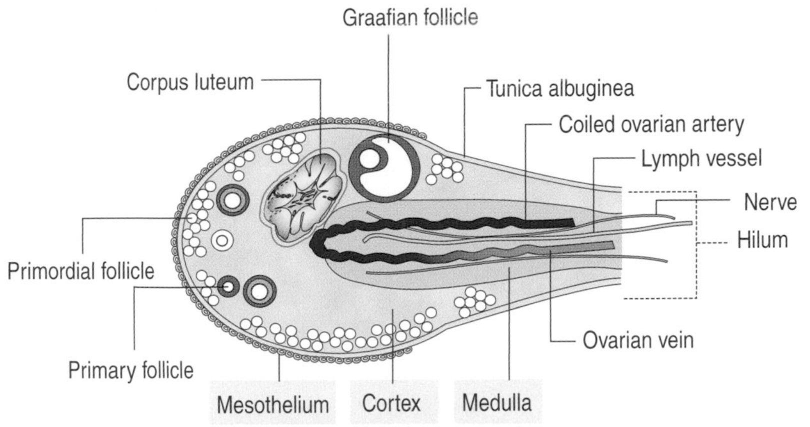

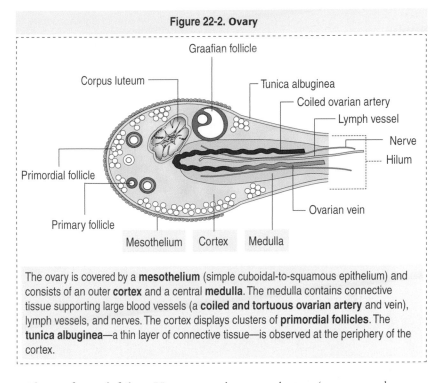

The ovary is covered by a **mesothelium** (simple cuboidal-to-squamous epithelium) and consists of an outer **cortex** and a central **medulla**. The medulla contains connective tissue supporting large blood vessels (a **coiled and tortuous ovarian artery** and vein), lymph vessels, and nerves. The cortex displays clusters of **primordial follicles**. The **tunica albuginea**—a thin layer of connective tissue—is observed at the periphery of the cortex.

evidence of growth failure. Hormone replacement therapy (estrogen and progesterone) compensates for ovarian atrophy.

Ovary

The ovary is lined by a **simple squamous-to-low cuboidal epithelium** and a subjacent connective tissue layer, the **tunica albuginea**. In a section, a **cortex** and a **medulla** without distinct demarcation can be visualized. The broad cortex contains connective tissue and **primordial follicles** housing **primary oocytes** (at the end of meiotic prophase I). The **medulla** consists of connective tissue, interstitial cells, nerves, lymphatics, and blood vessels reaching the ovary through the **hilum** (Figure 22-2).

The functions of the ovary are: (1) the production of the female gamete; (2) the secretion of estrogens and progesterone (steroid hormones); (3) the regulation of postnatal growth of reproductive organs; and (4) the development of secondary sexual characteristics.

Ovarian cycle

The three phases of the ovarian cycle are the **follicular phase**, **ovulatory phase**, and **luteal phase**.

The follicular phase consists of the development of a primordial follicle into a mature or graafian follicle (Figures 22-3 and 22-4)

The predominant and smallest follicle (25 μm in diameter) is the **primordial follicle**, which is surrounded by **squamous follicular** or **granulosa cells** (see Figure 22-3). Primordial follicles are retained in a resting phase from the time of their development in the fetal ovary.

Follicles leaving the resting stage are called **primary follicles**. There are two types:

1. **Unilayered primary follicles**, with a single layer of **cuboidal follicular cells**.

2. **Multilayered primary follicles**, lined by several layers of proliferating cuboidal follicular cells. The follicular cells are supported by a **basal lamina** separating the primary follicle from the stroma of the ovary.

In the primary follicle stage, the primary oocyte begins the synthesis of a

Figure 22-3. From primordial to primary follicle

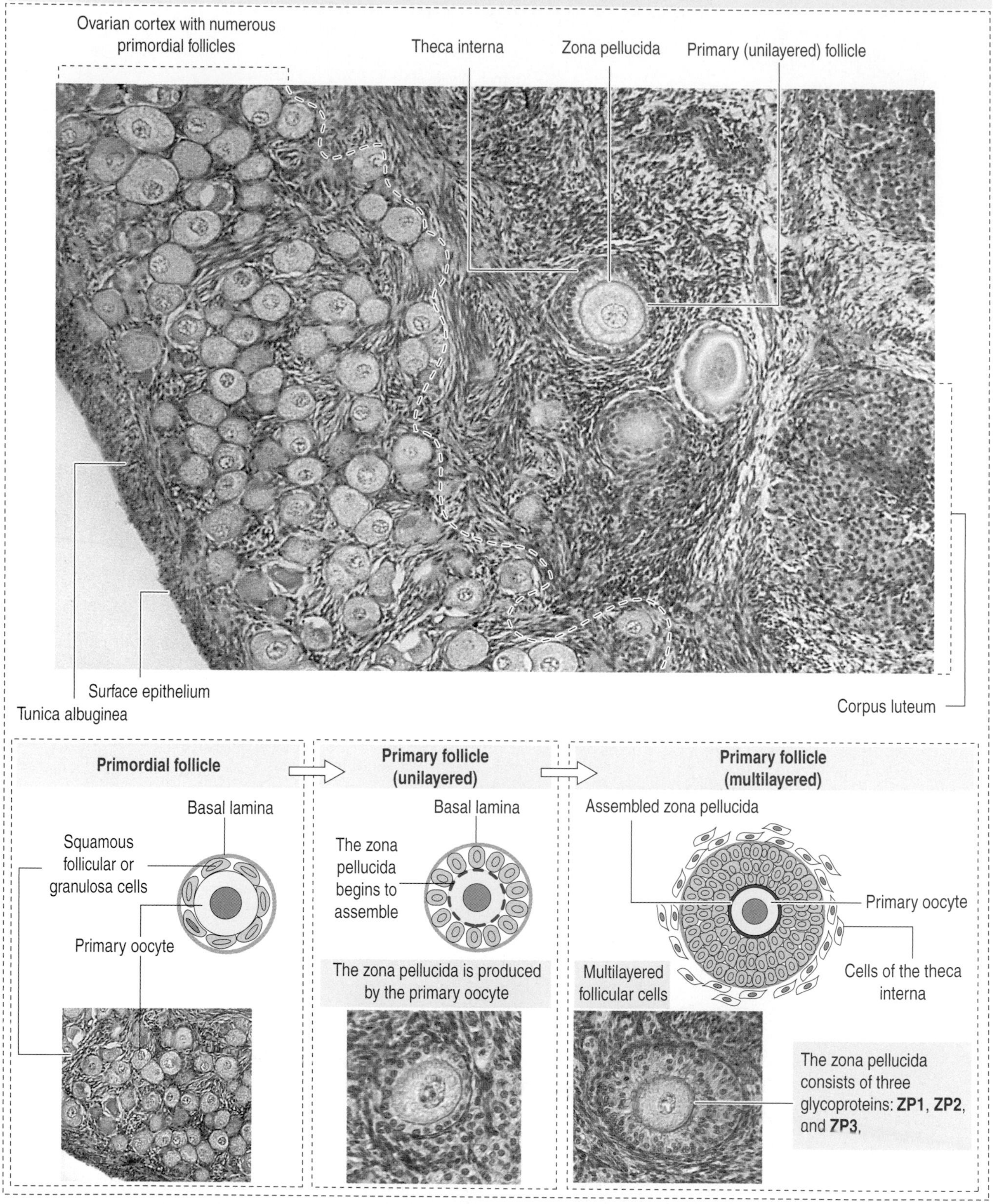

Ovarian cortex with numerous primordial follicles
Theca interna
Zona pellucida
Primary (unilayered) follicle
Surface epithelium
Tunica albuginea
Corpus luteum
Primordial follicle
Primary follicle (unilayered)
Primary follicle (multilayered)
Basal lamina
Squamous follicular or granulosa cells
Primary oocyte
Basal lamina
The zona pellucida begins to assemble
The zona pellucida is produced by the primary oocyte
Assembled zona pellucida
Primary oocyte
Multilayered follicular cells
Cells of the theca interna
The zona pellucida consists of three glycoproteins: **ZP1**, **ZP2**, and **ZP3**.

glycoprotein coat, the **zona pellucida**. The zona pellucida progressively separates the follicular cells from the oocyte. The zona pellucida is penetrated by thin cytoplasmic processes of the follicular cells that contact microvilli of the oocyte. **Gap junctions** are present at the contact sites.

The following stage, the **secondary follicle**, is characterized by the **continuous**

Figure 22-4. From a secondary to a graafian follicle

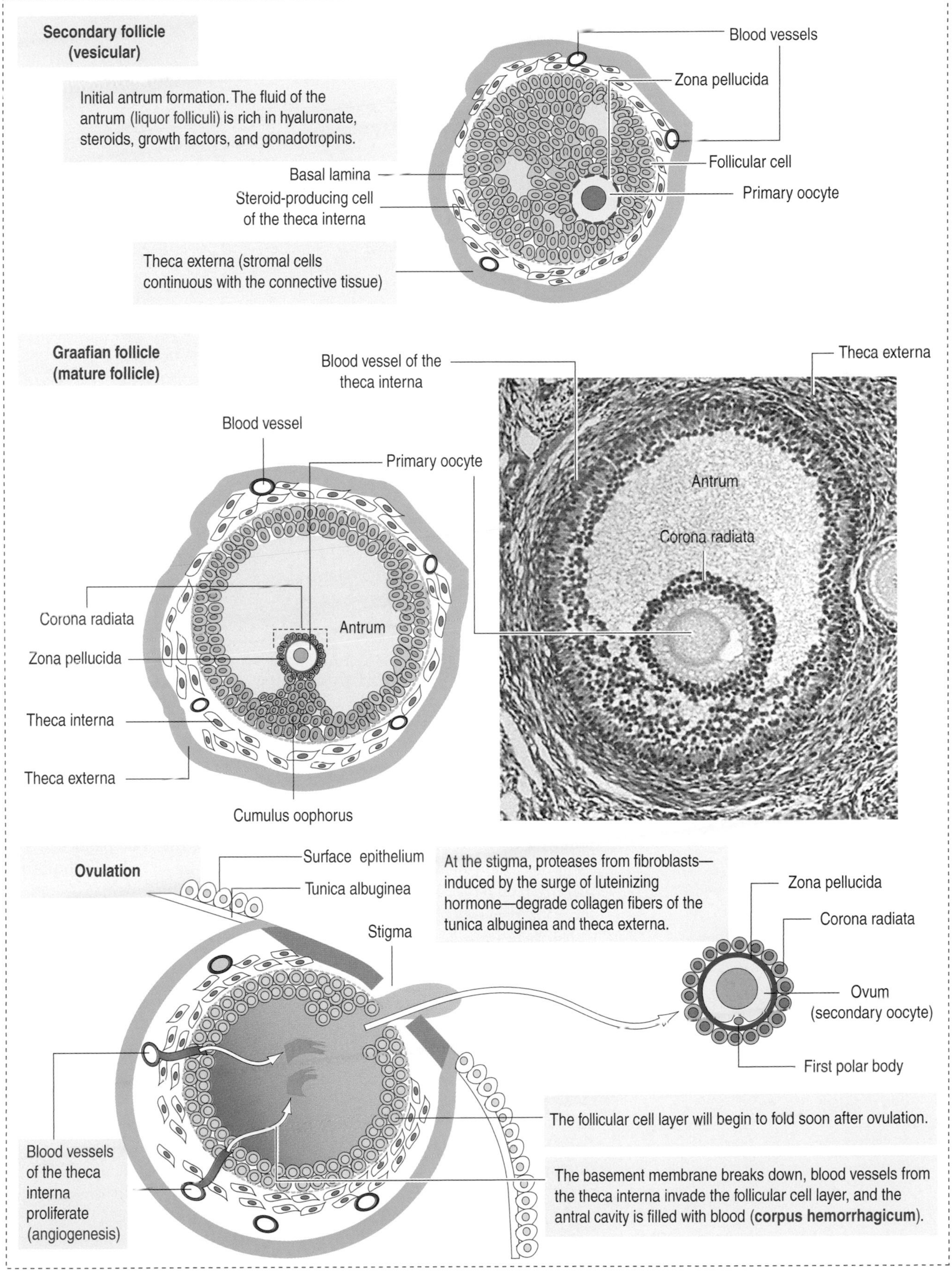
Secondary follicle (vesicular)
Initial antrum formation. The fluid of the antrum (liquor folliculi) is rich in hyaluronate, steroids, growth factors, and gonadotropins.
Blood vessels
Zona pellucida
Follicular cell
Primary oocyte
Basal lamina
Steroid-producing cell of the theca interna
Theca externa (stromal cells continuous with the connective tissue)
Graafian follicle (mature follicle)
Blood vessel of the theca interna
Theca externa
Blood vessel
Primary oocyte
Antrum
Corona radiata
Corona radiata
Zona pellucida
Antrum
Theca interna
Theca externa
Cumulus oophorus
Ovulation
Surface epithelium
Tunica albuginea
Stigma
At the stigma, proteases from fibroblasts—induced by the surge of luteinizing hormone—degrade collagen fibers of the tunica albuginea and theca externa.
Zona pellucida
Corona radiata
Ovum (secondary oocyte)
First polar body
The follicular cell layer will begin to fold soon after ovulation.
Blood vessels of the theca interna proliferate (angiogenesis)
The basement membrane breaks down, blood vessels from the theca interna invade the follicular cell layer, and the antral cavity is filled with blood (corpus hemorrhagicum).

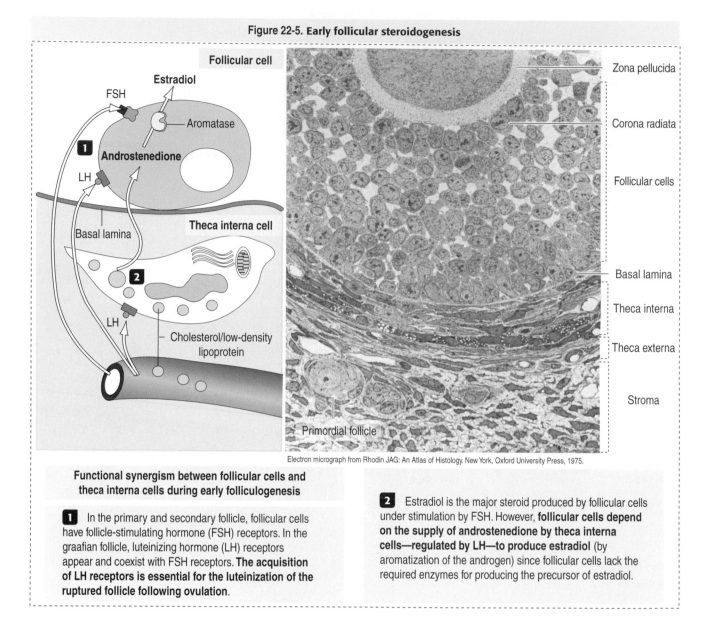

Figure 22-5. Early follicular steroidogenesis

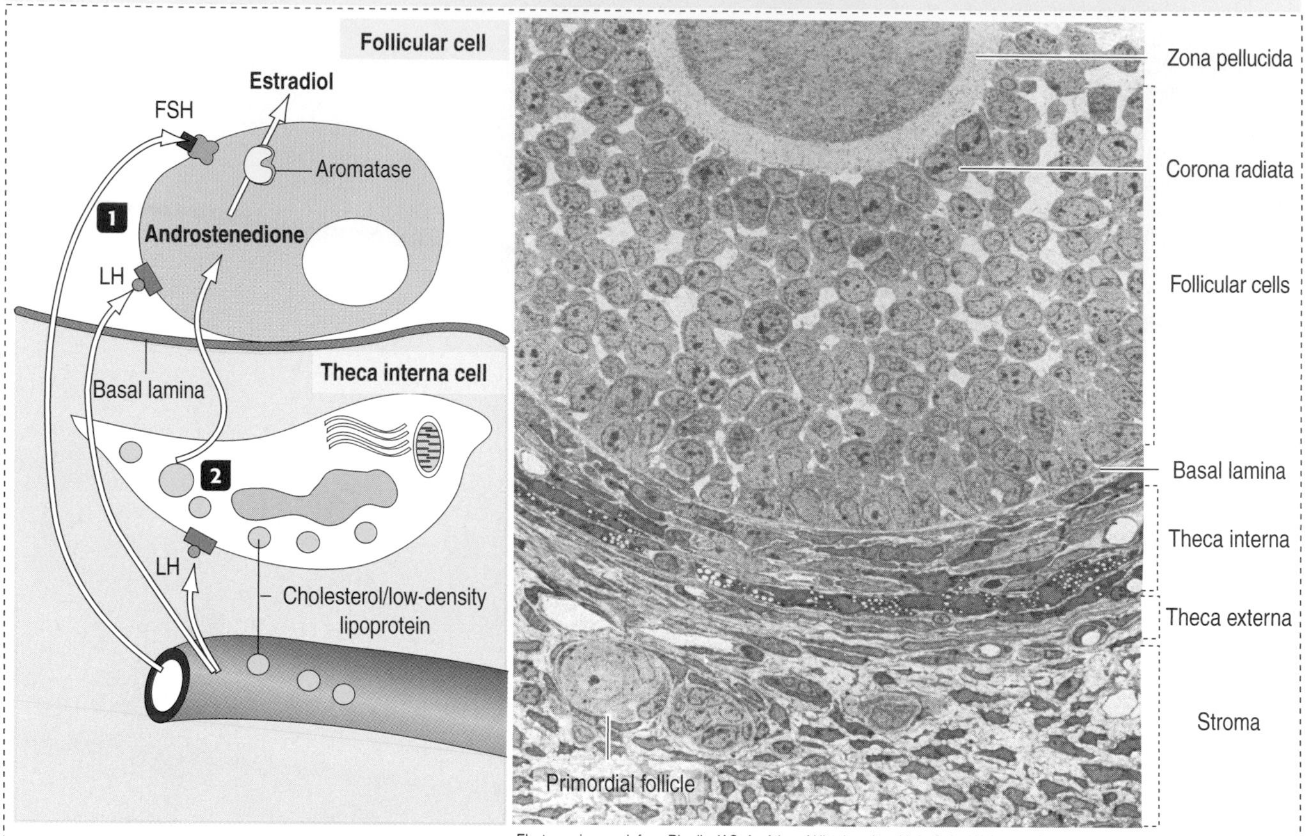

Follicular cell
Estradiol
FSH
Aromatase
1
Androstenedione
LH
Basal lamina
Theca interna cell
2
LH
Cholesterol/low-density lipoprotein
Zona pellucida
Corona radiata
Follicular cells
Basal lamina
Theca interna
Theca externa
Stroma
Primordial follicle

Electron micrograph from Rhodin JAG: An Atlas of Histology. New York, Oxford University Press, 1975.

Functional synergism between follicular cells and theca interna cells during early folliculogenesis

1 In the primary and secondary follicle, follicular cells have follicle-stimulating hormone (FSH) receptors. In the graafian follicle, luteinizing hormone (LH) receptors appear and coexist with FSH receptors. **The acquisition of LH receptors is essential for the luteinization of the ruptured follicle following ovulation.**

2 Estradiol is the major steroid produced by follicular cells under stimulation by FSH. However, **follicular cells depend on the supply of androstenedione by theca interna cells—regulated by LH—to produce estradiol** (by aromatization of the androgen) since follicular cells lack the required enzymes for producing the precursor of estradiol.

proliferation of follicular cells and the **thickening of the zona pellucida**. The stromal cells surrounding the follicle become arranged into a cellular capsule, the **theca** (Greek *theke*, box). The theca soon differentiates into two layers: (1) the **theca interna** and (2) the **theca externa**.

The **theca interna**, a well-vascularized cell layer adjacent to the basal lamina of the developing follicle, secretes **androstenedione**, an androgen precursor that is **transferred to the follicular cells** for the production of testosterone (Figure 22-5). Testosterone is then converted to **estradiol** by aromatase. Follicular cells lack enzymes required for the direct production of estrogens. As a result, **follicular cells cannot produce steroid precursors during folliculogenesis**.

The **theca externa** is a connective tissue capsule-like layer, continuous with the ovarian stroma.

Small intercellular spaces—**Call-Exner bodies**—appear between follicular cells. These spaces contain **follicular fluid** and coalesce later to form a large space, the **antrum**. The formation of the antrum soon dislocates the follicular cells with respect to the primary oocyte. A cluster of follicular cells, called the **cumulus oophorus**, is seen between the oocyte and the wall of the follicle.

The largest follicle is the **mature follicle** (also called the **graafian follicle** or **preovulatory follicle**). It measures 15 to 20 mm in diameter. Immediately before

Figure 22-6. Follicular cell–primary oocyte interaction through gap junctions

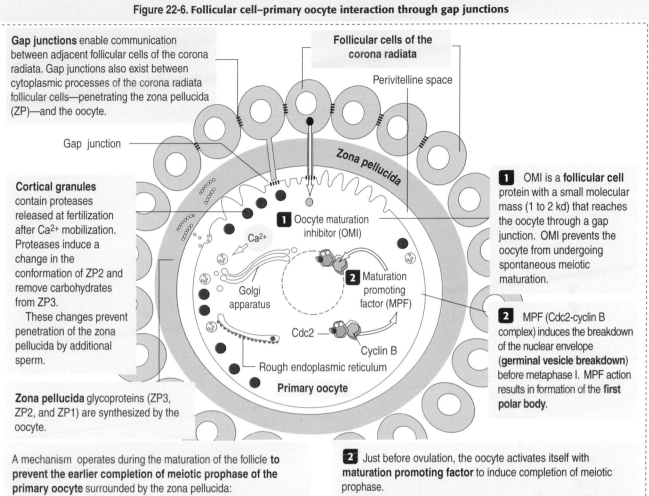

Gap junctions enable communication between adjacent follicular cells of the corona radiata. Gap junctions also exist between cytoplasmic processes of the corona radiata follicular cells—penetrating the zona pellucida (ZP)—and the oocyte.

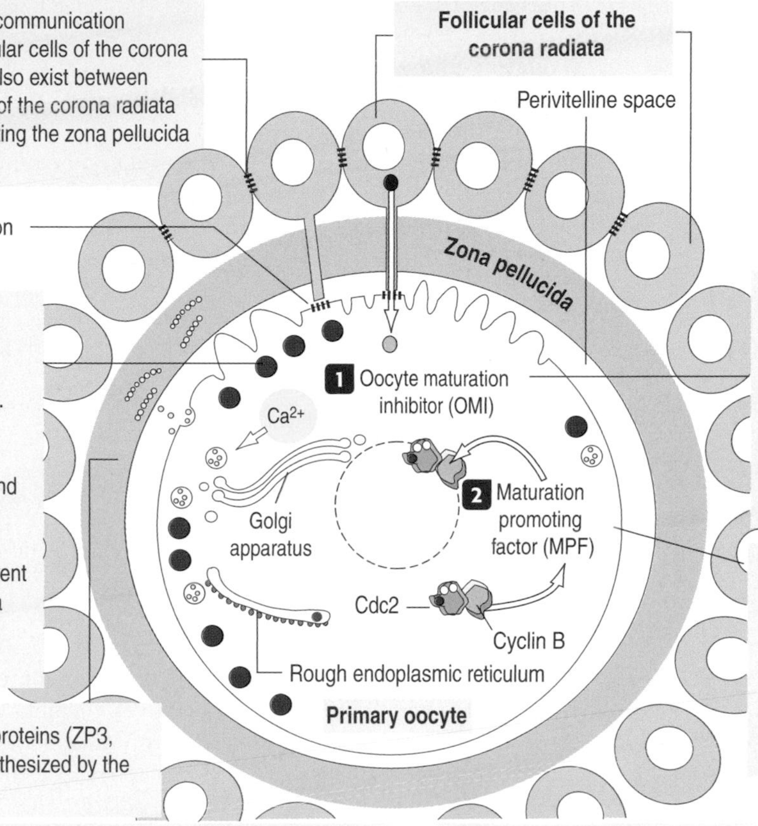

Cortical granules contain proteases released at fertilization after Ca^{2+} mobilization. Proteases induce a change in the conformation of ZP2 and remove carbohydrates from ZP3.

These changes prevent penetration of the zona pellucida by additional sperm.

Zona pellucida glycoproteins (ZP3, ZP2, and ZP1) are synthesized by the oocyte.

1 OMI is a **follicular cell** protein with a small molecular mass (1 to 2 kd) that reaches the oocyte through a gap junction. OMI prevents the oocyte from undergoing spontaneous meiotic maturation.

2 MPF (Cdc2-cyclin B complex) induces the breakdown of the nuclear envelope (**germinal vesicle breakdown**) before metaphase I. MPF action results in formation of the **first polar body.**

A mechanism operates during the maturation of the follicle **to prevent the earlier completion of meiotic prophase of the primary oocyte** surrounded by the zona pellucida:

1 This mechanism involves the transfer of **oocyte maturation inhibitor** from follicular cells to the oocyte through cell processes crossing the zona pellucida and establishing contact with the plasma membrane of the oocyte via gap junctions.

2 Just before ovulation, the oocyte activates itself with **maturation promoting factor** to induce completion of meiotic prophase.

Completion of meiosis I results in the formation of the first polar body—retained in the perivitelline space—and a secondary oocyte. At fertilization, proteases are released from the cortical granules in a Ca^{2+}-dependent manner. Proteases alter the structural conformation of the zona pellucida, preventing penetration of the egg by additional sperm.

ovulation, the primary oocyte occupies an eccentric position within the follicle, covered by a single layer of follicular cells—the **corona radiata**—firmly attached to the zona pellucida (Figure 22-6).

A mature follicle, or graafian follicle, is characterized by the following features: (1) a **large antrum**, containing follicular fluid; (2) the **zona pellucida**, invested by a single layer of follicular cells forming the **corona radiata**; (3) the **detachment of the oocyte and attached corona radiata from the cumulus oophorus**; the oocyte–zona pellucida–corona radiata complex floats free in the follicular fluid; (4) the **completion of meiosis I several hours before ovulation**, resulting in the formation of a **secondary oocyte** and the **first polar body**, which remains in a space—the **perivitelline space**—between the zona pellucida and the oocyte; and (5) **follicular cells acquire luteinizing hormone (LH) receptors** in addition to the already present follicle-stimulating hormone (FSH) receptors. This event is critical for **luteinization** or **development of the corpus luteum** (see Figure 22–5).

Box 22-A | Folliculogenesis

- The development of the ovarian follicle and steroidogenesis are controlled by gonadotropins (FSH and LH), in part by ovarian steroids and autocrine and paracrine secretions of the follicular cells.
- About 7 million primary oocytes are present in the fetal ovary by midgestation. There is a gradual loss of oocytes and, at birth, approximately 400,000 oocytes remain. Only 400 follicles ovulate after puberty. The remaining follicles degenerate and are called **atretic follicles**.
- The follicular phase begins with the development of 6 to 12 primary follicles. This development is FSH-dependent. By the sixth day of the cycle, one follicle predominates and the others become atretic.

Follicular atresia or degeneration

Several primary follicles initiate the maturation process (see Box 22-A), but only one follicle completes its development; the remainder degenerate by an apoptotic process called **atresia**. Follicles can become atretic at any stage of development.

Box 22-B | **Ovarian hormones**

- **Estradiol** (estradiol-17β) is the most abundant and most potent ovarian estrogen, produced mainly by granulosa and granulosa lutein cells. Significant amounts of **estriol**, a less potent estrogen, is produced from estrone in the **liver** during **pregnancy**. Most **estrone**, the least potent of the three estrogens, is predominant in the **postmenopausal woman** and is formed in **peripheral tissues** by the conversion of estradiol or androstenedione.
- **Progesterone**, a precursor of androgens and estrogens, is synthesized by follicular and luteal cells.
- Weak **androgens** (**dehydroepiandrosterone** and **androstenedione**) are produced by theca interna cells.
- Other ovarian hormones are **inhibin**, **activin**, and **relaxin**. **Relaxin**, produced by both the ovary and the placenta, induces **relaxation of the pelvic ligaments** and **softens the cervix to facilitate childbirth**.

Figure 22-7. **Atretic follicle**

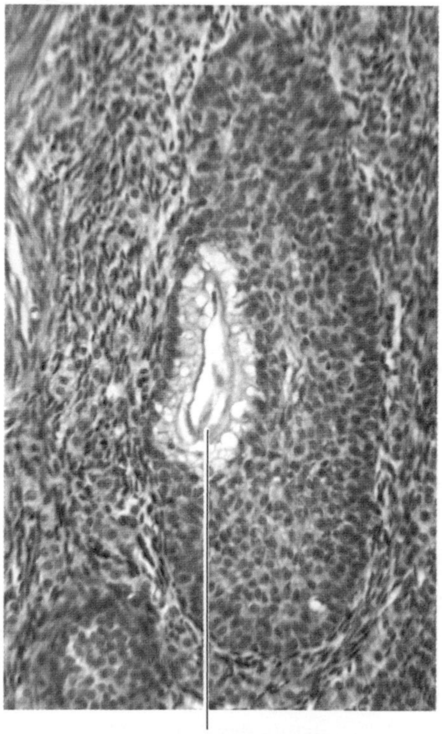

Initial stage of an atretic follicle with a collapsed zona pellucida

A woman ovulates about 400 oocytes during her reproductive years. During a reproductive cycle, a group of follicles starts the maturation process.

However, only one or two follicles complete folliculogenesis and are eventually ovulated. The others undergo—at any time of their development—a degenerative process called **follicular atresia**.

Atretic follicles (Figure 22-7) are identified by a thick folded basement membrane material, the **glassy membrane**, a relatively intact zona pellucida, remnants of degenerated oocytes and follicular cells, and invading macrophages.

Ovulatory phase

At the time of ovulation, the mature follicle protrudes from the ovarian surface, forming the **stigma**. Proteolytic activity within the theca externa and tunica albuginea, induced by a surge of LH, facilitates the rupture of the now mature graafian follicle. The released gamete enters the closely apposed uterine tube or oviduct. A few hours before ovulation, the **follicular cell layer** and the **theca interna** begin their transformation into a **corpus luteum**.

Luteal phase: Corpus luteum

Following ovulation, the residual follicular cell layer folds and becomes part of the **corpus luteum**, a major hormone-secreting gland.

This transformation (Figure 22-8) involves:

1. A **breakdown of the basement membrane of the follicle**.
2. **Invasion of blood vessels** into the formerly avascular follicular cellular mass. Blood flows into the former antral space and coagulates, forming a transient **corpus hemorrhagicum**. The fibrin clot is then penetrated by newly formed blood vessels (**angiogenesis**), fibroblasts, and collagen fibers.
3. A **transformation of follicular cells and theca interna cells**. Follicular cells change into **follicular lutein cells**, display the typical features of steroid-secreting cells (lipid droplets, a well-developed smooth endoplasmic reticulum, and mitochondria with tubular cristae) (Figure 22-9), and secrete **progesterone** and **estrogen in response to both FSH and LH stimulation**. Recall that the expression of LH receptors by follicular cells is a crucial step in the luteinization process. The theca interna cells change into **theca lutein cells**, which produce **androstenedione** and **progesterone in response to LH stimulation**.

Follicular lutein cells still lack the steroidogenic enzyme required for the complete synthesis of estradiol (see Box 22-B). Theca lutein cells cooperate with follicular cells by providing androstenedione, which is then converted into estradiol within follicular lutein cells (Figure 22-10).

The corpus luteum continues to enlarge and enters an involution stage about 14 days after ovulation unless fertilization occurs. If fertilization takes place, the corpus luteum continues to enlarge and produces **progesterone** and **estrogen** under the stimulatory action of **human chorionic gonadotropin** (**hCG**) produced by the **trophoblast** of the implanted embryo.

Progesterone and estrogen are required to maintain the endometrium until about the 9th to 10th week of gestation. At this time, the placenta, fetal adrenal cortex, and liver produce estrogens (see discussion of the adrenal gland in Chapter 19, Endocrine System, and Placentation in Chapter 23, Fertilization, Placentation, and Lactation).

Regression of the corpus luteum—**luteolysis**—leads to the formation of the **corpus albicans**, resulting from the stromal connective tissue replacing the mass of degenerating luteal cells of the corpus luteum (Figure 22-11). The corpus albicans remains in the ovary; it decreases in size but never disappears.

Luteal cells, remaining free in the stroma after involution of the corpus luteum, can retain their secretory activity and form the so-called **interstitial glands**. Such glandular interstitial cells are not abundant in the human ovary.

Hormonal regulation of ovulation and the corpus luteum

Two hormones of the anterior hypophysis regulate follicular growth (Figure 22-12):

1. **Follicle-stimulating hormone** stimulates folliculogenesis and ovulation as well as the production of estrogen.

Figure 22-8. Development, function, and involution of the corpus luteum

Formation of the corpus luteum (luteinization)

Following ovulation, the **follicular cell layer** (also called follicular membrane) of the preovulatory follicle becomes folded and is transformed into part of the **corpus luteum**. A surge in luteinizing hormone (LH) is correlated with luteinization.

This transformation includes the following:

The lumen, previously occupied by the follicular antrum, is filled with fibrin, which is then replaced by connective tissue and new blood vessels piercing the basement membrane.

Follicular or granulosa cells enlarge and lipid droplets accumulate. They become **follicular** or **granulosa lutein cells**.

The spaces between the folds of the follicular cell layer are penetrated by theca interna cells, blood vessels, and connective tissue. Theca interna cells also enlarge and store lipids. They are now **theca lutein cells**.

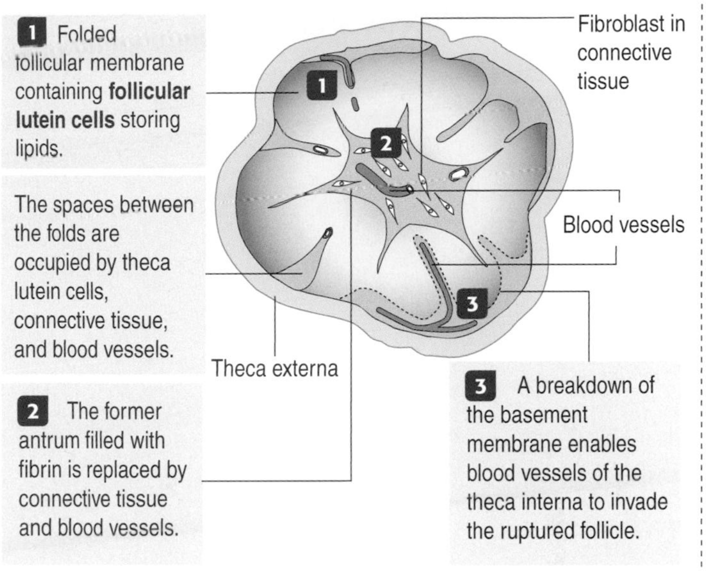

1 Folded follicular membrane containing **follicular lutein cells** storing lipids.
The spaces between the folds are occupied by theca lutein cells, connective tissue, and blood vessels.
2 The former antrum filled with fibrin is replaced by connective tissue and blood vessels.
Theca externa
Fibroblast in connective tissue
Blood vessels
3 A breakdown of the basement membrane enables blood vessels of the theca interna to invade the ruptured follicle.

Function of the corpus luteum

The function of the corpus luteum is regulated by two gonadotropins: FSH and LH.

Follicle-stimulating hormone (FSH) stimulates the production of **progesterone** and **estradiol** by follicular lutein cells.

LH stimulates the production of progesterone and androstenedione by theca lutein cells. Androstenedione is translocated into follicular lutein cells for aromatization into **estradiol**.

During pregnancy, **prolactin** and **placental lactogens** upregulate **the effects of estradiol** produced by follicular lutein cells by enhancing the production of estrogen receptors.

Estradiol stimulates follicular lutein cells to take up cholesterol from blood, which is then stored in lipid droplets and transported to mitochondria for progesterone synthesis.

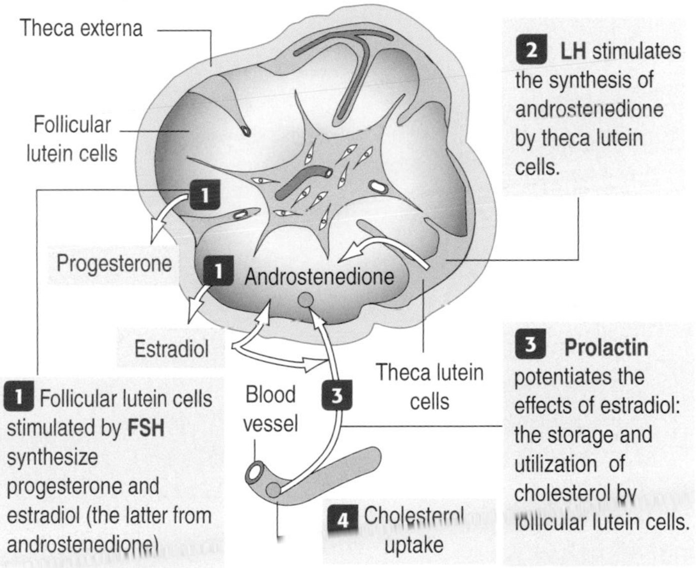

Theca externa
Follicular lutein cells
Progesterone
1 Androstenedione
Estradiol
2 **LH** stimulates the synthesis of androstenedione by theca lutein cells.
1 Follicular lutein cells stimulated by **FSH** synthesize progesterone and estradiol (the latter from androstenedione)
Blood vessel
3
Theca lutein cells
4 Cholesterol uptake
3 **Prolactin** potentiates the effects of estradiol: the storage and utilization of cholesterol by follicular lutein cells.

Regression of the corpus luteum (luteolysis)

If fertilization does not occur, the corpus luteum undergoes a process of regression called **luteolysis**.

Luteolysis involves a programmed cell death (apoptosis) sequence.

The following events take place:

A **reduction in the blood flow** within the corpus luteum causes a decline in oxygen (hypoxia).

T cells reach the corpus luteum and produce **interferon-**γ, which, in turn, acts on the endothelium to enable the arrival of macrophages.

Macrophages produce **tumor necrosis factor-**α and the apoptotic cascade starts.

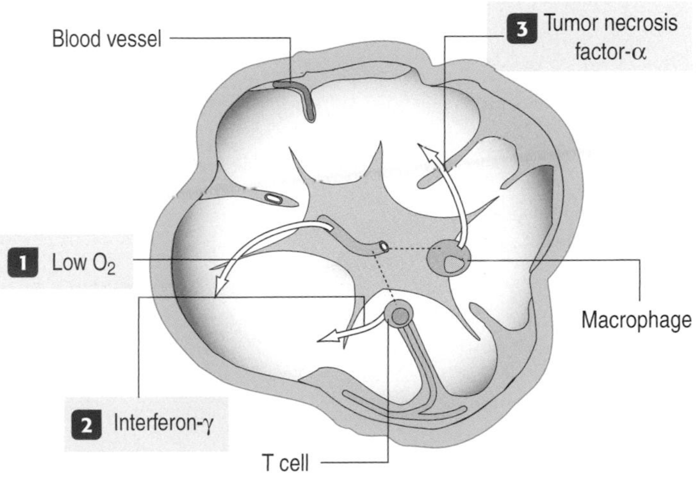

Blood vessel
3 Tumor necrosis factor-α
1 Low O$_2$
Macrophage
2 Interferon-γ
T cell

Figure 22-9. Lutein cell

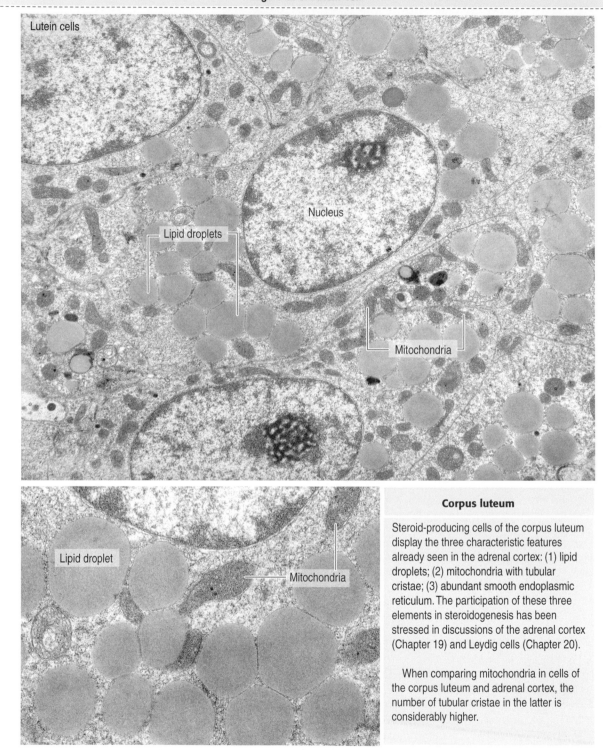

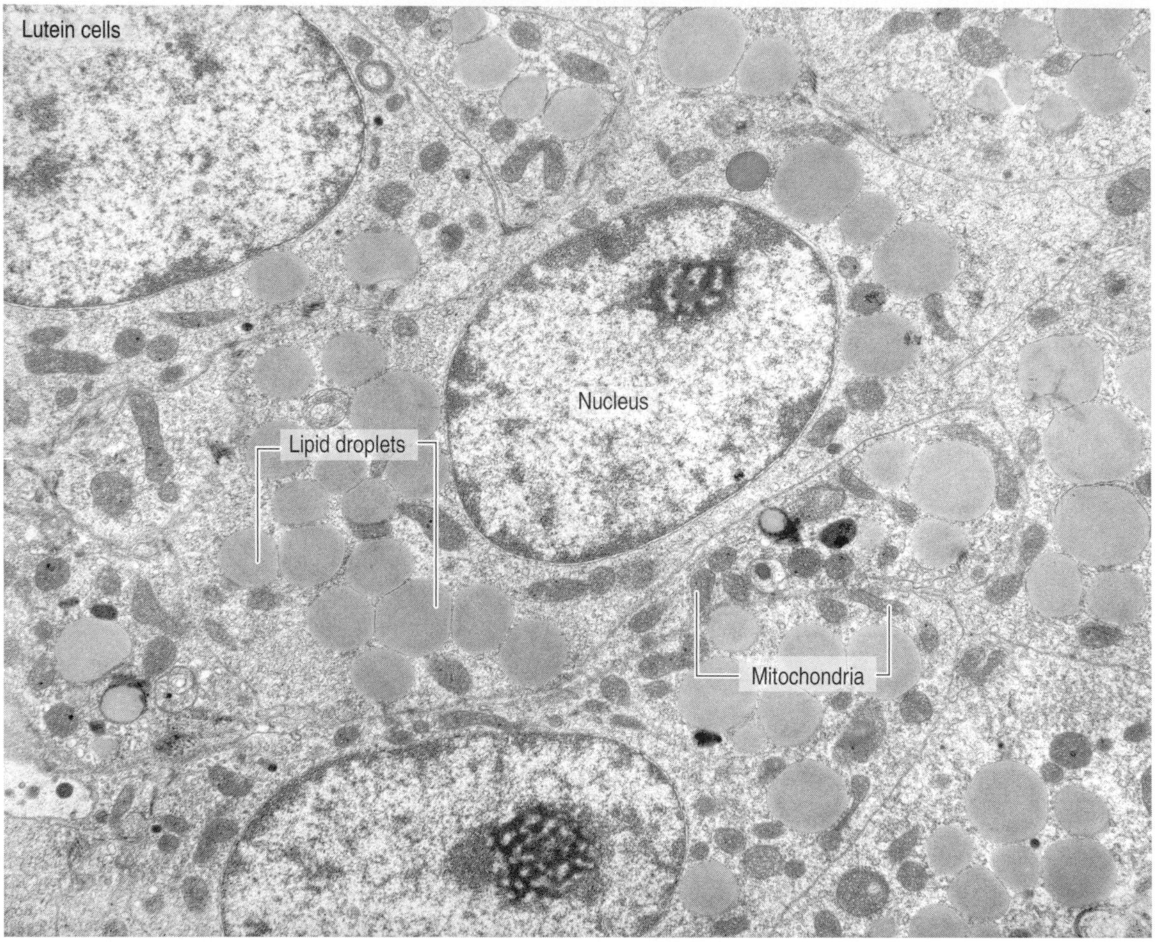

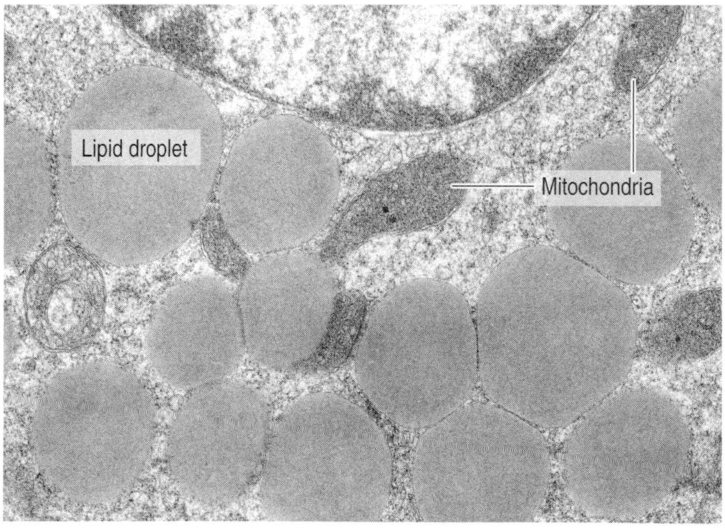

Corpus luteum

Steroid-producing cells of the corpus luteum display the three characteristic features already seen in the adrenal cortex: (1) lipid droplets; (2) mitochondria with tubular cristae; (3) abundant smooth endoplasmic reticulum. The participation of these three elements in steroidogenesis has been stressed in discussions of the adrenal cortex (Chapter 19) and Leydig cells (Chapter 20).

When comparing mitochondria in cells of the corpus luteum and adrenal cortex, the number of tubular cristae in the latter is considerably higher.

2. **Luteinizing hormone** stimulates the secretion of progesterone by the corpus luteum. A surge of LH immediately precedes ovulation. Continued LH secretion induces the **luteinization** of the residual follicular cell layer after ovulation. The production of FSH and LH ceases when the levels of progesterone and estrogen are high, and then the corpus luteum enters involution.

At the initiation of menstruation, estrogen and progesterone levels are low and increase gradually during the preovulatory period. Estrogen reaches maximum levels just before the LH peak precedes ovulation.

Figure 22-10. Follicular lutein–theca lutein cell cooperation

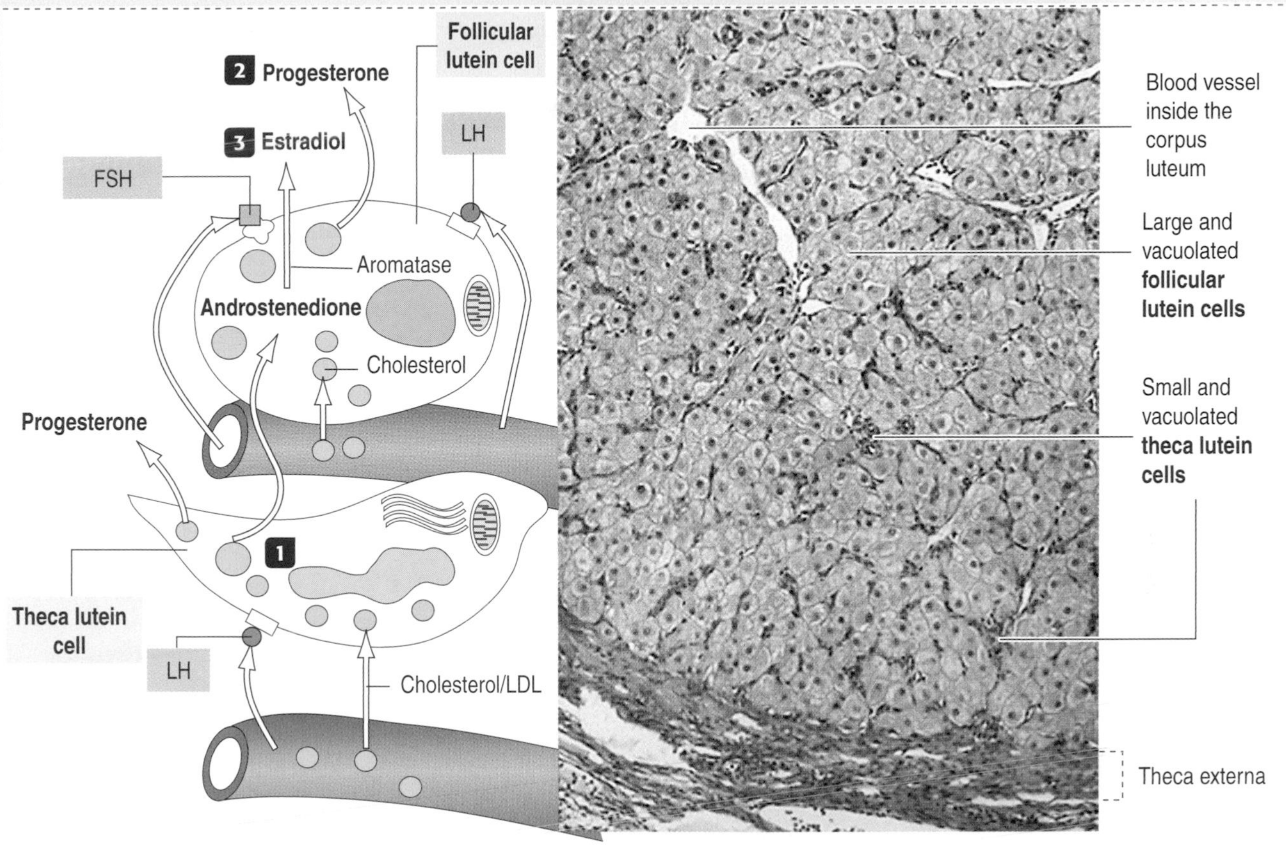

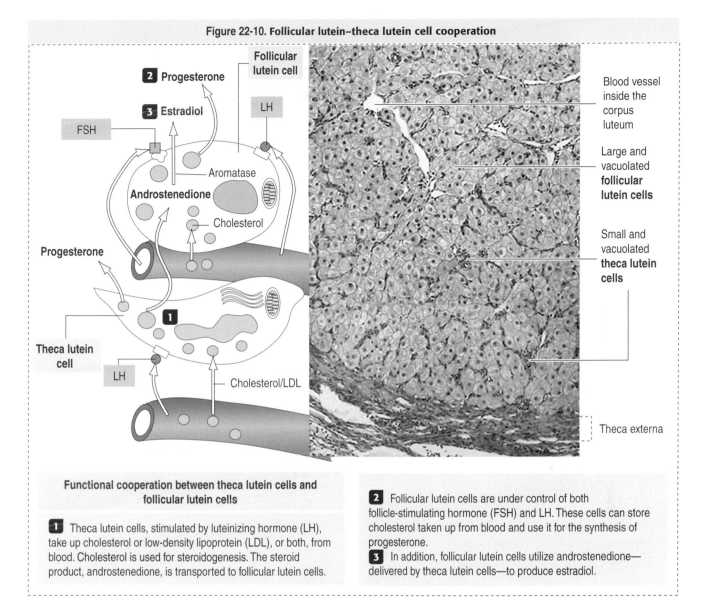

Functional cooperation between theca lutein cells and follicular lutein cells

1 Theca lutein cells, stimulated by luteinizing hormone (LH), take up cholesterol or low-density lipoprotein (LDL), or both, from blood. Cholesterol is used for steroidogenesis. The steroid product, androstenedione, is transported to follicular lutein cells.

2 Follicular lutein cells are under control of both follicle-stimulating hormone (FSH) and LH. These cells can store cholesterol taken up from blood and use it for the synthesis of progesterone.

3 In addition, follicular lutein cells utilize androstenedione—delivered by theca lutein cells—to produce estradiol.

Coinciding with the FSH and LH secretory pattern, the FSH-dependent synthesis of estrogen by follicular cells stimulates the **proliferation of the endometrial glands**. LH-dependent synthesis of progesterone by the corpus luteum **initiates and maintains the secretory activity of the endometrial glands**.

Figure 22-11. Corpus albicans

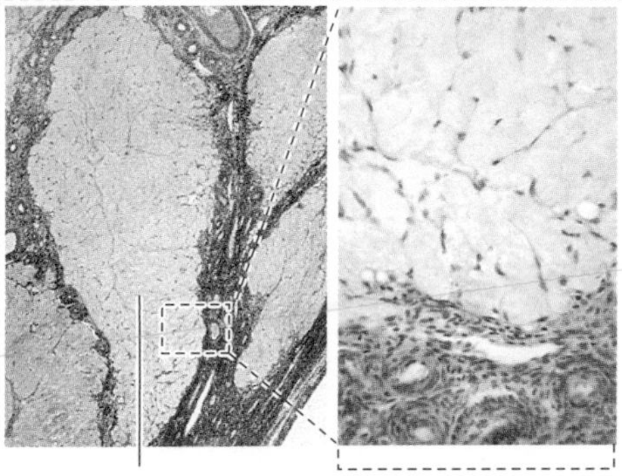

Oviduct, fallopian or uterine tube

The oviduct is the site of fertilization and early cleavage of the **zygote** (fertilized ovum). Each tube is divided into **four anatomic regions** (Figure 22-13): (1) the proximal fimbriated **infundibulum**; (2) a long and thin-walled **ampulla**; (3) a short and thick-walled **isthmus**; and (4) an **intramural** portion opening into the lumen of the uterine cavity.

The infundibulum consists of numerous finger-like projections of mucosal tissue called **fimbriae**. The ampulla and the isthmus are lined by **mucosal folds** projecting into the lumen of the tube. The isthmus has fewer mucosal folds than the ampulla.

The wall of the oviduct consists of three layers: (1) a **mucosa** supported by a **lamina propria**, (2) a **muscular layer**, and (3) a **serosa layer**.

The mucosa consists of a **simple columnar epithelium** with two cell populations (see Figure 22-13) under **hormonal control**:

1. **Ciliated cells**, which enlarge and produce cilia (**ciliogenesis**) as folliculogenesis

Figure 22-12. Ovarian cycle

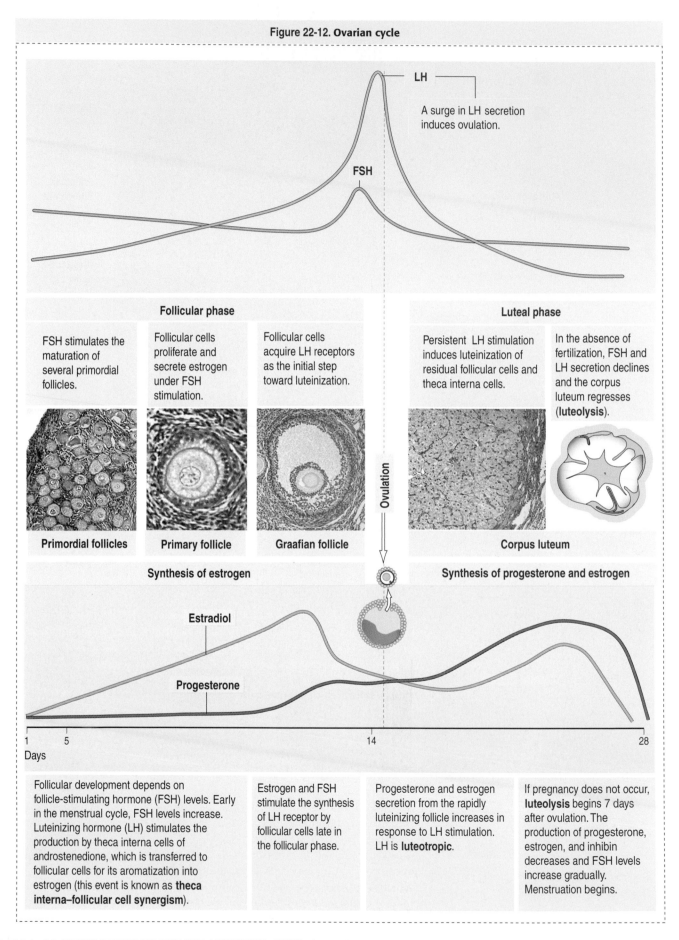

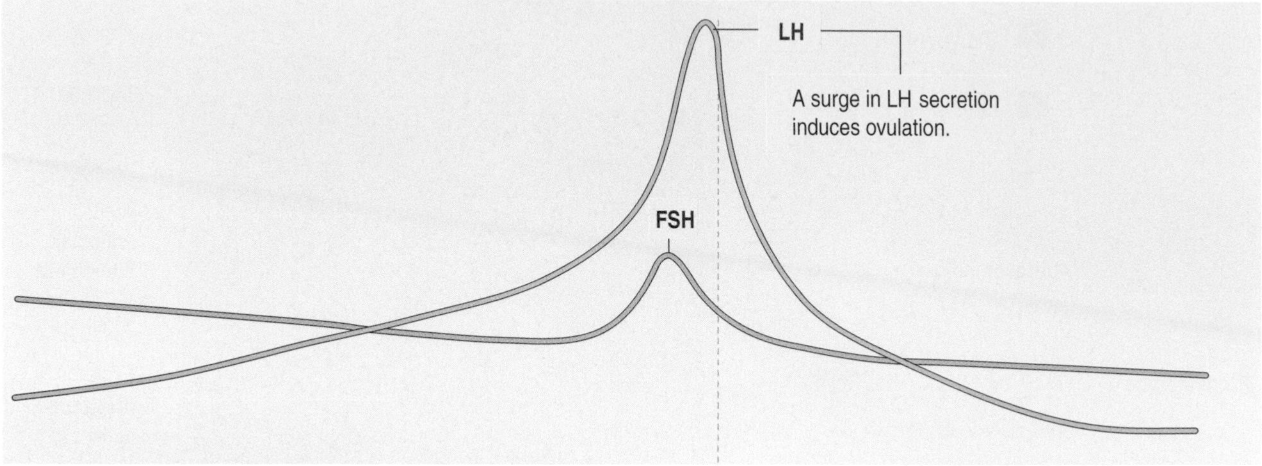

LH
A surge in LH secretion induces ovulation.
FSH

Follicular phase

FSH stimulates the maturation of several primordial follicles.

Follicular cells proliferate and secrete estrogen under FSH stimulation.

Follicular cells acquire LH receptors as the initial step toward luteinization.

Luteal phase

Persistent LH stimulation induces luteinization of residual follicular cells and theca interna cells.

In the absence of fertilization, FSH and LH secretion declines and the corpus luteum regresses (**luteolysis**).

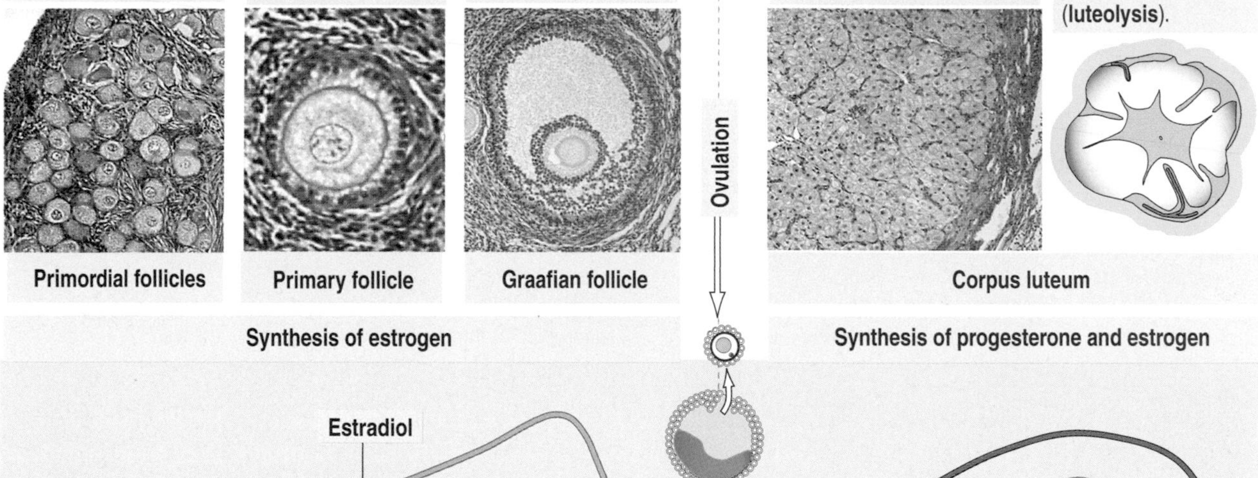

Ovulation

Primordial follicles | **Primary follicle** | **Graafian follicle** | **Corpus luteum**

Synthesis of estrogen

Synthesis of progesterone and estrogen

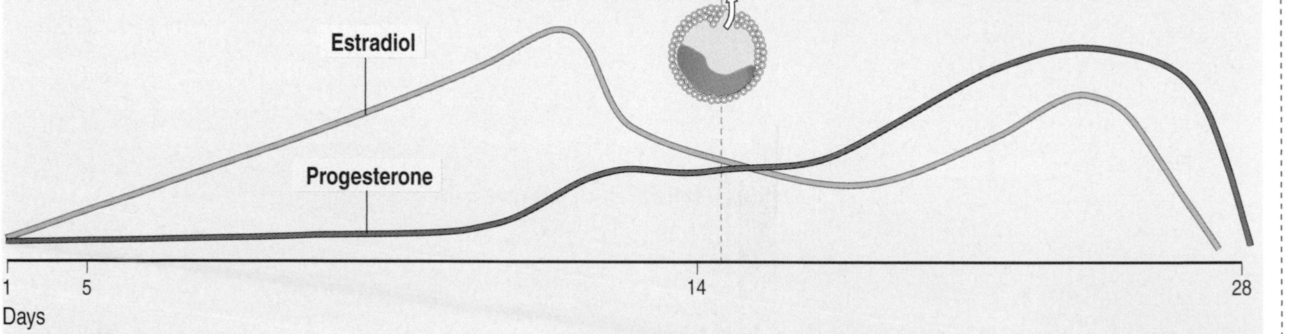

Estradiol
Progesterone
1
5
14
28
Days

Follicular development depends on follicle-stimulating hormone (FSH) levels. Early in the menstrual cycle, FSH levels increase. Luteinizing hormone (LH) stimulates the production by theca interna cells of androstenedione, which is transferred to follicular cells for its aromatization into estrogen (this event is known as **theca interna–follicular cell synergism**).

Estrogen and FSH stimulate the synthesis of LH receptor by follicular cells late in the follicular phase.

Progesterone and estrogen secretion from the rapidly luteinizing follicle increases in response to LH stimulation. LH is **luteotropic**.

If pregnancy does not occur, **luteolysis** begins 7 days after ovulation. The production of progesterone, estrogen, and inhibin decreases and FSH levels increase gradually. Menstruation begins.

Figure 22-13. Oviduct

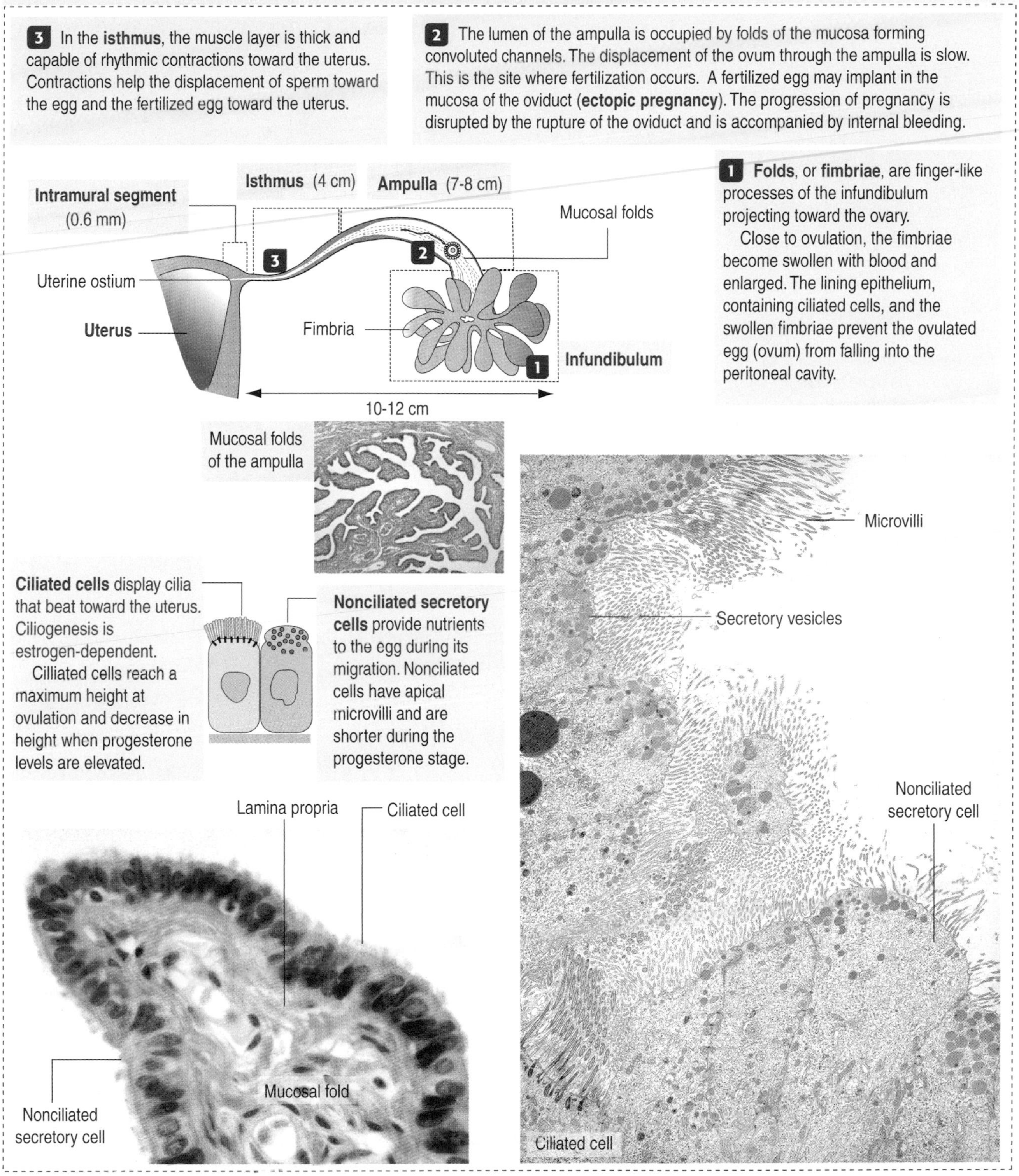

3 In the **isthmus**, the muscle layer is thick and capable of rhythmic contractions toward the uterus. Contractions help the displacement of sperm toward the egg and the fertilized egg toward the uterus.
2 The lumen of the ampulla is occupied by folds of the mucosa forming convoluted channels. The displacement of the ovum through the ampulla is slow. This is the site where fertilization occurs. A fertilized egg may implant in the mucosa of the oviduct (**ectopic pregnancy**). The progression of pregnancy is disrupted by the rupture of the oviduct and is accompanied by internal bleeding.
1 **Folds**, or **fimbriae**, are finger-like processes of the infundibulum projecting toward the ovary. Close to ovulation, the fimbriae become swollen with blood and enlarged. The lining epithelium, containing ciliated cells, and the swollen fimbriae prevent the ovulated egg (ovum) from falling into the peritoneal cavity.
Intramural segment (0.6 mm)
Isthmus (4 cm)
Ampulla (7-8 cm)
Mucosal folds
Uterine ostium
Uterus
Fimbria
Infundibulum
10-12 cm
Mucosal folds of the ampulla
Ciliated cells display cilia that beat toward the uterus. Ciliogenesis is estrogen-dependent. Cilliated cells reach a maximum height at ovulation and decrease in height when progesterone levels are elevated.
Nonciliated secretory cells provide nutrients to the egg during its migration. Nonciliated cells have apical microvilli and are shorter during the progesterone stage.
Lamina propria
Ciliated cell
Mucosal fold
Nonciliated secretory cell
Microvilli
Secretory vesicles
Nonciliated secretory cell
Ciliated cell

and estrogen production is in progress. Estrogens increase the rate of the ciliary beat. During luteolysis, ciliated cells lose their cilia (**deciliation**).

2. **Noncilated secretory cells** (called **peg cells**), whose secretory activity is also stimulated by estrogens. Nonciliated cells in some species have apical microvilli.

The **peristaltic contraction** of the muscular wall, with an **inner circular-spiral layer** and an **outer longitudinal layer**, as well as the ciliary activity of the lining epithelial cells, propels the oocyte or fertilized egg/embryo toward the uterus. The

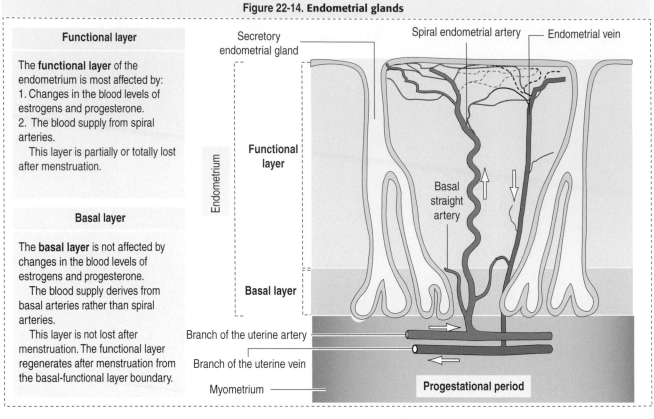

Figure 22-14. Endometrial glands

Functional layer

The **functional layer** of the endometrium is most affected by:
1. Changes in the blood levels of estrogens and progesterone.
2. The blood supply from spiral arteries.

This layer is partially or totally lost after menstruation.

Basal layer

The **basal layer** is not affected by changes in the blood levels of estrogens and progesterone.

The blood supply derives from basal arteries rather than spiral arteries.

This layer is not lost after menstruation. The functional layer regenerates after menstruation from the basal-functional layer boundary.

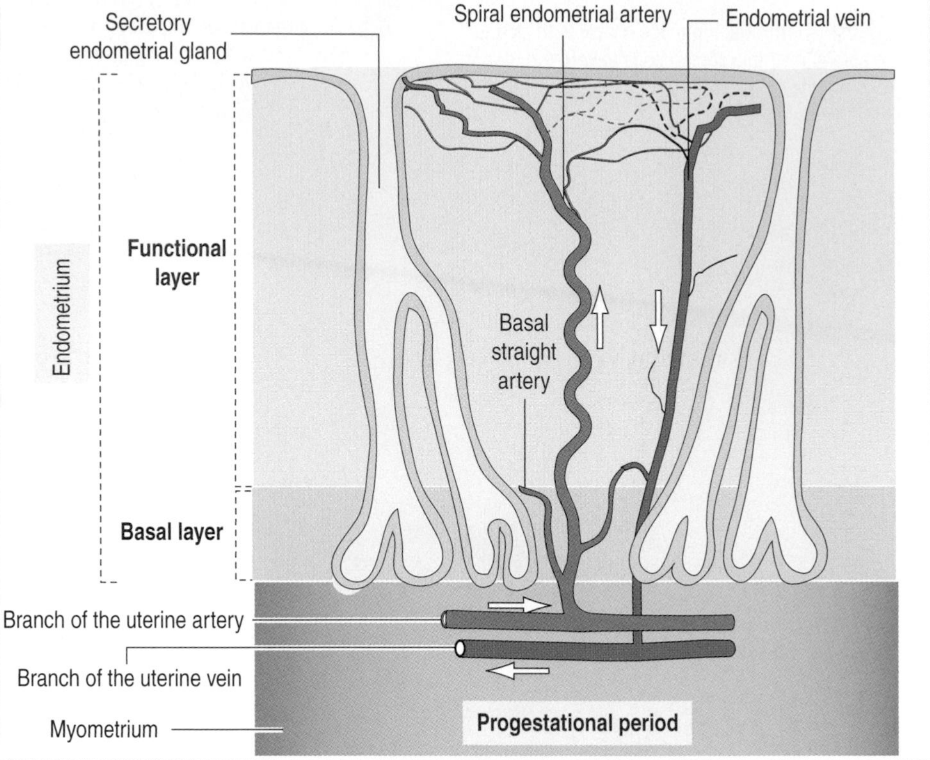

Secretory endometrial gland
Spiral endometrial artery
Endometrial vein
Endometrium
Functional layer
Basal straight artery
Basal layer
Branch of the uterine artery
Branch of the uterine vein
Myometrium
Progestational period

surface of the oviduct is covered by the peritoneal **mesothelium**. Large blood vessels are observed in the serosa.

Uterus

The uterus consists of two anatomic segments: (1) the **corpus** or **body** and (2) the **cervix**. The wall of the body of the uterus consists of three layers: (1) **endometrium** (Figures 22-14 and 22-15), (2) **myometrium**, and (3) **adventitia** or **serosa**. The major component of the wall is the **myometrium**, lined by a mucosa, the **endometrium**.

The **myometrium** has three poorly defined smooth muscle layers. The central layer is thick with circularly arranged muscle fibers and abundant blood vessels, which give the name **stratum vasculare** to this particular layer. The outer and inner layers contain longitudinally or obliquely arranged muscle fibers.

During pregnancy, myometrial smooth muscle enlarges (**hypertrophy**) and the fibers increase in number (**hyperplasia**). **Inhibition of myometrial contraction during pregnancy** is controlled by **relaxin**, a peptide hormone produced in the ovary and placenta. **Myometrial contraction during parturition** is under the control of **oxytocin**, a peptide hormone secreted from the neurohypophysis.

The **endometrium** consists of a **simple columnar epithelial lining**, associated with simple tubular endometrial glands, and the **lamina propria**, called the **endometrial stroma**.

Functionally, the endometrium consists of two layers (see Figure 22-14): (1) a superficial **functional layer**, lost during menstruation, and (2) a **basal layer**, retained as the source of regeneration of a new functional layer following menstruation.

The microscopic features of the functional layer change during the **menstrual cycle**, which lasts 28 days, with some slight variations in time. A menstrual cycle consists of four consecutive phases: **menstrual**, **proliferative**, **secretory**, and **ischemic phases** (see Figure 22-15).

The **menstrual phase** (4 to 5 days) is the initial phase of the cycle.

Figure 22-15. **Endometrial cycle**

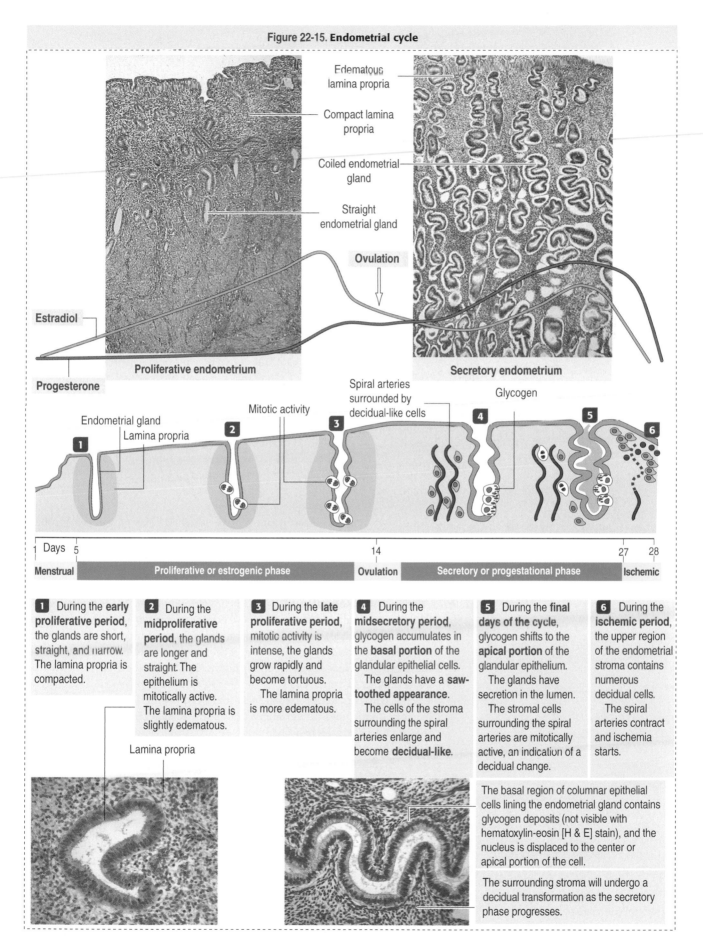

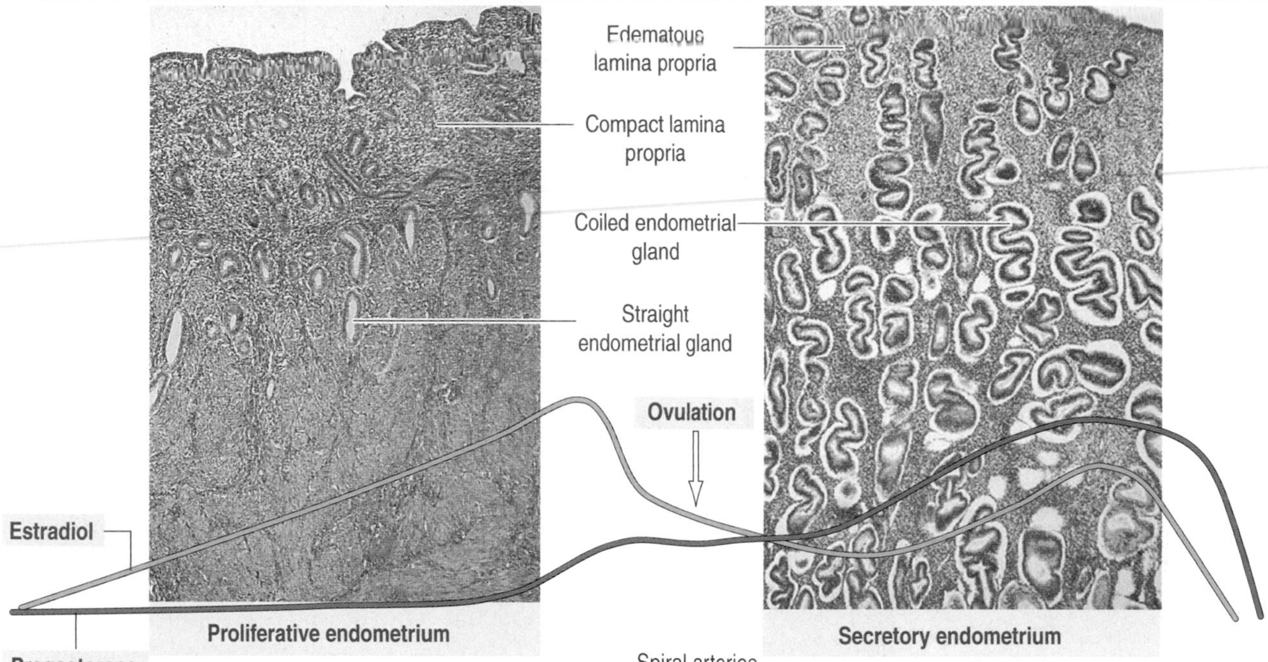
Edematous lamina propria
Compact lamina propria
Coiled endometrial gland
Straight endometrial gland
Ovulation
Estradiol
Progesterone
Proliferative endometrium
Secretory endometrium

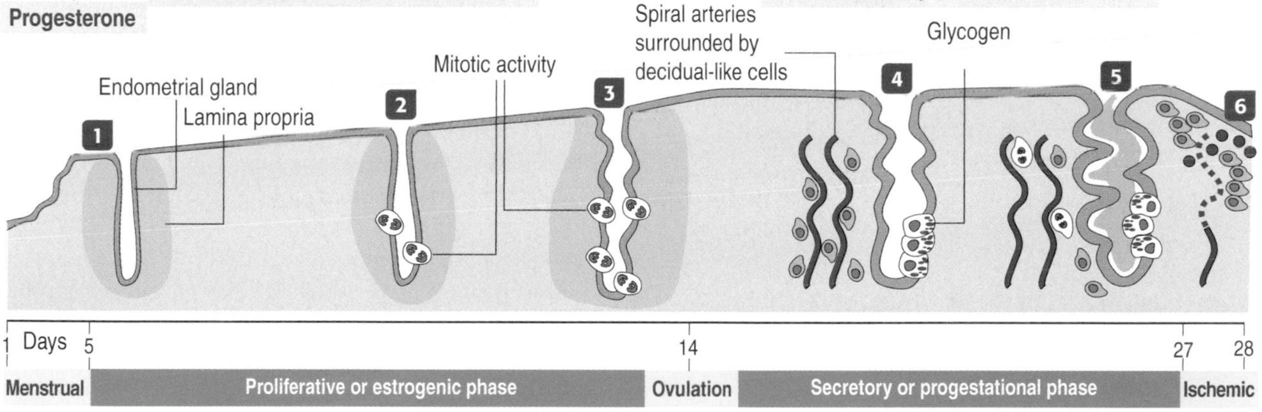
Spiral arteries surrounded by decidual-like cells
Glycogen
Mitotic activity
Endometrial gland
Lamina propria
1
2
3
4
5
6
Days
1
5
14
27
28
Menstrual
Proliferative or estrogenic phase
Ovulation
Secretory or progestational phase
Ischemic

1 During the **early proliferative period**, the glands are short, straight, and narrow. The lamina propria is compacted.

2 During the **midproliferative period**, the glands are longer and straight. The epithelium is mitotically active. The lamina propria is slightly edematous.

3 During the **late proliferative period**, mitotic activity is intense, the glands grow rapidly and become tortuous.

The lamina propria is more edematous.

4 During the **midsecretory period**, glycogen accumulates in the **basal portion** of the glandular epithelial cells.

The glands have a **saw-toothed appearance**.

The cells of the stroma surrounding the spiral arteries enlarge and become **decidual-like**.

5 During the **final days of the cycle**, glycogen shifts to the **apical portion** of the glandular epithelium.

The glands have secretion in the lumen.

The stromal cells surrounding the spiral arteries are mitotically active, an indication of a decidual change.

6 During the **ischemic period**, the upper region of the endometrial stroma contains numerous decidual cells.

The spiral arteries contract and ischemia starts.

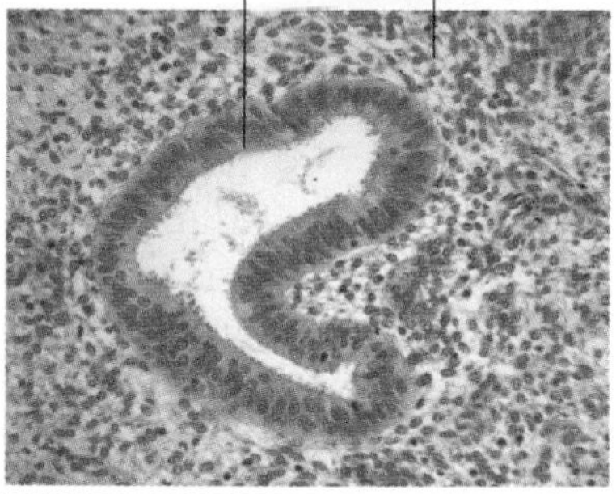
Lamina propria

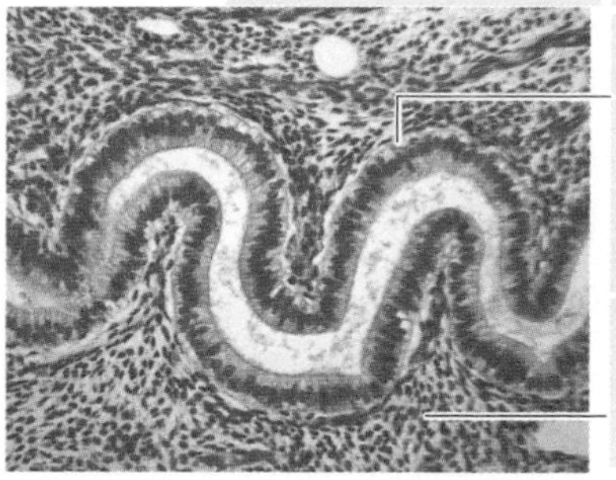

The basal region of columnar epithelial cells lining the endometrial gland contains glycogen deposits (not visible with hematoxylin-eosin [H & E] stain), and the nucleus is displaced to the center or apical portion of the cell.

The surrounding stroma will undergo a decidual transformation as the secretory phase progresses.

Figure 22-16. **Premenstrual endometrium**

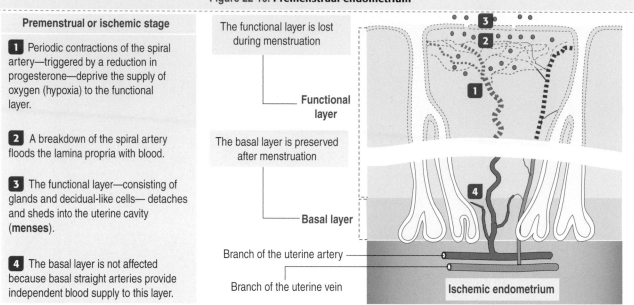

Premenstrual or ischemic stage

1 Periodic contractions of the spiral artery—triggered by a reduction in progesterone—deprive the supply of oxygen (hypoxia) to the functional layer.

2 A breakdown of the spiral artery floods the lamina propria with blood.

3 The functional layer—consisting of glands and decidual-like cells— detaches and sheds into the uterine cavity (**menses**).

4 The basal layer is not affected because basal straight arteries provide independent blood supply to this layer.

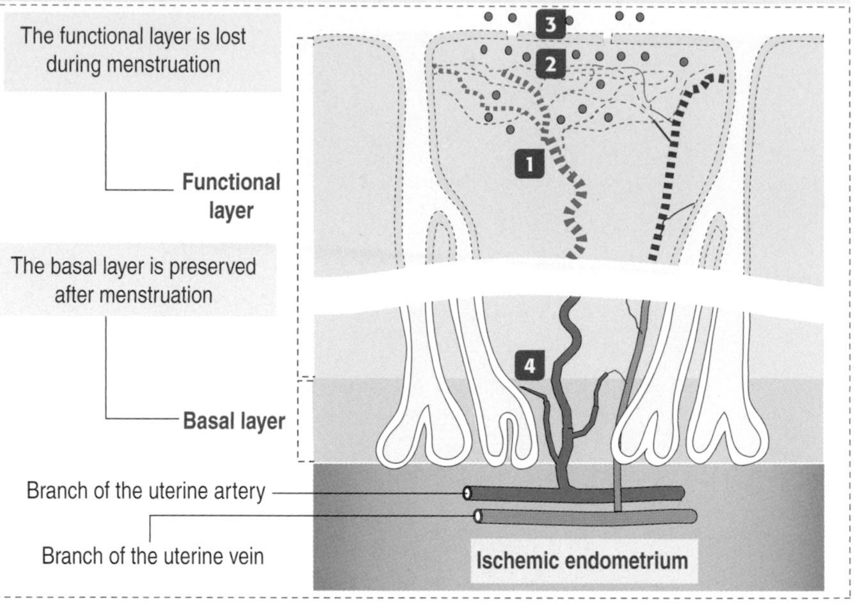

The functional layer is lost during menstruation
Functional layer
The basal layer is preserved after menstruation
Basal layer
Branch of the uterine artery
Branch of the uterine vein
Ischemic endometrium
1
2
3
4

The **proliferative phase** (also called the estrogenic or follicular phase) is of about 9 days duration. During the proliferative phase, the thickness of the endometrium increases as a result of the stimulatory activity of **estrogen** produced by maturing ovarian follicles. Mitotic activity is detected in both the lamina propria and the epithelium. Epithelial cells of the glandular epithelium migrate upward and the glands become straight and narrow.

After day 14, when ovulation occurs, the endometrium begins its third **secretory** or **progestational phase**, which lasts approximately 13 days. During this phase, endometrial glands initiate their secretory activity.

The outline of the tubular glands becomes irregular and coiled, the lining epithelium accumulates **glycogen**, and secretions rich in glycogen and glycoproteins are present in the glandular lumen. Blood vessels parallel to the endometrial glands increase in length and the lamina propria contains excessive fluid (edema). The secretory phase is controlled by both **progesterone** and **estrogen** produced in the corpus luteum.

At the end of the menstrual cycle, the involution of the corpus luteum results from a decrease in blood levels of steroid hormones, leading to an **ischemic phase** (duration of about 1 day). A reduction in the normal blood supply—causing intermittent **ischemia**—and the consequent hypoxia determine the necrosis of the functional layer of the endometrium, which sloughs off during the menstrual phase (Figure 22-16).

If pregnancy takes place, **stromal cells** in the endometrial lamina propria increase in size and store lipids and glycogen in response to increasing progesterone levels (Figures 22-17 and 22-18). This endometrial change is known as a **decidual reaction** (Latin *deciduus*, falling off) because the functional layer of the endometrium will be shed as the **decidua** at parturition.

Figure 22-17. **Decidual cells**

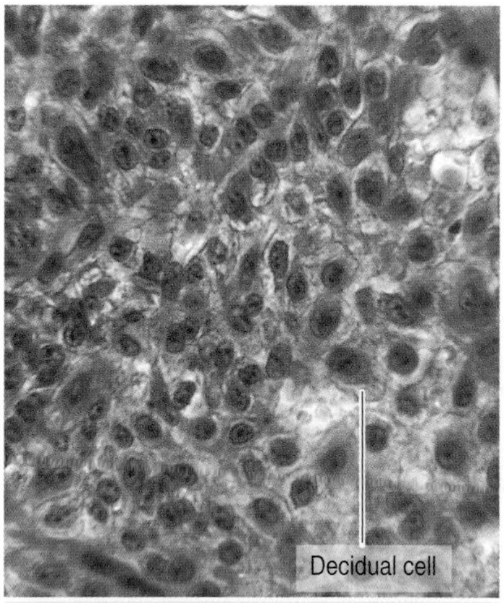

Decidual cell

The **decidual reaction** consists in the enlargement of endometrial stromal cells. Implantation of the fertilized egg depends on a hormonally primed endometrium (see Chapter 23, Fertilization, Placentation, and Lactation) consisting of secretory endometrial glands surrounded by decidual cells. In addition, high progesterone levels keep the myometrium relatively quiescent.

Vascularization of the endometrium and menstruation

The vascular supply to the endometrium is unusual. **Arcuate arteries** supply the endometrium. An arcuate artery has two segments (see Figure 22-14):

1. A **straight segment** (supplying the **basal layer** of the endometrium).
2. A **coiled segment** (supplying the **functional layer** of the endometrium).

The coiled segment stretches as the endometrium grows in thickness. Just before menstruation, **contraction of the artery at the straight-coiled segment interface reduces the blood flow and causes the destruction of the functional layer of the endometrium.**

Figure 22-18. **Decidual cell**

Decidual cells

Decidual cells derive from the epithelial-like transformation of endometrial **stroma cells** (**decidual reaction** in preparation for embryo implantation).

Decidual cells **modulate trophoblast cell invasion**.

Decidual cells **provide nutrients to the developing embryo**.

Together with trophoblast cells, decidual cells **prevent the immunologic rejection** of genetically different embryonic and fetal tissues.

Decidual cells have an **endocrine role**: the production of **decidual prolactin**—related to pituitary prolactin—with a trophic effect on the **corpus luteum**.

Decidual cell

Vascular changes
An increase in the permeability of endometrial blood vessels and angiogenesis occurs in response to embryo implantation.

Recruitment of inflammatory cells
Lymphocytes, macrophages, and eosinophils are attracted to the implantation site.

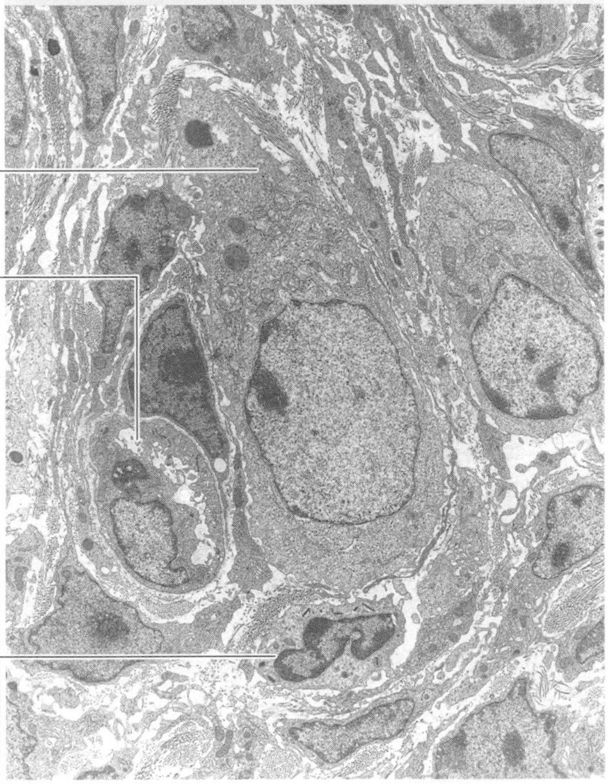

Electron micrograph from Cross PC, Mercer KL: Cell and Tissue Ultrastructure. New York, WH Freeman, 1993.

IGF-1 sequestered by IGF-bp prevents proliferation of endometrial glands.

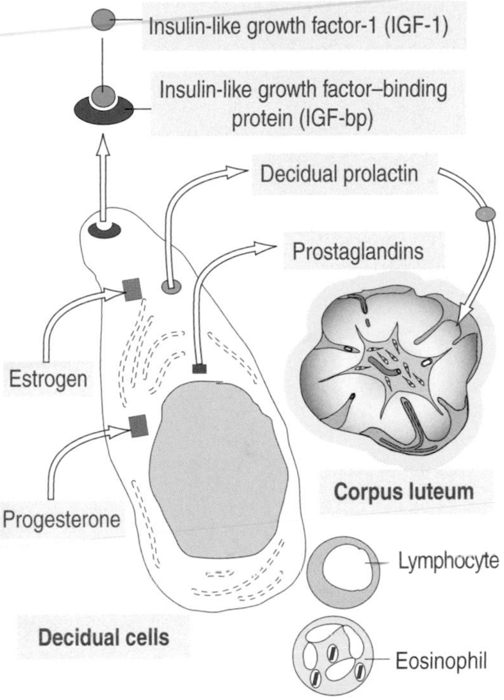
Insulin-like growth factor-1 (IGF-1)
Insulin-like growth factor–binding protein (IGF-bp)
Decidual prolactin
Prostaglandins
Estrogen
Progesterone
Corpus luteum
Lymphocyte
Eosinophil
Decidual cells

In addition to decidual prolactin, decidual cells produce **prostaglandins** and **relaxin**.

Decidual cells have receptors for **estrogens** and **progesterone**.

Decidual cells secrete **IGF-binding proteins** which bind IGFs to prevent their proliferative action on endometrial cells.

Clinical significance: Endometriosis

Endometriosis is a relatively common and painful disorder in which clusters of endometrium become implanted outside the uterus (predominantly in the oviduct, ovaries, and the peritoneal lining of the pelvis). During the menstrual cycle, the implanted endometrial tissue continues to proliferate, secrete, and bleed in relation to the hormonal levels as the endometrium does. Trapped bleeding can give rise to cysts, scar tissue, and adhesions.

Painful periods occur in the area of endometriosis during menstruation (**dysmenorrhea**). Excessive bleeding during the menstrual period (**menorrhagia**) or bleeding between periods (**menometrorrhagia**) can be seen. Endometriosis is commonly first diagnosed in patients seeking treatment for **infertility**.

The cause of endometriosis remains elusive. Possible causes include a flow back of endometrial tissue through the oviduct to the implanting site, the dissemination of endometrial cells through the bloodstream, and a familial predisposition to endometriosis.

Diagnosis is established by ultrasound and laparoscopy. A blood test to detect

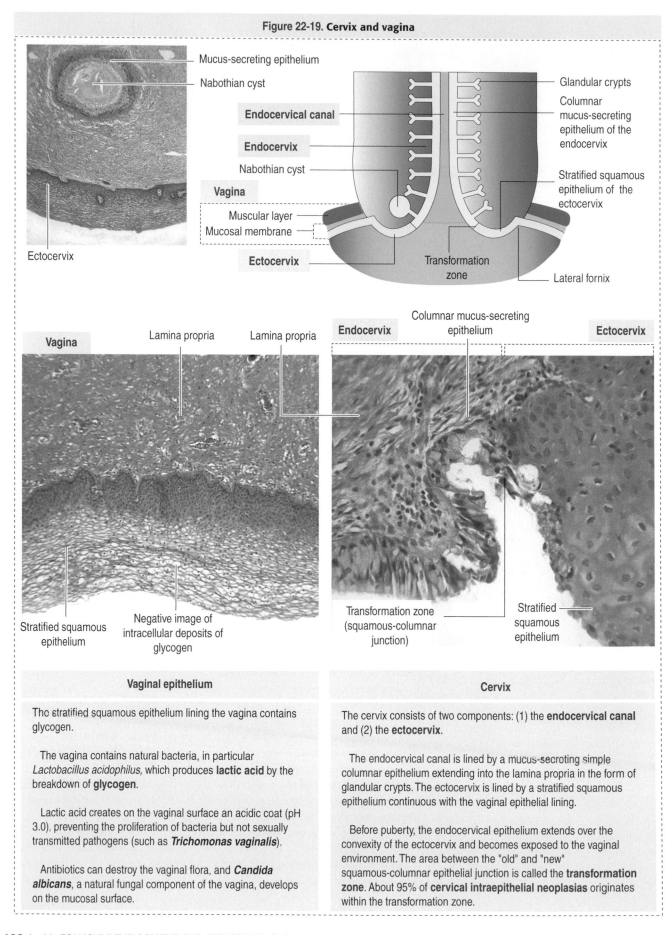

Figure 22-19. Cervix and vagina

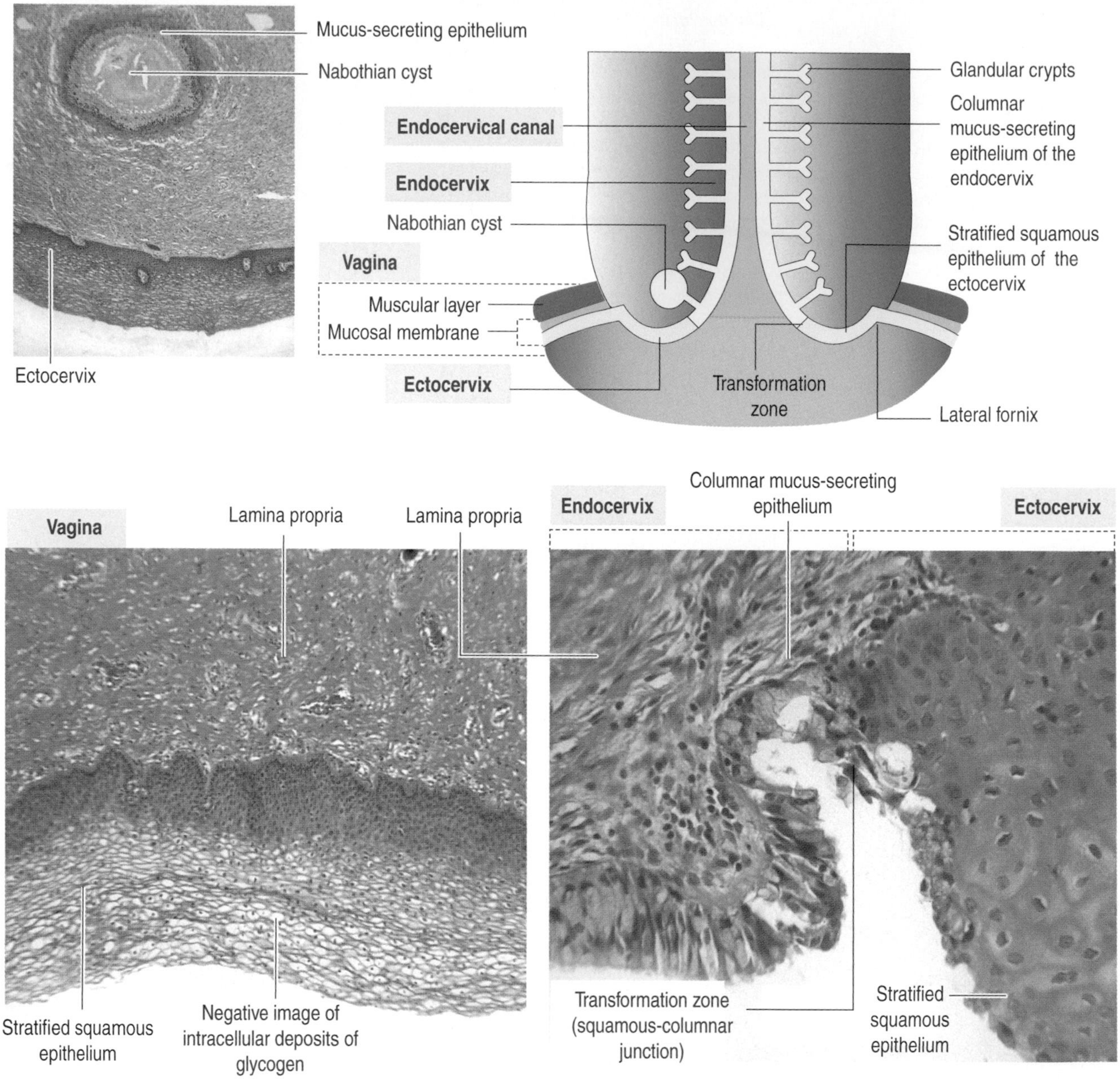

Mucus-secreting epithelium
Nabothian cyst
Ectocervix
Endocervical canal
Endocervix
Nabothian cyst
Vagina
Muscular layer
Mucosal membrane
Ectocervix
Glandular crypts
Columnar mucus-secreting epithelium of the endocervix
Stratified squamous epithelium of the ectocervix
Transformation zone
Lateral fornix
Vagina
Lamina propria
Lamina propria
Stratified squamous epithelium
Negative image of intracellular deposits of glycogen
Endocervix
Columnar mucus-secreting epithelium
Ectocervix
Transformation zone (squamous-columnar junction)
Stratified squamous epithelium

Vaginal epithelium

Tho stratified squamous epithelium lining the vagina contains glycogen.

The vagina contains natural bacteria, in particular *Lactobacillus acidophilus,* which produces **lactic acid** by the breakdown of **glycogen**.

Lactic acid creates on the vaginal surface an acidic coat (pH 3.0), preventing the proliferation of bacteria but not sexually transmitted pathogens (such as ***Trichomonas vaginalis***).

Antibiotics can destroy the vaginal flora, and ***Candida albicans***, a natural fungal component of the vagina, develops on the mucosal surface.

Cervix

The cervix consists of two components: (1) the **endocervical canal** and (2) the **ectocervix**.

The endocervical canal is lined by a mucus-secroting simple columnar epithelium extending into the lamina propria in the form of glandular crypts. The ectocervix is lined by a stratified squamous epithelium continuous with the vaginal epithelial lining.

Before puberty, the endocervical epithelium extends over the convexity of the ectocervix and becomes exposed to the vaginal environment. The area between the "old" and "new" squamous-columnar epithelial junction is called the **transformation zone**. About 95% of **cervical intraepithelial neoplasias** originates within the transformation zone.

protein CA-125, frequently found in women with endometriosis, can determine an elevation of this protein in advanced endometriosis but not in the incipient phase of the disease. The treatment includes pain medications, hormone therapy (oral contraceptives and gonadotropin-releasing hormone agonists and antagonists to block the production of ovarian hormones by creating an induced menopause), conservative surgery to remove implanted endometrial tissue, and, in the most severe cases, the surgical removal of the uterus (**hysterectomy**) and both ovaries.

Cervix

The cervix is the lower extension of the uterus. It communicates with the uterine cavity and the vagina through the **external os** of the **cervical canal** called the **endocervix**.

The endocervix contains mucus-secreting **tubular glands** lined by a columnar epithelium, and scattered ciliated cells (Figure 22-19). The endocervical glands are surrounded by a fibrocollagenous and smooth muscle stroma with abundant blood vessels. The endocervical tubular glands are deep invaginations (**crypts**) of the surface epithelium that increase the surface area of mucus-producing cells.

The secretory activity of the **endocervical glands** is regulated by **estrogens** and is **maximal at the time of ovulation**. The product of the glands lubricates the vagina during sexual intercourse and acts as a bacterial protective barrier blocking access to the uterine cavity.

During ovulation, the mucus is less viscous, is hydrated, and has an alkaline pH, conditions favorable for the migration of sperm. The high content of ions (Na^+, K^+, and Cl^-) is responsible for the **crystallization of the mucus** into a fernlike pattern in the ovulatory phase. This feature of cervical mucus is used clinically to assess the optimal time for fertilization to occur.

After ovulation, the mucus is highly viscous with an acidic pH, detrimental conditions for sperm penetration and viability. Endocervical glands may become obstructed, forming cysts called **cysts of Naboth** or **nabothian cysts**.

Clinical significance: Cervical intraepithelial neoplasia and human papilloma virus infection

The external segment of the cervix, the **ectocervix**, is lined by **stratified squamous epithelium**. There is an abrupt epithelial transition between the endocervix and the ectocervix, called the **transformation zone**.

At the transformation zone, **dysplasia**, an abnormal but reversible condition, may occur. Dysplasia is characterized by disorganized epithelial cells that slough off before reaching full stratified maturity.

However, dysplasia can progress into **carcinoma in situ**, a condition in which proliferation of epithelial cells is very active but within the limits of the basal lamina (**cervical intraepithelial neoplasia** or **CIN**). This condition can be reversible or can progress (if undetected) into an **invasive carcinoma** that breaks the continuity of the basal lamina and invades the underlying connective tissue. Dysplasia and carcinoma in situ can be detected by the routine **Papanicolaou smear** (Pap smear).

Various strains of the **human papillomavirus (HPV)**, a sexually transmitted infection, have been associated with the majority of cervical cancer cases. Like the Pap smear, cells collected from the cervix can be used to determine by an HPV test whether a patient is infected with any of the 13 types of HPV. This test can detect high-risk HPV strains (e.g., HPV-16 and HPV-18) in cell DNA before the development of CIN.

Vagina

The vagina is a fibromuscular tube consisting of three layers:

1. An inner **mucosal layer** (stratified squamous epithelium with a **lamina propria** usually infiltrated by neutrophils and lymphocytes; see Figure 22-19).
2. A middle **muscularis layer** (circular and longitudinal smooth muscle).

Figure 22-20. **Female urethra**

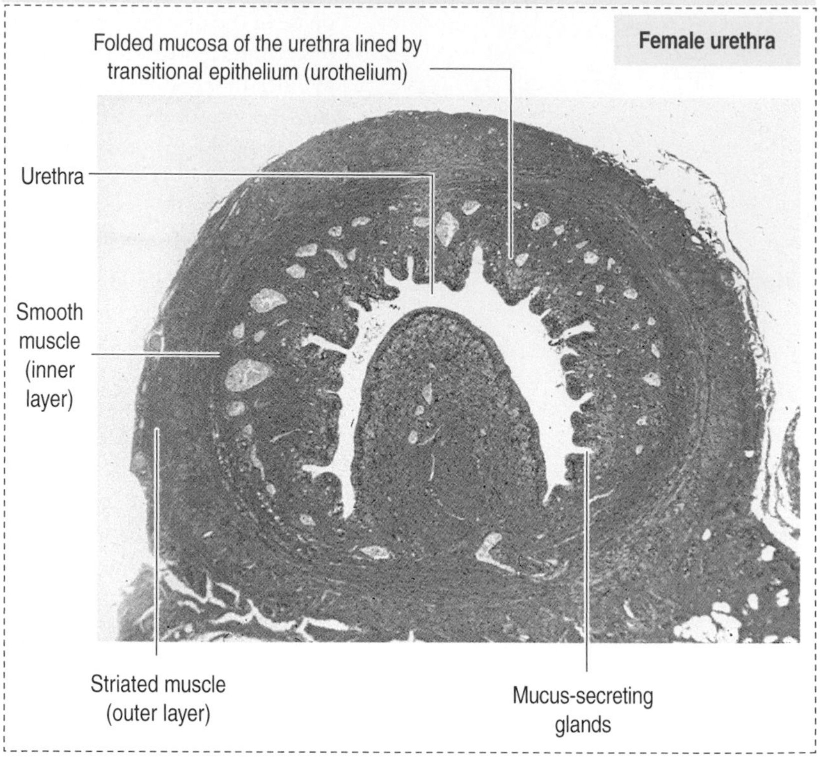
Female urethra
Folded mucosa of the urethra lined by transitional epithelium (urothelium)
Urethra
Smooth muscle (inner layer)
Striated muscle (outer layer)
Mucus-secreting glands

3. An outer **adventitial layer** (dense connective tissue).

The surface of the mucosa is kept moist by mucus secreted by uterine and endocervical glands and the **glands of Bartholin** in the vestibule. The wall of the vagina lacks glands.

The vaginal epithelium undergoes cyclic changes during the menstrual cycle. The **differentiation of vaginal epithelium** is stimulated by **estrogens**. At ovulation, the stratified epithelium is fully differentiated, and abundant acidophilic squamous cells can be seen in the Pap smear.

After ovulation, when **progesterone** predominates, the number of squamous cells declines and more basophilic cells appear, together with neutrophils and lymphocytes. The vaginal smear provides rapid information on estrogen and progesterone levels during the menstrual cycle and is also useful for monitoring the hormonal status during pregnancy.

Mons pubis, labia majora, and labia minora

The mons pubis, labia majora, and labia minora are modified skin structures. The **mons pubis** (mons veneris) is skin lined by **keratinized stratified squamous epithelium** with hair follicles covering subcutaneous fat overlying the symphysis pubis.

The **labia majora** are extensions of the mons pubis at each side of the vaginal introitus. In addition to skin with hair follicles and glands (**apocrine sweat glands** and **sebaceous glands**) covering the fat pad, smooth muscle fibers are detected in the subcutaneous fat. Hair follicles and fat accumulation are regulated by sex hormones at the onset of sexual maturity (by the age of 10 to 13 years old).

The **labia minora** are skin folds without adipose tissue and hair follicles but with abundant blood vessels, elastic fibers, and sebaceous glands opening directly onto the surface of the melanin-pigmented epidermis. Pigmentation of the epidermis of both labia majora and minora appears at the initiation of puberty.

The **hymen** is the limit between the internal and external genitalia. It consists of a thin fibrous membrane lining the lower vagina, covered on its external surface by a **keratinized stratified squamous epithelium** and on the internal surface by

nonkeratinizing stratified squamous epithelium with glycogen (like the vaginal epithelium).

The **clitoris**, located below the mons pubis, is the female equivalent of the penis. Like the penis, it consists of two side-by-side corpora cavernosa (erectile vascular tissue) separated by a septum, surrounded by a fibrous collagenous sheath. The clitoris is partially covered by skin containing rich sensory nerves and receptors but lacking hair follicles and glands.

Urethral meatus and glands (paraurethral glands and Bartholin's glands)

The urethral meatus communicates with the exterior close to the clitoris. **Paraurethral glands of Skene** are distributed around the meatus and are lined by **pseudostratified columnar epithelium**.

Bartholin's vulvovaginal glands are found around the lower vagina and consist of acini with mucus-secreting cells. A duct covered by a transitional epithelium connects these glands to the posterolateral side of the vagina.

The **female urethra** is covered by a **folded mucosa** lined by a **transitional epithelium** changing first to a pseudostratified columnar epithelium and, near the urethral meatus, to a nonkeratinizing stratified squamous epithelium. **Mucus-secreting glands** are observed in the **mucosa** (Figure 22-20).

The **muscular wall** consists of a **single longitudinal layer of smooth muscle (involuntary sphincter)**. A **circular striated muscle (voluntary sphincter)** is observed outside the smooth muscle layer. A connective tissue rich in elastic fibers provides support to the muscle layers.

Essential concepts | Follicle Development and Menstrual Cycle

• Development of the ovary. The cortical region of the indifferent gonad develops into an ovary. Primary sex cords (derived from the coelomic epithelium) are replaced by secondary sex cords surrounding oogonia, mitotically dividing cells derived from primordial germ cells with two X chromosomes. Oogonia complete mitosis and enter meiotic prophase I to become primary oocytes. Meiosis is arrested following crossing over, a state that will continue until puberty. Therefore, at the time of birth, primary oocytes at the diplotene stage are surrounded by follicular cells.

Turner's syndrome is caused by the absence of all or part of a second X chromosome (45,X). Atrophic ovaries, short stature, skeletal abnormalities, and lymphedema are characteristic features.

• Development of the female genital ducts. The cranial ends of the müllerian ducts remain separated to form the oviduct. The caudal segments fuse to develop into the uterovaginal primordium, which becomes the uterus and upper part of the vagina. The canalization of the vaginal plate (the contact point of the uterovaginal primordium with the urogenital sinus) results in the middle and lower part of the vagina. The genital tubercle (phallus) develops at the cranial end of the cloacal membrane. The labioscrotal swellings (that will give rise to the labia majora) and urogenital folds (that will give rise to the labia minora) develop at either side of the cloacal membrane. In the absence of androgens, the phallus develops into the clitoris.

Rokitansky-Küster-Hauser syndrome (absence of the uterus, cervix, and upper vagina; normal ovulation but no menstruation) is caused by the agenesis of the müllerian duct.

• The ovary is lined by simple squamous-to-low cuboidal epithelium supported by a layer of connective tissue, the tunica albuginea. The ovary has a cortex and a medulla. The cortex houses the primordial follicles; the medulla consists of blood vessels (ovarian artery and vein), nerves, and lymphatic vessels.

The ovarian cycle consists of three phases: (1) follicular phase (consisting of the development of a primordial follicle into a mature or graafian follicle); (2) ovulatory phase (rupture of the graafian follicle, completion of meiosis I [resulting in the formation of the first polar body], and release of the now secondary oocyte from the ovary); and (3) luteal phase (transformation of the residual follicular membrane and theca interna cells in a vascularized, steroid-producing corpus luteum).

The follicular phase (or folliculogenesis) results in the following sequence:

1. Primordial follicle (primary oocyte surrounded by a single layer of simple squamous epithelial follicular cells supported by a basement membrane).

2. Primary follicle. There are two substages: unilayered primary follicle (primary oocyte, which starts to produce glycoproteins of the zona pellucida, surrounded by a single layer of cuboidal follicular cells) and multilayered primary follicle (primary oocyte surrounded by several layers of follicular cells).

3. Secondary follicle (primary oocyte separated from the multilayered follicular cells by the zona pellucida). Cell processes of the follicular cells adjacent to the zona pellucida (the future corona radiata) penetrate the progressively thickening zona pellucida and establish contact with the plasma membrane of the primary oocyte. Gap junctions are present at the contact points and between adjacent follicular cells. In addition, spaces containing fluid (liquor folliculi; also named Call-Exner bodies) appear between the multilayered follicular cells. These spaces will coalesce to form the antrum in the mature follicle.

Stromal cells surrounding the developing follicle differentiate into two layers: the highly vascularized theca interna (producing androstenedione that is transferred to follicular cells across the basement membrane so they can produce estrogen), and the theca externa, a connective tissue continuous with the ovarian stroma.

4. Mature follicle (also called graafian follicle) consists of a primary oocyte surrounded by the zona pellucida. The follicular cells become displaced by the fluid in the antrum

and segregate into two distinct regions: the corona radiata, represented by follicular cells surrounding and anchored to the zona pellucida; and the cumulus oophorus, a cluster of follicular cells linking the primary oocyte–zona pellucida–corona radiata complex to the wall of the follicle. The cumulus oophorus prevents the cell complex from floating in the antrum fluid. However, at a later stage preceding ovulation, the cumulus oophorus will sever its relationship with the cell complex to facilitate the ovulation process.

A mechanism prevents primary oocytes to complete meiosis I while they remain inside the developing follicle. Follicular cells produce oocyte maturation inhibitor, which is transferred from follicular cells to the oocyte through cytoplasmic processes crossing the zona pellucida and connected to the oocyte by gap junctions. Just before ovulation, the oocyte produces maturation promoting factor (Cdc2-cyclin B complex), which induces completion of meiosis I and formation of the first polar body.

Follicular atresia is a physiologic apoptotic process consisting in a failure of ovarian follicles to complete folliculogenesis at any point in development.

The luteal phase occurs soon after ovulation and consists in the formation of the corpus luteum (a process called luteinization). Luteinization consists in the breakdown of the basement membrane of the follicle, the invasion of blood vessels from the theca interna, and the transformation of the remnant follicular cells into follicular lutein cells and of the theca interna cells into theca lutein cells. The secretion of estrogen and progesterone takes place in response to FSH (follicle strimulating hormone) and LH (luteinizing hormone) stimulation. Theca lutein cells cooperate with follicular lutein cells to produce estradiol; both cell types can independently synthesize progesterone.

If fertilization occurs, the secondary oocyte will complete meiosis II, produce the second polar body, and become a haploid pronucleus to fuse with the haploid sperm pronucleus to form a zygote. The trophoblastic cells of the implanted embryo produce chorionic gonadotropin, which will take over the control of corpus luteum estrogen and progesterone secretory function. If no fertilization occurs, the corpus luteum undergoes degeneration (a process called luteolysis) and changes into a connective tissue scar called corpus albicans.

• Oviduct (fallopian tube or uterine tube). The oviduct is a muscular tube divided into four anatomic regions: (1) Infundibulum (characterized by finger-like folds called fimbriae, responsible for capturing the ovulated complex from the ovary). (2) Ampulla (the site where fertilization takes place). (3) Isthmus (the site where the muscle layer of the tube thickens and muscle contraction helps the displacement of sperm toward the ovulated cell complex [called egg or ovum] and the movement of the fertilized embryo to the uterus). (4) Intramural segment (the oviduct-uterine junction). The wall of the oviduct consists of three layers: the mucosa, consisting of a simple columnar epithelium with ciliated and nonciliated cells supported by a lamina propria, a muscular layer, and a serosa layer.

• Uterus. The uterus consists of two anatomic segments: the corpus or body, and the cervix. The body of the uterus consists of three layers: the endometrium, the myometrium, and the serosa/adventitia.

The endometrium consists of a simple columnar epithelial cell lining and associated simple tubular endometrial glands surrounded by a lamina propria (the endometrial stroma). The endometrium has a superficial functional layer (lost during menstruation), and a basal layer (retained during menstruation as a reserve for tissue regeneration). The superficial functional layer is supplied by a spiral endometrial artery; the basal layer is supplied by a basal straight artery, an independent blood supply.

Four consecutive phases characterize the menstrual cycle: the menstrual phase (days 1 to 5), the proliferative or estrogenic phase (days 5 to 14), the secretory or progestational phase (days 15 to 27), and the ischemic phase (days 27 to 28). Contraction of the spiral endometrial artery during the ischemic phase reduces blood flow and triggers the destruction of the functional endometrial layer. Ovulation marks the end of the proliferative phase and the beginning of the secretory phase.

If pregnancy takes place, cells of the endometrial stroma change into an epithelial-like shape and become decidual cells. This change is called the decidual reaction. Decidual cells modulate trophoblast-driven embryo implantation, provide nutrients to the developing embryo, and, together with the trophoblast, prevent immunologic rejection of genetically different embryonic and fetal tissues.

Endometriosis is a disorder characterized by the implantation and growth of endometrial tissue in the oviduct, ovaries, and pelvic peritoneal surface. The ectopic endometrial tissue responds to hormonal stimulation, like the endometrium. Pain during menstruation (dysmenorrhea), excessive bleeding during menstruation (menorrhagia), or bleeding between periods (menometrorrhagia) are characteristic clinical findings. Infertility is associated with endometriosis.

• Cervix. The cervix consists of two components: the endocervical canal and the ectocervix.

The endocervical canal is lined by a mucus-secreting simple columnar epithelium extending into the lamina propria forming glandular crypts. During ovulation, the mucus is less viscous and alkaline, two conditions favoring sperm penetration. After ovulation, the mucus becomes viscous and acidic, two unfavorable conditions for sperm penetration. Occlusion of the glandular crypts gives rise to cysts, called nabothian cysts.

The ectocervix is lined by a stratified squamous epithelium. The simple columnar-stratified squamous epithelial junction is called the transformation zone, the site of origin of most cervical intraepithelial neoplasias. The Papanicolaou test (Pap smear) has played a significant role in the early detection of cervical cancer. **Human papillomavirus,** a sexually transmitted infection, has been associated with the origin of cervical cancer.

• Vagina. A fibromuscular tube consisting of three layers: an inner mucosa layer (stratified squamous epithelium, rich in glycogen, supported by a lamina propria), a middle smooth muscle layer, and an outer connective tissue adventitial layer. The differentiation of the vaginal epithelium is hormone-dependent and undergoes cyclic changes during the menstrual cycle. The breakdown of glycogen by *Lactobacillus acidophilus* into lactic acid creates an acidic vaginal coat preventing proliferation of bacteria but not sexually transmitted pathogens.

• Mons pubis, labia majora, and labia minora are modified skin structures. The mons pubis is skin lined by keratinized stratified squamous epithelium. The labia majora have, in addition to skin, apocrine sweat glands and sebaceous glands. Labia minora are melanin-pigmented epidermal skin folds with abundant blood vessels, elastic fibers, and sebaceous glands.

• Female urethra. The female urethra has a folded mucosa lined by transitional epithelium with mucosa glands. This epithelium changes into pseudostratified epithelium, and near the urethral meatus, to nonkeratinizing stratified squamous epithelium. The muscle wall consists of an inner smooth muscle layer (involuntary sphincter) and an outer striated muscle layer (voluntary sphincter).

Fertilization

Two events must occur before fertilization: (1) **sperm maturation** in the epididymis and (2) **sperm capacitation** in the female reproductive tract.

Sperm released from the testis and entering the epididymal duct have **circular motion**. After a 2-week **maturation process**, following epididymal transit and storage in the tail or cauda of the epididymis, sperm acquire **forward motility** necessary for fertilization. After ejaculation, sperm undergo a **capacitation process** in the uterus and fertilization of the ovum or egg takes place in the oviduct.

Essentially, **a fertilizing sperm must complete both maturation and capacitation before sperm-egg fusion**. Capacitation can be induced in vitro, a procedure that permits in vitro fertilization.

We have seen that the **sperm head** consists of three components: (1) the **condensed nucleus**, (2) the **acrosomal sac**, and (3) the **plasma membrane.**

The **condensed nucleus** consists of genomic DNA coated by very basic protamines. Nucleosomes are not present because somatic histones have been replaced by protamines.

The **acrosomal sac** is formed by three constituents (Figure 23-1): (1) the **outer acrosomal membrane**, (2) the **inner acrosomal membrane**, and (3) **hydrolytic enzymes** (mainly **hyaluronidase** and **acrosin**, the latter derived from the precursor **proacrosin**).

The thin portion of the acrosomal sac, extending toward the tail, is the **equatorial segment.**

Figure 23-1. Acrosome reaction

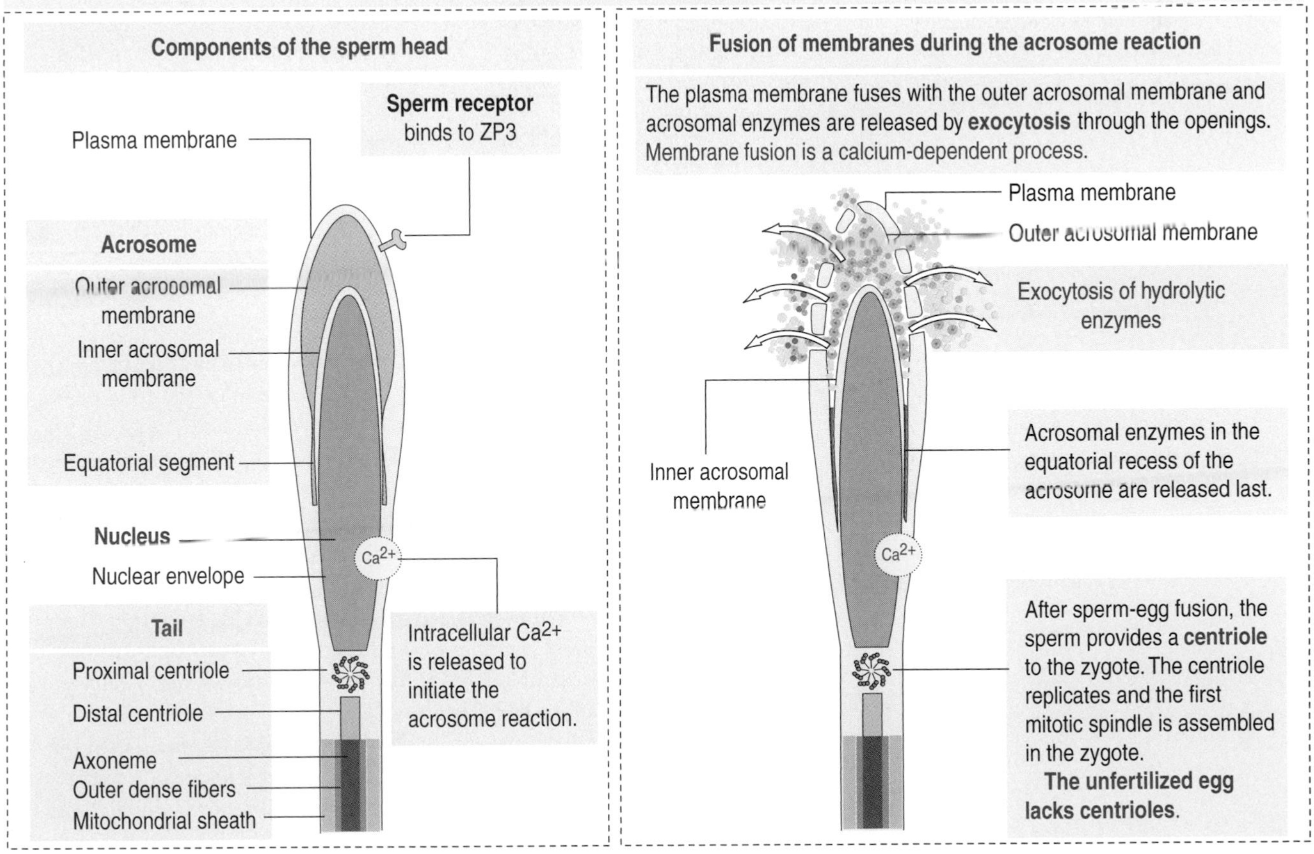

Components of the sperm head
Sperm receptor binds to ZP3
Plasma membrane
Acrosome
Outer acrosomal membrane
Inner acrosomal membrane
Equatorial segment
Nucleus
Nuclear envelope
Ca2+
Intracellular Ca2+ is released to initiate the acrosome reaction.
Tail
Proximal centriole
Distal centriole
Axoneme
Outer dense fibers
Mitochondrial sheath
Fusion of membranes during the acrosome reaction
The plasma membrane fuses with the outer acrosomal membrane and acrosomal enzymes are released by exocytosis through the openings. Membrane fusion is a calcium-dependent process.
Plasma membrane
Outer acrosomal membrane
Exocytosis of hydrolytic enzymes
Inner acrosomal membrane
Acrosomal enzymes in the equatorial recess of the acrosome are released last.
Ca2+
After sperm-egg fusion, the sperm provides a centriole to the zygote. The centriole replicates and the first mitotic spindle is assembled in the zygote.
The unfertilized egg lacks centrioles.

Figure 23-2. **Fertilization**

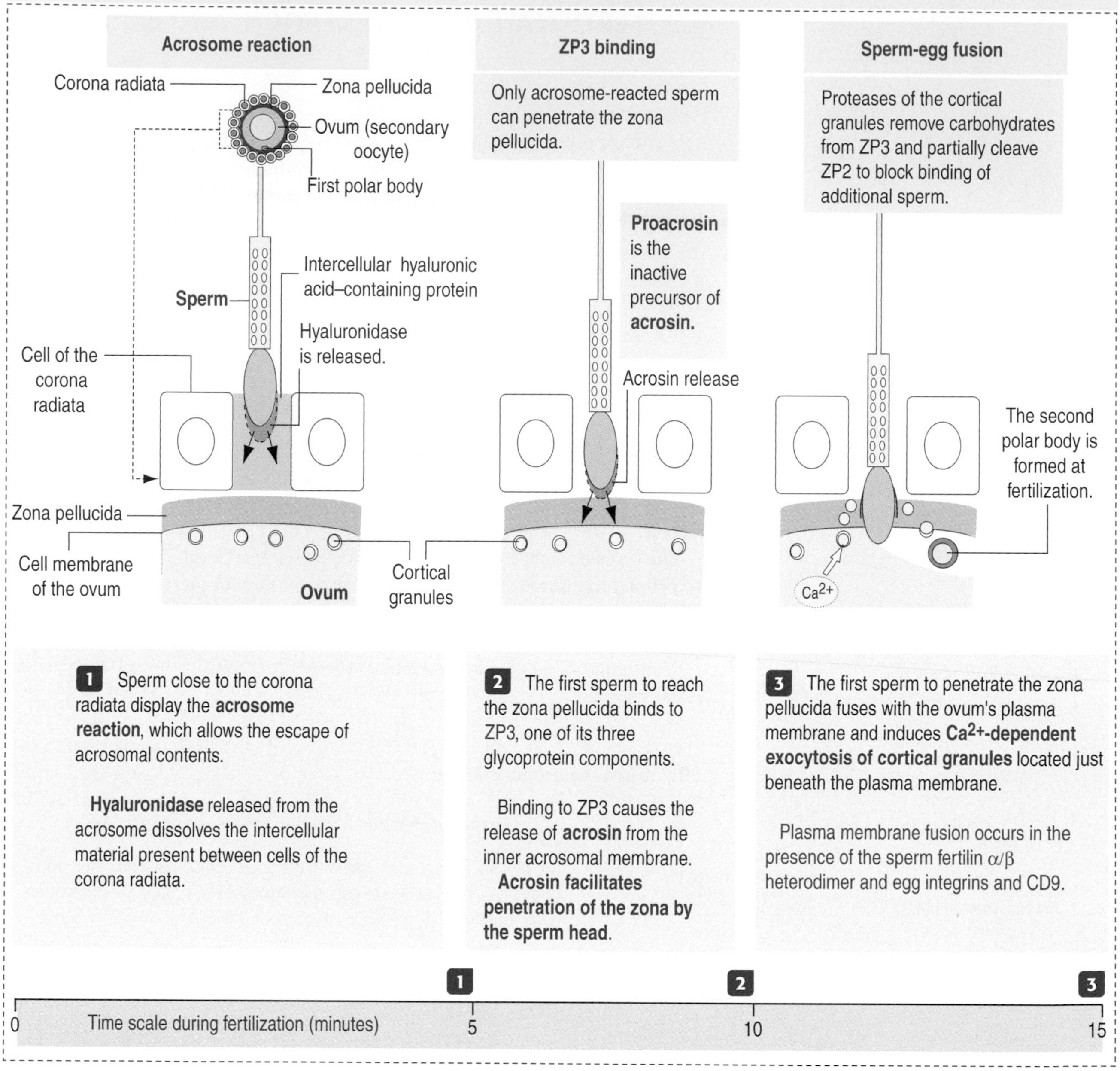
Acrosome reaction
Corona radiata
Zona pellucida
Ovum (secondary oocyte)
First polar body
Sperm
Intercellular hyaluronic acid–containing protein
Hyaluronidase is released.
Cell of the corona radiata
Zona pellucida
Cell membrane of the ovum
Ovum
Cortical granules
ZP3 binding
Only acrosome-reacted sperm can penetrate the zona pellucida.
Proacrosin is the inactive precursor of acrosin.
Acrosin release
Sperm-egg fusion
Proteases of the cortical granules remove carbohydrates from ZP3 and partially cleave ZP2 to block binding of additional sperm.
The second polar body is formed at fertilization.
Ca2+
1 Sperm close to the corona radiata display the acrosome reaction, which allows the escape of acrosomal contents.
Hyaluronidase released from the acrosome dissolves the intercellular material present between cells of the corona radiata.
2 The first sperm to reach the zona pellucida binds to ZP3, one of its three glycoprotein components.
Binding to ZP3 causes the release of acrosin from the inner acrosomal membrane.
Acrosin facilitates penetration of the zona by the sperm head.
3 The first sperm to penetrate the zona pellucida fuses with the ovum's plasma membrane and induces Ca2+-dependent exocytosis of cortical granules located just beneath the plasma membrane.
Plasma membrane fusion occurs in the presence of the sperm fertilin α/β heterodimer and egg integrins and CD9.
1
2
3
0
Time scale during fertilization (minutes)
5
10
15

The three main events during fertilization are, sequentially (Figure 23-2) the acrosome reaction, sperm binding to ZP3, a glycoprotein of the zona pellucida (Figure 23-3), and sperm-egg fusion (Figure 23-4).

The **sperm plasma membrane** harbors (see Figure 23-1) (1) **sperm receptors**, with binding affinity to the **zona pellucida**; and (2) **fertilin** α/β, a heterodimer member of a family of proteins called **ADAMs**, consisting of several domains, including a **metalloprotease** domain and a **disintegrin domain**. We have already discussed the structure of ADAM protein in Chapter 1, Epithelium (see Figure 1-10). The egg plasma membrane has $\alpha_3\beta_1$, $\alpha_6\beta_1$, and $\alpha_5\beta_1$ integrins, which associate with **CD9**, a protein member of the superfamily of **tetraspanins** (see Box 23-A). A lack of CD9 prevents sperm-egg fusion. The fertilin α and β heterodimer does not appear essential in sperm-egg fusion.

In the proximity of the ovum, and in the presence of Ca^{2+}, the sperm plasma membrane fuses with the outer acrosomal membrane. This event is known as the **acrosome reaction**. Small openings created by membrane fusion facilitate the release of hydrolytic enzymes (see Figures 23-1 and 23-2). The equatorial region of

Box 23-A | **Tetraspanins**

- **Tetraspanins,** first discovered on the human leukocyte surface, have four transmembrane domains, two extracellular loops (small and large), and short intracytoplasmic N- and C-terminal tails.
- The transmembrane domains enable the association of additional tetraspanins to assemble the tetraspanin web in which integrins are included. Tetraspanins function as surface organizers by grouping and interconnecting specific cell surface proteins.
- The large extracellular loop is involved in protein-protein interaction with laterally positioned proteins.
- The intracellular short tails are linked to intracellular cytoskeletal and signaling molecules.
- Tetraspanins behave as metastasis suppressor molecules. Decreased expression of tetraspanins correlates with an increased invasive and metastasis potential.

Figure 23-3. **Sperm binding to zona pellucida**

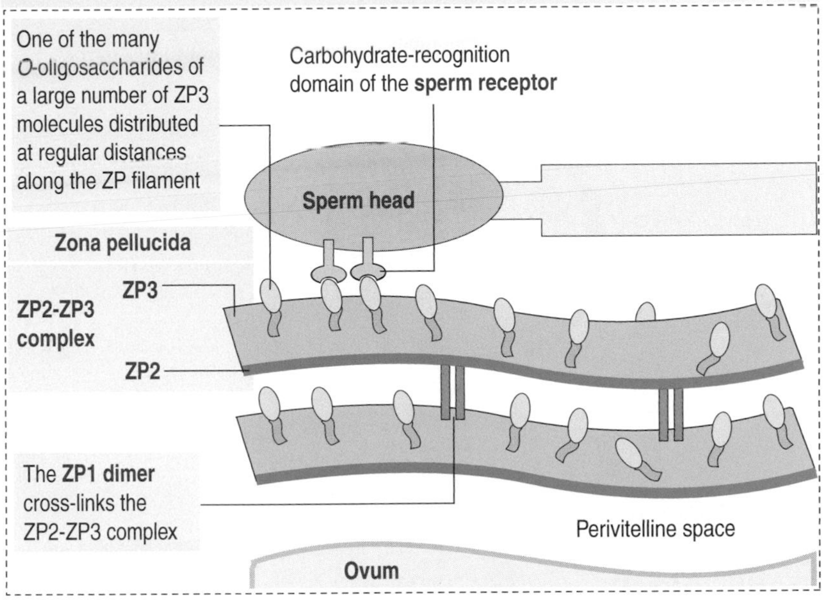

One of the many *O*-oligosaccharides of a large number of ZP3 molecules distributed at regular distances along the ZP filament
Carbohydrate-recognition domain of the **sperm receptor**
Sperm head
Zona pellucida
ZP3
ZP2-ZP3 complex
ZP2
The **ZP1 dimer** cross-links the ZP2-ZP3 complex
Perivitelline space
Ovum

the acrosome does not participate in the membrane fusion process at this time.

The zona pellucida

The plasma membranes of all mammalian eggs are surrounded by a 6- to 7-µm-thick zona pellucida produced by the egg. The zona pellucida is composed of only three glycoproteins (see Figure 23-3): **ZP1**, a dimer of 200 kd; **ZP2**, 120 kd; and **ZP3**, 83 kd.

ZP2 and ZP3 interact to form a long filament complex interconnected by ZP1 dimers at regular intervals. During sperm binding, ***O*-oligosaccharides** linked to ZP3 bind to sperm receptors. **Only acrosome-reacted sperm can interact with ZP3.**

Figure 23-4. **Sperm-egg fusion**

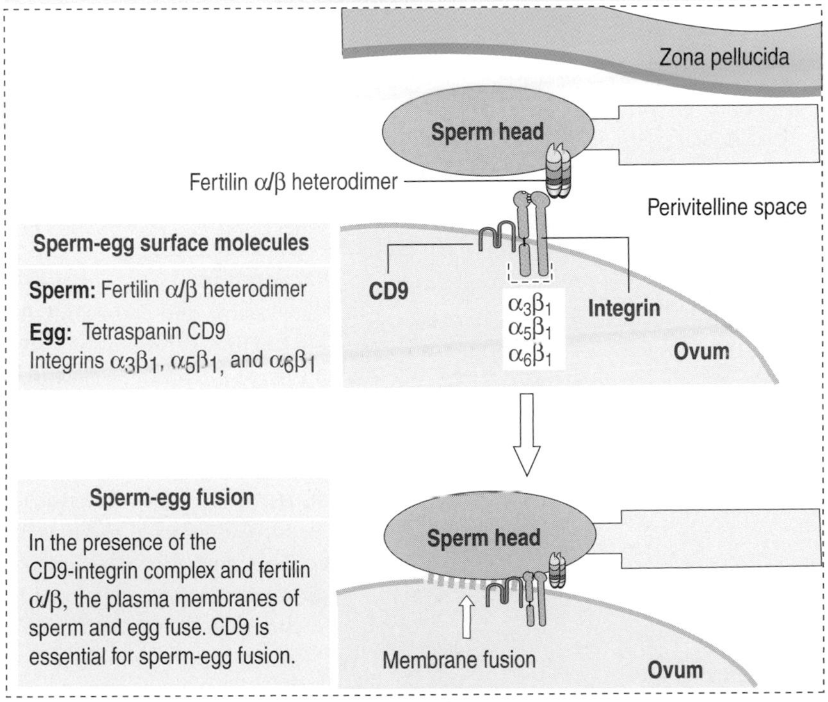

Zona pellucida
Sperm head
Fertilin α/β heterodimer
Perivitelline space
Sperm-egg surface molecules
Sperm: Fertilin α/β heterodimer
Egg: Tetraspanin CD9
Integrins $\alpha_3\beta_1$, $\alpha_5\beta_1$, and $\alpha_6\beta_1$
CD9
$\alpha_3\beta_1$
$\alpha_5\beta_1$
$\alpha_6\beta_1$
Integrin
Ovum
Sperm-egg fusion
In the presence of the CD9-integrin complex and fertilin α/β, the plasma membranes of sperm and egg fuse. CD9 is essential for sperm-egg fusion.
Sperm head
Membrane fusion
Ovum

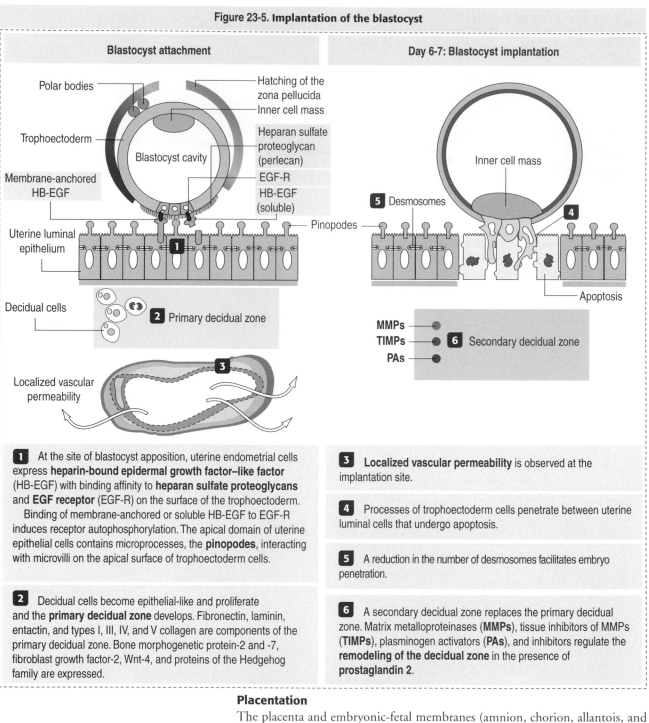

Figure 23-5. **Implantation of the blastocyst**

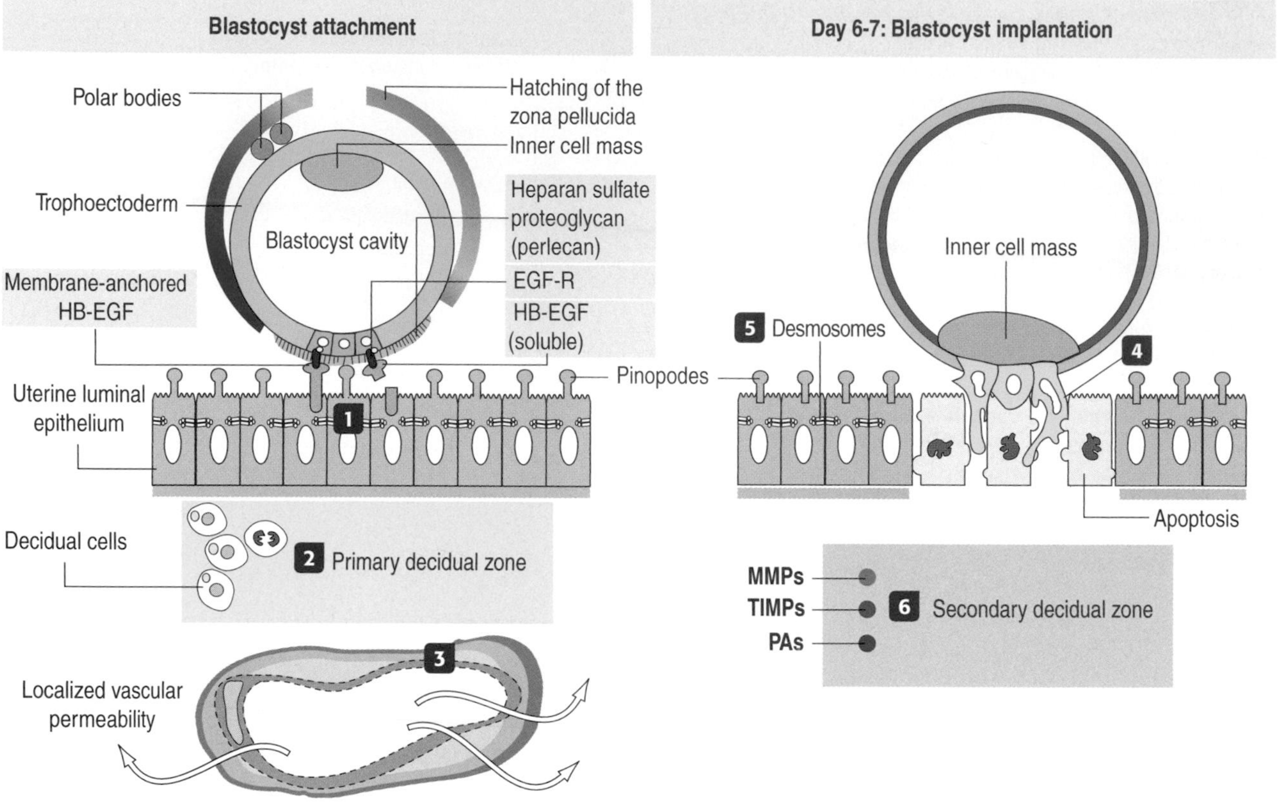

1 At the site of blastocyst apposition, uterine endometrial cells express **heparin-bound epidermal growth factor–like factor** (HB-EGF) with binding affinity to **heparan sulfate proteoglycans** and **EGF receptor** (EGF-R) on the surface of the trophoectoderm.

Binding of membrane-anchored or soluble HB-EGF to EGF-R induces receptor autophosphorylation. The apical domain of uterine epithelial cells contains microprocesses, the **pinopodes**, interacting with microvilli on the apical surface of trophoectoderm cells.

2 Decidual cells become epithelial-like and proliferate and the **primary decidual zone** develops. Fibronectin, laminin, entactin, and types I, III, IV, and V collagen are components of the primary decidual zone. Bone morphogenetic protein-2 and -7, fibroblast growth factor-2, Wnt-4, and proteins of the Hedgehog family are expressed.

3 **Localized vascular permeability** is observed at the implantation site.

4 Processes of trophoectoderm cells penetrate between uterine luminal cells that undergo apoptosis.

5 A reduction in the number of desmosomes facilitates embryo penetration.

6 A secondary decidual zone replaces the primary decidual zone. Matrix metalloproteinases (**MMPs**), tissue inhibitors of MMPs (**TIMPs**), plasminogen activators (**PAs**), and inhibitors regulate the **remodeling of the decidual zone** in the presence of **prostaglandin 2**.

Placentation

The placenta and embryonic-fetal membranes (amnion, chorion, allantois, and yolk sac) protect the embryo-fetus and provide for nutrition, respiration, excretion, and hormone production during development. The membranes are formed by the embryo. Both the embryo and the maternal endometrium begin to form the placenta as soon as the blastocyst implants in the endometrium.

Implantation of the blastocyst

The implantation of the blastocyst into a nurturing endometrium involves (1) the initial **unstable** adhesion of the blastocyst to the endometrial surface, called **apposition**, followed by a **stable** adhesion phase and (2) the **decidualization** of the endometrial stroma (Figure 23-5).

The timing of preimplantation and implantation is extremely precise (see Box 23-B). So is the preparation of the implantation site.

Box 23-B | **Timetable of fertilization**

- **Fertilization** occurs in the oviduct or fallopian tube within 24 to 48 hours after ovulation.
- The development of the fertilized egg, called **zygote**, to the **morula stage**, occurs as the embryo—surrounded by the zona pellucida—travels through the fallopian tube.
- The morula appears in the uterine cavity about 2 to 3 days after fertilization.
- The embryo, now a **blastocyst**, hatches from the zona pellucida 72 hours after entering the uterine cavity.
- Implantation occurs 6 or 7 days after fertilization. Implantation involves two stages: (1) **apposition** of the blastocyst to the endometrial surface and (2) **implantation** of the blastocyst mediated by penetrating **trophoblastic cells.**
- The blastocyst is entirely embedded in the receptive endometrium by day 10 after fertilization. **Uterine receptivity**—corresponding to days 20 to 24 of a regular 28-day menstrual cycle—is defined by the optimal state of endometrial maturation for the implantation of the blastocyst. Uterine receptivity consists in a vascular and edematous endometrial stroma, secretory endometrial glands, and apical microprocesses, the **pinopodes**, on the apical domain of the luminal endometrial lining cells.
- Differentiated syncytiotrophoblastic cells invade part of the myometrium (**interstitial invasion**), as well as local uterine blood vessels (**endovascular invasion**).
- The **uteroplacental circulation** is established when trophoblastic cells are in direct contact with maternal blood (see Box 23-C).

On day 4 of pregnancy, the embryo—at the blastocyst stage—is within the uterine cavity. The coordinated effect of ovarian estrogens and progesterone has already conditioned the endometrium for implantation, including an increase in endometrial vascular permeability at the implantation site.

The **blastocyst hatches from the zona pellucida** and exposes its trophoblast epithelial lining to the uterine luminal epithelium. If zona pellucida hatching fails to occur, the embryo will not implant. Failure of the uterine stroma to undergo decidualization can lead to spontaneous abortion.

Trophoblast-mediated attachment and subsequent implantation depend on (1) the uterine luminal epithelial cell membrane bound and soluble form of **heparin-bound epidermal growth factor-like factor** (HB-EGF), a member of the transforming growth factor-α family; and (2) strong binding affinity of HB-EGF for **epidermal growth factor receptor** (EGF-R), which autophosphorylates, and **heparan sulfate proteoglycan** (also called perlecan) present on the trophoectoderm surface.

At implantation (see Figure 23-5), cytoplasmic processes of trophoblastic cells interact with small processes on the apical surface of the uterine epithelial cells, called **pinopodes**, and penetrate the intercellular spaces of the endometrial luminal cells. Penetration is facilitated by a decrease in the number of desmosomes linking the endometrial cells that undergo apoptosis.

The **primary decidual zone** is remodeled by the action of metalloproteinases (see Figure 23-5), and a **secondary decidual zone** houses the implanting embryo.

The trophoblast differentiates into (1) an inner layer of mitotically active **mononucleated cytotrophoblastic cells** and (2) an outer layer of **multinucleated syncytiotrophoblastic cells** at the embryonic pole, facing the endometrium. The syncytiotrophoblast mass invades the endometrium (formed by glands, stroma, and blood vessels) and rapidly surrounds the entire embryo.

The blastocyst has a cavity containing fluid and the eccentric **inner cell mass**, which gives rise to the embryo and some extraembryonic tissues. The trophoblastic cells proximal to the inner cell mass begin to develop the **chorionic sac**. The chorionic sac consists of two components: the trophoblast and the underlying extraembryonic mesoderm.

Invasion of the endometrium and the inner third of the myometrium, a process called **interstitial invasion**, is determined by the action of secretory **proteolytic enzymes** released by the **syncytiotrophoblast.** Proteases erode the branches of the spiral uterine arteries to form spaces or **lacunae** of maternal blood within the syncytiotrophoblast mass. This endometrial eroding event, called **endovascular invasion**, initiates the **primitive uteroplacental circulation** and represents the starting point of the future **intervillous space**. Decidualization allows an orderly access of trophoblastic cells to the maternal nutrients by modulating the invasion of uterine spiral arteries.

The **syncytiotrophoblast** begins the secretion of **human chorionic gonadotropin (hCG)** into the maternal lacunae. The secretion of estrogens and progesterone by the corpus luteum is now under the control of hCG.

On the **maternal side**, **decidual cells**, close to the mass of invading syncytiotrophoblastic cells, degenerate and release **glycogen** and **lipids**, thus providing, together with maternal blood in the lacunae, the initial nutrients for embryonic development.

The **decidua** provides an immune-protective environment for the development of the embryo. The decidual reaction involves (1) the production of immunosuppressive substances (mainly prostaglandins) by decidual cells to inhibit the activation of **natural killer cells** at the implantation site and (2) infiltrating leukocytes in the endometrial stroma that secrete **interleukin-2** to prevent maternal tissue rejection of the implanting embryo. Syncytiotrophoblastic cells do not express **major histocompatibility complex class II**. Therefore, the syncytiotrophoblast cannot present antigens to maternal $CD4^+$ T cells.

Figure 23-6. **Primary and secondary chorionic villi**

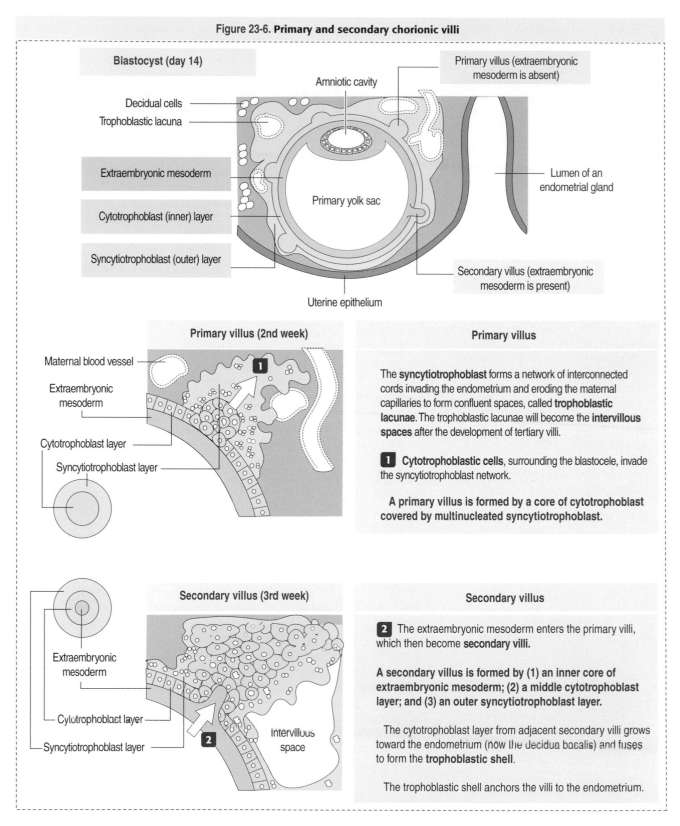

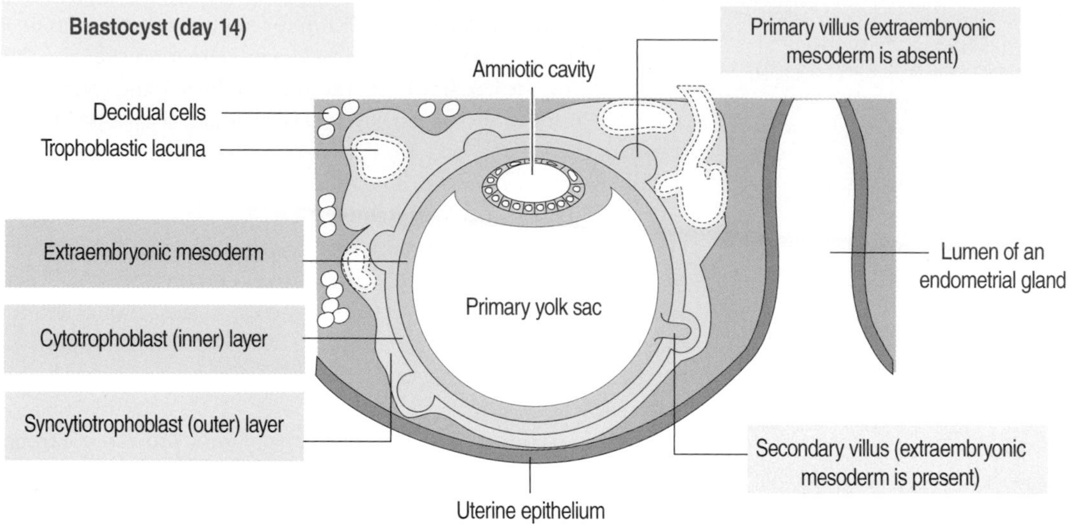

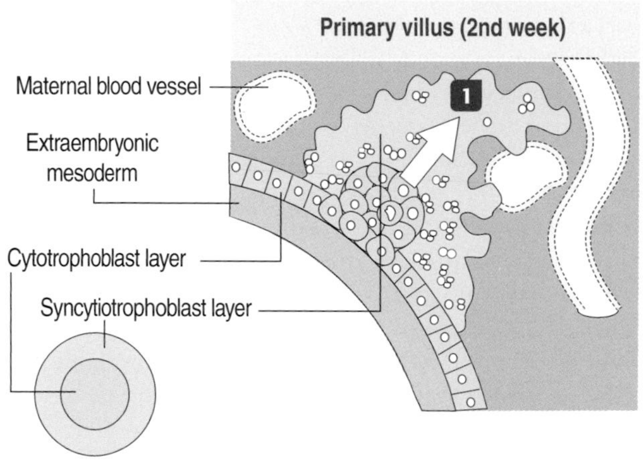

Primary villus

The **syncytiotrophoblast** forms a network of interconnected cords invading the endometrium and eroding the maternal capillaries to form confluent spaces, called **trophoblastic lacunae.** The trophoblastic lacunae will become the **intervillous spaces** after the development of tertiary villi.

1 **Cytotrophoblastic cells**, surrounding the blastocele, invade the syncytiotrophoblast network.

A primary villus is formed by a core of cytotrophoblast covered by multinucleated syncytiotrophoblast.

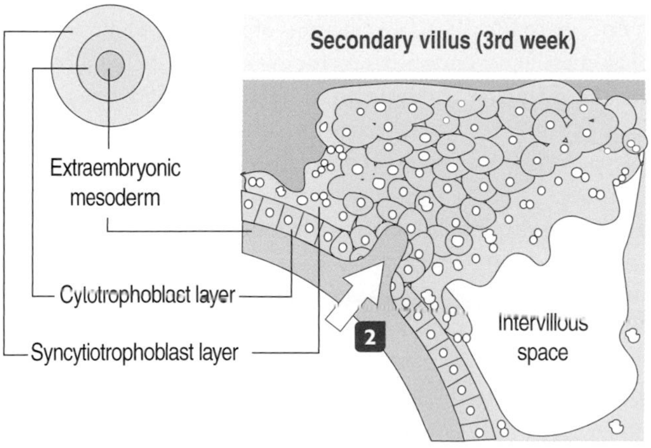

Secondary villus

2 The extraembryonic mesoderm enters the primary villi, which then become **secondary villi.**

A secondary villus is formed by (1) an inner core of extraembryonic mesoderm; (2) a middle cytotrophoblast layer; and (3) an outer syncytiotrophoblast layer.

The cytotrophoblast layer from adjacent secondary villi grows toward the endometrium (now the decidua basalis) and fuses to form the **trophoblastic shell**.

The trophoblastic shell anchors the villi to the endometrium.

Formation of primary, secondary, and tertiary villi

At the end of the second week, cytotrophoblastic cells proliferate under the influence of the extraembryonic mesoderm, and extend into the syncytiotrophoblast mass, forming the **primary villi** (Figure 23-6).

Primary villi represent the first step in the development of the chorionic villi of the placenta. In cross section, a primary villus is formed by a core of cytotro-

Figure 23-7. **Tertiary chorionic villi (3rd week, late)**

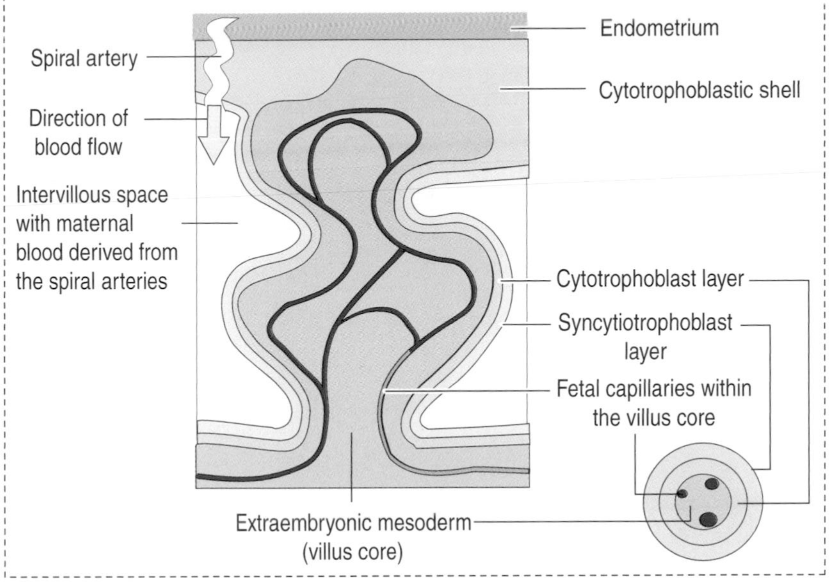
Endometrium
Spiral artery
Cytotrophoblastic shell
Direction of blood flow
Intervillous space with maternal blood derived from the spiral arteries
Cytotrophoblast layer
Syncytiotrophoblast layer
Fetal capillaries within the villus core
Extraembryonic mesoderm (villus core)

phoblastic cells covered by syncytiotrophoblast.

Early in the third week, the **extraembryonic mesoderm** extends into the cytotrophoblast-syncytiotrophoblast primary villi, forming the **secondary villi** (see Figure 23-6). Secondary villi cover the entire surface of the chorionic sac. In cross section, a secondary villus is formed by a core of extraembryonic mesoderm surrounded by a middle cytotrophoblast layer and an outer layer of syncytiotrophoblast.

Soon after, cells of the extraembryonic mesoderm differentiate into capillary and blood cells, forming the **tertiary villi** (Figure 23-7). The difference between the secondary and tertiary villus is the presence of capillaries in the latter. The capillaries in the tertiary villi interconnect to form **arteriocapillary networks** leading to the embryonic heart.

In cross section, a tertiary villus is formed by a core of extraembryonic mesoderm with capillaries, surrounded by a middle cytotrophoblast layer and an outer layer of syncytiotrophoblast.

The following events occur as the chorionic tertiary villi continue to develop:

1. Cytotrophoblastic cells extend beyond the syncytiotrophoblast to form the **cytotrophoblastic shell**, attaching the chorionic sac to the endometrium.

2. Some villi, the **stem** or **anchoring villi**, attach to the cytotrophoblastic shell.

3. **Branch** or **terminal villi** grow from the sides of the stem villi and are in direct contact with maternal blood in the intervillous space.

The chorionic villi cover the entire chorionic sac until the beginning of the eighth week. Then, villi associated with the decidua capsularis degenerate, forming a smooth chorion (**chorion laeve**).

Histologic features of the placenta

The mature placenta is 3 cm thick, has a diameter of 20 cm, and weighs about 500 g. The **fetal side** is smooth and associated with the amniotic membrane. The **maternal side** is partially subdivided into 10 or more **lobes** by **decidual septa** derived from the decidua basalis and extending toward the chorionic plate. The decidual septa do not fuse with the chorionic plate.

Each lobe contains 10 or more stem villi and its branches.

The 50- to 60-cm-long and 12-mm-thick and twisted **umbilical cord** is attached to the chorionic plate and contains **two umbilical arteries** (transporting deoxygenated blood) and **one umbilical vein** (transporting oxygen-rich blood).

Figure 23-8. **Differences between umbilical vein and umbilical artery**

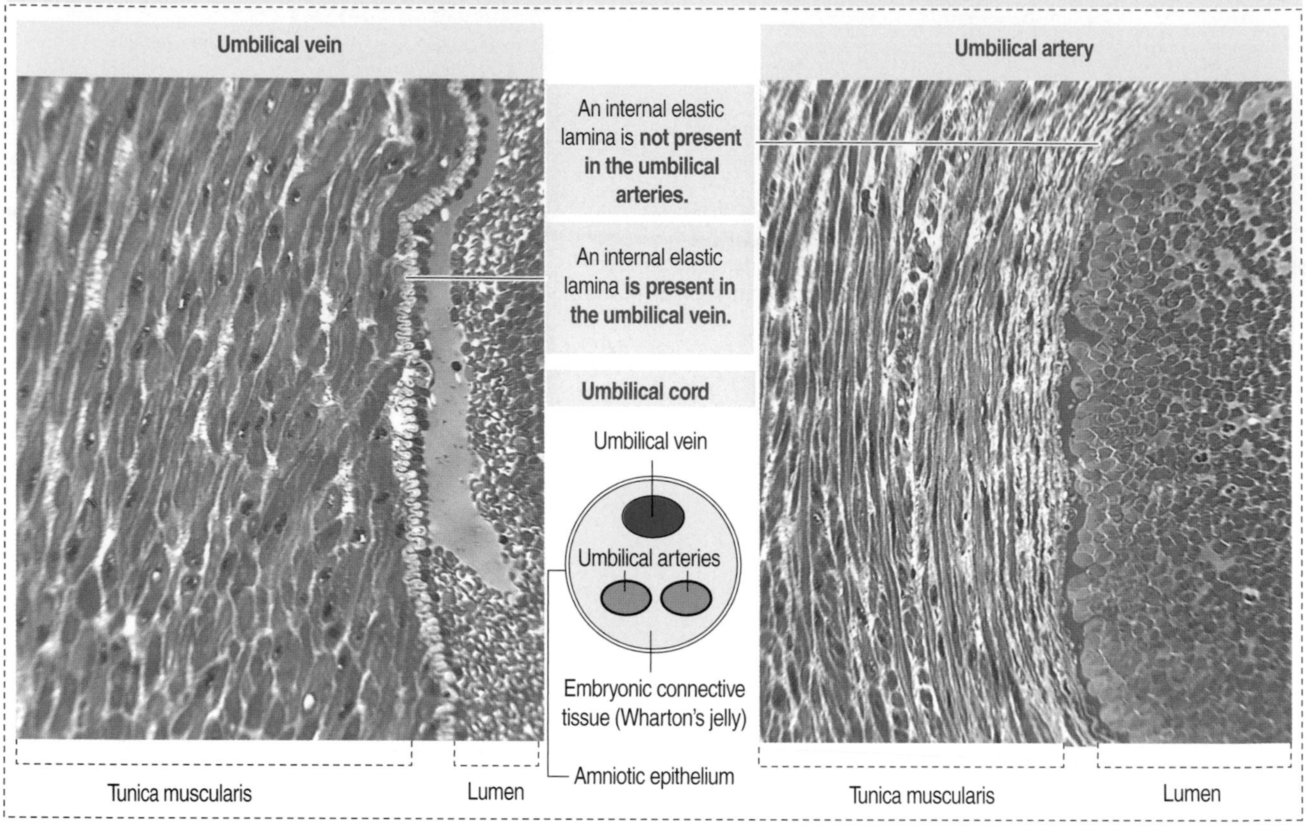

Umbilical vein
Umbilical artery
An internal elastic lamina is **not present in the umbilical arteries.**
An internal elastic lamina **is present in the umbilical vein.**
Umbilical cord
Umbilical vein
Umbilical arteries
Embryonic connective tissue (Wharton's jelly)
Amniotic epithelium
Tunica muscularis
Lumen
Tunica muscularis
Lumen

The umbilical vessels (Figure 23-8) are embedded in **embryonic connective tissue**, called **Wharton's jelly** (see Chapter 4, Connective Tissue). The cord is lined by amniotic epithelium.

Figure 23-9. **Uterine and fetal membranes**

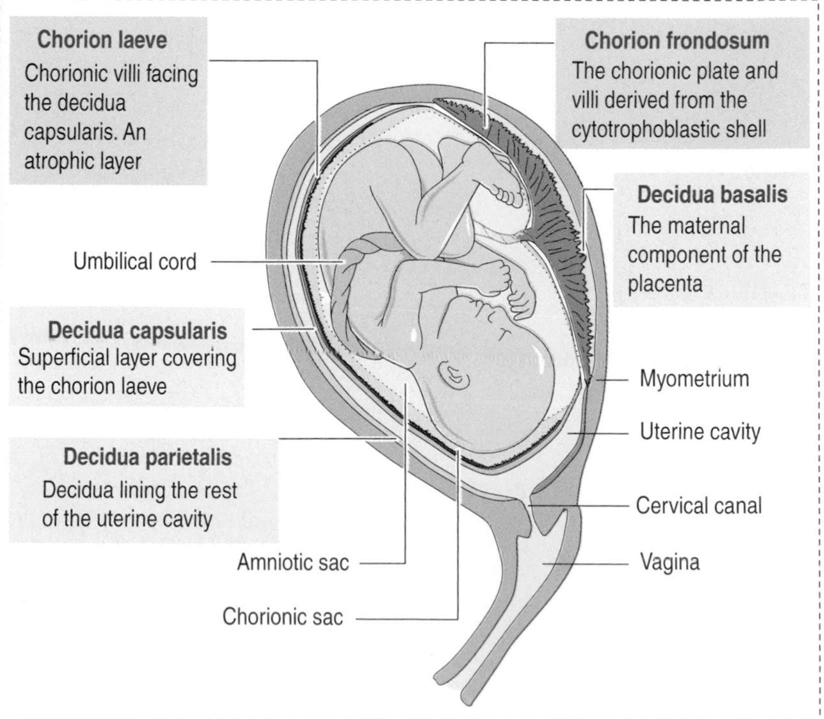

Chorion laeve
Chorionic villi facing the decidua capsularis. An atrophic layer
Chorion frondosum
The chorionic plate and villi derived from the cytotrophoblastic shell
Decidua basalis
The maternal component of the placenta
Umbilical cord
Decidua capsularis
Superficial layer covering the chorion laeve
Myometrium
Uterine cavity
Decidua parietalis
Decidua lining the rest of the uterine cavity
Cervical canal
Vagina
Amniotic sac
Chorionic sac

Figure 23-10. **Anatomy and histology of the placenta**

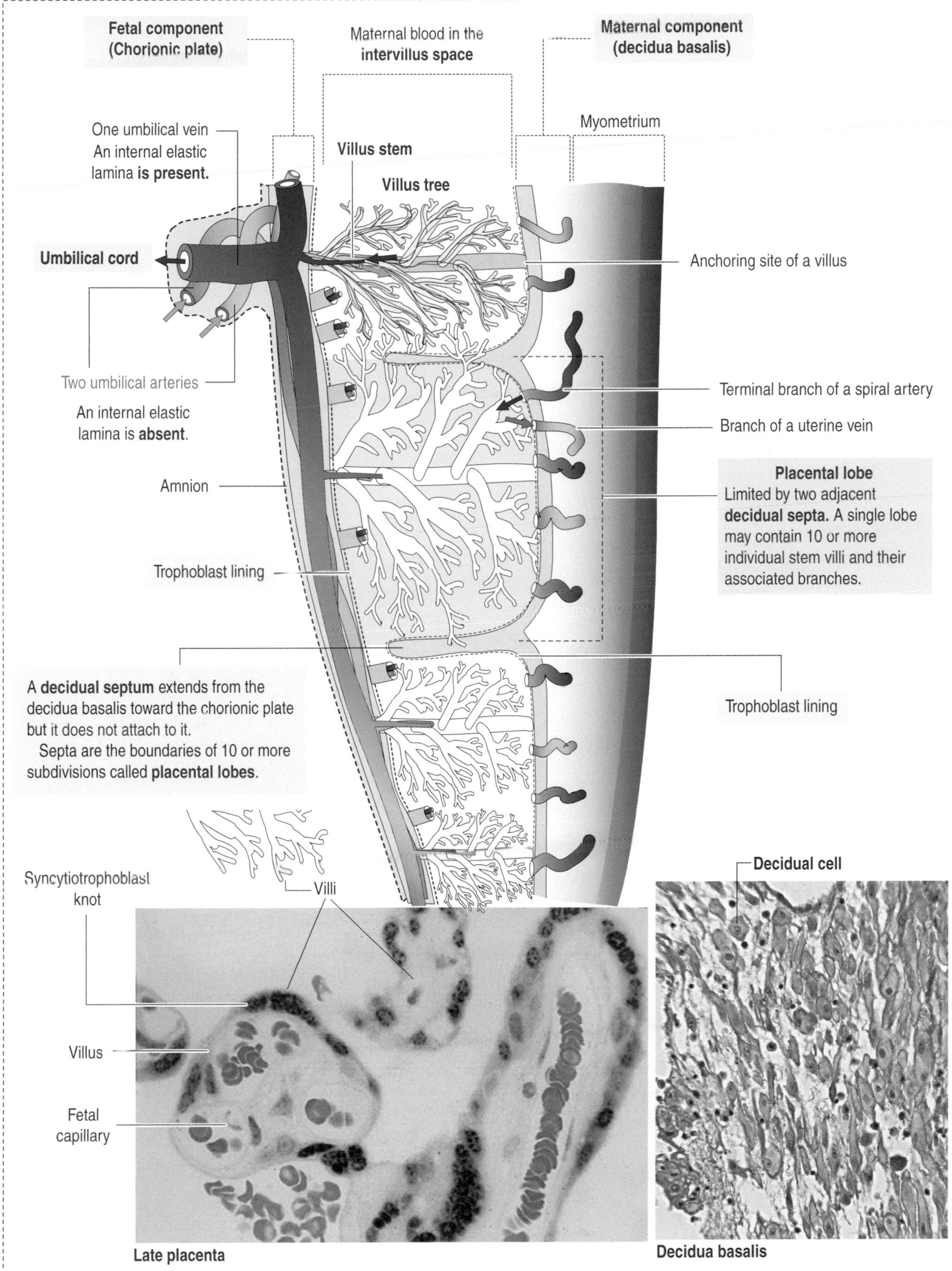

Fetal component (Chorionic plate)
Maternal blood in the intervillus space
Maternal component (decidua basalis)
Myometrium
One umbilical vein
An internal elastic lamina is present.
Villus stem
Villus tree
Umbilical cord
Anchoring site of a villus
Two umbilical arteries
An internal elastic lamina is absent.
Terminal branch of a spiral artery
Branch of a uterine vein
Placental lobe
Limited by two adjacent decidual septa. A single lobe may contain 10 or more individual stem villi and their associated branches.
Amnion
Trophoblast lining
A decidual septum extends from the decidua basalis toward the chorionic plate but it does not attach to it.
Septa are the boundaries of 10 or more subdivisions called placental lobes.
Trophoblast lining
Syncytiotrophoblast knot
Villi
Decidual cell
Villus
Fetal capillary
Late placenta
Decidua basalis

Maternal and fetal components

The placenta consists of a maternal and a fetal component (Figure 23-9). The **maternal component** is represented by the **decidua.** The decidua (Latin *deciduus*, falling off; a tissue shed at birth) is the endometrium of the gravid uterus.

There are **three regions of the decidua**, named according to their relation to the developing fetus:

1. The **decidua basalis** is the maternal component of the placenta. Chorionic villi facing the decidua basalis are highly developed and form the **chorion frondosum** (bushy chorion).

2. The **decidua capsularis** is the superficial layer covering the developing fetus and its chorionic sac.

3. The **decidua parietalis** is the rest of the decidua lining the cavity of the uterus not occupied by the fetus.

The **fetal component** is represented by the **chorion frondosum**. The chorion frondosum consists of the **chorionic plate** and derived **villi.** Chorionic villi facing the decidua capsularis atrophy, resulting in the formation of the **chorion laeve** (smooth chorion).

The **intervillous space** between the maternal and fetal components contains circulating maternal blood (Figures 23-10 and 23-11). Arterial blood, derived from the open ends of the spiral arteries, flows into the intervillous space and moves blood into the uterine veins. **A plug of cytotrophoblastic cells** and the **contraction of the smooth muscle wall** of the artery **control the flow of blood.**

Placental blood circulation

Placental blood circulation has two relevant characteristics: (1) the **fetal blood circulation** is **closed** (within blood vessels). (2) The **maternal blood circulation** is **open** (not bound by blood vessels). Maternal blood enters the intervillous space under reduced pressure, regulated by the cytotrophoblastic cell plugs, and leaves through the uterine veins after exchanges occur with the fetal blood in the terminal branched villi (see Box 23-C).

The **umbilical vein** has a **subendothelial elastic lamina**; the **two umbilical arteries lack an elastic lamina** (see Figure 23-8). The **umbilical vein carries 80% oxygenated fetal blood.** Although the partial pressure of oxygen in fetal blood is low (20 to 25 mm Hg), the higher cardiac output in organ blood flow, higher hemoglobin concentration in fetal red blood cells, and higher oxygen saturation provide adequate oxygenation to the fetus.

The **umbilical arteries return deoxygenated fetal blood to the placenta.**

Structure of the chorionic villus

The chorionic villus is the basic structure involved in maternal-fetal exchanges. It originates from the chorionic plate and is formed by a stem villus giving rise to villous branches. When you examine a histologic preparation of placenta, you are visualizing cross sections of villi corresponding to the villous branches. You may also be able to see a longitudinal section of a stem villus.

Each villus has a core of **mesenchymal connective tissue** and **fetal blood vessels** (**arterioles** and **capillaries**).

The mesenchymal core contains two major cell types (Figures 23-12 and 23-13):

1. **Mesenchymal cells**, which differentiate into **fibroblasts**, involved in the synthesis of various types of collagens (types I, III, V, and VI) and extracellular matrix components (see Figure 23-12).

2. **Hofbauer cells**, phagocytic cells predominant in **early pregnancy.**

The mesenchymal core is covered by two cell types:

1. **Syncytiotrophoblastic cells**, in contact with the maternal blood in the intervillous space.

2. **Cytotrophoblastic cells**, subjacent to the syncytiotrophoblast and supported

Box 23-C | Trophoblastic cells

- The blastocyst has two distinct cell populations: (1) **trophoblastic cells**, derived from the trophoectoderm and surrounding the blastocyst; and (2) the **inner cell mass**, which gives rise to the embryo.
- Trophoblastic cells (the collective designation of cytotrophoblastic cells and syncytiotrophoblastic cells) are always the outermost layer of fetal cells covering the mesenchyme and fetal capillaries of the chorionic villi.
- The wall of maternal blood vessels is infiltrated and ruptured by trophoblastic cells. Maternal blood is released into the intervillous space, and the outer layer of the chorionic villi (syncytiotrophoblastic cells) is immersed in maternal blood like a sponge in a container of blood.
- The uterine spiral arteries are converted to **uteroplacental arteries.** Trophoblastic cells replace the endothelium and tunica media of the uteroplacental arteries, which deliver blood, at low pressure, to the intervillous space. Basal straight arteries are not involved in these changes.
- When trophoblast cell replacement of spiral arteries is incomplete, the development of uteroplacental arteries is deficient and blood flow is reduced. Reduced development of the branches of the chorionic villus tree, and limited fetal growth, a manifestation of **preeclampsia**, occur.

Figure 23-11. Structure of the chorionic villus

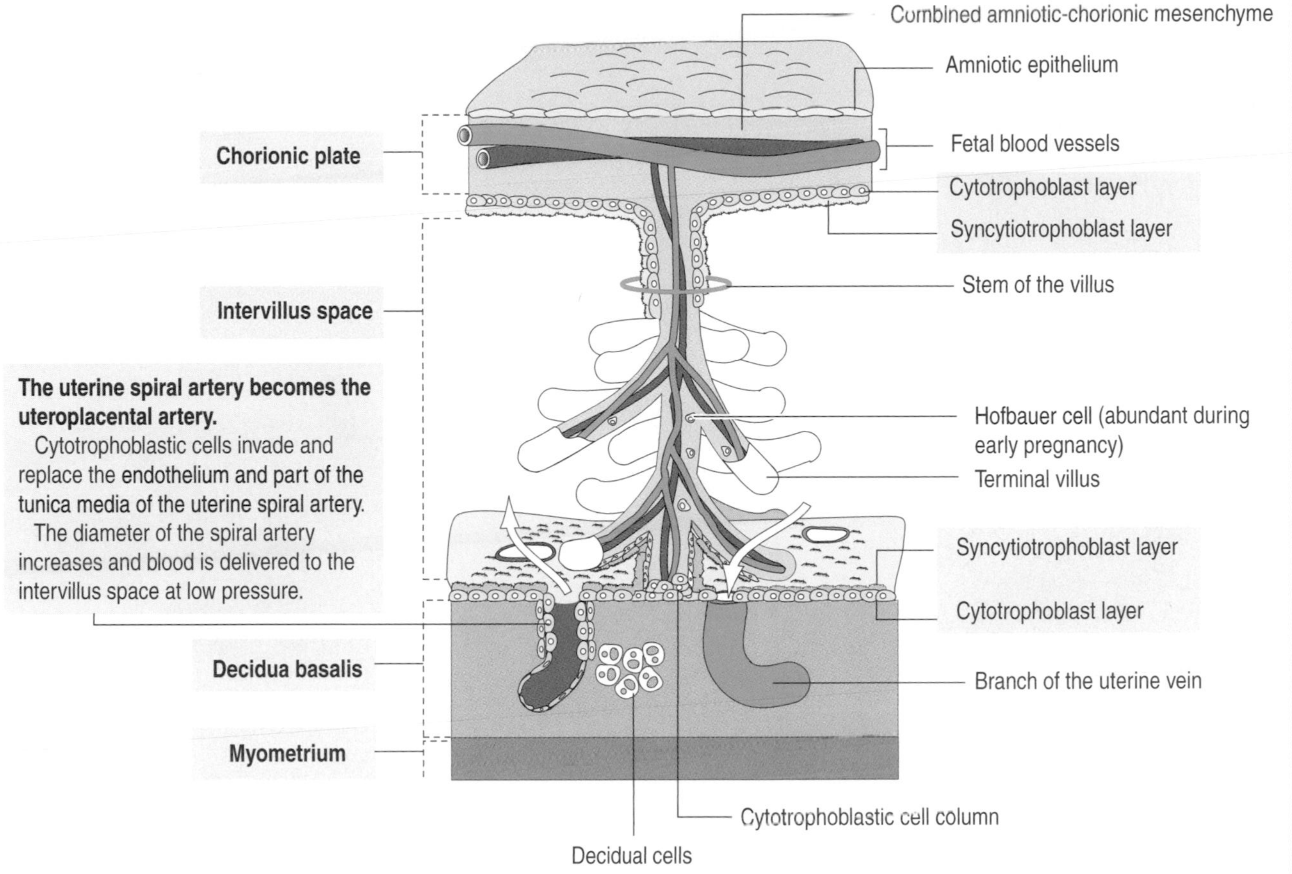
Combined amniotic-chorionic mesenchyme
Amniotic epithelium
Chorionic plate
Fetal blood vessels
Cytotrophoblast layer
Syncytiotrophoblast layer
Stem of the villus
Intervillus space
The uterine spiral artery becomes the uteroplacental artery.
Cytotrophoblastic cells invade and replace the endothelium and part of the tunica media of the uterine spiral artery.
The diameter of the spiral artery increases and blood is delivered to the intervillus space at low pressure.
Hofbauer cell (abundant during early pregnancy)
Terminal villus
Syncytiotrophoblast layer
Cytotrophoblast layer
Decidua basalis
Branch of the uterine vein
Myometrium
Cytotrophoblastic cell column
Decidual cells

by a basal lamina.

Several important structural characteristics define the cytotrophoblast and syncytiotrophoblast:

1. **Cytotrophoblastic cells divide by mitosis** and differentiate into syncytiotrophoblastic cells. In contrast, **the syncytiotrophoblastic cell is postmitotic**.

2. Cytotrophoblastic cells are linked to each other and to the overlying syncytiotrophoblast by **desmosomes**.

3. The apical surface of the syncytiotrophoblast contains numerous **microvilli**.

4. **Deposits of fibrin** are frequently seen on the villus surface on areas lacking syncytiotrophoblastic cells and preceding reepithelialization.

Fetal vessels are separated from maternal blood in the intervillous space by the **placental barrier** (see Figure 23-13), which is formed by (1) **endothelial cells and basal lamina of the fetal blood capillaries** and (2) the **cytotrophoblast** and **syncytiotrophoblast** and supporting **basal lamina**.

After the fourth month of pregnancy, the fetal blood vessels become dilated and are in direct contact with the subepithelial basal lamina. Cytotrophoblastic cells decrease in number and syncytiotrophoblastic cells predominate. The fetal connective tissue of the villus is not prevalent in the mature placenta.

Clinical significance: Disorders of the placenta

Ectopic pregnancy

The **implantation of the blastocyst outside the uterine cavity** is called ectopic pregnancy. About 95% of ectopic gestations occur in the oviduct (**tubal pregnancy**), mainly in the ampullary region. A predisposing factor is **salpingitis**, an inflammatory process of the oviduct.

Figure 23-12. **Fine structure of the chorionic villus**

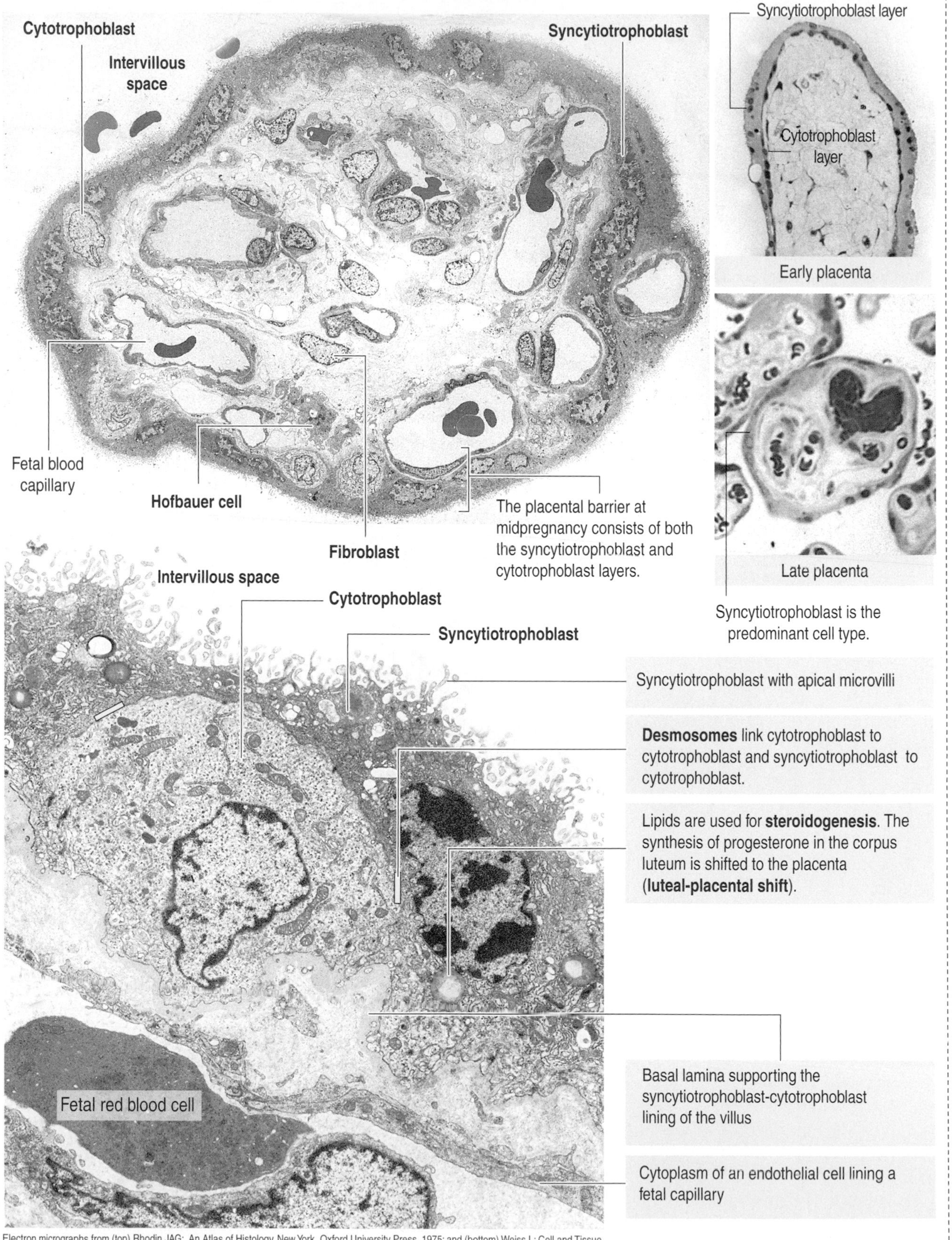
Cytotrophoblast
Intervillous space
Syncytiotrophoblast
Fetal blood capillary
Hofbauer cell
Fibroblast
The placental barrier at midpregnancy consists of both the syncytiotrophoblast and cytotrophoblast layers.
Syncytiotrophoblast layer
Cytotrophoblast layer
Early placenta
Late placenta
Syncytiotrophoblast is the predominant cell type.
Intervillous space
Cytotrophoblast
Syncytiotrophoblast
Syncytiotrophoblast with apical microvilli
Desmosomes link cytotrophoblast to cytotrophoblast and syncytiotrophoblast to cytotrophoblast.
Lipids are used for **steroidogenesis**. The synthesis of progesterone in the corpus luteum is shifted to the placenta (**luteal-placental shift**).
Basal lamina supporting the syncytiotrophoblast-cytotrophoblast lining of the villus
Fetal red blood cell
Cytoplasm of an endothelial cell lining a fetal capillary

Electron micrographs from (top) Rhodin JAG: An Atlas of Histology. New York, Oxford University Press, 1975; and (bottom) Weiss L: Cell and Tissue Biology, 6th ed. Baltimore, Urban & Schwarzenberg, 1988.

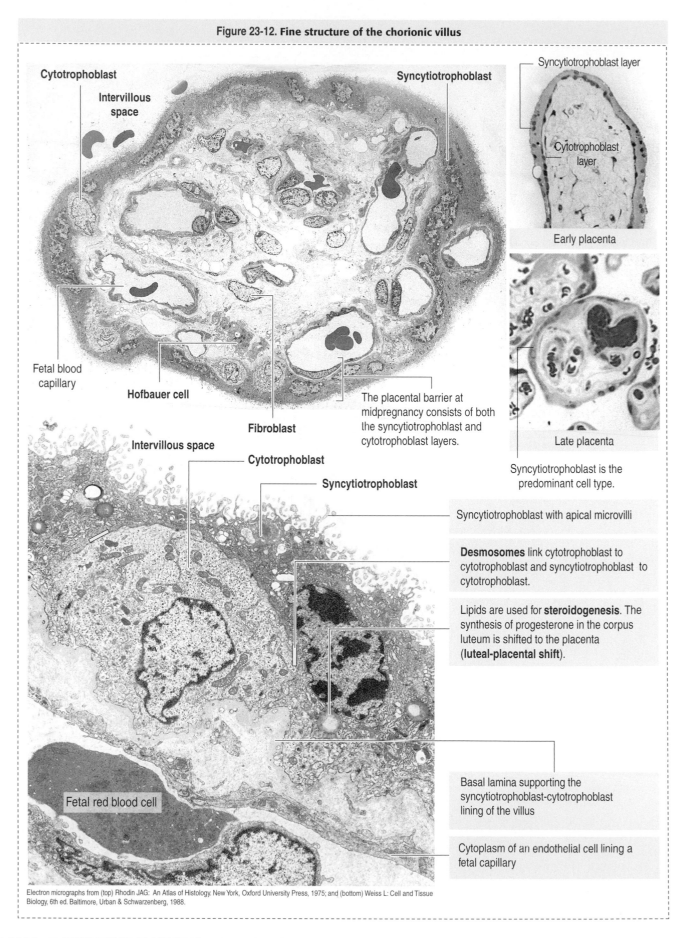

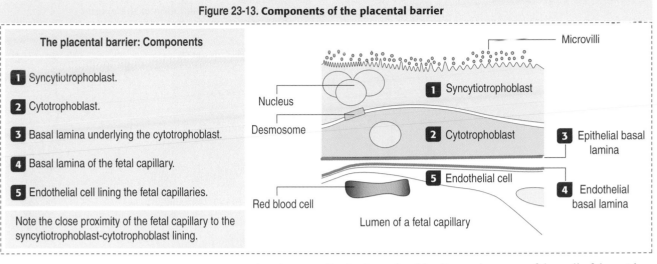

Figure 23-13. Components of the placental barrier

The placental barrier: Components
1 Syncytiotrophoblast.
2 Cytotrophoblast.
3 Basal lamina underlying the cytotrophoblast.
4 Basal lamina of the fetal capillary.
5 Endothelial cell lining the fetal capillaries.
Note the close proximity of the fetal capillary to the syncytiotrophoblast-cytotrophoblast lining.

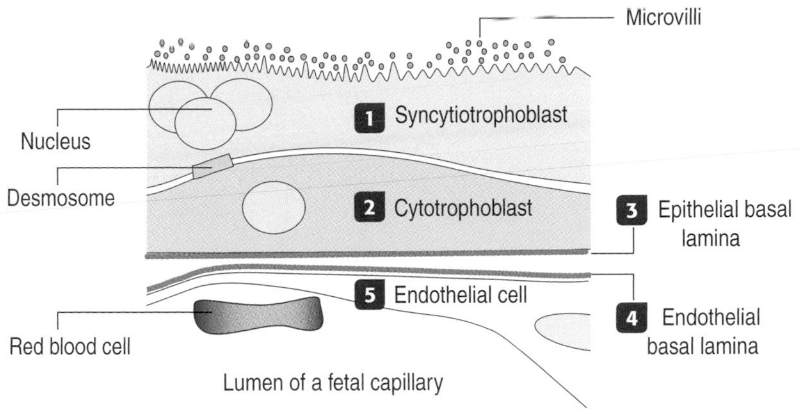
Microvilli
Nucleus
1 Syncytiotrophoblast
Desmosome
2 Cytotrophoblast
3 Epithelial basal lamina
5 Endothelial cell
4 Endothelial basal lamina
Red blood cell
Lumen of a fetal capillary

A major complication is profuse bleeding and rupture of the wall of the oviduct caused by the trophoblastic erosion of blood vessels and tissue layers. **Abdominal pain, amenorrhea,** and **vaginal bleeding** in a sexually active woman of reproductive age are symptoms of a suspected tubal pregnancy. A rapid and precise diagnosis of ectopic pregnancy is essential to reduce the risk of complications or death.

Placenta previa (second half of pregnancy)

The **abnormal extension of the placenta over or close to the internal opening of the cervical canal** is called **placenta previa**. A possible cause is **abnormal vascularization**.

There are three types of placenta previa (Figure 23-14): (1) **low implantation of the placenta**, when **the margin of the placenta lies close to the internal cervical os** (**marginal placenta previa**); (2) **partial placenta previa**, when **the edge of the placenta extends across part of the internal ostium**; and (3) **total placenta previa**, when the placenta **covers the internal cervical ostium**.

Spontaneous painless bleeding, caused by partial separation of the placenta from the lower portion of the uterus and cervix due to mild uterine contractions, is commonly observed.

Placental abruption, or abruptio placentae (second half of pregnancy)

The **premature separation of the normally implanted placenta** is called **placental abruption**. Hemorrhage into the decidua basalis leads to premature placental separation and bleeding. Separation of the placenta from the uterus impairs oxygenation of the fetus.

Possible causes include **trauma**, **maternal hypertension** (preeclampsia or eclampsia), **blood clotting abnormalities**, and **cocaine use** by the mother.

Spontaneous painful bleeding and **uterine contractions** are typical symptoms.

Uterine atony

The separation of the placenta from the uterus is determined by a cleavage at the decidua basalis region. After separation, the placenta is ejected by strong uterine contractions, which also constrict the spiral arteries of the vascular placental bed to prevent excessive bleeding.

In **uterine atony, the contractions of the uterine muscles are not strong enough and postpartum bleeding occurs.**

Predisposing factors of uterine atony include **abnormal labor**, **substantial enlargement of the uterus** (hydramnios), or **uterine leiomyomas** (benign tumors of the myometrium). Intravenous infusion of **oxytocin** stimulates uterine contractions and decreases the possibility of uterine atony.

Figure 23-14. Abnormal implantation of the placenta

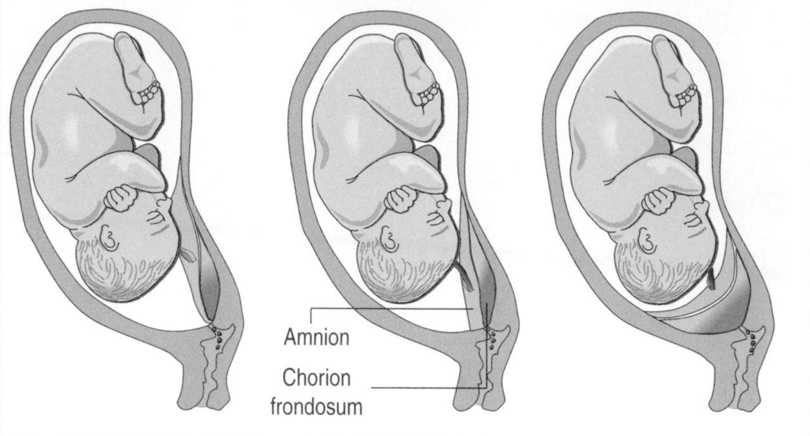
Amnion
Chorion frondosum
Low implantation of the placenta
Partial placenta previa
Total placenta previa

Placenta accreta

A placenta can be retained in the uterine cavity when the process of cleavage or ejection is incomplete. After expulsion, every placenta must be inspected **to detect missing lobes**, which may remain inside the uterus. When some placental tissue remains in the uterus, uterine contractions are deficient and excessive bleeding is observed. Curettage with a suction apparatus may remove the retained tissue.

The separation of the placenta from the uterus is defective **when placental villi penetrate deep into the uterine wall** to form a **placenta accreta**. No separation of the placenta occurs when the abnormal attachment involves the entire placenta.

Penetration of the placenta into the uterine muscle is called **placenta increta**. Extensive invasion of the placenta through the thickness of the uterine muscle is known as **placenta percreta**.

Clinical significance: Gestational trophoblastic disease

Hydatidiform mole designates the partial or complete replacement of normal trophoblastic tissue by dilated or hydropic (edematous) villi.

Complete moles are of **paternal origin** and result from the fertilization of a blighted (empty) ovum by a haploid sperm that reduplicates within the egg (Figure 23-15). The frequent karyotype of a complete mole is 46,XX, and no fetus is observed.

The fetus of a partial mole is usually 69,XXY (triploid): one haploid set of maternal chromosomes (23,X) and two haploid sets of paternal chromosomes (46,XY; arising from meiotic nondisjunction or two haploid fertilizing sperm). Extremely high levels of hCG are characteristic in patients with hydatidiform mole. Failure of high levels of hCG to regress after initial removal of intrauterine contents suggests a need for further treatment.

Choriocarcinoma is observed in about 20% of patients with molar pregnancies.

Clinical significance: Functions of the placenta

The main function of the placenta is the regulation of the fetal-maternal exchange of molecules, ions, and gases. This function is accomplished at specialized areas of the syncytiotrophoblast adjacent to fetal capillaries. The transfer of molecules across the placental barrier can follow intercellular and transcellular pathways. Figure 23-16 illustrates the main functional aspects of the placenta that are of clinical and physiologic relevance.

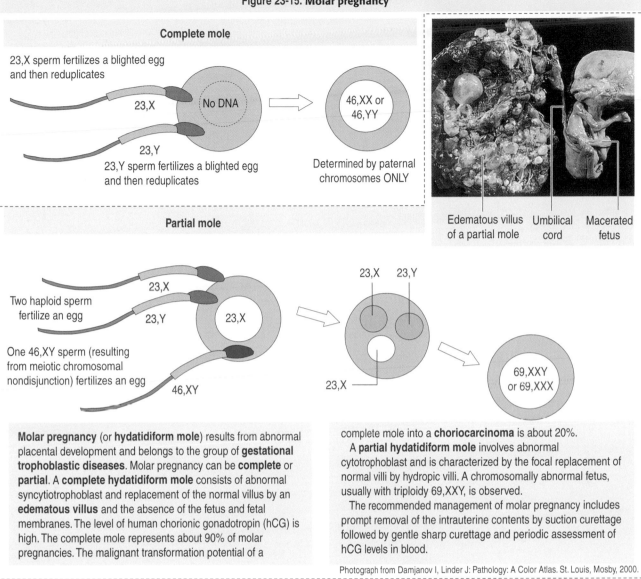

Figure 23-15. Molar pregnancy

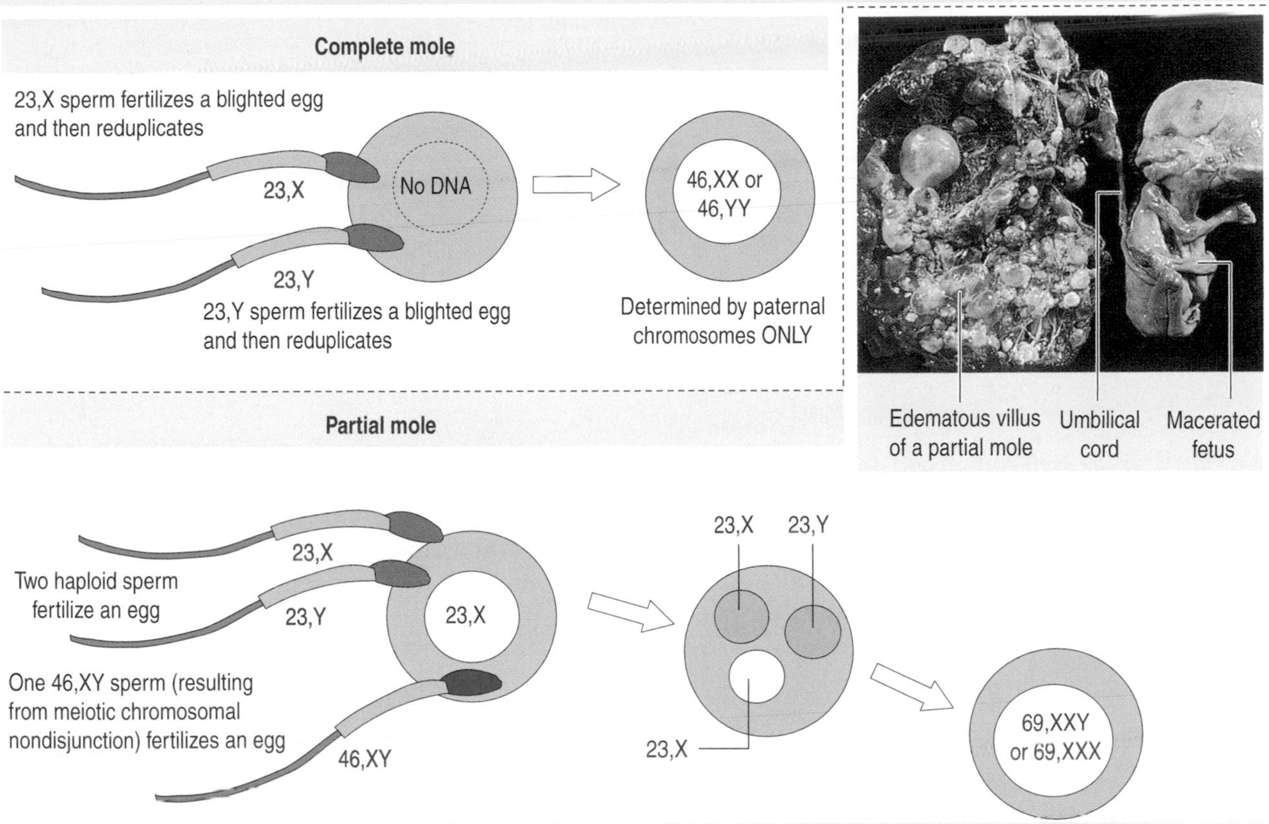
Complete mole
23,X sperm fertilizes a blighted egg and then reduplicates
23,X
No DNA
46,XX or 46,YY
23,Y
23,Y sperm fertilizes a blighted egg and then reduplicates
Determined by paternal chromosomes ONLY
Edematous villus of a partial mole
Umbilical cord
Macerated fetus
Partial mole
Two haploid sperm fertilize an egg
23,X
23,Y
23,X
One 46,XY sperm (resulting from meiotic chromosomal nondisjunction) fertilizes an egg
46,XY
23,X
23,Y
23,X
69,XXY or 69,XXX

Molar pregnancy (or **hydatidiform mole**) results from abnormal placental development and belongs to the group of **gestational trophoblastic diseases**. Molar pregnancy can be **complete** or **partial**. A **complete hydatidiform mole** consists of abnormal syncytiotrophoblast and replacement of the normal villus by an **edematous villus** and the absence of the fetus and fetal membranes. The level of human chorionic gonadotropin (hCG) is high. The complete mole represents about 90% of molar pregnancies. The malignant transformation potential of a complete mole into a **choriocarcinoma** is about 20%.

A **partial hydatidiform mole** involves abnormal cytotrophoblast and is characterized by the focal replacement of normal villi by hydropic villi. A chromosomally abnormal fetus, usually with triploidy 69,XXY, is observed.

The recommended management of molar pregnancy includes prompt removal of the intrauterine contents by suction curettage followed by gentle sharp curettage and periodic assessment of hCG levels in blood.

Photograph from Damjanov I, Linder J: Pathology: A Color Atlas. St. Louis, Mosby, 2000.

Exchange of gases

Oxygen, carbon dioxide, and carbon monoxide exchange through the placenta is by **simple diffusion.** Nitrous oxide anesthesia (used in the treatment of dental disease) should be avoided during pregnancy.

Transfer of maternal immunoglobulins

Maternal antibodies, mainly **immunoglobulin G (IgG)**, are taken up by the syncytiotrophoblast and then transported to fetal capillaries for **passive immunity.** The larger **immunoglobulin M (IgM)** molecules do not cross the placental barrier.

Rh (D antigen) isoimmunization

Maternal antibodies against D antigen (present in the Rh system of fetal red blood cells) cause hemolytic disease (**erythroblastosis fetalis**). The fetus is Rh-positive (Rh D antigen received from the father), but the mother lacks the D antigen (she is Rh-negative). **Isoimmunization** refers to maternal exposure and sensitization to fetal Rh^+ red blood cells, mainly during delivery. In a subsequent pregnancy, antibodies to D antigen (IgG) cross the placenta and cause hemolysis of fetal red blood cells (see Chapter 6, Blood and Hematopoiesis).

Figure 23-16. **Functions of the placenta**

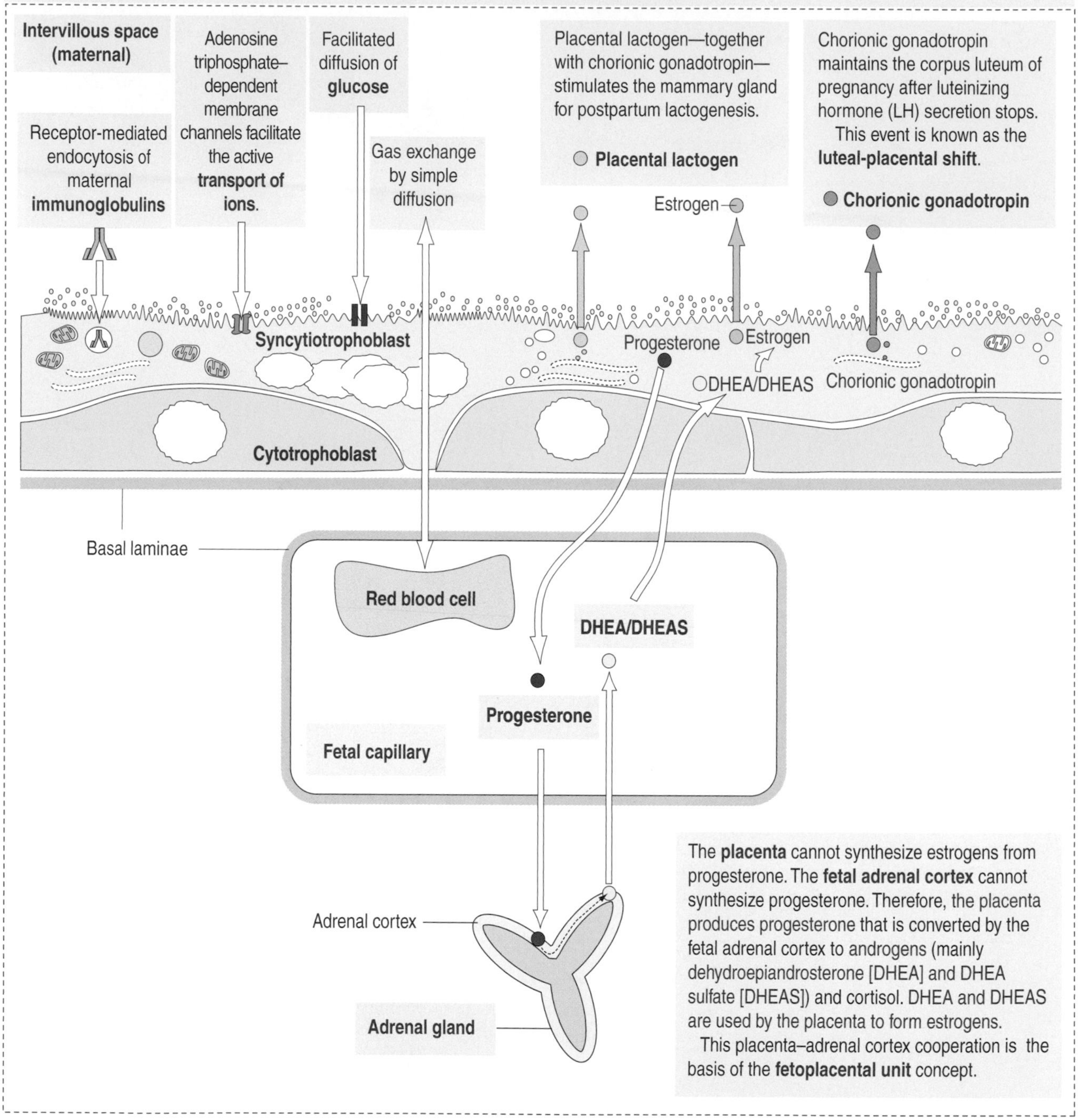

Intervillous space (maternal)
Receptor-mediated endocytosis of maternal **immunoglobulins**
Adenosine triphosphate–dependent membrane channels facilitate the active **transport of ions**.
Facilitated diffusion of **glucose**
Gas exchange by simple diffusion
Placental lactogen—together with chorionic gonadotropin—stimulates the mammary gland for postpartum lactogenesis.
Placental lactogen
Estrogen
Chorionic gonadotropin maintains the corpus luteum of pregnancy after luteinizing hormone (LH) secretion stops.
This event is known as the **luteal-placental shift**.
Chorionic gonadotropin
Syncytiotrophoblast
Progesterone
Estrogen
DHEA/DHEAS
Chorionic gonadotropin
Cytotrophoblast
Basal laminae
Red blood cell
DHEA/DHEAS
Progesterone
Fetal capillary
Adrenal cortex
Adrenal gland
The **placenta** cannot synthesize estrogens from progesterone. The **fetal adrenal cortex** cannot synthesize progesterone. Therefore, the placenta produces progesterone that is converted by the fetal adrenal cortex to androgens (mainly dehydroepiandrosterone [DHEA] and DHEA sulfate [DHEAS]) and cortisol. DHEA and DHEAS are used by the placenta to form estrogens.
This placenta–adrenal cortex cooperation is the basis of the **fetoplacental unit** concept.

Steroid hormone production: The fetoplacental unit

The placenta can synthesize progesterone but lacks 17-hydroxylase activity to synthesize estrogens from progesterone. The fetal adrenal cortex cannot synthesize progesterone.

A fetal-maternal cooperation—known as the **fetoplacental unit**—enables the transport of **placental progesterone** to the adrenal cortex and its conversion to dehydroepiandrosterone (DHEA), which can be sulfated to form DHEA sulfate (DHEAS). When DHEA and DHEAS are transported to the syncytiotrophoblast, the conversion to estrone (E_1) and estradiol (E_2) occurs. DHEA can be hydroxylated in the liver and serves as a substrate for the synthesis of estriol (E_3) by the syncytiotrophoblast.

Protein hormone production: The luteal-placental shift

Chorionic gonadotropin, instead of **maternal luteinizing hormone**, maintains the **corpus luteum** during pregnancy. This transition is called the **luteal-placental shift. Placental lactogen** (also called chorionic somatomammotropin) stimulates fetal growth and conditions the mammary gland for lactation. Placental lactogen has a **diabetogenic effect**: It increases the resistance of peripheral tissues and liver to the effects of **insulin.** Pregnancy is characterized by maternal **hyperglycemia, hyperinsulinemia**, and **reduced tissue response to insulin.**

Active transport of ions and glucose

The transport of ions is mediated by an adenosine triphosphate (ATP-dependent mechanism. **Glucose** enters the placenta by facilitated diffusion using a glucose transporter. Fetal glucose levels depend on maternal levels. The fetus does not depend on maternal insulin.

Fetal alcohol syndrome

The excessive ingestion of alcohol during pregnancy is the cause of **fetal mental retardation** and **craniofacial abnormalities**. Alcohol can cross the placenta and fetal blood-brain barrier causing direct toxicity. Indirect toxicity is mediated by the alcohol metabolite **acetaldehyde.**

Infectious agents

Rubella (German measles), cytomegalovirus, herpes simplex, toxoplasmosis, syphilis, and human immunodeficiency virus type 1 (HIV-1) are potential infectious agents. **Rubella** viral infection in the first trimester can cause spontaneous abortion or the **congenital rubella syndrome** (fetal congenital heart disease, mental retardation, deafness, and cataracts).

Lactation

The mammary gland

The breast, or mammary gland, develops as a downgrowth of the epidermis. The **nipple** is surrounded by the **areola**, a modified skin with abundant sebaceous glands. About 15 to 20 **lactiferous ducts** open at the tip of the nipple through individual **lactiferous sinuses.**

In the lactating mammary gland, each lactiferous duct drains one lobe. The nipple contains connective tissue and smooth muscle cells, forming a **circular sphincter.**

Structure of the mammary gland

Like most branched (compound) glands, the mammary gland contains a **duct system, lobes**, and **lobules** (Figure 23-17).

Each lobe contains a branching **lactiferous duct** that extends into the **fibroadipose tissue** of the breast. Each lactiferous duct is lined by a **simple columnar** or **cuboidal epithelium** and a discontinuous outer layer of **myoepithelial cells.** Each duct is surrounded by loose connective tissue and a capillary network.

In the **resting, nonpregnant state**, the mammary gland consists of lactiferous ducts, each ending in a group of blind, saccular evaginations (see Figure 23-17).

During **pregnancy**, the ducts branch and end in clusters of saccules (alveoli or acini), forming a **lobule.** Each lobule consists of various **secretory tubuloacinar units.** A **lobe** consists of a group of lobules drained by a **lactiferous duct. Lobules and lobes are not seen in the nonpregnant mammary gland.**

Development of the mammary gland

Placental lactogen and **estrogen** stimulate the development of the mammary gland. The development involves epithelial-mesenchymal interactions and consists of two phases (Figure 23-18): (1) the formation of the **nipple** and (2) the

Figure 23-17. **Structure of the mature female mammary gland**

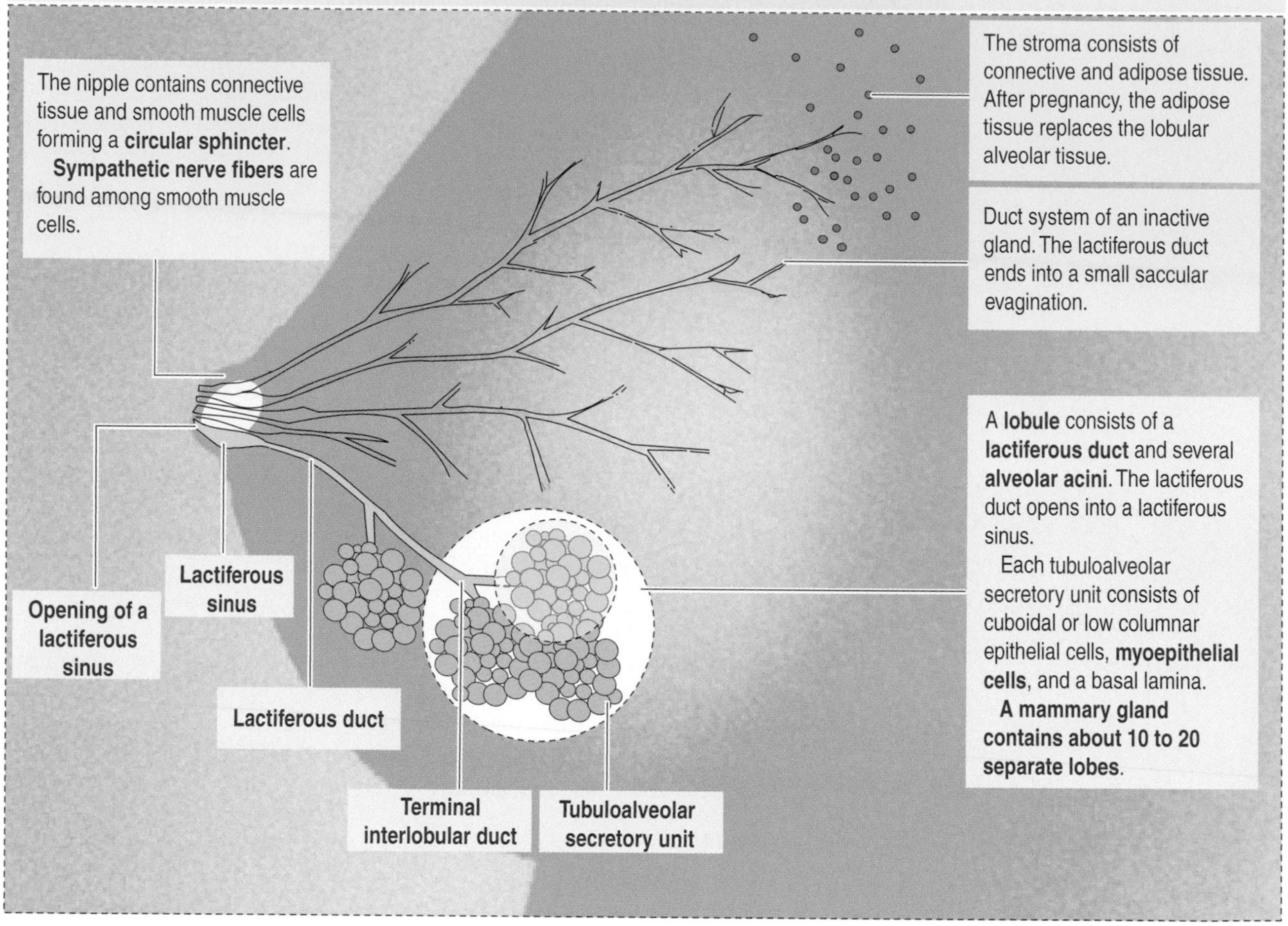
The nipple contains connective tissue and smooth muscle cells forming a **circular sphincter**.
Sympathetic nerve fibers are found among smooth muscle cells.
The stroma consists of connective and adipose tissue. After pregnancy, the adipose tissue replaces the lobular alveolar tissue.
Duct system of an inactive gland. The lactiferous duct ends into a small saccular evagination.
A **lobule** consists of a **lactiferous duct** and several **alveolar acini**. The lactiferous duct opens into a lactiferous sinus.
Each tubuloalveolar secretory unit consists of cuboidal or low columnar epithelial cells, **myoepithelial cells**, and a basal lamina.
A mammary gland contains about 10 to 20 separate lobes.
Opening of a lactiferous sinus
Lactiferous sinus
Lactiferous duct
Terminal interlobular duct
Tubuloalveolar secretory unit

development of the mammary gland.

The nipple is visible by week 6 as an accumulation of ectodermic epithelial cells along the **mammary line** (extending from the axilla to the groin), forming a depression, the **inverted nipple**. After birth, the nipple region protrudes and the areola becomes elevated as **areolar glands** develop around the nipple.

During development of the mammary gland, an ectodermic epithelial cell bud, the **mammary bud**, enters the underlying mesoderm. Epithelial buds sprout during the first trimester to give rise to 15 to 25 solid epithelial **mammary cords**. During the second trimester, the mammary cords become hollow, and alveoli develop by the end of the third trimester (see Figure 23-18). The **mammary ducts** become **lactiferous ducts**.

The mesoderm differentiates into a connective and adipose stroma as well as into the smooth muscle of the nipple. **Luminal epithelial cells of ducts and alveoli are precursors of the myoepithelial cells**, which migrate to the basal region of the lining epithelium. The epithelial-myoepithelial conversion also occurs in the mature mammary gland.

The epithelium of the lactiferous duct of the mammary glands of newborns of both sexes can respond to maternal hormones and may produce a secretion containing α-lactalbumin, fat, and leukocytes. This secretion is called "witch's milk." In most cases, the simple embryonic-fetal mammary duct system remains unchanged in the infant until the onset of puberty.

In the **male fetus**, the developing duct system undergoes **involution in the presence of testosterone**. The role of the mesoderm and testosterone receptors is well demonstrated in the **androgen insensitivity syndrome** (**testicular feminization syndrome**; see later).

At **puberty** (Figure 23-19), circulating **estrogen** (in the presence of prolactin)

Figure 23-18. Development of the mammary gland

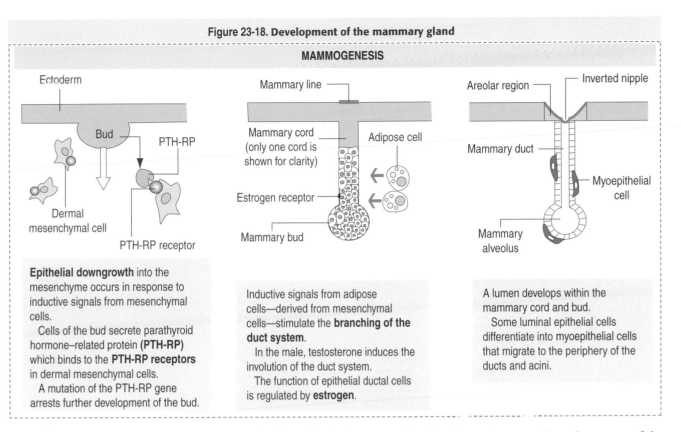

MAMMOGENESIS

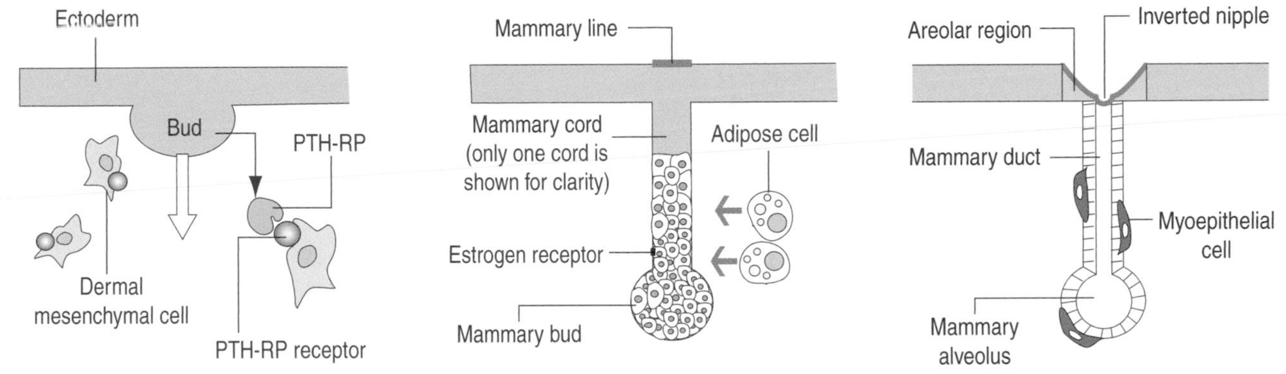

Epithelial downgrowth into the mesenchyme occurs in response to inductive signals from mesenchymal cells.

Cells of the bud secrete parathyroid hormone–related protein **(PTH-RP)** which binds to the **PTH-RP receptors** in dermal mesenchymal cells.

A mutation of the PTH-RP gene arrests further development of the bud.

Inductive signals from adipose cells—derived from mesenchymal cells—stimulate the **branching of the duct system**.

In the male, testosterone induces the involution of the duct system.

The function of epithelial ductal cells is regulated by **estrogen**.

A lumen develops within the mammary cord and bud.

Some luminal epithelial cells differentiate into myoepithelial cells that migrate to the periphery of the ducts and acini.

stimulates the development of the **lactiferous ducts** and the enlargement of the surrounding **fat tissue**.

Epithelial cells lining the lactiferous ducts contain cytosolic and nuclear **estrogen receptors. Progesterone** stimulates the formation of new alveolar buds, replacing old, regressing buds, which eventually disappear at the end of the ovarian cycle.

Figure 23-19. Mammary gland at puberty and during pregnancy

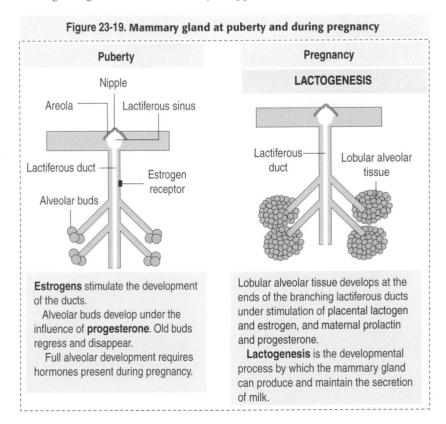

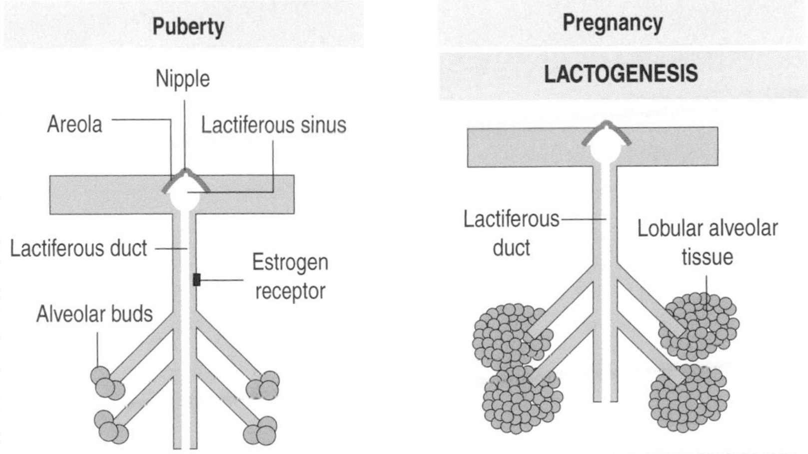

Estrogens stimulate the development of the ducts.

Alveolar buds develop under the influence of **progesterone**. Old buds regress and disappear.

Full alveolar development requires hormones present during pregnancy.

Lobular alveolar tissue develops at the ends of the branching lactiferous ducts under stimulation of placental lactogen and estrogen, and maternal prolactin and progesterone.

Lactogenesis is the developmental process by which the mammary gland can produce and maintain the secretion of milk.

Figure 23-20. **Histology of the inactive and active mammary gland**

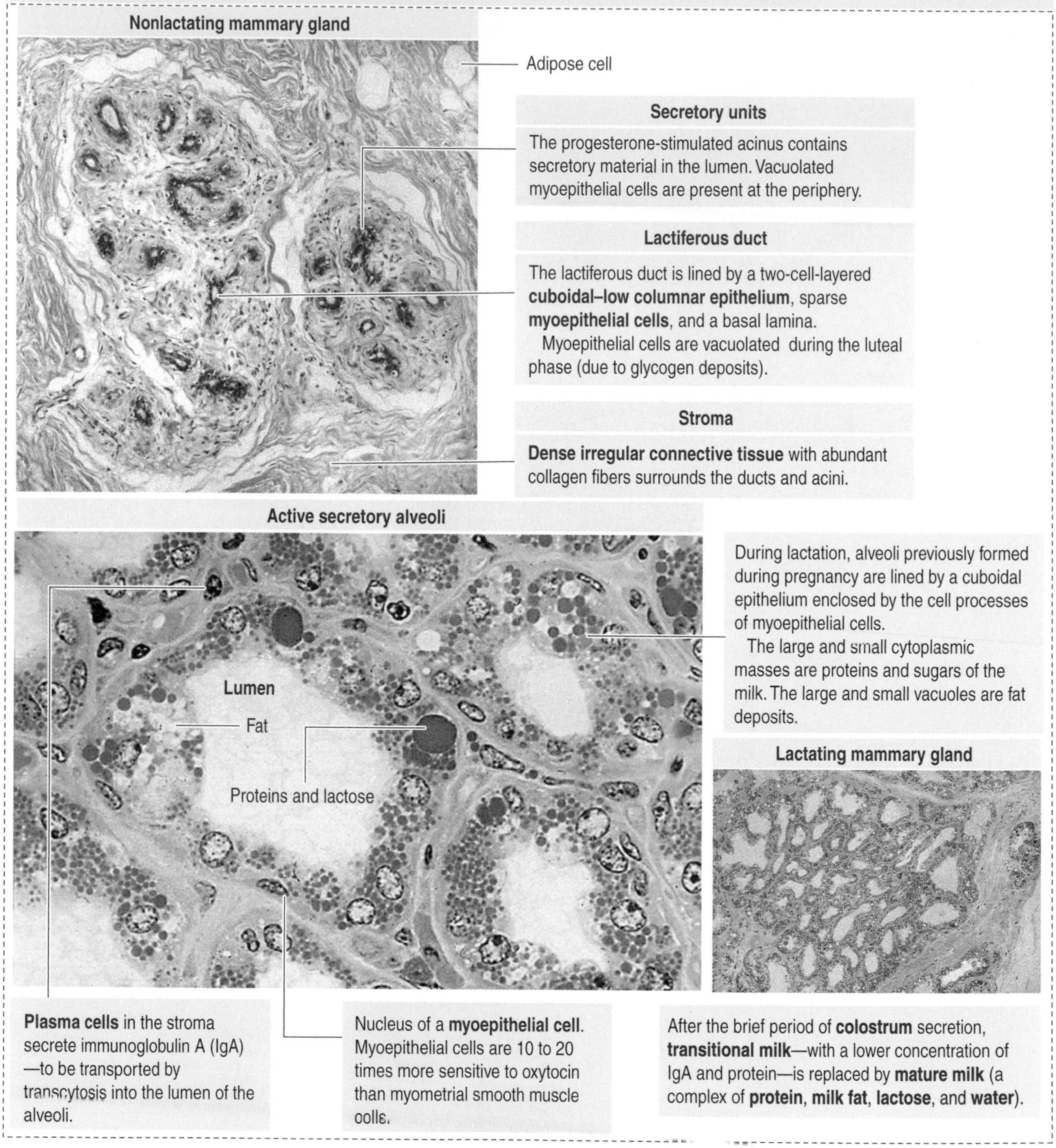

Nonlactating mammary gland
Adipose cell
Secretory units
The progesterone-stimulated acinus contains secretory material in the lumen. Vacuolated myoepithelial cells are present at the periphery.
Lactiferous duct
The lactiferous duct is lined by a two-cell-layered **cuboidal–low columnar epithelium**, sparse **myoepithelial cells**, and a basal lamina.
Myoepithelial cells are vacuolated during the luteal phase (due to glycogen deposits).
Stroma
Dense irregular connective tissue with abundant collagen fibers surrounds the ducts and acini.
Active secretory alveoli
Lumen
Fat
Proteins and lactose
During lactation, alveoli previously formed during pregnancy are lined by a cuboidal epithelium enclosed by the cell processes of myoepithelial cells.
The large and small cytoplasmic masses are proteins and sugars of the milk. The large and small vacuoles are fat deposits.
Lactating mammary gland
Plasma cells in the stroma secrete immunoglobulin A (IgA) —to be transported by transcytosis into the lumen of the alveoli.
Nucleus of a **myoepithelial cell**. Myoepithelial cells are 10 to 20 times more sensitive to oxytocin than myometrial smooth muscle cells.
After the brief period of **colostrum** secretion, **transitional milk**—with a lower concentration of IgA and protein—is replaced by **mature milk** (a complex of **protein, milk fat, lactose**, and **water**).

These cyclic changes are observed in each menstrual cycle.

During **pregnancy** (see Figure 23-19), prolactin and placental lactogen, in the presence of estrogen, progesterone, and growth factors, stimulate the **development of lactiferous ducts** and **secretory alveoli** at the ends of the branched ducts.

During **lactation**, the lactiferous duct system and the lobular alveolar tissue are fully developed and functional (Figure 23-20). **Prolactin** stimulates secretion by **alveolar cells**.

Suckling during lactation

A **neural stimulus** at the nipple resulting from **suckling** determines:

1. The ejection of milk by the release of oxytocin. Oxytocin causes contraction

Figure 23-21. Function of the mammary alveolar cell

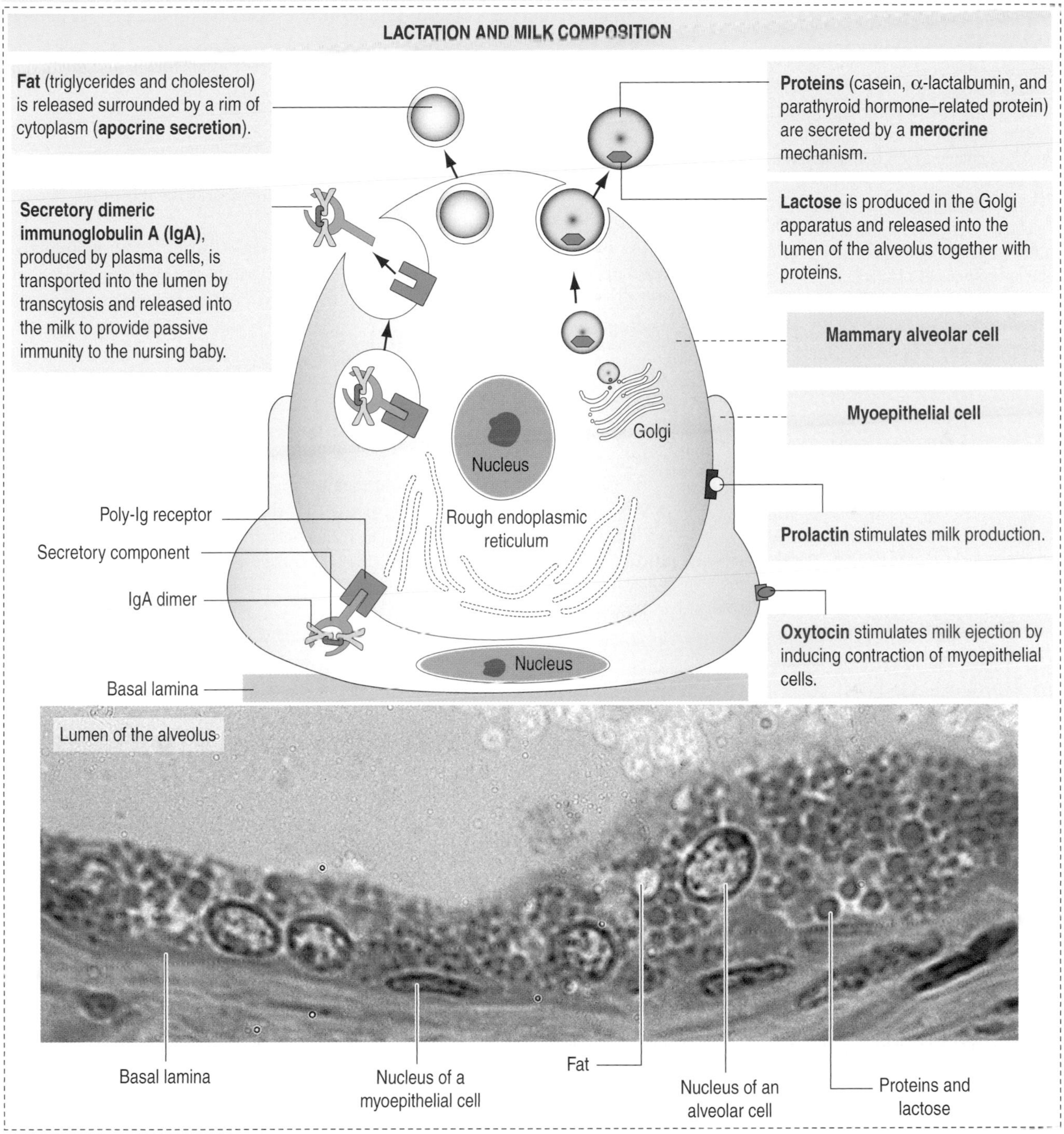

LACTATION AND MILK COMPOSITION
Fat (triglycerides and cholesterol) is released surrounded by a rim of cytoplasm (apocrine secretion).
Secretory dimeric immunoglobulin A (IgA), produced by plasma cells, is transported into the lumen by transcytosis and released into the milk to provide passive immunity to the nursing baby.
Proteins (casein, α-lactalbumin, and parathyroid hormone–related protein) are secreted by a merocrine mechanism.
Lactose is produced in the Golgi apparatus and released into the lumen of the alveolus together with proteins.
Mammary alveolar cell
Myoepithelial cell
Golgi
Nucleus
Rough endoplasmic reticulum
Poly-Ig receptor
Secretory component
IgA dimer
Prolactin stimulates milk production.
Oxytocin stimulates milk ejection by inducing contraction of myoepithelial cells.
Nucleus
Basal lamina
Lumen of the alveolus
Basal lamina
Nucleus of a myoepithelial cell
Fat
Nucleus of an alveolar cell
Proteins and lactose

of myoepithelial cells surrounding the alveoli.

2. The inhibition of the release of **luteinizing hormone–releasing factor** by the hypothalamus, resulting in the temporary **arrest of ovulation.**

Milk contains (Figure 23-21; see Box 23-D):

1. **Proteins** (**casein**, **α-lactalbumin**, and large amounts of **parathyroid hormone–related protein** [PTH-RP]), released by **merocrine secretion** together with lactose.

2. **Lipids** (**triglycerides** and **cholesterol**), released by **apocrine secretion.**

3. **Sugar** (in particular **lactose,** produced in the Golgi apparatus from glucose and uridine diphosphogalactose). Lactose osmotically draws water into secretory vesicles, a process that accounts for the large volume of milk.

Box 23-D | Lactation

- Colostrum: early milk (called fore milk) with a lower fat concentration but higher concentration of proteins and minerals. The fat content increases over the next several minutes (mature milk or hind milk).
- Milk: a unique species-specific fluid with nutritive, immunologic, and growth-promoting components.
- Lipids are surrounded by cytosol (called milk-fat globule). The cytosol becomes a stabilizing interface between fat and the aqueous components of the milk. The cytosol interface allows controlled lipolysis and formation of a micellar aqueous suspension useful for absorption in the small intestine. Lipids include cholesterol, triglycerides, short-chain fatty acids, and long-chain polyunsaturated fatty acids.
- Immunoglobulins: the most abundant immunoglobulin is secretory dimeric immunoglobulin A (IgA). It provides passive acquired defense for several weeks before the baby can produce its own secretory IgA in the small intestine.
- Protective functions of human milk: Milk contains lactoferrin, lysozyme, oligosaccharides, and mucins. These components enable some intestinal bacteria to become established while others are inhibited.

In addition, **plasma cells** present in the stroma surrounding the alveolar tissue secrete **dimeric IgA**. Dimeric IgA is taken up by alveolar cells and transported to the lumen by a mechanism similar to that discussed in Chapter 16, Lower Digestive Segment.

After nursing, prolactin secretion decreases, the mammary alveoli regress, and the lactiferous duct system returns to its normal nonpregnant stage within several months.

Clinical significance: Androgen insensitivity syndrome

In this genetic condition, genetic males (XY) lack **testosterone receptor**, encoded by a gene on the X chromosome.

In **normal males**, the lactiferous ducts undergo rapid involution by an **inductive mechanism** mediated by the **mammary mesenchyme**. Lactiferous ducts developing in the absence of testosterone or a functional androgen receptor, as in the androgen insensitivity syndrome, assume a female pattern of development.

Clinical significance: Benign breast diseases and breast cancer

Each of the tissues of the mammary gland (connective tissue, ducts, and acini) can be the source of a pathologic condition. Breast cancer is the most common malignancy in women.

Fibrocystic changes are the most common of all benign mammary gland conditions in 20- to 40-year-old patients. Hormonal imbalances are associated with fibrocystic changes. In this condition, a proliferation of the connective tissue stroma and cystic formation of the ducts are observed. Pain (**mastalgia**) tends to be cyclic as cysts expand rapidly.

Fibroadenoma, the second most common form of benign breast disease, occurs in young women (20 to 30 years old). Fibroadenomas are slow-growing masses of epithelial and connective tissues and are painless.

Gynecomastia, the enlargement of the **male breast**, is caused by a shift in the adrenal cortex estrogen-testis androgen balance. It may be observed during **cirrhosis**, since the liver is responsible for the breakdown of estrogens. Gynecomastia is a typical feature of **Klinefelter's syndrome** (47,XXY).

About 80% of **breast cancers** originate in the epithelial lining of the lactiferous ducts (Figure 23-22). **Epithelial cells lining the lactiferous ducts have estrogen receptors and about 50% to 85% of breast tumors have estrogen receptors.**

There are **two types of estrogen receptors**, α and β. The α receptor has a higher binding affinity for estrogen than the β receptor. The β receptor acts as a physiologic regulator of the α receptor. The expression of the α receptor is higher than the β receptor in invasive tumors than in normal breast tissue. This finding suggests that a balance between the receptors is important in determining the sensitivity of tissue to estrogen and the relative risk of breast tumor development. A large number of estrogen-dependent tumors regress after antiestrogen therapy (treatment with the antiestrogen **tamoxifen**).

The familial inheritance of two autosomal dominant genes, ***BRCA1*** and ***BRCA2***, has been determined in 20% to 30% of patients with breast cancer. *BRCA1* and *BRCA2* encode **tumor suppressor proteins** interacting with other nuclear proteins. Wild-type *BRCA1* can suppress estrogen-dependent transcription pathways related to the proliferation of epithelial cells of the mammary gland. A mutation of *BRCA1* can determine the loss of this ability, facilitating tumorigenesis. Women with *BRCA1* and *BRCA2* mutation have a lifetime risk of invasive breast and ovarian cancer. **Prophylactic bilateral total mastectomy** has been shown to drastically reduce the incidence of breast cancer among women with a *BRCA1* or *BRCA2* mutation.

Estrogen-replacement therapy in **postmenopausal** women has been implicated as a risk factor for breast cancer. In **premenopausal** women, the ovaries are the predominant source of estrogen. In **postmenopausal** women, estrogen derives predominantly from **aromatization** of adrenal (see Adrenal Gland in Chapter

Figure 23-22. Breast cancer

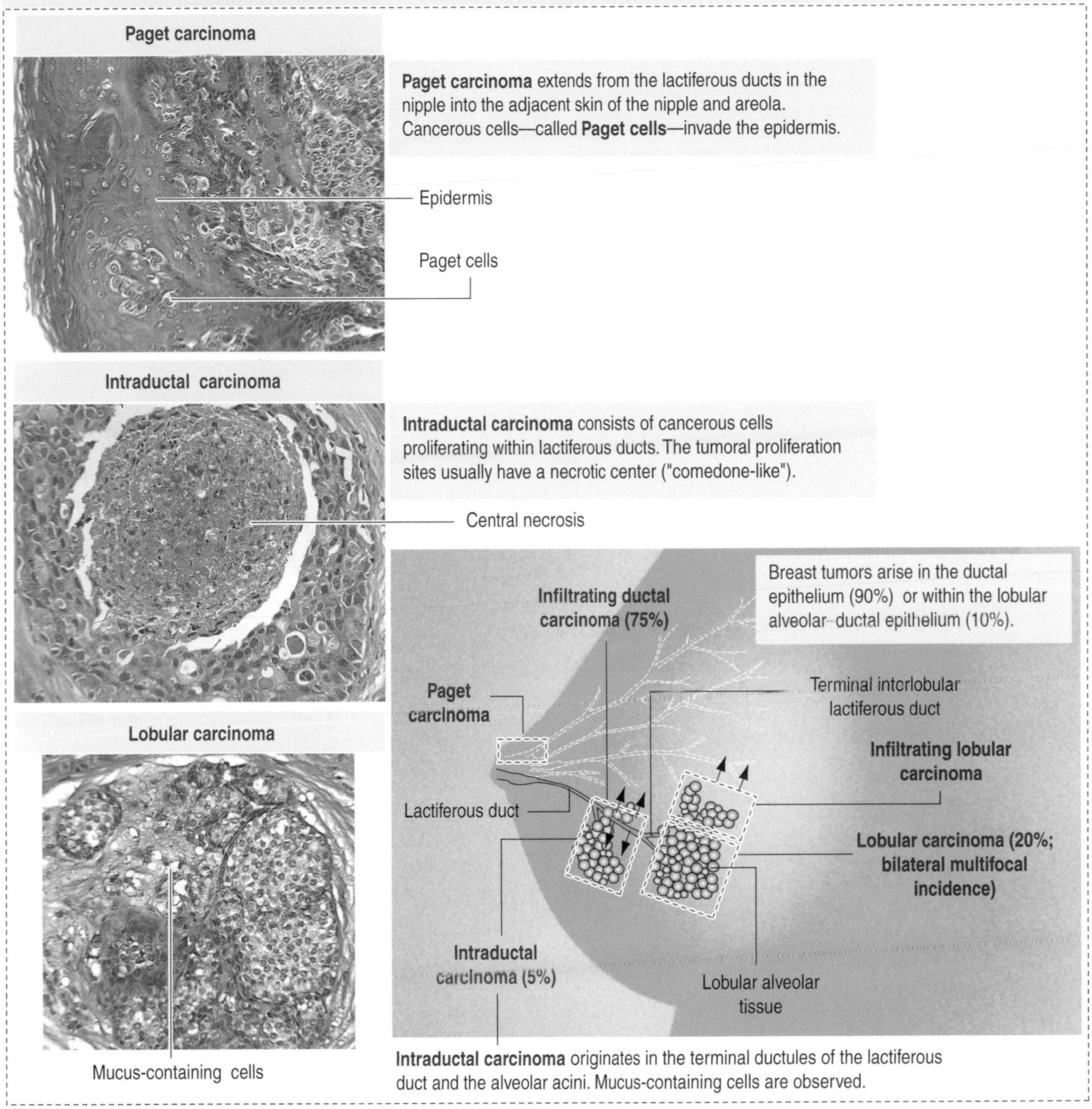
Paget carcinoma
Paget carcinoma extends from the lactiferous ducts in the nipple into the adjacent skin of the nipple and areola. Cancerous cells—called **Paget cells**—invade the epidermis.
Epidermis
Paget cells
Intraductal carcinoma
Intraductal carcinoma consists of cancerous cells proliferating within lactiferous ducts. The tumoral proliferation sites usually have a necrotic center ("comedone-like").
Central necrosis
Lobular carcinoma
Mucus-containing cells
Breast tumors arise in the ductal epithelium (90%) or within the lobular alveolar–ductal epithelium (10%).
Infiltrating ductal carcinoma (75%)
Paget carcinoma
Terminal interlobular lactiferous duct
Infiltrating lobular carcinoma
Lactiferous duct
Lobular carcinoma (20%; bilateral multifocal incidence)
Intraductal carcinoma (5%)
Lobular alveolar tissue
Intraductal carcinoma originates in the terminal ductules of the lactiferous duct and the alveolar acini. Mucus-containing cells are observed.

19, Endocrine System) and ovarian androgens in the liver, muscle, and adipose tissue.

The mammary gland has a rich blood and lymphatic system, which facilitates metastases. Axillary lymph node metastases are the most important prognostic factor.

• **Fertilization** encompasses three events: (1) acrosome reaction, (2) sperm binding to the egg zona pellucida, and (3) sperm-egg plasma membrane fusion.

The acrosome and the condensed nucleus are components of the sperm head. As discussed in Chapter 21 (Spermatogenesis), the sperm tail is attached to the head by a connecting piece derived from the centrosome (organized by the proximal and distal centrioles and pericentriolar matrix). The tail consists of a middle piece, a principal piece, and an end piece. The major components of the middle piece are the axoneme and the surrounding outer dense fibers and mitochondrial helical sheath. The major components of the principal piece are the axoneme surrounded by outer dense fibers and the concentric ribs of the fibrous sheath anchored to longitudinal columns.

The acrosome sac contains hydrolytic enzymes (mainly hyaluronidase and proacrosin; the latter gives rise to acrosin during the acrosome reaction). The sac consists of an outer acrosomal membrane facing the plasma membrane, and an inner acrosomal membrane facing the nuclear envelope of the condensed nucleus. The acrosome reaction occurs when the outer acrosomal membrane fuses at different points with the plasma membranes in the presence of Ca^{2+}.

Acrosomal-derived hyaluronidase facilitates sperm penetration between cells of the corona radiata. Acrosin enables sperm penetration of the zona pellucida. When the first sperm binds to the zona pellucida (consisting of three glycoproteins: ZP1, ZP2, and ZP3), proteases from the cortical granules in the egg cytoplasm are released. Consequently, the zona pellucida changes its molecular organization to prevent polyspermy.

The following molecules are involved in fertilization: The sperm plasma membrane contains receptors with binding affinity to *O*-oligosaccharides of ZP3 and fertilin α/β, a heterodimer of the family of ADAM proteins. The egg plasma membrane has several integrins ($\alpha_3\beta_1$, $\alpha_5\beta_1$, and $\alpha_6\beta_1$) and CD9, a member of the superfamily of tetraspanins, which interacts with integrins and other proteins to form a tetraspanin web.

• **Placentation** starts with the implantation of the blastocyst into the endometrium after the blastocyst hatches from the zona pellucida exposing the trophoblast layer.

Implantation consists in the adhesion of the blastocyst to the endometrial surface (a process called apposition) followed by implantation into the decidualized endometrial stroma with the help of the invasive trophoblastic cells (a process called interstitial invasion). Uterine receptivity is the optimal state of the endometrium for the implantation of the blastocyst. A primary decidual zone is remodeled into a secondary decidual zone by the action of local metalloproteinases and their inhibitors.

The trophoblast differentiates into an inner cell layer, the mitotically dividing cytotrophoblast, and an outer cell layer, the postmitotic syncytiotrophoblast. Proteolytic enzymes released by the syncytiotrophoblast erode the branches of the spiral uterine arteries, forming lacunae. This event, called endovascular invasion, initiates the uteroplacental circulation. Lacunae represent the starting point of the future intervillous space of the placenta.

A primary villus, the first step in the development of chorionic villi, is formed at the end of the second week. A primary villus consists of a cytotrophoblast core surrounded by the syncytiotrophoblast layer.

A secondary villus is formed early in the third week. A secondary villus consists of a core of extraembryonic mesoderm surrounded by the cytotrophoblast in the middle and an outer syncytiotrophoblast layer.

A tertiary villus is seen late in the third week. The tertiary villus has a structure similar to the secondary villus but it contains fetal arteriocapillary networks in the extraembryonic mesoderm.

The **placenta** consists of (1) the chorionic plate (fetal component) and (2) the decidua basalis (maternal component). These two components are the limits of the intervillous space containing maternal blood.

The intervillous space is subdivided by decidual septa into compartments, called lobes. The decidual septa, extending from the decidua basalis into the intervillous space, do not reach the chorionic plate. Therefore, the lobes are incomplete and the intervillous spaces are interconnected.

A chorionic villus consists of a stem giving rise to numerous villous branches. The core of the stem and villous branches contains extraembryonic mesoderm (mesenchymal cells), fetal blood vessels, and Hofbauer cells (a macrophage-like cell seen in early pregnancy). The surface of the stem and its branches is lined by an outer syncytiotrophoblast layer and an inner cytotrophoblast layer supported by a basal lamina. The apical domain of syncytiotrophoblastic cells displays short microvilli extending into the maternal blood space.

In late pregnancy, cytotrophoblastic cells decrease in number and disappear and syncytiotrophoblastic cells aggregate to form knots.

According to their relation to the fetus, the decidua consists of three regions: (1) decidua basalis, the maternal component of the placenta, (2) decidua capsularis, the superficial layer covering the developing fetus, and (3) decidua parietalis, covering the uterine cavity not occupied by the fetus.

The placental barrier is formed by the syncytiotrophoblast and cytotrophoblast layers supported by a basal lamina and endothelial cells and corresponding basal lamina of the fetal capillaries. Fetal capillaries become closely apposed to the trophoblastic layer. Recall that the population of cytotrophoblastic cells decreases with time and syncytiotrophoblast cells aggregate to form knots.

• **Functions of the placenta:** (1) exchange of gases by simple diffusion; (2) transfer of maternal immunoglobulins; (3) production of steroids. Syncytiotrophoblastic cells synthesize progesterone, which is transferred to the adrenal cortex for its conversion to weak androgens. Weak androgens are transferred to the syncytiotrophoblast for the conversion to estrogens. The placental–adrenal cortex cooperative mechanism represents the basis for the fetoplacental unit; (4) synthesis of chorionic gonadotropin (luteal placental shift to maintain the corpus luteum of pregnancy) and placental lactogen (to condition the mammary gland for lactation); and (5) active transport of ions and glucose.

• **Disorders of the placenta** include ectopic pregnancy, consisting in implantation in the ampulla of the oviduct. Uterine atony defines weak contractions of the uterine muscle during post partum. Placenta previa is defined by the abnormal extension of the placenta over or close to the cervical canal. Placental abruption corresponds to the premature separation of the normally implanted placenta. Placenta accreta consists in defective placental separation when placental villi penetrate deep into the uterine wall. Placenta increta defines placental villi extending into the uterine muscle (myometrium). An extensive invasion of placental villi through the thickness of the uterine muscle is known as placenta percreta.

Hydatidiform mole is the partial or total replacement of normal trophoblastic tissue by dilated grape-shaped villi. Total moles result from the fertilization of an empty egg by a haploid sperm that replicates within the egg. High levels of human chorionic gonadotropin are characteristic in patients with hydatidiform moles. Choriocarcinoma is the malignant transformation potential of a complete mole.

• **Lactation** includes the development, structure, and function of the mammary gland. The mammary gland is a branched (compound) organ with lactiferous ducts and tubuloalveolar secretory units forming a lobule in the lactating gland. A lobe consists of a group of lobules drained by a lactiferous duct. The resting, nonlactating gland is formed by lactiferous ducts, each ending in a group of blind saccular evaginations.

The lactiferous duct is lined by a simple columnar or cuboidal epithelium and a discontinuous layer of myoepithelial cells. Each secretory unit, the alveolus, is lined by the alveolar mammary epithelium and basal myoepithelial cells, both supported by a basal lamina.

Development of the mammary gland (mammogenesis). Placental lactogen, chorionic gonadotropin, and estrogen (produced by syncytiotrophoblast) stimulate the development of the mammary gland. The mammary bud, an ectodermic epithelial derivative, extends into the mesoderm. Mammary buds give rise to 15 to 25 solid epithelial mammary cords under the influence of estrogens. Mammary cords become hollow and change into mammary ducts. Alveoli develop at the end of the mammary ducts, the future lactiferous ducts. The mesoderm differentiates into connective and adipose tissue stroma.

In the male, the developing mammary duct system undergoes involution in the presence of testosterone.

During puberty, estrogens stimulate the development of the lactiferous ducts. Alveolar buds develop under control of progesterone and regress. Epithelial cells lining the lactiferous duct and alveolar buds are precursors of myoepithelial cells.

During pregnancy (lactogenesis), lobular alveoli develop at the end of the lactiferous ducts under control of placental lactogen and estrogen, and maternal progesterone and prolactin.

Milk production and ejection. The production of milk in the mammary alveolar cells is controlled by prolactin. The ejection of milk is controlled by oxytocin acting on myoepithelial cells.

Milk contains (1) proteins (casein, α-lactalbumin, parathyroid hormone–related peptide, and others) released by merocrine secretion; (2) fat (triglycerides and cholesterol) released by apocrine secretion; (3) lactose (produced in the Golgi apparatus and released together with proteins); and (4) secretory dimeric immunoglobulin A (produced by plasma cells and released in the alveolar lumen by transcytosis).

• **Tumors of the mammary gland.** Benign breast diseases include fibrocystic changes of the lactiferous ducts, and fibroadenoma (masses of epithelial and connective tissue). Gynecomastia is the enlargement of the male breast.

Breast cancer originates in the epithelial lining of the lactiferous ducts (80%). Estrogen receptors and the tumor suppressor genes *BRCA1* and *BRCA2* play an important role in breast tumors. The most frequent breast tumors are the infiltrating duct carcinoma (originating in lactiferous ducts) and lobular carcinoma (derived from the lobular alveolar tissue). Paget carcinoma extends from the lactiferous ducts to the nipple and areola. Intraductal carcinoma consists of tumor cells growing within the lactiferous duct lumen.

A

B

C

D

E

F

J

K

L

M

N

R

S

T

U

V

W

X

Y

Z